PERIANESTHESIA NURSING

A CRITICAL CARE APPROACH

FOURTH EDITION

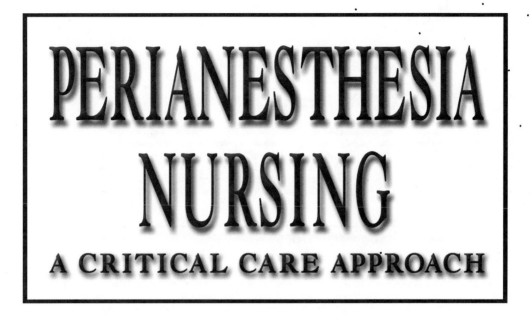

PERIANESTHESIA NURSING

A CRITICAL CARE APPROACH

CECIL B. DRAIN, PhD

Dean, School of Allied Health Professions
Virginia Commonwealth University
Richmond, Virginia

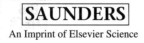

SAUNDERS

An Imprint of Elsevier Science

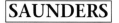

SAUNDERS

An Imprint of Elsevier Science

11830 Westline Industrial Drive
St. Louis, Missouri 63146

NOTICE

Perianesthesia nursing is an ever-changing field. Standard safety precautions must be followed, but as
new research and clinical experience broaden our knowledge, changes in treatment and drug therapy
may become necessary or appropriate. Readers are advised to check the most current product information
provided by the manufacturer of each drug to be administered to verify the recommended dose, the
method and duration of administration, and contraindications. It is the responsibility of the licensed
prescriber, relying on experience and knowledge of the patient, to determine dosages and the best
treatment for each individual patient. Neither the publisher nor the author assumes any liability for any
injury and/or damage to persons or property arising from this publication.

Previous editions copyrighted 1994, 1987, 1979

Library of Congress Cataloging-in-Publication Data

Perianesthesia nursing : a critical care approach / [edited by] Cecil B. Drain. – 4th ed.
      p. ;   cm.
   Rev. ed. of: The post anesthesia care unit. c1994.
   Includes bibliographical references and index.
   ISBN 0-7216-9257-5
   1. Post anesthesia nursing.   2. Recovery rooms.   I. Drain, Cecil B.   II. Post anesthesia care unit.
   [DNLM: 1. Postanesthesia Nursing—methods.   2. Anesthesia—nursing.   3. Anesthesia Recovery
Period.   4. Perioperative Nursing—methods.   5. Postoperative Care—nursing.   6. Recovery Room. WY
154 P441 2003]

   RD51.3.D73 2003
   617'.919–dc21

                                                                               2003041592

Executive Editor: Michael S. Ledbetter
Developmental Editor: Amanda Sunderman Politte
Editorial Assistant: Mary Parker
Publishing Services Manager: Pat Joiner
Project Manager: Keri O'Brien
Senior Designer: Mark A. Oberkrom
Cover Designer: Studio Montage

Printed in the United States of America

Last digit is the print number: 9   8   7   6   5   4   3   2   1

To my parents;

To my most treasured wife, Cindy, who has endured 4 editions of this book;

To my children for their love, support, and understanding—my son, Tim, and his wife, Holly; my son, Steve, and his wife, Christine; and my daughter, Katie, and her husband, Jeff;

To my grandchildren Peyton, Nathan, and Seth—always remember, anything is possible;

To the Virginia Commonwealth University family and, in particular, the faculty and staff of the School of Allied Health Professions;

To all my former colleagues in the Army Nurse Corps and, in particular, all my former students in the Anesthesiology for ANC Officers Course;

And finally, to all the perianesthesia nurses who have made the preparation of each edition so enjoyable.

CONTRIBUTORS

Kay Ball, RN, BSN, MSA, CNOR, FAAN
Consultant/Educator
K & D Medical, Inc.
Lewis Center, Ohio
Chapter 24: Transition from the Operating Room to the PACU

Nancy Burden, RN, MS, CPAN, CAPA
Director of Health Services
Morton Plant Mease Health Care
Largo, Florida
Chapter 43: Care of the Ambulatory Surgical Patient

Dennis M. Driscoll, PhD, RN, CCRN
Lieutenant Colonel
United States Army
Chapter 42: Care of the Thermally Injured Patient

Philip Hughston Ewing, MD
Resident in Pediatrics
Children's Medical Center of Dallas
University of Texas Southwestern Medical
    Center
Dallas, Texas
Chapter 28: Pain Management in the PACU

Michael D. Fallacaro, DNS, CRNA
Professor and Chair
Department of Nurse Anesthesia
Virginia Commonwealth University
Richmond, Virginia
Chapter 4: Crisis Resource Management in the PACU

Joanne L. Fletcher, EdD, CRNA
Clinical Assistant Professor
Department of Nurse Anesthesia
Virginia Commonwealth University
School of Allied Health Professions
Richmond, Virginia;
Staff Anesthetist
Commonwealth Anesthesia Associates
Midlothian, Virginia
Chapter 4: Crisis Resource Management in the PACU

Marie Fiascone Gerardo, MS, RN-C, ANP, CCRN
Adult Nurse Practitioner, Private Practice
Adjunct Faculty and Doctoral Student
Virginia Commonwealth University
Richmond, Virginia
Chapter 5: Managed Care and Its Impact on the PACU

Gordon Green, MD, MPH
Professor and Dean
Allied Health Sciences
The University of Texas Southwestern Medical
    Center
Dallas, Texas
Chapter 52: Bioterrorism and Its Impact on the PACU

Karen "Toby" Haghenbeck, PhD, RN, C, CCRN
Assistant Professor
Lienhard School of Nursing
Pace University
Pleasantville, New York
Chapter 32: Care of the Cardiac Surgical
  Patient

William Hartland, Jr., PhD, CRNA
Assistant Professor and Director of Education
Department of Nurse Anesthesia
Virginia Commonwealth University
School of Allied Health Professions
Richmond, Virginia
Chapter 53: Cardiopulmonary Resuscitation in the
  PACU

John K. Hawkins, PhD, RN, CRNA
Staff CRNA
Dwight David Eisenhower Army Medical
  Center
Fort Gordon, Georgia
Chapter 35: Care of the Neurosurgical Patient

Virginia C. Hawkins, MSN, RN, CCRN
Critical Care Educator
MCG Health Inc.
Medical College of Georgia Health System
Augusta, Georgia
Chapter 35: Care of the Neurosurgical Patient

Vallire Hooper, MSN, RN, CPAN
Clinical Nurse Specialist, Surgical Services
St. Joseph Hospital
Clinical Assistant Professor
School of Nursing
Medical College of Georgia
Augusta, Georgia
Chapter 44: Care of the Laser/Laparoscopic
  Surgical Patient

Melissa A. Hotchkiss, MSNA, CRNA
Assistant Professor,
Director, Center for Research in Human
  Simulation
Department of Nurse Anesthesia
Virginia Commonwealth University
Richmond, Virginia
Chapter 4: Crisis Resource Management in the
  PACU
Chapter 27: Assessment and Management of the
  Airway

Donna L. Johnson, RN, CRNA, MSNA
Adjunct Assistant Professor and Assistant
  Director of Education
Department of Nurse Anesthesia
Virginia Commonwealth University;
Staff Nurse Anesthetist
Virginia Commonwealth University Health
  Systems
Richmond, Virginia
Chapter 46: Care of the Pediatric Patient

Karen D. Keeler, RN, BSN, CCRN, CEN
Administrative Director of Patient Services
Hudson Valley Hospital Center
Cortlandt Manor, New York
Chapter 32: Care of the Cardiac Surgical Patient

**Kim Litwack, PhD, RN, FAAN, CPAN, CAPA,
CFNP**
Associate Professor of Nursing
Grand Valley State University
Grand Rapids, Michigan
Chapter 31: Care of the Thoracic Surgical Patient
Chapter 36: Care of the Thyroid and Parathyroid
  Surgical Patient

Stephen P. Long, MD
Medical Director
Commonwealth Pain Specialists;
Associate Clinical Professor of
  Anesthesiology
Virginia Commonwealth University
Richmond, Virginia
Chapter 28: Pain Management in the PACU

Charles H. Moore, PhD, CRNA
Medical College of Virginia Hospitals
Virginia Commonwealth University
Richmond, Virginia
Chapter 22: Local Anesthetics
Chapter 23: Regional Anesthesia

Carole Muto, RN, BSN, CPAN
Staff Nurse, PACU
Thomas Jefferson University Hospital
Wills Eye Hospital
Philadelphia, Pennsylvania
Member, ASPAN, PA PAN
Chapter 30: Care of the Ophthalmic Surgical
Patient

Denise O'Brien, MSN(c), RN, CPAN,
CAPA
Clinical Nurse II/Educational Nurse
   Coordinator
Perianesthesia Care Areas
Department of Operating Rooms/PACU
University of Michigan Health System
Ann Arbor, Michigan
Chapter 1: Space Planning and Basic Equipment
Systems
Chapter 26: Care of the Perianesthesia Patient
Chapter 37: Care of the Gastrointestinal,
Abdominal, and Anorectal Surgical Patient

Jan Odom, MSN, RN, CPAN, FAAN
Patient Care Manager, PACU
Forrest General Hospital;
Nursing Consultant
Hattiesburg, Mississippi
Chapter 3: Management and Policies

Donna M. DeFazio Quinn, BSN, MBA, RN,
CPAN, CAPA
Director
Orthopaedic Surgery Center
Concord, New Hampshire
Chapter 2: Perianesthesia Nursing as a
Specialty

Beverly Smith, BSN, RN, CPAN
Nurse Manager
Preoperative Holding Room/PACU
University of Michigan Health System
Ann Arbor, Michigan
Chapter 1: Space Planning and Basic Equipment
Systems

Judy Stevenson, RN, BSN, CCRN
Perianesthesia/Critical Care Educator
Cox Health Systems;
Staff Nurse, Trauma Emergency Center
St. Francis Hospital
Joplin, Missouri
Chapter 51: Care of the Shock Trauma Patient

Karen N. Swisher, MS, JD
Associate Professor
Health Law
Virginia Commonwealth University
Richmond, Virginia
Chapter 6: Legal Issues in the PACU
Chapter 7: Ethics of Health Care in the PACU

Peter Nash Swisher, MA, JD
Professor of Law
University of Richmond Law School
Richmond, Virginia
Chapter 6: Legal Issues in the PACU

Kenneth R. White, PhD, RN, FACHE
Associate Professor and Director
Graduate Program in Health Administration
Virginia Commonwealth University
Richmond, Virginia
Chapter 5: Managed Care and Its Impact on the
PACU

Wendy K. Winer, RN, BSN, CNOR
Center for Women's Care and Reproductive
   Surgery
Atlanta, Georgia
Chapter 39: Care of the Obstetric and Gynecologic
Surgical Patient

PREFACE

Since its initial publication in 1979, *The Recovery Room* has evolved into the standard text for perianesthesia nurses. I am so honored that the fourth edition will continue this tradition, providing perianesthesia nursing with the most comprehensive coverage available under one cover. The new title, *Perianesthesia Nursing: A Critical Care Approach*, reflects the evolving professionalism of the specialty. In 1983 under the aegis of the American Society of Post Anesthesia Nurses (ASPAN), the term *postanesthesia care unit (PACU)* was chosen to designate the postoperative work area and the term *postanesthesia nurse* was chosen to indicate the nurse specializing in that area of patient care. Now, in accordance with the advance practice concepts, the term *perianesthesia nurse* is accepted as defining the nursing practice to include the entire nursing care of the patient that is to undergo a surgical procedure.

This book is organized into five major sections. Section I, "The Postanesthesia Care Unit," focuses on the postanesthesia facilities and equipment, the specialty of postanesthesia nursing, and management and policy issues. The chapter on crisis resource management in the PACU is completely new and looks at the newest techniques in the care of the patient using technology such as anesthesia simulators. Because of the tremendous impact managed care has had on the health care system, and particularly, the PACU, a chapter devoted to managed care and its impact on the PACU has been added. Two other areas of interest that have had a deep impact on perianesthesia nursing are legal issues and ethics in health care. Hence, two chapters have been developed to provide the reader with the most current information on legal issues involving the PACU and ethics of health care in the PACU. The chapters in this section have been totally updated or newly written by recognized leaders in perianesthesia nursing and health care to provide the most up-to-date information in these areas for the nurse and nurse manager.

Section II deals with the physiologic considerations in the PACU. All of the chapters have been updated to reflect the current concepts in anatomy and physiology, including the most recent information available concerning the care and treatment of patients with acquired immunodeficiency syndrome. Because of numerous requests by readers, a chapter has been added in this section dealing with fluids and electrolytes.

Section III, Concepts in Anesthetic Agents, presents the reader with up-to-date pharmacologic considerations of postanesthesia care. The first chapter is completely new and presents an overview of pharmacology, including uptake and distribution, pharmacokinetic and pharmacodynamic principles, drug-drug interactions in the PACU and the influence of herbal medications on postanesthesia recovery. Also, this chapter contains an extensive table on most all of the drugs used in perianesthesia care. Because of advances in research and applications of intravenous anesthetic agents, this content has been divided into two separate chapters covering opioid and nonopioid intravenous anesthetic agents. Along with this, the regional anesthesia chapter, which was presented in a single chapter in the previous edition, has been divided into a chapter focusing on local anesthestics and another chapter discussing the use of regional anesthesia.

Section IV addresses the nursing care in the PACU for various surgical specialties. Many of the chapters in this section have been completely revised by guest authors. Chapter 24 looks at the transition of the patient from the operating room to the PACU. Chapter 25, "Assessment and Monitoring of the Perianesthesia Patient," includes an all-new section on monitoring equipment and data interpretation. This update is especially important owing to the many technologic advances in the PACU that have occurred in the last 5 years. Chapter 27 explores the art and science of airway management, with special attention to intubation and extubation of the trachea. This addition was in response to frequent requests by users of the previous edition for more information with a greater focus on the newest technology of airway management. Also updated in this text is Chapter 28, "Pain Management in the PACU," which includes discussions on related physiology and pharmacology. The advances in surgical technology has been immense and in particular the use of laser and laparoscopic surgery. Consequently, a new chapter has been added to review the use of this new technology and its implications to perianesthesia nursing care.

Section V, Special Considerations, has been revised and condensed in this edition. Two chapters are certainly worthy additions to this section: Chapter 50, "Care of the Patient with Thermal Imbalance," discusses the care of patients with hyperthermia and hypothermia, and Chapter 51 addresses the needs and care of the shock trauma patient, a topic currently receiving an exceptional amount of attention in professional meetings and literature. Because of the times we live in and the impact of perianesthesia nursing, a new chapter has been added to this section focusing on bioterrorism and its impact on the PACU.

The success of any multiauthored book is in large part dependent on the expertise and commitment of the contributors. The contributors to this book were invited because they are acknowledged authorities in their fields. With their help, I hope that this book will continue to inform and guide students, teachers, and clinicians in the critical care specialty of perianesthesia nursing. As in previous editions, I welcome all evaluations and suggestions for improvement.

CECIL B. DRAIN

CONTENTS

SECTION I The Postanesthesia Care Unit

1 Space Planning and Basic Equipment Systems, 1
2 Perianesthesia Nursing as a Specialty, 11
3 Management and Policies, 30
4 Crisis Resource Management in the PACU, 45
5 Managed Care and Its Impact on the PACU, 54
6 Legal Issues in the PACU, 64
7 Ethics of Health Care in the PACU, 77

SECTION II Physiologic Considerations in the PACU

8 The Nervous System, 93
9 The Cardiovascular System, 125
10 The Respiratory System, 150
11 The Renal System, 189
12 Fluid and Electrolytes, 201
13 The Endocrine System, 213
14 The Hepatobiliary and Gastrointestinal System, 221
15 The Integumentary System, 231
16 The Immune System, 238

SECTION III Concepts in Anesthetic Agents

17 Basic Principles of Pharmacology, 248
18 Inhalation Anesthesia, 276
19 Nonopioid Intravenous Anesthetics, 292
20 Opioid Intravenous Anesthetics, 304
21 Muscle Relaxants, 317
22 Local Anesthetics, 339
23 Regional Anesthesia, 346

SECTION IV Nursing Care in the PACU

24 Transition from the Operating Room to the PACU, 354
25 Assessment and Monitoring of the Perianesthesia Patient, 360
26 Care of the Perianesthesia Patient, 393
27 Assessment and Management of the Airway, 409
28 Pain Management in the PACU, 422
29 Care of the Ear, Nose, Throat, Neck, and Maxillofacial Surgical Patient, 433
30 Care of the Ophthalmic Surgical Patient, 452
31 Care of the Thoracic Surgical Patient, 465
32 Care of the Cardiac Surgical Patient, 473
33 Care of the Vascular Surgical Patient, 493
34 Care of the Orthopedic Surgical Patient, 506
35 Care of the Neurosurgical Patient, 517
36 Care of the Thyroid and Parathyroid Surgical Patient, 548
37 Care of the Gastrointestinal, Abdominal, and Anorectal Surgical Patient, 551
38 Care of the Genitourinary Surgical Patient, 566
39 Care of the Obstetric and Gynecologic Surgical Patient, 581
40 Care of the Breast Surgical Patient, 590
41 Care of the Plastic Surgical Patient, 600
42 Care of the Thermally Injured Patient, 607
43 Care of the Ambulatory Surgical Patient, 615
44 Care of the Laser/Laparoscopic Surgical Patient, 627

SECTION V Special Considerations

45 Care of the Patient with Chronic Disorders, **642**
46 Care of the Pediatric Patient, **661**
47 Care of the Geriatric Patient, **682**
48 Care of the Pregnant Patient, **688**
49 Care of the Substance Abuser, **697**

50 Care of the Patient with Thermal Imbalance, **706**
51 Care of the Shock Trauma Patient, **714**
52 Bioterrorism and Its Impact on the PACU, **730**
53 Cardiopulmonary Resuscitation in the PACU, **735**

PERIANESTHESIA NURSING

NURSING

A CRITICAL CARE APPROACH

1

SPACE PLANNING AND BASIC EQUIPMENT SYSTEMS

Beverly Smith, BSN, RN, CPAN
Denise O'Brien, MSN(c), RN, CPAN, CAPA

From the birth of the "Recovery Room" in the 1940s to the postanesthesia care unit (PACU) of the twenty-first century, the look and function of this room (or unit) has been in a constant state of evolution. Throughout the last six decades, surgical procedures have become more extensive and complicated, thus requiring more specially prepared nursing staff and equipment to care for the patients.

The first recovery rooms were established to centralize patients and personnel. The PACUs of today have evolved from general care to intensive care specialty providing a range of nursing care, from neonate to geriatric and outpatient/same-day surgery to inpatient. Today the PACU must be flexible to serve all perianesthesia phases and patient acuities. The design of the space is critical to the ability of the staff to care for a range of patients safely and efficiently.

SPACE

Many factors are considered in designing a PACU. Before the architect or design firm is consulted, the users of the space (i.e., perianesthesia nurses, anesthesiologists, and clerical staff) should come together to answer the following questions regarding the function of the space:

- Is this new construction or is the current space to be remodeled?
- How will the space be used?
- Is there a separate preoperative holding area? Or will those functions be carried out in this space?
- Is this space a PACU-Phase I and/or PACU-Phase II?

- What patient population will be served (i.e., outpatient, same-day admits, and/or inpatients)?
- What patient age groups will be served (i.e., neonatal, pediatric, adult only, or combined age groups)?

Another important area to consider besides the function of the space is the institutional demographics and current and future programs in the Department of Surgery. The following questions should be considered:

- How many operating rooms/suites will this area serve?
- How many operations will be done per day?
- How many different surgical services will be served?
- What types of procedures will be done?
- Will there be patients who will require prolonged monitoring/observation?
- What type of anesthesia practices will impact this area (i.e., regional anesthesia program, acute or chronic pain service)?
- What is the average patient acuity (i.e., American Society of Anesthesiologists [ASA] physical status classification)?
- Will nonsurgical or procedural patients who require anesthesia be recovered in this same space?

Define the Use

Flexibility is an important consideration. One of the first factors that needs consideration is how the space will be used. Are the bays strictly for postoperative care, or does the unit need the flexibility of preoperative use? Many institutions have a separate area dedicated to preadmission testing or screening. This area is best located near the surgical clinics and testing areas (i.e., blood draw station and radiology and cardiology [electrocardiogram] departments). However, consideration should be given to how the preoperative holding area will be designed and used. Because of the cost of construction and the limited hours of use, most administrators are reluctant to build space that has only a single function and that does not lend itself to change as the users or programs evolve. Therefore all disciplines using or anticipating using the area need to engage in the discussion related to space usage so that future needs can be anticipated. The department of anesthesia will have input regarding their preoperative needs—for example, a preadmission testing or screening area and day-of-surgery preoperative procedures.

Perianesthesia nursing will have knowledge of the entire process from preadmission testing to discharge the day of surgery. The department of surgery needs to have input regarding the types of operations, new surgical techniques, and the need for prolonged observation before the patient is discharged. Clerical services should have input related to the flow of patients and record/paperwork systems. Environmental services will have input related to needs of janitorial space to house cleaning supplies and equipment. Central supply personnel should be consulted regarding the space needed to store disposable supplies and linen so that it is readily available on the unit.

Taking adequate time to consult all of the potential users and ancillary personnel who will use or provide services in the space is wise. One needs only to talk briefly to someone who has been forced to "make do" with poorly designed space to understand the importance of this first step in the design process.

Determine the Location

The same factors that influence decisions to build a housing development or retail shops in one place versus another can be applied to our discussion of perianesthesia space needs. A new construction design typically offers greater probability of optimizing the design than remodeling does. Nevertheless, all of the factors should be considered to ensure that the end result best serves the unit's needs. Whether this is a free-standing ambulatory surgery center or an inpatient hospital setting, the first consideration should be ease of access for the patients and family. Parking should be easily accessible and plentiful, and the entrance should be located adjacent to the parking garage or lot. The patient reception and waiting area should be near the entrance to decrease patient anxiety and frustration that would result if they had to search for it.

The second consideration should be egress. A logical patient flow—with areas that naturally follow the patients' transit through the unit being adjacent—should be established. This will maximize staff efficiency and decrease steps between areas. The waiting area should be adjacent to the preoperative holding area. PACU Phase I and PACU Phase II should be adjacent but with separate entrances from the operating rooms (ORs) for safety and efficiency. In an inpatient setting, a separate elevator for OR patients to be transported to general care and intensive care units (ICUs) is essential. This is a matter of safety for patients going to an ICU and maximizes staff efficiency for patients going to general care.

If you are remodeling, great care should be taken to determine that the design has considered these factors and incorporates them whenever possible.

Components of the Space

Several key components must be incorporated into the design of the space. The first element that needs to be determined is the number of patient bays that will be needed. Before this number can be calculated, consideration must be given to several key factors that will influence the number. First, how will the bays be used? Other important questions include the following:

- Are they strictly PACU Phase I, or are they also PACU Phase II?
- Are they also going to be used for preoperative care, or is a separate space available for that function?
- How many ORs does the PACU service, and how many cases are done per day?
- Does the PACU service other procedure areas of the hospital (i.e., cardiac catheterization/electrophysiology lab, electroconvulsive therapy treatments, medical procedures [endoscopy, bronchoscopy], radiology and

angiography, anesthesia pain service [chronic and acute])? If so, how many cases per day and at what time of day?

- Are the patients adults, children, or both?
- What is the scheduling method used by the department of surgery? How many different surgical services are served?
- What is the hospital bed capacity and usual census?
- Do patients wait long periods for inpatient beds?
- Is the PACU used for ICU overflow?
- Does the department of anesthesia have a regional anesthesia program?
- What is the average patient acuity (i.e., ASA physical status classification)?

For an inpatient hospital PACU that services a combined patient population of inpatients and same-day admission patients, a ratio of 1.5 to 2 PACU bays per OR is necessary to safely care for the patients and not back up the OR. For an ambulatory surgery center with a limited number of surgical services and types of procedures, 2.5 to 3 PACU Phase I and PACU Phase II (combined) bays are necessary. The shorter surgical procedures require an increased number of PACU slots as the recovery time may be 2 to 3 times the length of the procedure. If pediatric cases are done in either setting, the number of bays may need to be increased because this patient population will be 1:1 nursing care for a longer time than a solely adult population.

Antibiotic-resistant organisms and tuberculosis infections have been on the rise over the past several years. The need for negative pressure isolation or body substance isolation should be considered in the design. Geographic location and patient population should be reviewed to determine the number of isolation rooms that will be needed. Every PACU should have at least one negative pressure room. However, if your institution services a more susceptible population, more rooms may be needed. It is advisable to consult with your institution's infectious diseases department to be sure that your design meets institutional policy and is prepared to serve your patient population.

Another consideration in the design of patient bays is the size and means of separation between them. Most states have building codes that define the minimum square footage of each bay (e.g., State of Michigan Health Care Facilities code is 80 square feet). However, consideration should be given to how the bays will be used. If they will be used strictly for PACU Phase I patients, the minimum required square footage may be adequate. If they will be used for anesthesia preoperative procedures or anesthesia pain procedures that require equipment such as fluoroscopy or bronchoscopy, the size may need to be increased (to as much as 150 square feet). Also, if the slots are to be used alternatively as PACU Phase I or PACU Phase II and then as observation for 23-hour admissions, they may need to be large enough to accommodate a patient bed, table, and/or lounge chair. Building some of the slots larger to accommodate these future needs—keeping in mind that the size of the slots will affect the configuration of the space—may also be wise.

Patient privacy needs to be considered in determining the means of separation between patient bays. Typically PACU bays are open spaces defined only by a curtain that can be pulled for privacy. The open floor plan maximizes patient safety and staff efficiency in the higher acuity PACU Phase I setting. Where preoperative and PACU Phase II care is provided, the patient acuity is typically lower, and the need to have continual observation of patients is usually not necessary. Patients are more alert, and families are generally present so the need for privacy is increased. Half walls may be considered in these spaces. A half wall (i.e., floor-to-ceiling wall one third to half the depth of the bay) gives more privacy to the patient and family from the sights and sounds of the adjacent bays. However, this still allows the clinicians to observe patients and be readily available for acute needs.

Care should be taken to arrange the bays to maximize staffing efficiency within the constraints of the American Society of PeriAnesthesia Nurses (ASPAN) staffing resource guidelines. The PACU Phase I staffing recommendation is a maximum of two patients per registered nurse (RN)—less if the patient is unstable or a pediatric patient. For PACU Phase II staffing, the recommendation is a maximum of 3 patients to 1 RN—less if the patient is unstable and requires transfer or is a pediatric patient without family/staff support. Grouping slots in multiples of two or three allows the most efficient, safe staffing. This also allows flexibility of the space; it can be used as PACU Phase I or PACU Phase II.

ASPAN standards do not define staffing ratios for preoperative patients. Ideal, safe staffing ratios will be determined by individual institutions based on their particular patient population, number of ORs, OR turnover time, and the number of preoperative procedures done by anesthesia. The amount of nursing time required to prepare a patient for surgery depends on the patient's age, amount of preparation done in the surgery clinic, and the patient's knowledgebase and anxiety level. Patients who are well prepared when they arrive for their surgery will require less preoperative nursing time. The number of ORs, the average length of procedures, and turnover time will affect how many patients are in the preoperative area at one time and how much time they will wait before going into the OR. In a small ambulatory surgery center, one or more rooms may do quick procedures that require little equipment or cleaning to ready the OR for the next patient. In this case two patients for that same OR may need to be in the preoperative area at the same time. Another factor that will affect preoperative staffing is the number and type of anesthesia preoperative procedures. Again, in a small ambulatory surgery center the majority of procedures may be done with a general anesthetic or sedation. Thus the preparation time is shorter. Conversely, a teaching institution may have a patient population with significant comorbid conditions that require monitoring lines (i.e., pulmonary artery catheters, arterial lines, central lines, etc.). Also many institutions have a pain service that offers patients epidural catheters or extremity blocks for postoperative pain management. These patients will occupy the preoperative holding area bay for a longer period and may require nursing assistance for sedation/monitoring during and after the procedure until they go into the OR. In these situations, a ratio of four to five patients to one RN would be safe and efficient with flexibility to decrease the number of patients per RN as the patient acuity increases.

To make the space flexible for any need, preoperative or postoperative care, all of the headwalls should be designed uniformly. This will allow flexibility day-to-day or in the future as institutional needs change. During new construction, when the walls are open, it is simple and cost-effective to pipe in medical gases, and vacuum for suction at each bay. To care for critically ill PACU Phase I patients, each bay should have two oxygen outlets, one air outlet, and three vacuum outlets for suction. A freestanding ambulatory surgery center that will never serve an inpatient population may be more prudent to decrease the number of oxygen and vacuum outlets. However, you must still consider the possibility of a patient who has a surgical or anesthesia complication that requires more intensive care. The other elements of the headwall design include electrical outlets and data and telephone jacks. Again, whether it is new construction or renovation, it is wise to plan for maximum care and future needs. Each bay should have adequate electrical outlets to service a variety of pieces of equipment—including a patient bed, forced air warming/cooling device, multiple infusion pumps, ventilator, physiologic monitor, computer, compression devices, and a patient-controlled analgesia machine. Telephone and data jacks should be installed to service the current standard of practice as well as future needs. Today most physiologic monitors are computers requiring a data jack. Technology development will bring online data entry to the bedside. Planning for enough data jacks to support this future need is wise and necessary.

Another important component of the design of the patient care bay is lighting. Adequate light needs to be available for admission assessment and emergency situations. Large overhead lights provide the best source of light to meet this safety need. Consideration should be given to the stable patient for whom bright lighting is not a safety concern. Wall-mounted lights or overhead canned lights on a dimmer or low-watt lighting provide the appropriate ambience for the patient and still allow the nurse to safely care for the patient.

Another important component of the patient bay is storage. It is essential to have some emergency equipment stored at each bay to be readily available to the practitioners. However, careful planning should take place to avoid clutter that hampers the nurses' ability to quickly access equipment. Many different systems are available to service this need. Before purchasing any

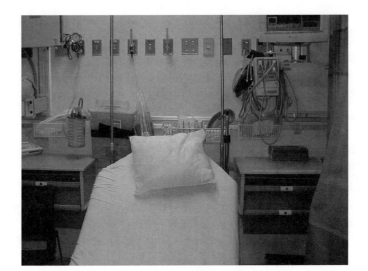

Fig. 1-1 An example of a preoperative and postanesthesia head-wall storage system with adjustable baskets and storage drawers.

system, one must plan the items that will be stored and how much space is needed. Another point to consider is what constitutes "emergent" equipment and what is at the bedside for convenience. Figure 1-1 shows one example of a storage system using a rail attached to the wall with a series of baskets that clamp onto the rail. The baskets are available in different shapes and sizes and can be moved along the rail to suit the user. A storage cart complements this system; it contains items that need to be readily available for efficiency but are not needed emergently.

The ability to care for patients in the PACU safely and efficiently is dependent on the layout of the room. Beyond the confines of the patient bay and its components, immediate access to supplies, equipment, and service areas is essential. Box 1-1 contains a list of the space and service areas needed for the preoperative holding area and PACU to function. Many of the supplies, pieces of equipment, and service areas overlap; this should be considered in the design. If service areas are strategically placed, they can service two units and thus increase staff efficiency while decreasing the cost of building and maintaining them.

To decrease the amount of duplication, determine the components that may be shared. Place these spaces between two units or in close proximity to one another. This careful, thoughtful planning will allow for safe, efficient care and minimize duplication and cost.

Staff needs are an important consideration in the design. Staff lounge and toilets adjacent to the unit(s) are essential. They allow staff the opportunity to take breaks consistent with the workflow. Because of the dynamic nature of the preoperative holding area and PACU, it is sometimes difficult to schedule breaks consistent with staff members' requests. Having facilities immediately adjacent to the units allows flexibility of scheduling and ensures availability of staff in the event of an emergency.

Ergonomics and efficiency are important elements to consider in the design of the space and the equipment. For patient safety the nurse must be able to visualize the patient from every point in the room. Essential equipment should be in the room so that the RN can constantly monitor the patient while the nurse is obtaining and using the equipment. A bedside table and chair should be available for every staff member so that he or she can sit at the patient's bedside and document while observing the patient. Tables, chairs, and computer monitors and keyboards should be adjustable to fit multiple users. With an aging workforce, the lack of adequate adjustable

Box 1-1 Support Areas and Equipment*

PREOPERATIVE HOLDING AREA
- Clean storage
- Dirty utility
- Patient toilet
- Equipment storage
- Procedure carts
- Blanket warmer
- Emergency cart
- Medication dispensing unit (e.g., Pyxis, Omnicell)
- Point-of-care testing (blood gas lab)
- Medical records storage
- Radiograph view box
- Bulletin board for patient education material

PACU PHASE I
- Clean storage
- Dirty utility
- Medication dispensing unit (e.g., Pyxis, Omnicell)
- Blanket warmer
- Emergency cart
- Equipment storage
- Point-of-care testing (blood gas lab)
- Radiograph view box
- Patient toilet

- Patient nourishment
- Medical records
- Procedure carts
- Patient education bulletin board
- Nursing station
- Physician dictation
- Staff toilet
- Staff lounge
- Staff locker room

PACU PHASE II
- Clean storage
- Dirty utility
- Medication dispensing unit (e.g., Pyxis, Omnicell)
- Patient toilet(s)
- Emergency cart
- Blanket warmer
- Patient nourishment
- Patient education bulletin board
- Nursing station
- Physician dictation
- Staff toilet
- Staff lounge
- Staff locker room

*This list is not meant to be all-inclusive. It should serve as a guide to help determine the needs of your institution.

Box 1-2 Contents of Anesthesia PACU Emergency Bag

PACU EMERGENCY BAG
MAIN COMPARTMENT
ET tubes with stylet and syringe (6.0, 7.0, and 8.0)
Extra ET tube (5.0, 5.5, 6.0, 6.5, 7.0, 7.5, 8.0)
Light wand with ET tube
Bougie
Blades (MAC 3 and 4, Miller 2 and 4)
Face mask, clear × 2
Pediatric ET tubes (2.5, 3.0, 3.5, and 4.0)
Succinylcholine
Sodium Pentothal

FRONT COMPARTMENT
Guedel airway (red, green, and yellow)
Disposable airway

Yankauer
Breathing circuit
Nasopharyngeal airway (6.5, 7.5, and 8.5)

SIDE POCKET
Syringes
Alcohol swabs

BACK POCKET EMERGENCY KIT
Cricothyrotomy
Nasal cannula
LMA 3, 4, 5
2 60-ml syringes

furnishings could lead to increased injury and exacerbate the growing nursing shortage.

Another component of the space is the reception and waiting area. This will vary depending on the location (i.e., inpatient hospital based versus free-standing ambulatory surgery center). In either location, several items need to be incorporated. If possible, preoperative patients/families should wait in a separate location than families of patients in the OR or PACU. Preoperative patient anxiety may be increased when patients see their physicians with another family or if a family is visibly upset. Also the sight and smell of food and drink is inconsiderate to a patient who has been fasting. Conversely, denying families of patients in the OR or PACU the ability to eat and drink in the waiting area so that they are not far from their loved ones and are readily available to clinical staff is unfair. The waiting areas should accommodate a variety of needs so that waiting patients and families can be entertained, distracted, or work if necessary. The waiting area should incorporate several smaller areas: an area dedicated to internet access with computer work stations and data connections for laptops, a television area, a quiet area for reading, and a children's play area with toys and furniture appropriate to the patient population served. Consult rooms should be available for private consultation between physicians and patients/families.

Standard Equipment

The type and amount of equipment needed to safely care for preoperative and postanesthesia patients will vary to some extent on the environment and patient population. However, some basic items are essential in any setting.

Types of equipment can be divided into three categories: emergent, readily available, and necessary. Emergencies in the PACU typically start as a result of airway compromise, so it is prudent to have supplies (e.g., resuscitation bag, oral/nasal airways, suction catheters, and lubricant) at the bedside to treat them. Intubation equipment should be readily available as part of the emergency cart or as a separate container/bag of anesthesia supplies. See Box 1-2 for a list of suggested items to stock in an anesthesia PACU emergency bag. Also the ASPAN Standards for PeriAnesthesia Nursing Practice 2002 Resource 6 is a list

of suggested emergency medications and equipment for a Preoperative Holding Area, PACU Phase I, and PACU Phase II.

Malignant hyperthermia (MH) is a rare but potentially fatal complication of general anesthesia. It is essential that the PACU Phase I has an MH box or cart or the equivalent supplies in the room. The Malignant Hyperthermia Association of the United States has a recommended list of supplies for MH emergencies (Box 1-3).

Institutions that recover intensive care patients in the PACU should have available a "travel box" of medications/supplies for use when transporting these patients. Table 1-1 lists the types of medications and supplies you may consider including in this box.

Readily available bedside supplies may vary between institutions depending on the types of patients and volume. However, some essential supplies should be at every patient bedside. Besides the aforementioned airway supplies, several means of oxygen delivery (see Chapter 26), a variety of suction catheters and tubing, gloves, emesis basins, and tissues should be immediately available at the bedside. Bedside supplies should be limited to only essential items to ensure they are stocked and easily retrievable by all personnel.

Other supplies that need to be readily available can be stored in a variety of ways. If the clean storage room is in close proximity to all patient bays and has a user-friendly system, equipment may be left there and retrieved at the time it is needed. If the room design does not allow for quick retrieval of supplies from the clean storage room, consideration should be given to a storage system that is located in the immediate proximity of patient bays. This system could be a cart that can be moved from bay to bay or built-in cupboards that service several bays. It is essential to involve the staff in the choice of a storage system so that it will meet their needs.

Institutions that have 24-hour equipment delivery service do not need to store such items as intravenous (IV) pumps, pneumatic compression devices, forced air warming devices, and IV poles for transport. However, if these items are not readily available, they should be stored on the unit.

Box 1-3   Malignant Hyperthermia Cart or Kit Supplies

An MH cart or kit containing the following drugs, equipment, supplies and forms should be immediately accessible to operating rooms.

DRUGS

1. Dantrolene sodium IV, 36 vials (each diluted with 60-ml sterile water)
2. Sterile water for injection USP (without a bacteriostatic agent) to reconstitute dantrolene, 1000 ml × 2
3. Sodium bicarbonate (8.4%), 50 ml × 5
4. Furosemide, 40 mg/amp × 4 ampules
5. D50, 50-ml vials × 2
6. Calcium chloride (10%) × 2
7. Regular insulin, 100 units/ml × 1 (refrigerated)
8. Lidocaine HCI (2%), 1 box = 2 grams or 20-ml vials × 5

GENERAL EQUIPMENT

1. Syringes (60 ml × 5) to dilute dantrolene
2. Mini spike IV additive pins × 2 and MultiAd fluid transfer sets × 2 (to reconstitute dantrolene)
3. Angiocaths: 20G, 2-inch; 22G, 1-inch; 24G, 3/4-inch (4 each) (for IV access and arterial line)
4. NG tubes: sizes appropriate for your patient population
5. Blood pump
6. Irrigation tray with piston syringe (× 1) for NG irrigation
7. Toomy irrigation syringes (60 ml × 2) for NG irrigation
8. Large clear plastic bags for ice
9. Bucket for ice
10. Disposable cold packs × 4

MONITORING EQUIPMENT

1. Esophageal temperature probes
2. CVP kits (sizes appropriate to your patient population)
3. Transducer kit

DRIP SUPPLIES

1. D5W, 250 ml × 1
2. Microdrip IV set × 1

NURSING SUPPLIES

1. Large sterile Steri-Drape (for rapid drape of wound)
2. Three-way irrigating Foley catheters: sizes appropriate for your patient population
3. Urine meter × 1
4. Toomy irrigation syringe (60 cc) × 2
5. Rectal tubes: sizes (Malecot Drain) 14 F, 16 F, 32 F, 34 F
6. Large clear plastic bags for ice × 4
7. Small plastic bags for ice × 4
8. Tray for ice

LABORATORY TESTING SUPPLIES

1. Syringes (3 ml) or ABG kits × 6
2. Blood specimen tubes (each test should have 2 pediatric and 2 large tubes): A for CK, myoglobin, SMA 19 (LDH, electrolytes, thyroid studies); B for PT/PTT, fibrinogen, fibrin split products; C for CBC, platelets; D for blood gas syringe (lactic acid level)
3. Urine cup × 2: myoglobin level
4. Urine dipstick: hemoglobin

FORMS

1. Laboratory request forms: ABG form × 6; hematology form × 2; chemistry form × 2; coagulation form × 2; urinalysis form × 2; physician order form × 2
2. Adverse Metabolic Reaction to Anesthesia (AMRA) Report form (obtained from Malignant Hyperthermia Association of United States)
3. Consult form

From Malignant Hyperthermia Association of United States.

Table 1-1 **Travel Box Contents**			
Contents	Quota	Contents	Quota
COMMON MEDICATIONS		Prochlorperazine 10 mg/2 ml 2-ml vial	1
Atropine 0.1-mg/ml syringe 10 ml	1	0.9% NaCl 50-ml IV bag	1
Atropine 0.4-mg/ml vial 1 ml	1		
Calcium chloride 10% 10-ml vial	1	**COMMON SUPPLIES**	
Dextrose 50% 50-ml vial	1	0.9% NaCl 20-ml vial	2
Diphenhydramine 50 mg/ml 1-ml vial	1	1-inch wide tape	1
Dopamine 400 mg/ml 5-ml vials	2	Alcohol prep	10
Epinephrine 1:10,000 10-ml syringe	2	Angiocath size 18, 20, 22, 24	1 of each size
Flumazenil 1 mg/10 ml 10-ml vial	1	Blood drawing butterfly needles	3
Furosemide 100 mg 10-ml vial	1	Gauze, Sterile 4 × 4	5
IV bags, 250 ml d5W	1	Hemostat	1
Labetalol 5 mg/ml 20-ml vial	1	Needle 21 g	4
Lidocaine 2% 5-ml syringe	1	Needle 18 g	4
Mannitol 25% 50-ml vial and filter needle	4	Oral airway	1
		Suction Catheter pediatric	2
NaHCO$_3$ pediatric bristoject 4.2% 10 ml	2	Suction Catheter adult 14 fr	2
		Syringe 1 ml	4
NaHCO$_3$ adult bristoject 8.4% 50 ml	1	Syringe 3-ml w needle	4
		Syringe 10 ml	4
Naloxone HCl 0.4 mg/ml 1 ml	1	Syringe 20 ml	4
Nitroglycerin SL 0.4 mg #25 tabs	1	Syringe pump tubing	1
		Tourniquet	1
Phenytoin 100-mg syringe 2 ml	10	Venoset, universal	1
		TPN filter	1
		Yankauer Suction Catheter	1

Pain management is an essential part of the patient care delivered in the PACU. If the institution uses IV patient-controlled analgesia pumps and epidural pumps for patient-controlled analgesia, a supply of these pieces of equipment should be kept in the PACU to be readily available. The PACU is an ICU and should therefore have a ventilator available at all times; individual institutional policy will govern what department is responsible for the set up and maintenance of any ventilators.

SUMMARY

Many changes in the care of postanesthesia patients have occurred in the last sixty years and changes are sure to continue. Thoughtful planning and interdisciplinary communication are essential for the space and equipment to continue to meet the patient care needs in perianesthesia care areas.

BIBLIOGRAPHY

American Society of PeriAnesthesia Nurses: Standards of perianesthesia nursing practice 2002, Cherry Hill, NJ, 2002.

Israel JS, DeKornfeld TJ: Recovery room care, ed 2, Chicago, 1987, Year Book Medical Publishers.

Malignant Hyperthermia Association of the United States, *http://www.mhaus.org*. American Society of PeriAnesthesia Nurses: Historical information, *http://www.aspan.org*.

Michigan State Government: Department of Consumer & Industry Services: Minimum design standards for health care facilities in Michigan, *http://www.cis.state.mi.us/bhs/hfes/pdfs/standard.pdf*.

2 PERIANESTHESIA NURSING AS A SPECIALTY

Donna M. DeFazio Quinn, BSN, MBA, RN, CPAN, CAPA

Recognition of perianesthesia nursing as a critical care specialty has been well established. This past decade has been witness to a number of significant factors that have influenced the practice of perianesthesia nursing. Among these are the emphasis on cost containment in health care, the aging and the increased acuity level of our population, the impact of human immunodeficiency viral infection, advances in technology, and fasttracking of patients through the postanesthesia care unit (PACU).

The emphasis on cost containment has stimulated the regionalization of health care and the development of tertiary care centers in major cities while primary care has increasingly moved to ambulatory settings. As a consequence, perianesthesia nursing is being practiced in a variety of settings, from the physician's office to recovery care centers to highly specialized postanesthesia care units (PACUs) in dedicated medical centers such as eye institutes and surgical hospitals. At the same time, in an effort to contain costs, many community hospitals have increased the use of the PACU for special procedures such as electroconvulsive therapy (ECT), elective cardioversion, and endoscopic examination. In addition, the PACU is being used for services such as pain clinics, preoperative holding areas (for both inpatients and outpatients), and overflow units when intensive care unit or inpatient beds are full. Although some of these changes seem to create less than optimal conditions for patient care, the creative collaboration of all health care practitioners is imperative to meet the challenges of the rapidly changing health care environment. PACUs have the unique opportunity to be innovative and creative in implementing methods to meet these changes.

The increasingly competitive business environment for health care and technologic advances has significantly increased the use of ambulatory surgical settings. The emergence of surgical hospitals has added to the equation. These multispecialty facilities provide surgical services for both inpatients and outpatients. By functioning much the same as an ASC, the surgical hospital operates in a cost-effective mode. Focus is on quick turnovers and a user-friendly atmosphere—hallmarks that make the ASC successful.

The acuity of inpatients has also greatly increased. In addition, the increasing age of the population in the United States means many surgical patients are presenting with a number of concomitant chronic problems, such as chronic obstructive lung disease, diabetes mellitus, and chronic heart conditions. The provision of quality care in the PACU requires a strong, knowledgeable leader with excellent skills and a highly skilled nursing staff. In addition to the promotion and support of the nursing staff, attention must be paid to the organizational and operational structure of the unit.

Fasttracking has become a popular concept in the PACU. Fasttracking involves admitting patients from the operating room directly to PACU Phase II and bypassing PACU Phase I. Policies and procedures on fasttracking should be developed collaboratively with involvement of nursing and anesthesia personnel. Policies should address patient selection, criteria for direct admission to PACU Phase II, patient monitoring, and discharge criteria. Nurses in the PACU Phase II unit must be competent to handle any unexpected outcome that may or may not be a direct result of fasttracking.

In an effort to define the role of the perianesthesia nurse, the American Society of PeriAnesthesia Nurses (ASPAN) has published a formal Scope of Practice document (Box 2-1), which addresses the core, dimensions, boundaries, and intersections of perianesthesia nursing practice.

ORGANIZATIONAL STRUCTURE

One person should be ultimately responsible for the management of the PACU. Typically, this person holds the title of nurse manager, director, supervisor, clinical leader, or head nurse. For the purpose of clarity, we will refer to this person as the nurse manager. The nurse manager is responsible for the administrative control of the PACU and may report directly to the surgical or the anesthesia service, depending on the institution's organizational structure.

The medical director of the PACU should be the chief of anesthesiology. In large institutions, if it is not possible for the chief of anesthesiology to fill this role because of other required duties, he or she may appoint a designee to this position. The medical director works closely with the nurse manager to develop policies and procedures and to assist with continuing education activities for the nursing staff. He or she may also be involved in the development and implementation of continuous quality improvement activities in the unit. Maintaining a good working relationship between the perianesthesia nurse manager and the medical director of the unit is essential. In this manner, areas of concern can be addressed in a collaborative, productive fashion.

STAFFING

Nurse Manager

The nurse manager of the PACU is responsible for planning, organizing, implementing, and evaluating the activities of both the nursing staff and the patient care functions. In addition, he or she is responsible for staff scheduling, assignments, performance evaluation, counseling, hiring and firing, educational program coordination (including the development and implementation of a unit-specific orientation program), and the unit budget formulation and monitoring. The nurse manager is also responsible for developing and implementing both standards of care and the unit's quality improvement program. He or she maintains responsibility for evaluating and monitoring the effectiveness of the quality improvement program as well.

The perianesthesia nurse manager needs to possess skills in time management, decision making, organization, financial management, communication, interpersonal relations, and conflict resolution. In addition, he or she should have the ability to negotiate and collaborate with other departments and healthcare team members. The nurse manager should also project a positive nursing image.

The nurse manager of the PACU should have a strong medical-surgical and perianesthesia background, preferably with critical care experience. He or she should also have previous management experience. The nurse manager should have, at minimum, a baccalaureate degree in nursing and, preferably, a master's degree in nursing or another health-related field, with emphasis on administration and business. A minimum of 5 years of experience in acute care nursing, with at least two of those years being in the PACU, is desirable. The nurse manager should also obtain certification as either a Certified Postanesthesia Nurse (CPAN) or a Certified Ambulatory Perianesthesia nurse (CAPA). Active involvement in the American Society of Perianesthesia nurses (ASPAN) will ensure that the unit is informed about the latest professional developments.

Selection of Nurses

The most important ingredient in a successful PACU is a well-educated, highly skilled, flexible nursing staff. The registered nurse must have not only a solid background in physiology, pathophysiology, and surgical procedures but also an understanding of medicine, pediatrics, geriatrics, and critical care. In addition, nurses must be thoroughly familiar with the pharmacodynamics of anesthesia and analgesia.

Selection of nursing personnel for the PACU is of the utmost importance. The nurse manager, in conjunction with the clinical nurse specialist, should establish qualifications for PACU nursing personnel. These qualifications should be written and used in all employment proceedings. This practice tends to preclude, or at least minimize, subsequent problems such as job dissatisfaction, unsatisfactory work performance, and staff

Box 2-1 Scope of Practice: Perianesthesia Nursing

The American Society of PeriAnesthesia Nurses (ASPAN), the professional organization for the specialty of perianesthesia nursing, is responsible for defining and establishing the scope of perianesthesia nursing. In doing so, ASPAN recognizes the role of the American Nurses Association (ANA) in defining the scope of practice for the nursing profession as a whole.

ASPAN supports the ANA Social Policy Statement 1997. This statement charges specialty nursing organizations with defining their individual scope of practice and identifying the characteristics within their unique specialty areas.

During the last decade, evolving professional and societal demands have necessitated a statement that clarifies the scope of perianesthesia nursing practice. Given rapid changes in healthcare delivery, trends, and technologies, the task of defining this scope is complex. This document allows for flexibility in response to emerging issues and technologies in healthcare delivery and the practice of perianesthesia nursing.

The Scope of Perianesthesia Nursing Practice involves the assessment and diagnosis of, intervention for, and evaluation of perceived, actual or potential, physical, or psychosocial problems that may result from the administration of sedation/analgesia or anesthetic agents and techniques. Our practice is systematic and includes nursing process, decision making, analytical and scientific thinking and inquiry. Our unique knowledge base regarding sedation/analgesia and anesthetic agents and techniques, the physiological and psychological bodily responses to them, and the vulnerability of the patient subjected to them is coupled with all the principles of medical surgical nursing.

The environment includes—but is not limited to—the following:

- Preanesthesia Phase
- Preadmission
- Day of Surgery/Procedure
- Postanesthesia Care Units (PACUs)
- Phase I Settings
- Phase II Settings
- Ambulatory Care Settings
- Phase III Settings

- Special Procedures Areas (i.e., Cardioversion, ECT, Endoscopy, Radiology, Oncology, etc.)
- Labor and Delivery Suites
- Pain Management Services
- Physician and Dental Offices

This specialty of perianesthesia nursing encompasses the care of the patient and family/significant other along the perianesthesia continuum of care— Preanesthesia, Postanesthesia Phase I, Phase II, and Phase III. Characteristics unique to perianesthesia practice are discussed in the following.

PREANESTHESIA PHASE

Preadmission: The nursing roles in this phase focus on preparing the patient/family/significant other physically, psychologically, socioculturally, and spiritually for his or her experience. Interviewing and assessment techniques are used to identify potential or actual problems that may result. Education and interventions are initiated to optimize positive outcomes.

Day of Surgery/Procedure: The nursing roles in this phase focus on validation of existing information and completion of preparation of the patient/family/significant other physically and emotionally for his or her experience.

Postanesthesia Phase I: The nursing roles in this phase focus on providing postanesthesia nursing care to the patient in the immediate postanesthesia period and transitioning him or her to Phase II in the inpatient setting or to an intensive care setting for continued care. Basic life-sustaining needs are of the highest priority, and constant vigilance is required during this phase because the needs of the patient are neither minimal nor episodic.

Postanesthesia Phase II: The nursing roles in this phase focus on preparing the patient/family/significant other for care in the home, Phase III, or an extended care environment.

Postanesthesia Phase III: The nursing roles in this phase focus on providing ongoing care for those patients requiring extended observation/intervention after discharge from Phase I or Phase II. Interventions are directed toward preparing the patient for self-care and/or the family/significant other for care in the home.

Continued

Box 2-1 Scope of Practice: Perianesthesia Nursing—cont'd

Perianesthesia nursing roles include those of patient care, research, administration, management, education, consultation, and advocacy. The specialty practice of perianesthesia nursing is defined through the implementation of specific role functions that are delineated in documents including ASPAN's Core Curricula for Postanesthesia and Ambulatory Surgery Nursing Practice, Standards of Perianesthesia Nursing Practice, and the Position Statement on Perianesthesia Advanced Practice Nursing. The scope of perianesthesia nursing practice is also regulated by policies and procedures dictated by the hospital/facility, state and federal regulatory agencies, national accreditation bodies, and the professional nursing organization.

Professional behaviors inherent in postanesthesia practice are the acquisition and application of a specialized body of knowledge and skills, accountability and responsibility, communication, autonomy, and collaborative relationships with others. Certification in perianesthesia nursing (Certified Postanesthesia Nurse: CPAN; Certified Ambulatory Perianesthesia nurse: CAPA) is recognized by ASPAN because it validates the defined body of knowledge for perianesthesia nursing practice. Resources to support this defined body of knowledge and nursing practice include ASPAN's Core Curricula for Postanesthesia and Ambulatory Nursing Practice, Standards of Perianesthesia Nursing Practice, Ambulatory Surgery

Core Curriculum, and Competency-Based Orientation and Credentialing Program.

ASPAN interacts with other professional groups within the domain of nursing such as the American Board of Perianesthesia Nursing Certification (ABPANC), American Nurses Association (ANA), the National League for Nursing (NLN), the American Association of Critical Care Nurses (AACN), the American Association of Nurse Anesthetists (AANA), the Federated Ambulatory Surgery Association (FASA), the National Student Nurses Association (NSNA), the Nursing Organization Liaison Forum (NOLF), and the Association of periOperative Registered Nurses (AORN). ASPAN also maintains an official liaison relationship with the American Society of Anesthesiologists (ASA), the American College of Surgeons (ACS), and the National Federation of Specialty Nursing Organizations (NFSNO). ASPAN interacts with these and other professional organizations to advance the delivery of quality care. The perianesthesia nursing scope of practice document defines the specialty practice of perianesthesia nursing. The intent of this document is to conceptualize practice and provide education to practitioners, educators, researchers and administrators and to inform other health professions, legislators, and the public about the participation in the contribution to health care by perianesthesia nursing.

Data from American Nurses Association: Nursing: a social policy statement (ANA Publication No. NP-63 20 M), Kansas City, Mo, 1997, and ANA Publishing and American Nurses Association: Code for nurses with interpretive statements, Kansas City, Mo, 1985, The Association.

turnover. It also helps ensure a smoothly functioning PACU.

The following characteristics should be considered in establishing selection criteria. The nurse considering employment in the PACU should have an interest in perianesthesia nursing. The candidate should also possess exceptional communications skills to communicate in a positive manner with all members of the healthcare team. In addition, the nurse should also have excellent patient teaching skills. He or she should be committed to providing high-quality, individualized patient care. The nurse should

have the ability to form good working relationships with all members of the healthcare team as well as to be a positive team player. The perianesthesia nurse should be capable of making intelligent, independent decisions and initiating appropriate action as necessary. He or she should be willing to accept the responsibility that accompanies working in a critical care unit. The ability to be flexible is of the utmost importance for nurses working in the PACU.

The nurse who seeks employment in the PACU should also express an interest in and ability to learn the scientific principles and theory underlying patient care as well as the technologic aspects of perianesthesia nursing. The person should be in good health, dependable, and motivated and should express an intention to stay at least 1 year in the PACU after completing the unit orientation. The orientation and training of a perianesthesia nurse requires significant time, energy, and money. Temporary assignment to the PACU is not worthwhile, except as a student learning experience.

The nurse manager should consider some professional qualifications when hiring for the PACU. The candidate should have a baccalaureate degree, and at least 1 year of general medical–surgical nursing is required. Critical care experience is suggested. The ability to coordinate care being rendered by a variety of health team members is a necessary skill, and the ability to function effectively in a crisis situation is essential.

Certification in basic cardiac life support (BCLS) and advanced cardiac life support (ACLS) should be required of all nurses working in the PACU. For units that treat a high volume of pediatric patients, certification in pediatric advanced life support (PALS) is also recommended. Application of BCLS in the PACU or ambulatory surgical unit helps sustain a patient in crisis until ACLS techniques can be instituted. ACLS includes training in arrhythmia recognition, intravenous infusion, blood gas interpretation, defibrillation, intubation, and emergency drug administration. If the perianesthesia nurse responds quickly and efficiently during crisis situations, the patient's chance of survival increases.

Certification by one of the professional nursing associations (Table 2-1) demonstrates commitment to professional excellence and should be considered positively when selecting perianesthesia nurses. Ideally, candidates for PACU positions who have attained a CPAN or CAPA credential should be given preference when hiring is done. Commitments to other professional nursing organizations should also help the candidate to be considered for a PACU position.

The perianesthesia nurse must also be able to adapt to changes in the healthcare setting. Continuous restructuring and reengineering of hospital practices has lead to turmoil in some

Table 2-1	**Certification by Professional Nursing Associations**	
Professional Association	**Credential**
American Nurses Association	Medical-surgical certification
American Association of Critical Care Nurses	CCRN
American Society of Postanesthesia Nurses	CPAN or CAPA
Association of Operating Room Nurses	CNOR
Emergency Nurses Association	CEN

institutions. Nurses must be able to accept and adapt to the constant changing environment of the future.

Nursing Personnel

Assignment of nursing personnel to the PACU should be permanent, and staff members should not be routinely rotated to other units. At least one registered professional nurse should be assigned for every 2.5 beds. Higher nurse-to-patient ratios are necessary for units that consistently deal with critical patients, such as those who have undergone open heart, thoracic, neurologic, and multiple trauma procedures. Optimal patient care is the goal of the unit. To accomplish this, continuous professional nursing judgment is required. Therefore only registered professional nurses ideally should be assigned patient care. Minimal numbers of ancillary personnel should be assigned to the unit to support the registered nurses.

Each PACU should have a registered nurse functioning in the position of clinical nurse specialist (CNS). This person may hold a title such as clinical leader, education coordinator, clinical expert, or preceptor. The CNS's role encompasses many spectra, including education, direct patient care, quality improvement, research, and consultation.

The role of education is filled by providing or arranging for continuing education of all PACU nursing staff. Support for continuing education activities increases satisfaction within the work environment, promotes stability of staff and, in turn, decreases turnover in the PACU. Perianesthesia nurses take pride in their competence to deliver safe patient care. Opportunities to broaden and expand the perianesthesia nurse's knowledge base should be fostered. Direct patient care is provided by working individually with staff members to ensure the necessary training, support, and guidance that will eventually enable the nurse to function efficiently and competently. This process allows for consistent teaching and evaluation on an individual level. In addition, the CNS becomes involved in ensuring the clinical competencies of each perianesthesia nurse as required by the Joint Commission on Accreditation of Healthcare Organizations.

The CNS's role should include involvement in quality improvement activities of the PACU. The CNS can play an important part in development of an effective monitoring and evaluation program. He or she is instrumental in implementing corrective action to correct deficiencies and improve patient outcome.

Research activities should be ongoing in the PACU. Research can serve to strengthen the identity of perianesthesia nursing as a specialty. The CNS can be invaluable in assisting staff members to develop and implement a research project.

The CNS is also the resource person for clinical problem solving and dissemination of information of an advanced nature. In addition, the CNS can ensure that standards of practice are implemented consistently throughout the organization. As a liaison, the CNS can work closely with units outside the PACU that are involved in recovering patients. These areas include labor and delivery, endoscopy, or special procedure units. The CNS could also be instrumental in collaborating with freestanding ASCs if the hospital is so affiliated.

The role of the CNS is an important one. Through skill and expertise, the CNS can offer support and encouragement to staff members, thereby promoting satisfaction and teamwork in the PACU. These factors ultimately lead to continued individual and professional growth among team members.

Licensed practical or vocational nurses (LPNs or LVNs) assigned to the PACU are restricted in their role. A registered nurse must be the primary nursing care provider in the PACU, thereby lim-

iting the role of the practical nurse in the PACU setting to one that does not allow the person to function to his or her fullest capacity. Therefore practical nurses should not be employed in the PACU. If the unit does have LPNs or LVNs, one role they could fill is assisting in the transport of patients from the PACU to the nursing unit. Orderlies and nurses' aides could be assigned to the unit to perform technical tasks that would be helpful to the nurse. These include tasks such as restocking supplies; assisting with transfer of patients; and running errands to the laboratory, central supply, or other locations.

The PACU may employ Unlicensed Assistive Personnel (UAP). When working with UAPs, the RN is responsible for knowing the policies and procedures as set forth by the individual institution. UAPs can be a valuable asset to the PACU, but the RN should remain cognizant of the fact that nursing care cannot be delegated to UAPs. UAPs can assist the nurse by performing nonnursing related tasks. Ultimately, the RN is responsible and accountable for the safe delivery of nursing care.

A skilled secretary–clerk is a definite asset to the PACU. A person adept at handling and redirecting the numerous phone calls to the PACU and proficient in clerical duties makes the job of the perianesthesia nurse much easier. The proficient secretary can assist the unit by being the liaison to family members. Providing frequent updates on the status of the patient helps reassure family members that the surgery is progressing as planned.

The secretary-clerk should possess excellent communication skills because he or she is the person who communicates to a wide spectrum of individuals—from patient and family members to physicians and other healthcare workers.

Because the patient's first contact is usually with the secretary-clerk, he or she must possess exceptional customer service skills—you don't get a second chance to make a good first impression. An individual who radiates with the impression that the patient is the most important contact that they will have that day is certainly the individual you want on the front line.

Staffing Patterns

Ideally, staffing patterns are developed based on the acuity of the patients who receive care in the PACU. Managers need to assess the acuity of the patients scheduled and staff accordingly. Historical data can also be used to predict staffing needs. Unfortunately, the operating room schedule and the PACU environment do not follow a predictable path. Unforeseen emergencies infiltrate daily operations, thus causing even the best-made plans to go awry. Having contingency staffing plans in place to deal with such fluctuations is thus the best practice. For example, a contingency plan could include bringing "on-call" or "per diem" staff members in to assist or calling on "cross-trained" nurses from other departments.

The staffing pattern developed for the PACU must include consideration for the length of patient stay, the type of surgical procedures performed, the type of anesthesia administered, and the patient population served. In addition, the skill level of the staff must be considered. According to ASPAN's Standards of Perianesthesia Nursing Practice (2000), two licensed nurses, one of whom is a registered nurse competent in PACU nursing, should be present whenever a patient is recovered in a PACU Phase I or II. Institutions unable to meet this ASPAN standard must have a policy that outlines the manner in which services are provided in their PACU and delineates how direct access to emergency assistance is accomplished. Other creative means to meet this standard include recovering the patient in an area where additional staff are present, such as the intensive care unit, or assigning the operating room staff nurse to remain available during the recovery process.

BASIC STAFF ORIENTATION PROGRAM

The orientation program for the PACU should be designed to specifically meet the needs of the nurse who works in the PACU. The program should include formal lectures and discussions as well as informal demonstrations and supervised practice. Each nurse being oriented to the PACU should have an individually assigned preceptor. The preceptor works closely with the orientee to ensure individual needs are met and deficiencies are promptly addressed. In addition, anesthesiologists, surgeons, the CNS, and other nurses in the PACU should be involved in the orientation program. Lectures should be geared toward the specific needs of the orientee.

It has been well established that nurses tend to "eat their young." In light of the national nursing shortage, experienced nurses must seek out opportunities to welcome new nurses into their specialty. Withholding valuable information and standing by as a new nurse falters does little to boost one's self esteem. Experienced staff members should support and encourage new staff members. Nurses who are made to feel a part of a team are certainly more likely to stay, whereas nurses who are unhappy will leave. Orienting a new staff nurse is costly and time-consuming; therefore implementing all possible measures to limit staff turnover is essential. Working to create a stable, cohesive staff will help with staff morale. This process begins at orientation. The orientation program should be structured to include objectives, content, and resources. It should also include the method used to evaluate the orientee's progress. The orientee should be provided with materials that clearly delineate the structure of the orientation program. The expectations the orientee faces should be absolutely clear to everyone.

Traditionally, nursing orientation programs used methods that focused on the new nurse acquiring the knowledge necessary to perform the job, but it lacked direct application to apply that knowledge. Competency-based orientation focuses on acquiring the knowledge necessary to perform the job and additionally encompasses applying that knowledge to real-life situations. Competency-based orientation is effective because it allows an expert clinician to transfer knowledge and skills to the novice learner. The learner now becomes responsible for his or her progress while the preceptor facilitates and guides the learner.

Objectives should be clearly stated, and methods for evaluating the achievement of the objectives should be clearly outlined. A notebook of the objectives, resources, evaluation forms, pertinent PACU policies and procedures, and other valuable resources should be given to each orientee. The notebook should be carefully reviewed with each orientee. A clear understanding of objectives and expectations in the beginning avoids problems in the long term.

Content of the Orientation Program

The content of the PACU orientation program should include the topics presented in Box 2-2. Additional material, as appropriate to the practice setting, should also be included.

Box 2-2   Suggested Topics for a PACU Orientation Program

REVIEW OF THE ANATOMY AND PHYSIOLOGY OF THE CARDIORESPIRATORY SYSTEM

- Pathophysiologic processes of the cardiorespiratory system
- Factors altering circulatory or respiratory function following surgery and anesthesia
- Position
- Type of incision
- Medication
- Blood loss and replacement; intake and output
- Anesthetic agent(s) used
- Type of operative procedure
- Monitoring techniques
- Hemodynamic monitoring
- Pulse oximetry
- Cardiac dysrhythmias
- Identification and treatment
- ACLS or PALS certification recommended
- Airway maintenance, equipment, and techniques pharmacological and non-pharmacological
  - Evaluation of treatment
  - Techniques to maintain a patent airway
  - Administration of oxygen
  - Use of suction equipment
- Ventilatory support, equipment, and procedures
  - Ambu bag
  - Airway insertion
- Cardiorespiratory arrest and its management
  - Use of monitor-defibrillator
  - Emergency medications
- Pain Management
  - Assessment of patient's pain level in all age groups
    - Use of pain scales
    - Documentation of pain level
  - Treatment modalities including patient education
- Treatment of hypotension or hypertension
- Interpretation of laboratory values
- Identification and treatment of malignant hyperthermia

REVIEW OF OTHER PHYSIOLOGIC CONSIDERATIONS IN THE PACU

- Neurologic system
- Musculoskeletal system
- Genitourinary system
- Fluid and electrolyte balance
- Fluid and electrolyte imbalance
- Gastrointestinal system
- Integumentary system
  - Identification of risk factors
  - Preventive measures
- Pediatric-adolescent physiology
  - Age-specific competencies
  - Patient education strategies
- Geriatric physiology
  - Age specific competencies
  - Patient education strategies
- Physiology of pregnancy

ANESTHESIA

- Administration and properties of selected agents (include all agents routinely used in the institution)
  - Intravenous agents
  - Muscle relaxants
  - Conduction anesthesia
  - Reversal agents
- Intravenous Conscious Sedation (IVCS)
  - Policies and procedures
  - Medications used
- Nursing implications

CARE OF THE PACU PATIENT

- Physical assessment of the postoperative patient
- General PACU care
  - Psychologic considerations
    - Anxiety
    - Coping responses
  - The stir-up regimen
  - Intravenous therapy and blood transfusion
  - Infection control
    - Universal precautions
    - Occupational Safety and Health Administration regulations
  - General comfort and safety measures
- Specific care required following surgical procedures
  - Ear, nose, and throat surgery
  - Ocular surgery
  - Cardiothoracic surgery
  - Neurosurgery
  - Orthopedic surgery

- Genitourinary surgery
- Gastrointestinal surgery
- Gynecologic and obstetric surgery
- Plastic surgery
- Vascular surgery
- Special considerations for the pediatric-adolescent patient
- Special procedures, such as ECT and pain blocks
- Postoperative medications
  - Pain control medications (intravenous, intramuscular, oral, epidural, patient-controlled analgesia, and pain pumps)
    - Age dependent assessment measures
    - Numerical, visual analog, or faces scale
  - Antiemetics
  - Others (antihypertensives, antiarrhythmics)
- Patient and family teaching
  - Preprocedure
  - Postprocedure
- Thermoregulation
  - Hypothermia
  - Hyperthermia (Malignant Hyperthermia)
- Department specifics
  - Layout
  - Policies and procedures
  - Preparation of patient units
- Documentation
  - Policies and procedures
  - Electronic charting
- Orientation program
  - Goals and expectations
  - Performance evaluation

The length of the orientation program should be tailored to meet the individual needs and previous experience of the orientees. Consideration should be given to the expectations placed on the orientees. Will they be expected to perform in a "call" situation at the conclusion of the orientation period, or will an experienced perianesthesia nurse be working with them for an indefinite period? The orientation period should be at least 3 months for nurses without previous PACU experience. During this time, the orientee should work fulltime. An experienced perianesthesia nurse should complete a 6-week orientation program before being placed in the position of functioning without special supervision.

Regardless of the orientation period, maintaining careful communication between the nurse manager, the orientee, and the preceptor is essential. Evaluation by the nurse manager and preceptor should be ongoing, and the orientee should receive a formal written evaluation at the end of the orientation. The orientee should clearly understand the expectations as set forth by the perianesthesia nurse manager, and the orientee and preceptor should discuss progress daily. If issues arise, the manager may need to step in and clearly review progress and expectations with the orientee. In some cases—for various reasons—an orientee may clearly not fit into the perianesthesia environment. In these circumstances, it is best to assist the orientee in gaining the required prerequisite skills rather than allowing him or her to flounder in an environment in which he or she will not succeed.

DEVELOPMENT OF EXPERTISE

Expertise in nursing involves the overlapping of three basic components of nursing: knowledge, skill, and experience. Mastering any one or two of these components will never equate with expertise. The expert nurse uses a complex linkage of knowledge, experience, skill, clue identification, gut feelings, logic, and intuition as he or she works through the problem-solving or the nursing process. As the nurse gains knowledge and experience through formal and informal programs, nursing intuition begins to develop. Intuition may be thought of as identifying a deviation from the expected, or the feeling that "something just doesn't seem right." Over time, with experience and practice, the nurse will become proficient. The accumulation of knowledge, along with the chance to practice the skills acquired, will lead to competence.

Once the nurse finishes the formal PACU orientation program, he or she should work continuously on improving background theory and skills. This may be accomplished by active participation in on-the-job training, nursing inservice programs presented on the unit, outside reading, membership in ASPAN and other state and local professional nursing organizations, and attendance at both in-house and outside-sponsored seminars and educational offerings. Constant review of basic knowledge and procedures is essential. Keeping abreast of new scientific information and innovations is necessary to ensure quality care.

Once the orientee has worked in the perianesthesia environment for at least a year and feels that he or she has gained sufficient knowledge and experience, certification as a CPAN or CAPA should be considered. Certification is one method of promoting to consumers that the quality of services they receive is enhanced because the nurses caring for them attained either a CPAN or CAPA credential.

Including funds to send nurses to important educational and information-sharing meetings in budgeting for the unit is essential. An investment made to stimulate the professional development of the nursing staff will be directly reflected in the level of nursing care provided to the patient.

COMPETENCY ASSESSMENT

Once the orientation period has ended, ensuring that staff members remain competent is essential. Integrating a competency checklist with the annual performance evaluation is one method to ensure competency. Assessing competency on an annual basis provides a number of benefits. Staff members are forced to review procedures and equipment that may not be routinely used.

Assessing competency can be divided into two aspects. The first aspect of assessing staff competence relates to policies and procedures. This could include facility standards as well as national standards as set forth by organizations such as ASPAN. Some competencies that managers may want to address include, but are not limited to, the following:

- Unit-specific administrative policies and procedures
- Patient confidentiality and patient rights
- Patient safety, including fire safety
- Environment of care issues

- Infection control practices
- Thermoregulation, including hypothermia and hyperthermia
- Variance reporting
- Compliance policies
- Medications commonly administered in the practice setting (including intravenous conscious sedation, anesthetic agents, antiemetics, and analgesics)
- Age-specific competencies (pediatric, adolescent, adult, geriatric)

The second aspect of assessing staff competence relates to equipment. Evaluation of staff members is essential to ensure their skills and knowledge in caring for equipment used in the practice setting. Specific equipment competencies include, but are not limited to, the following:

- Monitors, including EKG, pulse oximetry, and noninvasive blood pressure
- Defibrillator (defibrillation, cardioversion, external pacing)
- Warming devices
- Infusion pumps
- Ventilators

Managers should develop processes to assess the above named activities. To assess equipment competence, employees must be able to appropriately demonstrate proper use of the specific piece of equipment. To assess competence of policies and procedures, unit-specific tests can be developed.

In an effort to streamline processes, assessing competence of the new orientee and senior staff members should follow the same path. Competency assessment methods differ. The new orientee may be required to demonstrate the step-by-step process of defibrillation and to verbalize the rationale for each step. In contrast, the seasoned nurse may be required to just demonstrate the process.

It may also be helpful to incorporate competency assessments into monthly staff meetings. One method to accomplish this is to assign a staff member to present a short inservice on a specific piece of equipment or a specific policy to the staff. Competence can then be assessed using a follow-up posttest or return demonstration from the staff. Documentation can either be a checklist outlining the step-by-step return demonstration or the posttest, both of which can be filed in the employees' personnel files to document competence in the specific skill.

Quality management activities may uncover a specific deficiency. In this instance, developing a program to educate staff on the proper skills needed is important. After completing the education, the nurse manager can follow up with a competency assessment of the problem-prone activity.

THE GENERATION GAP

Finding individuals from two, three, or even four different generations in the work force today is unsurprising. Table 2-2 describes the diversity of the four different generations. Imagine the chaos that can erupt when individuals from four different generations are placed in an environment in which they have to work together.

The traditional, mature, veteran, GI, or silent generation, as they have been called, is the older generation. These individuals grew up in a time when the world was at war. They lived through the Depression and experienced hard times. They are usually hard-working, dedicated, and loyal in their values. The traditional generation of workers commonly respect authority and believe that rewards need to be earned. In the work force, they preferred to be managed in a hierarchical fashion.

The Baby Boomers are a competitive lot. Known as boomers or the sandwich generation, this group grew up in a time of educational and economic growth. As a result, they sought to find a solution to any problem they encountered. The fast-paced environment to which they are accustomed lead to many inventions that accommodate their lifestyle. They often place a high value on materialism and are not opposed to working long hours to get what they want. The Baby Boomers often do not trust those in power. Instead, they choose to have a love-hate relationship with the boss and sometimes would like it even better if they were the boss.

Individuals of generation X, also known as Xers, twenty-somethings, baby busters, or post-boomers, were the latchkey kids who grew up fending for themselves. This group adapts easily to change. Members of generation X cause chaos in the workplace because, in addition to being very upfront with their feelings, they often want flexible hours and don't want to work more than 40 hours a week. They are also the group that is most likely to have no problem doing ten things at once. They embrace the technologic advances presented to them.

The nexters, generation Y, generation next, millennial generation, and net generation, as they are known, often are the most educated group of individuals. They have been bombarded with learning since they were born. They are not afraid of technology but in fact have never known life without it. This group of individuals will seek out educational opportunities because they consider learning a lifetime endeavor.

What happens when staff members from two, three, or even four of these generations are required to work together as a team? The different values that each brings to the group are sure to cause conflict, yet when each group is nurtured appropriately, the end result of a cohesive team is not unrealistic. Finding creative ways to meld the group are sure to be each manager's challenge. Bridging the generation gap will require creative thinking on the manager's part.

The traditional group has a wealth of knowledge and experience that they bring to the group. Uncovering ways that allow the veterans to share their expertise will be key. Their knowledge can be channeled into inservice educational programs, preceptorships, and development of staff competencies. The traditional group operates in the "old-fashioned" mode. Remember common courtesies of "please" and "thank you" when communicating with this group. A written note of appreciation to the traditional member of the team will go a long way.

The Baby Boomers should also be valued for their knowledge and experience. Sometimes unlike the traditionals, they live in a competitive environment. The Baby Boomers will serve well as preceptors and educators. They also tend to like to be recognized for their accomplishments in a more public way. Publish achievements such as certifications in the organization's newsletter. Baby Boomers like to be in the spotlight and receive recognition for their accomplishments.

Generation Xers may have lived their early years with only one parent. They are in search of parental figures, and the traditional and Baby Boomers can fit well into this role. This group of individuals likes to control their own destinies.

Table 2-2 **Generational Diversity**				
	Mature (1922–1943)	Baby Boomers (1943–1960)	Generation X (1960–1980)	Nexters (1980–2000)
How many?	52 million	73.2 million	70.1 million	69.7 million
Popular names used for the generations	• Traditionalists • GI's • Mature • WWII generation • Silent generation • Seniors	• Baby Boomers • Sandwich generation	• Xers • Twenty-somethings	• Millenials • Generation Y • Generation 2001 • Nintendo generation • Generation Net • Internet generation • Dotcom generation • Generation "why"
Defining events	• Great Depression • WWII • Korean War • Radio • Rise of labor unions • Family • Patriotism	• Prosperity • Civil rights movement • Women's liberation • Vietnam • Television • Space race • Assassinations of JFK, MLK Jr. • Cold war • Suburbia • Birth control pill • Cuban missile crisis	• Watergate, Nixon resigns • Latchkey kids • Single-parent homes • AIDS • Computers • Challenger disaster • Fall of Berlin Wall • Persian Gulf • Exxon Valdez oil spill	• New millennium • Computers • School violence • Columbine High School • Oklahoma City bombing • It takes a Village • Girl's movement • Multiculturalism • 2000 political race • Stock market decline • September 11, 2001
Core values	• Hard work • Dedication • Loyalty • Detail-oriented • Conformity • Law and order • Respect for authority • Delayed reward • Duty • Adherence to rules • Honor • *Status quo* • Focus on family, country, others	• Optimism • Team orientation • Personal gratification • Health and wellness • Personal growth • Youth • Work • Involvement • Struggle with change • Seeking to find internal meaning • Struggle with self awareness • Materialistic	• Diversity • Thinking globally • Balance • Technoliteracy • Fun • Informality • Self-reliance • Pragmatism • Embrace change • Free time • Embrace self-awareness • Ecological awareness • Materialism not a driving factor	• Optimism • Civic duty • Confidence • Achievement • Sociability • Morality • Street smarts • Diversity • Change masters • Faster, faster

Table 2-2 **Generational Diversity**–*cont'd*				
	Mature (1922–1943)	Baby Boomers (1943–1960)	Generation X (1960–1980)	Nexters (1980–2000)
Education	• Institutions • Majority grade school or high school graduates	• Institutions • Majority high school graduates, increase in college graduates • Time to graduate from college, 4.5 years • SAT scores in 1965, 969 • Major: English literature, psychology, and sociology	• Institutions blended with virtual media • Majority college graduates • Time to graduate from college, 5.8 years • SAT scores in 1990, 900 • Major: business and computer science	• Multimedia in institutions, computer-based learning • Lifelong learning
Work	• Hierarchy • Seniority rules • Male breadwinner • Lifetime career or profession • Low risk takers • Diversity threatening • Externally motivated • Labor unions • Majority full-time workers • Honest day of work for honest day of pay • Grateful for a job • Large teams • Retirement age 62 to 64	• Shared leadership often just lip service • Value long-term employee • Increase of women in management and fulltime workers • Second career after age 50 • Struggle with diversity • Want wealth today • Tested on the job • Job defines them • 50–60 hour weeks • Many have two jobs • Benefit packages • Struggle with pleasing the boss and pleasing self • Commune-size teams • Pension plans	• Responsive competitive teams • Virtual teams • Brutally honest • Equal male and female workers and managers • Working at home—virtually • Decrease in unemployment • Work is just a job • Don't want to work more than 40 hours a week • Want flexible hours • Multitasking • Parallel processing • Technology wizards • Retirement age 67 to 70 • Increase in volunteers	• Civic-minded teams • Increase technologic conferencing • 50% work from home • Low unemployment • 8 careers in a lifetime • Resilient • Teamwork ethic • Can-do attitude • Technologically savvy • Expect to work 50 hour weeks • Confidence in the establishment • High productivity • Collective consensus driven • Will demand pay equity • Will reestablish the middle class • Will change the spirit from for-

Continued

	Mature (1922–1943)	Baby Boomers (1943–1960)	Generation X (1960–1980)	Nexters (1980–2000)
View of authority	• Distance between boss and worker	• Retirement age 65 to 67 • Untrustworthy • Not credible unless they are the boss • Love/hate	• Multiple careers in a lifetime • Disdain authority • Refuse to pay dues • Demand competent managers • Unimpressed	profit to not-for-profit sector • Retirement after 70 years of age • Trust in centralized authority • Will downgrade CEO and executive salaries • Polite
Rewards and recognition	Valued—to be earned	Valued, deserved	Valued, demand	Inclusively valued
Preferred leadership	Hierarchy	Consensus	Competence	Pulling together
Work ethic	Dedicated	Driven	Balanced	Determined

Table 2-2 Generational Diversity—cont'd

Adapted from Gerke ML: Understanding and leading the quad matrix: four generations in the workplace: the traditional generation, boomers, gen-x, nexters, Semin Nurse Manag 9(3):173–181, 2001.

Managers will do well if they just present the task to be accomplished and let the individual establish the means to accomplish the end goal. The generation Xers typically do not do well with politics in the work place. They also want to work in a positive, happy environment.

The nexters will thrive on new learning opportunities. Traditional nursing focused on one area of expertise—be it medical, surgical, or intensive care nursing. This group wants to learn it all. Establish opportunities for them to expand their knowledge base by allowing them to attend conferences and seminars.

Creating a work environment where all employees work together in harmony takes a great deal of work on the manager's part. Managers need to embrace this concept and employ strategies to build a work place in which all team members work in unity. The key is to find ways in which members from all the groups can work together and accept each other for what they are without trying to change each other's beliefs. Realistically, no work place will always be free of strife, but it certainly can be a place where conflict and low morale surfaces only on rare occasions.

AGING NURSING POPULATION

Unsurprisingly, the average age of a nurse is somewhere in the upper 40s. New career opportunities are steering prospective nurses toward what are seen as more appealing career paths. Seasoned nurses need to reexamine their views of their own profession and begin encouraging others to enter the field. After all, who will take care of this aging population if no new recruits join the field?

As the average age of a nurse increases, managers need to begin to find ways to accommodate staff members so they do not leave the profession. Many seasoned nurses feel they have "paid their dues" and do not want to work the "off-shifts" or be "on-call" any longer. Physically, they are getting tired.

Creative managers will develop mechanisms to keep this group in the work force. We can no longer afford to let their experience and expertise be tossed aside. Consider flexible staffing schedules for these individuals. Job-sharing and split shifts are other possibilities. If the individual tires easily because the environment is too fast-paced, consider another valued position in the department. Can he or she perform the required quality monitoring activities for which no one ever seems to have time? What about precepting that new nurse? Or developing required competency assessment of staff? Granted, there may not be enough of these positions for all the staff members, but being creative in how this issue is addressed will certainly impact retention.

The perianesthesia arena has been fortunate in that many nurses want to transfer in to this specialty. Many critical care nurses in need of a change frequently transfer into the specialty, expecting the perianesthesia unit to be slow-paced. This could not be farther from the truth! The PACU is not the place in which to transfer as one winds down one's career. In fact, many nurses, regardless of age, find the pace to be harried. Learning to prioritize and possessing good organizational skills are essential to avoid feeling overwhelmed. The current administrative strategy of using the PACU as a "dumping ground" when no beds are available in the hospital is also an issue that will impact staff morale. When morale gets low, staff retention becomes even more difficult.

Managers need to seek out what it is that will keep the older work force employed. Is it shorter hours or a more flexible schedule? Better lighting so that they can see? More ergonomically correct furniture? Better health care benefits? Whatever it is, methods to meet these needs should be investigated and implemented if at all possible.

Keeping the aging work force employed will be key to the future of our specialty. Being able to share the knowledge, experience, expertise, and wisdom that one has garnered over the years is crucial to the future of perianesthesia nursing.

STRESS AND BURNOUT IN THE PERIANESTHESIA NURSE

Stress is a word often too familiar to the perianesthesia nurse. It can be defined as the nonspecific response of the body to any demand, whether it is caused by or results in a pleasant or an unpleasant condition.

Stress can take the form of being either positive or negative (i.e., good or bad). The body responds to good or bad stress in essentially the same physiologic manner. The difference between the two responses is the body's ability to relax after encountering the stress. Left untreated, stress can act as a negative force that, in turn, can lead to physical ailments. Many adaptive methods are available to assist people who are dealing with stress. The real challenge, however, is successfully employing these adaptive measures.

Developing the ability to deal with daily stressors is essential, but before beginning to deal with daily stress, one must first be able to recognize it. Stress can manifest itself differently in each person. Being able to recognize your own individual response to stress is essential. Learning to recognize the individual message your body is sending you is a first step. Do you feel tightness in your chest? Heart palpitations? A nervous feeling in your gut? Something click in your head? Being able to recognize stress early will be of benefit in the long term because early detection makes stress easier to manage.

Stress in the Perianesthesia Setting

Behavioral symptoms of stress are exhibited in a number of ways (Box 2-3). These include behaviors such as temper outbursts, restlessness, impatience, forgetfulness, boredom, mood swings, and difficulty concentrating. When several people in the PACU exhibit symptoms of burnout, the unit will be faced with problems such as low morale, interpersonal conflict, decreased productivity, and lack of teamwork.

In the perianesthesia setting, burnout may result from the lack of positive feedback received from patients who do not remember the nurse

Box 2-3 **Behavioral Symptoms of Stress**
Temper outbursts
Restlessness
Impatience
Forgetfulness
Boredom
Mood swings
Difficulty concentrating

who took care of them. In the inpatient setting, the perianesthesia nurse rarely has the opportunity to see the positive results of care unless postoperative visits are a part of the PACU routine. Positive reinforcement by peers as well as the manager(s) aids in building self-esteem for the perianesthesia nurse. Perianesthesia nurses must learn to take care of themselves as well as they care for their patients. We as caregivers must be able to care for ourselves first if we are to remain productive.

Perianesthesia nurses are susceptible to burnout and experience many of the same frustrations as other nurses. In the past, the incidence of burnout in the PACU was very low. The reasons for this have not been fully explained, but it would seem that the regular hours as well as the social support gleaned from the close relationships developed with the entire surgical team assist in the prevention of burnout. Presently, nurses in the perianesthesia setting are under increasing stress. Perianesthesia nurses are being mandated to work long hours and extra shifts, many times to care for patients in the PACU who cannot be transferred to a hospital bed. The PACU is becoming a holding unit when no beds are available or nursing staff is insufficient to care for the patient on the nursing units. These same nurses are being "called in" to staff the PACU for an entire shift and then are required to work their designated shift. Therefore the nurses' feelings of being overworked and underappreciated are understandable. In these situations, it does not take long for the feelings of abuse to surface as stress, burnout, and resentment.

Managers need to be tuned in to how the staff is feeling. When stress is a factor, how does one deal with it at work, at home, and in everyday life? The nurse manager plays an important role in dealing with a staff that is overworked, understaffed, and stressed for any number of reasons. The manager must be able to offer support and guidance to nursing staff members so that they will be better able to deal with the numerous stressful situations they face every day.

The manager should reassure staff members that their concerns are legitimate (when they are). Listening to staff concerns with an active ear can also assist the staff nurse to deal with his or her own frustrations. Sometimes, just being able to vent concerns will help the situation.

Box 2-4 Causes of Stress in the PACU
Understaffing Critical patients Changes in policies Working overtime Lack of sleep Additional responsibilities

Managers should offer possible solutions to problems.

As stated previously, stress in the PACU can be caused by a number of factors (Box 2-4). Understaffing, critical patients, changes in policies, working overtime, lack of sleep, and additional responsibilities all contribute to stress. How does the perianesthesia nurse deal with the continuous evolution of change in the workplace? The perianesthesia nurse must first recognize the existence of the problem. Once this has been accomplished, the nurse can take three possible directions: (1) eliminate the stress; (2) resist or minimize it; or (3) accept the stress.

Eliminating the stress sometimes seems like the best way to go. Eliminating the stressor eliminates the need to face the problem. However, total elimination of the stress factor is not always possible. In circumstances in which the stress can be totally removed, the nurse may face undesirable consequences as a result of the elimination. For example, if working with a certain physician causes a great deal of stress, it may be possible to switch assignments with another nurse. The two nurses may be able to come to an agreement that one will care for all of Dr. X's patients if the other cares for all of Dr. Y's. Each nurse individually must weigh the consequences of always caring for Dr. X's patients. On the other hand, if the consequence is of no concern to the nurse, then eliminating the stressor through this option is the way to achieve the ultimate goal of avoiding Dr. Y. One must also consider that in reality the day may come when the nurse will have to care for Dr. Y's patients. This is especially true in a setting in which nurses are called in for emergencies.

The second approach is to minimize the stress element. Is there some way of reducing the stress factor so that its effect becomes minimal? Does accepting the responsibility to preceptor yet another staff nurse push a senior nurse over the edge? It may be that the nurse is already in the process of orienting two new staff members. As much as he or she enjoys this, the nurse may have to decline. The level of energy required to be a preceptor is high. In this instance, refusing the assignment may be the alternative to choose. When making choices that ultimately affect well-being, guilt should not be the deciding factor. Nurses tend to feel guilty when they make unpopular decisions. Overcoming the feeling of guilt is essential if true acceptance of the decision is expected.

Another part of reducing stress is to set priorities. Being able to look at one's current responsibilities and honestly assess what is important to accomplish at a particular time is a necessary step in reducing stress. Whenever possible, avoid procrastinating about tasks that you dislike but must be completed. Sometimes, getting the "dislikes" out of the way first will allow for thorough enjoyment of the work that remains.

The third approach to dealing with stress is to accept it. Some stress factors cannot be alleviated and must be accepted. These include realities such as divorce, death, or resignation of a favorite peer or manager. Although these events are difficult to manage, accepting them and moving ahead is one way to handle the stress. By managing the stressors that cannot be eliminated, the nurse will be able to achieve the goal of final acceptance.

Perianesthesia nurses must take time out to reward themselves and to set aside time for their personal needs. Too often nurses are absorbed in everyday activities and are too quick to give helpful advice to others yet neglect to follow their own advice. Set aside 30 minutes three times a week for exercise. No one says that nurses need to be world-class athletes, but a brisk 30-minute walk three times a week is certainly in order.

Take time to work on your favorite hobby or craft. Engage in an activity you enjoy, such as sports, cross-stitching, or sewing. Set aside some time to read that current bestseller you have been saving. Relaxation is an important element necessary to successfully reduce stress. Take time out to enjoy your free time. Do not fill every spare moment with work. It may be that the best way to relax is to just do nothing.

Activities such as bicycling, hiking, and swimming are also ways to reduce stress. When the body is physically fit, it is better able to handle stress. Nurses should also eat well and get plenty of rest. Nutrition plays an important part in maintaining a healthy lifestyle; avoidance of sugar, salt, caffeine, and alcohol is important. Eating well is essential for health maintenance, which, in turn, will assist the body in dealing with stress. Rest is vital for the rejuvenation of body cells.

Managing stress is important for the perianesthesia nurse. Once he or she has identified the stressors in his or her life, they require conscious responses. Take a moment to relax and "regroup." Eliminating, minimizing, and accepting the different stressors allow the opportunity to experience a more productive and enjoyable life.

SUMMARY

What makes perianesthesia nurses so special? It is the ability to blend expert clinical knowledge that is based on experience, education, and collegial sharing with caring practices that come from within and from being a nurse. This special ability to provide the highest level of quality care with the minimal amount of resources gives perianesthesia nurses pride.

The specialty of perianesthesia nursing is a little more than two decades in age. Perianesthesia nurses have expanded their roles to include all phases of postanesthesia care, from preadmission to discharge. Perianesthesia nurses work in a myriad of settings that include high-level trauma hospitals, ambulatory surgery centers, preadmission holding units, physician offices, and dental offices. The future will bring even more challenges for our specialty as we face reforms in healthcare delivery. The perianesthesia nurse must be flexible enough to handle competently and efficiently whatever situation he or she faces to allow the specialty of postanesthesia nursing to survive. The "specialness" of perianesthesia nursing will continue to develop and flourish as each individual nurse strives to gain that special expertise prevalent in PACUs across the country.

BIBLIOGRAPHY

American Society of PeriAnesthesia Nurses: Competency-based orientation credentialing program, Cherry Hill, NJ, 1997, The Society.

American Society of PeriAnesthesia Nurses: Standards of perianesthesia nursing practice, Cherry Hill, NJ, 2000, The Society.

Baker C et al: Transforming negative work cultures: a practical strategy, J Nurs Adm 30(7-8):357-363, 2000.

Barnes S: Pain management: what do patients need to know and when do they need to know it, J Perianesth Nurs 16(2):107-108, 2000.

Bartol GM: Creating a healing environment, Semin Perioper Nurs 7(2):90-95, 1998.

Berry PH, Dahl JL: The new JCAHO pain standards, Pain Manag Nurs 1(1):3-12, 2000.

Bickley JB: Care for the caregiver: the art of self-care, Semin Perioper Nurs 7(2):114-121, 1998.

Carley JM, Anderson FR: When a minute seems like a millennium, J Perianesth Nurs 14(5):275-277, 1999.

Carney DE, Nicolette LA, Ratner MH et al: Ketorolac reduces postoperative narcotic requirement, J Pediatr Surg 36(1):76-79, 2001.

Carter S, Ehrhardt J, Jurrus K, Sommerville S: The nursing shortage: implications for perianesthesia nursing in the 21st century, J Perianesth Nurs 15(3):169-174, 2000.

Castro B, Eshleman J, Shearer R: Using humor to reduce stress and improve relationships, Semin Nurs Manag 7(2):90-92, 1999.

Curtin LL: Autumn colors in the workplace might brighten the shortage, Semin Nurs Manag 9(3):188-194, 2001.

Dexter F, Rittenmeyer H: Measuring productivity of the phase I postanesthesia care unit, J Perianesth Nurs 12(1):7-111, 1997.

Gerke ML: Understanding and leading the quad matrix: four generations in the workplace: the traditional generation, boomers, gen-X, nexters, Semin Nurs Manag 9(3):173-181, 2001.

Helgadottir HL: Pain management practices in children after surgery, J Pediatr Nurs 15(5):334-340, 2000.

Huston CJ: Contemporary staffing-mix changes: the impact on perioperative pain management, Pain Manag Nurs 2(2):65-72, 2001.

Iacono M: Managing conflict/employee counseling, J Perianesth Nurs 15(4):260-262, 2000.

Iqbal Y, Taylor D: Surgical hospitals: where do they fit in? Outpatient Surgery Magazine 2(7):24-34, 2001.

Katz J, Wowk A, Culp D et al: Pain and tension are reduced among hospital nurses after on-site massage treatments: a pilot study, J Perianesth Nurs 14(3):128-133, 1999.

Kautzman L, Miller LH: Growing replacements for our 'graying' perioperative nurses, Today's Surgi Nurse 21(2):22-25, 1999.

Kline J: PACU staffing aided by point system, OR Manager 16(5):25-26, 2000.

Lindsay M: Is the postanesthesia care unit becoming an intensive care unit? J Perianesth Nurs 14(2):73-77, 1999.

Macready N: Burnout: an occupational hazard for manager, OR Manager 14(1):23-24, 1998.

Mamaril M: The official ASPAN position: ICU overflow patients in the PACU, J Perianesth Nurs 16(4):274-277, 2001.

Muller-Smith P: The problem with accountability, J Perianesth Nurs 12(2):109-112, 1997.

Muller-Smith P: How to keep cool in tough times, J Perianesth Nurs 14(1):31-34, 1999.

Murray-Calderon P, Connolly MA: Laryngospasm and noncardiogenic pulmonary edema, J Perianesth Nurs 12(2):89-94, 1997.

Odom J: Nursing shortage: impending doom or challenging opportunity, J Perianesth Nurs 15(5):348-349, 2000.

Odom J: Change: a matter of survival, J Perianesth Nurs 16(2):67-68, 2001.

Patel RI, Verghese ST, Hannallah RS et al: Fasttracking children after ambulatory surgery, Anesth Analg 92(4):918-922, 2001.

Patterson P: "Fasttracking" of patients through PACU: is it safe? OR Manager 14(6):1, 8-9, 1998.

Rittenmeyer H, Dolezal D, Vogel E: Pain management: a quality improvement project, J Perianesth Nurs 12(5):329-335, 1997.

Shertzer KE, Keck JF: Music and the PACU environment, J Perianesth Nurs 16(2):90-102, 2001.

Sigsby L: Effective learning about the concept of pain from a perioperative clinical rotation, Pain Manag Nurs 2(1):19-24, 2001.

Speers AT, Ziolkowski L: Preparing for the future: perianesthesia orientation, J Perianesth Nurs 11(3): 133-142, 1996.

Sullivan EE: A successful practice: Pre-Admiting test center, J Perianesth Nurs 16(3):198-200, 2001.

Summers S: Evidence-based practice part 3: acute pain management of the perianesthesia patient, J Perianesth Nurs 16(2):112-120, 2001.

Trossman, S: Stress!—It's everywhere! And it can be managed! Am Nurse 31(4):1-2, 1999.

Ulrich BT: Successfully managing multigenerational workforces, Semin Nurse Manag 9(3):147-153, 2001.

Watkins AC: Fasttracking after ambulatory surgery, J Perianesth Nurs 16(6):379-387, 2001.

Windle PE, Borromeo A, Robles H et al: The effects of accupressure on the incidence of postoperative nausea and vomiting in post surgical patients, J Perianesth Nurs 16(3):158-162, 2001.

3

MANAGEMENT AND POLICIES

Jan Odom, MSN, RN, CPAN, FAAN

All management procedures and policies of the postanesthesia care unit (PACU) should be established through joint efforts of the PACU staff, the nurse manager, and the medical director of the unit. These procedures and policies should be written and readily available to all staff working in the PACU and all physicians who use the area for postanesthesia care of their patients.

Policies are guidelines that give direction and have been approved by the administration of the institution. Procedures specify the way a policy is to be implemented and are either managerial in scope or specific to clinical nursing methods. The PACU policies and procedures should be reviewed periodically so that appropriate changes can be made when necessary. Policies and procedures must always reflect the actual practice of the unit.

Changes in the clinical situation of the hospital and advances in science and technology make revision of policies and procedures a continuous challenge. Some suggested areas that often require a written policy for the PACU are noted in Box 3-1. Policies and procedures must be tailored to meet the individual unit's needs.

PURPOSE OF THE PACU

The PACU is designed and staffed to provide intensive observation and care of patients following a procedure for which an anesthetic agent has been required. Criteria for admission to the PACU should be clearly outlined, and exceptions to the policy should be specifically delineated.

The effects on staffing and use of PACU beds have created a special concern—use of the PACU as a place to perform special procedures or to observe patients who have undergone special procedures, such as cardiac catheterization, arteriography or other specialized radiologic tests, and electroshock therapy. A recent development is use of the PACU to care for ICU or telemetry patients when no beds are available in those units in the hospital. Specific policies and procedures should address any of these special procedures performed in the unit or care of any patients under the care of the postanesthesia staff.

STAFF

Nursing staff should consist of registered professional nurses who provide direct patient care (see Chapter 2). Each unit also should have a clinical nurse specialist to provide for orientation and educational needs and to offer expertise in direct care of the patients. The clinical nurse specialist also functions in research and consultative roles. Licensed vocational or practical nurses may be employed in the area to assist the professional nurse, but they must be supervised by a registered nurse at all times. Some units use licensed vocational or practical nurses as members of their transport teams.

Student nurses should not be used to staff the PACU. Students are assigned to the PACU primarily to observe. Any patient care delivered by student nurses should be accomplished only under the direct supervision of a permanent staff nurse. No private duty or "float" nurses should be used to staff the PACU.

Retaining Nursing Staff in the PACU

Abundant information now alerts us to the existing nursing shortage—one that will only worsen over time. This shortage is multifaceted. One factor is the imminent retirements of baby boomer nurses. At the same time, fewer nurses

Box 3-1 Suggested Policies and Procedures for the PACU

Purpose and Structure of the Unit
  Unit philosophy of nursing
  Unit goals and objectives
  Patient population (scope of services)
  Admission and discharge criteria
  Admission and discharge procedures
  Staffing protocols
  Hours of operation
Job Descriptions
  Lines of authority
  Medical director
  Nurse manager
  Clinical nurse specialist
  Staff nurses
  Nursing assistants
  Unit clerks
Nursing Procedures
  All specific procedures
  Protocols
  Emergencies and code situations
  Fasttracking the ambulatory patient
  Care of the overflow patient: critical care, telemetry, medical
Special Procedures, Equipment, and Supplies
Maintenance and Safety
  Electrical safety
Control of radioactive materials

Role of biomedical engineers
Internal disaster plan
External disaster plan
Infection Control
  Standard precautions
  Transmission-based precautions
  Unit exposure control plan
  OSHA regulations
  Traffic control
  Visitors
  Attire
Laboratory Procedures
  Point of care testing
Physician's Orders
  Standing orders
  Intravenous medications
  Intravenous fluids
  Blood or blood component transfusions
Staff Education
  Orientation
  Continuing education
  Basic life-support programs and certification
  Advanced life-support programs and certification
  Certification of specialty skills
Quality Improvement
  Unit monitors
  Unit-based continuous quality improvement plan

are graduating, whereas demand for nurses is growing.

Nursing as a whole has begun to address the shrinking number of its practitioners. One issue is the professional image of nursing. Some believe that cost-cutting activities in health care that resulted in layoffs a few years ago discouraged some young people from entering a profession with an uncertain future. Other articles have mentioned the verbal abuse from physicians, low salary ceilings, inflexible working hours, and mandatory overtime as deciding factors. Also to be considered are the expanded options of female college students. Daughters of today can pursue more options than baby boomers could when

they were in college. These options have pulled some of the young people to other professions.

Recruitment into nursing and into specific hospitals is a widely discussed topic. Once staff is recruited into the perianesthesia setting, retention of experienced staff becomes a major issue. Some research has defined the nurse manager leadership behaviors had the most influence on retention of hospital staff nurse (Box 3-2).

Other factors linked to job satisfaction and retention have been flexible work schedules, appropriate pay scales, and shared governance. Flexible schedules and a shared governance philosophy are created and controlled by the manager. Creating an environment conducive to

Modified from The advisory board company: becoming a chief retention officer, Washington, DC, 2001, The Advisory Board Company: Nursing Executive Center.

Box 3-2 **Retention Practices for Nurse Managers**

- Peer interviews
  - Use appropriately educated staff to collaborate in interview process.
- Use of preceptors for new hires
  - Provides support for new hire and positive reinforcement for preceptor.
- High risk retention monitoring
  - Develop specific plans of action to retain those nurses at high risk for transfer.
- Supplies/resources available to do the job
  - Find out from staff any barriers to doing their jobs (e.g., supplies), and then take action.
- Individual career plan with each employee
  - Each employee should have an individualized career development plan.
- Regular feedback
  - Guarantee formal feedback to staff at least twice a year.
- Open communication in unit
  - Open communication a priority; staff with staff and manager with staff.
- Unit as a team
  - Make outside activities available for unit. Rely on staff input into unit goals.

staff growth and development is the manager's responsibility.

SHARED GOVERNANCE

Many units use a participative type of management. It is well documented that nurses want to be treated as professionals and desire autonomy and participation. A concept used by many hospitals to meet these needs is shared governance. In this form of management, the PACU nurse assumes more authority and responsibility and shares management skills with peers. The overall structure is that of self-management, with the staff involved in the decision-making processes that affect nursing practice and management.

Committees that address the needs of the unit, the employees, and the patients are established. Usually, a nursing practice committee is in charge of any decisions about policies and procedures or practice issues; a quality improvement committee is in charge of quality improvement in the unit; and an educational committee is responsible for meeting the educational needs of the unit. Other unit-specific committees that have been used are equipment supply, budget and finance, communications, and statistics.

The nurse manager becomes a facilitator and a resource person for the staff. Most nurse managers retain responsibilities such as employee evaluations, interviews, and liaison with administration or physicians. The challenge for the nurse manager within this system of management is to maintain a vision and to impart that vision to the staff.

SELF-SCHEDULING

One option for scheduling of staff is a system that is totally coordinated by the staff nurses. This is another method that recognizes professional nurses as capable of making crucial decisions about their practices. The schedule is developed and implemented by nurses and other staff in the unit. Advantages include decreased amount of time spent by the nurse manager on scheduling, increased team building by the staff, increased job satisfaction and autonomy of the staff, and decreased staff turnover.

PATIENT CLASSIFICATION

Most PACUs have some type of patient classification system (PCS). The most accurate PCSs seem to be those that base the patient classification on length of stay in the PACU and intensity of the care required. The PCS can be used to justify staffing and charges for the PACU stay. For example, a patient with a classification of 1 has a lower charge than a patient with a classification of 3.

Developing a PCS for the PACU is difficult at best. Many variables must be considered; for example, the length of stay of each patient varies, and the acuity of one patient can change within a short period. Moreover, patient populations can range from pediatric to geriatric and can require minor to extensive surgical procedures.

Advantages of a PCS include a more accurate assessment of the nursing time and energy required by each patient. This, in turn, allows a manager to estimate staffing requirements based on the next day's schedule. Other advantages may include knowledge of the peak workload each day and patient charges that reflect not only the length of stay but also the intensity of care required. PACU nurses also feel that the type of workload experienced in the PACU is acknowledged and that management is responsive to the staffing needs.

VISITORS

Visiting may be allowed if staffing and the physical structure of the unit permit. Traditionally, family visitation in the PACU has not been allowed. The restrictions have been due to lack of privacy, the acuity of the patients, and the fast turnover that is common to PACU patients. However, the value of allowing visitation in the PACU is a point of discussion among perianesthesia nurses. The catalyst behind the change has been, in part, the extended PACU stays many patients now require. For example, some patients may have a prolonged stay in the PACU while they wait for critical care or telemetry beds. As the incidence of morning admissions increases, the incidence of extended PACU stays also increases because of lack of postoperative bed availability. In some hospitals, the PACU is used to help with emergency department overflow.

The nursing care in the PACU has historically concentrated on the patient. However, family members also require nursing interventions. Because of this need, many PACUs are adapting critical care unit visiting policies, which may include a 5-minute visit each hour or 20-minute visit every 4 hours. Other criteria may include a limit of two family members at one time and visitation changes if warranted by the unit needs or patient condition. Privacy of other PACU patients must also be a priority.

Other situations in which visitation may be permitted include the following:

- Death of the patient may be imminent.
- The patient must return to surgery.
- The patient is a child whose physical and emotional well-being may depend on the calming effect of the parent's presence.
- The patient's well-being depends on the presence of a significant other. Patients in this category include the mentally retarded, the mentally ill, or persons with profound sensory deficits.
- The patient requires a translator because of language differences.

PATIENT RECORDS

A postanesthesia record should be kept on every patient admitted to the PACU. An example of a postanesthesia record is shown in Figure 3-1. The format may be modified to meet the needs dictated by specific procedures. Anecdotal notes should detail admission observations. The assessment, planning, and implementation phases of the nursing process should be documented as well as an evaluation of how the patient responded to the care provided. A discharge summary should also be included.

Patient records in some institutions are fully computerized. The computerized record may begin in the preoperative phase and follow the patient to the PACU. One advantage of a computerized patient record is that it is a valuable timesaver for nurses. Disadvantages may include the cost of installation and education and the time required to orient the staff to the system.

DISCHARGE OF THE PATIENT FROM THE PACU

Written criteria for discharge of the patient from the PACU must be available and should include (1) when the patient has regained consciousness and is oriented to time and place (provided he or she was oriented to time and place preoperatively); (2) when the airway is clear and the danger of vomiting and aspiration has passed; and (3) when circulatory and respiratory vital signs are stabilized. Criteria for discharge of a patient from the PACU vary by the unit or the location to which the patient will be going from the PACU, the anesthetic technique, and the physiologic status. Ultimately, the physician is in charge of the patient's discharge from the PACU. Predetermined criteria can be applied if the criteria have been approved by the physician staff.

Use of a numeric scoring system that assesses the patient's recovery from anesthesia is common. Many institutions have incorporated the postanesthesia recovery score as criteria for discharge (Box 3-3). This scoring system was introduced by Aldrete and Kroulik in 1970 and

FORREST GENERAL HOSPITAL
POST ANESTHESIA CARE UNIT RECORD

POST ANESTHESIA RECOVERY SCORE		MINUTES				
		in	30	60	90	out
Activity						
Able to move 4 extremities voluntarily or on command	= 2					
Able to move 2 extremities voluntarily or on command	= 1					
Able to move 0 extremities voluntarily or on command	= 0					
Respiration						
Able to deep breath and cough freely	= 2					
Dyspnea or limited breathing	= 1					
Apneic	= 0					
Circulation						
BP ± 20 of Preanesthetic level	= 2					
BP ± 20–50 of Preanesthetic level	= 1					
BP ± 50 of Preanesthetic level	= 0					
Consciousness						
Fully Awake	= 2					
Arousable on calling	= 1					
Not Responding	= 0					
O_2 Saturation						
Able to maintain O_2 Sat > 92% on room air	= 2					
Needs O_2 to maintain O_2 Sat > 90%	= 1					
O_2 Sat < 90% even with O_2	= 0					
TOTAL						

Pre-op B.P. _____
Allergy _____

Airway: On Adm.
Jawthrust _____
Chin Hold _____
Endotracheal _____
Oral Airway _____
Mask Oxygen _____
Nasal Oxygen _____
Trach _____
T-Tube _____
Nasal Airway _____
Ventilalor Settings _____

Addressogragh

Time In _____ Time Out _____
Accompanied by _____
Type of anesthesia _____
Surgical Procedure:

PULSE – RESPIRATION – BLOOD PRESSURE

	15	30	45		15	30	45		15	30	45		15	30	45	
240																
220																
200																
180																
160																
140																
120																
100																
80																
60																
40																
20																

O_2 Sat.
Pain Score
PAP

CODES	⊥ A-line T B.P.	V Manual or ∧ NBP	Pulse • Resp. ∘	Siderails: Yes No	Restraints:: Yes No

IV Type _____
Total IV in OR _____ cc
Blood in OR _____ units
Urinary Output in OR _____ cc
Est. Blood Loss _____ cc

Foley Cath. _____
Supra pubic _____
Ureteral _____
Levine _____

DRAINS

_____
RN Signature

RN Signature

MEDICATIONS AND TREATMENTS

	AMT.	ROUTE	TIME
Demerot			
Morphine			
Phenergan			
Droperidol			
Zotran			
Toradol			

Fig. 3-1 Postanesthesia care record. *(Courtesy of Forrest General Hospital, Hattiesburg, Miss.)*

FORREST GENERAL HOSPITAL

DATE	TIME	DESCRIPTIVE NOTES (SIGN EACH ENTRY)

Fig. 3-1 Postanesthesia care record. *(Courtesy of Forrest General Hospital, Hattiesburg, Miss.)—cont'd*

FORREST GENERAL HOSPITAL

DATE	TIME	DESCRIPTIVE NOTES (SIGN EACH ENTRY)

Report to Family: Time:	GU IRRIGANT	FOLEY OUTPUT
	TOTAL INFUSED:	TOTAL OUTPUT:

Fig. 3-1 Postanesthesia care record. *(Courtesy of Forrest General Hospital, Hattiesburg, Miss.)—cont'd*

PACU DISCHARGE SUMMARY

VITAL SIGNS ON DISCHARGE	PACU OUTCOME	COMFORT LEVEL
B/P: P: R: T:	UNEVENTFUL ☐	PAIN FREE ☐ PAIN CONTROLLED ☐
OXIMETER: PAR SCORE:	COMPLICATIONS ☐	SLEEPING BUT C/O PAIN WHEN AWAKEN ☐ Pain Score _____

REPORT TO: TIME:	SKIN CONDITION WARM COOL DRY MOIST	PINK	COLOR PALE JAUNDICED DUSKY

DRESSINGS/SURGICAL SITE/PUNCTURE SITE

X-RAYS TAKEN IN PACU	LABS DRAWN IN PACU	O₂ ORDERED YES NO _____ L/MIN PER _____ O₂ TRANSPORT YES NO

TOTAL IV IN PACU	TOTAL OUTPUT IN PACU		
	URINARY	LEVINE	DRAINS
TOTAL BLOOD IN PACU			
TOTAL PO INTAKE IN PACU	IV SITE:		
	_____ cc LTC		

ORDERS FAXED TO PHARMACY YES NO	EQUIPMENT ORDERED	TRANSPORT BY: AMBASSADOR
		RN LPN TECHNICIAN

DIAGNOSIS	GOAL	Goal Achieved	
(Circle number of any diagnosis made)		YES	NO
1 Alteration in neurological status			
2 Alteration in comfort level			
3 Alteration in emotional status			
4 Alteration in circulation			
5 Alteration in fluid volume			
6 Alteration in mobility			
7 Alteration in respiratory function			
8 Alteration in skin integrity			
9 Alteration in temperature			
10 Alteration in elimination			
11 Alteration in gastrointestinal function			
12 Alteration in injury			
13 Alteration in bleeding			
14 Other			

RHYTHM STRIPS

Fig. 3-1 Postanesthesia care record. *(Courtesy of Forrest General Hospital, Hattiesburg, Miss.)–cont'd*

Box 3-3 Postanesthesia Recovery Score (PARS)

ACTIVITY

0 = Unable to lift head or move extremities voluntarily or on command

1 = Moves two extremities voluntarily or on command and can lift head

2 = Able to move four extremities voluntarily or on command. Can lift head and has controlled movement. Exceptions: patients with a prolonged block such as bupivacaine (Marcaine) may not move an affected extremity for as long as 18 hours; patients who were immobile preoperatively

RESPIRATION

0 = Apneic; condition necessitates ventilator or assisted respiration

1 = Labored or limited respirations
Breathes by self but has shallow, slow respirations
May have an oral airway

2 = Can take a deep breath and cough well; has normal respiratory rate and depth

CIRCULATION

0 = Has abnormally high or low blood pressure; BP 50 mm Hg of preanesthetic level

1 = BP 20-50 mm Hg of preanesthetic level

2 = Stable BP and pulse. BP 2 mm Hg of preanesthetic level (minimum 90 mm Hg systolic). Exception: Patient may be released by anesthesia provider after drug therapy

NEUROLOGIC STATUS

0 = Not responding or responding only to painful stimuli

1 = Responds to verbal stimuli but drifts off to sleep easily

2 = Awake and alert; oriented to time, place, and person

O$_2$ SATURATION

0 = O$_2$ saturation <90% even with O$_2$ supplement

1 = Needs O$_2$ inhalation to maintain O$_2$ saturation >90%

2 = Able to maintain O$_2$ saturation >92% on room air

Modified from Aldrete J, Kroulik D: A post anesthetic recovery score, Anesth Analg 49:924-933, 1970; Aldrete JA: Discharge criteria, Baillieres Clin Anaesthesiol 8:763-773, 1994.

modified by Dr. Aldrete later to reflect oxygen saturation instead of color. The policy of the unit determines the appropriate score for discharge from the PACU. In most institutions, a patient with a score lower than 8 would require evaluation by the anesthesia provider and surgeon and possible disposition to a special care or critical care unit. A maximum score of 10 would indicate that the patient is in optimal condition to return to the nursing unit or to be discharged to home.

Clinical assessment must also be used in determining a patient's readiness for discharge from the PACU. This scoring system does not include detailed observations such as urinary output, bleeding or other drainage, changing requirements for hemodynamic support, temperature trends, or patient's pain management needs. All of these criteria should be considered when determining readiness for discharge.

Because patient conditions vary with surgical procedure, anesthesia used, use of analgesics, and patient response, no specific time required for the PACU stay can be stated. Professional judgment is required to determine when the patient is ready for discharge from the PACU. A complete, accurate report from the PACU nurse to the nurse who will be responsible for the care of the patient is required.

When ambulatory surgical patients are discharged to home, other criteria should be assessed. These criteria may include the following: control of pain acceptable to the patient, nausea controlled, patient ambulating in a manner consistent with the procedure and previous ability, a responsible adult present to accompany the patient.

Some PACUs require the patient to void or tolerate oral fluids before discharge to home.

Home care instructions should have been written and taught to the patient and responsible adult, both of whom have verbalized an understanding of the instructions. Emergency and routine phone numbers should be included with the instructions.

Patients should receive a follow-up visit by the anesthesia provider and be released as appropriate. In instances in which the nursing staff of the PACU is appropriately educated, a policy that defines discharge criteria and allows the nurse to discharge the patient may be in effect. Discharge criteria should be developed that meet appropriate standards but are individualized to each PACU.

FASTTRACKING

The practice of "fasttracking" refers to the practice of bypassing PACU Phase 1 and admitting the patient directly from the operating room (OR) to phase II PACU. Phase I bypass for the patient with general or regional anesthesia should only be practiced in the ambulatory setting. The patient is required to meet all Phase I discharge criteria in the OR before admission to Phase II PACU.

Contributing factors to the practice of fasttracking are technologic advancements in surgery, shorter-acting anesthetic agents, and improved pain management. Patients wake up faster and have fewer side effects and complications.

One advantage of bypassing care in PACU Phase 1 is that it decreases the expensive costs of a critical care area for patients who do not need those services and decreases total length of stay in the facility for the ambulatory surgery patient. Patients have reported higher satisfaction with the opportunity for earlier discharge.

Facilities so eager to begin a program of fasttracking that inappropriate patients bypass Phase I PACU have been reported. Anecdotes of patients admitted to Phase II in severe pain, respiratory distress, or emotional anxiety have been reported. ASPAN has developed a position on fasttracking because this practice has not been well defined (Box 3-4).

STANDARDS OF CARE

Standards of postanesthesia nursing practice have been published and are available from the

Box 3-4 **Collaborative Plan for Fasttracking**
Establish multidisciplinary workgroup—including anesthesia, Perianesthesia Phase I and II nurses, surgeons, perioperative nurses Define criteria for appropriate patient selection Develop a program to address preoperative education of patient and family Define appropriate selection and management of anesthetic agents Develop assessment criteria to evaluate patient Determine discharge criteria Develop a mechanism to monitor and report patient outcomes

Modified from American Society of PeriAnesthesia Nurses: A position statement on fast tracking, Cherry Hill, NJ, 2000, ASPAN.

American Society of PeriAnesthesia Nurses (ASPAN). These standards have been devised to stand alone or to be used in conjunction with other healthcare standards. They provide a basic framework for nurses practicing in all phases of postanesthesia care. A copy of these standards may be obtained by writing the ASPAN National Office, 10 Melrose Avenue, Suite 110, Cherry Hill, New Jersey 08003-3696 or ordered via the ASPAN website: www.aspan.org.

All preanesthesia, postanesthesia, and ambulatory surgical nurses should be familiar with these standards of practice, and a copy should be available on each unit. The PACU may develop its own standards specific to the hospital that uses the ASPAN standards as a reference or may adopt the ASPAN standards for use. If the PACU adopts ASPAN standards, they must be adopted in their entirety, or a policy must be added noting any exceptions. Any written standards must be attainable reflections of the actual practice.

Nurses must possess a minimum standard of knowledge and ability. Standards are objective and are the same for all persons. This is the reason that an inexperienced nurse in the PACU will be held to the same standard as an experienced nurse. Standards are commonly used today in legal proceedings to measure the care of patient received. The ASPAN standards have already been used in court proceedings, and many medical malpractice attorneys have a copy of the ASPAN Standards of Perianesthesia Nursing Practice in their libraries.

INFECTION CONTROL

Infection control has always been of importance in the perioperative process. It is even more significant now with the advent of multidrug-resistant tuberculosis (MDR-TB) and other drug-resistant organisms, the human immunodeficiency virus (HIV), and continued concerns with the hepatitis B (HBV) and hepatitis C (HCV) viruses.

The Centers for Disease Control and Prevention (CDC) and Hospital Infection Control Practices Advisory Committee have developed a two-level system of precautions to simplify isolation. The first level is called Standard Precautions. Standard Precautions combines what was formerly called Universal Precautions and Body Substance Isolation. Standard Precautions apply to blood, all body fluids except sweat, nonintact skin, and mucous membranes.

Transmission-Based Precautions are the second level of the system and are implemented when a patient is known or is suspected to be infected with highly transmissible pathogens (Box 3-5).

Tuberculosis

Tuberculosis (TB) is a communicable disease spread through droplets of bacteria in the air that are released when an infected person coughs, sneezes, or expectorates. TB has been about 98% curable since the 1950s with drug therapy. TB rates, however, have risen steadily since 1984, largely related to the HIV outbreak. Once infected with TB, HIV-infected persons quickly progress to an active state of the disease.

A newer and deadlier form of MDR-TB has become more common. This form of TB does not respond to the traditional treatments that are available. MDR-TB developed initially in patients who were noncompliant in taking their medication and has in turn spread to noninfected persons.

The CDC has recommended the following to healthcare settings:

| Box 3-5 | **Transmission-Based Precautions** |

Transmission-Based Precautions are applied based on method of transmission.

- Airborne—to reduce the risk of airborne transmission (e.g., dust particles that contain agents widely dispersed by air currents, special air handling, and ventilation).
- Droplet—contact of conjunctivae or mucus membranes of a susceptible person with large particle droplets that contain microorganisms that are airborne because of cough, sneeze, or suction and usually travel 3 feet or less.
- Contact—when transmission is skin-to-skin (e.g., healthcare worker-to-patient, patient-to-patient, host-to-inanimate object).

Other terminology has changed also. Nosocomial infections are a thing of the past and are now called healthcare associated infections. The rationale for this change is the stance that infections are now acquired and transmitted across a healthcare continuum—hospital, outpatient settings, and community settings. Healthcare associate infections are broken into surgical site infections and infections related to catheters.

---

1. Early identification and preventive treatment for those who have active TB and are at high risk for active TB.
2. Ventilation in the facility should be considered and designed so that air flows from clean areas to less clean areas.
3. Supplemental approaches can include high-efficiency filtration, germicidal ultraviolet irradiation, and disposable particulate respirators (PRs) to be worn by those caring for patients suspected of having TB. These PRs should also be worn by those performing procedures that are likely to produce bursts of droplet nuclei, such as bronchoscopy and endotracheal suctioning.
4. Any patient suspected or known to have active TB should be placed in respiratory isolation in a private room.

Multidrug Resistant Organisms

Vancomycin-Resistant *Enterocci* (VRE) and Methicillin-Resistant *Staphylococcus aureus* (MRSA) are the most well-known of the multidrug resistant organisms, of which a definite increase in percentage has occurred during the past few years.

The modes of transmission of these organisms are direct contact between patient and caregiver and patient and patient, and patient contact with contaminated surfaces. VRE can live for weeks on surfaces such as bedrails. MRSA can live for hours on a healthcare worker's hands.

Isolation precautions are transmission-based contact precautions. The patients can be placed in an isolation room in the PACU or placed away from other patients with a designated RN caregiver. The caregiver should wear gloves and a gown when caring for these patients. After care, gloves and gown should be removed and hands immediately washed with antiseptic soap. After removal of gown and gloves, potentially contaminated surfaces should not be touched.

Other multidrug resistant organisms of which to beware are VISA (*S. aureus* intermediately resistant to vancomycin), VRSA (*S. aureus* fully resistant to vancomycin), penicillin-resistant *Streptococcus pneumoniae* and *Neisseria gonorrhoeae*, and antibiotic-resistant mycobacterium tuberculosis.

Bloodborne Diseases

Prevention is the key to control of the bloodborne pathogens. Prevention of transmission includes three important elements: standard precautions, protective barriers, and sharps management. With standard precautions, blood and certain body fluids are considered potentially infectious for HIV, HBV, and other bloodborne pathogens. The protective gear used depends on the type of patient contact or procedure. Gloves are worn anytime that exposure to blood or body fluids is anticipated. Gloves should be changed and hands washed after each patient contact. If the procedure is likely to produce droplets or splashes of body fluid, appropriate gear would include gowns or aprons and protective eye wear and mask or face shield. Mouthpieces or artificial ventilation devices should be used instead of mouth-to-mouth resuscitation. Used needles should not be bent, broken, or otherwise manipulated. Needles should not be recapped; most facilities are using needle-less systems, which are much safer for the healthcare worker. Used needles and syringes should be placed in a puncture-resistant container immediately after use.

Despite an exposure rate of HIV of 0.3%, the CDC has documented 52 cases of HIV transmitted in the work setting to healthcare workers. HBV is transmitted more easily and has a transmission rate of 25% to 30% after hollow needle-stick injury. An estimated 12,000 to 18,000 healthcare workers contract HBV each year, and more than 250 die. The Occupational Health and Safety Administration (OSHA) mandates that employers offer health care workers HBV vaccine free of charge. HCV, which is associated with a high risk for chronic liver disease, is a growing threat to nurses. The exposure risk is only 3.5%, but the chronic disease rate is 50% to 80% after acute infection. No vaccine is currently available.

If an exposure occurs, several steps should be taken. The first step should be to decontaminate immediately with soap and water for the skin or a rinse with saline or water for the eyes, nose, or mouth. The exposure should then be reported as soon as the area is disinfected. A baseline HIV test is recommended, with a follow-up at 6 weeks, 12 weeks, and 6 months as well as frequent physical examinations when possible. A prophylaxis for HIV, such as zidovudine (AZT), should be considered and ongoing counseling support used.

OSHA: Final Rule

OSHA released guidelines regulating occupational exposure to bloodborne pathogens on December 6, 1991. Box 3-6 lists OSHA requirements that should be addressed by PACU policies.

QUALITY IMPROVEMENT

Each PACU should have a planned quality improvement program. Quality improvement programs differ from the quality assurance (QA) programs of the past in that the emphasis on inspection has changed to an emphasis on continuous improvement. Continuous quality improvement (CQI) is based on overall improvement of the system and includes the consumer in that process. A consumer is any person who uses output at any point in the system. Examples include the patient who receives care in the PACU or the PACU nurse who receives supplies from a central materials supply location.

The Joint Commission on Accreditation of Healthcare Organizations has established standards that focus on the role of the nursing staff in quality improvement. Every nurse is responsible for CQI. The result is that effective CQI will have a positive impact on the process and

outcome of care. Patient care problems can be prevented, or basic operating procedures or systems can be changed and improved.

One of the aspects of CQI is interdisciplinary participation in these activities. The common focus is on quality patient care and service. Departmental boundaries fade with a common focus on the patient. Figure 3-2 illustrates the way that QA was practiced in the past. Each department had its own QA plan developed with occasional interdepartmental and interdisciplinary participation. Figure 3-3 represents CQI as it must be practiced now, with no boundaries between departments and disciplines. The focus is on improved patient care and a seamless continuum.

CQI incorporates and uses QA but broadens its scope. Monitoring and evaluation are still parts of the process. Expansions include the role of leadership in improving quality, the scope of assessment from strictly clinical to other systems and processes that affect patients, and the focus on the processes, and not performance, of individual staff members.

Examples of CQI studies might include reducing the time it takes for the pharmacy to respond to PACU needs, improving the system to decrease the length of time patients remain in the PACU waiting for beds, changing staffing patterns in the PACU or ambulatory care areas to

---

Box 3-6   Suggested PACU Policies Based on OSHA Requirements

Exposure control plan
Engineering and work practice controls (including safer medical devices)
Handling of specimen and blood containers
Biohazard labeling
Needle use and disposal
Personal protective equipment
Housekeeping
Hepatitis B vaccination
Postexposure evaluation and follow-up
Employee education

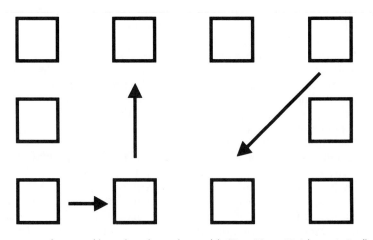

Fig. 3-2 Quality improvement demarcated intermittent interaction model. *(From Moran M, Johnson J: Quality improvement: the nurse's role. In Dienemann J, editor: Continuous quality improvement in nursing, Washington, DC, 1992, American Nurses Publishing.)*

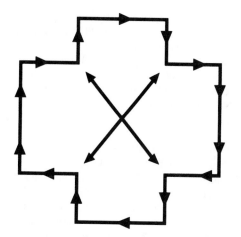

Fig. 3-3 Quality improvement seamless continuous interaction model. *(From Moran M, Johnson J: Quality improvement: the nurse's role. In Dienemann J, editor: Continuous quality improvement in nursing, Washington, DC, 1992, American Nurses Publishing.)*

meet patient care needs, or writing a patient education program for all outpatients discharged with a venous access device to ensure that all patients receive the same quality education.

SUMMARY

This chapter has focused on the management of a PACU and an ambulatory care setting involved in postanesthesia care. Important policies and management techniques were discussed along with aspects of infection control and quality improvement.

BIBLIOGRAPHY

American Society of PeriAnesthesia Nurses: Standards of Perianesthesia nursing practice, Cherry Hill, NJ, 2000, ASPAN.

Barnes SB: Are you watching the clock? Let criteria define discharger readiness, J Perianesth Nurs 15:174-176, 2000.

Buerhaus P, Staiger D, Auerbach D: Implications of a rapidly aging registered nurse workforce, JAMA, 283:2948-2954, 2000.

Burden N, editor: Ambulatory surgical nursing, ed 2, Philadelphia, 2000, WB Saunders.

Carter S et al: The nursing shortage: implications for perianesthesia nursing in the 21st century, J Perianesth Nurs 15:169-173, 2000.

Centers for Disease Control and Prevention, Hospital Infection Control Practices Advisory Committee: Recommendations for preventing the spread of vancomycin resistance, Infect Control Hosp Epidemiol 16:105-113, 1995.

Collett L, D'Errico C: Suggestions on meeting ASPAN standards in a pediatric setting, J Perianesth Nurs 15:386-391, 2000.

Department of Labor (January 18, 2001): Occupational exposure to bloodborne pathogens; needlestick and other sharps injuries: final rule, http://www.osha.gov/FedReg_osha_data/FED20010118A.html.

Dexter F, Rittenmeyer H: Measuring productivity of the phase I postanesthesia care unit, J Perianesth Nurs 12:7-11, 1997.

Health Care Financing Administration: Standards for privacy of individually identifiable health information: the HIPAA privacy rule, 2002, http://www.hcfa.gov/medicaid/hipaa/adminsim/privacy.htm.

Division of Healthcare Quality Promotion, Issues in Healthcare Settings. (August 27, 1999). MRSA, http:www.cdc.gov/ncidod/hip/aresist/mrsahcw.htm.

Feeley TW, Macario A: The postanesthesia care unit. In Miller R, editor: Anesthesia, ed 5, Philadelphia, 2000, Churchill Livingstone.

Jackson LB, Marcell J, Benedict S: Nurses' attitudes toward parental visitation on the postanesthesia care unit, J Perianesth Nurs 12:2-6, 1997.

Langley GJ et al: The improvement guide: a practical approach to enhancing organizational performance. New York, 1996, John Wiley & Sons.

Larson JL, Herrick C: Peer review in a shared governance model, J Perianesth Nurs 11:317-323, 1996.

Litwack K: Post anesthesia nursing care, ed 2, St Louis, 1995, Mosby.

Mamaril M: Fasttracking the postanesthesia patient: the pros and cons, J Perianesth Nurs 15:89-93, 2000.

Mamaril M: The official ASPAN position: ICU overflow patients in the PACU, J Perianesth Nurs 16:274-277, 2001.

Marshall SI, Chung F: Discharge criteria and complications after ambulatory surgery, Anesth Analg 88:508-517, 1999.

Muller-Smith PA: PACU management. In Litwack, K, editor: Core curriculum for perianesthesia nursing practice, ed 4, Philadelphia, 1999, WB Saunders.

Myers TA, Eichhorn DJ, Guzzetta CE: Family presence during invasive procedures and resuscitation, Am J Nurs 100(2):32-43, 2000.

Perry J: The bloodborne pathogens standard, 2001: what's changed? Nursing Management 32(6): 25-26, 2001.

Quinn DMD: Policies and procedures. In Quinn DMD, editor: Ambulatory Surgical nursing core curriculum, Philadelphia, 1999, WB Saunders.

Sandlin D: Take a bite out of high employee turnover, J Perianesth Nurs 16:109-111, 2001.

Schick L: Quality improvement. In Burden N, editor: Ambulatory surgical nursing, Philadelphia, 2000, WB Saunders.

Sheff B: (VRE & MRSA: putting bad bugs out of business, Nursing Management 30(6):44-49, 1999.

Smith S: Regulatory compliance. In Burden N, editor: Ambulatory surgical nursing, Philadelphia, 2000, WB Saunders.

Sullivan EE: Family visitation in PACU, J Perianesth Nurs 16:29-30, 2001.

Taunton RL et al: Manager leadership and retention of hospital staff, West J Nurs Res 19:205-226, 1997.

Taylor D: Decoding HIPAA: a 6-point guide, Outpatient Surgery 2(6):24-31, 2001.

Watkins AC, White PF: Fasttracking after ambulatory surgery, J Perianesth Nurs 16:379-387, 2001.

White PF, Song D: New criteria for fasttracking after outpatient anesthesia: a comparison with the modified Aldrete's scoring system, Anesth Analg 88:1069-1072, 1999.

4 CRISIS RESOURCE MANAGEMENT IN THE PACU

Joanne L. Fletcher, EdD, CRNA
Melissa A. Hotchkiss, MSNA, CRNA
Michael D. Fallacaro, DNS, CRNA

Emergency and urgent situations that necessitate immediate intervention are not uncommon in postanesthesia care units, but things do not always go smoothly as physicians and nurses care for the patient. Thus an innovative form of training may change the way patients receive care in the future. Crisis Resource Management (CRM) Training uses human factors, expertise, and patient simulators to better prepare medical teams to function effectively in their dynamic work environments.

Since WWII, aviation has used flight simulators to provide a safe yet very realistic training environment for pilots. Investigations into airline crashes have demonstrated that pilot technical skills were not usually the cause of accidents.[1] Teamwork and crew communication were often the cause of the incident. Airline crew team training was initiated in the 1980s as it became apparent that cockpit and cabin crews as well as the ground personnel and air traffic controllers needed to learn to work cohesively to prevent disasters. Although never empirically validated, simulation training has become the mainstay of aviation training. Pilots train extensively in all emergency procedures in the simulator to become proficient in the management before it occurs on an actual flight.

Since the introduction of full-sized patient simulators in the early 1990s, similar training in medicine is now possible. Dr. David Gaba and colleagues at Stanford University in Palo Alto, Calif., adapted the principles of Crew Resource Management training for the medical domain.[2] They found that the principles were as applicable in anesthesiology as they were in aviation. Both fields were dynamic, necessitated rapid decision making, and required that teams of individuals work together effectively to prevent loss of life. Since then, critical care medicine, emergency medicine and trauma teams have also begun using simulation and CRM training. Although the initial emphasis was on training physicians, the technique is now used to train nurse anesthetists and nurse practitioners, critical care nurses, paramedics, and other allied health personnel. Simulation has also been incorporated into many curricula for healthcare providers and continues to expand its role in education and training for improved patient care.

HUMAN FACTORS TRAINING AND THE SYSTEMS APPROACH TO MEDICAL ERROR

CRM training addresses the medical management of critical events with a strong emphasis on the human factors aspects. Its primary focus is on improving human performance in complex work environments: to promote better decision making, teamwork, and outcomes for the patient. This recently has become an area of intense interest in medicine. The Institute of Medicine's report on human error attracted media and public attention. Cooper et al[3] noted that more than 80% of incidents in anesthesia were preventable. Similar error rates have been found in other industries, such as aviation and nuclear power.[4]

Human error is an inevitable part of complex and rapidly changing work domains such as aviation, anesthesiology, or critical care medicine.

Human error in any discipline can lead to critical incidents with catastrophic outcomes. Major incidents such as the crash of the Concorde jet in 2000 gain media interest and prompt public attention and action primarily because of the drama and scope of the event in terms of lives altered or lost. Unfortunately, until more recently, human error–related accidents in health care tended to be less visible to the public, primarily because these events usually impact one patient at a time.

Human factors theorists have identified particular circumstances and error types and can help train individuals to recognize the signs of errant problem solving. Although human error can never be eradicated, it can certainly be managed better.[5] Aviation has tended toward teaching "error management" techniques rather than aiming for human perfection. Numerous organizations that focus primarily on patient safety measures and funding of research in this area have evolved. One such organization, the Anesthesia Patient Safety Foundation, has funded many studies[6] in recent years to facilitate human factors research and training in the field of Anesthesiology. Moreover, the recently organized National Patient Safety Foundation has broadened the study to all medical specialties. Both groups believe that further study and improved training can improve patient outcomes and safety.

Reason[7] operationalized error into three terms: slips, lapses, and mistakes. A slip is defined as an error of execution. It is observable and can simply involve the human action of picking up the wrong syringe or turning the wrong knob on an oxygen flowmeter. A lapse is not observable and involves the inability of a person to correctly recall something from memory—such as the mixture of a Lidocaine drip. Finally, a mistake is an error in planning instead of execution. Here a nurse may have planned to place a suction catheter down an endotracheal tube and extubate the patient while applying full suction. Although the execution was technically correct, it left the lungs devoid of oxygen in the process. This was a mistake in planning.

A common misconception is that errors only happen to lazy, incompetent individuals who lack vigilance. On the contrary, errors can happen to any individual despite vigilance and motivation.

When errors occur, we need to avoid placing blame on the individual(s); rather, we should strive toward a more enlightened view—to understand breakdown in the system and the resulting harm to a patient. Two compelling themes surface from human factors research: (1) humans are prone to err; and (2) the majority of errors are not the result of personal inadequacy or carelessness but instead are the product of defects in the design of healthcare environmental systems in which that work occurs. An illustrative case follows.

Sarah J, an experienced PACU nurse, was well into her double shift by the time her patient arrived in the unit at 2 AM. A 36-year-old woman involved in a motor vehicle accident had just undergone an exploratory laparotomy and splenectomy for intraabdominal bleeding. Thirty minutes after the patient's arrival, an alarm sounded. Sarah noted that her patient's heart rate was 36 beats per minute and dropping. Following unit protocol, Sarah quickly reached into the medication cart for atropine and intravenously administered a 0.4-mg dose. Almost instantly, the patient's blood pressure soared to 300 mm systolic on the arterial line monitor and the patient went into cardiac arrest. Despite full resuscitative efforts, the patient failed to respond.

Later, as Sarah was cleaning up the bedside stand of all the medications used in the code, she found an empty phenylephrine vial that had not been used during the resuscitation. It then became obvious to Sarah that she had inadvertently given her patient a 10-mg bolus of phenylephrine instead of the intended atropine.

A follow-up root cause investigation discovered that the pharmacy had recently stocked phenylephrine next to atropine in the medication drawer. Both the drugs were manufactured by the same company and came in exactly the same size vials, with the same color snap-off caps. The label for atropine was a light red color, and the phenylephrine label was pink. Instead of blaming the nurse in the case at hand, it was suggested to the pharmacy that the vials immediately be tagged with a black colored "A" atop the atropine and that the two drugs be physically separated from one another in the medication cart. The manufacturer was also notified and encouraged to change their labeling system.

Although one initially might question how a nurse would not read the label and give a wrong medication, in retrospect it is easy to see how an experienced nurse might slip while emergently reaching for a medication in a familiar vial. This slip is analogous to a once all-too-common error concerning gas flow meters among anesthetists. At one time, anesthesia gas delivery systems had two very similar gas control knobs—one to deliver oxygen and one for nitrous oxide. Slips would occur when anesthetists would inadvertently turn up the nitrous oxide when they had intended to turn up the oxygen, which resulted in a hypoxic gas mixture being delivered to the patient. A human factors approach was taken to remedy this problem. The oxygen knob was redesigned with deep indentations, whereas the nitrous oxide knob remained smooth. The anesthetist was then able to tell by touch alone that he or she had the correct knob in hand. The anesthesia machine was also given a built in fail-safe mechanism that would not allow the delivery of a hypoxic mixture regardless of how high the nitrous flow was set. This approach to the problem has effectively prevented any further patient from receiving a hypoxic mixture. Accidents and accident reporting were viewed in these examples as opportunities to design more robust systems that prevent the same type of injury from ever occurring again.

Historically, an adverse outcome results in blame toward the caregivers at the patient end—akin to the "pilot error" verdict after an airline disaster. Yet careful study of the larger system in which the incident occurs usually yields many factors that contributed to the event. Lack of training, improper equipment maintenance, poor staffing, or an illegible order transcribed incorrectly can individually or jointly contribute to a critical event.[8] In other words, a cascade of events—not just a single event—often results in the adverse outcome. CRM advocates this systems approach to adverse outcome investigations. It seeks answers from a broader perspective of the entire system to find the contributing factors. Looking at policies and administrative decisions that either supported or derailed a critical incident is a radical departure from the traditional "frame and blame" punitive approach used in medicine. This should not be interpreted as lessening the responsibility of the person who made an error but as gaining a better understanding of why it occurred. Only then can the system be adjusted to better prevent its reoccurrence. CRM training strives to make the practitioner aware of systemic factors and how to work effectively within the context of a large system that may not always be supporting their efforts.

CRISIS MANAGEMENT PRINCIPLES

"ERR WATCH" (Box 4-1) is an acronym developed by one of the authors to help the practitioner to recall the eight elements of crisis management and also remind him or her that the goal of crisis management is to reduce the element of human error in any given situation.[9] The human factor in performance is one of prime importance. Each of us has limitations in our ability to quickly and accurately process rapidly changing information during a crisis. We can do many things to improve our performances once we understand these limitations.

The role of PACU nurses is unique in the hierarchy of medicine. Not only must they be familiar with a wide variety of pathologies and their surgical treatment, but they must also be prepared to care for patients from neonates to older adults within a single shift. PACU nurses interact with staff and physicians from many disciplines and must be able to function with an often unpredictable workload. The following sections discuss the ERR WATCH principles in detail from the perspective of a PACU nurse.

Environment

The typical postanesthesia care unit presents a very complex work environment. Many pieces of sophisticated equipment are involved in the care of postoperative patients. Although nurses work with this equipment daily, they often rely on specialists such as respiratory therapists and perfusionists to maintain and regulate this equipment. Nursing staff may require additional training to deal with both routine troubleshooting and the catastrophic failure of ventilators, dialysis machines and intraaortic balloon pumps. Seconds can be critical if the patient becomes disconnected from any of these life support machines during routine patient care activities. The nursing focus can remain on the patient while the specialist concentrates on the equipment, but a crossover of skills is necessary. Inser-

---

Box 4-1   ERR WATCH Principles

Know Your **Environment**
Know equipment function, trouble-shooting, and plans for failure
Be aware of staffing levels throughout shift

Use Your **Resources**
Awareness of personal limitations
Use texts, references as resources
Plan ahead for probable problems

Frequent **Reevaluation**
Evaluate treatments for untoward effects or effectiveness
Gather information from all available sources
Maintain situation awareness

Manage Your **Workload**
Prioritize patient needs
Preload and offload tasks
Delegate tasks to others

Attention Allocation
Limited resource
Avoid fixation errors

Teamwork
Communicate changes and new information
Shared mental models

Communication
Closed loop communication
Avoid blame, criticism of others
Focus on patient needs

Call for **Help**
Global check before report
Clear concise report to incoming staff
Assign duties as needed

---

the admission is completed. Maintaining an awareness of staffing levels throughout a shift is important because these change frequently. What was adequate staffing at morning report can quickly become unsafe with staff leaving the bedside to transport patients for discharge or admission to a nursing unit, taking meal breaks, or attending meetings. As coverage decreases, so does the amount of help that will be available should an emergency arise. Be aware of how much coverage is safe in light of the patient acuity in the unit, and speak up if it is not adequate for patient safety.

Resources

Resources are assets that are available to help you care for patients safely but that may be overlooked in an emergency. Your primary resource is yourself. Your knowledge and skills are used daily in caring for your patients. But are they consistent? Human factors studies in aviation and medicine say they are not.[10] An honest self-appraisal may reveal multiple factors that can influence your performance and vigilance. Lack of sleep, boredom, concern over personal matters, coming to work with the flu, and taking medications can all adversely impact your work. No one is immune to these influences nor can consistently overcome them by sheer willpower. Being cognizant of these factors and communicating them to your coworkers can go a long way to overcome their deleterious effects. Requesting a lighter assignment, such as not taking the most critically ill patient in the unit, may be safer than trying to overcome fatigue after being up all night with a sick child. No one can perform at his or her peak level every day. Admitting to being at less than top form increases patient safety.

Critical care texts, drug formularies, and manuals provide reference for many of the drugs and dosages not used daily. Institutional protocols and procedure manuals should be kept on the unit for reference as needed. Previewing them is wise when caring for a patient whose condition is unfamiliar to you. Knowledge will be easier to recall if you have refreshed yourself on it. With the scope of nursing knowledge today, it is not possible to stay current in all areas without using these resources. Advanced Cardiac Life Support (ACLS) algorithm cards, for example, are invaluable in the event of a cardiac arrest when recall

vices can be provided to facilitate an exchange of information and contingency plans for major equipment failures. Familiarity with such emergency plans can save lives.

Unit staffing has a major impact on the nurse's role as a care provider. Open unit layouts facilitate nurses who watch multiple patients simultaneously. If one nurse is admitting a new patient, other nurses routinely cover for him or her until of the detailed protocols is difficult. Many practitioners carry a personal notebook of drugs, dosages, and protocols that can be readily available.

Taking a lesson from anesthesiology, planning ahead for emergencies that are likely to occur with your patients is prudent. Having a patient at risk for myocardial ischemia, you may benefit from precalculating dosages of various drugs used to treat ischemia before the need arises. If the problem actually occurs, you are ahead of the situation and can quickly initiate the planned intervention. You avoid the worry that you hastily miscalculated, and you probably will be extra vigilant for ischemic changes just because you are aware of a potential problem. Tactics such as this allow maximal use of mental resources without undue overload.

Reevaluation

The critical aspects of an emergency often cause nurses to lose sight of the whole patient. Thus reevaluation has a two-fold purpose: to reassess whether treatments were totally or partially effective or harmful and to look at the "big picture." Every intervention carries risks that may outweigh the benefit. Moreover, a nurse may become involved in initiating a cardiac arrest response and forget to turn the oxygen up to 100% on the ventilator. Scanning all the monitors and machines to see if anything else is changing is a benefit. Reevaluation helps draw the focus outward, to see whether additional parameters are changing that were not noted initially. With baseline data, you can then gain a better understanding of the trends in these parameters and be better able to judge the severity and direction the situation is taking. This ability to stand back and see the comprehensive situation is referred to as "situation awareness" in human factors literature.[11] It allows one to comprehend the impact of the changes and plan instead of merely reacting to the situation. It may well be what separates the "good nurse" from the "outstanding clinician." Having reevaluated the patient after initial treatment, one is better positioned to report to incoming help. He or she will be able to detail what has been done and to prioritize subsequent interventions. This helps new team members contribute positively and effectively.

Workload

A typical shift in any critical care unit is filled with many tasks. Most nurses quickly learn to distribute their workload throughout the shift and to prioritize the patient care needs as their conditions change. Experienced nurses frequently use tactics known as preloading and offloading to even out the demands of patient care. Preloading is preparing early for an upcoming procedure or medication that will be done at a busier time. Offloading is the opposite—catching up on the narrative chart after the care has been rendered. These two tactics can dramatically decrease the workload during busy periods in a shift.

An emergency dramatically increases workload. Additional help is essential to completing the many tasks required within a short period of time. When new staff arrives, they should be assigned a task appropriate to their training and experience. The charge nurse may page attending and house staff physicians and other support personnel and reassign patient care responsibilities to ensure coverage. Registered nurses can administer medications, change ventilator settings, and assist in procedures, while aides can run lab work, obtain blood from the blood bank, or get equipment.

Attention Allocation

Attention is a limited resource. It is possible to accurately follow only two to three rapidly changing variables at any time. Direct patient care activities further reduce the number of variables one can manage simultaneously. A crisis presents even greater opportunity for error. Often simply too many rapidly changing variables are in play for a single individual to comprehend and analyze accurately. Someone must be able to stand back from the direct care of the patient and be able to watch the "big picture." This is often the job of the leader in a code situation but may fall to the primary nurse until more help arrives.

Fixation and stalling in thinking are common for someone involved in a critical incident. Fixation errors occur commonly in dynamic situations and are often difficult events from which to recover. A nurse may note decreasing oxygen saturation levels and high peak pressures on the ventilator that lead him or her to treat a bronchospasm but fail to note the related hypotension, flushing, and rash that accompany an allergic reaction. This is an example of "this and only this" fixation error in which one has a reasonable diagnosis in mind and interprets any additional changes to fit that diagnosis. A second common pitfall is the "anything but this" error, in which treatment is delayed while seeking additional information in the face of a crisis. The nurse essentially knows what it is but continues to look for a more manageable diagnosis. The third type of fixation is called "everything's okay," wherein the healthcare professional denies that anything is happening or feels that he or she has a rapidly deteriorating condition under control when it is not. Any of these errors can happen to anyone faced with a critical event. They are the brain's method of signaling that it is overtaxed and cannot work effectively under the current workload. Cognitive overload is a very real phenomenon that can best be remedied by the use of additional help from colleagues. Often a fresh point of view that puts things back in perspective is gained.

Teamwork

PACU nurses routinely use teamwork to care for critically ill patients. Covering one another's patients when one nurse gets a new admission, assisting in turning, or preparing medications are just a few ways nurses work together to accomplish their many tasks.

During a critical event, teamwork needs change dramatically. Additional people join the team who may have different ways of doing things. Physicians and house staff arrive and begin ordering treatments, drugs, and tests. The previous team now becomes multidisciplinary and takes on a new character. New residents may be reluctant to take on a leadership role or several may attempt to be the leader simultaneously. Orders may be shouted into the air, directed at no one or everyone. What was well ordered may rapidly become chaotic. Studies in anesthesia and aviation have shown that the knowledge aspect rarely causes teams to perform poorly; teamwork and communication skills are lacking. Multidisciplinary team training at major institutions has had excellent results. Physicians are trained in leadership skills, and the other team members are taught to be productive and effective team members. Team members are encouraged to give

their input to the leader, to inform leaders of any changes they note as well as drugs and treatments that have been completed, and to critique their problem solving. Information from any source may provide the answer in an ambiguous situation. The team tries to help the leader to maintain good situation awareness and thus make better decisions. The leader should be willing to consider the input from all team members, communicate his or her diagnosis and plans for treatment, and keep them informed of progress. By doing so, he or she keeps the team focused on the immediate needs and further encourages their active role in the patient's management. A leader can only be as good as the team he or she leads.

Communication

Great leadership and teamwork cannot occur without the ability to communicate effectively. The military uses "closed loop" communication to ensure orders are received and understood. Address the person you are speaking to by name to attract their attention. Simply state your message and have them repeat it back to you to ensure they heard it correctly. "Give some Bicarb" should be "Sue, give one amp of Bicarb now." Sue, in turn, should state, "One amp of Bicarb now," and do it. When she completes the task, she should inform the leader that it has been done. This verifies that she was able to accomplish the task and that she is now free to do additional tasks.

Emergency situations often have very high noise levels as many people are trying to talk simultaneously. Speaking in a calm quiet voice does more to attract attention than another shout in the melee. Again, preceding the statement with the person's name will help gain his or her attention. Repeating the name may be necessary to divert them from other activities.

Conflict is common in these highly emotionally charged situations. The media have published several accounts of hostile interactions between healthcare providers that actually led to violence. To avoid escalating any existing hostility, speak in impersonal terms and avoid placing any blame on others. State facts clearly and avoid reacting to personal comments directed at you from others. Try to maintain the focus on the patient and leave the personal issues that arise for another time and place.

Call for Help

Nurses are used to working in teams and for using others to assist them. They rarely have trouble calling for additional help as needed for physical tasks, such as getting the crash cart, starting additional IVs, or hanging blood. However, many of us are reluctant to call for help when we need another opinion or to provide a different viewpoint on what is happening. Having a second person review the situation often brings out details that we have failed to notice or a diagnosis we had not considered because of our close involvement with the situation. Many of us feel that we will lose credibility with our colleagues if we call for assistance in this type of situation. However, this is precisely what must be done because recovering from a fixation error without outside help is difficult. Keep the adage "it's what's right for the patient, not who is right" in mind. Calling for a second opinion from someone with more expertise is a wise move—not a weak one.

Before help arrives, a global scan of the patient, the equipment, and the monitors is a good practice. This will provide a set of baseline data with which to compare as the treatment progresses and will allow the nurse to provide a full report to incoming assistants. When help arrives, they should receive a brief report on what has happened and any treatment that has begun. The pertinent information should be delivered succinctly, and they should be assigned specific tasks. Once the charge nurse or physician arrives, he or she should be informed of what has occurred, what is being done, and who is doing particular tasks. It need not be detailed, but it should convey the information necessary to assume the leadership role with a good understanding of the situation at hand.

These principles make good common sense. Most PACU nurses use them daily in their practices and will have them available when an emergency situation occurs. Recalling them and doing them in a rushed, stressful situation is often difficult. The principles are universal, and they have served many professions well. They can serve us as well if we use them effectively to improve our performance and positively influence the care we give our patients.

USE OF SIMULATION IN CRM TRAINING

Simulation has been an integral part of CRM training. Simulation participants are placed in a highly realistic simulated PACU environment in which they must manage common or rare critical events. CRM training for PACU staff usually uses a team approach in which a group of participants manages one crisis. Team training also allows participants to be trained in a multidisciplinary environment that is similar to the unit at work.

Simulated training consists of actual medical monitoring and resuscitative equipment normally located in the PACU. Each scenario comprises a very realistic clinical event as well as occasional interpersonal conflicts during the 20- to 30-minute session. Trainees rapidly become immersed in the situation and care for the patient as if he or she were real. Realtime feedback is given as the simulated patient responds realistically to medical interventions. The situation becomes more critical if it is mismanaged. Simulation allows participants to learn from their errors in judgment without putting an actual patient at risk.

Training Format

Simulation training sessions ideally comprise a brief introduction to the simulated environment, full-body patient simulator, and medical equipment as well as principles of CRM. After participants are oriented to the objectives of the course, they are then offered the opportunity to participate in at least one simulation session in which they are the primary care provider of the patient. The session is videotaped via multiple cameras for review after the scenario is completed. Microphones are strategically placed throughout the facility to facilitate videotape debriefing.

Immediately following the scenario, all participants proceed to a separate room in which the debriefing occurs. During the debriefing, the group is led by a trained CRM faculty facilitator who reviews the events of the scenario. The primary goal of the debriefing is to discuss the CRM principles as they related to the outcome. Focus is kept on issues such as communication, teamwork, and decision making. Trainees are often surprised at their performances as they view the videotape and are able to scrutinize their interaction with colleagues. Debriefing is a unique opportunity for participants to recognize how they became fixated on a small part of the problem or missed multiple cues which later led them to an incorrect diagnosis. Most importantly, the group discusses CRM strategies that may be used to prevent those errors in a similar situation. It is an "aha!" experience for the trainees. The key to the facilitated debriefing is a supportive atmosphere in which participants are allowed to come to their own understanding and awareness of their strengths and weaknesses. Most participants leave the course feeling they have been given information that may increase their performance in crisis situations in the PACU.

The Simulated Patient

A major component to this type of training is a realistic simulated patient. Several full-body patient simulators are commercially available in the United States and are capable of being used to teach crisis management. Currently more than 200 simulators are in operation worldwide; the majority in universities or major medical centers. Not only must the simulated patient be presented in a realistic manner; the setting must feel authentic as well. Participants must feel the environment realistically resembles the PACU because the unrealistic simulation of either the workplace or patient scenario may have a negative impact on the participant's performance.[12]

Although the simulator models have some differences, they have many common attributes. The "patient" is a life-sized computer-controlled adult mannequin. The patient's eyes open and close and its pupils respond to light, drugs, and hypoxia. The simulator can be programmed to demonstrate a wide variety of physiologic states as well as represent any age or gender. The simulated patient will react to intravenous or inhaled drugs according to the preprogrammed pathology and physiology. Standard monitoring equipment is used to display physiologically appropriate measurements of all invasive and noninvasive values. Simulators also have the ability to breathe spontaneously with measurable carbon dioxide exhalation and have heart and breath sounds appropriate to the prescribed condition. The

addition of props can make the patient a fullterm parturient, an elderly gentleman, or a young athlete. Placed within a realistic setting, the patient becomes very lifelike as the simulator converses with trainees via an instructor-speaker microphone.

The computer system that controls the simulator is often isolated in an adjacent room with a one-way mirror to allow instructor viewing. The computer models provide a range of critical events from hypotension to anaphylaxis, pulmonary emboli, and acute hemorrhage. Each event can be tailored to the expertise of the trainees—from obvious symptoms and easy treatment interventions for new graduates to subtle changes in clinical conditions with difficult treatment modalities for the more experienced practitioner. Regardless of experience level, the instructor's goal is still the same: to provide a realistic clinical situation to each trainee that will challenge (but not overwhelm) them.

Variety of Teaching Goals

Simulation centers provide a safe place to train healthcare providers. Mistakes made during sessions do not harm an actual patient. Procedures can be done repeatedly until the trainee gains a level of proficiency. New employees can learn the unit's routines or how to admit and care for various types of patients. PACU personnel can work with the actual unit equipment that they will use so that they may better understand its operation. Existing staff can use the simulator to practice rarely performed procedures, learn new skills, or orient to new equipment. Reviewing ACLS protocols is just one example of the potential use of simulation. Personnel can gain experience in the diagnosis and management of rare life-threatening medical crises that they may not see in any other setting. Several institutions have developed morbidity and mortality conferences using simulation to reenact real cases. Any of these topics can be taught either intermittently or as part of a comprehensive critical care course.

Most critical incidents require a team of physicians and nurses to be managed effectively. Simulation can provide an avenue for training these teams to work together to their maximum potential. Studies in aviation and medicine have found that lack of teamwork skills—not the personnel's technical knowledge—resulted in most disasters. Until the introduction of full-scale simulators, the training of teams was never formalized. Now actual teams of nurses, respiratory therapists, physicians and other health care providers can interact realistically to learn to communicate and function together as a cohesive unit. This type of training has been performed at various sites and been found to be very effective at improving team performance.[13,14]

SUMMARY

Technical knowledge and skills alone are not adequate to function in the complex environment of critical care. Patients today are sicker than ever before. With this increased acuity also comes an increasing number of critical events that need prompt and accurate management. Each problem has many possible outcomes that depend largely on the actions or inactions of caregivers. Every patient deserves to have well trained and knowledgeable care providers that can manage not only the usual events associated with their recovery but also the unexpected ones. CRM training and simulation offer a new approach to helping PACU nurses meet these challenges successfully.

REFERENCES

1. Helmreich RL, Foushee HC: Why crew resource management? Empirical and theoretical bases of human factors training in aviation. In Wiener EL, Kanki BG, Helmreich RL, editors: Cockpit resource management, San Diego, 1993, Academic Press.

2. Howard SK, Gaba DM, Fish KJ et al: Anesthesia crisis resource management training: teaching anesthesiologists to handle critical incidents, Aviat Space Environ Med 63(9):763-770, 1992.

3. Cooper JB, Newbower RS, Long CD et al: Preventable anesthesia mishaps: a study of human factors, Anesthesiol 49:399-406, 1978.

4. Cook RI, Woods DD: Operating at the sharp end: the complexity of human error. In Bogner MS, editor: Human error in medicine, Hillsdale, NJ, 1994, Lawrence Erlbaum Associates.

5. Helmreich RL: On error management: lessons from aviation, Br Med J 320:781-785, 2000.

6. Topics of Previous APSF Grants, retrieved October 3, 2001 from *http://www.gasnet.org/societies/apsf/foundation/topics/topics.html.*

7. Reason J: Human error, New York, 1990, Cambridge University Press.

8. Gaba DM, Fish KJ, Howard SK: Crisis management in anesthesiology, New York, 1994, Churchill Livingstone.

9. Fletcher JL: AANA journal course: update for nurse anesthetists. ERR WATCH: anesthesia crisis resource management from the nurse anesthetist's perspective, AANA Journal 66(6): 595-602, 1998.

10. Howard SK, Smith BE, Gaba DM et al: Performance of well-rested vs. highly-fatigued residents: a simulator study, Anesthesiol 87:A981, 1997.

11. Gaba DM, Howard SK, Small SD: Situation awareness in anesthesiology, Human Factors 37(1):20-31, 1995.

12. Hotchkiss MA, Mendoza SN: AANA Journal Course: update for nurse anesthetists. Full-body patient simulation technology: gaining experience using a malignant hyperthermia model, AANA Journal 69(1):59-65, 2001.

13. Lippert A, Ostergaard HT, White J et al: The knowledge and performance of the cardiopulmonary resuscitation team, Anesthesiol 90:A-1212, 2000.

14. Sexton B, Marsch S, Helmreich R et al: Participant evaluation of team oriented medical simulation, retrieved October 3, 2001 from http://www.Psy.utexas.edu/psy/Helmreich/evaltoms.htm.

5 | MANAGED CARE AND ITS IMPACT ON THE PACU

Kenneth R. White, PhD, RN, FACHE
Marie Fiascone Gerardo, MS, RN-C, ANP, CCRN

MANAGED CARE AND PERIANESTHESIA NURSING

The healthcare delivery system in the United States is a multifaceted, multipurpose organization that historically has emphasized care for acutely ill persons and relies on medical science and technology to solve healthcare problems. Therefore a healthcare system more accurately described as an "illness care" system has evolved. Today's healthcare system is influenced by health promotion and illness prevention strategies and gradually is shifting to wellness care and improving the health status of communities.

The healthcare financing system mirrors the healthcare delivery system in complexity and reflects its priorities. The financing of healthcare has also focused on acute care and critical conditions rather than the prevention of chronic, degenerative diseases and wellness. The healthcare financing structure includes both government (public) and private components and is increasingly challenged to meet the needs of a growing elderly population and access to healthcare for all those in need.

Healthcare is increasing in cost and complexity because of the advancement of technology and improved methods of diagnosis and treatment. The United States Center for Medicare and Medicaid Services (CMS) reports that national healthcare expenditures were $1.2 trillion in 1999, a six-year trend of growth below 6%.[1] Private spending for healthcare continued to grow more rapidly in 1999 than public spending. Private spending grew by 6.2%, whereas public spending grew 4.9%. The CMS estimates that national health expenditures are projected to reach 16.6% of the gross domestic product (GDP) by 2007[2] after having declined from 13.4% in 1993 to 13% percent in 1999.[1] However, access, affordability, and availability of the continuum of healthcare services for those who need it, remain critical issues that face healthcare providers and consumers.

Today, as a consequence of fundamental changes in the social and economic environment of healthcare, recognition that economic judgment is essential at all levels of decision making is widespread. Economic analysis is needed not only at the level of national health policymaking and the institutional level but also at the individual level as providers make decisions about the best way to use their time and resources for the best clinical outcomes for patients. This means that healthcare professionals must examine the services to ensure that decisions are worth the costs. Economic pressures demand this level of analysis to improve efficiencies while controlling costs and delivering quality services.

In addition to the federal government's role in regulating health services, a market system is controlling use, consumption, and availability of health services. In a market system the market rather than some other entity such as a national or state government determines the distribution of resources. One market force—managed care—refers to an organized system of care delivery that coordinates a broad range of patient services and monitors care to ensure that it is appropriate and provided in the most efficient and cost-effective way.[3] Managed care plans are health insurance products designed as a lower cost alternative to fee-for-service healthcare services. A fee-for-service (FFS) system asks providers—mainly physicians and hospitals—how much they spent

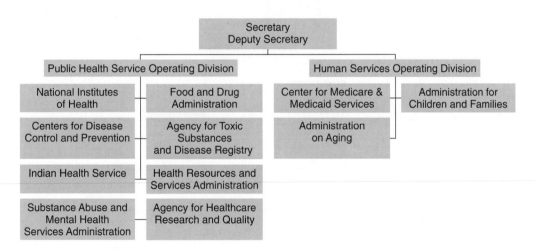

Fig. 5-1 Operating divisions of the U.S. Department of Health and Human Services.

and reimburses them for their costs. Alternatively, managed care plans selectively contract with hospitals and physicians for a prospective determination of how much will be reimbursed for healthcare services for the plan's enrollees. Thus through a stricter review of service use, various managed care plans (i.e., health maintenance organizations, preferred provider organizations, and others) provide alternative forms of less expensive healthcare.

The burgeoning enrollments in managed care plans significantly changed the health economy. Debates continue about the overall effects of managed care and whether healthcare costs have been "managed." One thing that is certain is the role of nurses has expanded to include a focus on managing the economical impact of care. Nurses more than ever are at the forefront of identifying less expensive ways to deliver quality healthcare services while integrating health promotion strategies. This chapter provides a broad overview of the ways that the healthcare delivery system is financed—including the aspects and trends of managed care—and the roles for nurses in economical decision making for the cost of care in the perianesthesia unit.

Healthcare Delivery Structure

The healthcare delivery system is a complex web of public and private services and programs devel-

oped to provide care at the federal, state, and local levels.

Role of the Federal Government

Federal healthcare activities are implemented by the Department of Health and Human Services (DHHS). This department oversees two divisions: the Public Health Service Division and the Human Services Division (Fig. 5-1). Within each division are several agencies, some of which have direct influence on healthcare delivery.

In the Public Health Service Division, the National Institutes of Health (NIH), the Food and Drug Administration (FDA), and the Centers for Disease Control and Prevention (CDC) are the primary federal agencies that conduct research and establish policy aimed at protecting the health and safety of the U.S. population.

In the Human Services Operating Division, the CMS plays a principal role in operating the multibillion dollar federal health insurance programs, Medicare and Medicaid, which provide health coverage to about one in every four Americans.[4] Medicare provides health insurance for 39.5 million elderly (over age 65) and disabled Americans. Medicaid, a joint federal-state program, provides health coverage for 33 million enrolled low-income persons, including 16.2 million children.[1]

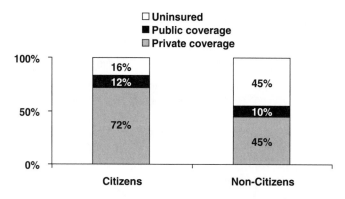

Source: Estimates by S. Glied et al., Columbia University, for The Commonwealth Fund Task Force, based on the March 1999 Current Population Survey.

Fig. 5-2 Distribution of insurance coverage based on citizenship status.

Another federal agency that contributes to the healthcare system is the Veterans Health Administration. This agency provides healthcare services to eligible veterans of military services in the Armed Forces.

Role of State and Local Governments

Although state programs vary greatly, state health departments are responsible for the oversight of a particular state's health needs. State and local health departments have responsibility for evaluating and regulating healthcare practices and coadministering the Medicaid program with the federal government. These agencies work closely in developing approaches and solutions to community health problems.

Role of Private Entities

Private healthcare organizations consist of (1) providers: hospitals, long term care facilities, hospices, home health agencies, ambulatory care centers, and others; and (2) payers: insurance companies, employers, and individuals. Healthcare provider organizations are concerned about the health status of the communities being served; thus they have a vested interest in keeping people healthy and providing healthcare services that are needed.

Insurance companies provide healthcare coverage for those who pay monthly premiums. Employers pay the majority of these premiums, although patients themselves pay copayments and must meet deductible amounts before

the insurance coverage begins to pay for services.

Who Pays for Health Care?

Health care is one of the most expensive necessities of life. Consequently, many approaches to financing the healthcare system, both public and private, exist. Financing health care may be categorized as the source of payment—direct personal payment, private insurance payment, or government health plan payment.

Direct Personal Payment

Direct personal payment pays for healthcare costs that are not covered by insurance plans and are paid out-of-pocket by consumers. In 1997, the average healthcare consumer spent 17.4% of their budgets in direct out-of-pocket expenditures for health care, as opposed to 15.1% on food and tobacco and 15.1% on housing.[5] This represents a major shift in spending patterns. Although consumers are paying more out-of-pocket, employers continue to pay the majority of the costs of health care, thus reflecting the increasing availability of private and government insurance plans.

Private Insurance Payment

The majority of healthcare consumers are covered by private insurance plans, many of which are paid all or in part by employers. In 1999, private insurance covered an estimated 72% of U.S. citizens[6] (Fig. 5-2). In addition to the 12% covered by public insurance, 16% of U.S. citizens at some point in any given year were left without health insurance and access to health care. The proportion of noncitizens without health insurance coverage jumps to 45%.[6]

The large and growing numbers of uninsured have been attributed to changes in the private insurance market, reductions in employer-sponsored health policies, and limited availability of dependent coverage.

Government Health Insurance

The two major health-related social insurance programs in the United States, Medicare and Medicaid, were enacted in 1965.

Medicare was designed to provide health care to individuals 65 years of age and older, the group with the greatest healthcare needs and fewest resources. Medicare is organized into three sections.

Part A of Medicare pays more than $100 billion to hospital and home health agencies. The Part A program is financed primarily through a mandatory payroll deduction (FICA tax). The FICA tax is 1.45% of earnings (paid by each employee and also by the employer) or 2.9% for self-employed persons.

Through Part B of Medicare, nearly $50 billion is paid to the facility operators and physicians in the outpatient setting. The Part B is financed (1) through premium payments ($45.50 per month in 1999), which are usually deducted from the monthly Social Security benefit checks of those who are enrolled in Part B; and (2) through contributions from general revenue of the United States Treasury. Beneficiary premiums are currently set to cover 25% of the average expenditures for aged beneficiaries.

When managed care plans receive premium payments from Medicare, they are obligated to pay for covered services for each enrolled beneficiary. This arrangement is known as Part C of Medicare.[7]

Medicaid is a financial aid program designed to provide medical assistance to low-income persons who are aged, disabled, blind, or members of families with dependent children. Jointly, the program is sponsored by the federal and state governments. Although the federal government provides broad guidelines for operation of Medicaid, states have wide latitude in determining eligibility and benefit criteria.

Changing Patterns of Financing Care

As the foregoing discussion has emphasized, the healthcare system in the United States is not meeting the needs of all its citizens and noncitizens, despite constantly increasing expenditures. Growth in spending persists; the number of uninsured continues to rise; and efforts to control rising costs have not given the desired outcome of stabilizing the healthcare expenditures as a percentage of the gross domestic product. Although many attempts have been made to reform the United States healthcare system, the most recent activity comes from the market system of purchasers and consumers. Controlling expenditures through a managed care strategy has slowed but not arrested the dramatic rate of cost escalation.

Managed Care Strategy

The impetus for managed care has arisen from the purchasers of health care—the government and employers—who are increasingly frustrated by escalating healthcare costs. Managed care works by shifting the financial risk of health care from the insurer (government or private insurance plans) to the individual providers (physicians, nurse practitioners, and others) and institutional providers (hospitals, nursing homes, home health agencies, and others). Providers are paid set, preestablished fees in a capitated or heavily discounted FFS arrangement. Capitation is a set dollar payment per patient per unit of time (usually per month) that is paid to cover a specified set of services and administrative costs without regard to the actual number of services provided. Discounting FFS pays for services rendered is another way of preestablishing fees. With either system, providers are held accountable for providing all health services necessary to the members or beneficiaries of the managed care plan for this set level of payment.

The advantage of managed care is primarily reducing costs while ensuring patients receive a standard level of quality healthcare services. However, criticisms of managed care are that the cost concerns may outweigh the quality concerns and that some patients may be restricted in their use of needed services merely to save money. Also, evidence is somewhat equivocal about the overall cost savings under managed care.[5] However, a preponderance of the evidence suggests that managed care is effective in controlling costs and excessive use of services without compromising quality.[7] For these reasons, managed care seems likely to remain an important aspect of the U.S. healthcare system for years to come.

Role of Case Managers

One way to reduce the fragmentation of healthcare delivery and to coordinate services so that patients are moved from more expensive to less expensive sites of care is the use of case managers. Case managers assess patients' overall needs for different health services, delineate comprehensive patient outcomes, identify and procure the most cost-effective means of meeting those outcomes, and evaluate the effectiveness of the provided services. Case managers oversee the complete continuum of care from preadmission through rehabilitation. Case managers also coordinate services through the continuum of care for patients with chronic conditions. Although nurses commonly fill this role, many different models of case management exist.

Implications for Perianesthesia Nurses

The spread of managed care has impacted the way that health care is delivered—not only for the nursing profession and healthcare provider organizations but also for the individual nurse at the bedside. Implications for nursing include facilitating access to care to those without health insurance, increasing collaboration with other healthcare providers for more prevention and education about health promotion and disease prevention, and increasing productivity and efficiency in providing direct and indirect patient care. For individual nurses, understanding the economics of health delivery and the advent of managed care is the first step in delivering cost-effective care without compromising—rather, perhaps, improving—quality.

Cost of Care in the PACU

Historically, surgical services were the most financially profitable area in the hospital. The advent of managed care and managed costs dramatically reduced the revenue generated by these areas. The majority of surgical cases are now reimbursed at a fixed rate regardless of the costs incurred by the facility. This shift in reimburse-ment strategy has caused hospitals and ambulatory surgery centers to look for ways to minimize their costs to maximize their revenues. Drugs, equipment—both reusable and disposable—prosthetics, linen use, and the numerous other incidental components have been examined to determine cost-effective procedures.

Charges do not necessarily reflect the cost incurred by the hospital to provide services to a patient. This is because charges often reflect the market forces of supply and demand and do not necessarily maintain a constant relationship with costs.[8] Charges may also be deliberately higher to cover costs for other departments that have no reimbursement, such as medical records and risk management.

The actual cost of providing services is much more difficult to calculate because of the wide array of items used to provide a service. Therefore most facilities use a charge structure that they believe reflects the cost of providing a service or procedure to patients. Total cost can be determined by adding together the cost of each component expended to complete a particular surgical case or procedure. The total cost is then compared with the charge for the surgery or the negotiated payer reimbursement; the difference determines the level of profit or loss for that procedure or surgery.[9] Costs are subdivided into fixed and variable categories.

Fixed Costs

Fixed costs are one-time costs, such as capital expenditures. Examples of this type of cost include monitors, stretchers, IV pumps, and the bricks and mortar of the facility itself. Fixed costs do not change in proportion to the number of procedures or surgeries performed.[8]

Variable Costs

Variable costs vary with the volume of patients who receive care. These costs are linked directly to the number of surgical cases.[8] Dressings, medications, laundry, oxygen/ventilator tubing, EKG electrodes, and the salaries of most staff members are variable costs. Labor (staff) costs are further subdivided into direct and indirect costs.

Direct labor costs represent the amount paid to employees for the length of time spent performing patient care. Direct labor costs for a PACU are calculated by multiplying the average hourly wage rate of each job class by the number of hours provided in each class and adding the results together.[9] These are variable costs because the number of patients cared for directly impacts the cost.

Indirect labor costs are made up of the salaries of those not involved in the provision of direct patient care. The nurse manager, unit secretaries, and any other staff who do not provide direct patient care are in this category. This category also contains any portion of staff salaries that are derived from attendance at meetings, inservice education, or other non–patient care activities.

How Nursing Contributes to Managing the Cost of Care

In the perianesthesia setting, labor represents the highest percentage of costs.[9] As revenues declined after the implementation of managed care, most facilities developed strategies that included reducing or eliminating paid time for meetings and education to reduce labor costs. In addition, facilities shifted away from hiring full-time employees, who carry higher benefit costs, to more parttime and hourly employees who have fewer—if any—benefit costs. Cost containment will always be an important strategy to ensure the financial viability of healthcare facilities. Nurses play important roles in identifying areas and process improvement opportunities that will result in cost savings for an organization while providing efficient, effective quality patient care.

Quality Versus Cost

When nurses talk about cost and quality, many seem to put the concepts on opposite ends of a spectrum, as if the two were mutually exclusive. This may be due to a knowledge deficit regarding the financial aspects of providing patient care. Nursing as a profession typically attracts individuals who value the capacity that the human touch has for promoting healing and a sense of well-being, which is not a quantifiable value. In addition, the concept of quality lacks a shared definition. "Quality" means different things to different people and organizations; however, the cost of providing care seems less important than ensuring patients have a positive experience of the healthcare system. Typically, once nurses

develop an understanding of how money flows through an organization, they become some of the best advocates for cost-reduction strategies. The individuals at the bedside usually know where money is wasted and how the system can be improved to benefit all parties involved. All they need is to be involved in the decision-making process.

Patient Education

The perianesthesia nurse can begin setting the tone of the patient experience during preoperative teaching. Discussing what the patient anticipates can help to guide care in the PACU. This exchange provides the opportunity for the nurse to explain the postoperative course and for the patient to share his or her expectations and concerns. In 1992, Orkin[10] found that patients were willing to tolerate a reduction in mental acuity and some degree of pain to avoid postoperative nausea. In addition, ambulatory surgery patients assume that their procedure and recovery will consume most of their operative day.[11] Discovering what is meaningful to the patient can help set expectations that are easily met by the PACU staff. This type of exchange and follow-through in care costs very little and can provide the patient and family with a better PACU experience.

Nurses who work in the ambulatory surgery setting have the additional challenge of providing extensive discharge teaching. Preprinted instructions are a necessity because patients will only remember about 10% to 15% of what they are told. Perianesthesia nurses must be involved in the creation of these materials and should serve on the patient education committee in their facility. In addition, nurses in this area are in a unique position to track the quality of care via the incidence of infections. Typically, ambulatory care centers call patients 24 hours after discharge to determine how the patient is progressing and to assess for any concerns. Some facilities have instituted a 72-hour callback to identify postoperative infections that may be related to quality issues at the hospital. These infections are typically underreported because most patients return to their primary care providers or surgeons for follow-up, and no tracking mechanism is in place to quantify this issue.

Using Clinical Guidelines

The American Society of PeriAnesthesia Nurses (ASPAN) is responsible for defining the practice of perianesthesia nursing.[12] Their mission is to advance nursing practice through education, research, and standards. Perianesthesia nurses should familiarize themselves with the mission and standards of this organization. Pain management, staffing, and intensive care unit (ICU) overflow guidelines are available on their web site and should be used by PACUs. These are some of the major issues that face perianesthesia nurses today and are some of the costliest issues. Appropriate use of these guidelines can aid in providing optimal patient care while controlling costs.

Evidence-Based Strategies

Evidence-based medicine refers to the way in which treatment options are chosen. Many traditional strategies for patient care are not supported by research. A simple example is the alcohol sponge bath that nurses in the past performed when a patient had a fever. We now know that this is actually detrimental in most cases because it promotes shivering, increases oxygen consumption, and increases carbon dioxide production which can be harmful to the patient. It made sense at the time, but research proved otherwise.

In the perianesthesia setting, a variety of research has been done on the prevention and management of nausea, returning patients to normothermia, and pain management. These studies provide necessary guidance to assist nurses in making care decisions regarding the patients entrusted to them.

A principal PACU nursing intervention is to assist patients' return to a normothermic state. Shivering increases oxygen demands and can cause airway obstruction and increased somnolence in postoperative patients. In 1997, Hershey, Valenciano, and Bookbinder[13] performed a study that examined different mechanisms for warming patients in the PACU. Patients were randomly assigned to one of three methods after a laparotomy. The first group received two warmed thermal blankets and a hospital bedspread; the second group received the same as the first group with the addition of a reflective blanket; and the third group received the same as the second group

as well as a reflective head covering. Normothermia was defined as an oral temperature of 96.8° Fahrenheit (36° Celsius). No significant differences were detected in the amount of time it took to reach normothermia. The authors found, however, that the warmer the patient upon arrival, the shorter time to normothermia. In addition, those patients that shivered reached normothermia significantly sooner. Both of these incidental findings were probably expected. Especially applicable is that the addition of reflective blankets provides no clinical benefit but increases the cost.

Pain management is equally important to restoring normothermia. Unfortunately, healthcare providers consistently use too little pain medication. This is becoming a growing concern for the consumer as studies typically prove this to be true. Perianesthesia nurses are in a unique position to initiate appropriate pain management and set the tone of the patient's experience. Nurses are educated to combine strategies to maximize pain relief. These other strategies cost very little but can be very effective and even reduce the need for pharmaceutical management. Chapter 28 will be devoted to the pharmacology of pain management.

In 1999, Medina[14] investigated the relationship between the sound level in a PACU and the use of analgesics. The study revealed that more analgesics were dispensed after periods of medium and high sound levels than were given in periods after low sound levels. This research supported findings from previous studies that sound influences the perception of pain and the use of analgesics.

Sound can easily be controlled in the PACU setting. Healthcare providers often become immune to the noise level in the care environment. Studies have demonstrated that minor modifications have the ability to improve the patient experience and decrease the cost of the PACU stay by reducing the need for medication.

Outcomes Research

Outcomes research is a rapidly growing field with enormous potential to provide critical information to the healthcare and pharmaceutical industries. The overall aim of outcomes research is to improve healthcare and to achieve optimal benefit from the available resources by assessing the outcomes of different medical treatments. The emphasis in this area of research is on the benefits to the patient. Economic, health, and clinical concerns combine to examine the influence of the treatment on the patient's quality of life, the functional status of the patient, and patient satisfaction with treatment.[15]

Cost-Benefit Analysis

Cost-benefit analysis is an economic principle used to evaluate outcomes. This approach promotes the efficient use of scarce resources by the methodology with which projects are evaluated and alternatives are compared.[5] The value of the project is determined in dollar amounts, and the consequences are measured in dollars.[16]

A common proposal to reduce PACU costs is to reduce the total length of time a patient stays in the PACU. Numerous studies on how much money can be saved if patients are moved through the system more rapidly have been conducted. Unfortunately, this is not a real cost savings to a facility. The delay in transferring patients out of the PACU arises in many administrative discussions. A 1999 study by Zollinger and associates[17] looked at patients delayed more than 15 minutes after being deemed ready for transfer. The authors concluded that the annual cost to the PACU was $138,000 to "board" transferable patients. The problem with this line of reasoning is that patients who are not treated in the PACU receive care in another unit of the hospital—at a cost to that unit. Unless the presence of these patients create the need for overtime, they present no real cost to the PACU because the staff would be there regardless. Nursing research needs to be done in areas that are within the scope of nursing to impact, improve, and innovate.

A cost-benefit analysis regarding PACU issues was conducted in 1995 by Dexter and Tinker.[18] They developed computer simulations to determine whether the cost of PACU care could be reduced. They examined three hypotheses. First, they looked at the influence of shorter-acting anesthetics. Secondly, they examined the hypothetical elimination of nausea and vomiting. Finally, they adjusted operating room scheduling practices to determine whether that could reduce PACU costs. They found that using drugs with "faster recovery" would only decrease PACU costs if operating rooms were scheduled to run later each day (not a popular concept with surgeons). Because all patients do not leave at the same time, the idea that decreasing the length of time in the PACU would decrease the cost is unlikely. If nausea and vomiting could be eliminated in the percent of patients that typically experience this phenomenon, the total time to discharge would have decreased by 4.8%. The largest impact on PACU costs was the distribution of admissions. Currently, as the day progresses, admissions increase. If the bulk of the admissions could occur in the earliest hours, personnel could leave sooner in the day and therefore reduce labor costs. This is not a likely scenario, given the other hospital systems and personnel involved in surgical services. This study also determined that supplies and medications account for only 2% of PACU charges, whereas personnel costs account for almost all the costs in the PACU.

Cost-Effectiveness Analysis

Placing monetary value on life and health in addition to valuing other intangible costs and benefits is difficult. Cost-effectiveness analysis is offered as a more practical approach to decision making than cost-benefit analysis.[5] In this type of analysis, one assumes that the objective is desirable, although the benefits cannot be measured in monetary terms. The cost is still determined in dollar amounts, but the consequences are measured in nondollar amount—such as life years gained or disability prevented.[16]

Anesthetic drugs can vary widely in cost. Newer, more expensive drugs are used for induction of anesthesia with the promise that they provide more rapid awakening as well as less nausea and vomiting. The choice for the newer drug is made based on the hope that it will allow patients to be discharged sooner. In reality, very little evidence suggests that earlier discharge is possible or that it decreases costs. Why do facilities switch to the more expensive drug? Typically they do so because they believe it will provide a better experience for the patient, something which is much more difficult to assign a dollar amount.

Nausea and vomiting can be a significant problem for some patients after anesthesia. The majority of individuals who have a surgical procedure would like to avoid those side effects. In a 1994 study by Watcha and Smith,[19] researchers demonstrated that the cost-effectiveness of an antiemetic drug depended on the incidence of emesis. Therefore the evaluation of the cost-effectiveness of an antiemetic must include the risk from any given anesthetic, the procedure performed, the patient-risk profile, and the value that the patient places on avoiding nausea.

Short-Term Outcomes

In the PACU, short-term outcomes would be those outcomes that are desirable for a patient to experience in the first 12 hours after surgery. Perianesthesia nurses can conduct cost-effectiveness research regarding nursing interventions that reduce the need for pain medication, reduce the incidence of nausea and vomiting, and promote a faster return to normothermia. The ability to positively alter these experiences for patients would result in improved short-term outcomes.

The impact of preoperative education can also be assessed as a short-term outcome. Identifying reductions in patient anxiety, the ability to perform certain postoperative maneuvers—such as incentive spirometry—correctly, and recalling home care instructions can help to evaluate the effectiveness of teaching.

Long-Term Outcomes

For the purposes of perianesthesia nursing, long-term outcomes can be defined as those that occur within 12 to 72 hours. These may include correctly following postoperative instructions for activity and pain management, the identification of wound problems by the patient, and the appropriate use of follow-up services. Nursing research can be directed to determine the effectiveness of discharge-teaching methodologies and strategies for PACU nurses.

SUMMARY

Our pluralistic healthcare system is designed to combine public and private healthcare delivery services and financing. Managing the economical issues related to patient care is necessary to control the costs of health care. Nurses are perfectly situated to assist with strategies that cut costs while simultaneously improving quality and health status of individuals.

Perianesthesia nurses should be part of education committees and policy and standards committees and should have a place on product committees. Perianesthesia nursing can make significant contributions to understanding the surgical experience of the patient. Many opportunities exist for research to determine the best practices of the art and science of nursing in this field.

REFERENCES

1. Center for Medicare & Medicaid Services: Highlights: national health expenditures, 1999, Accessed online October 8, 2001 from www.hcfa.gov/stats.htm, 2001.
2. Smith S et al: The next ten years of health spending: what does the future hold? Health Affairs 17:128-140, 1998.
3. White KR: Healthcare economics and delivery. In Berger KJ, Williams MB, editors: Fundamentals of nursing: collaborating for optimal health, ed 2, Stamford, Conn, 1999, Appleton and Lange.
4. Department of Health and Human Services: HHS Agencies. Accessed online October 22, 2001 from www.hhs.gov/agencies/, 2001.
5. Folland S, Goodman A, Stano M: Cost-benefit analysis and other tools of economic evaluation. In The economics of health and healthcare, ed 3, Upper Saddle River, NJ, 2001, Prentice Hall.
6. Glied SA: Challenges and options for increasing the number of Americans with health insurance, New York, 2001, The Commonwealth Fund.
7. Rossiter LF: Understanding Medicare managed care: meeting economic, strategic, and policy challenges, Chicago, 2001, Health Administration Press.
8. Macario A, Glenn D, Dexter F: What can the postanesthesia care unit manager do to decrease costs in the postanesthesia care unit? J Perianesth Nurs 14(5):284-293, 1999.
9. Kahl K, Preston B: Identifying the cost of patient care in the postanesthesia care setting, J Post Anesth Nurs 3(3):198-202, 1998.
10. Orkin F: What do patients want? Preferences for immediate postoperative recovery, Anesth Analg 74:S225-232, 1992.

11. Phillips B: Patients' assessment of ambulatory anesthesia and surgery, J Clin Anesth 4:355-358, 1992.
12. ASPAN: ASPAN mission statement. Accessed online September 23, 2001 from www.aspan.org/PosStmts5.htm, 1997.
13. Hershey J, Valenciano C, Bookbinder M: Comparison of three rewarming methods in a postanesthesia care unit, AORN Journal 65(3):597-601, 1997.
14. Medina M: The relationship between sound levels in the postanesthesia care unit and use of analgesics. Uniformed Services University of Health Sciences, 1999, unpublished master's thesis.
15. Rapier CM: An introduction to outcomes research, Surry, UK, 1996, Brookwood Medical Publications, Ltd.
16. Aday L et al: Efficiency: concepts and methods. In Evaluating the healthcare system, ed 2, Chicago, 1998, Health Administration Press.
17. Zollinger T, Saywell R, Smith C et al: Delays in patient transfer: postanesthesia care nursing, Nursing Economics 17(5):283-290, 1999.
18. Dexter F, Tinker J: Analysis of strategies to decrease postanesthesia care unit costs, Anesthesiol 82(1):94-101, 1995.
19. Watcha M, Smith I: Cost effectiveness analysis of antiemetic therapy for ambulatory surgery, J Clin Anesth 6:370-377, 1994.

6

LEGAL ISSUES IN THE PACU

Karen N. Swisher, MS, JD
Peter Nash Swisher, MA, JD

PUTTING MEDICAL MALPRACTICE IN PERSPECTIVE

A 61-year-old woman goes into a hospital for "routine" elective surgery on a deviated septum in her nose. Neither the attending surgeon nor the attending anesthesiologist was present when the patient was extubated by the nurse anesthetist. The extubation did not go well, and the patient was finally diagnosed in a persistent vegetative state. During the medical malpractice trial, the jury learned that both the surgeon and the anesthesiologist were in other operating rooms during the extubation and that each thought that the other was with this particular patient. In addition, the jury heard testimony that the anesthesiologist did not evaluate the patient between the operating room and the PACU unit. The jury was not pleased with this sequence of events and awarded the plaintiff $9.6 million in compensatory damages and an additional $3.5 million in punitive damages.[1]

Medical malpractice cases such as this with large jury verdicts are often widely publicized in the media and are used to illustrate medical malpractice that can be neatly categorized into risk management issues to be discussed by hospital attorneys during grand rounds. During this process, it becomes all too easy to play the so-called blame game. Is this a case of inappropriate medical supervision, or are other issues—such as the lack of informed consent—involved? Regardless of the cause and effect, jury verdicts this large are sure to get the attention of both the public and healthcare providers, and in doing so, the blame game is further perpetuated. Perhaps hospital employees will be fired, or physicians will lose their hospital privileges. Medical malpractice

insurance premiums may rise dramatically, and some may be unable to retain their professional malpractice coverage. Hospital administrators will tell everyone to "try harder" to avoid similar mistakes; otherwise, medical practice in the operating room often continues just about the same as before the tragic incident.[2,3] The important learning lessons from this—and from other medical mistakes—will often go undetected and unlearned. The reason for this unfortunate predicament is that we have too narrowly focused medical mistakes as being the result of individual error. As Dr. Lucian Leape aptly notes:

> Ironically, that unique nature of medical injury, or more precisely, our reaction to it, has been the major barrier to reducing medical errors and injury. Shame, guilt, and fear prevent many physicians from discussing their mistakes, being honest with patients, and being able to look beyond their individual errors to correct underlying systems failures. They can only try harder. For many lawyers, a sense of just cause, in some cases moral outrage, similarly blinds them to alternatives to tort litigation. Both are misplaced. And both have been manifestly unsuccessful in preventing medical injuries. We have created a monster.[4]

Analyzing medical malpractice issues therefore requires an understanding of the complex relationship between law and medicine as well as the role that both professions can play in developing healthcare policy in the United States. Medical malpractice has been an issue of intense public debate since the 1970s with periodic allegations that America is in a "malpractice crisis." Usually this perception of a malpractice "crisis" comes from many physicians dismayed at what they perceive to be excessively large jury verdicts against them, a growing number of legal claims against the medical profession, larger premium payments for professional malpractice insurance, the decreasing availability of malpractice insurance at any cost, and clinical practice changes physicians sometimes feel they must make in order to avoid litigation.[5,6] Physicians argued that they had to practice defensive medicine—including unnecessary tests and treatments—not to benefit their patients but to avoid potential liability.[7] This in turn created a significant increase in the cost of medicine to the consumer, often in the government's Medicaid and Medicare programs. Consequently, in 1970, the Secretary of Health, Education, and Welfare established a major Commission on Medical Malpractice to investigate the entire system. The results of this study, published in 1972, were not what many physicians expected to hear from the federal government:

> The Commission found that there were a large number of doctor-caused injuries for which claims were never made; that 75 percent of jury verdicts were for the defendant; that malpractice insurance was available, albeit at rising premiums; that most hospitals had experienced little litigation; that defensive medicine was widely believed to exist but impossible to measure, because of difficulties in identifying services provided solely or primarily to avoid legal liability; and that state licensing agencies had little authority, staff, or inclination to discipline incompetent or "impaired" physicians."[8]

Not achieving their desired results from this 1972 commission study, a number of medical organizations throughout the United States began a concerted effort to lobby state legislatures to create various statutory "tort reform" remedies in an effort to alleviate the societal costs of this perceived "malpractice crisis." Almost every state has passed some sort of medical malpractice "tort reform" legislation to date, although these state statutes vary considerably, and no particular pattern to them exists.

Examples of state "tort reform" remedies include imposing limits on the monetary amount received for pain and suffering or limiting the total amount recovered in a medical malpractice

action. Many states also require submission of a malpractice case to a medical screening board before a patient can bring a legal action in court, and other states require submission of a medical malpractice case to arbitration, as well as restricting attorney contingent fee systems.[9,10] The most contentious "tort reform" issue to date has been placing a statutory "cap" on total medical malpractices damages. Some state courts have held that these statutes are reasonable and constitutional under the circumstances to protect healthcare providers and healthcare services within a state, but other courts have held such statutes to be unconstitutional because they arbitrarily favor healthcare providers at the expense of other professionals and lay persons within a particular state.[11]

In practice, however, such "tort reform" has done little to alleviate the concerns of physicians and patients regarding the cost and quality of medicine.[12] Some evidence suggests that certain "tort reform" legislation such as those that directly limit physician liability through caps on medical malpractice damage awards, the limitation or abolition of punitive damages, and the abolition of mandatory prejudgment interest may reduce hospital expenditures somewhat, at least in certain populations.[13] However, if these "tort reform" remedies have done little to reduce the frequency and severity of malpractice cases, what else might work?

Traditionally, the medical malpractice liability system serves two principal roles: (1) it provides compensation for patients injured as the result of negligence on the part of players in the health care system; and (2) it provides an incentive for physicians and other healthcare providers to practice better quality medicine. Until recently, little empirical research had been published to demonstrate the prevalence of negligence within the healthcare system. This changed dramatically, beginning in the early 1990s, with the publication of a series of research results commonly called the Harvard Medical Practice Study. This was a population-based study of injuries that resulted from medical care during hospitalizations in New York. A review of thousands of medical records indicated that nearly 4% of patients suffered an injury that caused their hospital stays to be prolonged or resulted in measurable disability. Indeed, 14% of those identified as having suffered medical injury died as a result of their injuries.[14] Following up on the initial review of medical records, the authors identified patients who had filed claims against physicians and hospitals and discovered that only a fraction of those patients who were injured as the result of medical negligence filed claims and that compensation awarded was based primarily on the severity of injury rather than a finding of negligence. The authors concluded that:

> the civil justice system only infrequently compensates injured patients and rarely identifies and holds healthcare providers accountable for substandard medical care. Although malpractice litigation may fulfill its social objectives crudely, support for its preservation persists in part because of the perception that other methods of ensuring a high quality of care and redressing patients' grievances have proved to be inadequate.[15]

At about the same time that the Harvard Study was being conducted, the federal government was in the process of passing the Health Care Quality Improvement Act of 1986. One critical underlying assumption of this new law is that medical malpractice—not merely medical malpractice litigation—is increasing, and professional review can remedy this problem. Major portions of this act were designed to give immunity to physicians and others who participate in peer review processes, but the act also requires reporting medical malpractice payouts to the Secretary of Health and Human Services for inclusion into a national databank and also to state boards of medical examiners. The databank was created in large part to prevent unethical or incompetent healthcare practitioners from moving from state to state without any disclosure or discovery of their previous negligence or incompetent performance.[16,17] To date, little has been published on the efficacy of this databank, and little is known about the impact of this databank on physician practice or quality of health care to date.

Sources For Identifying Malpractice in the PACU

Despite this medical-legal conundrum, much can be learned in the area of risk management from individual malpractice claims. National malprac-

tice carriers, such as the St. Paul Fire and Marine Insurance Company, are able to give more detailed and "country-wide" data that involve medical malpractice claims, and a closed-claims study by the American Society of Anesthesiologists (ASA)—with a reported database of more than 4000 cases that represent 35 insurance companies—has substantially helped medical professionals understand and analyze the legal consequences of adverse outcomes.[18] This closed claim data, however, does not contain the "near misses" or bad outcomes without damages. The American Association of Nurse Anesthetists further examined adverse outcomes of anesthesia care provided by nurse anesthetists using the St. Paul databank.[19]

A claim is a demand for financial compensation for an injury resulting from medical care. On rare occasions hospitals or providers may pay for these claims out-of-pocket. Most claims are reported to the commercial malpractice insurance carrier who then investigates the claim; determines liability issues; and will either settle the case out of court, deny liability altogether, or go to trial. A few claims are dropped by the claimant before trial or are handled by arbitration or mediation. Trained reviewers using the professional Practice Manual for the Certified Registered Nurse Anesthetist (CRNA) along with available medical records and other information collected by the insurance carrier for investigative purposes are used to determine whether appropriate medical care was given as well as whether anyone on the treatment team could have prevented the adverse event.

The CRNA study found that "lack of vigilance contributed to 79% of damaging events and adverse outcomes and that in 62% of the incidents, the CRNA could have taken action to prevent harm to the patient. Vigilance was defined as state or quality of being watchful to detect any occurrences that might harm a patient during an anesthetic."[20] Most of the results of this study were predictable. For example, many of the claims involved inadequate preinduction of anesthesia activities, and almost half of all claims were deemed to have been preventable by the CRNA. The study concluded by noting that patients with PS I and II are at risk for damaging events and adverse outcomes and that just over half the claims provided inappropriate care, which indicates that filing a legal claim by the plaintiff/patient does not necessarily imply that substandard or inappropriate anesthesia care was provided.

As mentioned above, the National Practitioner Databank (NPDB) is a central source of information regarding malpractice payments for physicians, nurses, nurse anesthetists, and dentists. The databank became operational on September 1, 1990 and as of 1998 had more than 195,000 reports of malpractice payments, adverse licensure, clinical privileging, professional society membership, DEA actions, and Medicare/Medicaid exclusions actions concerning licensed professionals. Approximately 30,000 reports are added each year.[21] Nurse anesthetists are identified separately from other nursing specialties in the databank. Analysis of information in the databank is limited by the codes that the submitter must use. Anesthesia-related malpractice codes include assessment, monitoring, equipment testing, wrong agent or equipment, intubation, equipment use, improper technique/induction, positioning, consent issues, and "other." The most frequently reported malpractice reason code for both physicians and nurse anesthetists was "anesthesia not otherwise coded," followed by "failure to monitor."[22]

Understanding where and how medical mistakes happen is just half the picture. In hospitals patients sometimes have iatrogenic adverse outcomes induced in a patient through the effects of treatment by a physician, nosocomial infections, or other accidents. But is a bad outcome necessarily medical malpractice? Translating a medical mishap or mistake into medical malpractice takes a deeper understanding of how American laws define and prove medical malpractice.

Medical Malpractice Issues for the Nurse Anesthetist: A Traditional Overview

Many state laws that govern legal claims for medical malpractice specify that the actions or inactions of nurses and doctors may be the basis for a medical malpractice lawsuit.[23,24] The legal formula used in most medical malpractice cases is, that a physician, or other healthcare practitioner, must have and use the knowledge, skill, and care ordinarily possessed and employed by members of the profession in good standing and that a doctor or nurse will be liable if he or she does not have

them.[25,26] American states are split on whether the standard of care for a healthcare practitioner should be judged by practitioners in the "same or similar locality" or according to a "national standard" of medical care. A "national standard" is normally used in cases of medical specialists.[27,28] For example, a Louisiana court, in a medical malpractice case that involved a specialist nurse, stated the following:

> A nurse who practices [his or] her profession in a particular specialty owes to [his or] her patients the duty of possessing the degree of knowledge or skill ordinarily possessed by members of [his or] her profession actively practicing in such a specialty under similar circumstances. It is the nurse's duty to exercise the degree of skill ordinarily employed, under similar circumstances, by members of the nursing profession in good standing who practice their profession in the same specialty and to use reasonable care and diligence, along with his/her best judgment, in the application of his/her skill in the case.[29]

In deciding whether a nurse was negligent and legally liable for malpractice, the court therefore would need to compare the particular nurse's professional behavior with that of a "reasonably prudent nurse" under the same or similar circumstances. Thus in a case involving injury or death from a highly technical bad outcome involving anesthesia, the court's first question might be the following:

> whether the nurse was a nurse anesthetist or a general registered nurse specially tasked to work with anesthesia. A nurse anesthetist would probably be held to a higher standard [of care]. Nurse anesthetists are organized into a professional association (the American Association of Nurse Anesthetists) that has issued protocols for patient treatment. A nurse anesthetist would be expected to satisfy those standards, whereas a general registered nurse might not. . . . A court may agree that these specialist associations help define the appropriate standard of care for nurses regularly practicing within that specialty. . . . [In this scenario] the standard [of care] is implicitly national in application.[30]

Legal liability for nurse malpractice generally will fall on the responsible nurse or the nurse's employer (e.g., the hospital) and perhaps on the supervising physician as well under the legal doctrine of *respondeat superior*. American tort law generally assigns shared responsibility for the nurse's malpractice to his or her employer, the supervising physician, or all of the above under the doctrine of joint and several liability, which means that both the nurse and his or her *respondeat superior* codefendants are each liable for the full judgment against them, and this gives the plaintiff-patient the option of suing the nurse (and his or her liability insurance carrier), the nurse's co-defendant employer, and any other co-defendants (and their liability insurance carriers). However, a nurse who has committed malpractice is still primarily liable for damages to the patient-plaintiff:

> The mere fact that the plaintiff may focus collection efforts against a wealthier [or so-called "deep pockets"] codefendant, such as the nurse's employer, does not eliminate the nurse's liability (or the possibility that the nurse's employer will take some adverse job action, such as discipline or termination, or that the state licensing board will suspend or revoke the nurse's license). A nurse must be satisfied that he or she has [adequate] malpractice insurance, provided by either the self or the employer. In selecting the amount of coverage, the nurse should be aware of any caps or limits on damages that exist under state law.[31]

So under this traditional approach to medical malpractice actions, the blame game continues—for doctors, nurses, and other healthcare providers.[2]

A New Approach to Medical Malpractice

The continuing focus on "blaming" healthcare providers—and attorneys—for the current medical malpractice "crisis" has left little inclination for developing a more systematic analysis of medical malpractice. Sources of this perceived medical malpractice "crisis" certainly involve more than incompetent physicians or hungry attorneys ready to litigate at a moment's notice. First, a significant contribution to an increase in medical error is the simple fact that more people are receiving more complicated medical treatment than ever before, due in large part to new

Medicare and Medicaid programs beginning in the 1960s. Second, the increasing complexity of medical technology and drug advancements has created more injuries, which many times are considered a presumed risk of modern medicine. Third, an aggressive marketing of medical products and services directly to patient consumers often has created unrealistic patient expectations regarding favorable outcomes of medical treatment.[32] Finally, the role of insurance for both healthcare providers (in the form of liability insurance) and patients (in the form of health insurance) inadvertently insulates and cloaks the real financial risks involved in providing and receiving medical care.

Virtually all physicians carry some form of medical malpractice insurance, and because this insurance is loss-rated and not experience-rated and because it often provides no deductible, physicians often bear little knowledge or accountability of the costs of malpractice injuries. A majority of patients in the United States, on the other hand, have insurance that covers most costs of medical treatment. This leaves little incentive for patients to inquire about the costs and risks of medical treatment or otherwise shop around for the most "quality-oriented" healthcare providers.[33,34]

Although empirical research has contributed greatly to our understanding of medical malpractice, consideration should also be given to the outstanding qualitative research being conducted today. This research seeks information through questionnaires and opinions of what people believe to be reasonable behavioral conduct. Subjective in nature, such opinions often lead to hypotheses, which are eventually tested using quantitative methodologies. Few studies have questioned patients'/plaintiffs' motives for suing their healthcare providers because of the difficulty of conducting such research and the limitations involved in the results. These studies, however, are useful in demonstrating a serious breakdown in physician/patient communication, in individual perceptions on medical outcomes, and the stark reality that sometimes medicine does not have all the answers when bad things happen to good people. Clearly, more research is needed to better understand the complex interdependent nature of the doctor/patient relationship.[35,36]

One study published almost 10 years ago developed a questionnaire given to several hundred families in Florida who had filed malpractice claims that alleged that physicians and other healthcare practitioners who were providing medical care during the perinatal period and immediate postpartum period deviated from community and national medical standards and caused death or permanent injury to their infants. The families' responses were fascinating. Families were asked open-ended questions that led to multiple responses for each question. When asked, "What was wrong with the care you or your child received?" these families alleged that physicians failed to recognize fetal distress (53%), manage fetal distress appropriately (57%), perform a cesarean section (33%), or be available when needed (29%). In response to why families filed their medical malpractice lawsuits, many stated they did so on the advice of a family member or a close friend. Some filed a lawsuit because they needed money to pay for long-term care of their infants, and many filed when they realized that their physicians had failed to be completely honest and open with them about what had happened. Several others filed because they believed that the courtroom was the only forum in which they could find out what "had really happened" with the physicians who provided care. A good number responded that they filed legal action as a way to deter subsequent medical malpractice by the physician or to seek "revenge."

A central theme throughout this study was an apparent lack of communication and trust between the physician and the family. Respondents stated they believed their physicians would not talk with them or answer questions, that their physicians would not listen to them, that their physicians had misled them, or that no one involved in providing medical care during the perinatal period ever told them that their infants might have permanent medical problems.[37]

A review of current legal and medical literature revealed no end to the blame game. After all, tort liability depends on an identifiable victim and an identifiable wrongdoer, both connected by causation. Medicine, too, in its morbidity and mortality (M&M) conferences, grand rounds, physician credentialing, and the federal databank, all depend on identifying individual physicians, nurses, and other healthcare providers that cause individual medical mistakes. This all changed, however, with the publication of the 1999 report by the Institute of Medicine, *To Err is Human: Building a Safer Health System.*[38]

A Systematic Approach for Analyzing Medical Mistakes

Healthcare providers and the general public are familiar with the well-publicized statistics in the 1999 Institute of Medicine's report that medical errors kill between 44,000 and 98,000 people a year in American hospitals. If these statistics are true, medical mistakes today are the fifth leading cause of death in the United States. If true, this number is equivalent to the rate of three fully loaded jumbo jets crashing every other day. More importantly, if this is true, our prized American healthcare system, which is often cited as the finest in the world, may in reality constitute a public health menace of epidemic proportions.[39] Although the debate continues regarding exactly how many patients are actually harmed through medical error, those who work in the healthcare industry will find such statistics alarming but not unexpected. After all, the previously mentioned 1984 Harvard Study clearly demonstrated that the number of medical malpractice cases going through the courts was just the tip of the iceberg in sampling the true number of negligent incidents. The central message of this report—that errors are caused by faulty systems and not by faulty people—is nothing new or surprising to those in the medical field. Indeed, the whole focus of a management perspective to the delivery of health care has been written and researched for decades and is well established in the curriculum of any graduate hospital administration program.[40]

The major recommendations of this report were considered a number of years ago by anesthesiologists—long before "systems analysis" or "continuous quality improvement" became popular buzzwords—when consistent monitoring of anesthesia patients was established as a new "standard of care."[41-44] Anesthesiologists had found their own skyrocketing medical malpractice insurance was too expensive. To correct this imbalance, they took a number of steps to reduce their own liability by using a systems approach to anesthetic-related accidents.[45,46]

A systems approach to identifying and preventing medical errors gets away from the blame game, which tends to emphasize individual fault, and focuses instead on the underlying causes of medical error as part of a comprehensive process for managing patients and their medical care. Certainly, a nurse who gives a wrong medication to a patient is at fault because he or she did not read the label properly, but a closer examination of the process of giving medication to patients reveals that many medications have similar names, similar labels, and similar packaging formats and sometimes are stocked together, making it easier to commit the final medical error. Rather than emphasizing and focusing on the individual nursing error, a systems approach analyzes the entire process of ordering, stocking, delivering, and administering medications to patients. Rational redesign and evaluation of this systematic process must depend on sound empirical data of how, when, and where these medical mistakes occur. "Data collection must [then] be followed by careful epidemiological analysis and the dissemination of both anecdotal and statistical insights into prevention."[47]

If data collection on medical errors is critical for a systems approach to preventing future medical errors, it is also controversial. For one thing, a traditional malpractice litigation system largely depends on discovery of such reports to help substantiate medical error and assess legal "blame." Although laws designed to protect various medical documents and records from lawyer discovery and use in court exist, these laws have many loopholes and are often disregarded during actual litigation.[48] Moreover, many physicians do not believe that reporting medical errors contributes to the quality of medical care, and it appears that hospital administrators agree with this questionable philosophy, because the departments of risk management and quality improvement in many hospitals are substantively different enterprises.[49]

Reporting medical mistakes, whether voluntary or mandatory, requires a working definition of what a medical mistake encompasses. Reportable mistakes should include errors that resulted in no harm to the patient. For example, assume a physician writes a prescription for a 1% solution of a drug, but the pharmacist misreads the physicians' handwriting and prepares a 10%

solution instead. A nurse who is about to administer this medication notices this unusually high concentration and brings her concern to the attention of the prescribing physician, who corrects the dosage. This error, which does not injure the patient, is still an example of the kind of information that is essential for the development of a sound systems approach to prevent medication errors. Thus "if physicians, nurses, pharmacists, and administrators are to succeed in reducing errors in hospital care, they will need to fundamentally change the way they think about errors and why they occur."[50] As Palmer restates this systems approach to patient safety:

> Reaching the goal of patient safety requires a paradigm shift in the way we think about prevention of accidents in law. Rather than continue to debate about liability as instrumental or as an obstacle to increased safety in health care, we need to acknowledge that the single goal of preventing patient injuries requires a new and dynamic way of conceptualizing law so that knowledge about safety will continue to grow. In this new view, medical liability—the imposition of civil liability for damages on healthcare professionals and organizations—is acknowledged to be an imperfect system for enhancing patient safety. The goal is not to perfect or eliminate medical liability under the banner of efficiency or rationality. Rather, the goal of a new conceptualization of the role of law is to assess the capacity of the legal system to adopt new ways of viewing safety.[51]

A systems approach to patient safety therefore requires administrators, academics, and licensed professionals to look beyond individual mistakes and to analyze more closely the underlying goals of a healthcare system. Despite the efforts of many talented proponents and dedicated professionals in their attempts to "restructure" the healthcare system, improving patient safety has not been a major goal. Mergers, acquisitions, and affiliations have been commonplace within the health plan, hospital, and physician sectors. Yet all this organizational turmoil has resulted in very little change in the way health care is delivered to patients and with little evidence of improvement in either quality or cost in the United States. The discrepancy between what Americans should receive in health care and what they actually receive is so great that the Committee on Quality of Health Care in America published "Crossing the Quality Chasm: A New Health System for the 21ˢᵗ Century," which stresses that a redesign of the American healthcare system should include underlying goals focused on medical care that is safe, effective, patient-centered, timely, efficient, and equitable.[52] Although some medical errors are the result of poorly designed systems, some errors are the result of variances in physician practices. From this perspective, more focus should be placed on medical outcomes and clinical guidelines as a way of establishing the standard of care in medicine.

Individual Liability and the Standard of Care

In the past, nurses and physicians would attend continuing medical education lectures, sometimes presented by attorneys who would elaborate on the elements of medical malpractice negligence cases. These attorneys would normally analyze and discuss selected appellate court cases that were published in various trade journals.[53] Sometimes the attorneys would go into great detail about a particularly interesting medical malpractice case, similar to the case mentioned at the beginning of this chapter, and then conclude that medical providers need to "try harder" to avoid being sued.

As previously stated, healthcare providers owe their patients a duty to act in accordance with the specific norms or standards established by the profession, which are commonly called the standard of care. Whether the physician or nurse has performed at his or her full potential and in complete good faith may not matter. Instead the physician or nurse must have conformed to the standard of a "prudent physician" or "prudent nurse" under similar circumstances. Unfortunately, no clear definition of a standard of care for a particular patient during particular circumstances exists. The standards for evaluating the delivery of professional medical services are not normally established by either judge or jury. Instead, the medical profession itself sets the standards of practice, and the courts enforce these standards in tort suits. This requires that both plaintiff and defense attorneys present evidence of the standard of care by use of expert medical witnesses, almost always other physicians or nurses who practice medicine under similar circumstances as the defendant physician or nurse. No clear definitions of the standard of care for a particular situation exist. Medical expert witnesses rely heavily on their own personal experience from practice; they may use medical treatises or journals as evidence; they may cite from medical reference books; and because substantial regional variations exist in the use of many procedures, experts may rely more on anecdotal experiences with little regard for differences in outcome. Some experts comment that this is not a very good system because it generally boils down to a "battle of the experts" to determine which medical expert is more believable to the jury. Often attorneys on both sides will attempt to impeach the qualifications of the expert medical witness on the other side, questioning his or her qualifications, or perhaps attempting to prove that the expert medical witness is unqualified because he or she is not familiar with the practice of medicine in a particular locality or a particular area of expertise.

The development and proliferation of clinical practice guidelines is one of the transforming forces in current medical practice and has aided both plaintiff and defense attorneys in developing a more "objective" case on behalf of their clients. In this area clinical practice guidelines can be very useful.[54] As one author states:

> The consistent use of well-developed and medically appropriate practice guidelines has two potentially compelling benefits. First, scientifically reliable guidelines can improve medical practice by reducing the incidence of misdiagnoses and inappropriate treatment decisions. . . . Second, if major inroads are made into the process of creating and disseminating guidelines, their use may improve the process of malpractice litigation when the practice of medicine goes awry or when insurance coverage is denied. Clinical practice guidelines are being used by both plaintiff and defense attorneys as evidence of the standard of care in medicine. For this very reason, it may be more useful for practitioners, including nurse anesthetists, to review and implement guidelines rather than to review and analyze published malpractice cases on the same subject![55]

Several definitions of clinical practice guidelines exist, and the term itself has various synonyms—

including "clinical pathways," "critical pathways," "clinical paradigms," "practice parameters," "treatment protocols," and "evidence-based medicine standards." Regardless of the name, the definition includes "systematically developed statements to assist practitioners and patient decisions about appropriate health care for specific clinical conditions."[56] Most guidelines attempt to improve physician decision making by detailing appropriate indications for specific medical interventions.[57]

As in other areas of patient safety and quality of care, anesthesiologists have been leaders in embracing viable and realistic practice guidelines by developing practice parameters in pacemaker practice. The ASA has reviewed claims data from malpractice insurance carriers with the goal of ascertaining if there were common patterns to certain injuries. The ASA discovered that a high percentage of accidents could have been avoided by using equipment designed to measure the amount of oxygen in a patient's blood when he or she is under anesthesia. The challenges of developing such a practice parameter which could be considered the "standard of care" was described twelve years ago in the Journal of the American Medical Association (JAMA).[58]

Since the publication of this JAMA article, extensive research has been underway at federal, state, and private sector levels to develop viable practice guidelines and to disseminate such information on the Internet. Managed care organizations have embraced practice guidelines in the belief that their use would help control medical costs. A number of healthcare providers, feeling financial pressure to use such practice guidelines, have rebelled against their use believing that they would lead to a "cookbook" practice of medicine. Although this claim is partly valid, more compelling reasons for healthcare providers to embrace practice guidelines exist. American medicine is subject to too much variation in practice, according to some commentators, and physicians and nurses are now inundated with increased research on practice guidelines. Keeping up with all the medical advances made and published worldwide is simply impossible. Between 1966 and 1995, for example, the number of clinical research articles based on randomized clinical trials jumped from about 100 to 10,000 annually.[59,60]

Accordingly, the advantages of using evidenced-based guidelines in medical practice are gaining more widespread approval among healthcare providers. The Institute of Medicine declared that professional societies can contribute to improving patient safety through the promulgation and promotion of practice guidelines and that such guidelines can be written through a more interdisciplinary approach to medical care. Practice guidelines are among the most widely employed methods of modifying physician behavior and improving patient safety. Moreover, practice guidelines were cited in the most recent report on patient safety practices as evidence that guidelines are very effective in positively influencing the medical process and outcome of care .[61] Most significantly, medical practice guidelines are increasingly cited in court litigation and are used as evidence of a medical standard of care. They can also be raised as an affirmative defense by physicians and nurses in medical malpractice suits to show compliance with accepted medical practice. Several states have legislated the use of such medical practice guidelines and provide tort immunity for healthcare practitioners in exchange for their following such guidelines. Finally, because these medical practice guidelines are widely published on the Internet, failure to access such information is likely to become an important piece of evidence in a malpractice suit because it is evidence that a physician or nurse has failed to stay current in his or her field of practice. With more focus on practice guidelines based on medical outcomes, it is more important than ever for health care practitioners to understand the sources of medical malpractice to develop practice guidelines aimed at these patient safety areas.

SUMMARY AND RISK MANAGEMENT SUGGESTIONS

Healthcare providers remain deeply committed to the care and safety of their patients. However, focus on the blame game—singling out individuals for punishment and retribution—and reliance on the court system for compensation to injured patients have done little to increase patient care overall in American hospitals. The complex nature of the healthcare industry simply does not lend itself to this process of "blaming" individuals and allowing the courts to compensate injured patients. Instead, medical professionals should embrace and encourage a systematic approach to defining quality of patient care and improving patient safety. To this end, the blame game will hopefully give way to developing a root cause analysis of medical mistakes and a systematic approach for making patient safety a priority in hospitals. This is not to say that individual accountability or liability will disappear altogether—it will not. However, a systematic approach to individual liability will result in more focus on detailed credentialing processes, better assessment of professionals within certain job constraints, better licensing techniques, and better continuing educational programs—all geared to keep professionals competent and qualified for the particular tasks that they must do. With this new way of ascertaining how medical mistakes are made and how they can be avoided, healthcare attorneys can provide their clients valuable risk management. Some of the more important tips include the following:

- Report and investigate all "near misses." We can all learn from our mistakes, and mistakes that don't cause harm are just as important as understanding and investigating those that do cause harm.
- Be sure that your hospital has a system to report and investigate all medical mistakes by encouraging and rewarding those who report personal mistakes rather than punishing them. Develop a systematic process to question potential medical errors before they happen. Time and again, members of a healthcare team see problems coming, but are afraid to question the authority of the person who is about to make a mistake.
- Nurses are sometimes afraid to question physician's orders, yet their internal doubt can often save a patient's life. Develop a policy on questioning authority and use it. Every medical team member has the responsibility for patient outcome. You cannot hide behind the physician's cloak of authority any longer.
- Empower and actively involve your patients in the determination of their own standard of medical care. In an age of patient autonomy and informed consent, patient involvement is taking on new meaning. Informed consent no

longer is a signature on a piece of paper but a process of communication. The more patients know what to expect from their own treatment protocol, the better they will be able to help you do your job and improve their own safety during your care.
- Embrace medical protocols and electronic checklists into your practice. Human errors involving equipment misuse remain a big concern for anesthesia patients. Studies indicate that indexed electronic checklists are superior to either memorized or nonindexed paper checklists in reducing errors of omission.[58-63] Airline pilots would never fly without them, and neither should you.
- Embrace the use of clinical guidelines in your practice. Just as checklists and protocols can avoid many human mistakes made as the result of doing a repetitive task, clinical guidelines can avoid human mistakes made as the result of judgmental error. Guidelines are just that—guidelines—and are not a definitive standard of care. However, clinical guidelines will help you "armor plate" the medical record and justify in the record when you find it necessary to deviate from the guidelines. Untoward risks are part of medical care, but justifying what decision you made when you made it will really help in defending your medical actions later.
- Know what your malpractice insurance covers, excludes, and provides for you. Even if you have done all the previously listed recommendations, medical mistakes will happen and involvement in a legal claim is often the first time a medical professional learns what insurance he or she has or does not have. As an employee, you may be covered under a hospital "house" policy. Read that policy and know your coverage. If your job description changes dramatically, be sure to get written clarification of your coverage from your insurance carrier. All healthcare professionals should make appointments with their insurance agents to review their medical malpractice policies provision by provision. You may be surprised at the exclusions within your policy. Sexual misconduct with a patient is obviously excluded, but often, intentional acts are excluded as well. Know what this means; ask for examples; and know your coverage dollar amount limitation and your tail policy, if any.

In conclusion, focusing on patient safety rather than solely on medical malpractice must involve the coordinated efforts of several sectors of our society. First, it must involve the legal community to support and implement appropriate tort reform to protect medical incident reports from legal discovery, especially those that involve "near miss" medical incidents. If this is not feasible legal discovery should be limited in medical malpractice cases to encourage physicians and other healthcare providers to freely report and investigate all medical mistakes and near mistakes as they happen. Second, it must involve medical licensing boards and accreditation agencies to more closely monitor the quality of those licensed to practice in the various medical specialties. It is no longer acceptable for medical licensing boards to grant licenses to physicians and other healthcare providers and then fail to follow up with required continuing medical education as part of the license renewal process. Third, it will require real leadership on the part of hospital administrators, physicians, and nurse administrators to incorporate patient safety and the reduction of medical errors as a specific goal. This will require a real change in the way hospitals hire, monitor, and manage their human resources. Fourth, it must involve patients to take responsibility for their own medical care and treatment.

Most importantly, physicians and nurses need to accept the notion that error is an inevitable accompaniment of the human condition and that medical error must be accepted as evidence of a systems flaw—not a character flaw. Until this happens, that substantial progress in reducing medical errors is unlikely.

REFERENCES

1. Watkins vs. Cleveland Clinic Found, 719 N.E.2d 1052 (Ohio 1998).
2. O'Connell J: The blame game: injuries, insurance, and injustice, Lexington, Mass, 1987, Lexington Books.
3. Reason J: Human error: models and management, Br Med J 320, 2000.
4. Leape LL: Foreword: preventing medical accidents: is "systems analysis" the answer? Am J Law Med 27, 2001.
5. Law SA, Polan S: Pain and profit: the politics of malpractice, ed 1, New York, 1978, Harper & Row.
6. Robinson GO: The medical malpractice crisis of the 1970s: a retrospective, Law and Contemporary Problems 49:5, 1986.
7. Kessler D, McClellan M: Do doctors practice defensive medicine? The Quarterly Journal of Economics 353, 1996. (An excellent discussion of defensive medicine.)
8. Rosenblatt RE, Law SA, Rosenbaum S: Law and the American health care system, Westbury, NY, 1997, Foundation Press.
9. Sanders, J: Off to the races: the 1980s tort crisis and the law reform process, Houston Law Review 27:207, 1990.
10. Viscusi WK, Born P: Medical malpractice in the wake of liability reform, J Legal Studies, 24:463 1995.
11. Smith DR: Battling a tort frontier: constitutional attacks on medical malpractice laws, Oklahoma Law Review 38:195, 1995.
12. U.S. Congress Office of Technology Assessment: Impact of legal reforms on medical malpractice cases, Washington, 1993, US Government Printing Office.
13. Kessler DP, McClellan MB: Do doctors practice defensive medicine? The Quarterly J of Economics 111(2):353-359, 1996.
14. Harvard Medical practice study: Patients, doctors, and lawyers: medical injury, malpractice litigation, and patient compensation in New York, 1990. (copies available from the New York state department of health, Albany.)
15. Localio AJ, Lawthers AG, Brennan TA: Relation between malpractice claims and adverse events due to negligence, New Engl J Med, 325:245-251, 1991.
16. 42 U.S.C.A. section 1101 et seq.; 54 Fed. Reg. 42, 722.
17. Mullan F: The national practitioner databank: report from the first year, JAMA 268(1):73-80, 1992.
18. Caplan R: Adverse outcomes in anesthesia practice, 1995 annual refresher course lectures, Park Ridge, Ill, The American Society of Anesthesiologists, 254:17.
19. Jordan LM et al: Data-driven practice improvement: the AANA foundation closed malpractice claims study, AANA J 69(4):301-311, 2001.

20. Jordan LM et al: Data-driven practice improvement: the AANA foundation closed malpractice claims study, AANA J 69(4):304, 2001.

21. National Practitioner Data Bank: *www.npdb.com* (Accessed online Sept. 16, 2002).

22. Jordan LM, Oshel RE: Nurse anesthetist malpractice and the national practitioner databank, AANA J 66(6), 1998.

23. Andrews M: Nurse's legal handbook, ed 3, Spring House, PA, 1996, Springhouse Corp.

24. Gic J: Nursing and the law. In Legal medicine, ed 5, St Louis, 2001, Mosby.

25. William P, Keeton P: The law of torts, ed 5, St Paul, Minn, 1984, West Publishing Co.

26. Pegalis S, Wachsman H: American law of medical malpractice, ed 2, Deerfield, Ill, 1992, Clark Boardman Callaghan.

27. Annotation, 18 A.L.R. 4th 603, 1982.

28. Prosser WL, Keeton P: Prosser & Keeton on torts, ed 5, St. Paul, Minn, 1984, West Publishing Co.

29. King v. Department of Health and Hospitals, 728 So. 2d 1027, 1030 (La. Ct. App.) writ denied 741 So. 2d 656 (La. 1999).

30. Gic JA: Nursing and the law. In Legal medicine, ed 5, St Louis, MO 2001, Mosby.

31. Gic JA: Nursing and the law. In Legal medicine, ed 5, St Louis, MO 2001, Mosby.

32. Michael S: Do we really know anything about the behavior of the tort litigation system—and why not? U Penn Law Review 140(1147), 1992.

33. Danzon PM: Medical malpractice: theory evidence and public policy, Cambridge, Mass, 1985, Harvard University Press.

34. Kessler DP, McClellan MB: The effects of malpractice and liability reforms on physicians' perceptions of medical care, Law and Contemporary Problems 60:81, 1997.

35. Merz JF: On a decision-making paradigm of medical informed consent, J Leg Medicine 14(231), 1993. (A good discussion of the patient decision-making paradigm.)

36. May ML, Stengel DB: Who sues their doctors? How patients handle medical grievances, Law and Soc Rev 24(105), 1992.

37. Hickson GB: Clayton EW, Githens P et al: Factors that prompted families to file medical malpractice claims following perinatal injuries, JAMA 267:10, 1359-1363, 1992.

38. Kohn LT, Corrigan JM, Donaldson MS, editors: To err is human: building a safer health system, Washington, 2000, Academy Press.

39. Hayward RA, Hofer TP: Estimating hospital deaths due to medical errors: preventability is in the eye of the reviewer, JAMA 286(4):415-420, 2001.

40. Department of Health Administration, Virginia Commonwealth University. *http://www.had.vcu.edu* (accessed online Sept 15, 2002) (Program consistently rated in the top 10 programs in the United States with a focus on systems management in healthcare administration.)

41. Eichhorn JH et al: Standards for patient monitoring during anesthesia at Harvard Medical School, JAMA 256(1017), 1986.

42. Tinker JH et al: Role of monitoring devices in prevention of anesthetic mishaps: a closed claim analysis, Anesthesiol 71(541), 1989.

43. Cote CJ: A single blind study of combined pulse oximetry and capnography in children, Anesthesiol 74(980), 1991.

44. Cooper JP, Gaba DM: A strategy for preventing anesthesia accidents, Int Anesthesiol Clin 27, 1989.

45. Anesthesia Patient Safety Foundation: *www.gasnet.org/societies/apsf* (accessed online Sept 15, 2002).

46. Gellhorn W: Medical malpractice litigation (U.S.): medical mishap compensation (N.Z.), Cornell L Rev 73:170, 1988.

47. Studdert DM, Brennan TA: No-fault compensation for medical injuries: the prospect for error prevention, JAMA 286(2), 2001.

48. Scheutzow SO, Gillis SL: Confidentiality and privilege of peer review information: more imagined than real, J Law Health 7, 1992/3.

49. Brennan TA, Berwick DM: New rules: regulations, markets, and the quality of American health care, San Francisco, 1996, Jossey-Bass.

50. Lucian L et al: Promoting patient safety by preventing medical error, JAMA 280(16), 1998.

51. Palmer LI: Patient safety, risk reduction, and the law, Houston L Rev 36, 1999.

52. Institute of Medicine: Crossing the quality chasm: a new health system for the 21st century, Washington, 2001, National Academy Press.

53. Blumenreich G: The importance of following procedures in anesthesia, AANA Journal 68(2), 2000. (A regular feature in AANA Journal is "Legal Briefs," which details legal cases are detailed and risk management techniques.)

54. National Guidelines Clearinghouse: *www.guideline.gov/index.asp* (Accessed online Sept 15, 2002).

55. Finder JM: The future of practice guidelines: should they constitute conclusive evidence of the standard of care? Health Matrix 10:67, 2000.

56. Field MJ, Lohr KN, editors: Clinical practice guidelines: directions for a new program, Washington, 1990, National Academy Press.

57. Sheetz ML: Toward controlled clinical care through clinical practice guidelines: the legal liability for developers and issuers of clinical pathways, Brooklyn L Rev 63:1341, 1997.

58. Hirshfeld EB: Should practice parameters be the standard of care in malpractice litigation? JAMA 266:20, 2886, 1991.

59. Furrow BR: Broadcasting clinical guidelines on the Internet: will physicians tune in? American Journal of Law and Medicine 25:403-409, 1998.

60. Chassin MR: Is health care ready for six sigma quality? Milbank Q 76:565-574, 1998.

61. Agency for HealthCare Research and Quality, Pub. No. 01-E057: Making health care safer: a critical analysis of patient safety practices, Rockville, Md, 2001 (Available at www:ahrq.gov/clinic/ ptsafety).

62. Blike G, Biddle H: Preanesthesia detection of equipment faults by anesthesia providers at an academic hospital: comparison of standard practice and a new electronic checklist, AANA Journal 68(6):497-505, 2000.

63. Sheetz ML: Toward controlled clinical care through clinical practice guidelines: the legal liability for developers and issuers of clinical pathways, Brooklyn L Rev 63:134, 1997.

7

ETHICS OF HEALTH CARE IN THE PACU

Karen N. Swisher, MS, JD

MEDICAL ETHICS AND "WALKING THE FLOOR"

The study of medical ethics is well established in American academic medical institutions, hospitals, and within healthcare professions. Several medical journals are devoted solely to ethics.[1] Multidisciplinary treatises and monographs are available for those interested in the field.[2-4] Courses in ethics are prevalent at most academic institutions.[5-7] Many licensing boards require clinicians to have a minimal number of continuing education credits in medical ethics, but for those who want more, postgraduate fellowships and degreed programs at the Masters and Ph.D levels are available.[8] Ethics committees are prevalent in almost all hospitals, and are widely featured in popular television shows featuring hospital settings. Ethics newsletters, web sites, and textbooks abound. Grand round and other educational presentations continue to inform healthcare providers about the ethical dilemmas they might encounter.

However, with all these abundant resources, medical practitioners "walking the floor" and treating patients in the operating room (OR), emergency room (ER), postanesthesia care unit (PACU), or in medical offices still routinely debate about the right or wrong way to treat certain patients in particular situations. More importantly, they may debate how well these ethical resources actually serve the realities of everyday medical practice.

All too often bedside dilemmas end up as courtroom cases, thus further exasperating medical clinicians' ability to discriminate between an ethical dilemma and a legal issue. Many court cases involving end-of-life issues, physician-assisted suicide, conflicts of interest between a fetus and its mother—to name just a few—are often covered extensively in the public press. Physicians, nurses, and other healthcare providers know that the law is not developed only through rationally justified and formally articulated judicial opinions. The law also evolves out of political compromise, public policy debates, and lobbying by the many interest groups. More often than not, these court decisions do little to help guide most healthcare providers in determining what is ethically right from what is legally right.

Conflict between doing what is ethically right and what is legally right for patients is a rather recent mid-twentieth century phenomenon, brought on by the recent scientific and technologic advances in medicine and the "reorganization" of medicine into a business organization. They are the result of a society increasingly varied in cultures and mores. The rapidly changing culture of medicine has challenged many conceptions of traditional moral obligations that healthcare providers have toward their patients, their hospitals, and their payers. Now more than ever, a real need for understanding both the principles of ethical decision making and the process by which such decisions are made exists. Providers need to know: (1) where ethical problems should be resolved; and (2) what substantive principles should apply. Thus the questions become ones of process (who will decide ethical issues—and how) and substance (what principles must form the basis of a recognized decision).[9]

The study of clinical ethics deals mostly with four basic principles from which realistic guidelines for medical decision making can be made. These principles include the respect for patient autonomy, beneficence, nonmaleficence, and justice. The principle of respect for patient autonomy requires that one act toward others in a way that allows them to govern themselves and choose their own courses of action. A dynamic tension exists between patient autonomy and medical paternalism, which directs physicians to act in what they believe to be in the patient's best interest. A second element of respect for persons is truth-telling. Healthcare providers have an obligation of honesty with their patients in all activities. Confidentiality is the third element of the principle of respect for patient autonomy. It requires clinicians to keep what they learn about patients confidential. Like respect for persons, the principle of beneficence is rooted in Hippocratic tradition as well as in the long history of the caring professions. Beneficence is defined as acting with charity and kindness to patients. Beauchamp and Childress divide beneficence into providing benefits to patients while balancing benefits and harms that patients may receive from various treatment options. Nonmaleficence is an obligation for healthcare providers to "first of all, do no harm." Finally, the principle of justice requires fairness and equality for all patients and that all patients get what is due to them. It is easy to see that these principles can often conflict with each other under certain circumstances and that a process for prioritizing and determining which principles should prevail is an important part of any medical ethics course.

A chapter on medical ethics for nurse anesthetists could be organized in many ways. For professionals "walking the floor" and experiencing many ethical dilemmas, an understanding of the interaction between law and medicine as well as defining and resolving these ethical dilemmas, may be the most productive. This chapter therefore will present a brief history of the relationship between law and medicine and then describe the most common areas of ethical dilemmas that affect patients in hospitals and those who treat them. Finally, a model for mediating ethical dilemmas will be suggested, and the role of hospital ethics committees will be discussed.

At first blush, the relationship between law and ethics might appear to be an oxymoron. In recent years healthcare professionals seemed to view the role of law in determining ethical dilemmas in healthcare with cynicism. Although

lawyers suffer a certain amount of unpopularity by the general public, our basic laws, which they forcefully advocate and defend, still reflect society's ideal of what is right and just. Both law and ethics have emerged from the same philosophical roots and Judeo-Christian traditions, and both share a similar vocabulary in terms of rights, duties, responsibilities, and obligations alongside concepts such as justice, fairness, and equality.[10] In America, our legal history is a reflection of our moral history. America is—and prides herself on being—a pluralistic society. A pluralistic society values individual rights and respects differing ideas and values. At the same time, Americans have certain responsibilities concurrent with these rights that are often reflected in our laws defining and legislating morality. In this respect, law and ethics have much in common because both attempt to define and mandate what is morally correct in our society at any given time. Our laws regarding health care can be considered a subset of the larger study of medical ethics. It is often stated that our laws are the minimal expectation of what is moral and good. Where the two disciplines diverge, however, is significant. Although medical ethics seeks to define what is morally good, our laws have well-structured mechanisms to enforce various mandates. Indeed, looking at our laws is "like looking at a snapshot in time of our society's moral views about how people ought to behave towards each other."[11]

The practice of medicine is one of the most regulated industries in the United States. Licensing statutes govern entry into the licensed medical professions, disciplinary actions, and the delivery of healthcare services by unlicensed persons. Medical boards dominated by the regulated medical professions implement these statutes. In fact, the licensing of healthcare professionals is often described as a system of professional self-regulation. This form of regulation has been criticized by some as self-serving and as the foundation for a paternalistic philosophy of how medicine should be delivered to patients. Because physicians typically define and enforce the practice of medicine, examples of abuse have been numerous.

During the past century, for example, physicians often made unilateral or paternalistic decisions regarding information they would give patients. During the 1920s, many patients in mental hospitals were deemed "unfit" to have children and were routinely sterilized without their knowledge or consent.[12] Probably the most famous twentieth century American breach of medical ethics was the Tuskegee Syphilis Study.[13] In this study, hundreds of poor Southern African-American men were studied during the first half of the century, so that the United States Public Health Service could develop an understanding of the natural history of syphilis. But even when penicillin as the first effective treatment for syphilis became available, the Public Health Service physicians failed to offer that treatment to most of their subjects.

During the 1960s, the federally enacted "Seattle God Committee" routinely made "social worth" determinations as to which patients would be able to use hemodialysis machines that were in very short supply. Among the criteria used were income, net worth, marital status, educational and employment background, and the ability of the patient to contribute future potential to society. During the 1970s and 1980s as medicine became viewed more as a business, the federal government again began aggressive interventions to define morally acceptable medical practice. For example, physicians and hospitals had long practiced the right to treat whomever they chose. There was no duty to take in patients, as there was no fundamental "right" to health care in America. After numerous incidents of critically ill or fullterm labor patients being turned away from hospital emergency rooms because they could not afford the care, the federal government passed an "anti-dumping statute." This statute, entitled the Emergency Medical Treatment and Active Labor Act, requires most hospitals having emergency rooms to initially screen patients for an emergency medical condition and, if one exists, to stabilize the patient before transferring him or her to another facility.[14,15]

Federal legislation has been extensive in the arena of managed care. As physicians and hospitals combined financial resources to better compete for patients, now commonly called "insured lives" by the insurance industry, complaints of patients being referred to facilities owned by the referring physician for diagnostic tests, such as magnetic resonance imaging (MRI) or radiation therapy, arose. Such self-referrals were found to be profitable for physicians who owned these facilities. Moreover, many of these referrals were induced more for economic reasons than medical reasons. Thus the passage of the Ethics in Patient Referrals Act (commonly referred to as the Stark Act in recognition of the legislation's principal sponsor, Rep. Fortney Pete Stark).[16] Until recently, it was common practice for many managed care companies to prohibit its panel of selected physicians from informing patients of medical treatments and options that were not covered by the managed care contract. Gag orders, as these mandates were commonly called, were not unique to the public sector. Depending on the presidential administration, many examples of gag orders prohibiting physicians and clinics that receive federal Medicare and Medicaid monies from informing patients of their legal option for an abortion were found at the federal level.[17,18]

Recently, federal intervention was necessary after the well-known Nancy Cruzan case went before the United States Supreme Court. In that case, a young adult woman was in a car accident, resulting in severe injuries that rendered her in a persistent vegetative state. After several years in this condition, Nancy's family and physician decided to remove her feeding tube and let her die naturally. In this politically heated case, litigation went on for more than 4 years. The state of Missouri asserted its right to protect "all life" over the families' desire to discontinue treatment.[19] The outcome of this case resulted in the federally enacted Patient Self-Determination Act, which mandates that most hospitals and other entities give patients written materials on their right to create and enforce living wills.[20]

The preceding examples all illustrate federal laws that clarify acceptable medical practices and define new "illegal" medical practices. For the most part, however, health care is still primarily regulated at the state level. State licensing boards still define the practice of medicine, and state legislatures create many statutes guiding healthcare decisions. To better understand these ethical conflicts and how the courts address them is to better understand the practice of medicine in a contemporary American society.

ETHICAL ISSUES SURROUNDING INFORMED CONSENT AND REFUSAL

The principle of informed consent (i.e., that patients have the right—indeed the responsibility—to make decisions regarding their own medical treatments) is a relatively new concept in American medicine. Throughout most of the history of American medicine, the doctor-patient relationship has been founded on the principle of paternalism. The doctor decided what was best for the patient, and the patient impliedly accepted that decision without being given any options in medical treatment. Doing the right thing for the patient meant doing what doctors thought was the best thing for the patient.[21] In many respects, this model of paternalism was based on a power relationship between physician and patient. The balance of power and information was in the minds of well-educated physicians, and patients took the subordinate role of doing what their doctor thought best.[22] As America became more diverse and pluralistic, so did the attitudes of patients and their values regarding medical care and treatment. With the advent of the Civil Rights movement and the Consumer Rights movement, patients increasingly demanded a more active role in medical decision-making. The respect for patient autonomy thus became a well-established legal mandate in the requirement of patient consent for medical treatments.

In theory at least, consent is a process of communication that requires physicians to discuss with their patients the risks and benefits of the proposed medical treatment; alternatives, if any, to the proposed treatment; the prognoses of the proposed treatment; and the consequences of forgoing the proposed treatment.[23] Yet, in reality, patient autonomy does not seem to be as dominant a value as this rhetoric would suggest. This is not surprising for those physicians and nurses "walking the floor." Every day they see many exceptions to patient autonomy. For example, not all patients have the ability to make autonomous choices because of physical or mental impairments. Even with competent patients, physicians and nurses hear complaints that patients cannot understand the technical details of many proposed medical procedures. Some patients refuse to listen to medical details and prefer rather to defer the consent process to a family member. Patient autonomy necessarily assumes that physicians will offer rational viable choices and that patients will consent in a rational manner to these choices, yet exceptions to this rule abound.

On the floor of so many hospitals and doctors' offices, informed consent doctrine moves from the sublime to the ridiculous—from an active and constructive conversation to a multipage, incomprehensible consent document, from facilitating a dialogue to getting a signature for the files. Who is to blame? One may be tempted to say the law—or at least the lawyers.[24] But if lawyers or the law are to be "blamed," it is important to understand how the law interprets cases in informed consent and to understand that this blame is not so much with the law as it is with a break in the trust and foundation of the underlying doctor-patient relationship.

Difficult questions pervade all aspects of the consent process. How much information do patients need in order to give consent? Who makes decisions for patients if they cannot make decisions for themselves? What legal standard is used to determine the appropriateness of consent; should it be a doctor standard or a patient standard? What should be done when patients make wrong decisions?

A case in point is Arato v. Avedon. Mr. Arato was a 43-year old electrical contractor who had an operation to remove a nonfunctioning kidney. During surgery a tumor was found in the tail of his pancreas, and the tumor was removed. Several days later the surgeon met with Mr. Arato and his wife. He told them that he thought he had removed the entire tumor and then referred them to an oncologist. The surgeon did not tell them that only about 5% of patients with pancreatic cancer survive for 5 years, nor did the surgeon give Mr. Arato either a prognosis or a reasonable estimate of his life expectancy. The oncologist told the Aratos that a substantial chance of a recurrence existed and that it would mean the disease was incurable. He recommended experimental chemotherapy and radiation treatment and acknowledged that this might produce no benefit. During chemotherapy a recurrence was detected. Although the physicians believed Mr.

Arato's life expectancy could then be measured in months, they did not tell him so. Mr. Arato died approximately 1 year after his cancer had been diagnosed. After his death, his wife brought suit against the surgeons and oncologists, alleging that they had failed to tell Mr. Arato that approximately 95% of people with pancreatic cancer die within 5 years. The wife alleged that rather than consenting to experimental therapy, Mr. Arato would have put his "house in order," taken care of his business, and made better plans to provide for his family after his death. Instead, Mr. Arato put all his financial and psychologic efforts into the medical treatments.

At the trial, the treating physicians justified not disclosing statistical life expectancy data to their patient, Mr. Arato, on a variety of grounds. They believed such information would be too stressful for the patient to hear, as he had exhibited great anxiety over his condition—so much so that the surgeon determined that it would have been medically inappropriate to disclose this information to him. Other physicians indicated they did not want to give Mr. Arato a "cold shower" by informing him of such dismal information. Others stated that knowing the high mortality rates for his cancer would deprive Mr. Arato of any hope of a cure. The California court in this case declined to endorse a mandatory disclosure of life expectancy probabilities and refused to further intrude on the subtleties of the physician-patient relationship by requiring disclosure of information that might or might not be indicated in a given treatment context. The court did require that physicians must disclose such information, as a patient may need to make an informed decision. Mr. Arato was told that cancer of the pancreas is usually fatal and under those circumstances the court stated:

> In the contexts of clinical settings in which physician and patient interact and exchange information material to therapeutic decisions are so multifarious, the informational needs and degree of dependency of individual patients so various and the professional relationship itself such an intimate and irreducibly judgment-laden one, that we believe it is unwise to require as a matter of law that a particular species of information be disclosed . . . (I)n administering

the doctrine of informed consent each patient presents a separate problem, that the patient's mental and emotional condition is important and in certain cases may be crucial, and that in discussing the element of risk a certain amount of discretion must be employed consistent with the full disclosure of facts necessary to an informed consent.[25]

This case has been highly criticized in both legal and medical journals. The court, in agreeing with the physicians, noted that during all his visits, the patient had ample opportunity to bring up the subject of mortality if he chose to do so. However, numerous articles in medical literature for physicians discuss the fact that patients are often greatly intimidated by the medical process and are often too stressed to ask difficult questions such as those surrounding mortality. This process of communication therefore is best begun with the trained healthcare professional—not with the sick patient.

Another critique of this case lies in the emphasis the court imposed on the therapeutic privilege physicians use to justify withholding information from patients if the physician deems such information to be harmful to the well being of the patient.[26] Given general physician unhappiness with requirements of disclosure, this therapeutic privilege exception threatens in theory to eviscerate the informed consent doctrine. Little evidence in the literature suggests that patients are actually harmed by receiving negative information, although certainly they may become anxious.[27] On the other hand, the literature demonstrates that many patients with cancer tend to overestimate their probability of long-term survival.[28,29] Patients who do not have a good understanding of their prognosis have been shown to be unable to choose accurate treatments to best reflect their own internal values. Were Mr. Arato's physicians taking the easy alternative by recommending treatments with marginal effectiveness rather than focusing on the real needs of the patient and his family? Certainly this has been a major criticism of the consent process and its underlying focus only on the individual patient. It ignores all the other people who are so intimately tied to the patient, such as family members and other healthcare team members. Mr. Arato's choice left his family financially and emotionally devastated. Were the physicians assuming that Mr. Arato needed hope rather than the truth, or is the whole process of communication just too burdensome for busy physicians to confront?[30]

Most physicians agree that empowering patients with sufficient information to choose medical treatments best suited to their personal values is morally and ethically correct. Such information requires physicians to be trained in communication skills and to know their patients and the patients' families. Most importantly, it requires physicians who understand that their own internal values about what treatments to choose may indeed conflict with their patients' values. Arguably, then, the holding in the Arato case is reasonable; that physicians need to take patients individually and consider the circumstances to determine what information that patient can absorb at any particular time in the treatment regimen. The problem with this case, however, is that the court relied on a physician's determination about what information the patient needs to know rather than what a particular patient—or, indeed, most patients—would need to know. In the final analysis, if physicians would focus on treatment goals rather than treatment options then much of this litigation would be moot. Laws can only set minimal standards for the consent process. In the end, patients must make the final determination of what risks they are willing to take for the potential benefits of medicine.

Cases such as this one demonstrate how the courts interpret principles of patient autonomy, truth-telling, beneficence, and justice. These cases give healthcare practitioners legal guidelines to supplement ethical guidelines during the decision-making process; however, similar to all guidelines, the have exceptions. Nonetheless, following the general risk management rules given will help maintain trust between patient and the healthcare provider, respect for patient autonomy, and respect for medical autonomy as well.

Patients with capacity have the right—indeed, the responsibility—to consent to their own medical treatment. Consent is valid when given; therefore the determination of capacity should be made at the time consent is granted.

When in doubt, a second opinion should be sought.

Patients without capacity have the same right to consent to medical treatment. This is more difficult to ascertain because healthcare providers must confer with a surrogate, usually a family member, to obtain consent. When someone else makes a medical decision on behalf of a patient, two standards are used to determine the adequacy of this consent. First is the "substituted judgment" test. This means that the surrogate must make the decision based on what the patient would have wanted rather than on what the surrogate wants. Second is the "best interests" test and is used for patients who have never had capacity to let their wishes be known. Infants and mentally disabled patients are two examples of patients in this category. Because these patients have never been able to make their wishes known, surrogates and the healthcare team must determine whether the benefits of a medical procedure will outweigh the risks.

Concurrent with the right of informed consent is the right of informed refusal. When appraised of the risks, benefits, alternatives, and consequences of refusing treatment options, patients have the right to refuse medical treatments—even life-sustaining treatments. The general rule should be that when patients refuse medically indicated treatments, further inquiry into the refusal is best. Many times, patients simply need more information. For example, a patient may refuse blood for religious reasons, in which case a discussion of nonblood options is advisable. Patients need to know the consequences of their refusal, but in the final analysis, they must live or die with these consequences.

If the prognosis is dire and a fatal outcome a likely prospect, physicians should be guided by the strongest presumption in favor of disclosure and consent that can be modified only by clear and carefully documented evidence that patients do not wish to be fully informed. Therapeutic privilege should be a last resort for physicians to take.

The discussion of treatment options should include realistic options that will promote the medical treatment goals agreed on by both physician and patient. If patients are offered and accept marginally effective or futile medical treatment that will not change the outcome, they may be very disappointed with the final outcome. Litigation over futile treatment has been common when patients demand treatment that physicians believe will not benefit them. Patients who demand that physicians "do everything" should realize that physicians will do everything that is medically indicated but not everything that *can* be done. Most of these conflicts regarding futile medical treatment arise because physicians focus their discussion on medical modalities rather than on treatment goals. Treatment goals can be specific as dying at home, being discharged to the floor, increasing the patient's ability to be with family during the end, or providing aggressive pain management. Goals maintain trust between physician and patient. If an impasse is reached, physicians may want to consider transferring the patient to another physician who will provide the treatments demanded.

Ethical Considerations with Resuscitation

It may seem ironic that—with all the focus on patient autonomy and a consensus that patients do have the right to be informed of their medical treatments—cardiopulmonary resuscitation (CPR) is the only medical procedure routinely done in a hospital *without* express consent from the patient. The converse of this situation is that most hospitals have elaborate policies and procedures for withholding resuscitation, commonly called a do not resuscitate (DNR) order. From a legal point of view, this apparent twist in hospital policy makes sense. The law (which follows the medical mandate of beneficence) presumes that patients suffering an emergency condition would want all life-prolonging procedures to be applied.

From the early 1960s, CPR was first used as a curative intervention to revive healthy persons who nearly drowned or experienced lethal cardiac arrhythmia during general anesthesia. For these situations CPR has proven very beneficial.[31] Subsequently, CPR as a medical procedure moved almost exclusively into the hospital environment, where it was routinely given to all patients. Since many of these patients were extremely sick, terminally ill, very elderly, or severely and irreversibly incapacitated, it became clear that only a minority of patients who were successfully resuscitated survived until their hospital discharge. A growing number of physicians therefore viewed resuscitation on such patients as a violation of a physician's ethical principle of nonmalfeasance (first do no harm), and they supported developing clearer and more realistic hospital policies for DNR.[32] Typical DNR policies now require physicians to discuss the risks and benefits of treatment for patients who may wish to refuse resuscitation in the future.

Despite widespread adoption of hospital DNR policies, many troubling ethical dilemmas still occur in the use of resuscitation. For example, most patients are not routinely assessed on admission of their DNR status; thus resuscitation is still performed on patients who will receive no benefit from it. Moreover, because many of these patients are often mentally compromised, family members consent to a DNR order. When confronted with this choice of alternatives, families often demand that everything be done. When families are asked whether they want the medical team to try to restart the heart if the patient's heart stops beating, families most often respond with a resounding "yes." Even when patients have DNR orders, the orders are often considered "inactive" under certain circumstances. For example, DNR orders are oftentimes suspended during surgery. Medical personnel will often ignore DNR orders during transportation of a patient from one facility to another. DNR orders are often written for brief periods of time and require reassessment and new orders if the status of the patient changes. Finally, in some situations, patients themselves will not consent to a DNR order because they fear a DNR order will mean that they will be "abandoned" by the medical team and left to die.

As time went on, this situation only worsened. Many patients continued to receive very aggressive and invasive CPR procedure even when clearly contraindicated medically. As the medical community became increasingly aware of the serious harm caused by contraindicated use of CPR, healthcare providers developed elaborate mechanisms for avoiding CPR treatments they felt were futile or harmful to patients. Physicians did not openly discuss these procedures with their patients. These decisions often took the form of "slow codes."[33]

Slow codes are attempts by physicians and other healthcare providers to shield themselves from possible litigation that might arise from a written DNR order calling for the inaction of hospital personal.[34] Slow codes present many ethical and management problems.[35]

Consequently, a number of hospitals developed "resuscitation not indicated" (RNI) policies whereby a physician could make a unilateral decision that the patient was not a candidate for CPR and write a RNI note in the chart without getting "permission" from the patient. The purpose of an RNI policy is to give physicians an "out" for the requirement of discussing a "futile or harmful medical treatment" with the patient, when the physician believes that the patient would be harmed by such aggressive intervention.[36] Although it was well intended, this policy usually contained requirements to inform the patient's family that resuscitation would not be performed,[37] thus leaving physicians in an ethical dilemma as to what to do when family demanded resuscitation anyway. With resuscitation procedures commonly portrayed on television and with the belief that "miracles of medicine" might prevail over death, families often demand that everything be done to save the patient.[38,39]

Other ethical dilemmas are involved with the treatment of patients with DNR orders. For the most part, the use of DNR orders has been largely limited to hospital floors. Many physicians believe using expensive intensive care unit (ICU) beds for patients with a DNR status is inappropriate. This attitude changed somewhat when the Ethics Committee of the Society of Critical Care Medicine issued guidelines stating that a patient's resuscitation status should not preclude admissions to the ICU.[40] Problems still remain, however, in the operating room, in which patients with DNR orders undergo surgery and anesthesia. Many hospitals have policies that suspend DNR orders under these circumstances. Surveys of anesthesiologists found that the majority of them assume that DNR orders are always suspended during surgery and that informing patients of this fact is not necessary.[41] In 1993 the Ethics Committee of the American Society of Anesthesiologists (ASA) implemented guidelines to evaluate patient autonomy and the need to suspend DNR orders

during surgery. The statement published concluded the following:

> An institutional policy of automatic cancellation of the DNR status in cases where a surgical procedure is to be carried out, removes the patient from appropriate participation in decision-making, but automatic enforcement without discussion and clarification may lead to inappropriate perioperative and anesthetic management.[42]

With so much confusion regarding resuscitation procedures in hospitals, what can healthcare providers do to balance their concern and respect for patient autonomy, beneficence, nonmaleficence, and justice for all patients? Following a number of ethical principles and good old-fashioned common sense, healthcare providers can take specific steps to minimize ethical dilemmas with DNR orders.

All patients being admitted to a hospital should be assessed for the appropriateness of resuscitation. Whether patients are otherwise healthy (such as labor and delivery patients) or are extremely old, demented, or terminally ill, they all would benefit from a discussion of the risks and benefits of resuscitation for their particular circumstances.

Learn specific ways to communicate risks and benefits of resuscitation with patients. Asking patients or family members "if your heart stops, do you want me to try to start it again" is not sufficient information for an informed consent decision. Indeed, it is misleading. Resuscitation can be as specific as putting paddles on a patient or as complicated as the use of chemicals, open heart massage, intubation, and ventilator support. Depending on the patient's condition at admission, some or all of these procedures could be beneficial. However, they also might be harmful or futile. Developing good communication techniques with the patient is not difficult but unfortunately is taught very poorly in medical school.[43] In addition to developing individual communication skills, healthcare professionals should take advantage of written materials, videos, and the expertise of others, such as experienced nurses and other healthcare providers.[44]

Discuss the treatment goals of resuscitation with patients. Patients may be shocked to learn that a successful resuscitation is defined in the literature as only surviving for one hour after the procedure. Even if patients survive, they may be worse off than before—such as in a permanent coma with broken ribs and other painful complications. Even with resuscitation, many patients will not survive to discharge. This approach recognizes that patients are often less concerned with technical details of resuscitation than with more subjective and personal issues such as pain, neurologic damage, survival, and quality of life. A goal-directed approach would mean that some CPR procedures will be acceptable and that some will not. Most importantly, a goals approach will have patients, families, and healthcare team members working together to achieve these goals rather than getting into a "power play" while trying to decide who gets to select what treatment modalities are acceptable and who gets to define which medical treatments are futile.

Tell patients what medical procedures will be attempted when resuscitation is not indicated. Patients sometimes refuse to consent to a DNR because they believe the medical staff will abandon them. Tell them (and the rest of the medial team) exactly what procedures will be used. DNR patients often have very aggressive treatments, including surgery, to relieve pain and increase one's ability to do the activities of daily living. Discuss the treatments offered for palliative care. DNR patients are now in our ICUs; therefore focus on what is beneficial rather than what is futile.

Resolve ethical conflict internally. Use the resources available in your hospital. Do you have ethics consult services to help mediate differences in values and opinions? What other support services can you call on? Do you have trained social workers, clergy, patient advocates, or other physicians for second opinions? The object is not to put pressure on patients and families but to better clarify the issues and to help define a clear treatment plan that specifically helps to focus on treatment goals rather than treatment modalities.

If you reach an impasse with a patient or his or her family members, discuss the possibility of transferring the patient to another physician. Your relationship with your patient must be based on trust rather than conflict. Keep in mind, however, that in those few cases that have gone

to court, overwhelmingly the courts have upheld a patient's right to choose his or her own medical treatment. This also means that for patients and their families that are demanding treatment that the physician believes is futile or harmful to the patient, courts will probably support the patient's right to choose. On the other hand, in those cases in which patients received aggressive medical treatment including resuscitation despite being a clear "DNR" patient, courts generally have found no monetary damages, because assessing the value of life over not living is difficult.

Ethical Dilemmas During End of Life
Today, with most American patients dying in hospitals or nursing homes, the process of dying has become almost dehumanized. Over the last several years the law has been invoked regularly by physicians and other healthcare providers concerned about the ethical, legal, and medical propriety of discontinuing what is now generally called life-sustaining treatment. Typical issues the courts are asked to resolve include what medical modalities can be removed, whether treatment can be removed from nonterminal as well as terminal patients, whether physicians can prescribe "excessive" dosages of pain medication to terminally ill patients, and whether physicians can "assist" in the death of a patient. In addition, courts are asked to resolve family conflict as well, when some family members want aggressive treatment while others want to let the patient die naturally.

The Supreme Court ruled on a patient's right to forgo life-sustaining treatment when it rendered an opinion in 1990 on the fate of Nancy Cruzan. Cruzan was injured in an automobile accident in 1983. Doctors aggressively treated her when she arrived at the hospital because they were uncertain about her condition. After a few weeks, Nancy was diagnosed as in a persistent vegetative state—a state that the Supreme Court defined as "a condition in which a person exhibits motor reflexes but evinces no indications of significant cognitive function."[45] Nancy was kept alive by gastrostomy and hydration tubes. Six years after the accident, Nancy's parents requested that the state hospital where Nancy was being maintained discontinue her feeding tube and allow her to die. Either because the hospital administration and staff thought that this was an ethically and medically inappropriate action or because they were concerned about their potential legal liability, or both, they refused to allow the removal of the tube without a court order. Thus began several years of litigation culminating in a ruling by the Supreme Court. The issue before the Court was a narrow one. Can Missouri require "clear and convincing" evidence when family members make medical decisions on behalf of an incapacitated patient? Cruzan, 31 years old at the time of the accident, had no living will. It was a momentous decision. The Supreme Court ruled that although persons have a liberty right to refuse life-sustaining medical treatment, a state may apply a clear and convincing evidence standard in a proceeding in which a guardian seeks to discontinue nutrition and hydration of a person diagnosed to be in a persistent vegetative state. One of the issues thus resolved by the Cruzan case is the breadth permitted to state law by the United States Constitution: virtually any legal or medical procedure developed by a state to implement that state's substantively defined rights will be consistent with the U.S. constitutional requirements. However, the Supreme Court set outside limits on the states' use of these rights. First, the Court accepted the principle that competent persons have the right to forgo medical treatment, including nutrition and hydration. The Court also recognized that states may assert an "unqualified interest" in the preservation of human life, regardless of the quality of life the person may experience. Finally, the Court held that a state had the power to impose any reasonable procedural burden it wished in cases involving the right to forgo life-sustaining treatment.

As mentioned at the beginning of this chapter, the Cruzan ruling caused the federal government to pass the Patient Self-Determination Act.[46] This statute requires hospitals and other healthcare entities to provide patients with written information describing their rights under state law to make decisions concerning medical care, including the right to accept or refuse medical or surgical treatment and the right to formulate advance directives. The law, sometimes called a patient's "Miranda Rights" requires patients receive extensive information on living wills, medical durable power of attorney, and other state statutes on informed consent.[47]

One may assume that with this onslaught of state and federal legislation involving end-of-life decisions, most Americans would have living wills. However only 10% to 15% of Americans today have living wills, and most of those are the elderly. The burden is still on physicians and other healthcare providers to communicate with their patients regarding end-of-life treatment preferences, because these laws are relatively straightforward and give patients the right to choose their own medical treatments. At the same time, these laws clearly give physicians the responsibility to determine just what treatment choices patients want to make.[48]

Despite extensive legislation that clarifies patient rights to make end-of-life medical decisions, concern that physicians do not really listen to their patients or that physicians disregard provisions as expressed in living wills remained. More research was needed. From 1989 to 1994 the Robert Wood Johnson Foundation funded a study of medical care for patients with life-threatening conditions. The study, called SUPPORT,[49] followed 9105 patients admitted to five major medical centers in five states. SUPPORT was an ambitious study that cost $28 million and was executed in phases. Phase I revealed the shortfalls in patient-physician communication. The study found that although 31% of these patients wanted a DNR order, fewer than half the physicians treating these patients knew their patients' preferences. Pain management was undertreated, with about half the patients or their families reporting moderate to severe pain over the last few days of hospitalization.

Physicians and patients were interviewed to determine what changes the researcher could make to enhance better communication between healthcare provider and patient and to support patient autonomy. Physicians responded that they needed access to better information about their patients' preferences and would require trained nurses to intervene and give them reports on their patient's preferences based on interviews with the patients and their families. After extensive intervention during phase II, the results of SUPPORT were published and were dismal indeed:

> SUPPORT investigators reported that only 34% of the physicians acknowledged having received

a report . . . although a written report was provided in 78% of the cases. Fifty-nine percent of the doctors acknowledged having received the prognosis report, even though a written report was given to the doctor in 94% of the cases and had been placed in the patient's medical records 80% of the cases. Only 15% of the participating doctors reported having discussed the information on prognosis and preferences with their patients. The prevalence and timing of written DNR orders was the same for the control and intervention groups. There was an increase in reported untreated pain in the interviews conducted with patients themselves.[50]

In other words, most patients wanted information about living wills and resuscitation; they wanted to be treated for pain; and they wanted open discussions with their physicians about treatment options. Physicians replied that if they had better information about their patients, they would be able to give patients what they wanted. Despite massive interventions by highly trained nurses to obtain such information from the patients and to write this information up in a report placed in the patients' medical records, physicians still ignored this additional information and continued to treat their patients the same as always. The report concludes:

> SUPPORT joins a great body of evidence and analysis that proves that informed consent, conversation, and patient autonomy is ill suited to decision-making regarding medical interventions. Physicians simply will not talk with their patients, perhaps especially patients in terminal care, and will not yield control to the patients. Some argue that it is time to abandon the myth of individual patient autonomy, or consumer choice, and redesign the relationship between physician and patient along different and yet to be announced lines.[51]

Some may argue that the answer to patient autonomy lies not within living wills, medical durable power of attorney, hospital DNR policies, or thousands of court rulings on similar cases but with better training of healthcare providers during medical school, nursing school, and while they are "walking the floor" of every hospital in America. This important training is beginning to be implemented across the country, and includes the incorporation of many bioethical mandates, which have been further clarified by statutory and case law. These include the following:

- Patients have the right to refuse medical treatments, including all forms of life-sustaining medical treatments.
- Medical treatments mean anything done in the hospital environment, including feeding tubes and hydration.
- Patients have the right to appropriate pain management, especially during the end-of-life phase.
- Analgesics and sedatives may be titrated in whatever doses are necessary to ensure the patient's comfort.
- Physicians should focus their discussion on treatment goals rather than treatment modalities to ensure patient autonomy. Physicians should not offer "futile" treatments to patients unless the physicians are prepared to administer them.
- Patients have needs, but their families and the ICU treatment team have needs as well. By understanding all three sectors and anticipating their needs, potential conflicts are minimized.

Patient needs include the following:

- Aggressive pain management
- Company of family and friends
- Maintaining control and dignity over the dying process
- Fulfilling family and cultural expectations
- Attaining spiritual meaning

Needs of the family include the following:

- To be informed and to participate in the decision-making process if the patient is incompetent to do so himself or herself
- To be with the dying person
- To be helpful
- To be assured of the patient's comfort
- To express emotions
- To receive comfort and support from family and friends
- To receive comfort, support and reassurance from the healthcare team

Needs of the ICU team include:

- To receive clear communication on the treatment plan
- Cooperation among team members

- Competence in administering the treatment plan and in communication skills
- Administrative support
- Opportunity for debriefing and bereavement.[52]

In the final analysis, identifying and understanding typical ethical dilemmas in hospitals is important; understanding the ethical principals used to analyze dilemmas is also important; but having a mechanism to resolve ethical conflicts as they might arise with patients, families, or other medical team members is fundamental for those "walking the floor." For this, an institutional ethics committee can play an important role.

ROLE OF ETHICS COMMITTEES AND ETHICS CONSULT SERVICES

Ethics committees have become commonplace in hospitals. Since 1995, The Joint Commission on Accreditation of Healthcare Organizations requires that accredited facilities have in place a functioning process to address ethical issues. These functions might include ethics committees, the use of a formalized ethics forum, ethics consultations, or any combination of the above.[53] Estimates suggest that hospital and nursing home ethics committees attempt to resolve about 13,500 patient-physician dilemmas a year. Disputes overwhelmingly arise in one of two forms. The first involves the refusal of life-sustaining medical treatment, typically with terminally ill patients. The second involves patients who demand life-sustaining treatments that the patient's physician believes is futile or otherwise inappropriate.[54]

An ethics committee is a multidisciplinary committee that serves as a hospital resource for patients, families, and hospital staff by offering an objective process for resolving disputes involving ethical dilemmas. The goal of the ethics committee is to assist patients, families, physicians, nurses, and other hospital workers in coming to a consensus with the options that best meet the patient's goal for care.

Ethics committees have three major functions. First, they are a valuable resource for developing hospital policies and procedures in making difficult decisions. For example, ethics committees may play a substantial role in the development of DNR, informed consent, living will, and other related policies. Second, ethics committees provide education in the form of grand rounds on current issues of ethical dilemma. These programs are often provided as a community service in addition to an inhouse service. Third, ethics committees most often provide consultative services to patient, families, and health care workers to help mediate conflict and clarify alternative treatment options.[55]

Estimates indicate that 85% of all hospitals currently offer ethics consultation services. Except in rare instances, these services are not regulated in any manner. Members of the ethics committees, composed almost exclusively of a variety of hospital staff, usually perform the consult. Some ethics committees have outside community or lay persons as members. Some members are healthcare attorneys, although most prohibit attorneys and hospital administrators from being members because of a perceived conflict of interest.[56] Although anyone can request an ethics consult, patients generally have little or no knowledge of the existence of such committees, and requests are almost always from hospital staff. When assistance is requested the committee typically gathers information about the ethical dispute at hand, deliberates among its members, sometimes interviews other members of the healthcare team, and sometimes interviews the patient and family. The medical record is reviewed, and the committee will then issue a nonbinding recommendation about how the dispute should be resolved. The nature of this recommendation can be controversial because the ethics committee tends to take a stand in favor of one side over another. Sometimes this has the result of alienating the other side and forcing the unresolved ethics dilemma into court. As Gatter observes:

> Because ethics consultation results in a nonbinding decision by a third party rather than in a mutual agreement between the disputants, it is not well suited as mediation to prevent the unnecessary deterioration of the physician-patient relationship during efforts to resolve a physician-patient end-of-life treatment dispute. Like adjudication, ethics consultation . . . pits the physician and the patient . . . against each other. As adversaries, they compete for an ethics committee's opinion. Consequently, the fear is

that the ethics consultation will erode the trust of patients in their physicians and in the process by which end of life treatment disputes are resolved.[57]

In fact, ethics committees have become so popular in resolving disputes between physician, patient, family, and among medical team members that they risk alienating the very people they are trying to help. Ethics committees wield real power over the fate of real patients. But as Wolf notes:

> [Medical ethics] committees have thus far avoided taking responsibility for this power. Committees simultaneously seek power but offer assurances that they are merely advisory. They may exert a decisive influence over patients' legal and moral rights yet routinely offer no protection for those rights. They claim to benefit patients while serving healthcare professionals.[58]

Despite this potential conflict in the roles of ethics committees, many have advocated that ethics committees should be used as a resource for avoiding potential litigation. Annas claims, for example, that "good ethics committees begin where the law ends." He argues that setting up additional bureaucratic entities (or risk management or liability control committees, as he prefers to call ethics committees) to make legal pronouncements can only make medicine more legalistic and impersonal.[59] Other commentators, however, believe that medical ethics committees can act effectively as mediators of ethical disputes and can reduce costly, time-consuming, and the "adversarial" nature of litigating bedside dilemmas in the courtroom.[60] On the other hand, problems with medical ethics committees are also apparent. Because committee members are overwhelmingly employees of a hospital, they may internalize and perpetuate its parent hospital's dominant biases. Members of such ethics committees may also have conflicting views regarding their roles on the committee. Although some commentators argue that patient protection should be the primary purpose of the ethics committee, others argue that protecting institutional values and goals is a valid objective.

If medical ethics committees can't resolve these disputes, the courts are empowered to do so. However, as a final resort, the courts and the legal system—based on adversarial roles of attorneys that represent opposite sides in any legal dispute—present a new set of ethical, medical, and legal pitfalls. After all, judges lack expertise in medical matters and know less than doctors and other healthcare providers about the uncertainty surrounding death. But the trial court judge will be assisted by expert medical testimony in reaching his or her ultimate decision. Trial court judges also have been accused of imposing formidable costs on the family, in terms of money, time expended, and psychological stress.[61]

In the final analysis, however, the court system offers four major advantages: it encourages good bilateral decision making; it compensates persons who have been wrongfully harmed; it promotes social dialogue on questions of withdrawal and withholding of medical treatment; and it serves to guide the conduct of third parties and their subsequent conduct.[62]

Another significant reason why our legal system can reach a final resolution better than medical ethics committees is the fact that many physicians and other healthcare providers do not always follow these ethical canons while "walking the floor." Many research studies suggest that physicians do not follow the mandates of their patients living wills, that many physicians still make a distinction between withholding and withdrawing medical treatment, that physicians are sometimes afraid to give appropriate pain medication for fear of the "double effect," and that many physicians recommend futile or marginally effective medical treatments to their patients that they would not want for themselves.[63]

In other words, healthcare providers are human and are greatly influenced by their own codes of personal conduct, morality, and ethics. When a healthcare provider's personal code conflicts with a patient's personal rights and values, especially patients with different religious or cultural values, or a different ethnic diversity than the health care provider, then a relationship of trust may turn into an adversarial relationship that ultimately may have to be resolved in the courtroom.

SUMMARY

Medical science and technology are growing at an incredible rate, and at the same time they are creating new ethical dilemmas. The practice of medicine continues to evolve to involve conflicting values with medical access, equality of care, and market competition. Although increased education in medical ethics, more institutionalized hospital ethics committees, and a healthy debate on medical treatment options all attempt to resolve many of these ethical dilemmas, they cannot resolve them all.

Final resolution of these medical ethics issues ultimately must come from our legal system, a system which, being necessarily reactive to most legal and ethical disputes, is seldom in the forefront of this ethical debate. But it is just as well that the law does not change as rapidly as medical science and technology. Whereas the study and practice of medicine rapidly evolves at the speed of scientific discovery, law, on the other hand, embodies our basic underlying social principles and expectations of what is reasonably knowable, predictable, relatively consistent, equitable, and just in our society. Our legal system therefore must ultimately respond to the changing ethical rights, responsibilities, and obligations of all our citizens.

REFERENCES

1. Popular journals include Hastings Center Report; Journal of Law, Medicine, and Ethics; The Journal of Clinical Ethics; Journal of Medical Humanities and Bioethics; Journal of Medicine and Philosophy.
2. Beauchamp TL, Childress JF: Principles of biomedical ethics, ed 5, New York, 2001, Oxford University Press.
3. Beauchamp TL, Walters L: Contemporary issues in bioethics, ed 5, Belmont, Calif, 1999, Wadsworth Publishing.
4. Jecker NS (editor), Jonsen AR, Pearlman RA (contributors): Bioethics: an introduction to the history, methods, and practice, Sudbury, Mass, 1997, Jones & Bartlett Publishing.
5. Veatch RM, Flack HE: Case studies in allied health ethics, Upper Saddle River, NJ, 1997, Prentice Hall.
6. Harris, DM: Healthcare law and ethics: issues for the age of managed care, Chicago, 1999, Health Administration Press.
7. Pence GE: Classic cases in medical ethics, ed 3, 1999, McGraw Hill.
8. Kennedy Institute of Ethics, Georgetown University: www.georgetown.edu/research/kie (accessed online Sept 13, 2002); Center for Biomedical Ethics, University of Virginia: wwwmed.virginia.edu/bioethics (accessed online Sept 13, 2002.
9. Furrow BR, Greaney TL, Johnson SH et al: Health law cases, materials, and problems, ed 4, St Paul, Minn, 2001, West Group.
10. Bauman S: Clinical ethics: what's law got to do with it? Arch Fam Med 8:345-6, 1999.
11. Scott C: Why law pervades medicine: an essay on ethics in health care, Journal of Law, Ethics, and Public Policy, Notre Dame 14:245-248, 2000.
12. Buck v. Bell 274 US 2000 (1927).
13. Benedek T: The Tuskegee study of untreated syphilis: analysis of moral aspects versus methodological aspects, Journal of Chronic Diseases 31:1, 1978.
14. 42 USC 1395dd (1992).
15. Scaduto LH: Comment, the emergency medical treatment and active labor act gone astray: a proposal to reclaim EMTALA for its intended beneficiaries, UCLA L Rev 46:943, 1999.
16. Dechene JC, O'Neil KP: "Stark II" and state self-referral restrictions, J Health and Hospital Law, 29:65, 1996.
17. Martin JA, Bjerknes LK: The legal and ethical implications of gag clauses in physician contracts, Am J Law Med 22:433, 1996.
18. Sage WM: Physicians as advocates, Houston Law Review 35:1529, 1999.
19. Cruzan v. Director, Missouri Department of Health. 497 US 261, 314, 110 S. Ct. 2841 (1990).
20. 42 USCA sections 1395(a)(1)(Q), 1395cc(f), 1395mm(c)(8), 1396a(a)(57),(58).
21. Faden RR: A history and theory of informed consent, New York, 1986, Oxford University Press.
22. Katz J: The silent world of doctor and patient, 1986

23. Arabian A: Informed consent: from the ambivalence of Arato to the thunder of Thor, Issues in Law and Medicine 10:161, 1994.

24. Scott C: Why law pervades medicine: an essay on ethics in health care, Journal of Law, Ethics, and Public Policy, Notre Dame 14:245-248, 2000.

25. Arato v. Avedon, 4 Cal. 4th 1172, 23 Cal Rptr 2s 131, 858 P. 2d 598 at 606 (Supreme Ct California, 1993).

26. Sommervile M: Therapeutic privilege: variation on the theme of informed consent, Law, Med, and Health Care 12(4), 1984.

27. Rosoff AJ: Consent to medical treatment in treatise on health care law. In MacDonald MG, Kaufman RM, Capron AM, Birbaum IM, editors: Treatise on health law, New York, 1997, Matthew Bender & Co.

28. Siminoff LA, Fetting JH, Abeloff MD: Doctor-patient communication about breast cancer adjuvant therapy, J Clin Oncol 7:1192-2000, 1989.

29. Yellen SB, Cella DF: Ignorance is bliss? Beliefs about illness and perception of well-being. In Program and abstracts of the Fourth International Society of Behavioral Medicine, Washington, Abstract 45B, 1996.

30. Smith TJ, Swisher K: Telling the truth about terminal cancer, JAMA 1746(279):21, 1998.

31. Tucker KJ, Savitt MA, Idris A et al: Cardiopulmonary resuscitation: historical perspectives, physiology, and future directions, Arch Intern Med 154:2141-2150, 1994.

32. Mooney CA: Deciding not to resuscitate hospital patients: medical and legal perspectives, U Ill L Rev 1025, 1986.

33. Neher JO: The slow code: a hidden conflict, J Fam Prac 27:429-430, 1988.

34. Fowler MDM: Slow code, partial code, limited code, Heart and Lung 18:533, 1989.

35. Smith GP II: Euphemistic codes and tell-tale hearts: human assistance in end of life cases, Health Matrix 10:175, 2000.

36. Waisel DB, Truog RD: The cardiopulmonary resuscitation-not-indicated order: futility revisited, Ann Intern Med 122(4):304, 1995.

37. Hackler JC, Hiller FC: Family consent to orders not to resuscitate: reconsidering hospital policy, JAMA 264(10):1281, 1990.

38. Weil, MH, Weil CJ: How to respond to family demands for futile life support and cardio-

39. Diem S, Lantos J, Tulsky J: Cardiopulmonary resuscitation on television: miracles and misinformation, New England Journal of Medicine 334:1578-1582, 1996.

40. Society of Critical Care Medicine Ethics Committees: Consensus statement on the triage of critically ill patients, JAMA 271:1200-1203, 1994.

41. Robert DT, Waisel DB: Do not resuscitate orders: from the ward to the operating room; from procedures to goals, International Anesthesiology Clinics 30(3):53-55, 2001.

42. American Society of Anesthesiologists: Ethical guidelines for anesthesia care of patients with do not resuscitate orders or other directives that limit treatment (approved by the House of Delegates on Oct 17, 2001; can be found at www.asahq.org/standards/09.html).

43. Tulsky JA, Chesney MA, Lo B: See one, do one, teach one? House staff experience discussing do not resuscitate orders, Arch Intern Med 156:1285, 1996.

44. Jezewski MA: Obtaining consent for do not resuscitate status: advice from experienced nurses, Nursing Outlook 44, 114-119, 1996.

45. Cruzan v. Director, Missouri Department of Health, 497 US 261, 266, 11 S. Ct. 2841, 2845, 111 L. Ed. 2d 224 (1990).

46. Patient Self-Determination Act, 42 USCA, section 1395(a)(1)(Q).

47. Pope T: The mal-adaptation of Miranda to advance directives: a critique of the implementation of the patient self-determination act, Health Matrix 9:139, 1999.

48. Levinson W et al: Physician-patient communication: the relationship with malpractice claims among primary care physicians and surgeons, JAMA 277:533, 1997.

49. The SUPPORT Principal Investigators: A controlled trial to impede care for seriously ill hospitalized patients: the study to understand prognoses and preferences for outcomes and risks of treatment (SUPPORT), JAMA 274:1591, 1995.

50. Johnson SH: End of life decision making: what we don't know we make up; what we do know, we ignore, Indiana L Rev 31(13):44, 1998.

51. Johnson, SH: End of life decision making: what we don't know we make up; what we do

pulmonary resuscitation, Crit Care Med 28:3339-3340, 2000.

know, we ignore, Indiana L Rev 31(13):46-47, 1998.

52. Alexandra FM, Cist RD, Truog SE et al: Practical guidelines on the withdrawal of life-sustaining therapies, International Anesthesiology Clinics 39:87-90, 2001.

53. Joint Commission on Accreditation of Health Care Organizations: 1995 Manual for Hospitals 66, 1995.

54. Robert G: Unnecessary adversaries at the end of life: mediating end-of-life treatment disputes to prevent erosion of physician-patient relationship, Boston University Law Review 79:1091-1093, 1999.

55. Pozgar GD: Legal aspects of health care administration, ed 8, Gaithersburg, MD, 2002, Aspen.

56. When this author was invited to join a Veterans' Hospital ethics committee 12 years ago, her role was strictly that of the community member—not as a healthcare attorney.

57. Gatter R: Unnecessary adversaries at the end of life: mediating end of life treatment disputes to prevent erosion of physician patient relationship, 79 Boston University L Rev 1091 at 1118, 1999.

58. Wolf S: Ethics committees and due process: nesting rights in a community of caring, Md L Rev 50(798):844-849, 1991.

59. Annas G: Ethics committees: from ethical comfort to ethical cover, Hastings Center Report 21:18-21, 1999.

60. Fleetwood J, Unger SS: Institutional ethics committees and the shield of immunity, Ann Intern Med 120:320, 1994.

61. Wilson RF: Hospital ethics committees as the forum of last resort: an idea whose time has not come, North Carolina Law Review 76:353, 1998.

62. Wilson RF: Hospital ethics committees as the forum of last resort: an idea whose time has not come, North Carolina Law Review 76:394, 1998.

63. Dickerson DL: Are medical ethicists out of touch? practitioner attitudes in the US and UK towards decision at the end of life, J Med Ethics 26:254-260, 2000.

8

THE NERVOUS SYSTEM

The nervous system is affected not only by surgery carried out on it directly but also by regional anesthetics. Hence most patients in the postanesthesia care unit (PACU) are experiencing some alteration in central nervous system (CNS) function. Consequently, the perianesthesia nurse must have an understanding of some of the basic anatomic and physiologic principles that are operative in the CNS.

DEFINITIONS

Afferent: carrying sensory impulses toward the brain.
Autoregulation: an alteration in the diameter of the resistance vessels to maintain a constant perfusion pressure during changes in blood flow.
Cistern: a reservoir or cavity.
Commissure: white or gray matter that crosses over in the midline and connects one side of the brain or spinal cord with the other side.
Decussate: commonly refers to crossing of parts.
Dorsal: posterior.
Efferent: carrying motor impulses away from the brain.
Estrus: the cycle of changes in the female genital tract produced as a result of ovarian hormonal activity.
Inferior: beneath; also used to indicate the lower portion of an anatomic part.
Lower motor neurons: neurons of the spine and cranium that directly innervate the muscles (e.g., those found in the anterior horns or anterior roots of the gray matter of the spinal cord).
Metabolic regulation: a change in blood flow in response to the metabolic requirements of tissues.
Neuroglia: the supporting structure of nervous tissue, consisting of a fine web of tissue made up of modified ectodermal elements. It encloses branched cells known as neuroglia or glia cells but lacks nerve fibers itself. It performs less specialized functions of the nerve network.

Plexus: a network of nerves.
Postural reflexes: reflexes that are basically proprioceptive, being concerned with the position of the head in relation to the trunk and with adjustments of the extremities and eyes to the position of the head.
Proprioception: the awareness of posture, movement, and changes in equilibrium.
Ramus (rami): the primary division of a nerve.
Righting reflexes: reflexes that maintain the head in an upright position in relation to the environment, through use of the eyes, inner ears, and muscles of the neck and trunk.
Upper motor neurons: neurons in the brain and spinal cord that activate the motor system (e.g., the descending fibers of the pyramidal and extrapyramidal tracts).
Ventral: anterior.

CENTRAL NERVOUS SYSTEM

The CNS comprises the brain and spinal cord and is exceedingly complex, both anatomically and physiologically. None of the structures in the CNS function in an isolated manner. Neural activity at any level of the CNS always modifies or is modified by influences from other parts of the system. This accounts for the unique nature and extreme complexity of the CNS, much of which remains to be clearly understood.

The Brain

The human brain serves both structurally and functionally as the primary center for control and regulation of all nervous system functions. As such, it is the highest level of control and integration of sensory and motor information in the entire body.

The brain (encephalon) is divided into three large areas based on its embryonic development: (1) the forebrain (prosencephalon) contains the

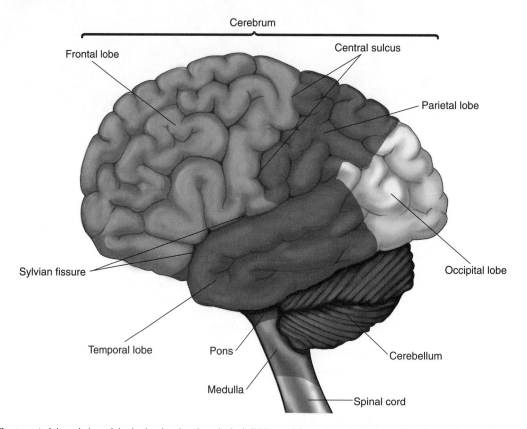

Fig. 8-1 Left lateral view of the brain, showing the principal divisions of the brain and the four major lobes of the cerebrum.

telencephalon (cerebrum) with its hemispheres; and the diencephalon; (2) the midbrain (mesencephalon) contains the cerebral peduncles, the corpora quadrigemina, and the cerebral aqueduct; and (3) the hindbrain (rhombencephalon) comprises the medulla oblongata, the pons, the cerebellum, and the fourth ventricle.

The Forebrain

The Telencephalon (Cerebrum)
The cerebrum is the largest part of the brain. It fills the entire upper portion of the cranial cavity and consists of billions of neurons that synapse to form a complex network of neural pathways.

The cerebrum consists of two hemispheres interconnected only by a large band of white fiber tracts known as the corpus callosum. Each hemi-

sphere is further subdivided into four lobes corresponding in name to the overlying bones of the cranium. These are the frontal, parietal, temporal, and occipital lobes (Fig. 8-1). Both hemispheres consist of an external cortex of gray matter, the underlying white matter tracts, and the basal ganglia (cerebral nuclei). Each hemisphere also contains a lateral ventricle, which is an elongated cavity concerned with the formation and circulation of cerebrospinal fluid (CSF).

The Cerebral Cortex
The cerebral cortex has an elaborate mantle of gray matter and is the most highly integrated area in the nervous system. It is arranged in a series of folds dipping down into the underlying regions. These folds greatly expand the surface area of the gray matter within the limited confines of the

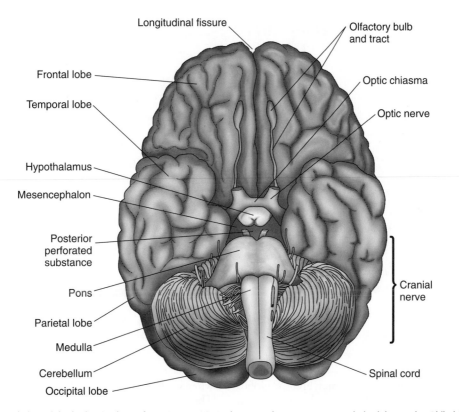

Fig. 8-2 Basal view of the brain. *(Redrawn from Guyton AC: Basic neuroscience: anatomy and physiology, ed 2, Philadelphia, 1991, WB Saunders.)*

skull. Each fold is known as a convolution or gyrus. Deeper grooves exist between these convolutions. A shallow one is known as a sulcus, whereas a deeper one is known as a fissure.

The cerebral hemispheres are separated from each other by the longitudinal fissure anteroposteriorly. The transverse fissure separates the cerebrum from the cerebellum beneath it.

Each hemisphere has three sulci between the lobes. The central sulcus (also known as the fissure of Rolando) separates the frontal and parietal lobes. The lateral sulcus (the fissure of Sylvius) lies between the frontal and parietal lobes above and the temporal lobe below. The small parietooccipital sulcus is located between its corresponding lobes (Fig. 8-2; see Fig. 8-1).

The white matter of the cerebrum is situated below the cortex and is composed of three main groups of myelinated nerve fibers arranged in related bundles or tracts. The commissural fibers transmit impulses between the hemispheres. The largest of these is the corpus callosum. The projection fibers ascend and descend to transmit impulses from one level of the CNS to another. A notable example is the internal capsule that surrounds most of the basal ganglia and connects the thalamus and the cerebral cortex. Finally, the association fibers disseminate impulses from one part of the cortex to another within the same hemisphere.

Basal Ganglia (Cerebral Nuclei)

A cerebral nucleus is a group of neuron cell bodies lying within the CNS. Four of these deep-lying masses of gray matter are located within the white matter of each hemisphere and are collectively known as the basal ganglia (Fig. 8-3). These are the caudate nucleus, the lentiform

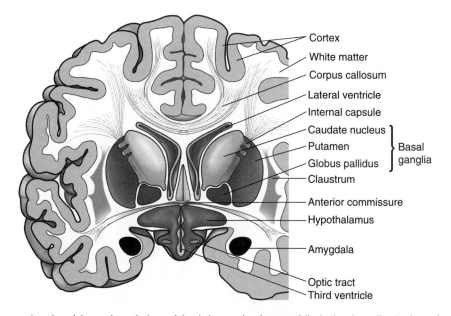

Fig. 8-3 A coronal section of the cerebrum in front of the thalamus, showing especially the basal ganglia. *(Redrawn from Guyton AC: Basic neuroscience: anatomy and physiology, ed 2, Philadelphia, 1991, WB Saunders.)*

nucleus (divided into the putamen and the globus pallidus), the amygdala, and the claustrum. Together, they exert a steadying influence on muscle activity. Along with that portion of the internal capsule that lies between them, the caudate and lentiform nuclei compose the corpus striatum, the most significant functional unit of the basal ganglia. The basal ganglia are an important part of the extrapyramidal motor pathway connecting nuclei with each other, with the cortex, and with the spinal cord. The ganglia also connect with areas in the hindbrain (the red nucleus and the substantia nigra) to assist in carrying out their role in smoothing and coordinating muscle movements. Disturbances in these ganglia result in tremor, rigidity, and loss of expressive and walking movements, as seen in Parkinson's syndrome.

Functional Aspects of the Cerebrum

Nearly every portion of the cerebral cortex is connected with subcortical centers, and no areas in the cortex are exclusively motor (expressive) or exclusively sensory (receptive) in nature. However, some regions are primarily concerned with the expressive phase of cortical functioning, whereas others are primarily receptive in nature. The activities of these areas are integrated by association fibers that compose the remainder of the cerebral cortex. Association fibers play important roles in complex intellectual and emotional processes.

Motor Areas

No single area of motor control exists within the brain because the integration and control of muscle activity depend on the harmonious activities of several areas, including the cerebral cortex, the basal ganglia, and the cerebellum.

Primary Motor Area.   The primary motor area of the cerebral cortex is located in the precentral gyrus of the frontal lobe, just anterior to the central sulcus, and is concerned mainly with the voluntary initiation of finely controlled movements, such as those of the hands, fingers, lips, tongue, and vocal cords. Skeletal muscles responsible for these discrete movements are largely represented by neurons in the motor cortex. Muscles of the arms, legs, and trunk are served by a comparatively small group of neurons, so that this part of the motor cortex controls

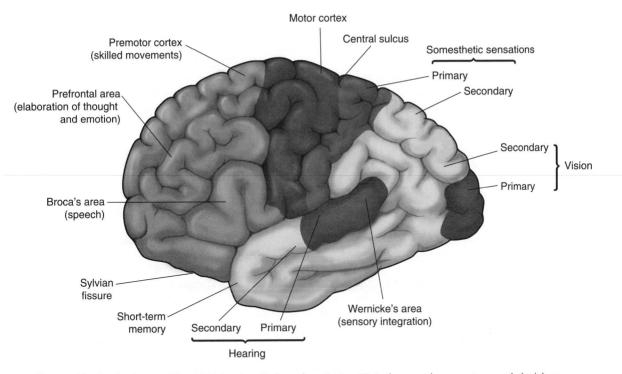

Fig. 8-4   The functional areas of the cerebral cortex. *(Redrawn from Guyton AC: Basic neuroscience: anatomy and physiology, ed 2, Philadelphia, 1991, WB Saunders.)*

larger groups of muscles and produces grosser movements (Fig. 8-4).

The axons of the pyramidal cell bodies in the primary motor area descend through the internal capsule, midbrain, and pons to the medulla, where most of them decussate, or cross, to the opposite side and continue down into the spinal cord, where they are known as the crossed pyramidal or lateral corticospinal tracts. Fibers that have not crossed are known as the uncrossed pyramidal or ventral corticospinal tracts. Most of these fibers eventually decussate at lower levels within the cord. Pyramidal cell axons also connect within the brain with the basal ganglia, the brainstem, and the cerebellum. All of the complex connections of the pyramidal cells play important roles in the overall coordination and control of skeletal muscle activity.

Premotor Area.   The premotor area of each hemisphere is located in the cortex immediately anterior to the precentral gyrus in the frontal lobe. On the whole, it is concerned with move-ment of the opposite side of the body, especially with control and coordination of skilled move-ments of a complex nature. In addition to its sub-cortical connections with the primary motor area, its neurons also have direct connections with the basal ganglia and related nuclei in the brainstem—for example, the reticular formation. Many of the axons from these subcortical centers cross to the opposite side before descending as extrapyramidal tracts in the spinal cord. Collec-tively, the connections from the premotor area to these related nuclei make up the extrapyramidal system, which coordinates gross skeletal muscle activities that are largely automatic in nature. Examples are postural adjustments, chewing, swallowing, gesticulating, and associated move-ments that accompany voluntary activities. Certain portions of the extrapyramidal tract also have an inhibitory effect on spontaneous move-ments initiated by the cerebral cortex. They serve to prevent tremors and rigidity. Complete struc-tural and functional separation of the pyramidal and extrapyramidal systems is impossible, because they are so closely connected in the harmonious work of executing complex coordinated movements (see Fig. 8-3).

Of interest to the PACU nurse is that drugs used to produce neuroleptanesthesia may cause extrapyramidal reactions. More specifically, the neuroleptics such as the phenothiazines, of which chlorpromazine (Thorazine) is the prototypal drug, and the butyrophenones, as typified by droperidol (Inapsine) and haloperidol (Haldol), are known to produce extrapyramidal reactions. Four types of extrapyramidal reaction exist: drug-induced parkinsonism, akathisia, acute dystonic reactions, and tardive dyskinesia.

Drug-induced parkinsonism, which can occur from 1 to 5 days after the administration of the neuroleptic drug, is typified by a generalized slowing of automatic and spontaneous movements (bradykinesia), with a masklike facial expression and a reduction in arm movements. The most noticeable signs of the drug-induced parkinsonism syndrome are rigidity and oscillatory tremor at rest. Treatment is with antiparkinsonian agents such as levodopa (Larodopa), trihexyphenidyl (Artane), and benztropine (Cogentin).

Akathisia, which can occur 5 to 60 days after the administration of a neuroleptic drug, is a term that refers to a subjective feeling of restlessness accompanied by a need on the part of the patient to move about and to pace back and forth. Treatment requires a reduction in the dosage of the responsible drug.

Acute dystonic reactions may occur after the administration of some psychotropic drugs and are characterized by torsion spasms such as facial grimacing and torticollis. These reactions are occasionally seen when a phenothiazine is first administered and are associated with oculogyric crises. Acute dystonic reactions may be mistaken for hysterical reactions or seizures and may usually be reversed by anticholinergic antiparkinsonian drugs such as benztropine or trihexyphenidyl.

Tardive dyskinesia is a late-appearing neurologic syndrome that is characterized by stereotypic, involuntary, rapid, and rhythmically repetitive movements, such as continual chewing movements and darting movements of the tongue. Treatment is not always satisfactory, because antiparkinsonian drugs sometimes exacerbate tardive dyskinesia. Tardive dyskinesia often persists despite discontinuation of the responsible drug.

Two important structural aspects of the premotor area are worth noting for those caring for neurosurgical patients. First, the fibers from both the primary motor and the premotor areas are funneled through the narrow internal capsule as they descend to lower areas of the CNS. This is significant because the internal capsule is a common site of cerebrovascular accidents. Second, lesions within one side of the internal capsule result in paralysis of the skeletal muscles on the opposite side of the body because of the crossing of fibers within the medulla.

Motor Speech Area. This area is only one point in the complicated network required to form spoken and written words. It lies at the base of the motor area and slightly anterior to it in the inferior frontal gyrus and is also known as Broca's area (see Fig. 8-4). In right-handed people (the majority of the population), the language and speech areas are usually located in the left hemisphere. In those who are left-handed, these areas may lie within the right or the left hemisphere.

Prefrontal Area. This area of the frontal lobe lies anterior to the premotor area. It has extensive connections with other cortical areas and is believed to play an important role in complex intellectual activities—such as mathematic and philosophic reasoning; abstract and creative thinking; learning; judgment and volition; and social, moral, and ethical values. The prefrontal area also influences certain autonomic functions of the body through the conduction of impulses directly or indirectly through the thalamus to the hypothalamus, which makes possible certain physiologic responses to feelings such as anger, fear, and lust.

Sensory Areas

Sensory information from one side of the body is received by the general sensory (or somesthetic) area of the opposite hemisphere. It is located in the parietal lobe in the area of the postcentral gyrus. Crude sensations of pain, temperature, and touch can be experienced at the level of the thalamus, but true discrimination of these sensations is a function of the parietal cortex. The activities of the general sensory area allow for propriocep-

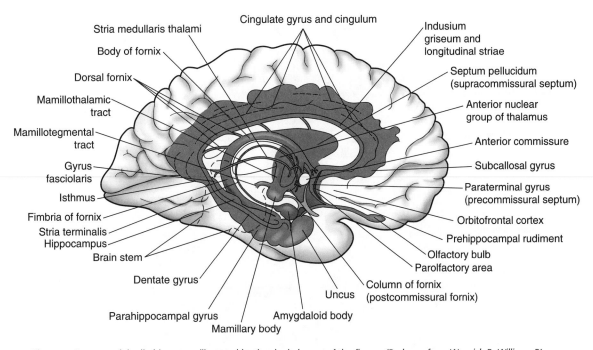

Fig. 8-5 Anatomy of the limbic system illustrated by the shaded areas of the figure. *(Redrawn from Warwick R, Williams PL: Gray's anatomy, ed 35, Philadelphia, 1973, WB Saunders.)*

tion; for the recognition of the size, shape, and texture of objects; and for the comparison of stimuli as to intensity and location.

The auditory area lies in the cortex of the superior temporal lobe. Each hemisphere receives impulses from both ears. The visual area is located in the posterior occipital lobe, where extremely complex transformations in the signals conveyed by the optic nerve occur. The right occipital cortex receives impulses from the right half of each eye, and the left occipital cortex receives impulses from the left half of each eye. The olfactory area (sense of smell) is believed to be located in the medial temporal lobe and that the gustatory area (sense of taste) is located nearby at the base of the postcentral gyrus.

Association Areas

Large areas of the cortex for which no discrete function is known remain. They are called association areas. They play a major role in the integration of the sensory and motor phases of cortical function by providing complex connections between them.

Limbic System

The principal structural and functional units of the limbic system are the two rings of limbic cortex and a number of related subcortical nuclei, the anterior thalamic nuclei, and portions of the basal nuclei (Fig. 8-5). The terms limbic system, limbic lobe, and rhinencephalon are often used interchangeably. In general, the limbic system is concerned with a wide variety of autonomic somatosensory and somatomotor responses, especially those involved with emotional states and other behavioral responses. Within the limbic system, the benzodiazepine and opiate receptors have been identified (see Chapters 19 and 20).

The limbic system, which acts in close concert with the hypothalamus, can evoke a variety of autonomic responses, including changes in heart rate, blood pressure, and respiratory rate. It plays an intimate role in the genesis of emotional states—particularly anxiety, fear, and aggression. Stimulation of the limbic system also evokes complex motor responses directly related to feeding behavior. The limbic system has been

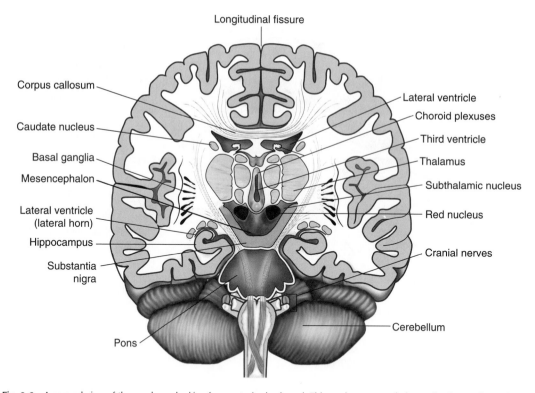

Fig. 8-6 A coronal view of the cerebrum looking from anterior backward. This section was made immediately anterior to the lower brainstem and through the middle of the thalamus. *(Redrawn from Guyton AC: Basic neuroscience: anatomy and physiology, ed 2, Philadelphia, 1991, WB Saunders.)*

demonstrated to have major relationships with the reticular formation of the brainstem and is presumed to have a role in the alerting or arousal process. It is also implicated in the hypothalamic regulation of pituitary activity. It may be associated somehow with the memory process for recent events as well. In addition, it is intimately concerned with complex phenomena such as the control of various biologic rhythms, sexual behavior, and motivation.

The Diencephalon

The second major division of the forebrain is the diencephalon (Fig. 8-6). It consists of the thalamus, the epithalamus, the subthalamus, and the hypothalamus. The diencephalon also contains the third ventricle and is almost completely covered by the cerebral hemispheres. This portion of the brain has a primary role in sleep, emotion, thermoregulation, autonomic activity, and endocrine control of ongoing behavioral patterns.

The thalamus consists of right and left egg-shaped masses, which make up the greatest bulk of the diencephalon and form the lateral wall of the third ventricle. Each thalamus serves as a relay center for all incoming sensory stimuli except taste and smell. These impulses are then grouped and transmitted to the appropriate area of the cerebral cortex. Because of its interconnections with the hypothalamus, the limbic system, and the frontal, temporal, and parietal lobes, this structure is also integrally involved with emotional activities, instinctive responses, and attentive processes.

The epithalamus contains the pineal body (or gland), which is known to secrete melatonin. Melatonin inhibits gonadal development and regulates estrus. Its most important function is to slow maturation. It is believed that melatonin has its greatest effect on brain tissue rather than on the gonads themselves.

Situated below the thalamus and above the midbrain, the subthalamus serves as a correlation center for the optic and vestibular impulses. Stimulation of centers in or around the subthalamic nuclei produce the excitation of appropriate patterns of action in the brainstem and spinal cord, which results in rhythmic motions of forward progression necessary in the act of walking. Damage to the subthalamic nuclei on one side is known to cause violent involuntary movements on the limbs of the opposite side of the body. These movements are brought about by contractions of their proximal muscles.

The hypothalamus is a group of bilateral nuclei that forms the floor and part of the lateral walls of the third ventricle. Extremely complex in function, it has extensive connections with the autonomic nervous system as well as with other parts of the CNS. It also influences the endocrine system by virtue of direct and indirect connections with the pituitary gland and the release of its own hormones. In association with these other structures, it participates in the regulation of appetite, water balance, carbohydrate and fat metabolism, growth, sexual maturity, body temperature, pulse rate, blood pressure, sleep, and aspects of emotional behavior. Because of the connection of the hypothalamus with the thalamus and cerebral cortex, it is possible for emotions to influence visceral responses on certain occasions.

The Midbrain

The midbrain, or mesencephalon, is a short, narrow segment of nervous tissue connecting the forebrain with the hindbrain (Fig. 8-7). The midbrain is vital as a conduction pathway and as a reflex control center. Passing through the center of the midbrain is the cerebral aqueduct, a narrow canal that serves to connect the third ventricle of the diencephalon with the fourth ventricle of the hindbrain for the circulation of CSF.

The cerebral peduncles are located in the anterior portion of the midbrain and consist of multiple projection fibers that connect the cerebral cortex with other structures in the brainstem. Their dorsal aspect (the tegmentum) contains the motor nuclei of the oculomotor, trigeminal, and trochlear nerves. The ventral

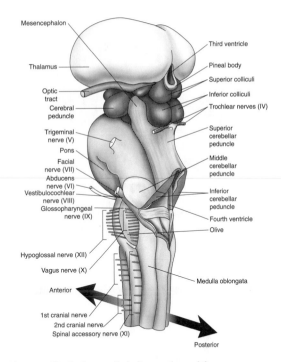

Fig. 8-7 The brainstem, including portions of the diencephalon, the midbrain, and the hindbrain. *(Redrawn from Guyton AC: Basic neuroscience: anatomy and physiology, ed 2, Philadelphia, 1991, WB Saunders.)*

aspect contains the red nucleus, a part of the reticular formation, and the origin of a portion of the extrapyramidal system.

The corpora quadrigemina is a group of cells divided in the midline and transversely to form four distinct areas, or colliculi. The inferior colliculi are vital components of the auditory pathway and are responsible for complex acoustic reflexes. The superior colliculi are optic reflex centers.

The centers for postural and righting reflexes are found in the midbrain. The dorsal, or posterior, portion of the midbrain is concerned with visual and auditory reflexes, such as movement of the eyes in accordance with changes in head position, the pupillary light reflex, and turning the head in the direction of a noise. Key structures of the reticular formation also originate in this area. Also, cranial nerves III (oculomotor) and IV (trochlear) originate in the ventral aspect of the midbrain.

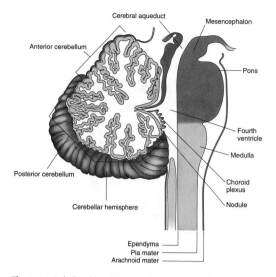

Cerebral aqueduct

Mesencephalon

Anterior cerebellum

Pons

Fourth ventricle

Medulla

Posterior cerebellum

Choroid plexus

Cerebellar hemisphere

Nodule

Ependyma
Pia mater
Arachnoid mater

Fig. 8-8 Relationship of the cerebellum to the brainstem. *(Redrawn from Guyton AC: Basic neuroscience: anatomy and physiology, ed 2, Philadelphia, 1991, WB Saunders.)*

The Hindbrain. The hindbrain, or rhombencephalon, consists of the pons, the medulla oblongata, the cerebellum, and the fourth ventricle (Fig. 8-8).

The Pons

Lying in front of the fourth ventricle and separating it from the cerebellum, the pons is literally the bridge between the midbrain and the medulla oblongata. It receives many ascending and descending fibers en route to other points in the CNS. It also contains the motor and sensory nuclei of cranial nerves V (trigeminal), VI (abducens), VII (facial), and VIII (acoustic). The pontine nuclei of the pons are composed of gray matter. White fiber tracts connect the medulla below with the cerebrum above. These are the so-called corticospinal tracts. White fiber (corticobulbar) tracts also connect the cerebellum with the pons. The roof of the pons contains a portion of the reticular formation, and the lower pons assists in the regulation of respiration.

The Medulla Oblongata

The medulla oblongata is an expanded continuation of the spinal cord and is located between the foramen magnum and the pons. It is anatomically complex and not usually amenable to surgery. Many of the white fiber tracts between the brain and spinal cord decussate as they pass through the medulla. Centers for many complex reflexes are located in the medulla oblongata and include those for swallowing, vomiting, coughing, and sneezing. The originating nuclei of cranial nerves IX (glossopharyngeal), X (vagus), XI (accessory), and XII (hypoglossal) are found in the medulla oblongata (Table 8-1; see Fig. 8-7). Because of this, the medulla plays an essential role in the regulation of cardiac, respiratory, and vasomotor reflexes. Injuries to the medulla, such as those accompanying basal skull fracture, often prove fatal.

The Cerebellum

Comprising two hemispheres and a constricted central portion, the cerebellum overlaps the pons and the medulla oblongata dorsally and is located just below the occipital lobes of the cerebrum. It is separated from the cerebrum by the tentorium above it and has a bilayered cortex composed of gray matter. Beneath the gray matter are white fiber tracts that extend like branches of a tree to all parts of the cortex. Deep within the white matter are masses of gray matter called the cerebellar nuclei. These connect the cerebellar hemispheres with each other and with areas in the cerebrum, the hindbrain, and the spinal cord.

The cerebellum has no sensory function and does not initiate movement as the cerebrum does. Functionally, it does coordinate muscle tone and voluntary movements through important connections via the spinal cord with the proprioceptor endings in skeletal muscles, tendons, and joints. In addition, the cerebellum is involved in reflexes necessary for the maintenance of equilibrium and posture, through its connections with the vestibular apparatus of the inner ear. The cerebellum also receives optic and acoustic information, but the anatomic pathways involved have not yet been discerned.

Damage to the cerebellum does not result in paralysis or sensory loss. The outcome of damage depends on which portion of the structure is involved. Damage to one part may result in loss of balance, nystagmus, and a reeling gait (cerebellar ataxia). Damage to another area may cause disturbances in the postural reflexes. Posterior lobe disturbances result in changes in voluntary movements such as discrepancies in force,

Table 8-1 Cranial Nerves and Their Functions

Number	Name	Type	Function
I	Olfactory	Sensory	Smell
II	Optic	Sensory	Vision
III	Oculomotor	Mixed—mainly motor	Motion of eye up, in, and down Raising of eyelid Constriction of pupil Accommodation of pupil to distance Proprioceptive impulses
IV	Trochlear	Mixed—mainly motor	Motion of eye down Proprioceptive impulses

V	Trigeminal:
	  Ophthalmic branch
	  Maxillary branch
	  Mandibular branch
		Mixed	Motor: muscles of mastication
			Sensory: face, nose, mouth
			Proprioceptive impulses from teeth sockets and jaw muscles

VI	Abducens	Mixed—mainly motor	Outward motion of eye Proprioception from eye muscles
VII	Facial	Mixed—mostly motor; some sensory and autonomic	Motor: movement of facial muscles, ear, nose, and neck Sensory: taste, anterior two thirds of tongue Autonomic: secretion of saliva, tears

VIII	Acoustic:
	  Cochlear branch
	  Vestibular branch
		Sensory	Cochlear: hearing
			Vestibular: maintenance of equilibrium and posturing of head

IX	Glossopharyngeal	Mixed—motor, sensory, and autonomic	Motor: muscles of swallowing Sensory: taste, posterior third of tongue; sensation from pharynx Autonomic: impulses to parotid glands; decrease blood pressure and pulse
X	Vagus	Mixed—motor, sensory, and autonomic	Motor, sensory, and autonomic: information to and from larynx, pharynx, trachea, esophagus, heart, and abdominal viscera
XI	Spinal accessory	Mixed—mostly motor	Cranial portion: motor and sensory information to and from voluntary muscles of pharynx, larynx, and palate (swallowing) Spinal portion: motor information to sternocleidomastoid and trapezius muscles May form components of cardiac branches of vagus
XII	Hypoglossal	Mixed—mostly motor	Motor and sensory information to/from tongue muscles Position sense

direction, and range of movements, lack of precision in movements, and, possibly, intention tremors.

The Fourth Ventricle

The fourth ventricle is a diamond-shaped space located between the cerebellum posteriorly and the pons and medulla oblongata anteriorly; it contains CSF.

The Brainstem

Authors disagree to some extent as to what structures collectively constitute the brainstem. All agree that it includes the midbrain, the pons, and the medulla oblongata. Some believe that the diencephalon rightly belongs in the group also. Whichever grouping is used, all functions of each structure within it may be considered to be basic activities of the brainstem. All of the cranial nerves are attached to the brainstem (if the diencephalon is included), with the exception of the olfactory nerve and the spinal portion of the accessory nerve.

The Reticular Formation

The reticular formation lies within the brainstem (including the diencephalon). An important function of the reticular formation is its action as an intermediary between the upper and lower motor neurons of the extrapyramidal system. In this way it facilitates or augments reflex activity as well as voluntary movements. Its motor neurons can be excitatory or inhibitory in action. For example, by inhibiting extensor muscles, it facilitates the action of flexor muscles.

Every pathway that carries information to the brain also contributes afferent fibers to the reticular formation, so that it is kept well informed about conditions of both the outside world and the internal organs. Efferent impulses that leave the reticular formation travel to the cerebral cortex and to the spinal cord. By virtue of its location in and connections with the brainstem and diencephalon, it participates integrally in their activities.

Another important function of the reticular formation is the activation and regulation of those brain activities related to attention-arousal and consciousness. For this reason, it is often called the reticular activating system (RAS).

Damage to the reticular formation results in greatly decreased levels of consciousness. When the cerebral cortex is isolated from the RAS by disease or injury of the upper portion of the midbrain, decerebrate rigidity occurs. This abnormal posturing results from the dominant effect of the extensor muscles and a lack of inhibition from opposing motor neurons and flexor muscles. This rigidity is accompanied by a profoundly reduced level of consciousness.

Protection of the Brain

The brain is protected by the cranial bones, the meninges, and the CSF (Figs. 8-9 and 8-10).

The Cranial Bones

Eight cranial bones encase the brain, supporting it and protecting it from most ordinary bumps and jarring. In the adult, immovable fibrous joints, or sutures, fuse these bones together to form the rigid walls of the box known as the cranium. The base of the cranium is both thicker and stronger than its roof or walls.

The bones of the cranium are the frontal, right and left parietal, occipital, sphenoid, ethmoid, and right and left temporal bones. The frontal bone forms the anterior roof of the skull and the forehead. Within the frontal bone are the frontal sinuses, which communicate with the nasal cavities. The parietal bones form much of the top and sides of the cranium. The occipital bone forms the back and a large portion of the base of the skull. The two temporal bones are complicated and form part of the sides and a part of the base of the skull. Their inner surfaces are not as smooth and regular as the bones previously mentioned. Parts of the temporal bones articulate with the condyles of the lower jaw, and air cells in the mastoid portions of the temporal bones communicate with the middle ear. The sphenoid bone occupies a central portion of the floor of the skull. It alone articulates with each of the other cranial bones. Its middle portion contains the sphenoid sinuses, which open into the nasal cavity. The upper portion of the sphenoid bone has a marked saddlelike depression, the sella turcica, which holds the pituitary gland. The ethmoid bone is light and has a spongy structure. It is located between the orbital cavities. It is a cribriform plate that forms the roof of the nasal cavity and part of the base of the cranium. The ethmoid sinuses open into the nasal cavities.

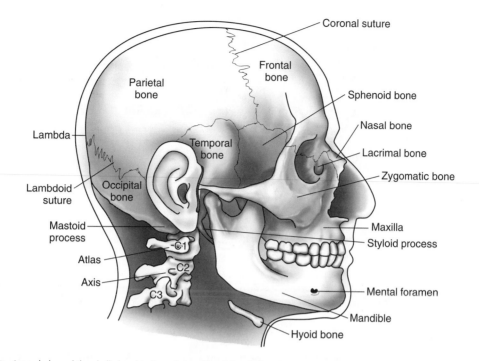

Fig. 8-9 Lateral view of the skull showing the relationship of the skull and cervical vertebrae to the face.

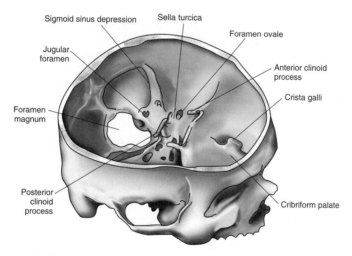

Fig. 8-10 Interior of the cranial cavity.

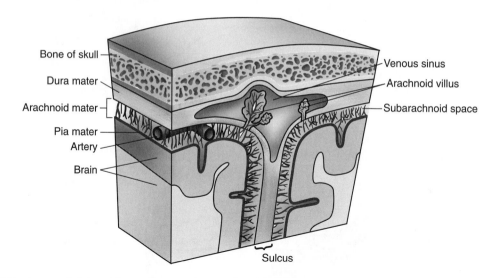

Fig. 8-11 An expanded view of the meninges covering a section of the brain. Note also the venous sinus with arachnoid villi protruding into it. *(Redrawn from Guyton AC: Basic neuroscience: anatomy and physiology, ed 2, Philadelphia, 1991, WB Saunders.)*

Several features of the cranial bones are particularly noteworthy for the PACU nurse. Among these is the fact that the air cells in the mastoid portion of the temporal bone may become infected secondary to otitis media or following surgery on the middle or inner ear. This mastoiditis may cause severe complications if it extends through the thin plate of bone that separates it from the cranial meninges. Another point of interest is that surgical access to the pituitary gland is commonly accomplished through the sphenoid bone via the nostrils; one example is transsphenoidal hypophysectomy. Finally, nasal suctioning is absolutely contraindicated in the cranial surgery patient because of the danger of perforating the cribriform plate of the ethmoid bone, which would result in leakage of CSF and would permit direct access to the brain by infectious organisms.

One main opening is located at the base of the skull and is called the foramen magnum. It marks the point at which the brainstem changes structure and becomes identified inferiorly as the spinal cord. Many smaller openings in the skull allow the cranial nerves and some blood vessels to pass through it to and from the face, the jaw, and the neck. The atlas of the vertebral column (the first cervical vertebra) supports the skull and forms a moveable joint with the occipital bone.

The Meninges

The meninges (Fig. 8-11) are three fibrous membranes between the skull and the brain and between the vertebral column and the spinal cord. The outer membrane is the dura mater; the inner one is the pia mater; and between them lies the arachnoid mater.

The Dura Mater. The dura mater is a shiny, tough, inelastic membrane that envelops and supports the brain and spinal cord and, by various folds, separates parts of the brain into adjoining compartments. The portion within the skull differs from the dura of the spinal cord in three ways. First, the cranial dura is firmly attached to the skull. The spinal dura has no attachment to the vertebrae. Second, the cranial dura consists of two layers; it not only covers the brain (meningeal dura) but also lines the interior of the skull bones (periosteal dura). Third, the two layers of the cranial dura are in contact with each other in some places but separate in others where the inner layer dips inward to form the protective partitions between parts of the brain. Also, the spaces or channels formed by these separations of dural layers are filled with venous blood that is leaving the brain and are called cranial venous

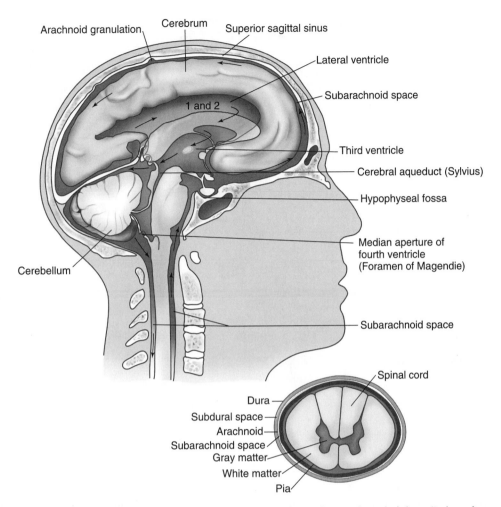

Fig. 8-12 Circulation of cerebrospinal fluid in the brain and the spinal cord. Note the superior sagittal sinus. *(Redrawn from Jacob SW, Francone CA, Lossow WJ: Structure and function in man, ed 5, Philadelphia, 1982, WB Saunders.)*

sinuses, an elaborate network unique to the brain (Fig. 8-12; see Fig. 8-11).

Three major partitioning folds of the meningeal dura exist. The falx cerebri separates the right and left hemispheres of the cerebrum. The tentorium cerebelli supports and separates the occipital lobes of the cerebrum from the cerebellum. The falx cerebelli separates the two cerebellar hemispheres. The tentorium separates the posterior cranial chamber from the remainder of the cranial cavity and serves as a line of demarcation for describing the site of a surgical procedure or a lesion as either supratentorial or infratentorial.

Encased between the two dural layers are two major groups of venous channels that drain blood from the brain. None of these vascular channels possesses valves, and their walls are extremely thin because of the absence of muscular tissue. The superior-posterior group consists of one paired and four unpaired sinuses. The anterior-inferior group consists of four paired sinuses and one plexus. The sinuses function to drain venous blood into the internal jugular veins, which are

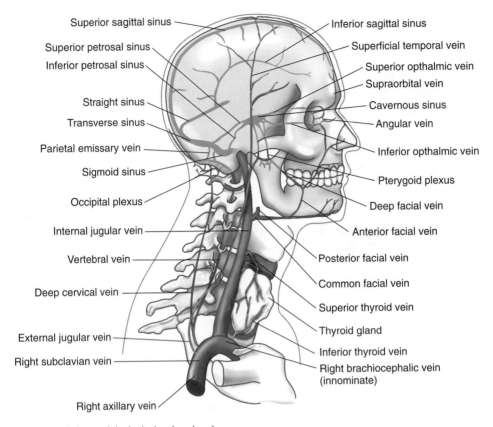

Superior sagittal sinus

Superior petrosal sinus

Inferior petrosal sinus

Straight sinus

Transverse sinus

Parietal emissary vein

Sigmoid sinus

Occipital plexus

Internal jugular vein

Vertebral vein

Deep cervical vein

External jugular vein

Right subclavian vein

Right axillary vein

Inferior sagittal sinus

Superficial temporal vein

Superior opthalmic vein

Supraorbital vein

Cavernous sinus

Angular vein

Inferior opthalmic vein

Pterygoid plexus

Deep facial vein

Anterior facial vein

Posterior facial vein

Common facial vein

Superior thyroid vein

Thyroid gland

Inferior thyroid vein

Right brachiocephalic vein
(innominate)

Fig. 8-13   Venous drainage of the brain, head, and neck.

the principal vessels responsible for the return of the blood from the brain to the heart (Fig. 8-13).

The Arachnoid.   The arachnoid is a fine membrane between the dura mater and the pia mater. Between the arachnoid and the dura is the subdural space, a noncommunicating space filled with CSF. The cerebral blood vessels traversing this space have little supporting structure, thus making them particularly vulnerable to insult at this point.

The arachnoid forms a type of roof over the pia mater, to which it is joined by a network of trabeculae in the subarachnoid space. It does not follow the depressions of the surface architecture. The arachnoid sends small, tuftlike extensions through the meningeal layer of the dura into the cranial venous sinuses. These are called the arachnoid granulations or arachnoid villi. The arachnoid villi serve as a pathway for the return of CSF to the venous blood system. Subarachnoid CSF is most abundant in the grooves between the gyri, particularly at the base of the brain, where the more freely communicating compartments form six subarachnoid cisternae, or reservoirs.

The Pia Mater.   The inner layer of the meninges, the pia mater, is a fine membrane rich in blood (choroid) plexuses and mesothelial cells. It is closely associated with the arachnoid and covers the brain intimately, following the invaginations and convolutions of the brain surface. The veins of the brain lie between threadlike trabeculae in the subarachnoid space. Branches of the cortical arteries in the subarachnoid space are carried with the pia mater and enter the brain substance itself (Fig. 8-14).

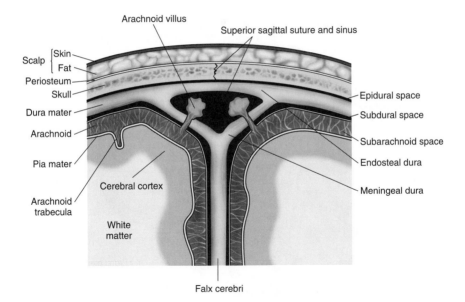

Fig. 8-14 Coronal section of the skull, brain, meninges, and superior sagittal sinus. *(Redrawn from Jacob SW, Francone CA, Lossow WJ: Structure and function in man, ed 5, Philadelphia, 1982, WB Saunders.)*

The Cerebrospinal Fluid System

The CSF is a clear, colorless, watery fluid with a specific gravity of 1.007. A principal function of this fluid is to act as a cushion for the brain. Because both brain tissue and CSF have essentially the same specific gravity, the brain literally floats within the skull. CSF also serves as a medium for the exchange of nutrients and waste products between the blood stream and the cells of the CNS.

CSF is found within the ventricles of the brain, in the cisterns surrounding it, and in the subarachnoid spaces of both the brain and the spinal cord (Figs. 8-15 and 8-16). Largest of the cisterns is the cisterna magna, which is located beneath and behind the cerebellum.

Although some CSF is formed by filtration through capillary walls throughout the brain's vascular bed, its primary site of formation is in the choroid plexuses within the ventricles. This is achieved by a system of secretion and diffusion. The choroid plexuses are highly vascular, tufted structures composed of many small granular pouches that project into the ventricles of the brain. CSF is formed continuously and is reabsorbed at a rate of approximately 750 ml per day.

The net pressure of the CSF is regulated in part by a balance between formation and reabsorption.

The four ventricles of the brain communicate directly with each other. The first and second (lateral) ventricles are elongated cavities that lie within the cerebral hemispheres. The third ventricle is a slitlike cavity beneath and between the two lateral ventricles. The fourth ventricle is a diamond-shaped space between the cerebellum posteriorly and the pons and medulla oblongata anteriorly.

The circulation of CSF is as follows. Each lateral ventricle contains a large choroid plexus that forms CSF. From the lateral ventricles, the fluid passes through an interventricular foramen (foramen of Monro) into the third ventricle. Together with the additional fluid formed there, the CSF travels posteriorly through the cerebral aqueduct (aqueduct of Sylvius) into the fourth ventricle, where more fluid is produced. The combined CSF volumes then pass through three openings leading from the fourth ventricle to the cranial subarachnoid space of the cisterna magna. These openings are the two lateral foramina of Luschka and the medial foramen of Magendie.

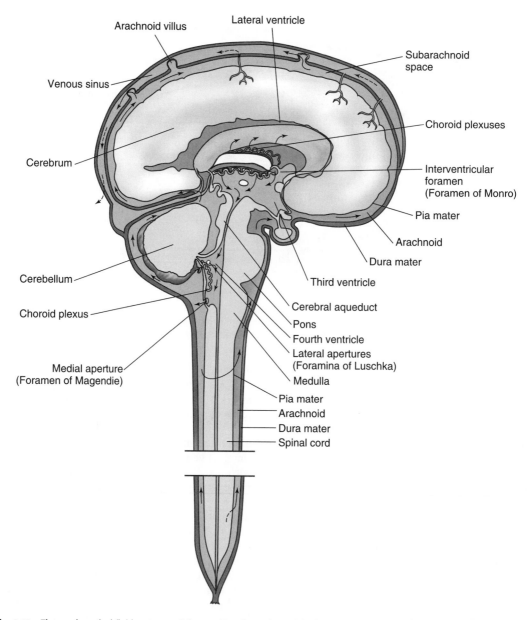

Fig. 8-15 The cerebrospinal fluid system and the meningeal coverings of the brain and spinal cord. Note the directions of flow of cerebrospinal fluid indicated by the arrows. *(Redrawn from Guyton AC: Basic neuroscience: anatomy and physiology, ed 2, Philadelphia, 1991, WB Saunders.)*

From the cisterna magna, CSF flows freely within the entire subarachnoid space of the brain and spinal cord.

The main route of reabsorption of excess CSF is through the arachnoid villi that project from the subarachnoid spaces into the venous sinuses of the brain, particularly those of the superior sagittal sinus. The arachnoid villi provide highly permeable regions that allow free passage of CSF, including protein molecules and some small par-

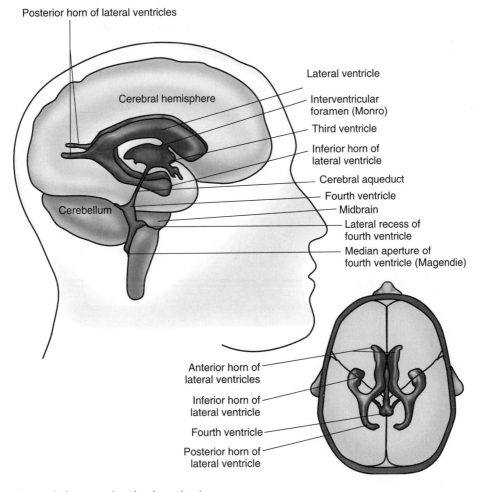

Posterior horn of lateral ventricles

Lateral ventricle

Cerebral hemisphere

Interventricular foramen (Monro)

Third ventricle

Inferior horn of lateral ventricle

Cerebral aqueduct

Fourth ventricle

Midbrain

Cerebellum

Lateral recess of fourth ventricle

Median aperture of fourth ventricle (Magendie)

Anterior horn of lateral ventricles

Inferior horn of lateral ventricle

Fourth ventricle

Posterior horn of lateral ventricle

Fig. 8-16   The ventricular system, lateral and superior views.

ticulate matter contained within it. The process of osmosis is believed to be mainly responsible for the reabsorption of the fluid.

Blood-Brain and Blood-CSF Barriers of the CNS

Throughout the body, the constancy of the composition of the extracellular fluid is maintained by multiple homeostatic mechanisms. Because of the exquisite sensitivity of the neurons in the CNS, additional mechanisms are necessary to prevent the far-reaching consequences that even minor fluctuations in their chemical environment would cause. In health, the unique blood-brain and blood-CSF barriers present in most regions of the CNS have evolved to accomplish this task. The development of the blood-brain barrier occurs gradually during the first several years of childhood.

The site of the blood-brain barrier is not at the surface of the neurons themselves. Rather, it is located between the plasma within the capillaries and the extracellular space of the brain. The exchange of many physiologically important substances within the capillaries of the CNS is generally believed to be slowed or practically prohibited by several anatomic factors rather than by any single factor alone. These structures likely also form a sequence of morphologic barriers acting in concert to prevent the rapid transport of substances from the blood to the nervous tissue. These include the tight intercellular junctions between the epithelial cells of the capillaries that appear to effectively reduce permeability. A substantial basement membrane surrounds the capillaries, and an external membrane is provided by the end-feet of the astrocytes between the neurons and the capillaries. These appear to have a major role in retarding or preventing the passage of foreign substances into the brain tissue.

Despite the uncertainty as to the ultimate site of the blood-brain barrier, it has been firmly established that the rapidity with which substances penetrate brain tissue is inversely related to their molecular size and directly related to their lipid solubility. Only water, carbon dioxide, and oxygen cross the blood-brain barrier rapidly and readily, whereas glucose crosses more slowly and by a facilitated transport mechanism. Water-soluble compounds, electrolytes, and protein molecules generally cross slowly. Most general anesthetics effectively cross the blood-brain barrier because of their high lipid solubility.

Of critical clinical importance is the fact that the effectiveness of the blocking mechanism of the blood-brain barrier may break down in areas of the brain that are infected, traumatized, or irradiated or that contain tumors. As effective as the blood-brain barrier is, no substance is completely excluded from reaching the central neurons. Instead, the rate of transport of substances through the barrier is of major significance in maintaining the constancy of the internal environment of the brain.

A limited number of structures in the brain have unique capillaries and are not restricted by the blood-brain barrier. These organs appear to function as chemoreceptors and as such must be in intimate contact with the chemical substances within the blood. The posterior pituitary gland is one of these structures. The blood-CSF barrier is located at the choroid plexus. As in the case of the blood-brain barrier, the rate of transport of substances across the blood-CSF barrier is controlled by molecular size and lipid solubility.

The routes whereby substances leave the CSF are different from those by which they enter.

They may leave rapidly via the arachnoid villi, regardless of their molecular size or lipid solubility. Alternatively, the bulk circulation of the CSF throughout the brain enhances the direct removal of certain lipid-soluble substances across the blood-brain barrier.

Arterial Blood Supply to the Brain

The entire arterial blood supply to the brain, with the exception of a small amount that flows in the anterior spinal artery to the medulla, is carried through the neck by four vessels: the two vertebral arteries and the two carotid arteries (Figs. 8-17 and 8-18).

The two vertebral arteries supply the posterior portion of the brain. They ascend in the neck through the transverse foramina on each side of the cervical vertebrae, enter the skull through the foramen magnum, and anastomose near the pons to form the basilar artery of the hindbrain. A relatively small volume of the total blood flow to the brain is carried by the vertebral or basilar artery. The circle of Willis, in turn, is formed by the union of the basilar artery and the two internal carotid arteries. Before they join the circle of Willis, these arteries send essential branches to the brainstem, cerebellum, and falx cerebelli.

The circle of Willis is a ring of blood vessels that surrounds the optic chiasm and the pituitary stalk. Three pairs of large arterial vessels that supply the cerebral cortex originate from the circle of Willis: the anterior, the middle, and the posterior cerebral arteries. Each pair of arteries supplies specific areas of the brain: (1) the anterior cerebral arteries supply about half of the frontal and parietal lobes, including much of the corpus callosum; (2) the middle cerebral arteries perfuse most of the lateral surfaces of the hemispheres and send off branches to the corpus striatum and the internal capsule; and (3) the posterior cerebral arteries supply the occipital lobes and the remaining portions of the temporal lobes that are not supplied by the middle cerebral arteries.

Regulation of Cerebral Blood Flow

The CNS has a complex and structurally diverse system to facilitate appropriate cerebral blood flow. With the advent of positron emission tomography (PET) and magnetic resonance imaging (MRI), studies are being conducted

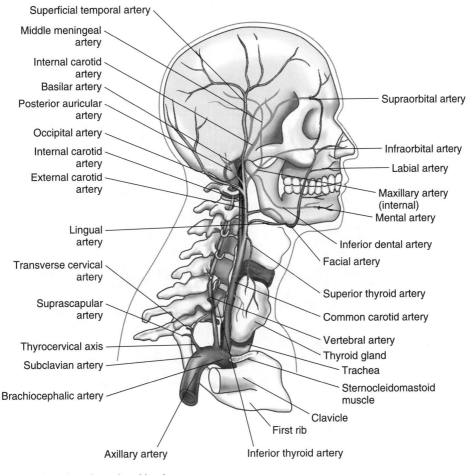

Fig. 8-17 Arterial supply to the neck and head.

Intracranial Pressure Dynamics

Intracranial pressure (ICP) is that pressure exerted against the skull by its contents: CSF, blood, and brain. The volumes of these contents may fluctuate slightly, but, despite variations, the total volume and ICP remain nearly constant. Compensatory mechanisms account for this stability in the overall ICP.

In health, the CSF pressure system is dynamic, allowing the pressure to vary only slightly by means of a compensatory mechanism that shunts CSF into the spinal subarachnoid space. The spinal dura covers the cord loosely and does not adhere to the vertebrae, which allows it to expand, whereas the cranial dura cannot. When CSF pressure becomes too great within the cranium because of an increase in volume of any of its contents, CSF is shunted out of the cranium, thus decreasing cranial volume and CSF pressure. In addition, CSF may be absorbed at an increased rate, which further aids in maintaining normal pressure.

Autoregulation of cerebral blood volume is another compensatory mechanism responsible for maintaining cerebral perfusion pressure (CPP) at a constant level. It is an alteration in the diameter of the resistance vessels aimed at maintaining

to investigate these most specialized vascular beds.

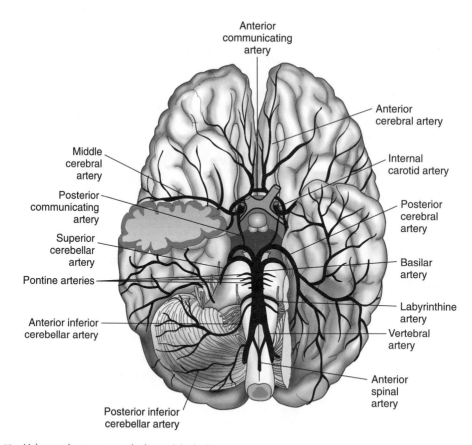

Fig. 8-18   Major arteries as seen on the base of the brain.

a constant perfusion pressure during changes in blood flow. When autoregulation is intact, vasodilatation occurs in response to moderate degrees of hypercapnia, hypoxia, hyperthermia, and increased ICP. The normal ICP ranges from 4 to 15 mm Hg. Normal CPP is 80 to 90 mm Hg.

Under normal conditions, CPP and resultant blood flow are determined by the difference between the inflow and the outflow pressures. Inflow pressures are represented by the mean systemic arterial pressure (MSAP), and under normal conditions the mean outflow pressure is equivalent to the mean venous pressure. In situ-

ations in which ICP is greater than venous pressure the following applies:

$$CPP = MSAP - ICP$$

It is readily apparent that any increase in ICP or reduction in MSAP will reduce CPP and the resulting cerebral blood flow.

Autoregulation is capable of maintaining a constant CPP only until the finite limit of CSF compensation is reached (Fig. 8-19). The spinal subarachnoid space is capable of holding only a limited amount of fluid, and, despite its inability to hold any additional displaced fluid, autoregulation continues. In this event, autoregulation

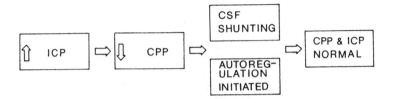

Fig. 8-19 CSF shunting and autoregulation as effective compensatory mechanisms. *ICP,* Intracranial pressure; *CPP,* cerebral perfusion pressure; *CSF,* cerebrospinal fluid.

ceases to be beneficial or effective in preventing further increases in ICP.

Spinal Cord

Protection of the Spinal Cord

Bones of the Spine

The spine is composed of a series of irregular bony vertebrae "stacked" one atop the other to form a strong but flexible column. They are joined by a series of ligaments and intervening cartilages and have two primary functions. Together these structures support the head and trunk. The spine also protects the spinal cord and its 31 pairs of spinal nerve roots by encasing them in a long canal formed by openings in the center of each vertebra. This vertebral canal extends the entire length of the spine and conforms to the various spinal curvatures as well as to the variations in size of the spinal cord itself.

There are 7 cervical, 12 thoracic, and 5 lumbar vertebrae. In the adult, the sacrum consists of five vertebrae fused to form one bone. Similarly, the coccyx results from the fusion of four or five rudimentary vertebrae.

Despite variations in their structure, all but two vertebrae share certain anatomic and functional aspects. With the exception of C1 and C2, all have a solid drum-shaped body that serves anteriorly as the weight-bearing segment. The posterior segment of the vertebra is called the arch, and each one comprises two pedicles, two laminae, and seven processes (four articular, two transverse, and one spinous). Projecting from the upper part of the body of each vertebra is a pair of short, thick pedicles. The concavities above and below the pedicles are the four intervertebral

notches. When the vertebrae are articulated, the notches in each adjacent pair of bones form the oval intervertebral foramina, which communicate with the vertebral canal and transmit the spinal nerves and blood vessels.

Arising from the pedicles are two broad plates of bone, the laminae, which meet and fuse at the midline posteriorly to form an arch. Projecting backward and downward from this junction is the spinous process, a knobby projection easily palpated under the skin of the back. Lateral to the laminae, near their junction with the pedicles, are paired articular processes, which facilitate movement of the vertebral column. The two superior processes of each vertebra articulate with the inferior processes of the vertebra immediately above it. The small surfaces where they articulate are called facets. The transverse processes are located somewhat anterior to the junction of the pedicles and the laminae. They are between the superior and inferior articular processes. These and the spinous processes provide sites for the attachment of muscles and ligaments. The hollow opening formed by the body of the vertebra and the arch is termed the vertebral foramen, a protected space through which the spinal cord passes.

Between each of the vertebrae and atop the sacrum is an intervertebral disk composed of compressible, tough, fibrous cartilage concentrically arranged around a soft, pulpy substance called the nucleus pulposus. Each disk acts as a cushionlike shock absorber between the vertebrae. When the intervertebral disk is ruptured, the soft nucleus pulposus may protrude into the vertebral canal, where it can exert pressure on a spinal nerve root, causing disturbances in motor and sensory functions. This herniated nucleus pulposus may

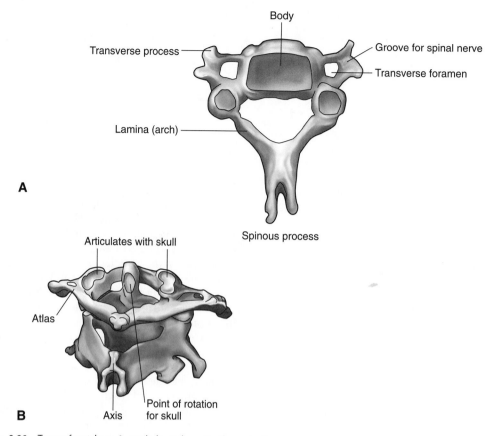

Fig. 8-20 Types of vertebrae. **A**, cervical vertebrae. **B**, atlas and axis.

require surgical excision through a laminectomy, if the herniation is severe enough.

Many important variations exist among the regional vertebrae. For example, the first cervical vertebra, or atlas, is ring-shaped and supports the cranium. It has no body or spinous process and allows for nodding motion of the head. The second cervical vertebra, or axis, is most striking because of the odontoid process, or dens, that arises perpendicularly to articulate with the atlas and allows rotation of the head. The cervical spine as a whole is extremely mobile and is therefore particularly susceptible to acceleration-deceleration and torsion injuries that hyperflex or hyperextend the neck. Also, the spinal cord is relatively large in this area and therefore sustains damage fairly easily after injury to the cervical spine (Fig. 8-20).

The 12 thoracic vertebrae increase in size as they approach the lumbar area. They are distinctive in that they have facets on their transverse processes and bodies for articulation with the ribs. The thoracic spine is fixed by the ribs, but the lumbar spine is not. This creates a vulnerability that is responsible for an increased incidence of fracture-dislocation at T12, L1, and L2. These injuries are typically found in motor vehicle accident victims who had been wearing lap seatbelts without shoulder restraints.

The five lumbar vertebrae are large and massive because of their prominent role in weight bearing. They have no transverse foramina. The sacrum, with its five fused vertebrae, is large, triangular, and wedge-shaped. It forms the posterior wall of the pelvis and articulates with L5, the coccyx, and the iliac portions of the hips. The triangular coccyx is formed by four small segments of bone, the most rudimentary part of the vertebral column.

Spinal Meninges

In addition to the bony vertebral column, the spinal cord is covered and protected by the continuous downward projection of the three meninges that perform the same protective function for the brain. The dura mater is the outermost membrane, a strong but loose and expandable sheath of dense, fibrous connective tissue that ends in a blind sac at the end of the second or third segment of the sacrum and protects the cord and the spinal nerve roots as they leave the cord. The dura does not extend beyond the intervertebral foramina. In contrast with the cranial dura, the spinal dura is not attached to the surrounding bone, consists of only one layer, and does not send partitions into the fissures of the cord.

The epidural space is located between the outer surface of the dura and the bones of the vertebral canal. It contains a quantity of loose areolar connective tissue and a plexus of veins. The subdural space is a potential space that lies below the inner surface of the dura and the arachnoid membrane. It contains only a limited amount of CSF.

The middle meningeal layer is the arachnoid membrane. Thin, delicate, and nonvascular, it is continuous with the cranial arachnoid and follows the spinal dura to the end of the dural sac. For the most part, the dura and arachnoid are unconnected, although they are in contact with each other.

The arachnoid is attached to the pia mater by delicate filaments of connective tissue. The considerable space between these two meningeal layers is called the subarachnoid space. It is continuous with that of the cranium and is largest at the lower end of the spinal canal, where it encloses the masses of nerves that form the cauda equina. The spinal subarachnoid space contains an abundant amount of CSF and is capable of expansion to the point of completely filling the entire space included in the dura mater. It plays a vital role in the regulation of ICP by allowing for the shunting of CSF away from the cranium. When spinal anesthesia is used, the local anesthetic agent is deposited into the subarachnoid space. Because the CSF in the subarachnoid space bathes the spinal nerves before they exit, the local anesthetic effectively blocks spinal nerve conduction.

The third and innermost meningeal layer of the spine is the delicate pia mater. Although it is continuous with the cranial pia mater, it is less vascular, thicker, and denser in structure than the pia mater of the brain. The pia mater intimately invests the entire surface of the cord and, at the point where the cord terminates, it contracts and continues down as a long, slender filament (central ligament) through the center of the bundle of nerves of the cauda equina and anchors the cord at the base of the coccyx.

Lumbar Puncture. The examination of CSF and determination of CSF pressure are frequently of great value in the diagnosis of neurologic and neurosurgical conditions. The collection of CSF is ordinarily accomplished through the insertion of a long spinal needle between L3 and L4 or L4 and L5, through the dura and arachnoid into the subarachnoid space. Because the spinal cord in adults ends at the level of the disk between L1 and L2, danger of injuring the cord through this procedure is minimal. In children, the spinal cord may extend below L3 so that the subarachnoid space is usually safely entered in the areas between L4 and L5. In both adults and children, flexion of the spine raises the cord superiorly somewhat farther, thus minimizing the risk of damage to the cord. Because the most superior points of the iliac crests are at the level of the upper border of the spine of L4, they are used as anatomic reference points in selecting the site for lumbar puncture. For a complete description of spinal and epidural anesthesia please see Chapter 23.

Structure and Function of the Spinal Cord and the Spinal Nerve Roots

The lowest level of the functional integration of information in the CNS takes place in the spinal cord. Here information is received in the form of afferent (sensory) nerve impulses from the periphery of the body. This information may be processed locally within the cord but more often is relayed to higher brain centers for additional processing and modification, thus resulting in sophisticated and elaborate motor (efferent) responses. A discussion of the spinal cord

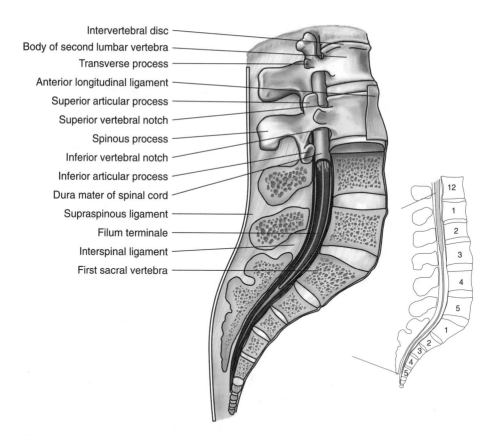

Intervertebral disc
Body of second lumbar vertebra
Transverse process
Anterior longitudinal ligament
Superior articular process
Superior vertebral notch
Spinous process
Inferior vertebral notch
Inferior articular process
Dura mater of spinal cord
Supraspinous ligament
Filum terminale
Interspinal ligament
First sacral vertebra

Fig. 8-21 Vertebral column showing the structure of vertebrae, filum terminale, termination of dura mater.

involves primarily the consideration of its function as a relay system for both afferent and efferent impulses.

The spinal cord is the elongated, slightly ovoid mass of central nervous tissue that occupies the upper two thirds of the vertebral canal. In the adult, it is approximately 45 cm (17 in.) long, although this varies somewhat from individual to individual depending on the length of the trunk. The cord is actually an inferior extension of the medulla oblongata and begins at the level of the foramen magnum of the occipital bone. From there it continues downward to the upper level of the body of L2, where it narrows to a sharp tip called the conus medullaris. From the end of the conus, an extension of the pia mater known as the filum terminale continues to the first segment of the coccyx, where it attaches (Fig. 8-21).

The small central canal of the spinal cord contains CSF. This cavity extends the entire length of the cord and communicates above directly with the fourth ventricle of the medulla oblongata.

The spinal cord (Fig. 8-22) is composed of 31 horizontal segments of varying lengths. It comprises 8 cervical, 12 thoracic, 5 lumbar, 5 sacral, and 1 coccygeal segment, each with a corresponding pair of spinal nerves attached.

During the growth of the fetus and young child, the spinal cord does not continue to lengthen as the vertebral column lengthens. Consequently, the cord segments, from which spinal nerves originate, are displaced upward from their corresponding vertebrae. This discrepancy becomes greater with each downward segment. For example, the cervical and thoracic nerve roots take an almost horizontal course as

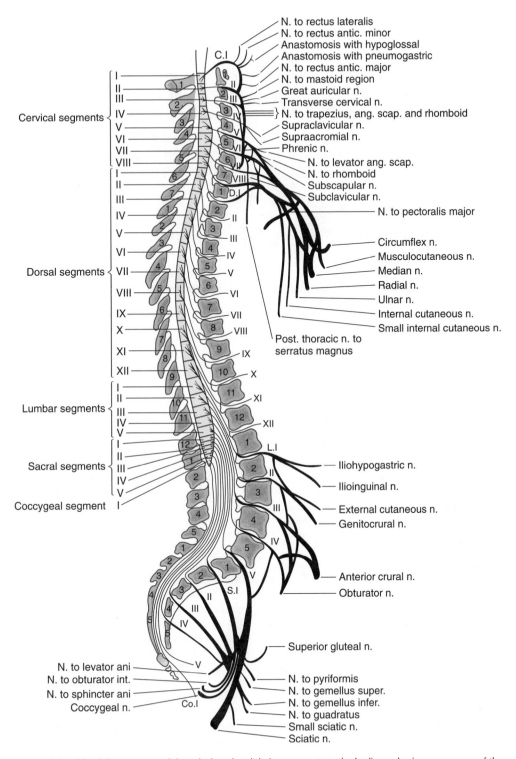

Fig. 8-22 Relationship of the segments of the spinal cord and their nerve roots to the bodies and spinous processes of the vertebrae.

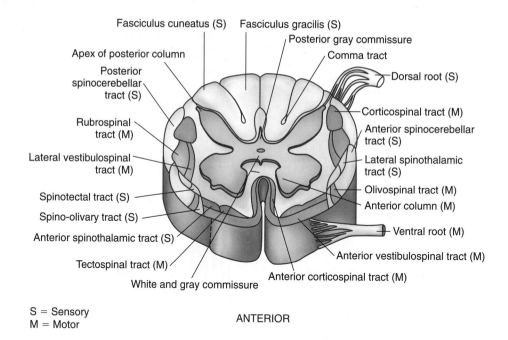

Fig. 8-23   Major ascending and descending tracts of the spinal cord.

they leave the spinal cord and emerge through the intervertebral foramina. The lumbar and sacral nerve roots, however, are extremely long and take an oblique, downward course before finally emerging from their appropriate lumbar or sacral intervertebral foramina. The large bundle of nerves lying within the inferior vertebral canal is called the cauda equina for its resemblance to a horse's tail (see Fig. 8-22). Several longitudinal grooves divide the spinal cord into regions. The deepest of these grooves is the anterior median fissure. Opposite this, on the posterior surface of the cord, is the posterior median fissure. These divide the cord into symmetric right and left halves that are joined in the central midportion (Fig. 8-23).

Like the brain, the spinal cord comprises areas of gray matter and areas of white matter. Unlike their locations in the brain, the gray matter of the cord is situated deep in its center, whereas the white matter is on the surface. The gray matter of the cord is composed of large masses of nerve cell bodies, along with dendrites of association and efferent neurons and unmyelinated axons, all embedded in a framework of neuroglia cells. It is also rich in blood vessels. The gray matter has two main functions: (1) synapses within the gray matter relay signals between the periphery and the brain, sometimes via the white matter of the cord; and (2) nuclei in the gray matter also function as centers for all spinal reflexes and even integrate some motor activities within the cord itself (such as the "knee-jerk" stretch reflex).

The white matter of the cord completely invests the gray matter. It consists primarily of long myelinated axons in a network of neuroglia and blood vessels. Its fibers are arranged into bundles called tracts, columns, or pathways that pass up and down, linking various segments of the cord and connecting the spinal cord with the brain, thus integrating and coordinating sensory and motor functions to or from any level of the CNS.

When viewed in cross section, the gray matter of the cord looks like the letter H, two crescent-shaped halves joined together by the gray commissure surrounded by white matter. For descriptive purposes, the four segments of the H are called right and left anterior (ventral) and posterior (dorsal) horns. The anterior motor (efferent) neurons lie within the anterior (ventral) gray horns and send fibers through the spinal nerves to the skeletal muscle. The nerve cell bodies that make up the posterior (dorsal) gray horns receive sensory (afferent) signals from the periphery via the spinal nerve roots. The lateral gray horns project from the intermediate portion of the H. The nerve cells in these horns (called preganglionic autonomic neurons) give rise to fibers that lead to the autonomic nervous system.

The white matter of each half of the cord is divided into three columns (or funiculi): the ventral, the lateral, and the dorsal. Each column is subdivided into tracts, which are large bundles of nerve fibers that are arranged in functional groups. The ascending or sensory projection tracts transmit impulses to the brain, and the descending or motor projection tracts transmit impulses away from the brain to various levels of the spinal cord. Some short tracts travel up or down the cord for only a few segments of the cord. These propriospinal (association or intersegmental) tracts connect and integrate separate cord segments of gray matter with one another and consequently have important roles in the completion of various spinal reflexes.

The 31 pairs of spinal nerves are symmetrically arranged. Each nerve contains several types of fibers and arises from the spinal cord by two roots: a posterior (dorsal) and an anterior (ventral) root (Fig. 8-24). The axons that make up the fibers in the anterior roots originate from the cell bodies and dendrites in the anterior and lateral gray horns. The anterior (ventral) root is the motor root, which conveys impulses from the CNS to the skeletal muscles. The posterior (dorsal) root is known as the sensory root. Sensory fibers originate in the posterior root ganglia of the spinal nerves. Each ganglion is an oval enlargement of the root lying just medial to the intervertebral foramen and contains the accumulated cell bodies of the axons making up the sensory fibers. One branch of the ganglion extends into the posterior gray horn of the cord. The other branch is distributed to both visceral and somatic organs and mediates afferent impulses to the CNS. The cutaneous (skin) area innervated by a single posterior root is called a dermatome. Knowledge of

dermatome levels is useful clinically in determining the level of anesthesia after spinal or regional anesthesia (see Chapter 23).

The lateral gray horns of the spinal cord give rise to fibers that lead into the autonomic nervous system that controls many of the internal (visceral) organs. Sympathetic fibers from the thoracic and lumbar cord segments are distributed throughout the body to the viscera, blood vessels, glands, and smooth muscle. Parasympathetic fibers, present in the middle three sacral nerves, innervate the pelvic and abdominal viscera. Hence, the ventral (anterior) root of the spinal nerve is often called the motor root, although it is also responsible for the preganglionic output of the autonomic nervous system.

The anterior and posterior roots extend to the intervertebral foramen corresponding to their spinal cord segment of origin. As they reach the foramen, the two roots unite to form a single mixed spinal nerve containing both motor and sensory fibers. As the nerve emerges from the foramen, it gives off a small meningeal branch that turns back through the same foramen to innervate the spinal cord membranes, blood vessels, intervertebral ligaments, and spinal joint surfaces. The spinal nerve then branches into two divisions that are called rami. Each ramus contains fibers from both roots. The posterior rami supply the skin and the longitudinal muscles of the back. The larger anterior rami supply the anterior and lateral portions of the trunk and all of the structures of the extremities. However, the anterior rami (except those of the 11 thoracic nerves) do not go directly to their destinations. Instead, they are first rearranged without intervening synapses to form intricate networks of nerve fibers called plexuses.

The five major plexuses are the cervical, brachial, lumbar, sacral, and pudendal. Peripheral nerves emerge from each plexus and are named according to the region that they supply.

The cervical plexus comprises the first four cervical spinal nerves. The phrenic nerve is the most important branch of the cervical plexus because it supplies motor impulses to the diaphragm. Any injury to the spinal cord above the origin of the phrenic nerve (C4) will result in paralysis of the diaphragm and death. Selective anesthesia of the brachial or pudendal plexuses is often used in regional anesthesia. By

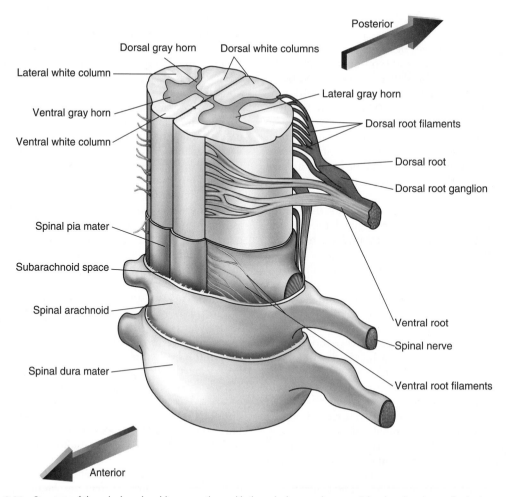

Fig. 8-24 Structure of the spinal cord and its connections with the spinal nerves by way of the dorsal and ventral spinal roots. Note also the spinal pia mater, spinal arachnoid, and spinal dura mater, which are known as the meninges, or coverings of the spinal cord. *(Redrawn from Guyton AC: Basic neuroscience: anatomy and physiology, ed 2, Philadelphia, 1991, WB Saunders.)*

depositing the local anesthetic at or near the brachial plexus, the musculocutaneous, median, ulnar, and radial nerves can be anesthetized, thereby allowing painless surgery from the elbow to the fingers. The pudendal nerve, which supplies motor and sensory fibers to the perineum, can be anesthetized by a pudendal plexus block. This type of nerve block is effective in relieving some of the pain of childbirth. Among the nerves given off by the lumbar plexus are the ilioinguinal, genitofemoral, obturator, and femoral nerves. Among those given off by the sacral plexus are the superior and the inferior gluteal nerves.

Anterior rami from the thoracic area do not form a plexus but lead instead to the skin of the thorax and to the intercostal muscles directly. The thoracic and upper lumbar spinal nerves also give rise to white rami (visceral efferent branches), or preganglionic autonomic nerve fibers. Parts of this ramus join the spinal nerves to the sympathetic trunk. The gray ramus is present in all spinal nerves.

The term "final common pathway" is often seen in literature. It refers to the motor neurons in the anterior gray horns. All excitatory or inhibitory impulses that control movement, from the cerebral cortex to the proprioceptors, influence the motor neurons of the anterior horn either directly or indirectly. Thus all neural impulses that arise in receptors—as well as in the brain and spinal cord—must ultimately converge in this area before movement of skeletal muscle can be integrated. Hence the term final common pathway.

Vascular Network of the Spinal Cord

The spinal cord derives its rich arterial blood supply from the vertebral arteries and from a series of spinal arteries that enter the cord at successive levels. Segmentally, the spinal arteries that enter the intervertebral foramina are given off by the intercostal vessels and by the lateral sacral, iliolumbar, inferior thyroid, and vertebral arteries.

The venous supply inside and outside the entire length of the vertebral canal is derived from a series of venous plexuses that anastomose with each other and end in intervertebral veins. The intervertebral veins leave the cord through the intervertebral foramina with the spinal nerves.

AUTONOMIC NERVOUS SYSTEM

The autonomic nervous system is made up of the sympathetic and parasympathetic nervous systems. These two divisions of the autonomic nervous system function to regulate and control the visceral functions of the body. In their regulation and control function, they usually work in opposition to each other.

Sympathetic Nervous System

The sympathetic nervous system originates from the thoracolumbar (T1 to L2) segments of the spinal cord. This system is mainly excitatory in physiologic function. Because the sympathetic nervous system involves the cardiovascular system and cardiovascular drugs, it is discussed in detail in Chapter 9.

Parasympathetic Nervous System

The parasympathetic nervous system basically functions as an inhibitor of the sympathetic nervous system. It originates in the cranium via cranial nerves III, V, VII, IX, and X. Cranial nerve X, or the vagus nerve, is the most important nerve because it carries about 75 percent of the parasympathetic nerve impulses. The parasympathetic nervous system also originates in the sacral portion of the spinal cord. Consequently, the parasympathetic nervous system uses the craniosacral outflow tracts. Because of the pharmacologic implications of the parasympathetic nervous system, it is discussed in detail in Chapters 9 and 21.

BIBLIOGRAPHY

Atlee J: Complications in anesthesia, Philadelphia, 1999, WB Saunders Company.

Barash P, Cullen B, Stoelting R: Clinical anesthesia, ed 4, Philadelphia, 2000, Lippincott Williams & Wilkins.

Benumof J, Saidman L: Anesthesia and perioperative complications, ed 2, St Louis, Mosby, 1999.

Benumof J: Anesthesia and uncommon diseases, ed 4, Philadelphia, 1998, WB Saunders.

Bickley L, Hoekelman R: Bates' guide to physical examination and history taking, ed 7, Philadelphia, 1998, Lippincott Williams & Wilkins.

Cottrell J, Smith D: Anesthesia and neurosurgery, ed 4, St Louis, 2001, Mosby.

Ganong W: Review of medical physiology, ed 20, New York, 2001, McGraw-Hill Professional.

Gray H, Williams P, Bannister L, editors: Gray's anatomy, ed 38, New York, 1995, Churchill Livingstone.

Guyton A, Hall J: Textbook of medical physiology, ed 10, Philadelphia, 2000, WB Saunders.

Hardman J, Limbird L: Goodman and Gilman's the pharmacological basis of therapeutics, ed 9, New York, 1996, McGraw-Hill.

Kaye A: Essential neurosurgery, ed 2, St Louis, 1997, Mosby.

Lake C, Hines R, and Blitt C: Clinical monitoring: practical applications for anesthesia and critical care, St Louis, 2001, Mosby.

Longnecker D, Murphy F: Dripps/Eckenhoff/Vandam introduction to anesthesia, ed 9, Philadelphia, 1997, WB Saunders.

Longnecker D, Tinker J, Morgan G: Principles and practice of anesthesiology, ed 2, St Louis, 1998, Mosby.

McIntosh L: Essentials of nurse anesthesia, New York, 1997, McGraw-Hill.

Miller R, editor: Anesthesia, ed 5, New York, 2000, Churchill Livingstone.

Nagelhout J, Zaglaniczny K: Nurse anesthesia, ed 2, Philadelphia, 2001, WB Saunders.

Stoelting R: Pharmacology and physiology in anesthetic practice, ed 3, Philadelphia, 1999, Lippincott-Raven.

Stoelting R, Miller R: Basics of anesthesia, ed 4, New York, 2000, Churchill Livingstone.

Stone D: Perioperative care: Anesthesia, medicine, and surgery, St Louis, 1998, Mosby.

Waugaman W, Foster S, Rigor B: Principles and practice of nurse anesthesia, ed 3, Norwalk, Conn, 1999, Appleton & Lange.

Weinberg G: Basic science review of anesthesiology, New York, 1997, McGraw-Hill.

9

THE CARDIOVASCULAR SYSTEM

Many drugs used for anesthesia depend on the cardiovascular system to produce their effects. Many of the same drugs also have effects on the cardiovascular system. It is therefore imperative for the perianesthesia nurse to understand the physiologic principles that relate to the cardiovascular status of the postanesthesia care unit (PACU) patient who has received an anesthetic.

The basic anatomy of certain structures of the cardiovascular system is not covered completely in this chapter, because basic nursing texts provide ample material on this subject.

DEFINITIONS

Adrenergic: a term describing nerve fibers that liberate norepinephrine.

Afterload: the impedance to left-ventricular ejection. The afterload is expressed as total peripheral resistance (TPR).

Angina pectoris: chest pain caused by myocardial ischemia.

Arrhythmia: an abnormal rhythm of the heart, also referred to as dysrhythmia.

Arteriosclerosis: degenerative changes in the arterial walls and resulting in thickening and loss of elasticity.

Automaticity: the ability of the cardiac pacemaker cells to undergo depolarization spontaneously.

Bathmotropic: affecting the response of cardiac muscle (or any tissue) to stimuli.

Bigeminy: a premature beat along with a normal heart beat.

Bradycardia: a heart rate of 60 beats per min. or less.

Cardiac arrest: ventricular standstill.

Cardiac index: a "corrected" cardiac output used to compare that of patients with different body sizes. The cardiac index (CI) equals the cardiac output (CO) divided by the body surface area (BSA).

Cardiac output: the amount of blood pumped to the peripheral circulation per minute.

Cholinergic: describing nerve fibers that liberate acetylcholine.

Chronotropic: affecting the rate of the heart.

Conduction: movement of cardiac impulses through specialized conduction systems of the heart that facilitate coordinated contraction of the heart.

Cor pulmonale: pulmonary hypertension due to obstruction of the pulmonary circulation and causing right-ventricular hypertrophy.

Cyanosis: bluish discoloration, seen especially on the skin and mucus membranes, due to a reduced amount of oxygen in the hemoglobin.

Diastole: the period of relaxation of the heart, especially of the ventricles.

Dromotropic: affecting the conductivity of a nerve fiber, especially the cardiac nerve fibers.

Ectopic: located away from a normal position; in the heart, a beat arising from a focus outside the sinus node.

Ectopic pacemaker: focus of ectopic pacemaker is demonstrated as premature contractions of the heart that occur between normal beats.

Electrolyte: an ionic substance found in the blood.

Embolism: a blood clot or other substance, such as lipid material, in the blood stream.

Excitability: the ability of cardiac cells to respond to a stimulus by depolarizing.

Fibrillation: an ineffectual quiver of the atria or ventricles.

Flutter: a condition, usually atrial, in which the atria contract 200 to 400 beats per min.

Heart block (complete): a condition that results when conduction is blocked by a lesion at any level in the atrioventricular junction.

Hypertension: persistently elevated blood pressure.

Hypervolemia: an abnormally large amount of blood in the circulatory system.

Infarction: a necrotic area due to an obstruction of a vessel.

Inotropic: affecting the force of contraction of muscle fibers, especially those of the heart.

Ischemia: local tissue hypoxia due to decreased blood flow.

Leukocytosis: increased number of white blood cells—a white blood cell count higher than 10,000 per mm³.

Leukopenia: decreased number of white blood cells—a white blood cell count lower than 5000 per mm³.

Murmur: an abnormal heart sound heard during systole, diastole, or both.

Myocardium: the muscular middle layer of the heart between the inner endocardium and the outer epicardium.

Normotensive: having a normal blood pressure.

Occlusion: an obstruction of a blood vessel by a clot or foreign substance.

Pacemaker: the area in which the cardiac rate commences, normally at the sinoatrial node.

Palpitation: an abnormal rate, rhythm, or fluttering of the heart experienced by the patient.

Paroxysmal tachycardia: a period of rapid heart beats that begins and ends abruptly.

Pericarditis: an inflammation of the pericardium.

Peripheral resistance: resistance to blood flow in the microcirculation.

Polycythemia: an excessive number of red blood cells, which is reflected in an abnormally high hematocrit level.

Preexcitation syndrome: when the atrial impulse bypasses the atrioventricular node to produce early excitation of the ventricle.

Preload: the left-ventricular end-diastolic volume (LVEDV).

Pulse deficit: the difference between the apical and radial pulses.

Re-entry (circus movement): re-excitation of cardiac tissue by the return of the same cardiac impulse using a circuitous pathway.

Syncope: fainting, giddiness, and momentary unconsciousness, usually caused by cerebral anoxia.

Systole: the period of contraction of the heart, especially the ventricles.

Thrombosis: the formation of a clot (thrombus) inside a blood vessel or a chamber of the heart.

THE HEART

The Cardiac Cycle

The heart is a four-chambered mass of muscle that pulsates rhythmically, pumping blood into the circulatory system. The chambers of the heart are the atria and the ventricles. The atria, which are pathways for blood into the ventricles, are thin-walled, have myocardial muscle, and are divided into the right and left atria by a partition. During each cardiac cycle, approximately 70% of the blood flows from the great veins through the atria and into the ventricles before the atria contract. The other 30% is pumped into the ventricles when the atria contract. On contraction of the right atrium, the pressure in the heart is 4 to 6 mm Hg. The contraction of the left atrium produces a pressure of 6 to 8 mm Hg.

Three pressure elevations are produced by the atria, as depicted on the atrial pressure curve. They are termed the a, c, and v waves (Fig. 9-1). The a wave is a result of atrial contraction. The c wave is produced by both the bulging of atrioventricular (AV) valves and the pulling of the atrial muscle when the ventricles contract. The v wave occurs near the end of the ventricular contraction as the amount of blood in the atria slowly increases and the AV valves close.

The ventricles receive blood from the atria and then act as pumps to move blood through the circulatory system. During the initial third of diastole, the AV valves open and blood rushes into the ventricles. This is called the period of rapid filling of the ventricles. The middle third of diastole is referred to as diastasis, during which a small amount of blood moves into the ventricles. During the final third of diastole, the atria contract, and the other 30% of the ventricles fills. As the ventricles contract, the AV valves contract and then close, thereby preventing blood from flowing into the ventricles from the atria.

As the ventricles begin to contract during systole, the pressure inside the ventricles increases, but no emptying of the ventricles occurs. During this time, called the period of isometric contraction, the AV valves are closed. As the right-ventricular pressure rises above 8 mm Hg and the left-ventricular pressure exceeds 80 mm Hg, the valves open to allow the blood to leave the ventricles. This period, termed the period of ejection, consumes the first three quarters of systole. The remaining fourth quarter is referred to as protodiastole, when almost no blood leaves the ventricles yet the ventricular muscle remains contracted. The ventricles then relax, and the pressure in the large arteries pushes blood back toward the ventricles, which forces the aortic and pulmonary valves to close. This is the period of isometric relaxation.

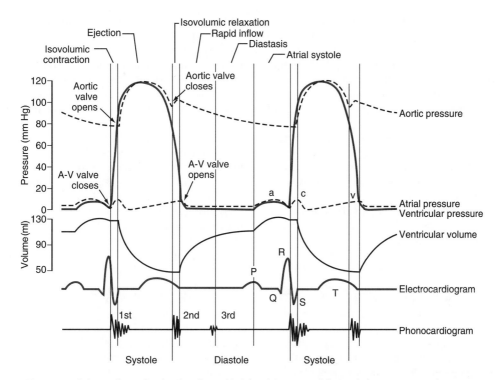

Fig. 9-1   The events of the cardiac cycle, showing changes in left atrial pressure, left ventricular pressure, aortic pressure, ventricular volume, the electrocardiogram, and the phonocardiogram. *(From Guyton A, Hall J: Textbook of medical physiology, ed 10, Philadelphia, 2000, WB Saunders.)*

At the end of diastole, each ventricle usually contains approximately 120 ml of blood. This is the end-diastolic volume. During systole, each ventricle ejects 70 ml of blood, which is the stroke volume. The blood that remains in the ventricle at the end of systole is end-systolic volume and amounts to approximately 50 ml.

Cardiac Output

Cardiac output is the amount of blood ejected from the left or right ventricle in 1 minute. In the normal adult with a heart rate of 70 beats per minute, the cardiac output is approximately 4900 ml. This estimate can be derived by taking the rate of 70 times the stroke volume of 70 ml. User-friendly sophisticated equipment is now available that makes it possible to monitor a patient's cardiac output in the PACU. The information derived from serial measurements of the cardiac output can be helpful in assessing the general status of the cardiovascular system as well as in the determination of the appropriate amount and type of fluid therapy for the patient.

The cardiac output is measured by a variety of techniques. Kaplan suggests that the thermodilution method, which employs the Swan-Ganz catheter, is the clinical method of choice. To facilitate a higher degree of reproducibility, Kaplan recommends a technique of standardization in which the injectate temperature and volume, as well as the speed of injection, should be carefully controlled and duplicated. The most reproducible results have been obtained using injections of 10 ml of cold (1°C to 2°C) 5% dextrose in water. It should be remembered that the thermodilution technique measures right-sided cardiac outputs. Hence patients with intracardiac shunts usually have unreliable measurements of their cardiac output when the thermodilution technique is used.

Other methods of calculating the cardiac output are the Fick and Stewart techniques. The

Fick technique involves calculations of the amount of blood required to carry oxygen taken up from the alveoli per unit of time. This technique is said to be accurate within a 10% margin of error. In the Stewart technique, a known quantity of dye is injected, and its concentration is measured after the dye is dispersed per unit of time.

Cardiac output can be influenced by venous return. As the Frank-Starling law of the heart states, "The heart pumps all the blood that it receives so that damming of the blood does not occur." If the heart receives an extra amount of blood from the veins ($\uparrow$ preload), the cardiac muscle becomes stretched, and the stretched muscle will contract with an increased force to pump the extra blood out of the heart. If the heart receives less blood than normal ($\downarrow$ preload), according to the Frank-Starling law of the heart, it will contract with less force. This concept is important to the perianesthesia nurse. For example, if a patient is receiving mechanical ventilation and too much positive end-expiratory pressure is overinflating his or her lungs, the increased pressure on the inferior vena cava will impede the venous return to the heart, thereby decreasing blood pressure. The blood pressure is derived from the following interacting factors: the force of the heart, the peripheral resistance, the volume of blood, the viscosity of blood, and the elasticity of the arteries. Thus it can be seen that cardiac output plays a major role in the maintenance of a normal blood pressure.

Arterial Blood Pressure

The arterial blood pressure consists of the systolic and diastolic arterial pressures. The systolic blood pressure is the highest pressure that occurs within an artery during each contraction of the heart. The diastolic blood pressure is the lowest pressure that occurs within an artery during each contraction of the heart. The mean arterial pressure is the average pressure that pushes blood through the systemic circulatory system. Methods of assessment and monitoring of the arterial blood pressure in the PACU are discussed in Chapter 25.

Some factors that affect the arterial blood pressure are the vasomotor center, the renal system, vascular resistance, the endocrine system, and chemical regulation. The vasomotor center, located in the pons and the medulla, has the greatest control over the circulation. This center picks up impulses from all over the body and transmits them down the spinal cord and through vasoconstrictor fibers to most vessels of the body. These impulses may be excitatory or inhibitory. One type of pressoreceptor that sends impulses to the vasomotor center is the baroreceptor. The baroreceptors are located in the walls of the major thoracic and neck arteries, in particular the arch of the aorta. When these vessels are stretched by an increased blood pressure, they send inhibitory impulses to the vasomotor center, which will lower the blood pressure. The aortic and carotid bodies located in the bifurcation of the carotid arteries and along the aortic arch can increase systemic pressure when stimulated by a low PaO_2.

The renal regulation of arterial pressure occurs through the renin-angiotensin-aldosterone mechanism (see Chapter 11).

The vascular resistance of the systemic vascular system can alter systemic pressure. As the total cross-sectional area of an artery decreases, the systemic vascular resistance increases. Therefore as the blood flows out of the aorta, a decrease in the arterial pressure in each portion of the systemic circulation is directly proportional to the amount of vascular resistance. This principle is the reason that the arterial pressure in the aorta is much higher than the pressure in the arterioles, which have a small cross-sectional area.

The nervous system, when stimulated by exercise or stress, elevates the arterial pressure via sympathetic vasoconstrictor fibers throughout the body.

When the radial artery is to be cannulated for direct monitoring of blood pressure and sampling of arterial blood gases in the PACU, an Allen test should be performed. This test is used to assess the risk of hand ischemia if occlusion of the cannulated vessel should occur. The Allen test is performed by having the patient make a tight fist, which will partially exsanguinate the hand. The nurse then occludes both the radial and the ulnar arteries with digital pressure. The patient is asked to open his or her hand, and the compressed radial artery is then released. Blushing of the palm (postischemic hyperemia) should be observed. After about a minute, the test should be repeated on the same hand with the nurse now releasing the ulnar artery while continuing to compress the radial artery. If the release of pressure over the ulnar artery does not lead to postischemic hyperemia, the contralateral artery should be similarly evaluated. The results of the Allen test should be reported as "refill time" for each artery.

Valves of the Heart

The semilunar valves are the aortic and pulmonary valves. They consist of three symmetric valve cusps, which can open to the full diameter of the ring yet provide a perfect seal when closed. During diastole, they prevent backflow from the aorta and pulmonary arteries into the ventricles.

The AV valves are the tricuspid and mitral valves. These valves prevent blood from flowing back into the atria from the ventricles during systole.

Attached to the valves are the chordae tendineae, which are attached to the papillary muscles, which in turn are attached to the endocardium of the ventricles. When the ventricles contract, so do the papillary muscles, thus pulling the valves toward the ventricles to prevent bulging of the valves into the atria (Fig. 9-2).

Heart Muscle

The heart muscle comprises three major muscle types: atrial muscle, ventricular muscle, and exci-

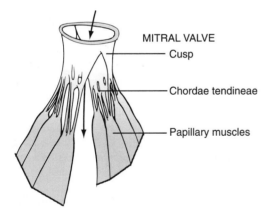

Fig. 9-2 The mitral valve and its attachments. *(From Guyton A, Hall J: Textbook of medical physiology, ed 10, Philadelphia, 2000, WB Saunders.)*

MITRAL VALVE
Cusp

Chordae tendineae

Papillary muscles

tatory and conductive muscle fibers. The atrial and ventricular muscles act much like skeletal muscles. The excitatory and conductive muscles function primarily as an excitatory system for the heart and a transmission system for conduction of impulses throughout the heart.

The cardiac muscle fibers are arranged in a latticework—they divide and then rejoin. The constriction of the cardiac muscle fibers facilitates action potential transmission. The muscle is striated, and the myofibrils contain myosin and actin filaments. Cardiac muscle cells are separated by intercalated disks, which are actually the cardiac cell membranes that separate the cardiac muscle cells from one another. The intercalated disks do not hinder conductivity or ionic transport between cardiac muscle cells to any great extent. When the cardiac muscle is stimulated, the action potential spreads to excite all the muscles. This is called a functional syncytium (Fig. 9-3). It can be divided into atrial and ventricular syncytia, which are separated by fibrous tissue. However, an impulse can be transmitted throughout the atrial syncytium and then via the AV bundle to the ventricular syncytium. The "all-or-none" principle is in effect—when one atrial muscle fiber is stimulated, all the atrial muscle fibers will react if the action potential is met. This principle applies to the entire ventricular syncytium as well.

The main properties of cardiac muscle are excitability (bathmotropism), contractility (inotropism), rhythmicity and rate (chronotropism), and conductivity (dromotropism). When cardiac muscle is excited, its action potential is reached and the muscle will contract. Certain chemical factors alter the excitability and contractility of cardiac muscle (Box 9-1).

Conduction of Impulses

The heart not only has a special system for generating rhythmic impulses but this system is able to conduct these impulses throughout the heart. This system for providing rhythmicity and conductivity consists of the sinoatrial (SA) node, the AV node, the AV bundle, and the Purkinje fibers (Fig. 9-4). The SA node is situated at the posterior wall of the right atrium and just below the opening of the superior vena cava. The SA node generates impulses by self-excitation, which is produced by the interaction of sodium and potas-

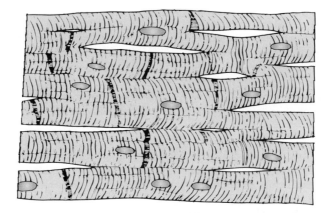

Fig. 9-3 The "syncytial" nature of cardiac muscle. *(From Guyton A, Hall J: Textbook of medical physiology, ed 10, Philadelphia, 2000, WB Saunders.)*

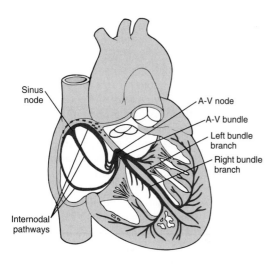

Fig. 9-4 The sinoatrial node and the Purkinje system of the heart. *(From Guyton A, Hall J: Textbook of medical physiology, ed 10, Philadelphia, 2000, WB Saunders.)*

Box 9-1	Chemical Factors that Affect Cardiac Muscle Excitability and Contractility

CAUSING INCREASE
High pH
Alkalosis
High calcium concentration

CAUSING DECREASE
High potassium concentration
High lactic acid concentration
Acidosis

sium ions. The SA node provides a rhythmic excitation approximately 72 times/min in the adult at rest. The action potential then spreads throughout the atria to the AV node.

The AV node is located at the base of the wall between the atria. Its primary function is to delay the transmission of the impulses to the ventricles. This allows time for the atria to empty before the ventricles contract. The impulses then travel through the AV bundle, sometimes called the bundle of His. The AV node is able to discharge

impulses 40 to 60 times/min if not stimulated by an outside source.

The Purkinje fibers originate at the AV node, form the AV bundle, divide into the right and left bundle branches, and spread downward around the ventricles. The Purkinje fibers can transmit the action potential rapidly, thus allowing immediate transmission of the cardiac impulse throughout the ventricles. The Purkinje fibers are able to discharge impulses between 15 and 40 times/min if not stimulated by an outside source.

The parasympathetic nerve endings are distributed mostly at the SA and AV nodes, over the atria, and, to a lesser extent, over the ventricles. If stimulated, they produce a decrease in the rate of rhythm of the SA node and slow the excitability at the AV node. The sympathetic nerves are distributed at the SA and AV nodes and all over the heart, especially the ventricles. Sympathetic stimulation increases the SA node rate of discharge, increases cardiac excitability, and increases the force of contraction.

Coronary Circulation

The coronary arteries furnish the heart with its blood supply. The main coronary arteries are on the surface of the heart, but smaller arteries penetrate the heart muscle to provide it with nutrients. The inner surface of the heart derives its nutrition directly from the blood in its chambers.

The coronary arteries originate at two orifices just above the aortic valve. The right coronary artery descends by the right atrium and ventricle and usually terminates as the posterior descending coronary artery. The left coronary artery is usually about 1 cm in length and divides into the anterior descending and the circumflex arteries. The anterior descending artery usually terminates at the apex of the heart and anastomoses with the posterior descending artery. The anterior descending artery supplies part of the left ventricle, the apex of the heart, and most of the interventricular septum.

The left circumflex artery descends posteriorly and inferiorly down to and terminates in the left marginal artery or communicates with the posterior descending coronary artery. Venous drainage is by superficial and deep circuits. The superficial veins empty into either the coronary sinus or the anterior cardiac veins, both of which drain into the right atrium. The deep veins drain into the thebesian or sinusoidal channels.

The regulation of coronary blood flow is determined primarily by the oxygen tension of the cardiac tissues. The most powerful vasodilator of the coronary circulation is hypoxemia. Other factors that may affect coronary blood flow are carbon dioxide, lactate, pyruvate, and potassium, all of which are released from the cardiac muscle. Coronary artery steal occurs when collateral perfusion of the myocardium is significantly reduced by an increase in blood flow to a portion of the myocardium that is normally perfused. More specifically, drug-induced vasodilation of normal coronary arterioles can then divert or steal blood flow from potentially ischemic areas of the myocardium being perfused by the vessels that have increased resistance (atherosclerotic vessels). Coronary artery steal can occur when arteriolar-vasodilating drugs, such as nitroprusside and isoflurane (Forane), are administered. This situation is especially likely to occur in "steal-prone" people, who constitute about 23% of the patients with coronary artery disease—especially those patients who have significant stenosis and occlusions to one or more coronary arteries.

Stimulation of the parasympathetic nervous system causes an indirect decrease in coronary blood flow. Direct stimulation is slight because of the sparse amount of parasympathetic nerve fibers to the coronary arteries. The sympathetic nervous system serves to increase coronary blood flow both directly (as a result of the action of acetylcholine and norepinephrine) and indirectly (caused by a change in the activity level of the heart). The coronary arteries have both alpha and beta receptors in their walls (see p. 139, adrenergic and cholinergic receptors).

Because so much cardiac disease involves the coronary arteries, the anesthetic risk increases in patients with cardiac disease. A functional classification of cardiac patients is based on their ability to perform physical activities (Box 9-2). Patients who are classes III and IV represent a significant risk for surgery and anesthesia and should be completely monitored when they receive care in the PACU.

Effect of Anesthesia on the Heart

Research now demonstrates that cardiac dysrhythmias are observed in about 60% of all patients who undergo anesthesia. The inhalation anesthetics—such as halothane, enflurane, and isoflurane—can evoke nodal rhythms or increase ventricular automaticity, or both. They also slow the rate of SA node discharge and prolong the bundle of His-Purkinje and ventricular conduction times. Along with these changes in rhythm, alterations in the balance of the autonomic nervous system between the parasympathetic and sympathetic systems caused by drugs such as anticholinergics and catecholamines or to light anesthesia can initiate cardiac dysrhythmias. Hence, in the immediate postoperative period cardiac dysrhythmias are likely because of light anesthesia during emergence or from the administration of drugs that alter sympathetic activity. Consequently, continuous monitoring of cardiac rate and rhythm is mandated in the PACU.

Myocardial Infarction

Acute myocardial infarction is a commonly encountered medical emergency that can occur in the PACU. The objectives in the management of a patient with an acute myocardial infarction are to relieve pain, control complications, salvage ischemic myocardium, and return the patient to a productive life. The diagnosis of a myocardial infarction is based on clinical findings, and therapy should be instituted immediately when it is suspected. (Cardiopulmonary resuscitation is discussed in Chapter 53.) An electrocardiogram performed in the PACU may reveal an injury pattern, but a normal electrocardiogram certainly does not exclude a diagnosis of myocardial infarction.

Physical assessment of a patient with a suspected myocardial infarction may include the following subjective findings: (1) pain or pressure, which is usually substernal but may be manifested in the neck, shoulder, jaws, arms, or other areas; (2) nausea; (3) vomiting; (4) diaphoresis; (5) dyspnea; and (6) syncope. The onset of pain may occur with activity but may also occur at rest. The duration may be prolonged, from 30 minutes to several hours. Objective findings may include hypotension, pallor, and anxiety. The blood pressure, pulse, and heart sounds may be normal in the patient who is experiencing an acute myocardial infarction. On auscultation of the chest, the abnormal cardiac findings may include atrial gallop, ventricular gallop, paradoxical second heart sound (S_2), friction rub, and abnormal precordial pulsations.

The electrocardiographic pattern may vary by the location and extent of the infarction, but myocardial damage may occur without changes in the electrocardiogram. Some typical features of a transmural infarction are acute ST-segment elevation in leads reflecting the area of injury, abnormal Q waves, and T-wave inversion.

The laboratory data usually reflect an elevated sedimentation rate and white blood cell count. The enzymes serum glutamic-oxaloacetic transaminase, lactic dehydrogenase (LDH), and creatine phosphokinase (CPK) may be elevated. Results of enzymatic studies in the patient with acute myocardial infarction do not indicate a specific cause, because other conditions and disease states may affect these enzymes. LDH and CPK isoenzyme studies may be necessary to differentiate the various disease abnormalities. Intramuscular injections may significantly elevate the level of CPK and therefore should be avoided. Along with this, surgical procedures that involve major trauma to muscle cause a postoperative increase in the CPK level. Because of the increase in the CPK level associated with surgical trauma, the perianesthesia nurse should use good judgment when evaluating enzyme studies in patients in whom acute myocardial infarction is suspected.

Research studies have demonstrated that patients who have had a myocardial infarction within 6 months before surgery will have a recurrence rate of 54.5% for a myocardial infarction that could occur during or after the surgical procedure. If the myocardial infarction occurred between 6 months and 2 years before surgery, the rate of recurrence of infarction is between 20% and 25%. Between the second and third years, the incidence of reinfarction is about 5%. Most studies indicate that 3 years after the original myocardial infarction, the recurrence rate is about 1%, which equals the normal rate of myocardial infarction in the general population. Hence, the chance of a patient's having an acute myocardial infarction in the PACU can be considered significant. This is especially true for PACU patients who have had a myocardial infarction within the last 3 years or who have a documented myocardial infarction risk factor—such as angina, hypertension, and diabetes—or for those with some combination of the above factors.

Perianesthesia Nursing Care

The perianesthesia nurse should be constantly alert for complications such as anxiety, arrhythmias, shock, left-ventricular failure, and pulmonary and systemic embolisms. Pain and apprehension may be relieved by morphine sulfate or meperidine hydrochloride (Demerol). Oxygen should be administered by nasal prongs because a face mask may increase the patient's apprehension. Continuous cardiac monitoring should be instituted, and the patient should be kept in a quiet area. Drugs such as atropine, lidocaine, digitalis, quinidine, sodium nitroprusside (SNP), phentolamine, and nitroglycerin should be available. A machine for countershock should be immediately available. Fluid therapy and urine output should be monitored completely to prevent fluid overload. A Swan-Ganz catheter or central venous pressure (CVP) monitor may be used to determine fluid replacement in patients with reduced intravascular volume and hypotension (see discussion of CVP catheters in the following section). A benign myocardial infarction does not exist—all patients with a diagnosed myocardial infarction require constant, competent perianesthesia care.

Central Venous Pressure Monitor

The CVP monitor enhances the assessment of venous return and hypovolemia. More specifically, the CVP monitor assesses the adequacy of central venous return, blood volume, and right-ventricular function. The actual pressure reading obtained from this monitor reflects of the pressure in the great veins when blood returns to the heart.

The left-ventricular end-diastolic pressure (LVEDP) serves as a good indicator of left-ventricular preload. Given that a patient has a good ejection fraction, the CVP measurement serves as an approximate value for the LVEDP. However, it should be remembered that the CVP has limited value in assessing left-ventricular hemodynamics.

In the immediate postoperative setting, the CVP remains an excellent parameter to indicate the adequacy of blood volume. In the hypovolemic state, the CVP is decreased. The administration of appropriate fluids and blood to expand the intravascular space increases the CVP toward the patient's baseline reading. In the clinical setting, no absolute, predetermined normal value for a CVP reading exists. The best use of this particular monitoring mode is to gather serial measurements to assess the patient's cardiovascular performance. See Chapter 25 for a complete discussion of the CVP monitor.

Pulmonary Artery Catheter

The pulmonary artery catheter monitors the central venous, pulmonary artery, and pulmonary capillary wedge pressures. This balloon-tipped catheter with four or five ports is discussed in detail in Chapter 25.

In the immediate postoperative period, the pulmonary artery catheter is usually used for patients with clinical shock, compromised ventricular function, and severe cardiac or pulmonary disease. Along with this, patients who have had extensive surgical procedures or major cardiovascular surgery can benefit from this monitor. Accurate monitoring of left-sided and right-sided preload along with the rapid determination of cardiac output makes this monitor an excellent parameter to determine mechanical and pharmacologic therapy, with the intended outcome of enhanced cardiac performance and tissue perfusion.

CIRCULATORY SYSTEM

Red Blood Cells (RBC)

The normal red blood cell (RBC) is in the form of a biconcave disk, which can change its shape to move through the microcirculation. The major function of the RBC is the transport of oxygen to the tissue cells; it is also an important factor in carbon dioxide transport. The RBC is responsible for approximately 70% of the buffering power of whole blood in maintaining acid-base balance.

RBCs are produced by the bone marrow. The normal rate of production is sufficient to form about 1250 ml of new blood per month. This is also the normal rate of destruction. The average life span of an RBC is 120 days. The hematocrit is the percentage of RBCs in the blood. The optimal range in adults is between 30% and 42%. When the hematocrit is reduced to lower than 30%, oxygen-carrying capacity declines steeply. Moreover, when the hematocrit rises higher than 55%, oxygen-carrying capacity will decline because the increase in blood viscosity causes increased work for the heart and decreased cardiac output. The normal amount of hemoglobin in the RBC ranges from 10 to 13.5 g. Indeed, the amount and type of hemoglobin determine the oxygen-carrying capacity. Recent evidence indicates that the cutoff value for risk of reduced oxygencarrying capacity and blood volume is a hemoglobin level of 9 g, a hematocrit of 27%, or both. Transfusion with blood or blood products to raise the level of hemoglobin should be strongly considered for any patient with values lower than the cutoff values.

White Blood Cells

White blood cells (WBCs), or leukocytes, are the body's major defense against infection. The two primary types of circulating leukocytes are polymorphonuclear leukocytes (PMNs) and lymphocytes. The role of the PMNs in combating infection is to migrate to the infectious site in large numbers and phagocytize the invading microbe. The role of the lymphocytes is to mediate immunoglobulin production and act in the delayed hypersensitivity in the type IV reaction (see Chapter 16). Evaluations of the WBC count should focus on the number of PMNs. When the PMN level is lower than 1000 per mm^3, incidence of infections is increased. Postanesthesia patients with a PMN level of 500 to 100 per mm^3 are at great risk of infection. Some of the major clinical situations that cause a reduction in PMNs (leukopenia) are viral infections—including human immunodeficiency virus—and cancer chemotherapy.

Blood Platelets

Normal hemostasis requires a proper interaction between blood vessels, platelets, and coagulation proteins. Any dysfunction in any one of the three components has a profound effect on hemostasis. When a tissue injury occurs, the vessel wall will vasoconstrict and activate the extrinsic pathway for coagulation proteins. Platelet adhesion and aggregation occur along with the activation of the intrinsic and extrinsic pathways for the coagulation proteins. The result of this interaction is a hemostatic plug.

Clinical evaluation for proper coagulation focuses on four tests: bleeding time (BT), platelet count (PC), prothrombin time (PT), and partial thromboplastin time (PTT). The BT and PC are tests to evaluate platelet function, and the PT and PTT are tests to evaluate the coagulation system.

A prolongation of the BT and surgically related hemorrhage seem to be correlated. The normal BT is between 2 and 9 minutes. The test results are considered abnormal when the BT is longer than 12 minutes. The template procedure should be used when the BT is performed, because it is more sensitive than older methods. The normal platelet count is between 200,000 and 450,000 per mm^3. More specifically, the patient will usually tolerate surgery and the postanesthesia phase quite well in regard to hemostasis with a platelet count of 100,000 per mm^3 or higher. Patients with a platelet count of 50,000 to 100,000 per mm^3 may experience ecchymoses due to tissue trauma. If the platelet count is lower than 50,000 per mm^3, many alterations in bleeding may occur. These patients require constant evaluation and therapy in the postoperative period.

The PTT is a test that evaluates the intrinsic and common coagulation pathways of the coagulation system. It is most commonly used to monitor heparin therapy. Normal results are considered to be 25 to 32 seconds, depending on the reagent. Abnormal results are considered to be longer than 35 seconds. The PT examines the extrinsic coagulation system. This test is used to evaluate oral anticoagulant therapy. Normal results are based on laboratory control for interpretation. Usually, the control is normal in patients with an appropriately functioning extrinsic coagulation system. When the value is more than 3 seconds above the control, the test results are considered to be abnormal.

Postoperative bleeding can occur when the patient's preoperative or intraoperative coagulation studies were abnormal. Bleeding tendencies are enhanced by the presence of postoperative hypertension. In addition, when hemostasis is lacking at the suture line or extensive surgical tissue trauma exists, the likelihood of postoperative bleeding is increased. Finally, the use of antibiotics intraoperatively and postoperatively can also increase bleeding tendencies. Therefore the perianesthesia nurse should evaluate the patient's preoperative and intraoperative coagulation studies and examine the surgical incision for bleeding during the initial assessment of the patient. Certainly, the postoperative trauma patient who has undergone extensive surgical trauma should be constantly monitored for bleeding tendencies, especially if he or she received intraoperative antibiotics. If the patient is receiving anticoagulant therapy, continued monitoring of the anticoagulant activity is mandated. Finally, in the patient in whom a bleeding tendency has been demonstrated, maintenance of a normal arterial blood pressure must be ensured. For a complete review of the fluid and electrolyte administration see Chapter 12.

Blood Vessels

The circulatory system can be divided into the systemic and the pulmonary circulation. The systemic or peripheral circulation comprises arteries, arterioles, capillaries, venules, and veins. The walls of the blood vessels, except the capillaries, are composed of three distinct coats: the tunica adventitia, the tunica media, and the tunica intima. The outer layer, the tunica adventitia, consists of white fibrous connective tissue, which gives strength to and limits the distensibility of the vessel. The vasa vasorum, which supplies nourishment to the larger vessels, is in this layer. The middle layer, the tunica media, consists of mostly circularly arranged smooth muscle fibers and yellow elastic fibers. The innermost layer, the tunica intima, is a fine transparent lining that serves to reduce resistance to the flow of blood. The valves of the veins are formed by the foldings of this layer. The capillaries consist of a single layer of squamous epithelial cells, which is a continuation of tunica intima.

The arteries are characterized by elasticity and extensibility. The veins have a poorly developed tunica media and are therefore much less muscular and elastic than arteries.

Microcirculation

Microcirculation is the flow of blood in the finer vessels of the body. It involves the arterioles, capillaries, and venules. The arteries subdivide to the last segment of the arterial system, the arteriole. The arteriole consists of a single layer of smooth muscle in the shape of a tube to conduct blood to the capillaries. As the arterioles approach the capillaries, they lack the coating of smooth muscle and are termed metarterioles. At the point at which the capillaries originate from the metarterioles, a smooth muscle fiber, the precapillary sphincter, encircles the capillary. At the other end of the capillary is the venule, which is larger but has a much weaker muscular coat than the arteriole.

The capillaries are usually no more than 8μ in diameter, which is barely large enough for corpuscles to pass through in single file. Blood moves through the capillaries in intermittent flow, caused by the contraction and relaxation of the smooth muscle of the metarterioles and the precapillary sphincter. This motion is termed vasomotion. The metarterioles and precapillary sphincter open and close in response to oxygen concentration in the tissues—a form of local autoregulation.

The microcirculation serves three major functions: (1) transcapillary exchange of nutrients and fluids; (2) maintenance of blood pressure and volume flow; and (3) return of blood to the heart and regulation of active blood volume.

ADRENERGIC AND CHOLINERGIC RECEPTORS

The cardiovascular system and the concept of adrenergic and cholinergic receptors are closely related. It is important for the perianesthesia nurse to understand the pharmacodynamics of these receptors.

Functional Anatomy: The Mediators

Cholinergic is a term used to describe the nerve endings that liberate acetylcholine. The cholinergic neurotransmitter, acetylcholine, is present in all preganglionic parasympathetic fibers, all preganglionic sympathetic fibers, all postganglionic parasympathetic fibers, and all somatic motor neurons. Two exceptions to the general rule are postganglionic sympathetic fibers to the sweat glands and to the vasculature of skeletal muscle. These are considered sympathetic anatomically but cholinergic in terms of their neurotransmitter (i.e., they release acetylcholine as their neurotransmitter).

The term adrenergic is used to describe nerves that release norepinephrine as their neurotransmitter. Epinephrine may be present in the adrenergic fibers in small quantities, usually representing less than 5% of the total amount of both epinephrine and norepinephrine. The adrenergic fibers are the postganglionic sympathetic fibers, with the exception of the postganglionic sympathetic fibers to the sweat glands and to the efferent fibers to the skeletal muscle (Box 9-3).

The adrenal medulla should be considered separately because it is innervated by a preganglionic sympathetic fiber liberating the neurotransmitter acetylcholine and because the postganglionic portion is the adrenal medulla, which behaves much like a postganglionic sym-

pathetic fiber. The adrenal medulla is therefore stimulated by acetylcholine, which causes the release of both epinephrine and norepinephrine from its chromaffin cells. As opposed to the usual finding of a preponderance of norepinephrine at the postganglionic nerve fiber terminals, the distribution in the adrenal medulla is 80% epinephrine and 20% norepinephrine. Therefore the neurotransmitter of the adrenal medulla is epinephrine.

Cholinergic Neurotransmitter: Biochemistry
The neurotransmitter acetylcholine is synthesized from choline and acetate through the enzymatic activity of choline acetylase to form acetylcholine (Box 9-4); it is then stored in vesicles. When acetylcholine is released from a preganglionic fiber, it may then act on the membrane of the preganglionic fiber with a positive feedback mechanism, thus enhancing the release of acetylcholine. The calcium ion facilitates this additional release of acetylcholine. This process is called excitation-secretion coupling through calcium.

Adrenergic Neurotransmitter: Biochemistry
The adrenergic neurotransmitter, epinephrine, begins in the body as phenylalanine. This is hydroxylated to tyrosine, which is again hydroxylated to form L-dopa, an amino acid. This process is probably the weakest step in the biosynthetic chain and may be a possible site of action of an autonomic drug. A soluble enzyme, L-dopa decarboxylase, acts on L-dopa to form dopamine, which in turn, is synthesized to norepinephrine. In the adrenal medulla, norepinephrine may be methylated in the cell to form the final product, epinephrine. This reaction is catalyzed by the enzyme phenylethanolamine-N-methyltransferase (see Box 9-4).

The storage site of norepinephrine in the adrenergic nerves appears to be in the intracellular granules. Depleting the total content of norepinephrine through continued nerve stimulation is difficult, but through continuous chronic drug administration, a clinical hypotensive state may be caused by the decreased sympathetic vasomotor tone.

The mechanism of release of norepinephrine from the adrenergic fibers and epinephrine from the adrenal medulla appears to be that of reverse

---

Box 9-3 Cholinergic and Adrenergic Nerves

MEDIATOR: ACETYLCHOLINE–CHOLINERGIC NERVES

Effects:

All preganglionic parasympathetic fibers

All preganglionic sympathetic fibers

All postganglionic parasympathetic fibers

All somatic motor neurons

Postganglionic sympathetic fibers to sweat glands

Postganglionic sympathetic vasodilator fibers innervating skeletal muscle vasculature

MEDIATOR: NONEPINEPHRINE–ADRENERGIC NERVES

Effects:

All postganglionic sympathetic fibers (except those to sweat glands and efferent fibers to skeletal muscle)

Modified from Drain CB: Current concepts on the pharmacodynamics of adrenergic and cholinergic receptors, AANA J 44:272, 1976.

Box 9-4 Synthesis of Neurotransmitters

Cholinergic

Choline + Acetate <u>Choline acetylase</u> Acetylcholine

Adrenergic

Phenylalanine ——————— Tyrosine <u>Tyrosine hydrolase</u> L-dopa

L-dopa <u>decarboxylase</u> Dopamine <u>Dopamine beta oxidase</u> Norepinephrine

Norepinephrine <u>Phenylethanolamine-N-methyltransferase</u> Epinephrine

---

Modified from Drain CB: Current concepts on the pharmacodynamics of adrenergic and cholinergic receptors, AANA J 44:272, 1976.

pinocytosis. Pinocytosis is a mechanism by which the membrane engulfs substances in the extracellular fluid. Under the influence of the appropriate stimuli, an opening—through which the soluble contents of a portion of the storage granules are released—is created. The major means of inactivation of norepinephrine is through a mechanism known as uptake, in which the released neurotransmitter is recaptured into the neuronal system by the neuron that released it or by neurons adjacent to it and, in some instances, by neurons associated with tissues some distance from the original site of release.

The norepinephrine that is not recaptured is metabolized eventually to vanillylmandelic acid. Epinephrine also undergoes a number of steps in its biodegradation to vanillylmandelic acid. An increase in vanillylmandelic acid concentration in the urine is useful in the diagnosis of conditions such as pheochromocytoma and neuroblastoma (Fig. 9-5).

When a patient is receiving a drug that is a monoamine oxidase inhibitor—such as isocarboxazid (Marplan), pargyline (Eutonyl), phenelzine sulfate (Nardil), or tranylcypromine sulfate (Parnate)—a buildup of epinephrine or norepinephrine can occur, thus leading to sympathetic hyperactivity. This is especially likely to occur when substances or drugs such as tyramine or indirect-acting vasopressors such as ephedrine are administered.

Cholinergic Receptors

The pharmacologic and physiologic actions of acetylcholine are apparently mediated by its com-

bination with specific cholinergic receptors. The actions of acetylcholine and drugs that mimic acetylcholine are mediated through two types of cholinergic receptors: nicotinic and muscarinic (see Chapter 21).

When the nicotinic receptors are stimulated, the following responses are observed:

1. Stimulation of autonomic ganglia—both parasympathetic and sympathetic.
2. Stimulation of the adrenal medulla, which results in the release of both epinephrine and norepinephrine.
3. Stimulation of skeletal muscle at the motor end-plate.

The muscarinic responses elicited by muscarine as well as acetylcholine are the following:

1. Stimulation or inhibition of smooth muscle in various organs or tissues.
2. Stimulation of exocrine glands.
3. Slowing of cardiac conduction.
4. Decrease in myocardial contractile force.

Nicotinic responses in terms of antagonism can be blocked by drugs such as ganglionic or neuromuscular blocking agents, or both, whereas muscarinic responses are blocked by the class of drugs best typified by atropine.

Muscarine is a specific agonist at muscarinic receptors, whereas nicotine is a specific agonist at nicotinic receptors; however, acetylcholine is capable of stimulating both receptor types (Table 9-1).

A series of compounds is specific in its ability to combine with acetylcholinesterase and inhibit

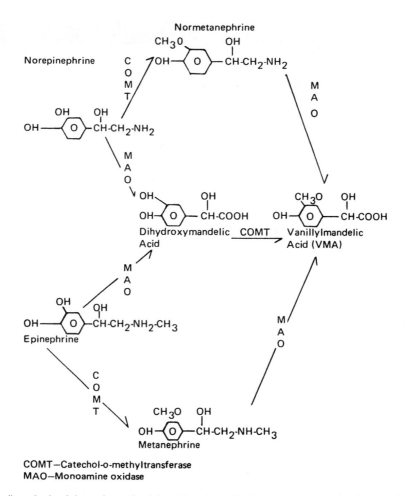

Fig. 9-5 Metabolism of epinephrine and norepinephrine. *(From Drain CB: Current concepts on the pharmacodynamics of adrenergic and cholinergic receptors, AANA J 44:272, 1976.)*

its activity through competitive inhibition. The prototype compounds in this category are neostigmine (Prostigmin), physostigmine salicylate (Antilirium), pyridostigmine (Regonol, Mestinon), and edrophonium (Tensilon, Enlon).

Belladonna alkaloids such as atropine have adverse effects that are peculiar to the PACU phase of the surgical experience. More specifically, belladonna alkaloids that cross the blood-brain barrier can cause disorientation, violent behavior, or somnolence. Physostigmine salicylate, an anticholinesterase that is capable of penetrating the blood-brain barrier, has been shown to be useful in reversing the adverse effects of bel-

ladonna alkaloids on the CNS. Physostigmine salicylate is also useful in reversing the disorientation or somnolence caused by drugs such as diazepam, the phenothiazines, the tricyclic antidepressants, the antiparkinsonian drugs, promethazine, droperidol, and, in some instances, halothane. Patients in the PACU who may benefit from treatment with physostigmine are those who have received a belladonna alkaloid or neuroleptic type of agent either preoperatively or intraoperatively, who have demonstrated disorientation or restlessness or both for more than 30 minutes after anesthesia, and who are difficult to arouse over an appropriate period. Patients who

Table 9-1 **Cholinergic Receptors**

Organ Stimulated by Cholinergic Agonist	Response	Type of Cholinergic Receptor Response
HEART		
SA node	Negative chronotropic effect	Muscarinic
Atria	Decreased contractility and increased conduction velocity	Muscarinic
AV node and conduction system	Decrease in conduction velocity—AV block	Muscarinic
EYE		
Sphincter muscle of the iris	Contraction (miosis)	Muscarinic
LUNG		
Bronchial muscle	Contraction	Muscarinic
Bronchial glands	Stimulation	Muscarinic
EXOCRINE GLANDS		
Salivary glands	Profuse, watery secretion	Muscarinic
Lacrimal glands	Secretion	Muscarinic
Nasopharyngeal glands	Secretion	Muscarinic
Adrenal Medulla	Catecholamine secretion	Nicotinic
Autonomic Ganglia	Ganglion stimulation	Nicotinic Muscarinic
SKELETAL MUSCLE		
Motor end-plate	Stimulation	Nicotinic (motor end-plate receptor)

Modified from Drain CB: Current concepts on the pharmacodynamics of adrenergic and cholinergic receptors, AANA J 44:272, 1976.

demonstrate any one of these dysfunctions qualify for treatment and can be given 1-mg increments of physostigmine intravenously at 15-minute intervals until they are conscious and oriented to time, place, and person. Once treatment has begun, the perianesthesia nurse should monitor the blood pressure and pulse immediately before and 5 minutes after the administration of physostigmine. Also, some patients may experience side effects from physostigmine, such as nausea, pallor, sweating, and bradycardia. Because glycopyrrolate (Robinul) does not cross the blood-brain barrier, treating the side effects of physostigmine is especially helpful. Finally, patients who have been treated with physostig-mine probably should remain in the PACU for about 1 hour after the administration of the anticholinesterase.

Adrenergic Receptors

The stimulation of the sympathetic nervous system can be both inhibitory and excitatory, which has caused considerable confusion. Originally, theories were postulated that this phenomenon handled the release of two different compounds. The variation in the effects of stimulation was later found to be related not to the differences in chemical release but rather to a difference in the receptors' responses to the transmitter.

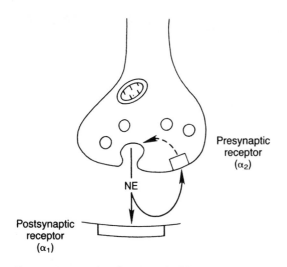

Fig. 9-6 Presynaptic and postsynaptic alpha receptors at the ending of a norepinephrine-secreting neuron. *(Adapted from Ganong WF: Review of medical physiology, ed 20, New York, 2001, Lange Medical Books/McGraw-Hill Medical Publications Division.)*

The adrenergic receptors, which respond to catecholamines, can be subdivided into three main types: the dopaminergic, the alpha, and the beta. The dopaminergic receptors are primarily in the CNS and the mesenteric and renal blood vessels. The agonist for these receptors is dopamine. The alpha receptors can be further divided into alpha$_1$ and alpha$_2$ receptors. The postsynaptic alpha$_1$ receptors are excitatory in action, except in the intestine. Stimulation of the alpha$_1$ receptors causes smooth muscle contraction, which results in a vasoconstriction or pressor response. Hence, the alpha$_1$ receptor is activated by the release of norepinephrine, and this released norepinephrine also activates the presynaptic alpha$_2$ receptors to inhibit the further release of norepinephrine. Thus the alpha$_1$ receptor is activated by the release of norepinephrine, and the released norepinephrine in turn stimulates the alpha$_2$ receptor, thus producing inhibition of the release of norepinephrine and resulting in a negative feedback loop (Fig. 9-6).

The drug clonidine (Catapres) is believed to stimulate the alpha$_2$ receptors, which lowers the sympathetic outflow of norepinephrine and ultimately leads to a hypotensive effect. In addition to lowering catecholamine levels, clonidine can reduce the plasma renin activity. This antihypertensive drug enjoys a significant degree of popularity, but it can have a negative impact on the patient in the PACU. More specifically, the "clonidine withdrawal syndrome" has been reported when the drug has been stopped abruptly. The sequelae of the syndrome resemble pheochromocytoma in that shortly after the withdrawal of the clonidine and in that the patient can experience hypertension, tachycardia, and increased blood levels of catecholamines. Treatment of this syndrome usually involves a reinstitution of the clonidine therapy and alpha-adrenergic blocking agents such as phentolamine.

Stimulation of the beta receptor causes vascular smooth muscle relaxation, which then leads to a decrease in blood pressure through a decrease in peripheral resistance. The beta receptor can be divided into two types: beta$_1$ and beta$_2$. Beta$_1$-subtype receptors are found in all cardiac tissue except the coronary vasculature and are responsible for characteristic effects noted after stimulation of the heart by epinephrine, including the following: (1) increase in heart rate; (2) increase in contractile force; (3) increase in conduction velocity; and (4) shortening of the refractory period. Beta$_1$-subtype receptors mediate effects elicited by catecholamines (Table 9-2).

The physiology of the beta receptor has many implications for the care of the PACU patient. Once the beta receptor has been activated by "first messengers"—which are endogenous catecholamines or exogenous beta agonists such as isoproterenol—certain biochemical events occur (Fig. 9-7). The enzyme adenylate cyclase, which is located on the plasma membrane, is stimulated by beta-receptor activation. Then, within the cell, adenosine triphosphate (ATP) is broken down to 3', 5'-adenosine monophosphate (cyclic AMP). The cyclic AMP is then released into the cytoplasm of the cell and acts to modulate cellular activities. Hence, the cyclic AMP is considered to be the "second messenger." Cyclic AMP is inactivated to 5-AMP by the enzyme phosphodiesterase.

Clinically, isoproterenol or terbutaline may be administered to increase the cyclic AMP levels in the beta$_2$ receptors in the bronchial airways with the intended result of bronchodilatation.

Table 9-2 **Adrenergic Receptors**	
Response	Type of Adrenergic Receptor
HEART	
Positive inotropic effect	$Beta_1$
Positive chronotropic effect	$Beta_1$
Cardiac arrhythmias	$Beta_1$
Positive dromotropic effect	$Beta_1$
VASCULAR	
Arterial and arteriolar constriction	$Alpha_1$
Coronary artery constriction	$Alpha_1$
Coronary artery dilatation	$Beta_1$
Arteriolar relaxation	$Beta_2$
GASTROINTESTINAL TRACT	
Intestinal relaxation	$Alpha_1$, $beta_1$
Sphincter contraction (usually)	$Alpha_1$
URINARY BLADDER	
Bladder relaxation (detrusor)	$Beta_2$
Bladder contraction (trigone and sphincter)	$Alpha_1$
EYE	
Contraction (mydriasis)	$Alpha_1$
Ciliary muscle of iris	$Beta_2$
Metabolic	$Alpha_1$, $beta_2$
Liver glycogenolysis (hyperglycemia)	$Beta_1$
Muscle glycogenolysis	$Beta_1$
Lipolysis	$Beta_1$, $beta_2$
Oxygen consumption (increases)	
OTHER SMOOTH MUSCLE	
Bronchial (relaxation)	$Beta_2$
Spleen (contraction)	$Alpha_1$
Ureter (contraction)	$Alpha_1$
Uterus (contraction)	$Alpha_1$
Uterus (relaxation)— nonpregnant condition	$Beta_2$

Modified from Drain CB: Current concepts on the pharmacodynamics of adrenergic and cholinergic receptors, AANA J 44:272, 1976.

Another way to increase the cyclic AMP levels is to inhibit the action of phosphodiesterase. Caffeine and the methylxanthines, such as aminophylline, are inhibitors of the enzyme phosphodiesterase and can be used alone or in combination (for synergistic effects) with the beta agonists to produce the desired bronchodilatation in the patient. It should be remembered that other catecholamine effects are produced by the increase in cyclic AMP levels. Consequently, although aminophylline is considered a bronchodilator, it increases the myocardial contractility and heart rate of the patient, thus mandating the perianesthesia nurse to monitor both respiratory and cardiac function when methylxanthines are administered.

The coronary arteries contain $alpha_1$ and $beta_1$ receptors and therefore also have the ability to vasoconstrict and vasodilate (see Table 9-2). The endogenous catecholamines, norepinephrine and epinephrine, are capable of stimulating both the alpha and the beta receptors.

Site of Action of Autonomic Drugs

Methyldopa (Aldomet) (the alpha-methylated analogue of L-dopa) is an antihypertensive drug. Methyldopa reduces the sympathetic nerve stimulation through the production of a selective agonist, alpha methylnorepinephrine.

Guanethidine has the ability to prevent nerve stimulation, thus inhibiting norepinephrine release. Guanethidine interferes with the storage of norepinephrine and, if given chronically, results in a decrease in the amount of norepinephrine stored in adrenergic nerves. Reserpine also shares this latter action with guanethidine. Thus chronic use of guanethidine and reserpine results in a relative depletion of the norepinephrine content from sympathetic nerves (Table 9-3).

The calcium channel blockers have been found to have considerable value in the treatment of supraventricular tachycardias, angina pectoris, and myocardial infarction. The prototype calcium channel blockers are verapamil (Isoptin), nifedipine (Procardia, Adalat), and diltiazem (Cardizem). All three drugs depress calcium entry into conduction tissue and cardiac muscle, which results in a depression of conduction and leads to a reduction of the circus movements. These calcium entry blockers produce

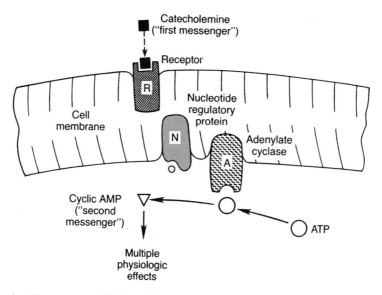

Fig. 9-7   Catecholamine ("first messenger") binds to the beta-receptor protein, which activates the enzyme adenylate cyclase via the nucleotide regulatory protein, which binds guanosine monophosphate. Via adenylate cyclase, ATP is broken down to cyclic AMP. The cyclic AMP, or "second messenger," then activates protein kinase, which ultimately produces a variety of physiologic effects. *(Modified from Catt KJ, Harwood JP, Clayton RN et al: Regulation of peptide hormone receptors and gonadal steroidogenesis, Recent Prog Horm Res 36:557–662, 1980.)*

Table 9-3   Drugs that Interfere with Specific Steps in the Process of Chemical (Neurohumoral) Transmission

	Adrenergic Nerves	Cholinergic Nerves
Synthesis of the mediator	Methyldopa	Hemicholinium
Storage of the mediator	Reserpine	—
Release of the mediator	Guanethidine	Botulinus toxin
Combination of the mediator with its receptor	Phenoxybenzamine (alpha receptor)	Atropine (muscarinic)
	Propranolol (beta receptors)	Nicotine (nicotinic)
Enzymatic destruction of the mediator	Pyrogallol (COMT inhibitor) Tranylcypromine (MAO inhibitor)	Physostigmine (cholinesterase inhibitor)
Prevention of inactivation of the mediator (blocks the uptake)	Cocaine	—
Repolarization of the postsynaptic membrane (persistent depolarization)	—	Succinylcholine

From Drain CB: Current concepts on the pharmacodynamics of adrenergic and cholinergic receptors, AANA J 44:272, 1976. MAO, Monoamine oxidase; COMT, catechol-O-methyl transferase.

hypotension by different mechanisms. Nifedipine, like SNP, decreases the systemic vascular resistance with a compensatory tachycardia, and verapamil and diltiazem lower the cardiac output by exerting a negative dromotropic effect. The effects of the calcium channel blockers may be enhanced by inhalation anesthesia agents such as halothane. Consequently, in the PACU, patients who received an inhalation of anesthetic and are being treated with a calcium channel blocker may experience some hypotension. Hence the perianesthesia nurse should vigorously monitor the cardiovascular parameters of these patients and report any confirmed hypotension to the attending physician.

Dopamine is a naturally occurring biochemical catecholamine precursor of norepinephrine. It exerts a positive inotropic effect and a minimal chronotropic effect on the heart. Therefore the contractility of the heart is increased without changing the afterload (total peripheral resistance), which leads to an increase in cardiac output. The increase is in the systolic and pulse pressures, with virtually no effect on the diastolic pressure. Dopamine is not associated with tachyarrhythmias and produces less of an increase in myocardial oxygen consumption than does isoproterenol. Blood flow to peripheral vascular beds may decrease while mesenteric flow increases. One of the major reasons for the increase in the use of dopamine clinically is its dilatation of the renal vasculature. This action is secondary to the inotropic effect and decreased peripheral resistance. Therefore the glomerular filtration rate is increased along with the renal blood flow and sodium excretion.

Dobutamine (Dobutrex) is synthetically derived from the catecholamine isoproterenol. Consequently, it produces a positive inotropic effect with specificity to the beta$_1$ receptors, thus resulting in an increase in cardiac output with minimal effects on blood pressure, heart rate, and systemic vascular resistance. The drug is usually administered intravenously in a dose range of 2 to 10 µg per kg per minute and is especially useful for patients who are recovering from cardiopulmonary bypass surgery. Dobutamine is sometimes combined with a vasodilator to reduce afterload in an effort to optimize the cardiac output.

Hypotension Therapy

Hypotension in the immediate postoperative period is of great concern, and it deserves the prompt attention of the perianesthesia nurse. When hypotension is detected in the postanesthesia patient, the nurse should first reaffirm the measurements. An incorrectly placed or sized blood pressure cuff or malfunction of the stethoscope can yield incorrect measurements (see Chapter 25). If an arterial catheter transducer system is being used, it should be appropriately zeroed and calibrated and the air bubbles should be removed to ensure that artificially low readings are not observed. Also, if the patient is hypothermic or receiving alpha-adrenergic agonists such as phenylephrine (Neo-Synephrine), he or she may have low blood pressures in the radial and brachial arteries, whereas the central blood pressure will be higher. This difference is because of the peripheral vasoconstriction produced by the alpha-adrenergic drugs.

If the hypotension is confirmed, hypovolemia should be considered as a possible cause. The clinical signs of hypotension due to hypovolemia include cold, pale, clammy, or diaphoretic skin; rapid, thready pulse; shallow, rapid respirations; disorientation, restlessness, or anxiety; decreased CVP; and oliguria. The nursing assessment of the hypotensive patient should include an inspection of the dressings for excessive bleeding and the evaluation of the clinical signs of hypovolemia. If the patient's circulating blood volume is reduced by more than 15% to 20%, hypotension can ensue. This usually happens when the patient has not received appropriate fluid volume replacement intraoperatively. Other factors in the development of postoperative hypovolemia are ongoing internal or external hemorrhage, sweating, insensible losses, and "third-space" losses. Third-space losses occur when an exudation of fluid into the tissues occurs (see Chapter 12). Other causes of hypotension include a high alveolar-inflating pressure when a patient is receiving mechanical ventilation, ventricular dysfunction, myocardial ischemia, and cardiac dysrhythmias. If the hypotension is 30% below preoperative baseline blood pressure readings or one or more of the clinical signs of hypovolemia is present, the attending physician should be notified.

Usual therapy for hypotension in the PACU includes the administration of a high fractional concentration of oxygen, fluid infusion, reversal of residual anesthetic depressant effects, repositioning of the patient to facilitate venous return, reduction in ventilator airway pressures, and administration of vasopressors or anticholinergics or both, such as glycopyrrolate or atropine, as indicated. More specifically, the first line of defense is to return the patient to normovolemia and, in this instance, administer a bolus of crystalloid solution of about 300 to 500 ml. The anticholinergics are indicated if sinus bradycardia accompanies the hypotension. The vasopressors exert their effect either directly or indirectly. The direct-acting vasopressor exerts its effect directly on the receptor. Conversely, the pharmacologic action of an indirect vasopressor facilitates the release of norepinephrine from its storage vesicles (primarily the terminal sympathetic nerve fibers), which stimulates the adrenergic receptor to achieve the desired effect. Therefore a direct-acting vasopressor is probably necessary to achieve a response in patients who are depleted of catecholamines by drugs such as reserpine and guanethidine (Table 9-4).

Another area of consideration when selecting a vasopressor is the cardiotonic action desired. Metaraminol (Aramine), by its action of norepinephrine release, causes improved cardiac function as a result of its beta-receptor activity. Conversely, phenylephrine and methoxamine (Vasoxyl) possess little or no cardiac effect and exert a pressor action by pure alpha stimulation. The alpha-adrenergic agonists are useful especially for patients that have received a "high" spinal or epidural anesthetic. High levels of regional anesthetics are associated with peripheral vasodilatation and bradycardia due to a sympathetic blockade. Consequently, an alpha-adrenergic agonist produces peripheral vascular vasoconstriction, or a mixed-action alpha and beta drug such as ephedrine can be administered.

A new category of drugs to combat hypotension is the cardiac inotropic agents. This class of drugs produces positive inotropic and vasodilating effects and can be considered to be related to digitalis in regard to pharmacologic effects. The major pharmacologic actions of these drugs include increased cardiac output and decreased LVEDP. These drugs are of benefit for the short-term management of congestive heart failure, especially in patients with congestive heart failure who do not respond adequately to digitalis, diuretics, or vasodilators. Along with this, the inotropic agents may be valuable in the treatment of cardiogenic shock. This class of drugs can be considered as an alternative to catecholamines for the treatment of low cardiac output in the postoperative period. Drugs in this category include amrinone (Inocor) and milrinone. As with other vasopressors, constant monitoring of the patient's vital signs is warranted when inotropic agents are administered.

Hypertension Therapy

A hypertensive emergency may occur in the PACU. The patient may arrive in a hypertensive state or become hypertensive during the postanesthesia phase. If the diastolic blood pressure rises to about 120 to 140 mm Hg and the patient complains of headache and blurred vision and has papilledema along with disorientation, the physician should be notified immediately.

Before any intervention can be instituted, the cause of the postoperative hypertension must be determined. First, the evaluation should focus on the equipment being used to determine the blood pressure; it may not be functioning correctly. For example, the blood pressure cuff may be too

Table 9-4	**Adrenergic Drugs According to Action**
Generic Name	Trade Name

DIRECT-ACTING ADRENERGIC AMINES

Epinephrine	Adrenalin
Norepinephrine	Levophed
Dopamine	Intropin
Dobutamine	Dobutrex
Isoproterenol	Isuprel
Methoxamine	Vasoxyl
Phenylephrine	Neosynephrine

INDIRECT-ACTING ADRENERGIC AMINES

Metaraminol	Aramine
Mephentermine	Wyamine
Ephedrine	Ephedrine

narrow; the transducer may not be calibrated correctly; or there may be transducer overshoot. Next, the evaluation should focus on preexisting diseases. More specifically, the patient may have essential hypertension, and the blood pressure readings may be "normal" for that patient.

Increased sympathetic nervous system activity causes postoperative hypertension. More specifically, pain, stimulation by an endotracheal tube, bladder distention, and preeclampsia are some of the clinical phenomena that may lead to hypertension. Postoperative pain should be assessed, because it can cause a significant degree of hypertension. Pain can be eliminated as a causative factor by determining whether adequate analgesia exists. If the patient is experiencing a significant amount of pain, an analgesic should be administered immediately. In addition, if the hypertension is caused by acute anxiety, the use of sedatives may dramatically reduce the blood pressure. Hypoxemia along with hypercarbia due to hypoventilation is also a common cause of postoperative hypertension. Hence during the evaluation of the patient, the patient's rate and depth of ventilation should be assessed. If the patient is experiencing hypoventilation, prompt use of the stir-up regimen is mandated. Another assessment tool to use in the evaluation of postoperative hypertension is the amount and degree of hypothermia. More specifically, if the patient is shivering, an accompanying increase in blood pressure will be seen. Prompt interventions to increase the patient's core temperature that will reduce shivering is warranted (see Chapter 50). Assessment of the patient's fluid volume status should be made to determine whether he or she is hypervolemic, because fluid overload can cause postoperative hypertension. Also, if the patient has acute pulmonary edema caused by hypertensive heart disease, correction of the pulmonary edema usually reduces the blood pressure to acceptable limits. Certainly, a determination should be made to see whether a hypertensive emergency exists—if it does, treatment must be started promptly.

If pharmacologic antihypertensive therapy is deemed necessary by the physician, the drugs listed in Table 9-5 usually are instituted. For severe postoperative hypertension, SNP is probably the drug of choice. While the SNP is being prepared, nifedipine (Adalat, Procardia) can be given sublingually. Nifedipine reduces the blood pressure and enhances coronary blood flow, especially in the presence of ischemic heart disease. Also, the use of nifedipine may preclude the use of a central venous catheter that is required when SNP is given. To give nifedipine sublingually, puncture a 10-mg capsule with a pin in several places and squeeze the contents under the tongue. Should SNP be required, the dose is 0.25 to 0.5 µg per kg per minute. Once the patient is stabilized, hydralazine 5 to 10 mg and propranolol 0.2 to 0.5 mg may be given in repeated doses intravenously to wean the patient off SNP. Propranolol should be titrated to maintain the heart rate at about 100 beats per minute. Other beta blockers, such as labetalol, metoprolol, and esmolol, may be used intravenously. Esmolol may be the drug of choice because of its short duration of action and rapid onset. The hydralazine can be given as intravenous boluses every 20 to 30 minutes to keep the patient normotensive. Because these drugs are extremely potent and have their own complications, they are discussed briefly in the following sections.

Diazoxide (Hyperstat)

Diazoxide is avidly bound to and inactivated by serum proteins and thus must be given as a rapid (within 15 seconds) intravenous bolus of 3 to 5 mg per kg every 5 minutes. After three bolus administrations, if the desired response is still not obtained, use of SNP should be considered. This is the major disadvantage of diazoxide as compared with SNP: diazoxide cannot be titrated in accordance with the patient's response. The onset of action of this drug is within 3 to 5 minutes, and its duration is between 5 and 12 hours. Its action is immediate and is achieved through its direct vasodilating effects. Because it has more effect on the resistance vessels than the capacitance vessels, it decreases the afterload and has no effect on the preload. It is usually advantageous to concurrently administer a loop diuretic, such as furosemide (40 to 80 mg intravenously), especially if the patient is edematous as a result of either cardiac or renal failure.

Sodium Nitroprusside (Nipride)

A compound of unusual chemical structure, SNP is immediately effective in all cases of severe hypertensive crises, including those resistant to

Table 9-5 Drugs Used to Treat Hypertensive Crisis

Drug*	Route	Initial Dose	Onset of Action (min)	Duration of Action	Comment
Diazoxide (Hyperstat)	IV	3-5 mg/kg slow bolus	3-5	5-12 hr	
Sodium nitroprusside (Nipride, Nitropress)	IV	0.25-0.5 µg/kg/min	1-2	<5 min	Titrate dose for desired effect
Nitroglycerin (Tridil, Nitrol IV, Nitrostat IV)	IV	0.25-3 µg/kg/min	2-5	<5 min	
Phentolamine (Regitine)	IV	5-15 mg bolus; 200-400 mg/L infusion	Immediate	<15 min	Titrate dose for desired effect
Hydralazine (Apresoline)	IV IM	5-10 mg 10-40 mg	15-20 30	4-6 hr	Given slowly when IV
Trimethaphan camsylate (Arfonad)	IV	10-20 µg/kg/min	1	2-4 min	
Propranolol (Inderal, Ipran)	IV	0.1-0.5 mg slowly, up to 2 mg	10	4-6 hr	May repeat dose
Esmolol (Brevibloc)	IV	50-300 µg/kg/min	5	20 min	Avoid concentration >10 mg/ml
Labetalol (Normodyne, Trandate)	IV	0.25 mg/kg	10	4-6 hr	Give slowly
Nifedipine (Procardia, Adalat)	SIV IV	10 mg 10 mg (slow)	3 5-10	7 hr	SIV dose while preparing nitroglycerin
Verapamil (Calan, Isoptin)	IV	2.5-5 mg	2-5	4-6 hr	

IV, Intravenous; *IM*, intramuscular; *SIV*, slow intravenous infusion.
*Listed by generic name, with trade name in parentheses.

diazoxide. Its action is thought to result from the peripheral arteriolar dilatory effect of the drug. Because it can lower blood pressure rapidly, it requires careful intravenous administration with constant bedside arterial pressure monitoring. The drug is extremely light-sensitive and must be administered through bottles and tubing that are wrapped and protected from the light. Only fresh solutions should be used. Solutions that are more than 4 hours old should be discarded because they may form thiocyanates. Treatment is started with a solution of 250 ml of 5% dextrose in water and 50 mg of SNP (200 µg per ml), using an infusion pump to ensure a precise flow rate. A dose of 1 to 2 µg/kg/min usually produces a prompt decrease in blood pressure, which will return to control levels within 5 minutes after the drug is stopped. Acute postoperative hypertension can be treated with a one-time single intravenous injection of 50 to 100 µg of SNP. The onset of action of this drug is 1 or 2 minutes, and its duration of action is 2 to 5 minutes. Because of its unique chemical structure, cyanide is released into the blood stream when the drug is used. The cyanide is quickly converted to thiocyanate by the liver. Thiocyanate toxicity (fatigue, nausea, anorexia, muscle spasms, and disorientation) may result from prolonged use or from high dosages; therefore monitoring of serum thiocyanate levels is advised when the drug is used longer than 24 hours. Toxic symptoms appear with serum thiocyanate levels of 5 to 10 mg per dl, and the compound can be rapidly removed by peritoneal dialysis. As with diazoxide, once blood pressure has been brought to control levels, concomitant use of an oral medication such as guanethidine or methyldopa allows the gradual tapering and discontinuance of SNP.

Phentolamine (Regitine)

Phentolamine mesylate, an alpha-receptor blocker, is specifically indicated for managing hypertensive crises associated with increased circulating catecholamines. These crises may result from pheochromocytoma or the sudden release of tissue catecholamine stores caused by certain drugs or foods containing tyramine in patients receiving monoamine oxidase (MAO) inhibitors (pargyline derivatives, primarily Eutonyl). The antipressor effect of a single intravenous injection is short lived, usually lasting less than 15 minutes. Therefore administering phentolamine by intravenous infusion (200 to 400 g per L) is desirable, along with titrating the dosage to achieve the desired pressure level after the blood pressure has been controlled initially by a rapid intravenous dose of 2 to 15 mg. Because the drug blocks only alpha receptors, beta-mediated effects of the circulating catecholamine on the heart must be controlled with the specific beta blocker, propranolol hydrochloride.

With rare exception, these three drugs (diazoxide, SNP, and phentolamine) can be considered the mainstays of modern therapy in acute hypertensive crises. The other drugs discussed here should be considered second-line drugs. Their primary disadvantages include slower onset of action, rapid development of tachyphylaxis, and marked central nervous system depressant effects. In most instances, they should be used to supplement and initiate long-term control once the acute crisis is resolved by the primary drugs.

Hydralazine (Apresoline)

Hydralazine is not effective in hypertensive encephalopathy complicating acute or chronic glomerulonephropathy; it is used in encephalopathy that has chronic essential hypertension as an underlying cause. Blood pressure is reduced through vasodilatation, which reduces vascular resistance. This results in a marked increase in cardiac output and heart rate that can aggravate underlying angina and cardiac failure. The determining factor in this situation is the net change in myocardial oxygen consumption achieved by lowering the elevated afterload. On the other hand, a decrease in blood pressure produced by hydralazine is not accompanied by a commensurate decrease in renal blood flow, so it is especially suited for managing hypertensive emergencies associated with renal insufficiency. The initial intravenous dose of 5 to 10 mg should be given. The onset of action of this drug is 15 to 20 minutes, and the duration is about 4 to 6 hours. Alternatively, the drug dosage may be increased in 5-mg increments up to 20 mg. The maintenance dose depends on patient response but is generally 5 to 10 mg intravenously every 4 to 6 hours.

Trimethaphan Camsylate (Arfonad)

Trimethaphan is a ganglionic vasodepressor that blocks both the sympathetic and parasympathetic systems at the autonomic ganglia. The effect is primarily orthostatic; therefore large doses must be employed to reduce blood pressure in supine patients. The head of the bed should be elevated (reverse Trendelenburg), if possible, to augment the antipressor action. The dose of this drug is 10 to 20 µg per kg per minute. The onset of action is about 1 minute, and the duration of action is 2 to 4 minutes. The 500-mg ampule of trimethaphan is mixed in 250 ml of normal saline, which results in a strength of 2 mg per ml. Complications of such ganglionic blockade include atony of the bowel and bladder and paralytic ileus, especially when the drug is used longer than 24 hours. Because of the commensurate decrease in the glomerular filtration rate when the blood pressure is lowered by the use of this agent, it is not recommended for use in patients for whom renal insufficiency complicates the hypertensive crisis. Its major disadvantage is that it rapidly loses effectiveness after 24 to 72 hours and another agent must be substituted. The drug requires extremely close monitoring by the perianesthesia nurse.

Nitroglycerin

Nitroglycerin is a potent vasodilator that produces relaxation of both arterial and venous smooth muscles. The pharmacologic effects of nitroglycerin are mainly on the venous circulation. It produces an increase in venous capacitance, which leads to a reduction in venous return and a decrease in right atrial and pulmonary capillary wedge pressures. Therefore the main effect of nitroglycerin is a reduction in the preload. Also, the myocardial oxygen demand is decreased because of the decrease in myocardial wall tension.

Intravenous nitroglycerin may be indicated to treat myocardial ischemia, to control hypertension, to relieve angina pectoris, and to produce vasodilatation for patients in severe congestive heart failure.

When intravenous nitroglycerin is administered in the PACU, an automated infusion pump should be used. The usual dosage is between 0.25 and 3 μg per kg per minute. The onset of action for this drug is 2 to 5 minutes, and the duration of action is between 3 and 5 minutes. The patient should be continuously monitored for hypotension. Should hypotension occur, an alpha agonist, such as methoxamine, may be used to ensure that the patient's coronary perfusion pressure is maintained. Nitroglycerin migrates into plastic; hence the perianesthesia nurse should periodically change the plastic tubing on the automated infusion pump and also ensure that only glass bottles are used for dilution.

Propranolol (Inderal, Ipran)

Propranolol is the prototype beta-blocking drug; consequently, all drugs in this class are compared with propranolol. This drug is known to be nonselective because it blocks both beta$_1$ and beta$_2$ receptors. After administration of this drug, decreased heart rate, contractility, and cardiac output occur. It can be administered in single intravenous doses of 0.1 to 0.5 mg, with a maximum dose of about 2 mg.

Esmolol (Brevibloc)

Esmolol is a cardioselective, ultrashort-acting, beta-blocking agent with a rapid onset and short duration of action. Because it is cardioselective, esmolol does not appear to affect bronchial or vascular tone at the doses required to reduce the heart rate. This drug has also been shown to blunt the response to endotracheal intubation and can be effective in treating postoperative hypertension. In the treatment of postoperative hypertension, a loading dose of 500 μg per kg should be administered over a 1-minute period. Then, a continuous infusion of 50 to 300 μg per kg per minute should be started. The peak response of esmolol occurs in 5 minutes, with a duration of action of about 20 minutes.

Labetalol (Normodyne, Trandate)

Labetalol is a drug that possesses antagonist activity at both the alpha and beta receptors. Given intravenously, it is about seven times more potent on the beta receptors than on the alpha receptors. More specifically, this drug is an alpha$_1$ antagonist and has antagonist activities on both the beta$_1$ and beta$_2$ receptors. For treatment of postoperative hypertension, a loading dose of 0.25 mg per kg should be administered over a 2-minute period. After this, intravenous titration to effect should be done at 10-minute intervals to a total of 300 mg. If a continuous infusion is required, a dose of 2 mg per minute can be used.

Metoprolol (Lopressor)

Metoprolol is a beta blocker that can be used in patients with reactive and obstructive lung disease. This is because this drug selectively blocks the beta$_1$ effects and consequently blocks the inotropic and chronotropic responses. This selective beta-adrenergic effect is dose related; at high doses, both beta$_1$ and beta$_2$ receptors become blocked and airway resistance may increase. For treatment of postoperative hypertension, an intravenous dose of 2 to 5 mg should be used.

BIBLIOGRAPHY

Alspach J: Core curriculum for critical care nursing, ed 5, Philadelphia, 1998, WB Saunders.

Atlee J: Complications in Anesthesia, Philadelphia, 1999, WB Saunders.

Barash P, Cullen B, Stoelting R: Clinical anesthesia, ed 4, Philadelphia, 2000, Lippincott Williams & Wilkins.

Benumof J, Saidman L: Anesthesia and perioperative complications, ed 2, St Louis, 1999, Mosby.

Benumof J: Anesthesia and uncommon diseases, ed 4, Philadelphia, 1998, WB Saunders.

Bickley L, Hoekelman R: Bates' guide to physical examination and history taking, ed 7, Philadelphia, 1998, Lippincott Williams & Wilkins.

Cottrell J, Smith D: Anesthesia and neurosurgery, ed 4, St Louis, 2001, Mosby.

DeFazio-Quinn D: Ambulatory surgical nursing core curriculum, Philadelphia, 1999, WB Saunders.

Ganong W: Review of medical physiology, ed 20, New York, 2001, McGraw-Hill Professional.

Guyton A, Hall J: Textbook of medical physiology, ed 10, Philadelphia, 2000, WB Saunders.

Hardman J, Limbird L: Goodman and Gilman's the pharmacological basis of therapeutics, ed 10, New York, 2001, McGraw-Hill Professional.

Jacobsen W: Manual of postanesthesia care. Philadelphia, 1992, WB Saunders.

Kaye A: Essential neurosurgery, ed 2, St Louis, 1997, Mosby.

Katzung B, editor: Basic and clinical pharmacology, ed 8, Los Altos, CA, 2000, Appleton Lange.

Lake C, Hines R, Blitt C: Clinical monitoring: practical applications for anesthesia and critical care, St Louis, 2001, Mosby.

Litwack K, editor: Core curriculum for postanesthesia nursing practice, ed 3, Philadelphia, 1994, WB Saunders.

Longnecker D, Murphy F: Dripps/Eckenhoff/Vandam introduction to anesthesia, ed 9, Philadelphia, 1997, WB Saunders.

Longnecker D, Tinker J, Morgan G: Principles and practice of anesthesiology, ed 2, St Louis, 1998, Mosby.

Martin J: Positioning in anesthesia and surgery, ed 3, St Louis, 1997, Mosby.

McIntosh L: Essentials of nurse anesthesia, New York, 1997, McGraw-Hill.

Murray J, Nadel J: Textbook of respiratory medicine, ed 3, Philadelphia, 2001, WB Saunders.

Nagelhout J, Zaglaniczny K: Nurse anesthesia, ed 2, Philadelphia, 2001, WB Saunders.

Stone D: Perioperative care: anesthesia, medicine, and surgery, St Louis, 1998, Mosby.

Stoelting R: Pharmacology and physiology in anesthetic practice, ed 3, Philadelphia, 1999, Lippincott-Raven.

Stoelting R, Miller R: Basics of anesthesia, ed 4, New York, 2000, Churchill Livingstone.

Townsend C, Beauchamp R, Evers B et al: Sabiston textbook of surgery: the biological basis of modern surgical practice, ed 16, Philadelphia, 2001, WB Saunders.

Traver G, Tremper Mitchell J, Glodquist-Priestley G: Respiratory care: a clinical approach, Gaithersburg, Md, 1991, Aspen Publishers, Inc.

Waugaman W, Foster S, Rigor B: Principles and practice of nurse anesthesia, ed 3, Norwalk, CT, 1999, Appleton & Lange.

Waxman SJ, Waxman SG: Correlative neuroanatomy, ed 24, Norwalk, Conn 1999, Lange Medical Publishers.

Weinberg G: Basic science review of anesthesiology, New York, 1997, McGraw-Hill.

Wood M, Wood A: Drugs and anesthesia: pharmacology for the anesthesiologist, ed 2, Baltimore, 1990, Williams & Wilkins.

The inhalation anesthetic agents depress respiratory function. They also depend largely on the respiratory system for their removal during emergence from anesthesia. The other anesthetic agents, such as intravenous agents, also depress respiration. Much of the morbidity and mortality that occurs in the postanesthesia care unit (PACU) can be attributed to an alteration in lung mechanics and a dysfunction in airway dynamics. In fact, it is postulated that 70% to 80% of the morbidity and mortality occurring in the PACU is associated with some form of respiratory dysfunction. Consequently, a detailed discussion of the many facets of respiratory anatomy and physiology is presented in this chapter. If the perianesthesia nurse incorporates this information into clinical practice, care of the surgical patient in the immediate postoperative period will be enhanced.

DEFINITIONS

Acidemia: lower than normal blood pH (increased hydrogen ion concentration).

Acidosis: the process leading to an increase in hydrogen ion concentration in the blood.

Adventitious sounds: abnormal noises that may be heard superimposed on the patient's breath sounds.

Alkalemia: higher than normal blood pH (decreased hydrogen ion concentration).

Alkalosis: the process leading to a decrease in hydrogen ion concentration in the blood.

Apnea: the absence of breathing.

Apneustic breathing: prolonged inspiratory efforts interrupted by occasional expirations.

Atelectasis: collapse of the alveoli.

Bradypnea: respiratory rate in the adult that is lower than 8 breaths per minute.

Bronchiectasis: dilatation of the bronchi.

Bronchospasm: constriction of the bronchial airways caused by an increase in smooth muscle tone in the airways.

Cheyne-Stokes respirations: periods of apnea alternating with rhythmic, shallow, progressively deeper and then shallower respirations that are associated with brain damage, heart or kidney failure, or drug overdose.

Compliance (lung): a measure of distensibility of the lungs, the amount of change in volume per change in pressure across the lung.

Cyanosis: a sign of poor oxygen transport, characterized by a bluish discoloration of the skin produced when more than 5 grams of hemoglobin per deciliter of arterial blood is in the deoxygenated, or reduced, state.

Dyspnea: a patient's perception of shortness of breath.

Epistaxis: hemorrhage from the nose.

FIO$_2$: fractional inspired concentration of oxygen.

Hypercapnia: increased tension of carbon dioxide (PaCO$_2$) in the blood.

Hyperoxemia: increased tension of oxygen (PaO$_2$) in the blood.

Hyperpnea: increased rate of respirations.

Hyperventilation: overventilation of the alveoli in relation to the amount of carbon dioxide produced by the body.

Hypocapnia: decreased tension of carbon dioxide (PaCO$_2$) in the blood.

Hypoventilation: underventilation of the alveoli in relation to the amount of carbon dioxide produced by the body.

Hypoxemia: decreased tension of oxygen (PaO$_2$) in the blood.

Hypoxia: inadequate tissue oxygen levels.

Kussmaul respirations: rapid, deep respirations associated with diabetic ketoacidosis.

Methemoglobin: hemoglobin that has the iron atom in the ferric state.

Minute ventilation (V$_E$): the volume of air expired during a period of 1 minute.

Orthopnea: severe dyspnea that is relieved when the patient elevates his or her head and chest.

Oxyhemoglobin: hemoglobin that is fully oxygenated.

Paroxysmal nocturnal dyspnea (PND): a sudden onset of severe dyspnea when the patient is lying down.

Partial pressure: the pressure exerted by each individual gas when mixed in a container with other gases.

PEEP: positive end-expiratory pressure.

Polycythemia: increased number of red blood cells (RBCs) in the blood.

Rales: short, discontinuous, explosive adventitious sounds, usually called crackles.

Reduced hemoglobin: hemoglobin in the deoxy state (not fully saturated with oxygen).

Respiration: the process by which oxygen and carbon dioxide are exchanged between the outside atmosphere and the cells in the body.

Rhonchi: continuous musical adventitious sounds.

Torr: units of the Torricelli scale, the classic mercury scale, which is used to express the same value as mm Hg.

Ventilation: the mechanical movement of air in and out of the lungs.

Wheeze: a high-pitched, sibilant rhonchus usually produced on expiration.

RESPIRATORY SYSTEM ANATOMY

The Nose

The nose, which is the first area in which inhaled air is filtered (Fig. 10-1), is lined with ciliated epithelium. Cilia move mucus and particles of foreign matter to the pharynx to be expectorated or swallowed (Fig. 10-2). Other functions of the nose include humidification and warming of the inhaled air and the olfactory function of smell.

Dry gases are often administered during anesthesia. These gases dry the mucus membranes and

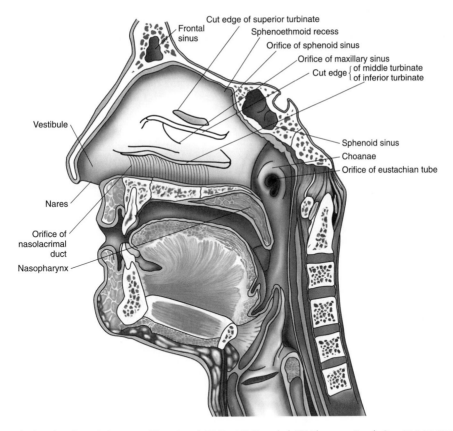

Fig. 10-1 Sagittal section through the nose. (*From Lough M, Boat T, Doershuk CF: The nose, Respir Care 20:844, 1975.*)

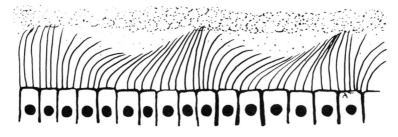

Fig. 10-2 Mucus blanket of the nasal airways. The outer (gel-like) layer rests on the tips of the beating cilia, and the inner (water) layer bathes the cilia. Particles are trapped on the sticky outer blanket and carried posteriorly into the nasopharynx by the organized beating of cilia. *(From Lough M, Boat T, Doershuk CF: The nose, Respir Care 20:845, 1975.)*

slow the action of the cilia. The administration of moist gases in the PACU by various humidification and mist therapy devices keeps this physiologic filter system viable.

A tracheostomy precludes the functions of the nose, and it is important that proper tracheostomy care, including the administration of humidified oxygen, be instituted.

The blood supply to the nose is provided by the internal and external maxillary arteries, which are derived from the external carotid artery, and by branches of the internal carotid arteries. The venous plexus of the nasal mucosa is drained into the common facial vein, the anterior facial vein, the exterior jugular vein, or the ophthalmic vein. A highly vascular plexus of vessels is located in the mucosa of the anterior nasal septum. This plexus is called Kiesselbach's plexus or Little's area. In most instances, this area is the source of epistaxis.

Epistaxis may occur in the PACU after trauma to the nasal veins from nasotracheal tubes or to nasal airways during anesthesia. If epistaxis occurs, prompt action should be taken to prevent aspiration of blood into the lungs. The patient should be positioned with his or her head up and flexed forward toward the chest. Cold compresses applied to the bridge of the nose and neck may be effective in slowing or stopping the bleeding. If the bleeding is profuse, the oral cavity should be suctioned carefully and the attending physician notified. A nasal pack or cautery with silver nitrate or electrical current may be necessary to stop the bleeding.

The Pharynx

The pharynx originates at the posterior aspect of the nasal cavities. It is called the nasopharynx until it reaches the soft palate, where it becomes the oropharynx. The oropharynx extends to the level of the hyoid bone, where it becomes the laryngeal pharynx, which extends caudally to below the hyoid bone.

The Larynx

The larynx, or voice box (Fig. 10-3), is situated anterior to the third, fourth, and fifth cervical vertebrae in the adult male. It is situated higher in women and children. Nine cartilages held together by ligaments and intertwined with many small muscles constitute the larynx. The thyroid cartilage, the largest, is V-shaped; its protruding prominence is commonly referred to as the Adam's apple. The thyroid cartilage is attached to the hyoid bone by the hyothyroid membrane and to the cricoid cartilage. The cricoid cartilage is situated below the thyroid cartilage and anteriorly forms a signet-shaped ring. The "signet" lies posteriorly as a quadrilateral lamina joined in front by a thin arch. The inner surface of the cricoid cartilage is lined with a mucus membrane. In children younger than 10 years of age, the cricoid cartilage is the smallest opening to the bronchi of the lungs.

The epiglottis, a cartilage of the larynx, is an important landmark for tracheal intubation that serves to deflect foreign objects away from the trachea. This cartilage is leaf-shaped and projects outward above the thyroid cartilage over the entrance to the trachea. The lower portion is attached to the thyroid lamina, and the anterior surface is attached to the hyoid bone and thereby to the base of the tongue. The valleys on either side of the glossoepiglottic fold are termed the valleculae.

The arytenoid cartilages are paired and articulate with the lamina of the cricoid through the

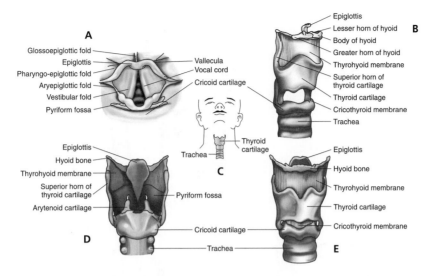

Fig. 10-3 The larynx as viewed from above (A) and the side (B) in relation to the head and neck (C), from behind (D), and from the front (E). *(A through E redrawn from Jacob SW, Francone CA, Lossow WJ: Structure and function in man, ed 5, Philadelphia, 1982, WB Saunders.)*

articular surface on the base of the arytenoid. The anterior angle of the arytenoid cartilage projects forward to form the vocal process. The medial surface of the cartilage is covered by a mucus membrane to form the lateral portion of the rima glottis—that is, the split between the vocal cords. The rima glottis is completed anteriorly by the thyroid cartilage and posteriorly by the cricoid cartilage.

The corniculate cartilages are two small nodules that are located at the apex of the arytenoid. The cuneiform cartilage is a flake of cartilage within the margin of the aryepiglottic folds. It probably serves to stiffen the folds.

The larynx has nine membranes and extrinsic or intrinsic ligaments. Extrinsic ligaments connect the thyroid cartilage and the epiglottis with the hyoid bone and the cricoid cartilage with the trachea. Intrinsic ligaments connect the cartilages of the larynx with each other.

The fissure between the vocal folds—or true cords—is termed the rima glottidis or glottis. In the adult, this opening between the vocal cords is the narrowest part of the laryngeal cavity. Any obstruction in this area leads to death by suffocation if not promptly relieved. The rima glottidis divides the laryngeal cavity into two main compartments: 1) the upper portion is the

vestibule, which extends from the laryngeal outlet to the vocal cords and includes the laryngeal sinus—sometimes called the middle compartment; and 2) the lower compartment, which extends from the vocal cords to the lower border of the cricoid cartilage and thereafter is continuous with the trachea.

The muscles of the larynx are also either intrinsic or extrinsic. The intrinsic muscles control the movements of the laryngeal framework. They open the cords on inspiration, close the cords and the laryngeal inlet during swallowing, and alter the tension of the cords during speech. The extrinsic muscles are involved in the movements of the larynx as a whole, such as in swallowing.

The nerve supply to the larynx is from the superior and recurrent laryngeal nerves of the vagus. The superior laryngeal nerve passes deep to both the internal and the external carotid arteries and divides into a small external branch that supplies the cricothyroid muscles that tense the vocal ligaments. The larger internal branch pierces the thyrohyoid membrane to provide sensory fibers to the mucosa of both sides of the epiglottis and the larynx above the cords.

The recurrent laryngeal nerve on the right side exits from the vagus as it crosses the right

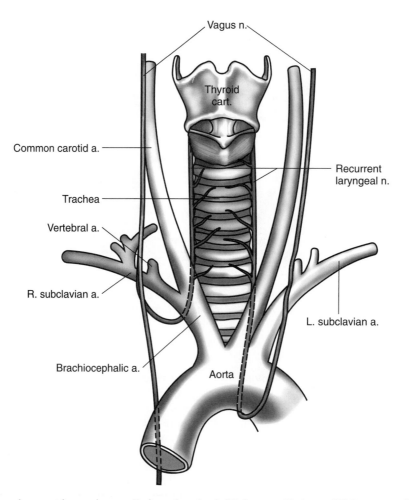

Fig. 10-4 Course of recurrent laryngeal nerve. *(Redrawn from Jacob SW, Francone CA, Lossow WJ: Structure and function in man, ed 5, Philadelphia, 1982, WB Saunders.)*

subclavian artery and ascends to the larynx in the groove between the trachea and esophagus (Fig. 10-4). Once it reaches the neck, it assumes the same relationships as on the right. This nerve provides the motor function to the intrinsic muscles of the larynx, with the exception of the cricothyroid. It also provides sensory function to the laryngeal mucosa below the vocal cords.

Laryngospasm, a spasm of the laryngeal muscle tissue, may be complete—when there is complete closure of the vocal cords—or incomplete—when the vocal cords are partially closed. Patients who experience partial or complete airway obstruction, such as laryngospasm, usually have a paradoxical, rocking motion of the chest wall. This motion can be misinterpreted as normal abdominal breathing. Hence the perianesthesia nurse should always auscultate the patient's lungs to determine the degree of ventilation and should not rely on just a visual assessment of the motion of the chest.

When a laryngospasm occurs in the PACU, prompt emergency treatment is necessary to save the patient's life. The perianesthesia nurse should have someone on the PACU staff summon the anesthetist or anesthesiologist when laryngospasm is suspected. Treatment consists of mask ventilation with sustained moderate pressure on

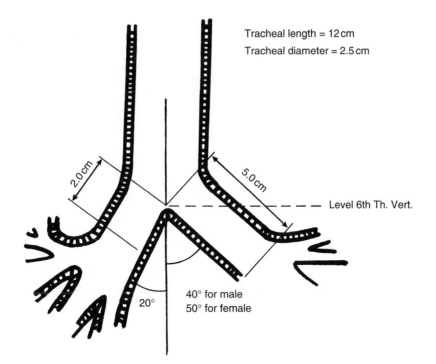

Tracheal length = 12 cm

Tracheal diameter = 2.5 cm

2.0 cm

5.0 cm

Level 6th Th. Vert.

40° for male
50° for female

20°

Fig. 10-5 Bifurcation of the trachea into the main stem bronchi. *(From Collins VJ: Principles of anesthesiology, ed 2, Philadelphia, 1976, Lea & Febiger.)*

the reservoir bag. This maneuver usually helps overcome the partial laryngospasm. Complete laryngospasm not relieved by positive pressure within at least 1 minute requires more aggressive treatment. Intravenous (0.5 mg per kg) or intramuscular (1 mg per kg) succinylcholine may be administered to relax the smooth muscle of the larynx. Endotracheal intubation may be necessary. The nurse must remember that ventilation of the patient should be continued until complete respiratory functioning has returned.

The Trachea

The trachea is a musculomembranous tube surrounded by 16 to 20 incomplete cartilaginous rings. These C-shaped rings prevent the collapse of the trachea, thereby maintaining free passage of air. The trachea is lined by ciliated columnar epithelium, which aids in the removal of foreign material.

The area at the distal end of the trachea at the point of bifurcation into the right and left main stem bronchi is called the carina (Fig. 10-5). The carina contains sensitive pressoreceptors, which on stimulation (i.e., an endotracheal tube) cause the patient to cough and "buck." The angle created at the point of bifurcation into the right and left main stem bronchi is clinically significant to the perianesthesia nurse. This angle varies according to the age and gender of the person (Table 10-1). The angle at the right main

Table 10-1	**Variations of Bronchial Bifurcation Angles in Adults and Children**	
	Right Bronchus (Degrees)	Left Bronchus (Degrees)
Newborn	10-35	30-65
Adult male	20	40
Adult female	19	51

stem bronchus is smaller than the angle at the left main stem bronchus. Foreign material can easily enter the right main stem bronchus at this point. Endotracheal tubes, if advanced too far, usually enter the right main stem bronchus, thereby occluding the left main stem bronchus. Thus the left lung cannot be ventilated. Signs of this complication include decreased or absent breath sounds in the left side of the chest, tachycardia, and uneven expansion of the chest on inspiration and expiration.

The Bronchi and Lungs

Each primary bronchus supplies a number of lobar bronchi (Fig. 10-6). Humans have an upper, middle, and lower lobe bronchus on the right and only an upper and lower lobe bronchus on the left. Within each pulmonary lobe, a lobar (secondary) bronchus soon divides into tertiary branches that are remarkably con-stant as to their number and distribution within the lobe. The segment of a lobe aerated by a ter-tiary bronchus is usually well delineated from adjoining segments by complete planes of con-nective tissue. These areas of the lung are well defined; therefore pulmonary diseases may be limited to a particular segment or segments of a lobe.

The bronchi bifurcate 22 or 23 times from the main stem bronchus to the terminal bronchi. These bronchi have connective tissue and carti-laginous support. The terminal bronchi branch to the bronchioles with a diameter of 1 mm or smaller and lack cartilaginous support. Bronchi-oles have thin, highly elastic walls composed of smooth muscle, which is arranged circularly. When the circular smooth muscle is contracted, the bronchiolar lumen is constricted. This circu-lar smooth muscle is innervated by the parasym-pathetic nervous system (vagus nerve), which

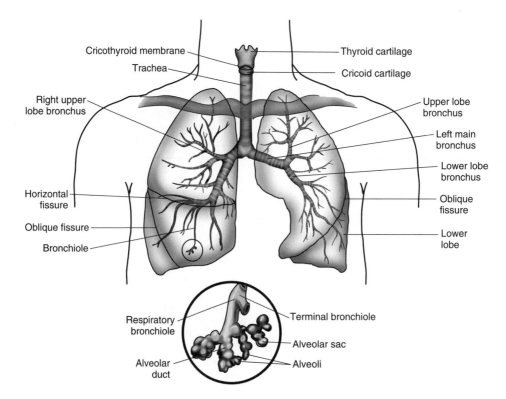

Fig. 10-6   Distribution of bronchi within the lungs. Enlarged inset shows detail of an alveolus. (*Redrawn from Jacob SW, Francone CA, Lossow WJ: Structure and function in man, ed 5, Philadelphia, 1982, WB Saunders.*)

causes constriction, and the sympathetic nervous system, which causes dilatation. The patency of the terminal bronchioles therefore is determined by the tonus of the muscle produced by a balance between the two components of the nervous system. Bronchospasm occurs when the smooth muscles constrict or experience spasm, ultimately leading to airway obstruction.

The terminal bronchioles divide into the respiratory bronchioles in which actual gas exchange first occurs. The respiratory bronchioles bifurcate to form alveolar ducts, and these, in turn, terminate in spherical enclosures called the alveolar sac. The sacs enclose a small but variable number of terminal alveoli.

The number of alveoli in an average adult's lungs is estimated to be about 750 million. The surface area available for gas exchange is approximately 125 m². Alveoli are shaped like soap bubbles in a glass. The interalveolar septum has a supporting latticework composed of elastic collagenous and reticular fibers. The capillaries are incorporated into and supported by the fibrous lattice. The capillary networks in the lungs are the richest in the body.

The lungs receive unoxygenated blood from the left and right pulmonary arteries, which originate from the right ventricle of the heart. The divisions of the pulmonary artery tend to follow the bifurcations of the airway. Typically, two pulmonary veins exit from each lung, and all four veins empty separately into the left atrium. The blood arriving in the rich pulmonary capillary network from the pulmonary arteries provides for the metabolic needs of the pulmonary parenchyma. Other portions of the lungs, such as the conducting vessels and airways, require their own private circulation. The bronchial arteries, which arise from the aorta, provide the oxygenated blood to the lung tissue. The blood of the bronchial arteries returns to the heart by way of the pulmonary veins.

Each lung is contained in a thin, elastic membranous sac called the visceral pleura, which is adherent to the external surface of the lung. Another membrane, the parietal pleura, lines the chest wall. These two membranes normally are quite close to each other. A few milliliters of viscous fluid is secreted between them to provide lubrication. The visceral pleura continuously absorbs this fluid.

RESPIRATORY SYSTEM PHYSIOLOGY

Lung Volumes and Capacities

Care of the perianesthesia patient is based largely on knowledge of the physiology and pathophysiology of the respiratory system. Dysfunction in lung volumes and capacities that occur in the postoperative patient is the compelling reason for instituting the stir-up regimen in the PACU. Accordingly, the physiology of the lung volumes and capacities as well as lung mechanics will be described in detail. Table 10-2 provides the definition and normal value for each lung volume and capacity. As shown in Table 10-2 and Figure 10-7, a lung capacity comprises two or more lung volumes.

The Lung Volumes. The tidal volume (V_T) represents the amount of air moved into or out of the lungs during a normal ventilatory excursion. It is an important lung volume to monitor when the patient is receiving ventilatory support. Because the V_T measurement is highly variable, it is not an extremely helpful parameter in pulmonary function tests. Clinically, the V_T can be estimated at 7 ml per kg. For example, a man weighing 70 kg has a V_T of approximately 490 ml ($7 \times 70 = 490$).

The expiratory reserve volume (ERV) is the maximum amount of air that can be expired from the resting position following a normal sponta-

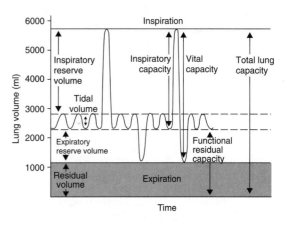

Fig. 10-7 Graphic representation of normal lung volumes and capacities. *(From Guyton A, Hall J: Textbook of medical physiology, ed 10, Philadelphia, 2000, WB Saunders.)*

Table 10-2	Lung Volumes and Capacities		
Terminology	Definition	Normal Male*	Normal Female*
Tidal volume (V_T)	Volume of air inspired or expired at each breath	660 (230)	550 (160)
Inspiratory reserve volume (IRV)	Maximum volume of air that can be inspired after a normal inspiration	2240 —	1480 —
Expiratory reserve volume (ERV)	Maximum volume of air that can be expired after a normal expiration	1240 (410)	730 (300)
Residual volume (RV)	Volume of air remaining in the lungs after a maximum expiration	2100 (520)	1570 (380)
Vital capacity (VC)	Maximum volume of air that can be expired after a maximum inspiration	4130 (750)	2760 (540)
Total lung capacity (TLC)	Total volume of air contained in the lungs at maximum inspiration	6230 (830)	4330 (620)
Inspiratory capacity (IC)	Maximum volume of air that can be inspired after a normal expiration	2900 —	2030 —
Functional residual capacity (FRC)	Volume of gas remaining in the lungs after a normal expiration	3330 (680)	2300 (490)

Adapted from Wylie WB, Churchill-Davidson HC, editors: A practice of anaesthesia, ed 4, London, 1978, Lloyd-Luke Medical Books.
*Data are mean values, with the standard in milliliters deviation in parentheses.

neous expiration. The ERV reflects muscle strength, thoracic mobility, and a balance of forces that determine the resting position of the lungs and chest wall following a normal expiration. It is a lung volume that is usually decreased in patients who are morbidly obese (see Chapter 45). It is also a lung volume that is decreased in the immediate postoperative period in patients who have had an upper abdominal or thoracic operation.

The residual volume (RV) is the volume of air that remains in the lungs at the end of a maximum expiration. This lung volume represents the balance of forces of the lung elastic forces and thoracic muscle strength. Patients who did not have their skeletal muscle relaxant adequately reversed at the end of the anesthetic may experience an elevated RV, because they are unable to generate enough muscle strength to force all the air out of their lungs. As the RV

increases, more air will remain in the lungs, so that it will not participate adequately in gas exchange and will become dead-space air. As the dead-space volume of air increases, it can impinge on the V_T, and hypoxemia can ensue. The importance of the RV is that it allows for continuous gas exchange throughout the entire breathing cycle by providing air to most of the alveoli and that it aerates the blood between breaths. Consequently, the RV prevents wide fluctuations in oxygen and carbon dioxide concentrations during inspiration and expiration.

The inspiratory reserve volume (IRV) reflects a balance of the lung elastic forces, muscle strength, and thoracic mobility. It is the maximum volume of air that can be inspired at the end of a normal spontaneous inspiration. Physiologically, the IRV is available to meet increased metabolic demand at a time of excess physical exertion. It assists in moving a larger volume of air into the alveoli through each ventilatory cycle to increase the overall performance and efficiency of the respiratory system.

The Lung Capacities. The inspiratory capacity (IC) is the maximum volume of air that can be inspired from the resting expiratory position. The IC is the sum of the V_T and the IRV.

The functional residual capacity (FRC) represents the previously mentioned resting position. The FRC is the volume of air remaining in the lungs at the end of a normal expiration when no respiratory muscle forces are applied. At FRC, the mechanical forces of the lung and thorax are at rest, and no air flow is present. Because the FRC is usually reduced in patients who are recovering from anesthesia, this particular lung capacity is of great importance to the perianesthesia nurse when intensive nursing care is rendered to such patients. For this reason, breathing maneuvers such as the sustained maximum inspiration (SMI) are instituted in the PACU—to raise the FRC (see next section on lung mechanics). The FRC represents the sum of the ERV and the RV. A severe increase in the FRC is often associated with pulmonary distention, which is technically a state of hyperinflation of the lung. This state of hyperinflation can be caused by two abnormal conditions: airway obstruction and loss of elasticity. Airway obstruction is exemplified by an episode of acute bronchial asthma; a loss of lung elasticity is usually associated with emphysema. A severe decrease in FRC is associated with pulmonary fibrosis and can be the sequela of postoperative atelectasis.

The vital capacity (VC) is the amount of air that can be expired following the deepest possible inspiration. It is the sum of the V_T, the ERV, and the IRV. The VC measures many factors that simultaneously affect ventilation, including activity of respiratory centers, motor nerves, and respiratory muscles, as well as thoracic maximum, airway and tissue resistance, and lung volume.

The total lung capacity (TLC) is simply the total amount of air in the lung at a maximum inspiration. The TLC is the sum of the VC and the RV.

The TLC, FRC, and RV are difficult to measure clinically because they include a gas volume that cannot be exhaled. Therefore the measurements require sophisticated pulmonary function testing equipment with gas dilution techniques or plethysmography. As will be seen, measurements of lung volumes and capacities are useful in the evaluation of lung function.

Lung Mechanics

Mechanical Features of the Lungs. Mechanical forces of the respiratory system actually determine the lung volumes and capacities. To understand how these lung volumes and capacities are determined and how they are affected by anesthesia and surgery, the perianesthesia nurse should become familiar with the "balance of forces" concept of the respiratory system (see section on the combined mechanical properties of the lungs and chest wall, p. 165). The PACU stir-up regimen is designed to increase the postoperative patient's lung volumes and capacities by enhancing the mechanical forces of the respiratory system.

The lungs and chest wall are viscoelastic structures, one within the other. Because they are elastic, the lungs always want to collapse or recoil to a smaller position. Therefore, as can be seen in the pressure-volume (P-V) curve of the lungs alone (Fig. 10-8), below RV the lungs are collapsed, and no pressure is transmitted across the lungs (i.e., no transpulmonary pressure). When the lungs are inflated to a volume halfway

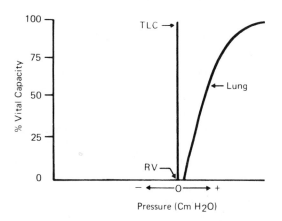

Fig. 10-8 Static deflation pressure-volume curve for the lung. The positive pressures represent pressures that tend to decrease lung volume. *TLC,* Total lung capacity; *RV,* residual volume. *(From Drain C: Physiology of the respiratory system related to anesthesia, CRNA: The Clinical Forum for Nurse Anesthetists 7(4):163-180, 1996.)*

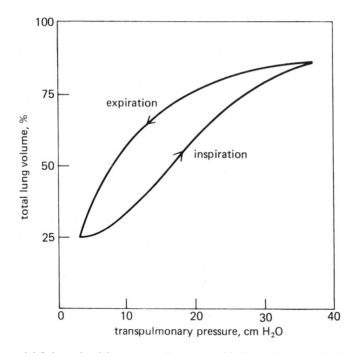

Fig. 10-9 The inflation and deflation paths of the pressure-volume curve of the lungs. *(From Levitzky M: Pulmonary physiology, ed 5, New York, 1999, McGraw-Hill.)*

between RV and TLC, the lungs seek to recoil or collapse back to the resting position at or actually below RV; this is reflected by an increase in transpulmonary pressure. When the lungs are fully inflated at TLC, a maximum transpulmonary pressure is also exhibited. By analogy, when a balloon is completely deflated, the pressure measured at the mouth of the balloon is zero. When the balloon is partially inflated, the pressure increases as the elastic forces of the balloon try to make the balloon recoil to its resting position. If the balloon is maximally inflated, the elastic recoil of the balloon is greater, as is the pressure measured at the mouth of the balloon.

Pulmonary Hysteresis.   Inflation and deflation paths of the P-V curve of the lung are not aligned on top of each other (Fig. 10-9). The path of deformation (inspiration) to TLC is different from the path followed when the force is withdrawn (expiration) from TLC to RV. This phenomenon is known as pulmonary hysteresis. The factors that contribute to pulmonary hysteresis are 1) properties of the tissue elements (a minor

factor); 2) recruitment of lung units; and 3) the surface tension phenomenon (surfactant).

Elastic Properties of the Lung.   The elastic properties of the lung tissue contribute only a small part to the phenomenon of hysteresis.

Recruitment of Lung Units.   Recruitment of lung units has an important part in pulmonary hysteresis. To understand recruitment of lung units, the nurse must be familiar with the concept of airway closure. In the lung, there is an apex-to-base gradient of alveolar size (Fig. 10-10). This gradient occurs because of the weight of the lung, which tends to "pull" the lung toward its base. As a result, the pleural pressure is more negative at the apex than at the base of the lung. Ultimately, at low lung volumes, the alveoli at the apex are inflated more than the alveoli at the base. At the base of the lungs, some alveoli are closed to ventilation because the weight of the lungs in that area causes the pleural pressure to become positive. Airways open only when their critical opening pressure is achieved during inflation, and the lung units peripheral to them are recruited to participate in volume exchange. This is called

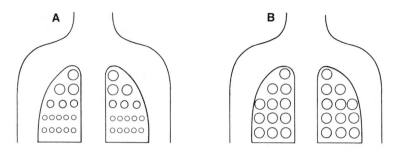

Fig. 10-10 Alveolar size from apex to base of lungs, as a subject inhales from residual volume (A) to total lung capacity (B).

radial traction or a tethering effect on airways. An analogy of a nylon stocking may aid in explaining this concept—when no traction is applied to the nylon stocking, the holes in the stocking are small. As traction is applied to the stocking from all sides, each nylon filament pulls on the others, which will spread apart all the other filaments; and the holes in the stocking will enlarge. Similarly, as one airway opens, it produces radial traction on the next airway and pulls the next airway open; in other words, it recruits airways to open. The volume of air in the alveoli behind the closed airways is termed the closing volume (CV). The CV plus the RV is termed the closing capacity (CC). The CC normally occurs below the FRC.

During the early emergence phase of anesthesia, patients usually have low lung volumes, which can lead to airway closure. Consequently, a postoperative breathing maneuver that has a maximum alveolar inflating pressure, a long alveolar inflating time, and high alveolar inflating volume—such as the SMI or yawn maneuver—should facilitate the maximum recruitment of lung units. With the recruitment of lung units, the FRC could be raised out of the closing volume range, and ultimately hypoxemia would be reduced.
Surface Tension Phenomenon. The surface tension phenomenon relates to the action of surfactant on lung tissue. Surfactant is a phospholipid rich in lecithin that is produced by the type II alveolar cells. Surfactant lines the alveolus as a thin, surface-active film. This film has a physiologic action of reducing the surface tension of the alveoli and terminal respiratory airways. If the surfactant were not present, the surface tension would be fixed and greater pressure would

be required to keep the alveolus open. As a result, small alveoli would empty into larger ones; atelectasis would regularly occur at low lung volumes; and large expanding pressures would be required to reopen collapsed lung units. Surfactant is also an important factor in alveolar inflation because it provides uniformity in the inflation of lung units. In these ways, surfactant helps impart stability to alveoli in the normal lung. In addition to playing a major role in pulmonary hysteresis, surfactant also contributes to lung recoil and reduces the workload of breathing.

Lung Compliance

Several other terms relating to the P-V curve of the lung deserve attention. One is lung compliance (C_L), which is defined as the change in volume for a given change in pressure, or the pressure required to maintain a given volume of inflation. The normal value for C_L is 0.1 L per cm H_2O.

$$C_L = \frac{\Delta V}{\Delta P}$$

C_L is a measure of the distensibility of the lungs during breathing. According to convention, C_L means the slope on the static deflation portion of the P-V curve over the V_T range. Therefore it can be said that C_L is the slope of the P-V curve, and it may remain unchanged even if marked changes in lung elastic properties cause a shift of the P-V curve to the left or right. Hence when the compliance of the lung is measured clinically, it is done over the V_T range, during deflation. Measuring the C_L over any other portion of the P-V curve may result in an inaccurate reading as compared with normal. Lung elastic recoil (Pst$_L$) is the pressure exerted by the lung (transpulmonary pressure) because of its tendency to recoil or collapse to a smaller resting state. At low lung volumes the Pst$_L$ is low, and at high lung volumes the Pst$_L$ is high. This elastic retractive force (Pst$_L$) is the result of the overall structural elements of the lung combined with the lung surface tension forces. As mentioned earlier, the C$_L$ represents the slope of the P-V curve, and the Pst$_L$ represents the points along the P-V curve. Changes in C$_L$ and Pst$_L$ have dramatic implications in the alteration in lung volumes that occurs in the immediate postoperative period (see section on postoperative lung volumes, p. 183).

The Equal Pressure Point. The equal pressure point (EPP) has many clinical implications to perianesthesia practice. More specifically, intraoperative and postoperative mechanical ventilation, along with pursed lips and abdominal breathing of the patient with compliant airways, are based on this concept.

One can imagine the alveoli and airways as a balloon in a box (Fig. 10-11). Flow out of the balloon is facilitated by the recoil of the balloon, forcing the air out of the balloon through the neck and out into the atmosphere. Adding pressure all over the box will force the air out of the balloon at a higher rate of flow. Physiologically, the balloon recoil is analogous to the alveolar recoil pressure (Palv). The pressure pushing down on the balloon and its neck corresponds to a positive pleural pressure (Ppl) that is generated on a forced expiratory maneuver. To move the air out of the alveoli, the alveolar pressure must exceed the pressure at the mouth (Pao). The pressure inside the neck of the balloon corresponds to the intraluminal airway pressure. Consequently, the alveolar pressure comprises the recoil pressure of the alveoli and the plural pressure. Also, the pressure to generate air flow decreases down the airway to the mouth (see Fig. 10-11). During a forced expiratory maneuver, the plural pressure pushes down on the alveoli and the airways. If the alveolar recoil pressure was 30 and the plural pressure was 20, the alveolar pressure would be 50. The pressure inside the airway (intraluminal pressure) decreases progressively downstream toward the mouth. The EPP occurs when the intraluminal pressure is equal to the plural pressure (20 = 20); from that point on, the plural

pressure exceeds the intraluminal pressure, and dynamic compression of the airway occurs. Total collapse of the airways from the EPP and the mouth does not normally occur because of the compliance of the airways. Physiologically, the dynamic compression will reduce the airways radius, thus resulting in an increase in flow rates in the compressed area that will aid physiologic mechanisms, such as the cough maneuver, to sheer and expel secretions and mucus out of the airways.

In the patient with highly compliant airways (i.e., chronic obstructive pulmonary disease), the dynamic compression can completely close the airways. The air that is trapped will increase the FRC and becomes dead space. The harder the patient tries to expel air, the greater the plural pressure will become, and more dynamic compression will occur; thus a vicious cycle ensues. Interventions to help these patients move air out of their lungs are focused on reducing the amount of dynamic compression on the airways. The interventions are to increase the expiratory time and provide physiologic positive end-expiratory pressure (PEEP). Lengthening the expiratory time will aid in reducing the amount of positive plural pressure on the airways, and physiological PEEP will enhance the airway's intraluminal pressure in the highly compliant airways. In the awake patient who has highly compliant airways, abdominal breathing will prolong the expiratory time, and pursed lips breathing will provide physiologic PEEP. In the anesthetized patient, prolonging the expiratory time (i.e., I:E ratio of 1:3) on the ventilator and using physiologic PEEP (i.e., 5 cm/H$_2$O) will aid in moving air out of the airways.

The Pulmonary Time Constant. The pulmonary time constant is similar to the half-life used to assess the pharmacokinetic activity of drugs. A time constant represents the amount of time required for flow to decrease by a rate equal to one half the initial flow. A time constant equals the resistance multiplied by the compliance. Therefore the time required to reach each time constant depends on the individual values of resistance and compliance. Under normal conditions, the decrease in flow at the first time constant is about 37% of the initial flow, or about 63% of the total volume added or removed from the lungs. The first time constant represents the time required to remove or add 63% of the total

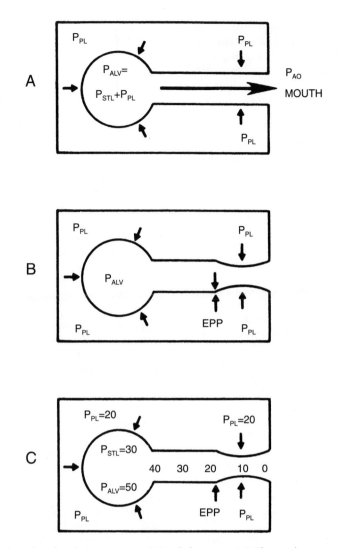

Fig. 10-11 The EPP during a forced expiratory maneuver. **A,** Bag-in-box concept. **B,** The equal pressure point added to model. **C,** Conceptual numbers used to illustrate the concept of the EPP. *PALV,* Alveolar pressure; *PSTL,* elastic recoil pressure; *PPL,* plural pressure; *PAO,* pressure at mouth. *(From Traver G: Respiratory nursing: the sience and the art, New York, 1982, John Wiley & Sons.)*

volume of air in the lungs. The decrease in flow rate at the second time constant is about 14%, and the percent volume of air added or removed from the lungs is 86%. The decrease in flow at the third time constant is 5%, with a corresponding 95% volume added or removed. Hence the higher the time constant, the more air that is removed or added to the lungs.

The clinical implications of time constants are extremely important in the care of perianesthe-

sia patients who have received an inhalation anesthetic. Patients who have increased airway resistance or increased C_L, or both, experience a prolonged time necessary for filling and emptying of the lungs. The lung units in this situation are referred to as "slow lung units." The type of patient with slow lung units usually has chronic obstructive pulmonary disease. Patients with a significant amount of increased secretions also have some slow lung units. Consequently, patients who have slow lung units usually expe-rience a slow emergence from inhalation anes-thesia. Patients with a low C_L, such as patients with pulmonary fibrosis, have "fast lung units." Hence these patients can fill or empty their lungs rather rapidly and experience a rapid emergence from inhalation anesthesia.

Mechanical Features of the Chest Wall. Because of the elastic properties of the chest wall, it always springs out or recoils outward, seeking larger resting volume. The resting volume of the lungs alone is below RV, and the resting volume of the chest wall is about 60% of the VC.

Action of the chest wall can be illustrated by the analogy of a wire screen attached around a balloon. The wire screen tends to spring outward, so at lower balloon volumes the screen pulls the balloon open. A measure of the pressure at the mouth of the balloon would reflect a negative number. At about 60% of the total capacity of the balloon, the screen no longer tends to spring outward. At that point, the addition of air causes the screen to push down on the balloon—a reflection of a positive pressure at the mouth of the balloon. The screen around the balloon can be likened to the chest wall. As shown in Figure 10-12, it is clear that at lower lung volumes the chest wall is inclined to recoil outward—thus cre-ating a negative pressure—and at about 60% of the VC the chest wall starts to push down on the lungs—thus creating a positive pressure. The result of the interplay between the chest wall's strong tendency to spring outward and the lung's strong tendency to recoil inward is the subat-mospheric pleural pressure.

Pleural pressure can become positive during a cough or other forced expiratory maneuvers. Pneumothorax can occur when the chest wall is opened or when air is injected into the pleural cavity. When this occurs, the lungs collapse because they naturally recoil to a smaller posi-tion; the ribs flare outward because of their natural inclination to recoil outward. Clinically, inspection of a patient with a pneumothorax may reveal protuding ribs on the affected side.

There are two types of pneumothorax—open (simple) and closed (tension). Simple pneu-mothorax occurs when air flow into the pleural space results in a positive pleural pressure. The lungs collapse because their recoil pressure is not counterbalanced by the negative pleural pressure.

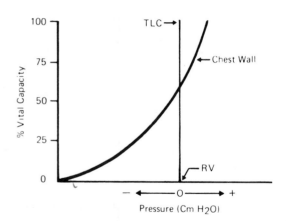

Fig. 10-12 The pressure-volume curve of the chest wall during deflation going from TLC to RV. Positive pressures of the chest wall represent pressures tending to decrease lung size, and the negative pressures represent the pressure tending to increase lung volume because of the outward recoil tendency of the chest wall at about 60% of the vital capacity or less. *TLC,* Total lung capacity; *RV,* residual volume. *(From Drain C: Physiology of the respiratory system related to anesthesia, CRNA: The Clinical Forum for Nurse Anesthetists 7(4):163-180, 1996.)*

Treatment for a pneumothorax can be conserva-tive or more aggressive, depending on the type and amount of pneumothorax. Aggressive treat-ment consists of the insertion of chest tubes into the pleural space to recreate the negative pleural pressure. This maneuver reestablishes normal ventilatory excursions. In most instances, the air leak between the lung and the pleural space will seal after the chest tubes have been removed. If air continues to flow into the intrapleural space but cannot escape, the intrapleural pressure will continually increase with each succeeding inspi-ration. Like a one-way valve, pressure increases and a tension pneumothorax develops. In a brief period, as the intrapleural pressure increases, the affected lung is compressed and puts a great amount of pressure on the mediastinum. Hypox-emia and reduction in cardiac output result, and if treatment is not instituted immediately, the patient may die. Treatment consists of immediate evacuation of the excess air from the intrapleural space either by chest tubes or by a large-bore needle. A tension pneumothorax is truly a medical emergency.

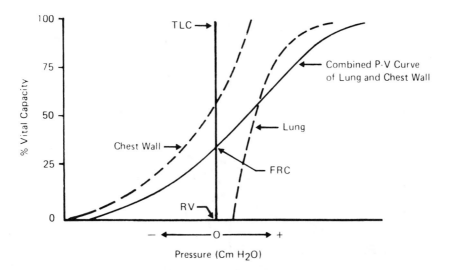

Fig. 10-13   The combined P-V curves of the lungs and chest wall. The individual P-V curves of the lungs and chest wall are represented by dashed lines. They are transposed from the static deflation P-V curves of the lungs (see Fig. 10-8) and chest wall (see Fig. 10-12). The combined P-V curve is the algebraic sum of the deflation curves of the lungs and chest wall. In the combined P-V curve, it can be seen that the FRC is determined by the balance of elastic forces of the lungs and chest wall when no respiratory muscles are applied. *P-V,* Pressure-volume; *TLC,* total lung capacity; *RV,* residual volume; *FRC,* functional residual capacity. *(From Drain C: Physiology of the respiratory system related to anesthesia, CRNA: The Clinical Forum for Nurse Anesthetists 7(4):163-180, 1996.)*

Combined Mechanical Properties of the Lungs and Chest Wall.   The combined P-V characteristics of the lungs and the chest wall have many implications for the perianesthesia nurse. The combined P-V curve is the algebraic sum of the individual P-V curves of the lungs and chest wall. When no muscle forces are applied to the respiratory system, the FRC is determined by a balance of elastic forces between the lungs and the chest wall (Fig. 10-13). Any pathophysiologic or pharmacologic process that affects the elasticity of either the lungs or the chest wall affects the FRC.

Alterations in the Balance of Pulmonary Forces in the Perianesthesia Patient.   During the induction of anesthesia, the shape of the P-V curve of the chest wall is altered. This agent-independent phenomenon is probably the result of loss of chest wall elasticity. Thus the P-V curve of the chest wall of a patient with normal lung function is shifted to the right; the balance of forces occurs sooner; and the FRC decreases (Fig. 10-14). This shift to the right affects the P-V curve of the lung; it also shifts to the right, and secondary changes

occur in the lung. More specifically, the changes consist of an increase in lung recoil ($\uparrow$Pst$_L$) and a decrease in C_L ($\downarrow C_L$). Ultimately, the lung becomes stiffer, and the FRC decreases and may drop into the closing capacity range. Hence during tidal ventilation, some airways are closed to ventilation, and ventilation-perfusion mismatching occurs ($\downarrow V_A/Q_C$), which ultimately leads to hypoxemia. Research indicates that this phenomenon, coupled with sighless breathing patterns in the PACU, can cause patients to experience hypoxemia in the recovery phase of the anesthetic (see section on postoperative lung volumes, p. 183).

Pulmonary Circulation
The basic functions of the pulmonary circulation are exchanging gas, providing a reservoir for the left ventricle, furnishing nutrition, and protecting the lungs.

Gas Exchange.   The major aspects of gas exchange are discussed in the section on blood gas transport (p. 169), but because of the implications for perianesthesia nursing care, the con-

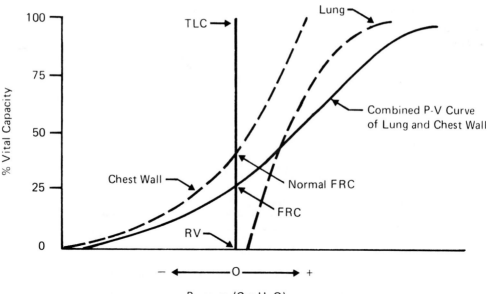

Fig. 10-14 P-V curve representing the lung mechanics of a patient in the immediate postoperative period who has undergone an upper abdominal or thoracic surgical procedure. This patient has a loss of chest wall elastic recoil that cause the lungs to become less compliant. Consequently, the combined P-V curve shifts to the right, thus leading to a decline in FRC because the balance of forces occurs at lower lung volumes. *P-V*, Pressure-volume; *FRC*, functional residual capacity; *TLC*, total lung capacity; *RV*, residual volume. *(From Drain C: Pathophysiology of the respiratory system related to anesthesia, CRNA: The Clinical Forum for Nurse Anesthetists 7(4):181-192, 1996.)*

cepts of transit time and pulmonary vascular resistance are presented here.

Of the 5 L of blood that flows through the lungs every minute, only 70 to 200 ml is active in gas exchange at any one time. The time it takes an RBC to cross the pulmonary capillary bed is 0.75 second, yet it takes the RBC only 0.25 second to become saturated with oxygen—that is, until all the oxygen-bonding sites on the hemoglobin molecule are occupied. Because the transit time is 0.75 second and the saturation time is only 0.25 second, the body has a tremendous back-up of 0.5 second for hemoglobin saturation with oxygen. If the RBCs move across the pulmonary capillary bed at an accelerated pace (decreased transit time), the amount of time available for oxygen to saturate the RBCs is decreased; during stress or exercise, however, the complete saturation of the hemoglobin can still be accomplished because the transit time of a RBC rarely decreases below 0.25 second.

However, this is not true for patients with interstitial fibrosis who have a thickened respiratory exchange membrane. They may have a normal PaO_2 at rest, but exercise or exertion of surgery increases the cardiac output and decreases the RBC transit time. Therefore the hemoglobin will not become completely saturated during its passage through the pulmonary capillary bed. This phenomenon occurs because more time is needed for oxygen to pass through the diseased membrane. For these patients, the lower limit for complete saturation may be 0.5 second, not 0.25 second. Hence, patients with disorders of the respiratory exchange membrane can demonstrate a lower oxygen saturation (SaO_2) on the pulse oximeter when they experience any exertion that could decrease RBC transit time. Clinically, this phenomenon is sometimes called desaturation on exercise. Therefore PACU patients who are suspected of having this problem should be given low-flow oxygen and closely monitored for desaturation via a pulse oximeter. Because of the possibility of desaturation, the low-flow oxygen should not be discontinued until the patient stabilizes, which may include continued administration after the patient is discharged from the PACU. Measures should be started to reduce the extrinsic factors—such as stress, elevated body temperature, and anxiety, which increase the cardiac output.

The pulmonary and systemic circulations have the same pump—the heart. The pulmonary system receives the same cardiac output as the systemic circulation—approximately 5 L per min. The pulmonary circulation—in comparison to the systemic circulation—is a low-pressure system with low resistance to flow, distensible vessels with extremely thin walls, and a small amount of smooth muscle. Many stimuli affect pulmonary vascular resistance. Probably the most potent vasoconstrictor of the lung is alveolar hypoxia. Research indicates that neuroendothelial bodies, which respond to a low PAO_2, may exist close to the pulmonary vascular bed. Also, the neuroendothelial bodies may liberate prostaglandins or histamine, or both, when alveolar hypoxia is present. Pulmonary vascular resistance does not seem to be affected by the volatile anesthetics such as halothane, enflurane, and isoflurane. However, nitrous oxide can increase pulmonary vascular resistance, especially in patients with preexisting pulmonary hypertension. Neonates who may or may not have preexisting pulmonary hypertension are prone to develop increased pulmonary vascular resistance when nitrous oxide is administered. If a PACU patient is prone to develop increased pulmonary vascular resistance, the effect of nitrous oxide on pulmonary vascular resistance will almost be dissipated due to the rapid excretion from the lungs of nitrous oxide because of its low blood-gas coefficient.

In the postoperative period, if a patient experiences atelectasis in some portion of the lungs, the PaO_2 in that particular area of the lungs will be reduced. As a result, the neuroendothelial bodies are stimulated to produce increased pulmonary vascular resistance in that area of the lungs. Eventually, the blood is redirected or shunted to areas of the lungs that are adequately ventilated. Because of this, the SaO_2 in a patient with atelectasis may indicate hypoxemia (<90%).

After about 5 to 10 minutes, the SaO_2 may be slightly improved because of the increased pulmonary vascular resistance in the area of atelectasis. Therefore the perianesthesia nurse should continue to use an aggressive stir-up regimen on a patient with atelectasis, even though the patient's SaO_2 values indicate a slight improvement.

Reservoir for the Left Ventricle.　In regard to their functioning as a reservoir for the left ventricle, the pulmonary veins are considered extensions of the left ventricle.

Nutrition.　The pulmonary circulation can be divided into the bronchial circulation and the actual pulmonary circulation. The bronchial circulation carries nutrients and oxygen down to the respiratory bronchioles in the lungs. The bronchial circulation empties its deoxygenated blood via the pulmonary veins to the left heart. The pulmonary circulation carries nutrients to the respiratory bronchioles and the alveoli.

Protection.　The role of the lungs in protection is vital for the preservation of the human organism. For example, on the surface of the pulmonary epithelium are invaginations called caveoli. Bradykinin and angiotensin I are enzymatically converted on the surface of the caveoli. Ninety percent of the bradykinin is deactivated in the caveoli during each pass through the lungs, and angiotensin I is converted to angiotensin II by angiotensin-converting enzyme in the lungs. In the presence of hypoxia, the conversion of angiotensin I to angiotensin II is inhibited. Also, in the hypoxemic state, less than 10% of the bradykinin is deactivated by the lungs. In the hypoxemic state, the liberated bradykinin then becomes prostaglandins. Interestingly, the inappropriate levels of prostaglandins due to hypoxemia in the chronic state are thought to produce the clubbing of the fingers in patients who experience long-standing chronic hypoxemia. Finally, the pulmonary epithelium also deactivates norepinephrine and serotonin. Serotonin plays an important part in platelet aggregation. Increased levels of serotonin due to decreased lung function caused by hypoxia or lung disease lead to a high risk for venous thrombus. The implications for PACU care are that patients who are immobile and hypoxemic ($SaO_2 < 90\%$) should be monitored for pulmonary and systemic thromboemboli.

Water Balance in the Lung

The alveoli stay dry by a combination of pressures and lymph flow (Fig. 10-15). The forces tending to push fluid out of the pulmonary capillaries are the capillary hydrostatic pressure (P_{cap}) minus the interstitial fluid hydrostatic pressure (P_{is}). The forces tending to pull fluid into the pulmonary capillaries are the colloid osmotic pressure of the proteins in the plasma of the pulmonary capillaries (π_{pl}) minus the colloid osmotic pressure of the proteins in the interstitial fluid (π_{is}). The Starling equation describes the movement of fluid across the capillary endothelium:

$$Q_f = K_f(P_{cap} - P_{is}) - \sigma_f(\pi_{pl} - \pi_{is})$$

in which

Q_f = net flow of fluid

K_f = capillary filtration coefficient. This describes the permeability characteristics of the membrane to fluids.

σ_f = is the reflection coefficient. This describes the ability of the membrane to prevent extravasation of solute particles.

Thus the membrane is permeable to fluid, and in normal circumstances, σ_f is equal to 1.0 in the equation.

Substituting normal values into the Starling equation,

$$Q_f = K_f[10 \text{ torr} - (-3 \text{ torr})]$$
$$- \sigma_f(25 \text{ torr} - 19 \text{ torr})$$

in which K_f and σ_f are dropped out of the equation because they are considered normal and do not affect the outcome of the example; therefore

$$Q_f = (13 \text{ torr}) - (6 \text{ torr})$$
$$Q_f = +7 \text{ torr}$$

Thus the pressure favors flow out of the capillaries to the interstitium of the alveolar wall tracts through the interstitial space to the perivascular and peribronchial spaces to facilitate transport of the fluid to the lymph nodes. Hence a net pressure of +7 torr pushes fluid to the interstitial space. The lymph flow draining the lungs is about 20 ml per hour in rate of flow. Thus the lungs depend on a continuous net fluid flux to remain in a consistently "dry" state.

Pulmonary edema, defined as increased total lung water, is associated with dysfunction of any parameter of the Starling equation. Examples of conditions that produce an overwhelming

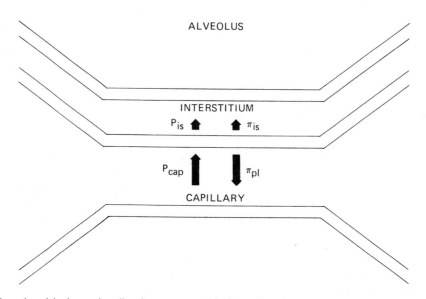

Fig. 10-15 Illustration of the factors that affect the movement of fluid from the pulmonary capillaries. P_{cap}, Capillary hydrostatic pressure; P_{is}, interstitial hydrostatic pressure (assumed to be negative); p_{pl}, plasma colloid pressure; p_{is}, interstitial colloid osmotic pressure. *(From Levitzky M: Pulmonary physiology, ed 5, New York, 1999, McGraw-Hill.)*

amount of fluid to be drained by the lymphatic system are elevated pulmonary capillary pressure (due to left-sided heart failure), decreased capillary colloid osmotic pressure (due to hypoproteinemia or overadministration of intravenous solutions), and extravasation of fluid through the pulmonary capillary membrane (due to adult respiratory distress syndrome). The earliest form of pulmonary edema is characterized by engorgement of the peribronchial and perivascular spaces and is known as interstitial edema. If interstitial edema is allowed to continue, alveolar pulmonary edema develops.

Pulmonary edema is difficult to assess in the early stages. As the fluid volume increases in the interstitium that surrounds the blood vessels and airways, reflex bronchospasm may occur. A chest radiograph at this time would reveal Kerley's B lines, which denote fluid in the interstitium. Once the lymphatics become completely overwhelmed, fluid will enter the alveoli. In the beginning of this pathophysiologic process, fine crackles are heard on auscultation. As pulmonary edema progresses into the alveoli, coarse crackles are heard, especially at the base of the lungs. Because of the direct stimulation of the J-receptors in the interstitium, the patient has a tachypneic ventilatory pattern. Initial arterial blood gas values demonstrate a low PaO_2 and $PaCO_2$. As the pulmonary edema progresses, the $PaCO_2$ increases because hyperventilation (tachypnea) is not able to counterbalance the rise in the carbon dioxide in the blood. Finally, when the pulmonary edema becomes fulminant, the sputum becomes frothy and blood-tinged.

Treatment of pulmonary edema is based on the Starling equation. If edema is cardiogenic, the focus of the treatment is to lower the hydrostatic pressures within the capillaries. Noncardiogenic pulmonary edema is usually treated with the infusion of albumin to increase the osmotic forces. Diuretics and dialysis also may be used in noncardiogenic edema in an effort to lower the vascular pressures. Positive end-expiratory or continuous positive airway pressure is used with high oxygen concentrations to correct the hypoxemia.

Blood Gas Transport

Respiration is the gas exchange between cellular levels in the body and the external environment. The three phases of respiration are the following:

1) ventilation, the phase of moving air in and out of the lungs; 2) transportation, which includes diffusion of gases in and out of the blood in both pulmonary and systemic capillaries, reactions of carbon dioxide and oxygen in the blood, and circulation of blood between the lungs and the tissue cells; and 3) gas exchange, in which oxygen is utilized and carbon dioxide is produced. Blood gas transport is the important link in carrying gas to or from the cell.

At sea level the barometric pressure is 760 torr. Air contains approximately 21% oxygen, which exerts a partial pressure of 159 torr. As described by Dalton's law of partial pressure, the total pressure of a given volume of a gas mixture is equal to the sum of the separate or partial pressures that each gas would exert if that gas alone occupied the entire volume. Therefore the total pressure is equal to the sum of the partial pressures of the major gases in the atmosphere. For example:

$$P_{TOTAL} = PN_2 + PO_2$$

in which P_{TOTAL} = total atmospheric pressure and PN_2 = partial pressure of nitrogen. If the actual numeric quantities are then substituted into the formula, 760 torr = 601 torr + 159 torr.

Expressed in percentages, 100% (total atmospheric pressure) is equal to 79.07% (nitrogen) plus 20.93% (oxygen). Thus nitrogen is 601 torr (0.7907×760), and oxygen is 159 torr (0.2093×760). In the lower airways, water vapor exerts a pressure that can be accounted for by Dalton's law. At the body temperature of 37°C, the water vapor pressure in the lower airways is 47 torr. Because the water vapor pressure affects the partial pressures of both nitrogen and oxygen, it is subtracted from the atmospheric pressure of 760 torr, which results in a pressure of 713 torr (760 torr − 47 torr = 713 torr). To determine the PO_2 in the lower airways, the percent oxygen (20.93) is multiplied by 713 torr, with a resultant PO_2 of 149.2 torr. The respiratory exchange ratio can be used to understand how the alveolar partial pressure of oxygen is determined. This ratio represents carbon dioxide production divided by oxygen consumption. The normal respiratory exchange ratio is 0.8. Theoretically, then, for every 10 torr of carbon dioxide that is added to the alveolus, 12 torr of oxygen is displaced. Therefore with no respiratory pathophysiology present, if the $PaCO_2$ is 40 torr, 48 torr of oxygen will be removed from the alveolus, in which: $4 \times 10 = 40$ torr (carbon dioxide) and thus $4 \times 12 = 48$ torr (oxygen).

This results in a PAO_2 of 101 torr (149 torr − 48 torr = 101 torr). This is called the 12-10 concept and is very helpful in assessing arterial blood gas determinations in the PACU (see section on causes of hypoxemia, p. 177).

As oxygen diffuses across the pulmonary membrane, the PO_2 is further decreased to 95 torr by a venous admixture. This effect occurs because of vascular shunts that normally redirect 1% or 2% of the total cardiac output either to nonaerated areas in the lungs themselves or directly through the heart, bypassing the lungs.

Oxygen Transport

Oxygen is carried in the blood in two forms: in combination with hemoglobin or in simple solution. About 98% of oxygen transported from the lungs to the cells is carried in combination with hemoglobin in the RBC; it is a reversible chemical combination. The remaining 2% is dissolved in the plasma and in the cytoplasm of the RBC. The amount of oxygen transported in both forms is directly proportional to the PO_2.

When the blood passes through the lungs, it does not normally become completely saturated with oxygen. Usually, the hemoglobin becomes about 97% saturated. Hemoglobin that is saturated with oxygen is called oxyhemoglobin.

Normally, the oxygen content of the arterial blood is 19.8 ml per dl of blood. This total oxygen content in the arterial blood (CaO_2) is equal to the oxygen-carrying capacity of hemoglobin, which is 1.34 times the number of grams of hemoglobin. That number divided by 100 is the oxygen content carried by the hemoglobin. To determine the total amount of oxygen in the blood, the oxygen content that is dissolved in the plasma must be added to the oxygen content of the hemoglobin. The amount of oxygen dissolved in the plasma is determined by multiplying the PaO_2 by the solubility coefficient for oxygen in plasma, which is 0.003.

Therefore the equation for the total oxygen content in the blood is:

$$CaO_2 = \frac{(Hb \times 1.34 \times \%Hb \text{ saturation})}{100} + (PaO_2 \times 0.003)$$

in which Hb = hemoglobin. If the normal values of Hb = 15 g, percent Hb saturation = 97, and PaO_2 = 95 torr are substituted into the equation:

$$CaO_2 = \frac{(15 \times 1.34 \times 97)}{100} + (95 \times 0.003)$$

$$CaO_2 = 19.497 + 0.285$$

$$CaO_2 = 19.782 \text{ ml of oxygen per dl of blood}$$

It must be remembered that oxygen content is different from oxygen partial pressures. Content refers only to the amount of oxygen carried by the blood—not to its partial pressure (PO_2).

In the lungs, venous blood is oxygenated or arterialized. The oxygen bond with hemoglobin is loose and reversible. The bond is also PO_2-dependent—that is, the higher the PaO_2, the more oxygen saturation of the hemoglobin. However, the hemoglobin cannot be supersaturated, because when all the bonding sites on the hemoglobin molecule are occupied by oxygen, no matter how much more oxygen is presented to the hemoglobin, it will not be able to bond to hemoglobin.

The oxygen-hemoglobin dissociation curve relates the percentage of oxygen saturation of hemoglobin to the PaO_2 value. Note in Figure 10-16 that the curve is sigmoid in shape with a very steep portion between the 10- and 50-torr PaO_2 range, with a leveling off above 70 torr. The flat portion of the curve indicates the capacity to oxygenate most of the hemoglobin despite wide variations in the PO_2 (70 to 98 torr). This flat portion of the curve can be called the association portion of the curve, and it corresponds to the external respiration that is taking place in the lungs. The steep portion of the curve indicates the capacity to unload large amounts of oxygen in response to small tissue PO_2 changes. This part of the curve is called the dissociation portion of the oxygen-hemoglobin dissociation curve.

As discussed, the normal oxygen content at the association portion of the curve is about 19.8 ml of oxygen per dl of blood. At the venous dissociation portion of the curve, the content of oxygen is 15.2 ml of oxygen per dl of blood. The following formula is used to derive the content of oxygen in the mixed venous blood (CvO_2):

$$CvO_2 = \frac{(Hb \times 1.34 \times \%Hb \text{ saturation})}{100} + (PvO_2 \times 0.003)$$

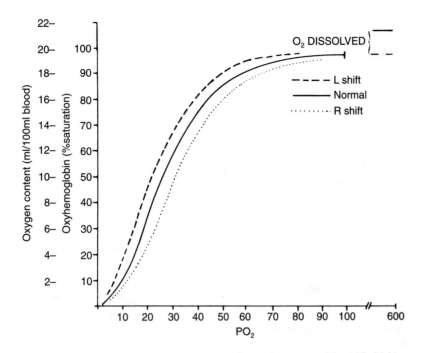

Fig. 10-16 Oxyhemoglobin dissociation curve. *(From Guenter C, Welch M: Pulmonary medicine, Philadelphia, 1977, JB Lippincott.)*

Substituting normal values for mixed venous blood of Hb = 15 g, percent Hb saturation = 75, and PvO_2 = 40 into the formula:

$$CvO_2 = \frac{(15 \times 1.34 \times 75)}{100} + (40 \times 0.003)$$

$$CvO_2 = 15.08 + 0.12$$

$$CvO_2 = 15.20 \text{ ml of oxygen per dl of blood}$$

Therefore in this example the net delivery of oxygen to the tissues is 4.6 ml of oxygen per dl of blood (19.8 − 15.2 = 4.6).

Factors that Affect Oxygen Transport. The association portion of the oxygen-hemoglobin dissociation curve is not necessarily a fixed line determined solely by the PaO_2. The height and the slope of the curve are dependent on many factors, including pH and temperature. Generally, a decrease in pH (an increase in hydrogen ions) or an increase in body temperature causes a shift of the curve to the right, which leads to a decrease in the height and slope of the curve. Ultimately, there will be less saturation (loading) of the hemoglobin for a given PaO_2. Hence patients who have a low pH or high tempera-

ture—or both—will probably benefit from a higher fraction of inspired oxygen (FIO_2) than normal to facilitate an appropriate level of saturation of their hemoglobin. However, before changes in the FIO_2 are made, arterial blood gas determinations should be analyzed.

At the dissociation portion of the oxygen-hemoglobin dissociation curve, the same is true. It is not a fixed line, because it also changes position in response to physiologic processes. At the tissue level, metabolically active tissues produce more carbon dioxide and more acid (↓pH) and have an elevated temperature. All these products of metabolism shift the curve to the right. The curve shifts far more in response to physiologic processes in the dissociation portion than in the association part. Metabolically active tissues produce more carbon dioxide and need more oxygen. The effect of carbon dioxide on the curve is closely related to the fact that deoxyhemoglobin binds hydrogen ions more actively than does oxyhemoglobin. As a result, at the tissue level, increased carbon dioxide decreases the affinity of hemoglobin for oxygen. Thus the dissociation portion of the curve is shifted to the right, and more oxygen is given to the tissue. This effect of carbon dioxide on oxygen transport is called the Bohr effect.

2,3-Diphosphoglycerate (2,3-DPG) regulates the release of oxygen to the tissue. It is a glycolytic intermediary metabolite that is more concentrated in the RBC than anywhere else in the body. High concentrations of 2,3-DPG shift the oxyhemoglobin dissociation curve to the right, making oxygen more available to the tissues. Lower concentrations of 2,3-DPG cause a shift of the curve to the left, ultimately leading to the release of less oxygen to the tissues. The clinical implications of these observations involve the administration of outdated whole blood. Whole blood stored longer than 21 days has low levels of 2,3-DPG. Therefore if outdated blood were administered to a patient, the tissues would not receive an appropriate amount of oxygen due to the shift to the left of the oxygen-hemoglobin dissociation curve.

Pulse Oximetry and the Oxygen Dissociation Curve.

Oxygen delivered to the tissues is determined by the cardiac output and the CaO_2. Most of the oxygen is bound to the hemoglobin, and the percentage of the oxygen bound to the hemoglobin is expressed as the SaO_2. The amount of oxygen that is dissolved in simple solution in the arterial blood is the PaO_2. A gradient is set from the lung to the tissues in regard to oxygen delivery and is represented by the oxygen dissociation curve. A normal curve, without any shifts left or right, is determined by the $PaCO_2$, pH, body temperature, and hemoglobin and 2,3-DPG levels. A normal curve is therefore set at values of $PaCO_2$ of 40 torr, pH of 7.4, temperature of 37°C, and hemoglobin of 15 g per dl. Using the oxygen dissociation curve (see Fig. 10-16), the PaO_2 can be determined by the SaO_2 reading on the pulse oximeter. For example, an SaO_2 of 90% corresponds to a PaO_2 of 60 torr. Looking at the curve, below an SaO_2 of 90%, the PaO_2 drops rapidly (the dissociation portion of the curve). Clinically, an SaO_2 of 90% can be considered to be hypoxemia, and severe hypoxemia occurs when the PaO_2 is less than 40 torr or the SaO_2 is 75%.

Carbon Dioxide Transport

The transport of carbon dioxide begins within each cell in the body. Carbon dioxide is a main byproduct of the energy-supplying mechanisms of the cell. Approximately 200 ml per minute of carbon dioxide is produced within the body at rest. Carbon dioxide is 20 times more soluble in water than oxygen; therefore it traverses the fluid compartments of the body rapidly. The intracellular partial pressure of carbon dioxide is 46 torr. A 1-torr gradient exists between the cell and the interstitial fluid. Carbon dioxide will diffuse out of the cell to the interstitial fluid and have a new partial pressure of 45 torr. When the tissue capillary blood enters the venules, the partial pressure of the carbon dioxide is 45 torr.

Carbon dioxide is transported in the blood in three forms: (1) physically dissolved in solution; (2) as carbaminohemoglobin; and (3) as bicarbonate ions.

Carbon Dioxide in Simple Solution.   About 10% of the total amount of carbon dioxide transported in the body is physically dissolved in solution.

Carbaminohemoglobin.   Approximately 30% of carbon dioxide is transported as carbaminohemoglobin, a chemical combination of carbon dioxide and hemoglobin that is reversible because the binding point on the hemoglobin is on the amino groups and is a very loose bond. This chemical bonding of carbon dioxide with hemoglobin can be graphically described by the use of the carbon dioxide dissociation curve. There are two differences between the carbon dioxide dissociation curve (Fig. 10-17) and the oxygen-hemoglobin dissociation curve. First, over the normal operating range of blood PCO_2 from 47 (venous) to 40 (arterial) torr, the slope of the carbon dioxide dissociation curve is nearly linear and not sigmoid like the oxygen-hemoglobin dissociation curve. Second, the total carbon dioxide content is about twice the total oxygen content. Oxygen has a definite effect on carbon dioxide transport. On the upper curve, or venous portion of the carbon dioxide curve, note that the point for the $PvCO_2$ is 47 and the PvO_2 is 40. On the lower curve, or arterial carbon dioxide curve, observe the points for the $PaCO_2$ of 40 torr and the PaO_2 of 100 torr. Notice how the venous carbon dioxide curve is shifted to the left and is above the arterial curve. This description is the effect of oxygen on carbon dioxide transport, or the Haldane effect. In terms of physiologic significance, the Haldane effect plays a more important role in gas transport than does the Bohr effect. Specifically, in the lungs, the binding of

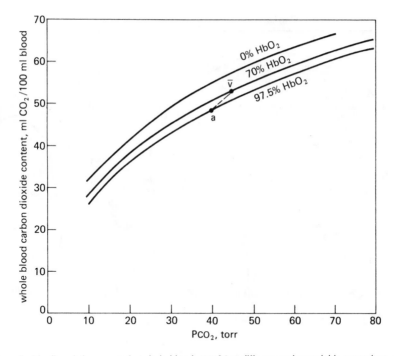

Fig. 10-17 Carbon dioxide dissociation curves for whole blood at 37°C at different oxyhemoglobin saturations. *a*, Arterial point (code; am); $\bar{v}$, mixed venous point. *(From Levitzky M: Pulmonary physiology, ed 5, New York, 1999, McGraw-Hill.)*

oxygen with hemoglobin tends to displace carbon dioxide from the hemoglobin (oxyhemoglobin is more acidic than deoxyhemoglobin). At the tissue level, oxygen is removed from the hemoglobin (due to a pressure gradient), reducing the acidity of the hemoglobin and enabling it to bind more carbon dioxide. In fact, because the hemoglobin is in the reduced state (deoxygenated), the hemoglobin can carry 6 volumes percent more carbon dioxide than the amount of carbon dioxide that could be carried by oxyhemoglobin.

Bicarbonate.   Sixty-five percent of carbon dioxide is transported as bicarbonate, which is the product of the reaction of carbon dioxide with water. When the carbon dioxide and water join, they form carbonic acid. Almost all the carbonic acid dissociates to bicarbonate and hydrogen ions, as seen in the following equation:

$$CO_2 + H_2O \xrightarrow{\text{Carbonic anhydrase}} H_2CO_3 \rightarrow$$
$$H^+ + HCO_3$$

This reaction occurs mostly within the RBCs, because carbonic anhydrase accelerates the hydration of carbon dioxide to carbonic acid 220 to 300 times faster than if carbon dioxide and water were joined without this enzymatic catalyst.

When the bicarbonate produced in this reaction in the RBCs exceeds the bicarbonate ion level in the plasma, it will diffuse out of the cell. The positively charged hydrogen ion tends to remain within the RBC and is buffered by hemoglobin. Because of ionic imbalance, chloride, a negatively charged ion that is abundant in the plasma, diffuses into the RBC to maintain electrical balance. This movement is called the chloride shift. Because of the increase in osmotically active particles within the cell, water from the plasma diffuses into the RBC. This process explains why the RBCs in the venous side of the circulation are slightly larger than the arterial RBCs (Fig. 10-18).

As the venous blood enters the pulmonary capillaries, the carbon dioxide in simple solution freely diffuses to the alveoli. The carbaminohemoglobin reverses to free the carbon dioxide, which diffuses across the alveoli and is then

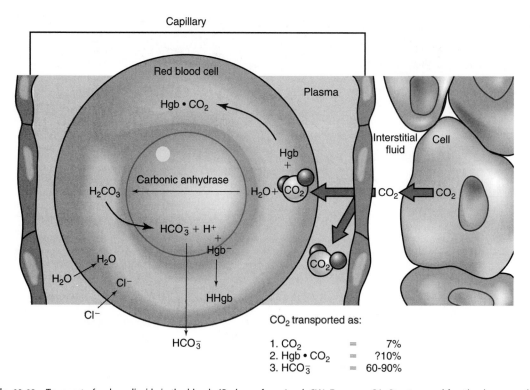

Fig. 10-18 Transport of carbon dioxide in the blood. *(Redrawn from Jacob SW, Francone CA: Structure and function in man, ed 3, Philadelphia, 1974, WB Saunders.)*

expired. The hydrogen and the bicarbonate combine to form carbonic acid, which is rapidly broken down by carbonic anhydrase to form carbon dioxide and water. The carbon dioxide then diffuses through the alveoli and is expired.

Not all carbon dioxide is eliminated by pulmonary ventilation. Other buffer systems that remove excess carbon dioxide are acid-base buffers and urinary excretion by the kidneys. The respiratory system can adjust to rapid fluctuations in carbon dioxide, whereas the kidneys may require hours to restore a normal carbon dioxide tension.

Acid-Base Relationships

A buffer is a substance that causes a lesser change in hydrogen ion concentration to occur in a solution on addition of an acid or base than would have occurred had the buffer not been present. The buffers can respond in seconds to fluctuations in carbon dioxide tension. Buffers include the carbonic acid–bicarbonate system, the proteinate-protein system, and the hemoglobinate-hemoglobin system.

The pH is a measure of alkalinity or acidity and depends on the concentration of hydrogen ions. Acidic solutions have more hydrogen ions, and alkaline solutions have fewer hydrogen ions. The pH is described in logarithmic form. Acid solutions have more hydrogen ions and a lower pH (which would indicate acidity). If, on the other hand, the hydrogen ion concentration is low, then the pH is high, which indicates alkalinity. The pH range is from 1 to 14, with 7 being equilibrium (pK). The normal pH in extracellular fluid is 7.35 to 7.45, which is slightly alkaline.

The normal bicarbonate level in the extracellular fluid is 24 mEq. Base excess is used to describe alkalosis or acidosis. If a positive base excess number is noted, this indicates more base in the extracellular fluid. If a negative number is

---

Box 10-1 **Common Causes of Carbon Dioxide Retention and Respiratory Acidosis (Hypoventilation)**

Normal lungs
Anesthesia
Sedative drugs (overdose)
Neuromuscular disease
Poliomyelitis
Myasthenia gravis
Guillain-Barré syndrome
Obesity (pickwickian syndrome)
Brain damage
Cardiac arrest
Pneumothorax
Pulmonary edema
Bronchospasm
Laryngospasm

Abnormal lungs
Chronic obstructive pulmonary disease (chronic bronchitis, asthma, and emphysema)
Diffuse infiltration pulmonary disease (advanced)
Kyphoscoliosis (severe)

Box 10-2 **Common Causes of Excessive Carbon Dioxide Elimination and Respiratory Alkalosis (Hyperventilation)**

Normal lungs
Anxiety
Fever
Drugs (aspirin)
Central nervous system lesions
Endotoxemia

Abnormal lungs
Pneumonia
Diffuse infiltrative pulmonary disease (early)
Acute bronchial asthma (early)
Pulmonary vascular disease
Congestive heart failure (early)

---

reported, the base is being used to neutralize the acid to a point of encroaching on the amount of available base, which is demonstrated by a negative value for the base excess (acidosis).

Respiratory Acid–Base Imbalances. Respiratory acidosis is characterized by a $PaCO_2$ above the normal range of 36 to 44 torr. All other primary processes that tend to cause acidosis are metabolic. Some common causes of carbon dioxide retention and respiratory acidosis are summarized in Box 10-1.

Respiratory alkalosis is characterized by a reduced $PaCO_2$. Hyperventilation frequently causes this disorder. Common causes of excessive carbon dioxide elimination and respiratory alkalosis are summarized in Box 10-2.

In respiratory alkalosis or acidosis, a linear exchange takes place between the carbon dioxide and bicarbonate concentrations, which is summarized as follows:

1. In acute respiratory acidosis, bicarbonate concentration is approximately 1 mEq per L for each 10-torr change in $PaCO_2$.

2. In chronic respiratory acidosis, the change in actual bicarbonate concentration is approximately 2 mEq per L for each 10-torr change in $PaCO_2$.

3. The change in actual bicarbonate concentration with a chronic change in $PaCO_2$ above the range of 40 torr change is approximately 4 mEq per L for each 10-torr change in $PaCO_2$. This rule holds true for 1 or 2 days after the onset of the disorder because of the slow renal buffer system.

Another rule of thumb to determine whether the acid-base disorder is entirely respiratory in origin is that an acute increase in $PaCO_2$ by 10 torr produces a corresponding decrease in pH by 0.07 pH units. In chronic hypercapnia, each increase in $PaCO_2$ by 10 torr results in a corresponding decrease in pH by 0.03 pH units. $PaCO_2$ and pH changes that deviate significantly from these standards suggest that the acid-base disorder is not completely respiratory in origin. For example, if a patient who is recovering from a spinal anesthetic in the PACU has blood gases (room air) of PaO_2 = 92 torr, $PaCO_2$ = 30 torr, and pH = 7.47 as compared with preoperative arterial blood gas values (room air) of PaO_2 = 80 torr, $PaCO_2$ = 40 torr, and pH = 7.40, the rule of thumb can be applied. Because the $PaCO_2$ decreased by 10 torr and the pH increased by 0.07 pH units, it is clear that the patient is experi-

Box 10-3	**Common Causes of Metabolic Acidosis**

Increased nonvolatile acids
Diabetes mellitus
Uremia
Severe exercise
Hypoxia
Shock
Idiopathic
Methyl alcohol ingestion (formic acid)
Aspirin ingestion (salicylic acid)
Excessive loss of bases (usually $NaCO_3$ from lower gastrointestinal tract)
Severe diarrhea (e.g., cholera, diarrhea in infants)
Fistulas (e.g., pancreatic, biliary)

Table 10-3 Summary of Blood Gas Discrepancies in Acidosis and Alkalosis

Condition	HCO_3^-	PCO_2	pH
Metabolic acidosis	↓	↓	↓
Respiratory acidosis	↑	↑	↓
Metabolic alkalosis	↑	↑	↑
Respiratory alkalosis	↓	↓	↓

encing respiratory alkalosis, not a metabolic disorder. Moreover, using the 12-10 concept, one can determine that this patient is probably suffering from acute hyperventilation. This is because the $PaCO_2$ decreased by 10; thus the PaO_2 should increase by 12—or from 80 to 92 torr.

Metabolic Acid–Base Imbalances. Metabolic acidosis usually results when there is an increase in nonvolatile acids or a loss of bases from the body. The usual result is a deficit in buffer, base excess, and bicarbonate. Because acidosis stimulates respiration, the $PaCO_2$ will usually decrease. The magnitude of the ventilatory response usually differentiates between acute and chronic metabolic acidosis. Some of the common causes of metabolic acidosis are summarized in Box 10-3.

Metabolic alkalosis is produced by an excessive elimination of nonvolatile acids (such as in vomiting, gastric aspiration, and hypokalemic alkalosis) or by an increase in bases (such as in alkali administration or hypochloremic alkalosis caused by some diuretics). A summary of blood gas discrepancies in each condition is provided in Table 10-3.

Matching of Ventilation to Perfusion

Distribution of Ventilation. A gravity-dependent gradient of pleural pressure in the upright lung exists at resting lung volumes. The weight of the lung tends to pull the lung tissue toward the base of the lung. As a result, the intrapleural pressure is more negative at the apex of the lung in comparison to the intrapleural pressure at the base and over the V_T range (the alveoli at the apex being more fully inflated as compared with the alveoli at the base). Consequently, the alveoli at the base have a greater capacity for volume change during inspiration, whereas the alveoli at the apex are already "stretched," or distended. In a normal subject who breathes out to RV and then inspires in small steps, the initial inspired air (a small portion) goes to the apex and the base remains completely underventilated. After a certain lung volume is attained, the base of the lung will receive almost all of the air because of the capacity of the alveoli at the base of the lung for volume change. Therefore because of the mechanical properties of the lung, the greatest volume change during inspiration from RV to TLC occurs near the base of the lungs.

Distribution of Perfusion. A gravity-dependent gradient for perfusion in the lungs exists; approximately 80% to 90% of blood flow occurs from the middle portion to an area near the base of the lungs. Therefore the blood flow per unit of lung volume increases down the lung from the apex to the base.

Matching. Matching of alveolar ventilation (V_A) to perfusion (Q_C) is defined in terms of a certain volume of alveolar gas that is required to arterialize a given volume of mixed venous blood. The normal alveolar ventilation ratio is:

$$\frac{V_A}{Q_C} = \frac{4000 \text{ ml/min}}{5000 \text{ ml/min}} = 0.8$$

If blood and gas were matched equally throughout the lung, the V_A/Q_C would be 1. However, in the normal lung, the matching of ventilation to perfusion is not proportional, which results in varying V_A/Q_C throughout the lung. More specifically ventilation at the apex is high as opposed to perfusion, and perfusion is higher than ventilation at the base of the lung. Finally, if all the V_A/Q_C relationships were added together, the mean ratio would be 0.8.

Causes of Hypoxemia

Hypoventilation. The PaO_2 and $PaCO_2$ are determined by the balance between the addition of oxygen and the removal of carbon dioxide by the alveolar ventilation and the removal of oxygen and the addition of carbon dioxide by the pulmonary capillary blood flow. If the alveolar ventilation is decreased (with no other lung pathologic changes present), the PaO_2 will decrease, and the $PaCO_2$ will increase. In fact, the PaO_2 will decrease almost proportionally to the increase in the $PaCO_2$. Recall the calculations made in the 12-10 concept. At any specific inspired oxygen tension, a 10-torr increase in the $PaCO_2$ causes an approximate 12-torr decrease in the arterial oxygen tension. For example, if the normal $PaCO_2$ is equal to 40 torr and the PaO_2 is equal to 95 torr and the patient's alveolar ventilation decreases because of narcotics given in the PACU, the $PaCO_2$ will increase to 60 torr. The new PaO_2 should be 71 torr (change of 20 torr in the $PaCO_2$, so 12 + 12 = 24 − 95 = 71). Therefore when one is assessing blood gas data and the 12-10 relationship is determined to be present, hypoventilation should be suspected. Remember, the 12-10 relationship does not have to be exact, but if the numbers are close to the 12-10 relationship, hypoventilation is the probable cause. An increased F_IO_2 will affect the 12-10 relationship. However, most patients in the PACU receive low-flow oxygen therapy, and therefore the F_IO_2 is usually between 25% and 50%. Consequently, if the values seem to change proportionally, hypoventilation can still be suspected. Hypoventilation is the most common cause of hypoxemia in the PACU. Nursing interventions should include administration of a higher F_IO_2 via low-flow oxygen therapy, stimulation of the patient, use of an aggressive stir-up regimen, and possible pharmacologic reversal of narcotics or muscle relaxants.

Ventilation/Perfusion Mismatching. If the 12-10 relationship is not present during the analysis of the arterial blood gases, V_A/Q_C mismatching is probably the cause. However, determining whether the mismatching problem is the result of increased or decreased V_A/Q_C is difficult. As seen in Figure 10-19, normal V_A/Q_C exists when appropriate matching of ventilation to perfusion occurs. Decreased V_A/Q_C occurs when the matching ventilation is reduced in comparison to perfusion of the alveoli, and increased V_A/Q_C is caused by increased ventilation as compared with perfusion.

Decreased Ventilation to Perfusion ($\downarrow V_A/Q_C$). Reduced ventilation, in comparison to perfusion, may be caused by excessive secretions or partial bronchospasm. When atelectasis or airway closure occurs, intrapulmonary shunting results. In these situations, oxygen cannot diffuse properly across to the pulmonary capillary blood. In decreased V_A/Q_C, some oxygen diffuses across from the alveoli to the pulmonary capillary blood. Thus the alveolar-arterial oxygen difference (PAO_2-PaO_2) will be slightly reduced. If there is a large gradient in the PAO_2-PaO_2, intrapulmonary shunting is probably present. For a

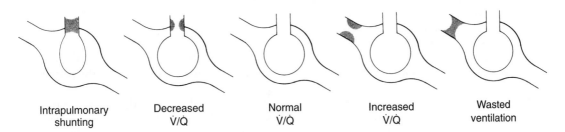

| Intrapulmonary shunting | Decreased $\dot{V}/\dot{Q}$ | Normal $\dot{V}/\dot{Q}$ | Increased $\dot{V}/\dot{Q}$ | Wasted ventilation |

Fig. 10-19 Graphic representation of normal and abnormal matching of ventilation (V_A) to perfusion (Q_C). *(From Harper R: A guide to respiratory care: physiology and clinical applications, Philadelphia, 1981, JB Lippincott.)*

patient breathing room air, the normal PAO_2-PaO_2 is between 5 and 15 torr. When a patient is breathing oxygen at a FIO_2 of 0.5 (50%), the PAO_2-PaO_2 should be about 50 torr. A gradient greatly in excess of 50 torr suggests V_A/Q_C mismatching. The focus of the nursing interventions to improve decreased V_A/Q_C is on airway clearance, reinflation of alveoli, and enhanced patency of the airways. The newly advocated stir-up regimen of turn, cascade cough, and SMI should improve the decreased V_A/Q_C. Percussion or vibration, or both, may also need to be instituted to facilitate secretion clearance. Also, if partial bronchospasm (expiratory wheeze) is suspected, the attending physician should be consulted about instituting appropriate bronchodilator therapy.

At this point, a clarification of terms used to describe decreased V_A/Q_C and shunt is in order. Basically, intrapulmonary shunts result in the mixing of venous blood that has not been properly oxygenated into the arterial blood (pulmonary vein). Anatomic shunts, which occur normally, are attributed to the 2% or 3% of the cardiac output that bypasses the lungs. The shunted, unoxygenated venous blood comes mainly from the bronchial circulation, which empties into the pulmonary veins, and from the thebesian vessels that drain the myocardium into the left heart. Intrapulmonary shunts occur when mixed venous blood does not become oxygenated when it passes by underventilated, unventilated, or collapsed alveoli. Absolute intrapulmonary shunts—sometimes called true shunts—are associated with totally unventilated or collapsed alveoli. Shuntlike intrapulmonary shunts are the areas of low V_A/Q_C in which blood draining the partially obstructed alveoli has a lower arterial oxygen content than the alveolar capillary units that are well matched. As a result, the presence of anatomic shunts is normal. Abnormal shunts can be classified as physiologic shunts. Physiologic shunts are made up of the anatomic shunts plus intrapulmonary shunts (absolute and shuntlike intrapulmonary shunts).

Increased Ventilation to Perfusion.

According to Figure 10-20, compromise of the circulation to the individual alveolocapillary unit creates an excess of ventilation in comparison to perfusion. If the flow of blood in the pulmonary capillary is

partially obstructed, increased V_A/Q_C results. If the flow of blood is completely obstructed—such as by a pulmonary embolus—only ventilation continues and produces wasted or dead space. Wasted ventilation is the total amount of inspired gas that does not contribute to carbon dioxide removal; it is also known as physiologic dead space ($V_D$physio). $V_D$physio is that volume of each breath that is inhaled but does not reach functioning terminal respiratory units. $V_D$physio has two components: alveolar and anatomic dead space. Alveolar dead space ($V_D$alv), as depicted in Figure 10-20, is that volume of air contributed by all those terminal respiratory units that are overventilated relative to their perfusion. Anatomic dead space ($V_D$anat) consists of the volume of air in the conducting airways that does not participate in gas exchange. This category includes all air down to the respiratory bronchioles. The following formula depicts $V_D$physio:

$$V_D physio = V_D alv + V_D anat$$

Normally, $V_D$physio consists mainly of $V_D$anat, with the $V_D$alv component being minute. This explains why the normal $V_D$physio volume in milliliters is approximately equal to the weight of a person in pounds. For example, a person who weighs 150 lb has a $V_D$physio of 150 ml. When alveoli become overventilated in comparison to perfused, the $V_D$alv increases, which in turn increases the $V_D$physio.

The amount of $V_D$physio can be determined by the Bohr equation. Clinically, the Bohr equation is commonly referred to as the V_D/V_T. The ratio of dead space (V_D) to V_T can be used to determine whether the obstruction to pulmonary capillary blood flow is partial V_A/Q_C or complete (wasted ventilation). The V_D/V_T can be derived from the following equation:

$$V_D/V_T = \frac{PaCO_2 - P_E CO_2}{P_E CO_2}$$

In which the $PaCO_2$ is the arterial carbon dioxide partial pressure and the $P_E CO_2$ is the partial pressure of the expired carbon dioxide. The V_D/V_T ratio is normally 0.3. If the V_D/V_T increases to 0.6, more than half of the V_T is dead space. Most patients can double their minute ventilation V_E, but beyond that amount the effort is too exhausting, and a V_D/V_T ratio of more than 0.6 usually

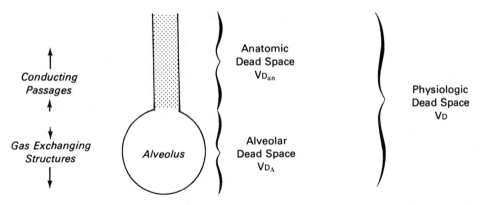

Fig. 10-20 Graphic representation of dead space. The physiologic dead space represents the sum of the anatomic dead space in the conducting passages (shaded area) and alveolar dead space in the alveoli (circle). *(From Harper R: A guide to respiratory care: physiology and clinical applications, Philadelphia, 1981, JB Lippincott.)*

mandates that the patient's ventilation be assisted mechanically.

Implications for Perianesthesia Care

In the early postoperative period (including the transport of the patient from the operating room to the PACU), the patient should be considered to have a reduced FRC and hypoventilation and to experience some ventilation-perfusion mismatch. All these factors lead to a reduction in arterial oxygenation as reflected by a low SaO_2 and PaO_2. Research now demonstrates that hypoxemia exists during transport to the PACU. Consequently, all patients should receive supplemental oxygenation during transport to the PACU and certainly throughout their stay there. In addition, because these respiratory alterations occur in almost all patients recovering from anesthesia, pulse oximetry should be used on each patient during transport and in the PACU.

REGULATION OF BREATHING

In the past, medullary control of breathing was thought to be a function of reciprocal inhibition between the inspiratory and expiratory centers. Research now indicates a more discrete regulatory process occurring at two levels: the sensors and the controllers. Patients with altered regulation and control of breathing present a significant challenge to the perianesthesia nurse. Also, anesthesia, surgery, and medications administered in the PACU can have a profound impact on the patient's regulatory processes of breathing.

The Sensors

Peripheral Chemoreceptors. The carotid and aortic bodies are the peripheral chemoreceptors and are located at the bifurcation of the common carotid arteries and at the arch of the aorta, respectively. The carotid and aortic bodies are responsible for the immediate increase in ventilation due to lack of oxygen. These peripheral chemoreceptors are made up of highly vascular tissue and glomus cells. The carotid and aortic bodies monitor only the PaO_2, not the CaO_2 of the hemoglobin. Therefore the receptors are not stimulated in conditions such as anemia and carbon monoxide and cyanide poisoning.

The carotid bodies are much more important physiologically than the aortic bodies. The carotid bodies respond, in order of degree of response, to low PaO_2, high $PaCO_2$, and low pH. The carotid bodies respond to a low PaO_2, and the response is augmented by a high $PaCO_2$, a low pH, or both. The physiologic responses to the stimulation of the carotid sinus are hyperpnea, bradycardia, and hypotension. The aortic bodies, on the other hand, respond to a low PaO_2 and high $PaCO_2$ but not to pH. The results of stimulation of the aortic bodies are hyperpnea, tachycardia, and hypertension.

The carotid and aortic bodies mainly respond to a low PaO_2. This response is commonly called the hypoxic or secondary drive. The impulse activity in these chemoreceptors begins at a PaO_2 of about 500 torr. A rapid increase in impulses occurs at a PaO_2 lower than 100 torr. The impulses are greatly increased as the PaO_2 falls below 60 torr. Below 30 torr, the impulse activity from the chemoreceptors decreases because of the direct oxygen deficit in the glomus cells. In addition, these peripheral arterial chemoreceptors are stimulated by low arterial blood pressure and increased sympathetic activity.

Central Chemoreceptors. The central chemoreceptors lie near the ventral surface of the medulla. Specifically, these chemosensitive areas are near the choroid plexus (venous blood) and next to the cerebrospinal fluid (CSF). The central chemoreceptors respond indirectly to carbon dioxide. This is because the blood-brain barrier allows lipid-soluble substances (e.g., carbon dioxide, oxygen, and water) to cross the barrier, whereas water-soluble substances (e.g., sodium, potassium, hydrogen ion, and bicarbonate) pass through the membrane at very slow rates. Bicarbonate requires active transport to cross the barrier. Therefore carbon dioxide enters the CSF and is hydrated to form carbonic acid. The carbonic acid rapidly dissociates to form hydrogen ion and bicarbonate. The hydrogen ion concentration in the CSF parallels the arterial PCO_2. Actually, the hydrogen ion concentration stimulates ventilation via hydrogen receptors located in the central chemoreceptor area. In summary, carbon dioxide has little direct effect on the stimulation of the receptors in the central chemoreceptor area but does have a potent indirect effect. This indirect effect is due to the inability of hydrogen ions to easily cross the blood-brain barrier. For this reason, changes in hydrogen ion concentration in the blood have considerably less effect in stimulating the chemoreceptor area than do changes in carbon dioxide. Consequently, the central chemoreceptor area precisely controls ventilation and therefore the $PaCO_2$. For that reason, the index to the adequacy of ventilation is the $PaCO_2$.

Bicarbonate is the only major buffer in the CSF. The pH of the CSF is a result of the ratio between bicarbonate and carbon dioxide in the CSF. Carbon dioxide is freely diffusible in and out of the CSF via the blood-brain barrier. However, bicarbonate is not freely diffusible and requires

active or passive transport to enter or leave the CSF. When an acute increase in the $PaCO_2$ occurs, carbon dioxide enters the CSF and is hydrated, and hydrogen ions and bicarbonate are formed. The hydrogen ion stimulates the chemoreceptors, and the bicarbonate decreases the pH of the CSF. The resultant hyperpnea lowers the blood $PaCO_2$, thus creating a gradient that favors the diffusion of carbon dioxide out of the CSF. The blood $PaCO_2$ and pH will be corrected immediately, but the pH in the CSF requires some time to reestablish a normal carbon dioxide–bicarbonate level because of the poor diffusibility of bicarbonate. This is usually not a problem for the person with normal respiratory function. However, for the patient with chronic carbon dioxide retention (chronic hypercapnia) who is hyperventilated to a "normal" $PaCO_2$ of 40 torr, serious deleterious effects may occur. Patients with a chronically elevated $PaCO_2$ have a higher amount of carbon dioxide and bicarbonate in the CSF, but the ratio is maintained in a chronic situation. In this instance, the patient will be breathing at a higher set point. That is, instead of being maintained at 40 torr, the normal $PaCO_2$ for this patient might be maintained at 46 torr, and near-normal sensitivity to changes in the $PaCO_2$ would be present. If this patient were aggressively ventilated in the PACU with the goal of lowering the $PaCO_2$ to 40 torr, significant negative repercussions could occur. With a lower $PaCO_2$ the carbon dioxide in the CSF diffuses out and the bicarbonate remains because of its inability to diffuse out of the CSF. Thus an excess of bicarbonate in comparison to carbon dioxide ($\uparrow$bicarbonate pool) exists in the CSF and causes the primary stimulus to ventilation to cease. Because the patient was hyperventilated, the $PaCO_2$ decreases and the PAO_2 increases (because of the 12-10 concept; see p. 169, blood gas transport). Therefore the secondary (hypoxic) drive may also become extinguished; thus this patient will have no effective drive for ventilation. If patients with chronic hypercapnia are acutely hyperventilated, they must be monitored for apnea once the accelerated ventilation is discontinued. It is more appropriate to maintain the $PaCO_2$ at the level that is normal for that patient to avoid an apneic situation. Thus for the patient with chronic carbon dioxide retention who is emerging from anesthesia, an overaggressive stir-up regimen (hyperventilation) should be avoided. The patient should perform the SMI at normal intervals, and the arterial blood gas values should be closely monitored.

In some patients with chronic carbon dioxide retention (chronic hypercapnia), the sensitivity to hydrogen ions via the carbon dioxide may be effectively decreased to the point at which the primary stimulus to ventilation becomes the low PaO_2 at the carotid and aortic bodies. The low PaO_2 becomes an effective stimulus to ventilation, especially when the $PaCO_2$ is elevated. The high $PaCO_2$ augments the response to the low PaO_2 by the peripheral chemoreceptors. For this reason, the patient is breathing via his or her hypoxic drive. Because the carotid bodies are the major peripheral chemoreceptors, patients using the hypoxic drive may also experience bradycardia and hypotension. For that reason, patients with abnormally high preoperative $PaCO_2$ values who have bradycardia and hypotension should be suspected of using the hypoxic drive as their primary drive to ventilation. In the PACU, patients suspected of primarily using this drive should be monitored closely and given oxygen to attain adequate oxygen content (a hemoglobin saturation of between 80% and 90%). The primary goal is to keep the patient oxygenated without extinguishing his or her main control of ventilation. High-flow techniques that use a Venturi mask that works on the Venturi principle to ensure precise FIO_2 values (i.e., 24% to 50%) can be used with these patients.

The Response to Carbon Dioxide. Carbon dioxide is the primary stimulus to ventilation. The carbon dioxide response test is used to assess the ventilatory response to carbon dioxide. In this test, the subject inhales carbon dioxide mixtures (with the PaO_2 held constant) so that the inspired $PaCO_2$ gradually increases. Normally, the V_E increases linearly as the $PaCO_2$ increases (Fig. 10-21). Some disease states and drugs cause the carbon dioxide response curve to shift to the left or the right. If the curve shifts to the left, the subject is more responsive to carbon dioxide. Factors such as thyroid toxicosis, aggressive personality, salicylates, and ketosis shift the curve to the left. A decreased ventilatory response to carbon dioxide occurs when the curve is shifted to the right. This is called a blunted response. Patients who have a blunted response to carbon

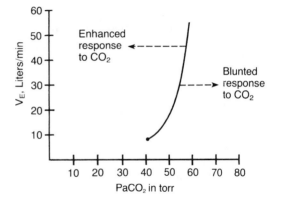

Fig. 10-21 Carbon dioxide response curve. *(From Traver G: Respiratory nursing: the science and the art, New York, 1982, John Wiley & Sons.)*

dioxide require intensive perianesthesia nursing care. The ventilatory response to an increased concentration of inspired carbon dioxide is blunted by hypothyroidism, mental depression, aging, general anesthetics, barbiturates, and narcotics. Many patients in the PACU either have these conditions or have received these drugs intraoperatively. This blunted response to carbon dioxide is one of the main justifications for giving supplemental oxygen to all patients who are emerging from anesthesia in the PACU. It is also the rationale behind the need for critical perianesthesia nursing care that includes frequent assessment and interventions such as the stir-up regimen to prevent respiratory depression.

Upper Airways Receptors. Receptors that are sensitive to mechanical stimulation and chemical agents and have afferent pathways via the trigeminal and olfactory nerves are located in the nose. Activation of these receptors can cause apnea, bradycardia, and, most commonly, a sneeze. When a patient is to be intubated nasally, the perianesthesia nurse should monitor for bradycardia and apnea and be prepared for necessary interventions. Atropine or glycopyrrolate (Robinul) may be required for their vagolytic effect; succinylcholine may facilitate the intubation. Finally, to provide positive-pressure ventilation, a bag-valve–mask system should be immediately available should apnea occur.

Receptors located in the epipharynx are sensitive to mechanical stimulation. Their activation is associated with the sniff or aspiration reflex. Mechanical stimulation of these receptors causes deep inspiration, bronchodilatation, and hypertension. This is a protective reflex that allows material in the epipharynx to be brought down to the pharynx, clearing the nasal airways. In the larynx are irritant receptors that respond to both mechanical and chemical stimulation. Afferent pathways from these receptors travel along the internal branch of the superior laryngeal nerve. Stimulation invokes many responses, including coughing, slow deep-breathing, apnea, bronchoconstriction, and hypertension. In addition, the trachea possesses irritant receptors. Stimulation of these receptors can cause responses such as coughing, bronchoconstriction, and hypertension.

During any procedure that involves the intubation of the trachea, the perianesthesia nurse should be prepared to assess the appropriate cardiorespiratory parameters and implement nursing care as required.

Lung Receptors. Pulmonary stretch receptors (PSRs) lie within the smooth muscle of the small airways. These receptors are activated by marked distention or deflation (atelectasis) of the lungs. On marked inflation of the lungs, the activation of the PSR leads to a slowing of inspiratory frequency because of an increase in expiratory time. Bronchodilatation and tachycardia also may result from activation of these receptors. The PSRs are thought to be part of the Hering-Breuer reflex. The low threshold for the PSR is present for approximately the first 3 months of life; after that the threshold is high throughout adulthood. Hence for the adult, the Hering-Breuer reflex is not important in the control of ventilation except in the anesthetized state. When an adult is under general anesthesia and ventilated with prolonged maximum lung inflations, a prolonged expiratory time can result because of activation of the PSR.

Of great interest in regard to the pathogenesis of asthma are the irritant receptors that lie between the airway epithelial cells. These receptors respond to chemical irritants (e.g., histamine) and mechanical irritants (e.g., small particles and aerosols) that irritate the pulmonary epithelium. The irritant receptors are mediated by vagal afferent fibers, and, on receptor stimulation, bronchoconstriction and hyperpnea occur.

It is suggested that the pathogenesis of asthma revolves around the sequence of histamine release, which stimulates the irritant receptors and ultimately leads to bronchoconstriction mediated via the vagus nerve.

The J, or juxtapulmonary capillary, receptors are located in the wall of the pulmonary capillaries. Like the irritant receptors, J-receptors' afferent impulses are transmitted to the central nervous system by the vagus nerve. Normal stimuli of the J-receptors include pneumonia, pulmonary congestion, and increased interstitial fluid pressure. Stimulation of these receptors by interstitial or pulmonary edema results in tachypnea, bradycardia, and hypotension. Therefore when assessing patients who are at risk for developing pulmonary edema, the nurse should always evaluate the rate of ventilation. Knowing that interstitial edema usually precedes pulmonary edema and that increased interstitial congestion stimulates the J-receptors, the nurse should consider a rapid, shallow breathing pattern to be a danger signal and report it to the attending physician.

Located in the walls of the large systemic arteries, especially in the aortic and carotid sinuses, are stretch receptors called baroreceptors. These receptors help to control the systemic blood pressure. They also affect ventilation. When the systemic blood pressure increases, a reflex hypoventilation will occur because of stimulation of the baroreceptors. On the other hand, a low systemic blood pressure causes the baroreceptors to produce a reflex hyperventilation. Hence if a patient in the PACU experiences a significant amount of hypertension or hypotension, a reflex ventilatory response will usually occur because of the stimulation of the baroreceptors in the large systemic arteries.

The Controllers

The controllers of breathing are located in the central nervous system. They comprise two functionally and anatomically separate components. Voluntary breathing is controlled in the cortex of the brain. Automatic breathing is controlled by structures within the brainstem. The spinal cord functions to integrate the output of the brainstem and the cortex. The cortex can override the other controllers of breathing if voluntary control is desired. Examples of voluntary control include voluntary hyperventilation and breath-holding.

The Brainstem. Located bilaterally in the upper pons is the pneumotaxic center. This center functions to fine-tune the respiratory pattern by modulating the activity of the apneustic center and regulating the respiratory system's response to stimuli such as hypercarbia, hypoxia, and lung inflation. Near the pontomedullary border is the apneustic center. This center is probably the site of the inspiratory cutoff switch that terminates inspiration. In fact, apneusis, which consists of prolonged inspirations with occasional expirations, results when the apneustic center has been deactivated. Consequently, the apneustic center is also a fine-tuner of the rhythm of breathing.

Located in the medullary center, above the spinal cord, are two groups of neurons: the dorsal respiratory group (DRG) and the ventral respiratory group (VRG). The DRG is composed of inspiratory neurons and is the initial intracranial processing site for many reflexes that affect breathing. It is probably the site of origin of the rhythmic respiratory drive. The DRG sends motor fibers via the phrenic nerve to the diaphragm. It sends inspiratory fibers to the VRG, which is also part of the medullary center. However, the VRG does not send fibers to the DRG; therefore the reciprocal inhibition theory of the regulation of breathing seems unlikely. The VRG is made up of both inspiratory and expiratory cells. The VRG neurons are driven by the cells of the DRG; therefore respiratory rhythmicity and the processing of sensory inputs do not occur initially within the VRG. The major function of the VRG is to project impulses to distant sites and drive either spinal respiratory motor neurons (primary intercostal and abdominal) or the auxiliary muscles of breathing innervated by the vagus nerve.

The DRG receives information from almost all the chemoreceptors, the baroreceptors, and the other sensors in the lung. In turn, the DRG generates a breathing rhythm that is fine-tuned by the apneustic center (inspiratory cutoff switch) and the pneumotaxic center. The inspiratory motor impulses are sent to the diaphragm and to the VRG. The VRG then drives spinal respiratory neurons (innervating the intercostal and abdominal muscles) or the auxiliary muscles

of respiration innervated by the vagus nerve. Again, the cerebral cortex can override these centers if voluntary control of breathing is desired. Also, the vagus nerve has a profound effect on many aspects of the control of breathing, because the afferent pathways of the vagus nerve from the stretch, J, and irritant receptors serve to modulate the rhythm of breathing. Thus any dysfunction that includes transection of the vagi results in irregular breathing patterns, depending on the level of dysfunction (pons or medulla).

POSTOPERATIVE LUNG VOLUMES

Postoperative pulmonary complications are the most common single cause of morbidity and mortality in the postoperative period. The reported incidence of postoperative pulmonary complications ranges from 4.5% to 76%.

Patients with Abnormal Pulmonary Function

When patients undergo anesthesia and surgery, certain risk factors predispose them to develop postoperative pulmonary complications. Patients at the highest risk are those with preexisting pulmonary problems with abnormal pulmonary function before surgery. The other major risk factors associated with postoperative pulmonary complications are chronic cigarette smoking, obesity, and advanced age.

Preexisting Pulmonary Disease. Patients with preexisting pulmonary disease can have clinical or subclinical manifestations of their disease state. Consequently, preoperative pulmonary function tests are valuable in assessing the presence or absence of pulmonary pathophysiology as well as in determining operative risk. Obstructive lung disease (i.e., asthma, emphysema, and chronic bronchitis)—the most common category of lung disease—can be assessed by flow-volume measurements. Burrows and associates suggest that a maximum voluntary ventilation that is less than 50% of what is predicted, a maximum expiratory flow rate below 220 L per min, or a forced expiratory volume in 1 second below 1.5 L indicates an increased operative risk for pulmonary complications. These flow-volume measurements are valuable predictors of the patient's ability to generate an adequate cough, which is a pulmonary defense mechanism rendered ineffective in the immediate postoperative period by anesthesia and surgery. Consequently, these patients require vigorous, informed nursing care in the immediate postoperative period. Priorities of nursing care should include frequent use of the stir-up regimen of turn, cascade cough, and SMI, along with the use of appropriate nursing interventions designed to enhance secretion clearance, which ensures airway patency.

Patients with restrictive lung disease (i.e., pulmonary fibrosis and morbid obesity) represent a significant risk for postoperative pulmonary complications when their pulmonary function test reveals a VC or a diffusion capacity of less than 50% of predicted values, or exercise arterial blood gas values that demonstrate slight hypoxemia on exertion. In the PACU, these patients require a vigorous stir-up regimen with attention to tissue oxygenation via monitoring for hypoxemia. This is needed because during the surgical experience and in the PACU, physiologic stress can occur. One of the major products of physiologic stress is an increase in cardiovascular parameters, which reduces the transit time of the RBCs across the respiratory gas exchange membrane. Because of the pathologic changes in the respiratory membrane, patients with restrictive lung disease can desaturate on exertion, such as in the stress reaction.

Cigarette Smoking. Chronic cigarette smoking has been shown to increase the incidence of postoperative pulmonary complications. Morton suggests that patients who smoke only 10 cigarettes a day have a sixfold increase in pulmonary morbidity in the postoperative period. The incidence of pulmonary embolism is higher in the smoker because of increased coagulability produced by chronic cigarette smoking. The ciliated epithelium of the lungs is damaged by chronic cigarette smoking. This damage can cause some blockage of the mucociliary transport system, which finally results in bronchiolar obstruction, infection, and atelectasis. Patients who smoke should be encouraged to stop smoking for at least 2 weeks before surgery to allow the mucociliary transport system to return to a nearly normal level of function. The focus of nursing care for the active chronic cigarette smoker should be similar to the interventions discussed for the patient with obstructive lung disease.

Obesity. The markedly overweight patient has a significant chance of developing postoperative pulmonary complications. This is caused by the altered lung volumes and capacities caused by the excess adipose tissue. Expansion of the lungs is hindered by an enlarged abdomen, which elevates the diaphragm and adds weight on the chest wall, thereby hindering the outward recoil of the chest wall. This leads to a decreased thoracic wall compliance and ultimately to a reduced FRC. Finally, these complications result in hypoxemia from increased airway closure and V_A/Q_C abnormalities (see Chapter 45). The goal of nursing interventions in the PACU is to prevent further airway closure. Thus a vigorous stir-up regimen, including early ambulation, should help prevent further reduction in the FRC. That measure reduces the amount of airway closure, alleviates the hypoxemia, and ultimately improves the outcome of the patient.

Advanced Age. Patients of advanced age (older than 70 years of age) have a slightly higher risk of developing postoperative pulmonary complications. A greater decrease in the FRC after surgery in patients of advanced age has been demonstrated. Because the closing volume increases with age, significant airway closure can occur postoperatively during tidal ventilation. Although advanced age is not associated with the same degree of risk as the factors previously discussed, it can increase the danger of the other risk factors. However, patients of advanced age should receive a vigorous stir-up regimen in the PACU if only because of the alterations in their lung mechanics.

Physiology of Perianesthesia Pulmonary Nursing Care

Because of the change in the mechanical properties of the lungs and chest wall, patients emerging from anesthesia experience a decrease in their lung volumes and capacities (Fig. 10-22). This is especially true of the patient who has undergone a thoracic or upper abdominal surgical procedure. In the PACU, a further reduction in lung volumes and capacities may be seen. The major factor that contributes to this reduction in lung volumes in the postoperative patient is a shallow, monotonous, sighless breathing pattern that is caused by general inhalation anesthesia, pain, and narcotics. Sighless ventilation may result in an uneven distribution of surfactant and a loss of stability of the small airways and alveoli, which

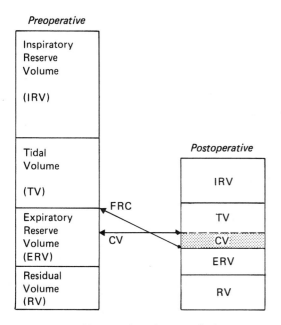

Preoperative

Inspiratory Reserve Volume (IRV)

Tidal Volume (TV)

Expiratory Reserve Volume (ERV)

Residual Volume (RV)

FRC

CV

Postoperative

IRV

TV

CV

ERV

RV

Fig. 10-22 Graphic comparison of preoperative lung volumes to the probable lung volumes in the immediate postoperative period in a patient who has undergone an upper abdominal surgical procedure. *FRC,* Functional residual capacity; *CV,* closing volume. *(From Drain C: Pathophysiology of the respiratory system related to anesthesia, CRNA: The Clinical Forum for Nurse Anesthetists 7(4):181-192, 1996.)*

can then lead to alveolar collapse and ultimately to atelectasis. Normally, adults breathe regularly and rhythmically, spontaneously performing a maximum inspiration that is held for about 3 seconds at the peak of inspiration. This physiologic process, or SMI, is commonly called a sigh or a yawn.

In normal lungs, the closing volume is less than the resting lung volume (i.e., the FRC), and airways remain open during tidal breathing. In the immediate postoperative period, patients who have a sighless, monotonous, low V_T ventilatory pattern usually have a reduced FRC. When the FRC plus V_T is within the closing volume range, the airways leading to dependent lung zones may be effectively closed throughout tidal breathing (see Fig. 10-22). Inspired gas is then distributed mainly to the upper or nondependent lung zones. Perfusion continues to follow the

normal gradient, with higher flows to the dependent areas of the lung.

In the immediate postoperative period, as airway closure occurs, gas is trapped behind closed airways. This sequestered air can become absorbed and the alveoli then become airless (atelectasis). The atelectasis, as it becomes more widespread, leads to a decrease in ventilation as compared with perfusion (low V_A/Q_C), which results in a widening of the PAO_2-PaO_2 and ultimately to hypoxemia. In addition, atelectatic areas in the lung provide an excellent culture medium in which pneumonia can develop.

Various investigators have demonstrated a decrease in lung volumes in the postoperative period. Patients who have undergone an upper abdominal surgical procedure experience an immediate postoperative decrease in the FRC from hour 1 to hour 2 (Fig. 10-23). The FRC then seems to return to near the baseline value by about the fourth postoperative hour. A second subsequent decrease in the FRC is then seen after hour 4, and baseline values are not restored until 5 days postoperatively. A possible explanation of the "peaks and valleys" in the FRC during the postoperative period may be that the first reduction in the FRC is associated with anesthesia and the latter reduction may be due to pain. General inhalation anesthesia and pain can dampen the physiologic sigh mechanism. Consequently, all patients who have undergone a surgical procedure—especially those who have their incision sites near the thorax or diaphragm—should be strongly encouraged to perform the SMI maneuver both in the PACU and on the surgical unit. The incentive spirometer, a device designed to encourage the patient with positive feedback to perform the SMI maneuver, can be used by the patient on the surgical unit.

OXYGEN ADMINISTRATION IN THE PACU

Administration of oxygen to the patient in the PACU is an important facet in the emergence phase of anesthesia. Oxygen is given to the PACU patient primarily because of the blunted or depressed response to carbon dioxide and low lung volumes. It is especially important that the patient who has received a general or spinal anesthetic be given supplemental oxygen during the recovery phase of anesthesia. The methods of

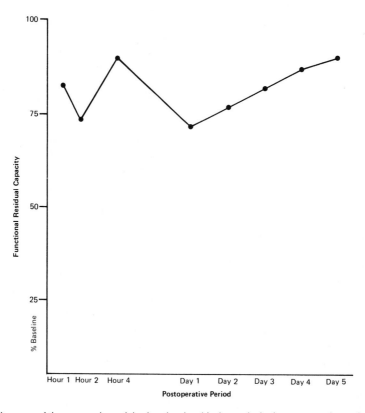

Fig. 10-23 Composite curve of the mean values of the functional residual capacity in the postoperative period. *(From Drain C: Anesthesia care of the patient with reactive airways disease, CRNA: The Clinical Forum for Nurse Anesthetists 7(4):207-212, 1996.)*

oxygen administration are summarized in Chapter 26.

Perianesthesia Nursing Care

A patent airway must be maintained throughout the administration of oxygen. The patient should be encouraged to cascade cough, perform the SMI, and change positions according to the stir-up regimen discussed in this chapter and in Chapter 26. If a nasal catheter is used, the catheter should be removed every 6 hours to be cleaned and reinserted into the other nostril. Also, the nasal mucosa should be inspected periodically for dryness when a nasal catheter or prongs are used. Oxygen given in the dry gas form can cause drying and irritation of the mucosa, impair the ciliary action, and thicken secretions; therefore oxygen should always be administered with humidity.

It is imperative for the perianesthesia nurse to receive a report from the anesthesiologist or anesthetist or both as to the patient's preoperative pulmonary status. It is especially important to ascertain whether the patient has a history of chronically retaining carbon dioxide, as occurs in chronic obstructive pulmonary disease. As described in this chapter, the patient with carbon dioxide retention who is receiving oxygen in the PACU should be monitored carefully for any signs of hypoventilation, confusion, or becoming semicomatose. If any of these signs appear, the surgeon and anesthesiologist or anesthetist should be notified immediately.

Oxygen Toxicity

When excessive concentrations of inspired oxygen (>60%) are administered to patients for a prolonged period, the eyes, lungs, and central nervous system can be damaged.

Eyes. Premature infants who have a high PaO_2 longer than 24 hours are at risk for developing retrolental fibroplasia, which is caused by vasoconstriction of the blood vessels of the retina as a result of high oxygen concentrations in the blood. It presents in an acute form as vascular retinopathy at the developing edge of blood vessels in the premature infant's eye. This is followed by perivascular exudation, tissue hyperplasia, and scar tissue that exerts traction on the retina and leads to retinal detachment and destruction of the infant's vision. Research indicates that the incidence of acute retrolental fibroplasia is inversely proportional to birth weight. Most of the clinical research indicates that to minimize the risk of development of retrolental fibroplasia, the infant's PaO_2 should be maintained between 60 and 90 torr. The perianesthesia nurse should use his or her best-informed judgment when caring for these infants. As with the adult, the infant who needs a high-inspired oxygen concentration to provide adequate oxygenation should not be denied oxygen because of fear of complications.

Lungs. Concentrations of oxygen higher than 60% damage the lungs within 3 or 4 days. A 100% oxygen concentration administered for 24 to 48 hours also causes pulmonary damage, the signs of which are manifested by type II cell dysfunction in the lung. The type II cells secrete surfactant, and the lack of surfactant in the alveoli leads to alveolar collapse. The hyperoxic environment also stops the ciliary action in the lungs. The early symptoms of this disorder include cough, nasal congestion, sore throat, reduced VC, tracheobronchitis, and substernal discomfort. The early signs of airway irritation may appear when a patient has received 80% to 100% oxygen continuously for 8 hours or longer. The lung appears to indefinitely tolerate oxygen concentrations lower than 40%.

Central Nervous System. Headache is an early indicator of oxygen toxicity. As oxygen toxicity continues to develop, the patient will demonstrate some confusion. When a patient is receiving a high concentration of oxygen and has these signs and symptoms, the attending physician should be notified. Convulsions usually are not seen in the PACU but may occur when oxygen

is delivered in above-normal atmospheric pressure, such as in hyperbaric oxygen chambers.

BIBLIOGRAPHY

Atlee J: Complications in anesthesia, Philadelphia, 1999, WB Saunders.

Barash P, Cullen B, Stoelting R: Clinical anesthesia, ed 4, Philadelphia, 2000, Lippincott Williams & Wilkins.

Benumof J, Saidman L: Anesthesia & perioperative complications, ed 2, St Louis, 1999, Mosby.

Benumof J: Anesthesia and uncommon diseases, ed 4, Philadelphia, 1998, WB Saunders.

Berge K, Warner D: Anesthetic effects on respiratory muscles, Seminars in Anesthesia 15(4):321-327, 1996.

Bickley L, Hoekelman R: Bates' guide to physical examination and history taking, ed 7, Philadelphia, 1998, Lippincott Williams & Wilkins.

Bowdle T, Horita A, Kharasch E: The pharmacologic basis of anesthesiology, New York, 1994, Churchill Livingstone.

Drain C: Providing appropriate anesthesia outcomes in the managed care environment, CRNA: The Clinical Forum for Nurse Anesthetists 7(4):162, 1996.

Drain C: Physiology of the respiratory system related to anesthesia, CRNA: The Clinical Forum for Nurse Anesthetists 7(4):163-180, 1996.

Drain C: Pathophysiology of the respiratory system related to anesthesia, CRNA: The Clinical Forum for Nurse Anesthetists 7(4):181-192, 1996.

Drain C, Robinson S: The pharmacology of respiratory disorders related to anesthesia, CRNA: The Clinical Forum for Nurse Anesthetists 7(4):193-199, 1996.

Drain C: Anesthesia care of the patient with reactive airways disease, CRNA: The Clinical Forum for Nurse Anesthetists 7(4):207-212, 1996.

Gal T: Physiologic and therapeutic concerns in anesthesia for patients with reactive airways, Seminars in Anesthesia 15(4):363-375, 1996.

Ganong W: Review of medical physiology, ed 20, New York, 2001 McGraw-Hill Professional.

Geiger-Bronsky M: Pulmonary rehabilitation and self-care after ambulatory surgery, J Perianesth Nurs 13:382-393, 1998.

Greensmith J, Aker J: Ventilatory management in the postanesthesia care unit, J Perianesth Nurs 13(6):370-381, 1998.

Guyton A, Hall J: Textbook of medical physiology, ed 10, Philadelphia, 2000, WB Saunders.

Hoffman C, Nakamoto D, Okal R et al: Effect of transport time and FIO$_2$ on SpO$_2$ during transport from the OR to the PACU, Nurse Anesth 2(3):119-125, 1991.

Lake C, Hines R, Blitt C: Clinical monitoring: practical applications for anesthesia and critical care, St Louis, 2001, Mosby.

Levitzky M: Pulmonary physiology, ed 5, New York, 1999, McGraw-Hill.

Longnecker D, Murphy F: Dripps/Eckenhoff/Vandam introduction to anesthesia, ed 9, Philadelphia, 1997, WB Saunders.

Longnecker D, Tinker J, Morgan G: Principles and practice of anesthesiology, ed 2, St Louis, Mosby, 1998.

Lustik S, Henson L: Preoperative evaluation of patients at risk for postoperative pulmonary complications, Seminars in Anesthesia 15(4):353-362, 1996.

Marienau M, Buck C: Preoperative evaluation of the pulmonary patient undergoing nonpulmonary surgery, J Perianesth Nurs 13(6):340-348, 1998.

Marley R: Postoperative oxygen therapy, J Perianesth Nurs 13(6):394-412, 1998.

Martin J: Positioning in anesthesia and surgery, ed 3, St Louis, 1997, Mosby.

McIntosh L: Essentials of nurse anesthesia, New York, 1997, McGraw-Hill.

Miller R, editor: Anesthesia, ed 5, New York, 2000, Churchill Livingstone.

Murray J, Nadel J: Textbook of respiratory medicine, ed 3, Philadelphia, 2000, WB Saunders.

Newton N: Supplementary oxygen—potential for disaster, Anaesthesia 46:905-906, 1991.

Nagelhout J, Zaglaniczny K: Nurse anesthesia, ed 2, Philadelphia, WB Saunders, 2001.

Ogunnaike B, Whitten C: Anesthetic management of morbidly obese patients, Seminars in Anesthesia, Perioperative Medicine and Pain 21(1):46-58, 2002.

Ownby D: Pathophysiology of immediate allergic reactions, Anesthesia Today 7(3):1-5, 1996.

Rau J: Recent developments in respiratory care pharmacology, J Perianesth Nurs 13(6):359-369, 1998.

Shapiro B, Peruzzi W, Kozlowski-Templin R: Clinical applications of blood bases, ed 5, St Louis, 1994, Mosby.

Stoelting, R: Pharmacology and physiology in anesthetic practice, ed 3, Philadelphia, 1999, Lippincott Raven.

Stoelting R, Miller R: Basics of anesthesia, ed 4, New York, 2000, Churchill Livingstone.

Stone D: Perioperative care: anesthesia, medicine, and surgery, St Louis, 1998, Mosby.

Taylor L, Stephens D: Arterial blood gases: clinical application. J Post Anesth Nurs 5(4):264-272, 1990.

Traver G, Mitchell J, Flodquist-Priestley G: Respiratory care: a clinical approach, Gaithersburg, MD, 1991, Aspen Publications.

Waugaman W, Foster S, Rigor B: Principles and practice of nurse anesthesia, ed 3, Norwalk, Conn, 1999, Appleton & Lange.

Weinberg G: Basic science review of anesthesiology, New York, 1997, McGraw-Hill.

11

THE RENAL SYSTEM

Most of the drugs used in anesthesia are excreted unchanged or as a metabolic byproduct by the kidneys. Homeostasis is maintained by proper kidney function, because the kidneys regulate the balance of acid-base, electrolyte, and fluid volumes and remove waste materials and toxic substances from the body.

Kidney function is sometimes difficult to assess in the postanesthesia care unit (PACU), especially in the uncatheterized patient. In patients who have urinary catheters in place after surgery, assessment of kidney function should be part of the perianesthesia nursing care. It is important to understand renal anatomy and physiology to enhance the outcomes of the patient who is suffering from renal dysfunction.

DEFINITIONS

Acetonuria: the appearance of acetone in the urine. It is present when excessive fats are consumed or when an inadequate amount of carbohydrates is metabolized.
Albuminuria: the presence of protein in the urine, also called proteinuria. Albumin is the most common protein found in the urine. This condition usually indicates malfunction in glomerular filtration.
Azotemia: the presence of nitrogenous products in the blood, usually because of decreased kidney function.
Cystitis: an inflammation of the bladder.
Dysuria: painful or difficult urination.
Enuresis: involuntary discharge of urine.
Glycosuria: the presence of glucose in the urine.
Hematuria: the presence of blood in the urine.
Nephritis: inflammation of the kidney; called Bright's disease.
Nephrosis: degeneration of the kidney without the occurrence of inflammation.
Oliguria: a decrease in the normal amount of urine formation.

Pyelitis: an inflammation of the renal pelvis and calices.
Stricture: an abnormal narrowing; in the urinary tract, a narrowing of the ureter or urethra.
Uremia: the toxic condition usually caused by renal insufficiency and retention of nitrogenous substances in the blood.
Urinary incontinence: the inability to retain urine in the bladder.
Urinary retention: failure to expel urine from the bladder.

ANATOMY OF THE KIDNEYS

The kidneys are two bean-shaped organs in the retroperitoneal spaces near the upper lumbar area. The right kidney is at a slightly lower level than the left. Each kidney weighs approximately 150 g. The notched portion of the kidney is called the hilum, which is where the ureter, the renal vein, and the renal artery enter the kidney (Fig. 11-1).

The ureter opens into a large cavity called the pelvis. From the pelvis, two to five major calices project deeper into the kidney. The major calices branch out to form six to ten minor calices. The ends of the minor calices are capped by the renal papillae.

The medulla is the inner portion of the kidney. It comprises several pyramids, which correspond to the number of minor calices. The base of the pyramid projects toward the outer portion of the kidney, which is termed the cortex. The apex of the pyramid forms the papillae, which cap each minor calix.

Blood is supplied to the kidney by the renal artery. The rate of blood flow through both kidneys of a man who weighs 70 kg is about 1200 ml per minute, or about 21% of the cardiac output. As the renal artery enters the kidney at the hilum, it divides into the interlobar arteries in the medulla; then, as they enter the cortex,

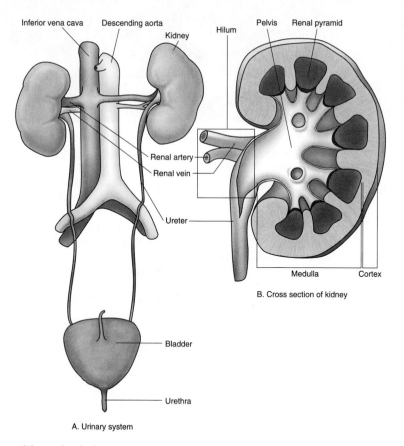

Fig. 11-1 Anatomy of the renal and urinary systems.

they divide into the arciform (arcuate) arteries. The afferent arteries project from the interlobar arteries and go to the nephron, where they divide into capillaries. The capillaries form the efferent arterioles, which then divide to form the peritubular capillaries, which help supply the nephron, a portion of the tubular capillaries, and the vasa recta, which descend around the loop of Henle, in the case of juxtamedullary nephrons. These nephrons, which are close to the renal medulla, have a long, extended loop of Henle that dips deep into the medulla. They then return to the venules, as do the tubular capillaries (Figs. 11-2 and 11-3).

The nephron is the functional unit of the kidney. The two kidneys contain approximately 2.4 million nephrons. Each nephron can be divided into three major portions: the renal corpuscle, the renal tubule, and the collecting ducts. The blood enters the afferent arteriole and goes into the glomerulus in the cortex. It consists of a network of 50 parallel capillaries encased in Bowman's capsule. This structural component is the renal capsule.

The renal tubules begin in Bowman's capsule. A pressure gradient forces fluid to leave the glomerulus and enter Bowman's capsule. The fluid then flows into the proximal tubule, which is still in the cortex of the kidney, and then into the loop of Henle. The loop of Henle is at first thick-walled but becomes thin-walled at the distal segment in the medulla of the kidney. The fluid then flows into the distal tubule, located in the cortex of the kidney, and passes into the collecting ducts, which go from the cortex to the medulla where they form papillary ducts (ducts of

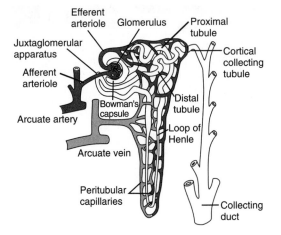

Fig. 11-2 The functional nephron. *(From Guyton A, Hall J: Textbook of medical physiology, ed 10, Philadelphia, 2000, WB Saunders.)*

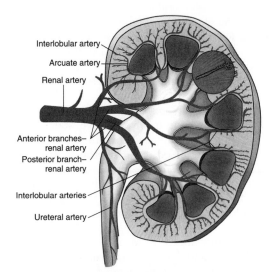

Fig. 11-3 Arterial supply to the kidney. Soon after entering the hilum of the kidney, the renal artery divides into several anterior and posterior branches. The branches divide into interlobar arteries, which course between the medullary pyramids. The interlobar arteries then give off the arcuate arteries, which course between the cortex and the medulla. From this arcuate complex arise the interlobar arteries, which give off the afferent arterioles to the glomeruli.

Bellini) and into the renal pelvis by way of the renal calices. At this point the fluid in the renal pelvis is termed urine.

RENAL PHYSIOLOGY

The constituents of urine are formed by filtration, reabsorption, and secretion. Filtration occurs as the blood passes through the glomerulus. The force of filtration is a pressure gradient pushing fluid through the glomerular membrane. Approximately 180 L of water every 24 hours is filtered out of plasma with other substances (Table 11-1). Blood cells and colloidal substances are usually retained in the blood because they are too large to pass through the epithelium. The presence of red blood cells or protein in the urine usually indicates a pathologic process in the kidney.

Reabsorption occurs in the proximal and distal tubules. Approximately 99% of the water is reabsorbed. Many substances in the water are reabsorbed by active or passive transport. Active transport requires energy for movement of the substance across the membrane. Passive transport can be regarded as simple diffusion that is devoid of energy.

Substances such as glucose, amino acids, sodium, potassium, calcium, and magnesium—those that are important constituents of body fluids—are almost entirely reabsorbed. Certain substances are reabsorbed in limited quantities and consequently appear in the urine in considerable amounts. Some of these substances are urea, creatinine, and the phosphates.

The last mechanism in the formation of urine is secretion. Various substances, including hydrogen and potassium ions, are secreted directly into the tubular fluid through the epithelial cells lining the renal tubules.

REGULATION OF KIDNEY FUNCTION

The formation of urine and the retention of substances needed for proper body function are aided by three physiologic mechanisms: the countercurrent mechanism, autoregulation, and hormone control.

Countercurrent Mechanism

The countercurrent mechanism is used by the kidneys to concentrate urine. This mechanism is aided by the anatomic arrangement of the loops of Henle of the juxtamedullary nephrons, which

Table 11-1	**Measure of Reabsorption by the Kidney** Excreted		
Substance	Filtered (mEq/24 hr/170 L)	Reabsorbed (mEq/24 hr/169 L)	Excreted (mEq/24 hr/45 L)
Sodium	24,500	24,350	150
Chloride	17,800	17,700	150
Bicarbonate	4,900	4,900	1
Potassium	700	600	24
Glucose	780	780	0
Urea	870	460	410
Creatinine	12	0	12
Uric acid	50	45	5

go deep into the medulla, and the peritubular capillaries, which are called the vasa recta. The osmolality of the interstitial fluid increases as it moves more deeply into the medulla; this greater osmolality results in active transport of solutes into the interstitial fluid. This countercurrent mechanism is useful when the body needs to excrete a large amount of waste products yet reabsorb the normal amount of solutes. This is also true when the water in the body needs to be conserved, as in conditions of inadequate water supply. Therefore water is conserved while waste products are eliminated.

Autoregulation

Autoregulation helps to keep the glomerular filtration at a near normal rate, despite fluctuations in arterial pressure. In fact, within the blood pressure range of 60 to 160 torr, little change in either renal plasma flow or glomerular filtration rate occurs. Consequently, as the arterial pressure increases, the sympathetic innervation to the afferent arterioles causes constriction, thus keeping the glomerular filtration rate constant. The reverse is also true. When the arterial pressure is low, dilatation of the afferent arterioles serves to keep the glomerular filtration rate constant.

Hormone Control

The antidiuretic hormone (ADH) is secreted by the posterior pituitary gland. The secretion of this hormone is influenced by plasma osmolality. If hypertonicity of the blood occurs, ADH is secreted, and water is retained by the kidneys. If the blood is hypotonic, less ADH is formed, and the kidneys release water. This hormone acts on the distal tubule and collecting tubules by altering their permeability to water.

The juxtaglomerular apparatus is located just before the glomerulus. If the sodium concentration is low, if the pressure in the afferent arteriole is low, or if a reduced glomerular filtration rate or increased sympathetic stimulation exists, an enzyme—renin—will be released from the juxtaglomerular cells.

Renin probably plays an important role in conserving sodium in hypotensive states and controlling fluid volume excretion. Renin, when released in the blood, catalyzes the splitting of angiotensin I from a renin substrate. As angiotensin I passes through the lungs, it is converted to angiotensin II (Fig. 11-4). Angiotensin II is a highly effective pressor agent and a major stimulus to the secretion of aldosterone. Aldosterone, a mineralocorticoid, appears to act on the distal tubule and the thick segment of the ascending loop of Henle. When secreted, it controls the reabsorption of some of the sodium and water. Because the renin-angiotensin system causes this reabsorption of water and sodium, it plays a role in the control of arterial blood pressure.

RENAL ROLE IN REGULATION OF BODY HOMEOSTASIS

The kidneys play a role in regulation of body fluids. For the most part, they determine the adjustment of blood volume, extracellular fluid

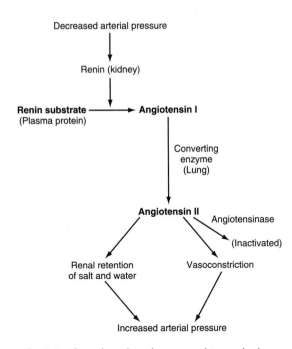

Decreased arterial pressure

↓

Renin (kidney)

↓

Renin substrate ———→ **Angiotensin I**
(Plasma protein)

Converting
enzyme
(Lung)

↓

Angiotensin II   Angiotensinase

(Inactivated)

Renal retention   Vasoconstriction
of salt and water

Increased arterial pressure

Fig. 11-4   The renin-angiotensin-vasoconstrictor mechanism for arterial pressure control. *(From Guyton A, Hall J: Textbook of medical physiology, ed 10, Philadelphia, 2000, WB Saunders.)*

Table 11-2	**Average Water Loss per 24 Hours at Average Temperature and Humidity**
Route	**Amount (ml)**
Through the skin	500
Through the lungs	350
Through the kidneys	1500
Through the feces	150

volume, and osmolality of the extracellular fluids, electrolytes, and ions; they remove waste products and toxic substances; and they maintain the acid-base balance.

The kidneys regulate blood volume in the following manner. When the circulating blood volume is excessive, the cardiac output and arterial pressure increase, thus causing stimulation of volume receptors located in the left and right atria and the baroreceptors located in the carotid, aortic, and pulmonary regions. The net effect is an increase in urine formation, returning blood volume to a normal range. Aldosterone and ADH also have a role in improving the economy of blood volume and electrolytes.

If the patient is hypovolemic, the kidney will conserve fluid and thus return the blood volume to normal limits.

The normal intake of water into the body in 24 hours is 2500 ml. Of this, 1200 ml is ingested liquids, and 1000 ml is water in solid food. The remaining 300 ml is water derived from oxidation of food in the tissue cells. Table 11-2 shows the avenues by which water is lost in a 24-hour period.

The extracellular fluid volume is controlled by the kidneys as they control the blood volume. The relative ratio of the extracellular fluid volume to blood volume depends on the physical properties of the circulation and of the interstitial spaces, including their compliances and their dynamics.

The kidney maintains the osmolality of the extracellular fluid mainly by regulating the extracellular sodium concentration. Extracellular sodium controls 90% to 95% of the effective osmotic pressure of extracellular fluid.

The kidneys also control the extracellular concentration of other electrolytes, such as potassium, calcium, magnesium, and phosphate ions.

COMPONENTS OF URINE

The end product of excretion by the kidneys is urine, which is 95% water and 5% solids. The solids, which account for approximately 60 g per L of urine, are listed in Table 11-3. Urea is derived mostly from the catabolism of amino acids. Creatinine is thought to be derived from creatine, a nitrogenous substance found in muscle tissue. Because it is not reabsorbed by the tubular mechanism of the kidney, creatinine is a good indicator of kidney function. Creatinine and sulfates are considered nonthreshold substances because they are excreted in their entirety. Uric acid is an end product of purine metabolism, formed from purines ingested as food and from those formed in the body.

High-threshold substances are almost entirely reabsorbed in the kidney. They are an important

Table 11-3	**Principal Constituents of Urine**
Constituents	Amount (g/L)
ORGANIC	
Urea	20-300
Uric acid	0.6-0.75
Creatinine	1.5
Others	2.6
INORGANIC	
Sodium chloride	9.0
Potassium chloride	2.5
Sulfuric acid	1.8
Phosphoric acid	1.8
Ammonia	0.5-15
Calcium	0.2
Magnesium	0.2

portion of the blood and are excreted only if they are in an excess concentration. Some of the high-threshold substances are glucose, potassium, calcium, and magnesium. Low-threshold substances, such as urea, uric acid, and phosphates, are only minimally reabsorbed by the kidney.

In considering the substances found in urine, knowing the characteristics of normal urine is useful. Normal urine should be amber in color because of the pigment urochrome, and it should also be clear and transparent. It usually is acidic, with a pH of about 6, because of the presence of sodium acid phosphate. The specific gravity is between 1.003 and 1.025. The volume of urine excreted every 24 hours is about 1500 ml.

ACID-BASE BALANCE

The kidneys play a major role in acid-base balance. Although they are the most powerful acid-base regulators, they require several hours to 1 day to return the hydrogen ion concentration to a normal range. The buffer systems (bicarbonate, phosphate, and protein) can react within a fraction of a second to alterations in hydrogen ion concentration. In contrast, the respiratory system usually takes 1 to 3 minutes to react.

The pH is a negative logarithmic expression of the hydrogen ion concentration in the body fluids (see Chapter 6). Bicarbonate and carbon dioxide are also factors. The bicarbonate is mainly under renal control, whereas the carbon dioxide is under respiratory control. The 20:1 ratio exists because approximately 20 times more bicarbonate than carbon dioxide is in the plasma. Thus any change in the 20:1 ratio affects the pH. Any change that negates the functioning of the kidneys or the rest of the body may affect the bicarbonate portion of the ratio and is a metabolic problem. Conversely, any change in the function of the lungs, which usually affects the carbon dioxide portion of the ratio, is a respiratory problem.

If, for example, a large amount of a bicarbonate solution were rapidly infused into a patient and his or her ventilation did not change (PCO_2 stays constant), the result would be a higher value for the bicarbonate and no change in the PCO_2. The net result would be a higher pH, which would constitute alkalosis, in this case termed metabolic alkalosis. On the other hand, if an acid were infused, the ratio would become smaller and the pH would fall, indicating acidosis, which would be termed metabolic acidosis.

Respiratory acidosis occurs when the PCO_2 is increased, as in acute hypoventilation, for example. The pH will be lowered because the ratio will become smaller. Conversely, if the patient hyperventilates, the PCO_2 will drop and the ratio will rise, thus increasing the pH and producing respiratory alkalosis.

The kidneys regulate pH by increasing or decreasing the bicarbonate ion concentration in the body fluid. This is done by a complex series of reactions, which begins with hydrogen ions being secreted into the tubular fluid. Carbon dioxide, an end product of tubular cell metabolism, combines with water to form carbonic acid (H_2CO_3). The carbonic acid dissociates to form hydrogen (H^+) and bicarbonate (HCO_3). The hydrogen ion is taken by active transport to the renal tubule and usually exchanges in the tubule with sodium. By active transport the sodium moves to the extracellular fluid, where it combines with the bicarbonate that was reabsorbed into the extracellular fluid to form sodium bicarbonate ($NaHCO_3$). In the tubules, the hydrogen ion that was actively transported to the tubule combines with the filtrate bicarbonate to form carbonic acid. The carbonic acid dissociates to form carbon dioxide and water. The carbon dioxide is reabsorbed into the extracellular fluid and eventually excreted by the lungs; the water is excreted as part of the urine.

The kidneys correct alkalosis by decreasing the bicarbonate in the extracellular fluid. This occurs because fewer hydrogen ions enter the tubules because of a low carbon dioxide concentration and because a high bicarbonate concentration exists in the tubules. The bicarbonate cannot be reabsorbed without first combining with the hydrogen; therefore the excess bicarbonate ions are lost to the urine as are other positive ions such as sodium and hydrogen. Cellular potassium may exchange with the sodium instead of the cellular hydrogen to conserve the hydrogen, which may help return the pH to normal limits.

Renal correction of acidosis is achieved by increasing the amount of bicarbonate in the extracellular fluid. An excess of hydrogen ions in comparison to the bicarbonate filtration into the tubules exists. The excess hydrogen ions are secreted into the tubules, where they combine with the phosphate or the ammonia buffer systems. The sodium ions in the tubules move by active transport to the extracellular fluid and combine with the bicarbonate ion to form sodium bicarbonate, which helps correct the acidosis. The urine is acidic because the kidney is excreting the excess hydrogen ions.

DIURETIC THERAPY IN THE PACU

In the PACU, diuretics are commonly used to reduce brain size and intracranial pressure, to treat hypervolemia, to prevent oliguria, or to help in diagnosing the cause of the oliguria. The major side effects of diuretic therapy are related to the contraction of the extracellular fluid volume and the alterations in potassium concentrations. Diuretics are categorized according to their site of action on renal tubules and their mechanism of altering the secretion of urine. The major categories of diuretics are osmotic diuretics, thiazide diuretics, potassium-sparing diuretics, loop diuretics, aldosterone antagonists, and carbonic anhydrase inhibitors. Because the use of diuretics is so important in the PACU, a brief review of the major types of diuretics will be presented.

Osmotic Diuretics

Osmotic diuretics are used to evaluate the cause of oliguria, to reduce intracranial pressure and brain size, and to protect the kidneys against the development of acute renal failure. Urea is an effective osmotic diuretic; however, this drug does have some disadvantages that limit its use as compared with mannitol. The major disadvantage of urea is that it causes a significant amount of rebound increase in intracranial pressure and a high incidence of venous thrombosis. Mannitol, a six-carbon sugar, is the prototype of the osmotic diuretics. This high-molecular-weight drug, when given intravenously, increases the plasma osmolality, with a resulting expansion of the intravascular volume by means of drawing fluid from the intracellular space into the extracellular space. In the kidneys, mannitol's osmotic effect on the tubules leads to a diuretic effect. The major concern with mannitol therapy is an increased extracellular fluid volume. This can be of grave consequence in patients with impending pulmonary edema. Hence the perianesthesia nurse should frequently assess the pulmonary parameters in patients who receive mannitol and in whom pulmonary edema is possible. An early sign of pulmonary edema is wheezing. Wheezing usually indicates interstitial edema. If wheezing is detected in a nonasthmatic patient, the attending physician should be notified immediately. As the edema formation progresses, wet basilar rales or crackles may be heard during auscultation of the chest. The crackles become coarser as the pulmonary edema worsens.

Thiazide Diuretics

Thiazide diuretics are mainly used in the treatment of hypertension, edema, and diabetes insipidus. These diuretics are secreted in the proximal convoluted tubule and have their major effect in the loop of Henle, where chloride reabsorption is inhibited. This results in diluting defects and increased distal delivery of salt and water. Patients on long-term thiazide diuretic therapy can experience increased urinary losses of water, sodium, chloride, and potassium and some loss of bicarbonate. Hence these patients are particularly susceptible to hypochloremic, hypokalemic metabolic alkalosis. Some of the common thiazide diuretics are chlorothiazide (Diuril), benzthiazide (Exna), and hydrochlorothiazide (Esidrix, HydroDiuril, Oretic).

The most common untoward effect of thiazide diuretics is hypokalemia. Hypokalemia, which is a reduced serum potassium level, can cause paralytic ileus, severe weakness or flaccid paralysis, hypotension, atrial and ventricular dysrhythmias, and potentiation of digitalis toxicity. If it is determined that treatment for hypokalemia should be instituted, intravenous potassium replacement may be given in the PACU. If the infusion rates of the potassium replacement exceed 40 mEq per hr or if the concentration of potassium in the individual intravenous container is greater than 40 mEq per L, continuous electrocardiographic (ECG) monitoring should be instituted to detect any dysrhythmias. Also, if potassium chloride is added to solutions in flexible plastic bags in the PACU, the nurse should ensure that it is properly mixed in the infusion solution to prevent the patient from receiving an inadvertent bolus of potassium chloride. Other untoward side effects of thiazide diuretics are dermatitis, bone marrow depression, and reduced liver function.

Potassium-Sparing Diuretics

This class of diuretics acts on the distal convoluted tubule. The product of their actions is an increased urinary output without potassium loss. The most popular potassium-sparing diuretics include triamterene (Dyrenium) and amiloride (Midamor). A fixed-dose combination of triamterene and hydrochlorothiazide, which is marketed under the trade name of Dyazide, can also be considered to be in this category of diuretics. The major side effect of this class of diuretics is hyperkalemia, which can occur because of excess usage along with overusage of potassium supplementation. The symptoms of hyperkalemia include muscular weakness, conduction defects, ventricular dysrhythmias, and ileus. To reduce the effects of hyperkalemia, calcium gluconate or calcium chloride may be administered. Also, to reduce the high potassium levels, sodium bicarbonate, glucose, or insulin in combination with glucose may be given.

Loop Diuretics

The loop diuretics, of which ethacrynic acid (Edecrin), bumetanide (Bumex), and furosemide (Lasix) are the prototype drugs, are used primarily in the treatment of pulmonary edema and general edema and in the diagnosis of acute renal failure. The loop diuretics are secreted into the tubule and have their major action on the medullary concentrating segment where chloride transport is inhibited. Consequently, they interfere with the concentrating and diluting mechanisms of the kidneys, which results in the production of isotonic urine. In addition, because of the increased delivery of salt with these drugs, potassium secretion is increased. Hence the major problems with these drugs are in the realm of deafness (caused by ethacrynic acid), hepatic dysfunction, hypokalemia, alkalosis, extracellular fluid volume contraction, and electrolyte imbalance. Because of their high potency and their ability to act rapidly, loop diuretics are usually the diuretic of choice when indicated for the patient in the PACU. The two major concerns when one of these drugs is administered are hypokalemia and hypovolemia. The effects and treatment of hypokalemia were discussed in the section on thiazide diuretics. The objective findings that indicate hypovolemia (contraction of the extracellular fluid volume) are hypotension, tachycardia, and low right- and left-ventricular filling pressures. Treatment can include repositioning the patient with the legs elevated or the administration of intravenous salt-containing solutions, or both.

Aldosterone Antagonists

Drugs in this category, of which spironolactone (Aldactone) is the prototype drug, act on the aldosterone receptors in the conducting ducts. Spironolactone acts to antagonize the effects of aldosterone. Aldosterone enhances the reabsorption of sodium and chloride and increases the excretion of potassium in the renal tubules. Consequently, when spironolactone is administered, sodium and chloride reabsorption are increased, and potassium excretion is decreased. Because of this decrease in potassium excretion in the conducting ducts, hyperkalemia, especially when renal dysfunction is present, is a serious side effect of the drug. Spironolactone is indicated for patients with fluid overload due to cirrhosis of the liver, nephrotic syndrome, and congestive heart failure.

Carbonic Anhydrase Inhibitors

Drugs in this class bind to the carbonic anhydrase enzyme in the proximal renal tubules. The outcome is to inhibit the actions of carbonic anhydrase, which results in the diminished excretion of hydrogen ions and increased excretion of bicarbonate with an ionic exchange with potassium and sodium. The net result is a diuresis of alkaline urine. The prototype drug in this category is acetazolamide (Diamox). This drug is indicated for the reduction of intraocular pressure and the management of seizures. If this drug is administered to a patient with chronic obstructive pulmonary disease, careful monitoring of the patient's rate of ventilation and $PaCO_2$ is mandated because excessive bicarbonate is lost in the urine and because hypercarbia can result, which can ultimately lead to central nervous system (CNS) depression.

EFFECTS OF ANESTHESIA ON RENAL FUNCTION

In patients with normal renal function who receive general inhalation anesthesia, some depression of renal function occurs. This effect arises because all of the general anesthetics depress functions such as glomerular filtration rate, renal blood flow, and urinary flow. The depression in renal function is the result of direct and indirect effects of the general anesthetic agents. In regard to the vascular effects, during general anesthesia the renal blood flow may be depressed because of renal vasoconstriction, systemic hypotension, or both. Of interest is that droperidol, the tranquilizer component of Innovar, has the smallest effect on the changes in renal function. In most instances, the renal depression caused by the anesthetic agents is completely reversible at the end of the operative procedure.

Patients who are anesthetized in lighter planes of anesthesia may experience some manifestations of the stress response. One of the hormones that is released in response to a stressor is ADH. This hormone is the most important regulator of urine volume. When ADH is released, it promotes an increase in tubular reabsorption of water, which results in a decrease in urine volume and an increase in urine concentration. Other biochemical products of the stress response, namely epinephrine, norepinephrine, and the renin-angiotensin system, also affect the renal system. More specifically, when these amines are liberated, renal blood flow is decreased. Because some patients can undergo a stress response under anesthesia, it is important for the perianesthesia nurse to monitor renal function during the emergent phase of the anesthesia. It is not uncommon for patients who have undergone major abdominal or thoracic surgery to experience some diuresis during the immediate postoperative period. Hence urine volume and concentration should be monitored in all patients who 1) have undergone a major surgical procedure; 2) have received general anesthesia for more than 2 hours; (3) have a compromised cardiovascular or renal system, or both; and (4) have had a significant blood volume replacement during the preoperative or intraoperative phase of the anesthetic experience.

EFFECTS OF DRUGS IN PATIENTS WITH COMPROMISED RENAL FUNCTION

Patients with severe renal disease usually have anemia, body fluid relocation, abnormal cell membrane activity, and alterations in blood albumin and electrolytes. In addition, these patients are usually debilitated, and—if they are uremic—CNS depression is usually present. Drugs that are not metabolized in the body and are therefore excreted unchanged by the kidneys should be avoided in patients with severe renal disease. Hence the long-acting barbiturates barbital and phenobarbital and the skeletal muscle relaxants decamethonium and gallamine, along with digoxin and lanatoside C, should be avoided in these patients. Because about half of the administered dose of the belladonna alkaloids atropine and hyoscyamine is excreted unchanged, the dosage should be modified by the degree of severity of the renal impairment. When CNS depression is present in the patient with renal impairment, the actions of narcotics are intensified and prolonged. Along with this, diazepam, which has a 24-hour half-life, is probably not a good choice because of its additive effect on the CNS depression. In patients with mild to moderate renal dysfunction, all inhalation anesthetics except methoxyflurane and possibly enflurane can be used in the usual clinical dose range. Because thiopental depends on redistribution for the termination of its action, it may be used in patients with renal impairment. However, the sleeping time is increased in proportion to the degree of uremia. Along with this, the skeletal muscle relaxants succinylcholine, curare, and pancuronium are also acceptable for use in the patient with compromised kidney function. Neuroleptanalgesia, which derives from the combination of a narcotic and a tranquilizer, when achieved with nitrous oxide and oxygen, is an acceptable technique for the uremic patient. If a patient has received Innovar, which is the prototype neuroleptanalgesic drug, the perianesthesia nurse should monitor the patient for prolonged depressant effects of the drug. More specifically, the tranquilizer component of Innovar, droperidol, has a very long half-life; therefore its prolonged effects, coupled with CNS depression from the uremia, may cause the patient to be slow to arouse in the immediate postoperative emergence phase. Consequently, airway patency and the cardiovascular parameters should be monitored closely for an extended period when droperidol has been administered to the patient in either the preoperative or the intraoperative phase of the anesthetic experience.

RENAL SHUTDOWN OR FAILURE

Acute renal failure can occur in the PACU for a variety of reasons—such as hemorrhage and circulatory failure from trauma or extensive surgery, acute glomerulonephritis, vascular occlusions, or toxicity from drugs.

The most common cause of acute renal failure is acute tubular necrosis. Oliguria produces the clinical setting in which renal cell necrosis may develop. Persistent oliguria—less than 25 ml of urine per hour for more than 2 hours—constitutes a medical emergency, and the surgeon should be notified immediately. The urine volume may be abnormally high in conditions in which the glomerular filtration rate is reduced to the point of renal failure, and the increased urine volume represents a supplemental failure of tubular function. In patients with mild to moderate renal dysfunction, enflurane may potentially cause nephrotoxicity. This is because enflurane is metabolized to inorganic fluoride. However, clinical studies have not been able to demonstrate this pos-

sibility. Nephrotoxicity is characterized by polyuria and azotemia. Therefore the accurate and continuous measurement of urine volume is essential in the postoperative nursing care of the patient with suspected renal failure.

Creatinine clearance is a laboratory test that provides an excellent index to measure the quantity of glomerular filtrate. Creatinine is a component of urine not reabsorbed by tubular mechanisms. Hence every milliliter of glomerular filtrate should contain precisely the same quantity of creatinine as 1 ml of plasma.

Measurement of urinary sodium yields information about sodium absorption. The urine plasma osmolar ratio provides an index of water reabsorption in the collecting tubules and is an excellent measurement of tubular function. The quality rather than the quantity of the urine provides useful information about the renal state of the patient (Fig. 11-5).

PERIANESTHESIA NURSING CARE

Perianesthesia nursing care centers on recognition and care of the patient in impending renal failure. Urinary output should be monitored by an indwelling urethral catheter. This monitoring provides moment-to-moment information concerning urine output and its constituents that can be measured. Modern collecting devices provide a closed system between the catheter and a graduated measuring flask that can be emptied from the bottom without disconnecting the catheter. In this way, the danger of gross contamination is minimized while the necessary monitoring facility is still provided.

Continuous ECG monitoring should be done because the patient in acute renal failure probably has hyperkalemia, which can lead to cardiac arrest. The ECG changes indicative of hyperkalemia are initially high-peaked T waves and depressed S-T segments. Subsequent disappearance of T waves, heart block, and diastolic cardiac arrest occur with increasing levels of potassium (Fig. 11-6).

Osmotic diuretics, such as mannitol, or one of the loop diuretics, such as ethacrynic acid and furosemide, may be used in the treatment of tubular necrosis. A central venous pressure monitor may be inserted to measure blood volume. If renal failure continues, dialytic therapy will probably be necessary.

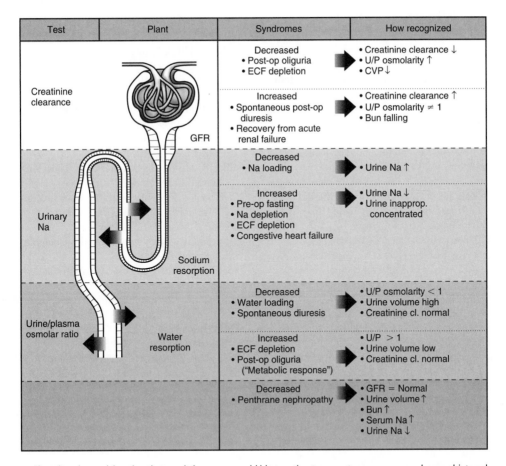

Test	Plant	Syndromes	How recognized
Creatinine clearance	GFR	Decreased • Post-op oliguria • ECF depletion	• Creatinine clearance ↓ • U/P osmolarity ↑ • CVP ↓
		Increased • Spontaneous post-op diuresis • Recovery from acute renal failure	• Creatinine clearance ↑ • U/P osmolarity ≠ 1 • Bun falling
Urinary Na	Sodium resorption	Decreased • Na loading	• Urine Na ↑
		Increased • Pre-op fasting • Na depletion • ECF depletion • Congestive heart failure	• Urine Na ↓ • Urine inapprop. concentrated
Urine/plasma osmolar ratio	Water resorption	Decreased • Water loading • Spontaneous diuresis	• U/P osmolarity < 1 • Urine volume high • Creatinine cl. normal
		Increased • ECF depletion • Post-op oliguria ("Metabolic response")	• U/P > 1 • Urine volume low • Creatinine cl. normal
		Decreased • Penthrane nephropathy	• GFR = Normal • Urine volume ↑ • Bun ↑ • Serum Na ↑ • Urine Na ↓

Fig. 11-5 Alterations in renal function that result from a normal kidney acting to correct or preserve an abnormal internal environment. The quantity and quality of urine are appropriate for preserving the entire organism, but alterations, if uncorrected, may result in renal damage. *GFR,* Glomerular filtration rate; *ECF,* extracellular fluid; *U/P,* urine/plasma; *CVP,* central venous pressure; *BUN,* blood urea nitrogen; *CL,* clearance; *VOL,* volume. (*Redrawn from Kinney JM, Egdahl RH, Zuidema GD: Manual of preoperative and postoperative care, ed 2, Philadelphia, 1971, WB Saunders*)

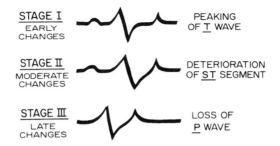

STAGE I EARLY CHANGES	PEAKING OF T WAVE
STAGE II MODERATE CHANGES	DETERIORATION OF ST SEGMENT
STAGE III LATE CHANGES	LOSS OF P WAVE

Fig. 11-6 Stages of electrocardiographic evidence of hyperkalemia. (*From Kinney JM, Egdahl RH, Zuidema GD: Manual of preoperative and postoperative care, ed 2, Philadelphia, 1971, WB Saunders.*)

BIBLIOGRAPHY

Alspach J: Core curriculum for critical care nursing, ed 5, Philadelphia, 1998, WB Saunders.

Atlee J: Complications in anesthesia, Philadelphia, 1999, WB Saunders.

Barash P, Cullen B, Stoelting R: Clinical anesthesia, ed 4, Philadelphia, 2000, Lippincott Williams & Wilkins.

Benumof J: Anesthesia and uncommom diseases, ed 4, Philadelphia, 1998, WB Saunders.

Benumof J, Saidman L: Anesthesia & perioperative complications, ed 2, St Louis, 1999, Mosby.

Bickley L, Hoekelman R: Bates' guide to physical examination and history taking, ed 7, Philadelphia, 1998, Lippincott Williams & Wilkins.

Ganong W: Review of medical physiology, ed 20, New York, 2001, McGraw-Hill Professional.

Guyton A, Hall J: Textbook of medical physiology, ed 10, Philadelphia, 2000, WB Saunders.

Hardman J, Limbird L: Goodman and Gilman's the pharmacological basis of therapeutics, ed 10, New York, 2001, McGraw-Hill.

Katzung B, editor: Basic and clinical pharmacology, ed 8, Los Altos, Calif, 2000, Appleton & Lange.

Lake C, Hines R, Blitt C: Clinical monitoring: practical applications for anesthesia and critical care, St Louis, 2001, Mosby.

Longnecker D, Murphy F: Dripps/Eckenhoff/Vandam introduction to anesthesia, ed 9, Philadelphia, 1997, WB Saunders.

Longnecker D, Tinker J, Morgan G: Principles and practice of anesthesiology, ed 2, St Louis, 1998, Mosby.

Martin J: Positioning in anesthesia and surgery, ed 3, St Louis, 1997, Mosby.

McIntosh L: Essentials of nurse anesthesia, New York, 1997, McGraw-Hill.

Miller R, editor: Anesthesia, ed 5, New York, 2000, Churchill Livingstone.

Nagelhout J, Zaglaniczny K: Nurse anesthesia, ed 2, Philadelphia, 2001, WB Saunders.

Stoelting R: Pharmacology and physiology in anesthetic practice, ed 3, Philadelphia, 1999, Lippincott-Raven.

Stoelting R, Miller R: Basics of anesthesia, ed 4, New York, 2000, Churchill Livingstone.

Stone D: Perioperative Care: Anesthesia, medicine, and surgery, St Louis, 1998, Mosby.

Walsh S, Retik A, editors: Campbell's Urology, ed 8, Philadelphia, 2002, WB Saunders.

Waugaman W, Foster S, Rigor B: Principles and practice of nurse anesthesia, ed 3, Norwalk, Conn, 1999, Appleton & Lange.

Weinberg G: Basic science review of anesthesiology, New York, 1997, McGraw-Hill.

12

FLUID AND ELECTROLYTES

M any improvements have been made in the methods and types of fluids and electrolytes that are administered to patients in the perioperative period. The maintenance of appropriate concentrations of body fluid and electrolytes are essential to normal physiologic function of all body systems. A clear understanding of the basic physiology in this area along with a brief introduction to the many types and regimes of fluid management of the patient will be presented.

DEFINITIONS

Anions: ions that carry a negative charge and migrate to the anode (+ terminal) in an electrical field.

Autologous: originating within the same person, such as an autotransfusion.

Cations: ions that carry a positive charge and migrate to the cathode (– terminal) in an electrical field.

Chvostek's sign: an abnormal spasm of the facial muscles elicited by light taps on the facial nerve and which indicates hypocalcemia.

Colloids: compounds such as red blood cells (RBCs), albumin, or dextran that, due to size, are retained within a specific fluid compartment and increase the oncotic pressure of that compartment.

Cryoprecipitate: a precipitate that results from cooling, such as the antihemophilic factor in blood plasma.

Crystalloids: Balanced electrolyte solutions that are in isotonic solutions of water or dextrose and can move between the intravascular and interstitial compartments.

Edema: accumulation of fluid in the interstitial spaces.

Isotonic solutions: solutions that have the same osmolality as plasma.

Hemolysis: a disruption of the integrity of the red cell membrane, thus causing release of cell contents to include hemoglobin.

Hemostasis: the arrest of bleeding by the interaction of the platelet with the blood vessel wall and the formation of the platelet plug.

Hypercalcemia: increased plasma concentration of calcium (>5.6 mEq/L).

Hyperkalemia: greater than 6 mEq/L blood concentration of potassium.

Hypermagnesemia: an increase in the plasma concentration of magnesium (>2.6 mEq/L).

Hypernatremia: an increase in sodium in the plasma above 145 mEq/L.

Hypertonic solutions (hyperosmotic): solutions that have an osmolality greater than that of plasma.

Hypocalcemia: reduced plasma concentration of calcium (<4.4 mEq/L)

Hypokalemia: less than 3 mEq/L blood concentration of potassium.

Hypomagnesemia: a decrease in the plasma concentration of magnesium (<1.6 mEq/L).

Hyponatremia: a decrease of sodium in the plasma below 135 mEq/L.

Hypotonic solutions (hypoosmotic): solutions that have an osmolality less than that of plasma.

Osmolality: a physical property of a solution, one that is dependent on the number of dissolved particles in the solution.

Tetany: a condition characterized by cramps, muscle twitching, sharp flexion of the wrist and ankle joints, and convulsions.

Third space: losses of fluid and electrolytes from the extracellular fluid (ECF) to a nonfunctional "space"–an acute sequestered space that accompanies surgery.

Trousseau's sign: a test for latent tetany in which carpal spasm is induced by inflating a sphygmomanometer cuff on the upper arm to a pressure exceeding systolic blood pressure for three minutes.

BODY FLUID BALANCE

Water is the most abundant component of the body. It represents approximately 60% of adult body weight and as much as 75% to 77% of body weight in infants under one month of age. By approximately age 17, the adult percentage is attained, and in a 154 pound or 70 kilogram person, the total body water will be about 42 liters. Because women have higher fat content in their bodies and because fat is essentially water-free, they have a lower water content than men do. Older adults and obese individuals also have a lower proportion of water in their bodies. Water is essential to the body. It is the medium within which metabolic reactions takes place to facilitate the ionization of electrolytes; it acts as a reagent in many chemical reactions; it transports nutrients to cells and removes waste products; and its high specific heat and heat of vaporization make it especially suitable as a temperature regulator.

The total amount of body water remains very stable, as its intake usually equals its output. Water intake includes not only the water consumed in beverages but also the fluids obtained from the metabolism of solid foods. The water taken in by beverages and food is referred to as exogenous water. Although variance does occur on a day-to-day basis, overall the average adult living in a moderate climate and receiving a mixed diet consumes about 2500 to 3000 ml daily. Approximately 1000 ml is obtained from beverages and 1500 ml from solid and semisolid foods. The water formed during metabolism of organic foodstuffs is called endogenous water. Because metabolism varies with body temperature, the amount of exercise being performed, and other factors, the amount of endogenous water available will also vary on a day-to-day basis. In a healthy adult who performs a moderate amount of exercise, an average of 300 to 350 ml of endogenous water will be available daily. Intake is influenced by the "thirst" center in the hypothalamus. If the fluid volume inside the cells decreases, salivary secretion is reduced, thereby causing a dry mouth and the sensation of thirst. Under normal circumstances, an individual will then drink and restore the fluid volume (Box 12-1).

Water output also remains quite stable and usually approximates the total body water intake. Removal or output of water from the body is through four types of excretion. They are the lungs, gastrointestinal tract, skin, and kidney.

Lungs

Expired air is nearly saturated with water. The amount lost through the lungs varies with the

Box 12-1	Normal Intake and Output of Water per Day

INTAKE	
Water	2150 ml
Endogenous Water	250 ml
Total water intake	2400 ml

OUTPUT	
Insensible loss	
Skin	350 ml
Respiratory tract	350 ml
Urine	1400 ml
Sweat	100 ml
Feces	100 ml
Total water output	2300 ml

humidity and the temperature of inspired air as well as with the rate and depth of respiration. As a rule, about 300 to 400 ml of water is thus lost daily. This loss of water via the respiratory tract is termed insensible loss of water, so named because one is not aware of this loss. The water content of inhaled gases decreases as the ambient temperature decreases. Consequently, the insensible water loss from the lungs is higher in cold environments. Hence patients with respiratory dysfunction require a greater water intake to offset the increased insensible water loss when they are in cold environments. Also, an increase in the respiration rate can increase the water loss to as much as 2000 ml—which is very significant in patients suffering from chronic obstructive pulmonary disease (see Chapter 45).

Gastrointestinal Tract

The amount of water lost via the feces averages to be about 100 ml daily. However, with vomiting or diarrhea, this loss may be greatly increased. Up to 7000 ml can be lost by diarrhea and 6000 ml by vomiting. The implications to the perianesthesia nurse are great because this can significantly impact the volume status of the patient who is actively vomiting. In cases such as this, fluids should be increased in rate, and the anesthesia practitioner should be notified.

Skin

Water lost via the skin can be considered under two categories: insensible perspiration and sensible perspiration. The skin is not impervious to water, and a constant diffusion of moisture from its deeper layers to the dry surface where the water evaporates occurs. Insensible loss depends largely on environmental humidity. Sensible perspiration refers to loss of water by production of sweat. Sweating is an emergency mechanism for regulating body temperature when the heat produced by metabolic processes is excessive. The amount of sweat will therefore vary with exercise and with body temperature. In a moist atmosphere, sweat may be more visible than in a dry atmosphere, but the amount of water lost is the same. Despite its role as a safety factor, sweating can become a hazard when body water supplies are low, because the body continues to lose sweat to maintain its temperature. In the normal adult who performs moderate exercise in a comfortable environment, approximately 500 ml of water is lost in both sensible and insensible perspiration.

Kidneys

Water loss via the kidneys varies with the supply of body water. The kidneys are able to concentrate the urine, and the specific gravity may approach 1.040. On the other hand, if the amount of excess water is great, such as might occur when a large quantity is administered intravenously, the kidneys will excrete very dilute urine, the specific gravity of which might approach 1.002. Under normal conditions, the kidneys excrete about 1.2 liters per day. In patients that are experiencing vomiting or diarrhea, less water is available, and the kidneys respond promptly to curtail most of the water loss via urine. The two hormones responsible for controlling the volume of urine are antidiuretic hormone (ADH) from the posterior pituitary and aldosterone from the adrenal cortex. ADH, by increasing the permeability of the renal distal convoluted tubule and collecting ducts, increases the amount of water reabsorbed and thus decreases the urine volume. Aldosterone increases the renal reabsorption of sodium and secondarily of water. Both hormones are secreted in response to lowered blood volume and serve to control output to balance intake. However, a minimal loss of fluids is obligatory. It is therefore critical to monitor fluid balance.

DISTRIBUTION OF BODY FLUIDS

The fluids in the body can be divided into two compartments along with a potential third compartment. The total body water is equal to about 60% of the total body weight, or about 42 L in the average 70 kg man. The two compartments are normally divided relative to the location of the cell membrane—intracellular (inside the cell) and extracellular (outside the cell). The intracellular fluid (ICF) is estimated to be about 40% of the body weight, or about 28 liters of fluid, and represents about two thirds of the total body water. It provides a medium for all intracellular activities. The other compartment, the extracellular fluid (ECF), is approximately 20% of the body weight and ranges from 12 to 14 liters of fluid. The extracellular fluid compartment includes the blood plasma or intravascular fluid, the interstitial fluid (ISF) that bathes the cells, the lymph, cerebrospinal fluid (CSF), and the transcellular fluids. The transcellular fluids include the synovial fluid, peritoneal fluid, digestive fluids, and fluids of the eye and ear. The lymph, CSF, and the transcellular fluids normally constitute only about 1% of the body mass. Blood constitutes 4% and the interstitial fluid 15.7% of the body weight.

The third compartment, which is commonly called the "third space," is a concept that is defined as a compartment that includes the interstitial spaces that are swollen by local responses to tissue trauma and hormonal influx due to the stress of surgery. This third space can occur even when patients have undergone massive surgical procedures and their fluid loss, to include insensible loss, are appropriately replaced. This accumulation of fluid in the third space compartment usually occurs during and immediately after the surgical procedure and is difficult to clinically differentiate from actual blood loss. Clinically, the signs of hypovolemia will reflect third space loss and actual blood loss. The treatment includes infusion of fluids in the range of 3 to 10 ml/kg/hour and is usually adequate along with establishing the underlying cause. The third space loss will usually resolve in several postoperative days, and the nurse on the unit that receives the patient after the PACU should be alert for signs of possible fluid overload as the fluid postoperatively returns to the ECF.

Fluid balance involves not only maintenance of the total amount of body water but also the maintenance of a relatively constant distribution of that water in the different compartments. Circulation of fluid between compartments depends on the relative hydrostatic and osmotic pressures in each compartment. Hydrostatic pressure is the force "pushing" fluid from one compartment to the other. For example, if the hydrostatic pressure in the capillaries (blood pressure) exceeds the pressure in the interstitial space, fluid moves from the capillary into the interstitial space. Osmotic pressure is the "pull" of fluids into the compartment. It is a function of the number of dissolved molecules in the solution and is not influenced by weight or size of the molecule. Because of the relatively large quantities, the electrolytes are the major contributors to the osmotic pressure of the fluids. The electrolytes are a group of compounds that dissociate in solution to form ions. These ions carry an electrical charge. The cations are positively charged electrolytes and include sodium, potassium, calcium, and magnesium. The anions are negatively charged ions and include chloride, bicarbonate, phosphate, sulfate, and ions of inorganic acids such as lactate. Protein also carries a negative charge at physiologic pH. Each of the fluid compartments of the body contains electrolytes, and although the concentration and specific composition of electrolytes in each compartment varies, the number of cations in each compartment balances the number of anions to maintain electrical neutrality.

The major ions found in the extracellular fluid are sodium and chloride, whereas potassium and phosphate are predominately intracellular ions. The preponderance of sodium outside the cell and potassium inside the cell is the result of a cell membrane "pump" that exchanges sodium and potassium ions. This active transport mechanism requires energy from ATP. Sodium represents almost half the osmotic strength of the plasma.

The major difference between the two major compartments that make up the extracellular fluid is the much higher protein content in the plasma than in the interstitial fluid. Because capillary membranes are not selectively permeable to small particles, ions and small molecules can exchange rapidly between the plasma and the ISF. However, because proteins are too large to cross the capillary barrier, they remain in the plasma. As a result, the electrolyte composition differs slightly from the plasma and the interstitial fluid. Specifically, the sodium concentration in plasma is slightly greater, whereas the chloride concentration is slightly less than in the interstitial fluid and the sum of the diffusible ions. Thus the osmotic pressure in the plasma is greater. The osmotic pressure caused by plasma colloids is called the colloid osmotic pressure (COP) or oncotic pressure. Protein molecules are responsible for the COP or oncotic pressure. The proteins that exert a COP help to retain the plasma water in the intravascular compartment. Albumin is the major protein in the plasma that contributes to the COP.

The extracellular fluid is regulated carefully by the kidneys to facilitate the cells being bathed in fluid containing appropriate concentrations of electrolytes to include sodium, potassium, and nutrients. A patient who is experiencing major abdominal surgery will usually excrete about 100 mEq of potassium during the first 48 postoperative hours and about 25 mEq each day thereafter. As a result, the potassium is usually administered intravenously in the immediate postoperative period. It should be noted that plasma potassium measurements do not exactly predict total body potassium because potassium is primarily an intracellular ion. From a clinical chemistry point of view, the international standard unit is called a milli mole (mmol)—commonly called the milli equivalant (mEq). The clinical implications for the perianesthesia nurse is that patients undergoing major surgery should routinely have their potassium levels checked and evaluated preoperatively to determine whether they are receiving any non-potassium-sparing diuretics (see Chapter 11).

EDEMA

A delicate balance of pressures keeps fluids passing between compartments. A dynamic equilibrium exists between the plasma and the interstitial fluid because proteins are too large to cross the capillary barrier. This creates a colloid osmotic pressure between the two components. The hydrostatic pressures of the blood and the interstitial fluid tend to oppose each other, which is called the effective filtration pressure. Similarly, the colloid osmotic (or oncotic) pressures is the opposition between the blood and the interstitial fluid. The final common pathway is that these pressures result in a pulling in opposite directions when in appropriate physiologic equilibrium that will not allow fluid to accumulate into the interstitial spaces. Edema then results when either of the two pressures are in dysfunction.

ELECTROLYTES

The electrolytes, which only constitute a small fraction of the body weight, are essential to facilitate normal body function. The electrolytes maintain electroneutrality and chemical conditions in the body fluids, equilibrium between ECF and ICF, and regulation of neuromuscular activity.

Sodium

Sodium, a cation, is primarily found in the extracellular fluid. The blood plasma sodium averages about 142 mEq/L and usually does not vary more then 5 mEq/L. Variations greater than this can affect many physiologic activities; thus mechanisms for regulating sodium concentration are of prime importance in maintaining balance. Basically, the body regulates sodium by conservation mechanisms when the sodium is low, and if body stores of sodium are high, the body will excrete sodium via sweat, feces, and—in large part—the kidneys.

The body fluids are maintained in an isotonic state by regulating the concentration of sodium and its most abundant anion, chloride. Concentration of sodium and chloride in the fluids is maintained primarily by loss or retention of water. Loss of salt is accompanied by loss of water and retention of salt by retention of water. Hence it can be said that water goes where the salt is in higher concentration. This is why patients are often placed on a low salt diet in an effort to reduce fluid overload on the heart and other major organs. However, it should be noted that patients who receive magnesium sulfate will have impaired fluid excretion.

Of clinical interest is that patients who have undergone urologic surgery that require the use of irrigation fluids in the bladder are very susceptible to hyponatremia. The most common surgical procedure that can have this complication is a transurethral resection of the prostate (TURP). The irrigation fluids typically consist of sorbitol and mannitol in 100 ml of water—called Cytal—and—also commonly—glycine in a 1.5% solution. The amount of irrigation solution absorbed through the venous sinuses in the bladder averages about 10 to 30 ml per minute of resection time. For this reason the resection time is usually limited to less than an hour. This absorption of the irrigating fluid results in the fluid entering the vascular system, which leads to volume overload and ultimately in dilutional hyponatremia.

The resulting lowering of the serum sodium concentrations can cause serious cardiac and neurologic consequences. Concentrations of sodium at 120 mEq/L are usually associated with the development of cardiac dysrhythmias and progressive neurologic symptoms such as restlessness, confusion, nausea, vomiting, coma, and convulsions.

Hypernatremia is most often caused by a loss of body fluids that results in sodium excess. The clinical signs of this resemble the signs of hypovolemia, and many times edema will also be present because of the sodium excess.

Potassium

Potassium is the most important intracellular ion. It is very difficult to measure intracellular potassium; therefore only extracellular potassium is measured. The normal values are between 3.5 and 5.5 mEq/L. Potassium is important in the maintenance of cardiac rhythm, deposition of glycogen in liver cells, and transmission and conduction of nerve impulses. It also contributes to cellular energy production.

Potassium depletion may or may not be accompanied by changes in plasma potassium concentration. True depletion develops only with a net loss of potassium, whereas a decrease in plasma potassium—hypokalemia—may occur with a shift of potassium from the ECF to the ICF. Decreased intake can cause a mild deficit, because the mechanisms for potassium conservation are not as efficient as those for sodium. Severe depletion results from abnormal losses rather than decreased intake. Most common causes of severe potassium loss are usually associated with diuretics (see Chapter 11), acute blood loss, and lack of replacement over time (e.g., NPO plus a long surgical procedure). Cardiac arrhythmias and weakness of skeletal muscle are commonly observed in mild hypokalemia, which reflecst potassium's role in neuromuscular function. Severe depletion can cause widespread damage to cell function and structure.

If the patient has low potassium—a serum level between 3.5 and 2.6 mEq/L—the rate of potassium infusion is usually about 40 mEq/hour. Treatment of hypokalemia for potassium concentrations below 2.5 mEq/L requires the administration of 0.5 mEq/kg of potassium chloride. This will usually raise the serum potassium concentration by 0.6 mEq/L. If the patient was receiving catecholamine drugs, the increase would only be about 0.1 mEq/L; if the patient was receiving beta-adrenergic antagonists, the serum concentration would increase by about 0.9 mEq/L. It should be noted that correction of hypomagnesemia may be needed to avoid the increased loss of potassium by the kidneys.

Hyperkalemia is associated with situations in which cells are injured or destroyed. Usually, the administration of succinylcholine, a depolarizing skeletal muscle relaxant, can produce hyperkalemia and is discussed in Chapter 21. However, accidental lethal doses have been administered to patients by rapid intravenous infusion in the PACU. Cases have been recorded in which death occurred within five minutes of the rapid injection of just 25 mEq of potassium. Hence under no circumstance should the perianesthesia nurse administer potassium chloride IV push.

Calcium

Calcium is deposited in the bone tissue as crystalline salts composed primarily of calcium and phosphate; the remainder is in the plasma, ISF, and soft tissues. The major fraction of calcium that accounts for its physiologic effects is the ionizable calcium in plasma, of which the normal plasma concentration is maintained between 4.5 to 5.5 mEq/L. The remainder is bound to protein and other substances in nonionizable form. Calcium has an important function in neuromuscular transmission, skeletal muscle contraction, blood coagulation, and exocytosis necessary for release of neurotransmitters and autocoids.

When the calcium ion concentration in the plasma becomes reduced, it can be severe enough to cause extreme immediate effects. The nervous system becomes progressively more excitable as the membrane becomes increasingly permeable to sodium, and at a certain critical level of calcium, the nerve fibers become so excitable that they begin to discharge spontaneously. Impulses pass to skeletal muscles and cause severe tetanic spasms called tetany. Severe hypocalcemia rarely gives rise to other acute responses because the tetany may be rapidly fatal. An increased secretion of parathyroid hormone, most commonly caused by a parathyroid tumor, can cause hypercalcemia. In this situation, nervous system depression results in reduced reflex activity, and depression of muscle contractility results in skeletal muscle weakness, constipation, and loss of appetite. Because some calcium is excreted in the urine, a mild hypercalcemia can induce kidney stones as the calcium combines with phosphate or other anions and precipitates.

Hypocalcemia occurs when the serum calcium concentration is lower than 4.5 mEq/L and is usually due to hypoparathyroidism, pancreatitis, or renal failure. In this case, the neuromuscular function becomes impaired and there is decreased myocardial contractility, increased central venous pressure, and hypotension. Because the skeletal muscle spasms, laryngospasm is quite possible (see Chapter 27). Hence when caring for patients with hypocalcemia, the perianesthesia nurse should have appropriate airway equipment readily available for resuscitation.

Phosphate

Inorganic phosphate ions normally range from about 3.0 to 4.5 mg/dl. However, the major portion of phosphate ions are found within the cells, and these ions regulate phosphate function. They are, in fact, the major anions in the ICF and probably represent the single most important mineral constituent in cellular activity. Phosphates serve many functions—including forming RBCs and acting as an intermediary in the metabolism of carbohydrates, proteins, and fats. Phosphate promotes deposition of calcium in the bone and is essential for the delivery of oxygen via the RBCs to body tissues. The small number of phosphate ions in the plasma is important in acid-base balance by way of the phosphate buffer system. Phosphate is also important in regulating energy metabolism, such as in adenosine triphosphate (ATP).

Magnesium

Magnesium is an essential element that is found primarily in muscle and bone. It apparently has an effect on tissue irritability and is a cofactor in various enzyme reactions. It has a large impact on cardiac cell membrane ion transport and is essential for activating many enzyme systems. Magnesium is an essential regulator of calcium within cells and is the natural physiologic antagonist of calcium. In regard to skeletal muscle contraction, the presynaptic release of acetylcholine (ACh) depends on the actions of magnesium.

Hypomagnesemia is many times overlooked as an electrolyte deficiency: chronic alcoholics, persons with poor diets, patients with high renal loss of magnesium, and patients with protracted vomiting or diarrhea may experience this syndrome. Subsequently, patients who have had cardiopulmonary bypass may be susceptible because of the dilutional effects of the pump-priming solutions. Symptoms of acute hypomagnesemia may include Chvostek's and Trousseau's signs, carpopedal spasm, stridor, skeletal muscle weakness, seizures, and coma. In the perianesthesia period, ventricular dysrhythmias are usually the most common symptom of hypomagnesemia. Treatment for this syndrome is magnesium 1 to 2 g IV over 5 to 60 minutes or a continuous infusion of magnesium at 0.5 to 1.0 g/hour. In severe life-threatening hypomagnesemia an infusion of magnesium of 10 to 20 mg/kg is usually administered over 10 to 20 minutes.

Hypermagnesemia is a rare clinical phenomena. The most common cause of hypermagnesemia is the parenteral administration of magnesium as a treatment for pregnancy-induced hypertension. Symptoms of hypermagnesemia include sedation, myocardial depression, relaxed skeletal muscles and—when severe—paralysis of the muscles of ventilation. Treatment of the life-threatening hypermagnesemia is with calcium gluconate, 10 to 15 mg/kg given intravenously followed by increased fluid loading to produce diuresis in an effort to enhance the excretion of the excess magnesium.

PERIOPERATIVE BLOOD AND FLUID REPLACEMENT

Because of many factors—such as NPO, insensible fluid loss, and the surgical stresses of hemostatic function—fluid status, past medical/ surgical history, and medication regimes should be assessed. If problems with hemostasis are envisioned, coagulation function should be assessed preoperatively to ensure appropriate intraoperative and postoperative coagulation.

Assessment of Coagulation

The coagulation function for hemostasis is usually viewed in two separate events. The first event is platelet function, which includes aggregation, adhesion, and release of platelet contents and the coagulation cascade of events, which results in the deposition of a fibrin network to form a clot.

Routine screening tests are commonly performed preoperatively and particularly on any patient that expresses a history of bleeding problems. These tests include the platelet count and bleeding time to assess platelet function as well as the PT and PTT to assess the coagulation cascade.

The normal platelet count is 130,000 to 370,000/mm^2. Interestingly, patients that experience hemostatic stress of a major surgical procedure begin to experience bleeding during the operation when the platelet counts become less than 100,000/mm^2. Moreover, certain drugs—such as aspirin, plavix, and the nonsteroidal anti-inflammatory drugs (NSAIDs)—will potentially increase surgical bleeding.

Bleeding times measure the primary phase of hemostasis. Based on the standardized method, the normal bleeding time is 3 to 10 minutes. It will be elevated in individuals with qualitative platelet abnormalities. In this instance, patients bleeding times are helpful diagnostically in that they provide data to determine whether to proceed with procedures involving bleeding into closed spaces. A bleeding time greater than 1.5 times the normal predicts significant hemostatic abnormality.

The prothrombin time (PT) and the activated partial thromboplastin time (APTT) tests are reliable and accurate. The PT evaluates the extrinsic system of coagulation (requiring a tissue factor to initiate clotting) and is sensitive to defects in fibrinogen and to the clotting factors V, VII, and X. The APTT evaluates the intrinsic system of coagulation (all factors found in the circulation) and is sensitive to defects in fibrinogen; prothrombin; and the factors V, VIII, IX, X, XI, and XII. The PT is evaluated during management of coumadin therapy. The APTT monitors heparin therapy. The normal PT values are between 11 to 13.2 seconds, and the normal APTT is between 22.5 to 32.2 seconds.

Another test, fibrinogen, is also helpful in the prediction of coagulation problems—particularly DIC (disseminated intravascular coagulation). The normal value for this test is 195 to 365 mg/dL.

Disseminated intravascular coagulation (DIC) is discussed in detail in Chapter 9. As an overview, it is an uncontrolled activation of the coagulation system, with consumption of platelets and clotting factors. Diagnosis is based on such factors as the presence of thrombocytopenia, prolongation of the prothrombin time and partial thromboplastin time, and increased circulating concentrations of fibrin degradation products in the presence of diffuse hemorrhage. Treatment is focused on removing the cause such as hemolytic transfusion reactions, low cardiac output, hypovolemia, and sepsis. The other parameters of treatment include the administration of platelet concentrates and fresh frozen plasma.

CRYSTALLOID AND COLLOID ADMINISTRATION

The use of crystalloid or colloid fluid administration in the PACU is usually based on the purpose of the fluid therapy and replacement, an attempt to maintain the patient as normal volemic as possible during and after the surgical procedure. Research on these two types of fluid administration cites many advantages and disadvantages for each type. However, no definitive data seems to support significant differences in outcomes. Hence the choice of fluid type should be based on the immediate short-term needs of the patient and not by personal preferences and availability of the particular fluid. Some of the factors on which to base the decision are the amount of volume loss, the type of loss amount, and whether the patient has autologous blood available.

Crystalloid fluids are electrolyte solutions dissolved in water or dextrose and water. These electrolytes are impermeable to the cellular membrane, and dextrose will cross cell membranes. However, crystalloids are freely permeable to the vascular membranes. Crystalloid solutions help determine the total osmotic pressure or osmolality that helps balance water

between the extracellular and the intracellular compartments. Osmolality reflects the number of dissolved particles in solutions. An isotonic solution has the same osmolality as plasma, whereas a hypertonic solution has an elevated concentration of particles and a hypotonic solution has fewer dissolved particles than plasma does. Administration of hypertonic solutions would promote movement of water from the cells into the plasma and shrink the brain, whereas hypotonic solutions will expand the brain.

Isotonic crystalloid solutions have a sodium concentration of between 130 to 150 mEq/L and an osmolality of 280 to 310 mOsm/L. The isotonic fluids remain in the extracellular fluid, and the sodium-free solutions are distributed throughout the total body water. Hypertonic crystalloid solutions have a sodium concentration of greater than 150 mEq/L and an osmolality of greater than 310 mEq/L.

The amount of crystalloid required to replace 1 ml of blood loss is about 5 ml of saline or Ringer's solution. The ratios certainly depend on the circumstances. For example, in patients that are suffering from major hemorrhage, the ratio can be 1 ml of blood volume replaced with 1 ml of Ringer's solution. The ratio can go as high as 10 ml of Ringer's to 1 ml of blood volume in the massively traumatized patient who has received large amounts of fluid.

The advantages of using crystalloids are that they are inexpensive, promote urinary flow, and restore third-space losses. The disadvantages of using crystalloids are that they can dilute plasma proteins, decrease the colloid pressure, and lead to a filtration from the intravascular to the interstitial compartment—which could result in interstitial pulmonary edema. However, crystalloids are an excellent choice for use as maintenance fluids for compensation for insensible losses, as replacement for body fluid deficits, and for special replacements of specific fluids and electrolytes.

Colloids are solutions that contain natural or synthetic molecules that are usually impermeable to the vascular membrane. Hence they remain predominately in the intravascular space. By doing so, colloids determine the colloid oncotic pressure that helps to balance the water distribution between the intravascular and interstitial spaces. Albumin is the prototype natural colloid and accounts for about two-thirds of the plasma oncotic pressure. Dextrans 40 and 70, along with hetastarch 6% with an osmolality of 310 mEq/L, are the major synthetic colloids in clinical use. The advantages of using colloids are that the solution tends to remain in the intravascular compartment, thus causing less peripheral edema and rapidly restoring the circulating volume. Along with this, smaller volumes of colloids as compared to crystalloids can be used for fluid resuscitation, and the colloids will restore the patients volume status sooner and create a sustained increase in plasma volume. Finally, because colloids increase the plasma colloid oncotic pressure, they prevent pulmonary edema. Some of the disadvantages with colloids include their expense, potential to cause coagulation problems and anaphylactic reactions, and interference with blood-typing and crossmatching procedures. Although colloids will improve the circulating volume, they redistribute into the third space and can exacerbate edema after 24 hours.

Perioperative Replacement for Crystalloid and Colloid Administration

An intravenous line is started preoperatively, and maintenance fluids are infused to replace the insensible loss from the last intake of oral fluids. The usual rate is 2 ml/kg/hr. Intraoperatively, the insensible loss rate of 2 ml/kg/hr is continued along with an increase in rate according to the surgical trauma. For minimal trauma, 4 ml/kg/hr is added. For moderate trauma, 6 ml/kg/hr and for severe trauma, 8 ml/kg/hr is added. A colloid solution is added if the blood loss is greater than 20% of the patient's total blood volume. Total blood volume is equal to approximately 5,000 ml. PACU monitoring to ensure appropriate fluid support should include vital signs and urine output.

BLOOD COMPONENT THERAPY

Blood is a viscous fluid medium that contains white blood cells (leukocytes), RBCs (erythrocytes), platelets, and plasma. The RBCs are biconcave disks that contain hemoglobin, which transports oxygen and acts as a buffer to help maintain acid-base balance. The membrane of the RBC has antigens, and the plasma contains circulation antibodies. The ABO and Rh classification systems are two of the common blood group systems. ABO/Rh blood-typing is extremely important to prevent incompatibility between donor and recipient. A person with blood type AB is termed a universal recipient because AB blood has no A or B antibodies in the plasma. An individual with type O is termed a universal donor because no A or B antigens are present on their RBCs. During the screening process for compatibility, the ABO/Rh blood-typing normally is performed; then an antibody screen is performed to detect the presence of the various antibodies in the recipient's and the donor's blood. The last test is the crossmatch, in which a trial transfusion is simulated.

Donated blood can be stored as whole blood or centrifuged and separated into RBCs, leukocytes, platelets, and plasma. Whole blood less than 24 hours old is considered fresh whole blood. A unit of blood contains 450 ml of blood and 63 ml of anticoagulant. If the blood is over 24 hours old, it will contain no viable platelets, and a reduced content of factors V and VIII. Along with this, there will be a decrease in RBC adenosine triphosphate and 2,3-diphosphoglycerate levels, which usually resolve by dilution with the patients blood during transfusion. Blood lactate increases the longer the blood is stored—which can be problematic if multiple blood transfusions are given. Usually sodium bicarbonate is administered to offset the lactate (acid). The patient's potassium also should be monitored because the potassium can be released off the RBC. The patient's pH and PCO_2 are used to evaluate the need for the sodium bicarbonate. Normal blood storage does not exceed 35 days. Generally, 1 unit of whole blood will increase the hematocrit about 3% to 4%, and the hemoglobin level will rise by 1 to 1.5 g/dl. The whole blood should be administered via a large-gauge needle, and a blood filter and warmer should be used. A standard blood filter removes degenerated platelets, leukocytes, and fibrin accumulation. The standard filter has pores between 170 to 230 microns and can be used for up to 2 to 4 units.

The use of autologous blood for transfusions is very popular because it reduces the chances for disease transmission and incompatibility and saves the use of banked blood. In this case the patient donates his or her own blood within 21 to 42 days of operation, depending on the anticoagulant used in the blood storage. The autologous patients are usually given iron supplements and erythropoietin in an effort to keep their hemoglobin within normal limits.

Another type of autologous blood transfusion is the use of acute isovolemic hemodilution during the operative procedure. In this situation, a portion of the allowable blood loss is collected with a large bore intravenous cannula. Usually an equal amount of crystalloid is administered to dilute and subsequently reduce the number of RBCs during the operation. Near the end of the operation, the autologous blood is reinfused to provide more RBCs and fresh platelets.

The last type of autologous blood transfusions is the use of intraoperative blood scavenging systems that collect the blood lost from the operation, which is then reinfused into the patient. Commercial products are available to perform this scavenging and collecting. They use anticoagulants and either provide washed RBCs or the entire blood products back to the patient. Because of the risk of reinfusing bacteria or tumor cells, this procedure is not used on patients who are having surgical procedures performed on the bowel or on malignancies.

The role of the perianesthesia nurse in the administration of blood and blood products is critical to the well-being of the patient. The importance of the nurse's checking and rechecking the blood and following all hospital procedures on the appropriate administration of blood or blood products cannot be overstated.

Perioperative Fluid Therapy—An Example

Usually, for most healthy patients, blood loss is replaced with crystalloid in which for every ml of blood lost, 3 ml of crystalloid is administered. If a colloid solution is chosen, the blood loss is replaced ml for ml. That is, for each ml of blood loss, 1 ml of colloid solution is administered. If the anemia due to blood loss continues, the administration of blood therapy may need to be started.

With the very serious consequences of HIV and other blood borne diseases, the basis for the determination of when to administer blood has been revised. Formerly, if a patient had a hematocrit of 30 or less and/or a hemoglobin of less than 10 grams/dl, blood was usually administered. Now, the major factor in the determination of the administration of blood is the hemoglobin.

Usually a patient with a hemoglobin of 7 grams/dl or less, blood is usually administered. The formula used in calculating the approximate allowable loss of blood is that the allowable loss (AL) is equal to the estimated blood volume (EBV) times the preanesthesia hemoglobin ($Hb_{initial}$) minus the target hemoglobin (Hb_{target}), which is divided by the $Hb_{initial}$.

$$AL = EBV \times \frac{Hb_{initial} - Hb_{target}}{Hb_{initial}}$$

For example, for a 70-kg male patient, his estimated blood volume would be 5180 ml. For adult men, the total blood volume is equal to 74 ml times the weight in kg. In adult women, total blood volume would be 70 ml times the weight in kg. Our adult male in this example has a hemoglobin before anesthesia of 13 gm/dl. It was determined that the patient should not have his hemoglobin drop below 7 grams/dl before blood should be administered. Hence his target hemoglobin is 7.0 gm/dl. Therefore the equation would be the following:

$$AL = 5180\,ml \times \frac{13\,gm/dl - 7\,gm/dl}{13\,gm/dl}$$

Thus this adult male patient's acceptable blood loss is 2391 ml. Therefore the first 2391 ml of blood loss could be replaced by crystalloid or colloids. After that, blood or blood component therapy is usually instituted.

TYPES OF BLOOD COMPONENT THERAPY

Packed Red Blood Cells

These RBCs are "packed" in 200 ml and contain only 50 ml of plasma. They are indicated in older adults, patients with increased oxygen demand, and patients that will not compensate with an increased cardiac output. The packed RBCs will help to restore oxygen transport but will not facilitate blood coagulation. Packed RBCs should be diluted with 100 ml of normal saline to reduce the amount of hemolysis and enhance the flow rate during administration before they are administered. Along with this, no medications or other blood products should be added to the packed RBCs before or during administration. The potential for fluid overload exists during the administration of packed RBCs, especially in older adults. The perianesthesia nurse should monitor these patients' respiratory status. Respiratory dysfunction in this situation may include dyspnea and arterial hypoxemia.

Fresh Frozen Plasma

Fresh frozen plasma (FFP) is used to used to treat bleeding or documented coagulation problems. It should not be used for volume expansion or for replacing large deficiencies in coagulation factors. FFP is separated from whole blood usually within 6 hours of collection. It can be stored for up to one year.

Single Donor Plasma

This plasma is collected from whole blood and is rich in vitamin K–dependent factors II, VII, IX, X, and XI. It has lower levels of the labile factors V, VIII, and fibrinogen than does FFP. Single donor plasma is used for volume expansion and reversal of warfarin (coumadin) effects.

Platelets

Platelet concentrate is usually suspended in 50 ml of plasma. It is indicated for thrombocytopenia due primarily to massive blood transfusion and for thrombocytopathies that are usually drug-induced. One unit of platelets will usually increase the platelet concentration in the adult by 5000 to 10,000/mm^3 and for the newborn 75,000 to 100,000/mm^3. The platelets are administered via a large-gauge needle with a filter (170 to 220-micron) that is in line.

Cryoprecipitate

Cryoprecipitate is produced by thawing fresh frozen plasma and collecting the precipitate. It can be frozen and stored for up to a year. Cryoprecipitate is used for the specific treatment of bleeding associated with deficiencies in fibrinogen, factor XIII, von Willebrand's factor, and factor VIII. The cryoprecipitate should be administered within 6 hours after thawing through a standard blood or special component infusion set with an inline 170-micron filter.

Albumin

Albumin is used for acute volume expansion and is considered a colloid. It does not contain any cellular products and is available in 5% or 25% solutions in saline. Albumin is heat-treated, which eliminates the possibility of transmission of hepatitis and other diseases.

TRANSFUSION REACTIONS

First, the appropriate procedures for obtaining the blood sample for type and crossmatch should be followed. The patient who is receiving the blood should be identified by name and hospital number. Then the unit of blood should be checked against that patient by checking the name of the patient and hospital number as written on the unit of blood. Two PACU nurses should conduct this identification process.

During the administration of the blood or blood products, the patient should be monitored for acute hemolytic reactions. Although the symptoms of a transfusion reaction may be masked by the depressant effects of the anesthetic, usually an acute hemolytic transfusion reaction is signaled by cardiovascular instability such as severe hypotension. Another excellent parameter for which to monitor is any unexplained bleeding at the operative site. Other signs include pain at the infusion site, anxiety, chills, headache, an increase in temperature, and decreased renal function. If it is an allergic transfusion reaction, the patient will have signs of urticaria, stridor, hypotension, and pruritus. A delayed type of hemolytic transfusion reaction may be seen in the PACU. The signs and symptoms include fever and malaise. Laboratory tests that reflect this include an increased direct bilirubin, decreasing hematocrit, and increased urine urobilinogen.

If a hemolytic transfusion reaction is suspected, the PACU nurse should stop the transfusion immediately and attach normal saline to the intravenous catheter. The attending physician and the blood bank should be notified, and a specimen of blood should be drawn and sent to the blood bank along with the blood unit and administration set. A specimen of urine should be obtained to send to the laboratory to be evaluated for hemoglobin content. Finally, the other units of blood for that patient should be rechecked.

VOLUME STATUS ASSESSMENT OF THE PATIENT IN THE PACU

Assessment of hypovolemia in the PACU can be difficult because vasoconstriction due to such things as surgical stress, intraoperative catecholamine administration, and hypothermia can sometimes compensate for the hypovolemia. Other assessment tools include poor skin perfusion—such as cool, pale, and clammy skin particularly in the feet—oliguria, hypotension, tachycardia, and tachypnea. Along with this, the estimated blood loss as well as the type and amount of replacement fluids recorded on the anesthesia record should be evaluated for excessive blood loss. Once these symptoms are demonstrated, the PACU nurse should check the patient for excess bleeding and the IV infusion sites for infiltration. The nurse should also notify the attending physician immediately.

BIBLIOGRAPHY

Alspach J: Core curriculum for critical care nursing, ed 5, Philadelphia, 1998, WB Saunders.

Atlee J: Complications in anesthesia, Philadelphia, 1999, WB Saunders.

Barash P, Cullen B, Stoelting R: Clinical anesthesia, ed 4, Philadelphia, 2000, Lippincott Williams & Wilkins.

Benumof J, Saidman L: Anesthesia & perioperative complications, ed 2, St Louis, 1999, Mosby.

Benumof J: Anesthesia and uncommon diseases, ed 4, Philadelphia, 1998, WB Saunders.

Cottrell J, Smith D: Anesthesia and neurosurgery, ed 4, St Louis, 2001, Mosby.

DeFazio-Quinn D: Ambulatory surgical nursing core curriculum, Philadelphia 1999, WB Saunders.

Estafanous F, Barash P, Reves J: Cardiac anesthesia, ed 2, Philadelphia, 2001, Lippincott Williams & Wilkins.

Ganong W: Review of medical physiology, ed 20, New York, 2001, McGraw-Hill Professional.

Guyton A, Hall J: Textbook of medical physiology, ed 10, Philadelphia, 2000, WB Saunders.

Lake C, Hines R, Blitt C: Clinical monitoring: practical applications for anesthesia and critical care, St Louis, 2001, Mosby.

Litwack K: Perioperative fluid administration: colloid or crystalloid, J PeriAnesth Nurs 8(2):15-18, 1997.

Longnecker D, Murphy F: Dripps/Eckenhoff/Vandam introduction to anesthesia, ed 9, Philadelphia, 1997, WB Saunders.

Longnecker D, Tinker J, Morgan G: Principles and practice of anesthesiology, ed 2, St Louis, 1998, Mosby.

Murray D: Coagulopathies: current perioperative evaluation and management, Anesthesia Today 8(2):1-6, 1997.

Nagelhout J, Zaglaniczny K: Nurse anesthesia, ed 2, Philadelphia, 2001, WB Saunders.

Roizen M, Miller R, Miller E et al, editors: Anesthesia, ed 5, New York, 1998, Churchill Livingstone.

Rose B, Post T: Clinical physiology of acid-base and electrolyte disorders, ed 5, New York, 2001, McGraw-Hill Professional.

Stoelting R: Pharmacology and physiology in anesthetic practice, ed 3, Philadelphia, 1999, Lippincott-Raven.

Stoelting R, Miller R: Basics of anesthesia, ed 4, New York, 2000, Churchill Livingstone.

Stone D: Perioperative care: anesthesia, medicine, and surgery, St Louis, 1998, Mosby.

Townsend C, Beauchamp R, Evers B et al: Sabiston textbook of surgery: the biological basis of modern surgical practice, ed 16, Philadelphia, 2001, WB Saunders.

Waugaman W, Foster S, Rigor B: Principles and practice of nurse anesthesia, ed 3, Norwalk, Conn, 1999, Appleton & Lange.

Waxman SJ, Waxman SG: Correlative neuroanatomy, ed 24, Norwalk, Conn, 1999, Lange Medical Publishers.

Weinberg G: Basic science review of anesthesiology, New York, 1997, McGraw-Hill.

Weiskopf R: The rational perioperative use of blood and blood components, Anesthesia Today 8(2):7-10, 1997.

13

THE ENDOCRINE SYSTEM

The essence of physiology is regulation and control. Physiologic functions of the body are regulated by two major controls: the nervous system and the endocrine system. Many interrelationships exist between the endocrine and the nervous systems. Dysfunction of the endocrine system is associated with overproduction or underproduction of a single hormone or multiple hormones. This dysfunction may be the primary reason for surgery, or it may coexist in patients requiring surgery on other organ systems. To ensure the provision of appropriate nursing interventions for the patient with endocrine dysfunction in the postanesthesia care unit (PACU), the perianesthesia nurse must understand the physiology and pathophysiology of the endocrine system.

DEFINITIONS

Endocrine gland: a group of hormone-secreting and hormone-excreting cells.
Gluconeogenesis: the conversion of amino acids into glucose.
Glycogenesis: the deposition of glycogen in the liver.
Hormone: a biochemical substance secreted by a specific endocrine gland and transported in the blood to distant points in the body to regulate rates of physiologic processes.
Lipolysis: the mobilization of deposited fat.
Releasing factor (RF): a hormone of unknown chemical structure secreted by the hypothalamus.
Releasing hormone (RH): a hormone secreted from the hypothalamus.
Stress: a chemical or physical disturbance in the cells or tissues produced by a change either in the external environment or within the body that requires a response to counteract the disturbance.
Target organ: a gland whose activities are regulated by tropic hormones.

Tropic hormone: a hormone that regulates the blood level of a specific hormone secreted from another endocrine gland.

MEDIATORS OF THE ENDOCRINE SYSTEM: THE HORMONES

A hormone is a biochemical substance synthesized in an endocrine gland and secreted into body fluids to regulate or control physiologic processes in other cells of the body. Biochemically, hormones are either proteins (or derivatives of proteins or amino acids) or steroids.

Protein hormones—such as the releasing hormones, catecholamines, and parathormone—fit the fixed-receptor model of hormone action. In this model, the stimulating hormone, called the first messenger, combines with a specific receptor for that hormone on the surface of the target cell. This hormone-receptor combination activates the enzyme adenylate cyclase in the membrane. That portion of the adenylate cyclase that is exposed to the cytoplasm causes the immediate conversion of cytoplasmic adenosine triphosphate into cyclic adenosine monophosphate (AMP). The cyclic AMP then acts as a second messenger and initiates any number of cellular functions.

In the mobile receptor model, a steroid hormone, because of its lipid solubility, passes through the cell membrane into the cytoplasm, where it binds with a specific receptor protein. The combined receptor protein-hormone either diffuses or is transported through the nuclear membrane and transfers the steroid hormone to a smaller protein. In the nucleus, the hormone activates specific genes to form the messenger ribonucleic acid (RNA). The messenger RNA then passes out of the nucleus into the cytoplasm, where it promotes the translation process in the ribosomes to form new proteins. Hormones that fit the fixed-receptor model produce an almost instantaneous response on the part of the target organ. In contrast, because of their action on the genes to cause protein synthesis, when the steroid hormones are secreted a characteristic delay in the initiation of hormone response varies from minutes to days.

PHYSIOLOGY OF THE ENDOCRINE GLANDS

The Pituitary Gland

The pituitary gland rests in the sella turcica of the sphenoid bone at the base of the brain. This gland is divided into the anterior and posterior lobes. Because of its glandular nature, the anterior lobe is called the adenohypophysis; the posterior lobe, which is an outgrowth of a part of the nervous system—the hypothalamus—is called the neurohypophysis. The pituitary gland receives its arterial blood supply from two paired systems of vessels: (1) the right and left superior hypophyseal arteries from above; and (2) the right and left inferior hypophyseal arteries from below. However, the anterior lobe receives no arterial blood supply. Instead, its entire blood supply is derived from the hypophyseal portal veins. This rich capillary system facilitates the rapid discharge of releasing hormones that have target cells in the anterior hypophysis.

Although the pituitary gland is called the master gland, it is actually regulated by other endocrine glands and by the nervous system. The secretion of the hormones of the anterior hypophysis is primarily influenced and controlled by the higher centers in the hypothalamus. Releasing hormones are secreted by the hypothalamic nuclei through the infundibular tract to the portal venous system of the pituitary gland to their respective target cells of the adenohypophysis. Consequently, the hypothalamus brings about fine regulation of the action of the anterior pituitary, and still higher nervous centers apparently further modulate the production of the releasing factors. Hence the many influences coming into the brain and central nervous system impinge on the anterior pituitary gland either to enhance or to dampen its activity.

Hormonal control of the pituitary involves certain feedback systems. For example, corticotropin-releasing hormone stimulates the production and release of adrenocorticotropin (ACTH). The increased concentration of ACTH causes the hypothalamus to decrease its production of corticotropin-releasing hormone, which in turn reduces ACTH production, ultimately reducing the blood level of ACTH. Therefore when exogenous corticoids are administered chronically, ACTH secretion decreases and the adrenal cortex atrophies. On the other hand, the removal of endogenous corticoids by a bilateral adrenalectomy can result in a tumor of the pituitary gland because of the absence of the feedback depression of the corticotropin-releasing hormone.

The posterior lobe of the pituitary gland has an abundant nerve supply. Nerve cell bodies in the posterior lobe produce two neurosecretions (antidiuretic hormone and oxytocin), which are stored as granules at the site of the nerve cell bodies. When the hypothalamus detects a need for either neurohypophyseal hormone, nerve impulses are sent to the posterior lobe, and the hormone is released by granules into the neighboring capillaries. Consequently, the hormonal function of the posterior lobe is under direct nervous system regulation.

Hormones of the Adenohypophysis

Growth Hormone, or Somatotropin.   The growth hormone is unique because it has no target gland to stimulate but acts on all tissues of the body. Its primary functions are to maintain blood glucose levels and to regulate the growth of the skeleton. Growth hormone conserves blood glucose by increasing fat metabolism for energy. It enhances the active transport of amino acids into cells, increases the rate of protein synthesis, and promotes cell division. In addition, growth hormone enhances the formation of somatomedin, which acts directly on cartilage and bone to promote their growth. The active secretion of growth hormone is regulated in the hypothalamus via growth hormone–releasing hormone. Stimuli such as hypoglycemia, exercise, and trauma cause the hypothalamus to secrete growth hormone–releasing hormone, which is transported to the anterior lobe of the pituitary gland and released into the blood. Secretion of growth hormone can be inhibited by somatostatin, also called growth hormone-inhibiting hormone, which is secreted by the hypothalamus and the delta cells of the pancreas.

Hyposecretion of the growth hormone before puberty leads to dwarfism, or failure to grow. After puberty, growth hormone hypofunction may result in the condition known as Simmonds' disease. This disease is characterized by premature senility; weakness; emaciation; mental lethargy; and wrinkled, dry skin. Giantism is the result of growth hormone hyperfunction before puberty. After puberty, when the epiphyses of the long bones have closed, growth hormone hyperfunction leads to acromegaly. In this disease, the face, hands, and feet become enlarged. Patients with acromegaly are prone to airway obstruction caused by their protruding lower jaws and enlarged tongues. Hence in the PACU, constant vigilance as to the respiratory status of these patients is essential.

Thyroid-Stimulating Hormone (TSH), or Thyrotropin. The follicular cells of the thyroid are the target for TSH. This hormone promotes the growth and secretory activity of the thyroid gland. Production of TSH is regulated in a reciprocal fashion by the blood levels of thyroid hormone and the formation of thyrotropin-releasing hormone in the hypothalamus.

Adrenocorticotropin (ACTH). ACTH promotes glucocorticoid, mineralocorticoid, and androgenic steroid production and secretion by the adrenal cortex. This hormone is released in response to stimuli such as pain, hypoglycemia, hypoxia, bacterial toxins, hyperthermia, hypothermia, and physiologic stress. More specifically, the hypothalamus monitors for these various stressors, and on excitation corticotropin-releasing hormone (CRH) is secreted, which stimulates ACTH secretion from the adenohypophysis. Levels of adrenocortical hormones in the blood regulate secretion of ACTH by a hypothalamic feedback mechanism.

Gonadotropic Hormones. Gonadotropic hormones regulate the growth, development, and function of the ovaries and testes. The gonadotropic hormones are the follicle-stimulating hormone and the luteinizing hormone. Secretion of the gonadotropic hormones is stimulated by gonadotropin-releasing hormone and secreted by the hypothalamus.

Lactogenic Hormone, or Prolactin. Prolactin stimulates postpartum lactation. Unlike other pituitary hormones, the hypothalamic control of prolactin secretion is predominantly inhibitory.

Melanocyte-Stimulating Hormone. Melanocyte-stimulating hormone exerts its effect on the melanin granules in pigmented skin.

Hormones of the Neurohypophysis
Antidiuretic Hormone (ADH), or Vasopressin. During normal activities of daily living, ADH is secreted in small amounts into the blood stream to promote reabsorption of water by the renal tubules, which leads to a decreased excretion of water by the kidneys. When ADH is secreted in large quantities, vasoconstriction of the smooth muscles occurs, which ultimately elevates the blood pressure. The pressor effects of ADH are produced only by large doses that are not in the usual physiologic range. The secretion of ADH is regulated by several feedback loops, one of which involves plasma osmolality. Within the hypothalamus are osmoreceptors, whose function is to secrete ADH when plasma osmolarity is increased. On the other hand, dilution of plasma inhibits ADH secretion. The second feedback loop or major stimulus of ADH secretion is the volume or stretch receptors located in the left atrium. These receptors are activated when the extracellular fluid volume is increased, and when this happens, ADH secretion is inhibited. The baroreceptors, which are located in the carotid sinus and aortic arch, are the receptors for the third feedback loop. A decrease in the arterial blood pressure stimulates the baroreceptors, which in turn stimulate a release of ADH. Both the stretch receptors and the baroreceptors transmit their neuronal input to the brain by way of the vagus nerve.

Lack of ADH leads to a condition called diabetes insipidus. This condition is characterized by the output of a large volume of dilute, sugar-free urine.

Oxytocin. Oxytocin produces contraction of uterine muscle at the end of gestation and has a role in milk excretion—that is, in stimulating the contraction of the surrounding myoepithelial cells of the mammary glands.

Pituitary Dysfunction
Hyperfunction rarely involves more than one endocrine gland. On the other hand, hypofunction does usually involve more than one endocrine gland, although instances of isolated deficiencies have been reported. A common

cause of pituitary hypofunction is compression of glandular cells by the expansion of a functional or nonfunctional tumor. In this situation, an excess of one hormone may coexist with a deficiency of another.

The Pineal Gland

The pineal gland is situated in the diencephalon just above the roof of the midbrain. This gland is considered an intricate and highly sensitive biologic clock, because the secretory activity of the pineal gland is greatest at night. The pineal gland secretes melatonin, which affects the size and secretory activity of the ovaries and other organs. The production and release of melatonin are regulated by the sympathetic nervous system. In fact, the pineal gland is considered a neuroendocrine transducer because it converts nervous system input into a hormonal output.

The Thyroid Gland

The thyroid gland is located in the anterior middle portion of the neck immediately below the larynx. The gland consists of two lobes that are attached by a strip of tissue called the isthmus. Structurally, this gland is made up of tiny sacs called follicles. Each follicle is formed by a single layer of epithelial cells surrounding a cavity that contains a secretory product known as colloid. This colloid fluid consists mainly of a glycoprotein-iodine complex called thyroglobulin.

On stimulation by TSH, thyroid hormones are produced in the following steps: (1) iodide trapping; (2) oxidation and iodination; (3) storage of the hormones in the colloid as part of the thyroglobulin molecules; and (4) proteolysis (which can be inhibited by iodide) and release of the hormones. The two hormones released from the thyroid gland are triiodothyronine (T_3) and thyroxine (T_4). T_4 represents more than 95% of the circulating thyroid hormone and is considered to be relatively inactive physiologically in comparison to T_3. Consequently, although T_3 has a relatively low concentration, it passes out of the blood stream faster than T_4, has a more rapid action, and is probably the major biologically active thyroid hormone. After these hormones are secreted by the thyroid gland, they are transported to all parts of the body by means of plasma proteins, in the form of protein-bound iodinated compounds. Hence the laboratory test for protein-bound iodine is useful in determining the amount of circulating thyroid hormone in the blood.

T_3 and T_4 regulate the metabolic activities of the body. More specifically, they regulate the rate of cellular oxidation. Along with this, they are essential for the normal growth and development of the body. Other metabolic activities that are influenced by T_3 and T_4 are the promotion of protein synthesis and breakdown, increase of glucose absorption and utilization, facilitation of gluconeogenesis, and maintenance of fluid and electrolyte balance. The thyroid hormones are also involved in a feedback mechanism. The concentration of T_3 and T_4 in the blood regulates the secretion of TSH by the anterior pituitary gland. TSH regulates the growth and secretory activity of the thyroid gland.

The thyroid gland also secretes thyrocalcitonin, or calcitonin, to maintain the proper level of calcium in the blood. More specifically, calcitonin decreases the serum concentration of calcium by counteracting the effects of parathormone and inhibiting the resorption of calcium from the bones.

The Parathyroid Glands

The parathyroid glands are located on the posterior portion of the thyroid gland. In most instances one parathyroid gland is present on each of the four poles of the thyroid gland. The parathyroid glands release a polypeptide hormone called parathormone. This hormone is the principal regulator of the calcium concentration in the body. Parathormone is released into the circulation by a negative feedback mechanism that depends on the serum concentration of calcium. Hence, a high serum concentration of calcium suppresses the synthesis and release of parathormone and a low serum calcium concentration stimulates the release of the hormone. Normal serum calcium concentrations depend on the regulatory mechanisms, which include parathormone, calcitonin, phosphorus, magnesium, and vitamin D. In fact, the serum calcium concentration is maintained by these regulatory mechanisms within narrow and constant limits. The normal serum calcium level is 9 to 10.3 mg per dl for men and 8.9 to 10.2 mg per dl for women. Serum levels of calcium expressed in milliequivalents per liter are one half the value given in milligrams per deciliter.

Parathormone influences the rate at which calcium is transported across membranes in the bone, the gastrointestinal tract, and the kidneys. More specifically, calcium release from bone is facilitated by parathormone-induced stimulation of osteoclastic activity. The absorption of calcium by the gastrointestinal tract is enhanced by the parathormone-induced synthesis of vitamin D. Parathormone activates the synthesis of vitamin D, which leads to increased tubular reabsorption of calcium and enhanced renal tubular clearance of phosphorus. This results in more calcium entering the circulation.

The Adrenal Glands

The adrenal glands are located on the apex of each kidney. Each gland consists of an outer portion called the cortex and an inner portion called the medulla. The medulla is responsible for the secretion of catecholamines (see Chapter 9). The preganglionic fibers of the sympathetic nervous system provide the stimulation that facilitates the liberation of the catecholamines by the medullary cells. The cortex makes up the bulk of the adrenal gland and is responsible for the secretion of the steroids. The cortex is divided anatomically and physiologically into three zones: the zona glomerulosa, the zona fasciculata, and the inner zona reticularis. These are the sites of secretion of the three major steroid hormones: the mineralocorticoids, the glucocorticoids, and the androgens, respectively.

The mineralocorticoids are responsible for the maintenance of fluid and electrolyte balance. Aldosterone is, physiologically, the most important mineralocorticoid. The basic action of aldosterone is to promote the reabsorption of sodium by stimulating cellular sodium pumps in the target tissue. Overall, aldosterone causes increased tubular reabsorption of sodium and excretion of potassium. This decreases urinary excretion of sodium and chloride and increases urinary secretion of potassium, consequently expanding the extracellular fluid compartment. Aldosterone secretion is increased by ACTH, a depletion in sodium, and an increase in potassium. The secretion of aldosterone is also regulated by the renin-angiotensin system. Thus when the blood supply to the kidneys is low, the juxtaglomerular cells are stimulated to release renin. Renin, which is an enzyme, enters the blood and converts the plasma protein angiotensinogen to angiotensin I. In the lungs and elsewhere, angiotensin I is converted enzymatically to the physiologically active form, angiotensin II. One of the basic actions of angiotensin II is to stimulate the adrenal cortex to secrete aldosterone. Thus aldosterone secretion is regulated by the blood pressure and volume, and because it causes retention of sodium and a rise in blood pressure, aldosterone also acts as a feedback mechanism to shut off the further release of renin.

The glucocorticoids are secreted in the zona fasciculata. Cortisol (hydrocortisone) constitutes about 95% of the total glucocorticoid activity, with corticosterone and cortisone making up the remaining 5%. These hormones function to preserve the carbohydrate reserves of the body. They do this by promoting gluconeogenesis, glycogenesis, lipolysis, and oxidation of fat in the liver. Because they conserve carbohydrates, these hormones serve as functional antagonists to insulin. Finally, these hormones possess an excellent anti-inflammatory action. The major regulator of their secretion is ACTH, which is secreted by cells in the anterior pituitary gland. ACTH is, in turn, modulated by CRH, which is secreted by the hypothalamus. Cortisol serves as a negative feedback mechanism to inhibit both ACTH and CRH production. Physical and mental stresses stimulate the release of CRH from the hypothalamus. Hence in addition to the catecholamines, cortisol and ACTH are considered to be the major stress hormones.

The androgens, or sex hormones, are actively involved in the preadolescent growth spurt and the appearance of axillary and pubic hair.

The Pancreas

Islet of Langerhans cells are scattered throughout the pancreas. There are three islet cell types—alpha, beta, and delta—which secrete glucagon, insulin, and somatostatin, respectively. Glucagon has several functions that are diametrically opposed to those of insulin. Glucagon is commonly referred to as the hyperglycemic factor, and its most important function is to increase the blood glucose level. This increased glucose level in the blood is due to the effects of glucagon on glucose metabolism—that is, glycogenolysis (in the liver) and increased gluconeogenesis. When the blood glucose concentration decreases lower than 70 mg/dl, the alpha cells secrete glucagon to protect against hypoglycemia. Along with this, amino acids enhance the secretion of glucagon. In this instance, the glucagon helps prevent the hypoglycemia that can result, because amino acids stimulate insulin release, which tends to reduce the blood glucose concentration. The secretion of glucagon appears to be inhibited by the release of somatostatin from the delta cells of the pancreas, and, because it is a polypeptide, glucagon is rapidly destroyed by proteolytic enzymes.

Insulin is a protein secreted by the beta cells of the islets of Langerhans in response to elevated levels of blood glucose. Its secretion is inhibited by low blood glucose levels and somatostatin. In addition, insulin secretion can be inhibited by epinephrine, glucocorticoids, and thyroxine. When insulin is secreted by the beta cells, a metabolic state favoring the storage of nutrients is set into action. These physiologic actions include (1) retention of glucose by the liver; (2) slowing of hepatic glucose release; (3) increase in uptake of glucose by muscle (stored as glycogen) and adipose tissue (stored as triglycerides); (4) translocation of amino acids and neutral fats into muscle and adipose tissue; and (5) retardation of lipolysis and proteolysis. Hence insulin seems to "open the door" of most of the cell membranes of the body to facilitate the movement of glucose, amino acids, and fatty acids into the cells. Diabetes mellitus, which is a disease involving the synthesis, storage, and release of insulin, is discussed in detail in Chapter 45.

The Gonads

The hormone testosterone is produced in the interstitial cells of the testes. The synthesis and secretion of this hormone are regulated by luteinizing hormone, which is secreted by the anterior pituitary gland. Testosterone regulates the development and maintenance of the male secondary sexual characteristics as well as produces some metabolic effects on bone and skeletal muscle. Another action of this hormone is the modulation of male behavior by limbic system stimulation. Estrogen, another gonadal hormone, is secreted by the ovarian follicles in response to the follicle-stimulating hormone and the luteinizing hormone of the anterior pituitary gland and is responsible for the development and maintenance of the secondary sexual characteris-

tics in the female. Estrogen, along with progesterone, which is produced by the cells of the corpus luteum, plays an important role in the menstrual cycle.

SELECTED SYNDROMES AND DISEASES ASSOCIATED WITH THE ENDOCRINE SYSTEM

Hypoadrenocorticism

A reduction in function of the hormones associated with the pituitary-adrenal axis can develop as a result of (1) the destruction of the adrenal cortex by degenerative disease, neoplastic growth, or hemorrhage; (2) a deficiency of ACTH; or (3) a prolonged administration of corticosteroid drugs. Primary adrenal insufficiency (Addison's disease) results from destruction of the adrenal cortex. At present, most cases of Addison's disease are caused by idiopathic atrophy that is probably the result of an autoimmune disease. Other causes include tuberculosis, histoplasmosis, bilateral hemorrhage due to anticoagulation therapy, surgical removal of the adrenal glands, tumor chemotherapy, metastasis to the adrenal glands, and sepsis.

A deficiency of ACTH is associated with panhypopituitarism. Patients who have been administered frequent "bursts" of exogenous steroid preparations such as prednisone can experience a suppression of their output of endogenous corticosteroids because of augmentation of the feedback mechanism to the anterior pituitary gland. Concern about the development of hypoadrenocorticism should be shown in the case of any patient who has received 20 mg of prednisone per day for more than 2 weeks in the preceding 12 months (although authors vary on dosage and length of time). The recovery of the normal function of the pituitary-adrenal axis may require as long as 12 months following the discontinuation of steroid therapy. Patients who are even remotely suspected of having hypoadrenocorticism are usually administered steroids preoperatively, intraoperatively, and postoperatively.

The reason for this perioperative steroid coverage is that infection, injury, operation, or other stressors activate the pituitary-adrenal axis. If this axis is suppressed (i.e., hypoadrenocorticism), acute adrenal insufficiency (Addisonian crisis) can develop. This is a life-threatening situation that requires prompt action by the PACU nurse. Clinical manifestations of the Addisonian crisis include dehydration, nausea and vomiting, muscular weakness, and hypotension, which are followed by fever, marked flaccidity of the extremities, hyponatremia, hyperkalemia, azotemia, and shock. Therefore the PACU nurse should monitor patients who are even remotely likely to develop the Addisonian crisis. If some of the signs and symptoms appear, the attending physician should be notified immediately. The severely ill patient must be treated while the diagnosis is being confirmed. Two to 4 mg of dexamethasone is usually administered intravenously along with intravenous therapy of 5% dextrose in normal saline. Dexamethasone is the drug of choice because it does not interfere with the diagnostic tests and yet does provide the needed glucocorticoid. If dexamethasone is not available, it would be advantageous to administer a single 100-mg dose of hydrocortisone intravenously to obtain both the glucocorticoid and the mineralocorticoid activity. This can be followed by 50 to 100 mg of hydrocortisone administered parenterally every 6 hours. During the administration of the treatment, the PACU nurse should continuously monitor the patient's cardiorespiratory status.

Syndrome of Inappropriate Secretion of ADH

The syndrome of inappropriate secretion of antidiuretic hormone (SIADH) occurs in the event of continued secretion of ADH in the presence of serum hypoosmolality. More specifically, the feedback loops that regulate ADH secretion and inhibition fail. Usually, both dilution and expansion of the blood volume serves to stimulate a suppression of the release of ADH. However, in SIADH, the feedback loops do not respond appropriately to the osmolar or volume change, and a pathologic positive feedback loop continues, thus resulting in continued production of ADH.

When hemorrhage and trauma occur during a surgical procedure, ADH secretion is appropriately elevated, and in this situation SIADH can be induced as a result of overzealous fluid administration. Because of the urinary sodium loss occurring along with the water retention, the syndrome of acute water intoxication may be seen in the PACU. The symptoms of water intoxication derive from increased brain water, inoperative sodium pump, and hyponatremia. The symptoms begin with headache, muscular weakness, anorexia, nausea, and vomiting and progress to confusion, hostility, disorientation, uncooperativeness, drowsiness, and terminal convulsions or coma. These symptoms usually do not occur if the serum sodium level is higher than 120 mEq/L. Therefore in patients who have experienced major vascular surgery, trauma, or hemorrhage, the PACU nurse should assess frequently for the symptoms of SIADH and notify the attending physician if the symptoms become evident. The focus of treatment for SIADH is fluid restriction, diuresis with mannitol or furosemide, and administration of sodium chloride. Along with this, the PACU nurse should frequently assess the neurologic signs and cardiorespiratory status of the patient with SIADH and measure and record accurately the intake and output of all fluids.

BIBLIOGRAPHY

Alspach J: Core curriculum for critical care nursing, ed 5, Philadelphia, 1998, WB Saunders.

Atlee J: Complications in anesthesia, Philadelphia, 1999, WB Saunders.

Barash P, Cullen B, Stoelting R: Clinical anesthesia, ed 4, Philadelphia, 2000, Lippincott Williams & Wilkins.

Benumof J, Saidman L: Anesthesia & perioperative complications, ed 2, St Louis, 1999, Mosby.

Benumof J: Anesthesia and uncommom diseases, ed 4, Philadelphia, 1998, WB Saunders.

Bowdle T, Horita A, Kharasch E: The pharmacologic basis of anesthesiology, New York, 1994, Churchill Livingstone.

Brown B: Anesthesia and the patient with endocrine disease, Philadelphia, 1980, FA Davis.

Butterworth J: Atlas of procedures in anesthesia and critical care, Philadelphia, 1992, WB Saunders.

Coursin DB, Coursin DB, Unger B: Endocrine complications in intensive care unit patients, Seminars in Anesthesia, Perioperative Medicine and Pain 21(1):59-74, 2002.

Degroot LJ, Jameson L: Endocrinology, ed 4, Philadelphia, 2000, WB Saunders.

Ganong W: Review of medical physiology, ed 20, New York, 2001, McGraw Hill Professional.

Greenspan F, Gardner D: Basic and clinical endocrinology, ed 6, Los Altos, Calif, 2000, Appleton & Lange.

Guyton A, Hall J: Textbook of medical physiology, ed 10, Philadelphia, 2000, WB Saunders.

Hardman J, Limbird L: Goodman and Gilman's the pharmacological basis of therapeutics, ed 10, New York, 2001, New York, McGraw-Hill Professional.

Katzung B, editor: Basic and clinical pharmacology, ed 8, Los Altos, Calif, 2000, Appleton & Lange.

Longnecker D, Murphy F: Dripps/Eckenhoff/Vandam introduction to anesthesia, ed 9, Philadelphia, 1997, WB Saunders.

Longnecker D, Tinker J, Morgan G: Principles and practice of anesthesiology, ed 2, St Louis, 1998, Mosby.

McIntosh L: Essentials of nurse anesthesia, New York, 1997, McGraw-Hill.

Nagelhout J, Zaglaniczny K: Nurse anesthesia, ed 2, Philadelphia, 2001, WB Saunders.

Roizen M, Miller R, Miller E et al, editors: Anesthesia, ed 5, New York, 1998, Churchill Livingstone.

Stoelting R: Pharmacology and physiology in anesthetic practice, ed 3, Philadelphia, 1999, Lippincott-Raven.

Stoelting R, Miller R: Basics of anesthesia, ed 4, New York, 2000, Churchill Livingstone.

Waugaman W, Foster S, Rigor B: Principles and practice of nurse anesthesia, ed 3, Norwalk, Conn, 1998, Appleton & Lange.

14

THE HEPATOBILIARY AND GASTROINTESTINAL SYSTEM

Because so many surgical procedures involve the gastrointestinal tract, it is important for the perianesthesia nurse in the postanesthesia care unit (PACU) to understand some functions of the organs of this system. This chapter discusses the overall function of each organ and the possible postoperative complications that may involve the gastrointestinal tract.

DEFINITIONS

Achalasia: a condition in which the lower esophageal sphincter fails to relax during the swallowing mechanism and food transmission from the esophagus to the stomach is impeded or prevented. This condition is also called megaesophagus.

Achlorhydria (hypochlorhydria): a condition in which hydrochloric acid is not secreted by the stomach.

Biliary: pertaining to the gallbladder and bile ducts.

Cholelithiasis: the presence of a common bile duct stone. Also called chronic cholangitis.

Chyme: food that has become mixed with the secretions of the stomach and is passed down the gut.

Deglutition: the act of swallowing.

Diarrhea: rapid movement of fecal matter through the large intestine.

Enteric system: the gastrointestinal tract.

Gastritis: inflammation of the gastric mucosa.

Lithotripsy: a procedure for treating upper urinary tract stones.

Nausea: conscious recognition of subconscious excitation in an area of the medulla closely related to the vomiting center.

Oxyntic glands: gastric glands that secrete hydrochloric acid, pepsinogen, intrinsic factor, and mucus.

Pancreatitis: inflammation of the pancreas.

Peptic ulcer: an excoriated area of the mucosa caused by the digestive action of gastric acid; frequently located in the first few centimeters of the duodenum.

Pyrosis: heartburn, of which gastroesophageal reflux is usually the cause.

Vomiting: a method for the gastrointestinal tract to rid itself of its contents when almost any part of the upper gastrointestinal tract becomes overirritated, distended, or excitable. The physical act of vomiting results when the muscles of the diaphragm and abdomen contract so that the gastric contents can be expelled.

THE ESOPHAGUS

The esophagus is a muscular tube extending from the pharynx to the stomach (Fig. 14-1). It is located behind the trachea and in front of the thoracic aorta and traverses the diaphragm to enter the esophagogastric junction, sometimes called the cardia. Approximately 5 cm above the junction with the stomach is the gastroesophageal sphincter, which functions to prevent the reflux of stomach contents into the esophagus. The resting pressure is normally about 30 torr. This pressure is maintained by the vagus nerve as well as by the nervous system. Ordinarily, the sphincter remains constricted except in the act of swallowing. Anticholinergic drugs, such as atropine, and pregnancy decrease the resting pressure of the lower esophagus. Drugs that increase the lower esophageal pressure include metoclopramide (Reglan) and antacids. Another factor preventing reflux of gastric contents into the esophagus is physiologic compression by intra-abdominal pressure on the esophagus just below the diaphragm. This mechanism is referred to as a flutter valve closure. The main function of the esophagus is to conduct ingested material to the stomach. The innervation of the esophagus appears to originate from the vagus.

Disorders of the Esophagus

Esophageal achalasia, a disease of unknown origin, is characterized by an absence of

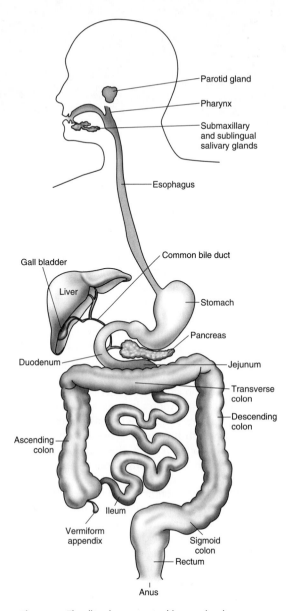

Fig. 14-1 The digestive system and its associated structures.

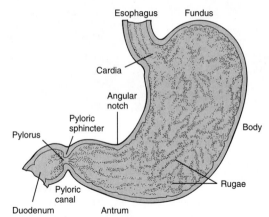

Fig. 14-2 Anatomy of the stomach. *(From Guyton A, Hall J: Textbook of medical physiology, ed 10, Philadelphia, 2000, WB Saunders.)*

peristalsis in the esophagus and by constriction of the cardiac sphincter. The patient with this disorder usually has hypermotility and diffuse spasms of the esophagus.

Hiatal hernia can occur where the esophagus traverses the diaphragm. Ultimately, a lower esophageal stricture may occur that can cause symptoms such as heartburn, pain, and vomiting. Patients with a hiatal hernia require constant observation for active and passive vomiting during the emergent phase of anesthesia. This is especially important if the surgery was performed on an emergency basis when the patient had a full stomach.

THE STOMACH

The stomach can be anatomically divided into three sections: the fundus, the body, and the pyloric portion (Fig. 14-2). The fundus is the dome of the stomach, where peptic juice is secreted. The body is the middle portion of the stomach and is lined with parietal cells that secrete hydrochloric acid. The pH of the solution as secreted is approximately 0.8, which is extremely acidic. The total gastric secretion on a 24-hour basis is about 2 L. This volume normally has a pH of about 1 to 3.5. Histamine has a major role in hydrochloric acid production by the parietal cells in the stomach. This is an effect mediated by histamine$_2$ (H$_2$) receptors, vagal stimulation, and the hormone gastrin. Activation on any one of these receptors potentiates the response of the other to stimulation. Blockade of the activated receptor produces a reduction in acid response because the potentiating effect of the stimulation is reduced. The third portion of the stomach is the pyloric portion, sometimes called the pyloric antrum. Here, a thick, viscous mucus and the hormone gastrin are secreted. At the end of the antrum is the pylorus, an opening surrounded by a strong band of sphincter muscle that controls the amount of gastric contents entering the duodenum.

The vagus nerve (parasympathetic nervous system) provides the nerve supply to the stomach. When the vagus is stimulated, it causes increased motility of the stomach and the secretion of acid, pepsin, and gastrin. Thus a vagotomy is sometimes performed during gastric surgery to decrease gastric motility and acid production. However, it should be stated that the H_2 receptor is a major pathway for stimuli of acid secretion.

Nervous and hormonal stimulation have profound effects on gastric volume and pH. More specifically, stimulation of the parasympathetic nervous system causes increased gastric secretion, and stimulation of the sympathetic nervous system causes decreased gastric secretion. Consequently, pain and fear, which activate the sympathetic nervous system, decrease gastric emptying. In addition, the administration of opioids and active labor prolong gastric emptying. Food, depending on the type and amount, passes through the stomach at a variable rate. For example, foods rich in carbohydrates pass through the stomach in a few hours, whereas proteins exit more slowly. The emptying time for fats is the slowest. Fluids, on the other hand, pass through the stomach rather rapidly. In fact, 90% of 750 ml of ingested saline exits the stomach within 30 minutes. Also, 150 ml of fluids taken 1 or 2 hours before induction of anesthesia stimulates peristalsis and facilitates gastric emptying. Consequently, the small "sips" of water taken with the preoperative oral medications may in fact contribute to lower intraoperative and postoperative gastric volumes. Finally, a prolonged period of fasting does not completely ensure that the stomach is completely empty of fluids or food.

Effect of Pregnancy on Gastric Motility and Secretions

During pregnancy, many alterations occur as a result of the enlarged uterus and altered hormonal state. Because of the enlarged uterus, the stomach and intestine are moved cephalad, and the axis of the stomach is shifted to a more horizontal position. The gastric emptying time is increased in women who are at least 34 weeks pregnant. In regard to the gastric volume and pH, no difference between pregnant and nonpregnant states seems to exist. Consequently, pregnant patients who have been NPO for elective surgery do not present any additional risk of aspiration pneumonitis than do nonpregnant patients. However, research does suggest that pregnant patients who have pyrosis (heartburn) may be at greater risk for regurgitation and subsequent development of aspiration pneumonitis. In addition, if intramuscular narcotics are given during labor, gastric emptying time will be substantially delayed. Epidural anesthesia with local anesthetics does not seem to affect gastric volume or pH; however, if narcotics are introduced into the epidural space, a delay in gastric emptying will occur.

Vomiting and Regurgitation

Vomiting and regurgitation with subsequent aspiration of gastric contents into the airways and lungs are an important cause of morbidity and mortality in the PACU. Various reports have indicated a 4% to 27% risk of this phenomenon. Patients with a gastric pH lower than 2.5 and a gastric volume of more than 25 ml are at high risk of serious pulmonary complications should they experience vomiting and regurgitation with subsequent aspiration.

Various methods of increasing the pH and decreasing the volume of the gastric contents can be used. Anticholinergic agents, such as atropine and glycopyrrolate, inhibit the production of gastric juice—but only to a highly variable degree. These drugs also have side effects of tachycardia, reduced gastric sphincter tone, and delayed gastric emptying. Antacid prophylaxis with the administration of oral antacids has had mixed success, because the subsequent aspiration of the antacid particles, which are nonabsorbable, can have devastating effects on the lungs. The oral antacid sodium citrate (Bicitra) has become popular because it has soluble particles that produce less severe hypoxia and lung abnormalities if aspirated. This drug has been used with great success in patients who require cesarean section.

H_2 receptor–blocking drugs have met with some success in the treatment of gastric hypersecretory states. Cimetidine (Tagamet) is an H_2 receptor–blocking agent that is used as a premedication regimen to control gastric acid production before the induction of anesthesia. The length of action of this drug is 3 hours, with a peak action of about 60 to 90 minutes. Cimetidine does not change the lower esophageal pressure, the rate of gastric emptying, or the volume of gastric juice. Cimetidine can cause a dose-related neuropsychiatric disturbance that is characterized by confusion, slurred speech, hallucinations, delirium, and coma. These symptoms dissipate once the blood level of cimetidine is reduced to $1.5 \mu g$ per ml or lower. Because cimetidine inhibits the metabolism of any drug that is biotransformed by the cytochrome P-450 microsomal enzyme system in the liver, drugs such as propranolol, metoprolol, lidocaine, bupivacaine, diazepam, midazolam, theophylline, and warfarin are potentiated when given in conjunction with cimetidine. Hence cimetidine can prolong the length of action of these drugs.

Ranitidine (Zantac) is an H_2 receptor–blocking agent that is gaining wide popularity as a premedication. By virtue of its H_2 receptor–blocking actions, ranitidine inhibits gastric secretion in response to acetylcholine, histamine, and gastrin. It is more potent than cimetidine, and it is administered in about half the dose of cimetidine, with a peak of 90 minutes and a length of action of about 10 hours. This drug is usually given orally about 1 hour before anesthesia. The usual dose is 150 mg. Ranitidine has a small, clinically insignificant effect on the cytochrome P-450 system. Two new H_2-receptor antagonists, famotidine and nizatidine, have been introduced into clinical practice. These drugs are similar to cimetidine and ranitidine. Unlike cimetidine, neither drug binds to the cytochrome P-450 system; hence they do not interfere with the hepatic metabolism of other drugs.

Metoclopramide (Reglan) is a drug that is often included in the premedication regimen. This drug is a dopamine antagonist that increases the lower esophageal sphincter pressure; speeds gastric emptying, thereby reducing the gastric volume; and prevents or alleviates nausea and vomiting. Metoclopramide can be given orally in a 10 mg-dose as part of a premedication regimen. It also can be given intravenously at 0.15 mg per kg to produce its antiemetic properties. Metoclopramide has minimal side effects.

A problem for which every perianesthesia nurse should watch is regurgitation after anesthesia. When a patient is under the influence of a general anesthetic, the swallowing mechanism is abolished. Foodstuffs or fluids can be passively or actively vomited. The vomitus may then be aspirated into the trachea and lungs. In some instances, this type of aspiration is called Mendelson's syndrome. Inspiring vomitus can lead to aspiration pneumonia. It can occur during the induction of anesthesia, during the operation, or in the immediate PACU phase as the patient emerges from anesthesia.

If a patient begins vomiting, he or she should be placed in a head-down position and given oxygen immediately. The purpose of the head-down position is to allow fluid to flow *away* from the lungs rather than *into* the lungs. Consequently, if at all possible, the patient should be placed in this position if aspiration is suspected. Fluid should be suctioned rapidly while administration of oxygen continues. If the patient's airway is obstructed by large particles, finger or forceps should be used to clear the debris, and then oxygen should be administered. The physician or anesthetist should be notified immediately.

Further treatment may include intubation and instillation of a weak solution of bicarbonate or saline through the endotracheal tube to aid in the neutralization of acidic gastric fluid in the respiratory tract. Steroids and antibiotics may also be administered.

A patient recovering from a general anesthetic should be assessed for possible passive regurgitation, especially if the patient was not intubated during surgery. Clinical signs include dyspnea, cyanosis of varying degrees, and tachycardia. On auscultation of the lungs, abnormal sounds are usually heard. If the assessment indicates the possibility of this syndrome, oxygen should be administered and the physician notified at once.

Patients who had a "full stomach" at induction of anesthesia, who have had intestinal or emergency surgery, or who have a suspected hiatal hernia have a higher incidence of this syndrome. The best treatment is prevention. These patients should have a complete return of consciousness before the endotracheal tube is removed. If the endotracheal tube is to be removed in the PACU, the patient should be placed in a lateral position with the head down. Oxygen should be administered, and suction should be available for immediate use before the extubation is performed.

THE INTESTINE

The duodenum, which is a part of the small intestine, arises at the pylorus of the stomach and ends at the duodenojejunal junction. The duodenum is divided into four segments: superior, descending, transverse, and ascending. The common bile duct and the main pancreatic duct empty into the descending duodenum. The main function of the stomach and the first portion of the duodenum is to alter the form of food and to supply enzymes for digestion.

The jejunum begins at the descending duodenum at the duodenojejunal angle. It constitutes the first two fifths of the small intestine, and the ileum occupies the distal three fifths of the small intestine. The mesentery, which contains blood vessels, nerves, lymphatics, lymph nodes, and fat, stabilizes the small bowel and prevents it from twisting and constricting its blood supply.

The digestive glands secrete large quantities of water to aid in the digestive process. It has been estimated that between 5 and 10 L of water enters the small intestine and that only about 500 ml leaves the ileum and enters the colon. Among the important materials absorbed from the small intestine are sodium, bicarbonate, chloride, calcium, iron, carbohydrates, fats, and amino acids.

Sodium is absorbed by the small intestine at a rate of 25 to 35 g per day. This accounts for approximately 14% of all the sodium in the body. When a patient is experiencing extreme diarrhea, sodium can be depleted to a lethal level within a few hours.

THE COLON AND RECTUM

At the end of the small intestine is the ileocecal valve, which functions to prevent backflow of fecal material from the colon into the small intestine.

The colon is divided anatomically into the cecum, ascending colon, transverse colon, and descending and sigmoid colon. The functions of the colon are the absorption of water and electrolytes, which occurs principally in the proximal half of the colon, and the storage of fecal material, which occurs in the distal colon. The contents of the cecum are mainly liquid, as compared with the solid material contained in the sigmoid colon. Therefore if a patient has had a colostomy, it is important to know from which portion of the colon the stoma originates, so as to determine whether the excreted fecal material has the normal amount of water content.

Of surgical importance is the appendix, which arises from the cecum at its inferior tip. It represents a special type of intestinal obstruction when it becomes inflamed by hyperplasia of submucosal lymphoid follicles, fecaliths, foreign bodies, or tumors.

The rectum functions entirely as an excretory canal and has no digestive function. It begins anatomically at the distal end of the sigmoid colon and ends at the anus. It is tubular and has two layers. The innermost layer is the lumen of the intestinal tract, and the outermost layer is skeletal muscle of the pelvic floor. The muscle is innervated by the parasympathetic nervous system.

THE ANUS

The anus is the termination of the alimentary canal. It is encircled by striated muscle and innervated by somatic sympathetic and parasympathetic fibers. Because of the parasympathetic innervation of the rectum and anus, parasympathetic stimulation may occur during a rectal examination or surgical procedure. This parasympathetic reflex can also occur when a patient is recovering from a general anesthetic. If a physician deems it necessary to perform a rectal examination, the perianesthesia nurse should be prepared to monitor the patient for bradycardia and laryngospasm because they may result from stimulation of the anus and rectum.

THE LIVER

The importance of the liver is generally underestimated. In Chinese medicine, the liver is considered the most important organ of the body. It is one of the basic homeostatic organs, because it maintains the consistency of the blood on a minute-to-minute basis.

The liver is located in the right upper quadrant of the abdomen. It has a dual blood supply, consisting of the hepatic artery and the portal vein. Both carry oxygen and nutrients to the liver for assimilation. The sinusoids, which surround the hepatocytes (liver cells), empty into a venous system that eventually forms the hepatic vein and empties into the inferior vena cava. About 1400 ml of blood per min flows through the liver; this amount is about 30% of the cardiac output. The hepatocytes absorb nutrients from the portal venous blood; store and release proteins, lipids, and carbohydrates; excrete bile salts; synthesize plasma proteins, glucose, cholesterol, and fatty acids; and metabolize exogenous and endogenous compounds. Along with this, hepatocytes have alpha$_1$-, alpha$_2$-, and beta$_2$-adrenergic receptors on their plasma membranes. The preponderance of adrenergic receptors seems to be alpha$_1$, and on stimulation of these receptors, an increase in intracellular calcium ions has been demonstrated.

The liver is the body's most important storage organ. It is able to absorb glucose in the form of glycogen, and it maintains a normal glucose concentration in the body. The liver also stores amino acids, iron, and vitamins. The liver can store up to 400 ml of blood in the sinusoids. If a person loses an appreciable amount of blood, the liver can release stored blood into the circulation to replace what was lost.

The liver performs many vital physiologic functions that have a significant impact on the pharmacologic actions of many of the drugs used in the perioperative period. More specifically, the liver performs biotransformation of drugs by the cytochrome P-450 microsomal enzyme system. Consequently, knowledge of bilirubin metabolism, protein synthesis, and drug biotransformation is of critical importance to the perianesthesia nurse.

Bilirubin Metabolism

Bilirubin is made from one of the byproducts of red blood cell hemolysis—hemoglobin. The reticuloendothelial system converts hemoglobin to unconjugated bilirubin. The bilirubin is transported to the liver via serum albumin. In the liver, the bilirubin is then removed from the albumin and is conjugated with glucuronic acid. Conjugated bilirubin is highly water-soluble and easily excreted in the urine. The other type of bilirubin, which is unconjugated, is lipid-soluble and not excreted in the urine. Conditions such as sickle cell disease, thalassemia minor, drug-induced hemolysis, and breakdown of red blood

cells (RBCs) after massive transfusions can increase unconjugated bilirubin levels. This eventually leads to an increase in bilirubin production. Jaundice, a yellowish tint to the body tissues, can be caused by a high concentration of bilirubin in the extracellular fluids. Consequently, diseases that are considered prehepatic cause an increase in unconjugated bilirubin and eventually lead to what is known as hemolytic jaundice. Obstructive jaundice occurs when the outflow of bile is blocked by an obstruction such as gallstones, stricture, and compression from external masses. In this instance, the conjugated bilirubin level increases in the serum. The third type of jaundice, toxic jaundice, usually follows damage to the liver cells. Use of chloroform can cause this type of jaundice, as can use of carbon tetrachloride.

Protein Synthesis

The liver is responsible for the synthesis of most of the proteins found in the plasma. Albumin is the most notable of the plasma proteins synthesized by the liver. Albumin synthesis is regulated by the state of nutrition; therefore a nutritional deficit results in reduced albumin production. Because many drugs used in anesthesia are protein-bound, a reduction in the albumin level can have a significant impact on the pharmacologic action of the drugs. Because the protein-binding sites are reduced, the unbound fraction of the drug is increased, which ultimately leads to an increased sensitivity to the drug or a prolonged action. This is particularly true for the highly protein-bound barbiturates. Hence in the PACU, hyponatremic patients who intraoperatively have received thiopental should be closely monitored for respiratory and cardiovascular depression due to the prolonged action of the ultra–short-acting barbiturate. The liver also synthesizes the enzyme pseudocholinesterase (plasma cholinesterase). This protein is the principal enzyme in the metabolism of succinylcholine and the ester-type local anesthetics. Succinylcholine, which is the principal depolarizing skeletal muscle relaxant in use, demonstrates an inverse correlation between duration of action and pseudocholinesterase levels. Therefore any patient with suspected liver dysfunction who intraoperatively has received succinylcholine should be closely monitored for respiratory depression in the immediate postoperative period. Finally, the liver produces a large proportion of the protein substances used in coagulation.

Drug Biotransformation

The enzymes required for oxidation and conjugation in the liver are called the microsomal enzymes. These enzymes are part of the cytochrome P-450 microsomal system. Exposure to certain drugs, including barbiturates and some anesthetics, can lead to an increase in the microsomal enzymes. This process is commonly called enzyme induction. Enzyme induction increases the rate of drug biotransformation. Patients with severe liver disease may have reduced microsomal activity in the liver. Hence drugs such as thiopental, diazepam, and meperidine have a prolonged action caused by a decreased rate of drug biotransformation by the microsomal enzymes. Consequently, patients with severe hepatic disease should be closely monitored for respiratory and cardiovascular depression in the PACU phase of their anesthetic experience.

Acute Hepatic Failure

Acute hepatic failure is a rare syndrome that may be seen if the patient has undergone a period of severe hypotension (40 mm Hg systolic) during anesthesia. Because of the hypotension, the liver cells die, and the patient postoperatively appears lethargic and drowsy. Persistent oliguria, which leads to anuria within 24 to 48 hours, is the cardinal symptom of this syndrome. The signs of liver damage ensue and include headache, anorexia, malaise, vomiting, and pyrexia. The syndrome progresses to persistent vomiting and, by the end of the first week, jaundice may be present. The final stages of this disease are marked by delirium, coma, and death.

Treatment of this syndrome is entirely symptomatic and includes maintenance of fluid and electrolyte balance, treatment of the anuria, and a high carbohydrate diet.

THE GALLBLADDER

The gallbladder is a thin-walled, pear-shaped organ attached to the inferior surface of the liver (Fig. 14-3). It is 7 to 10 cm long and 3 to 5 cm wide. It has a capacity of 30 to 60 ml of fluid. Anatomically, it is divided into the fundus; the distal tip; the corpus (body), the middle body

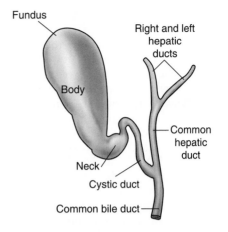

Fig. 14-3 Gallbladder showing right and left hepatic ducts coming from the liver, common hepatic duct, cystic duct, and common bile duct. (Redrawn from Jacob S, Francone C, Lossow WJ: Structure and function in man, ed 5, Philadelphia, 1982, WB Saunders.)

portion; the infundibulum, a pouchlike structure; and the neck, which leads to the cystic duct. The cystic duct joins the common hepatic duct to form the common bile duct. The common bile duct and the main pancreatic duct of Wirsung usually join at the choledochoduodenal junction, which is a passageway through the duodenal wall. The muscle of the choledochoduodenal junction is the sphincter of Oddi, which regulates the flow of bile into the duodenum. Many common narcotic analgesics can produce spasm of the sphincter of Oddi and the duodenum and can increase the pressure in the biliary tree.

Cholelithiasis is a common occurrence in patients with chronic gallbladder disease. As many as 20 million people suffer from some form of cholelithiasis. Gallstones are composed of cholesterol, which is almost insoluble in pure water. The causes of gallstones include too much cholesterol in the bile, chronic inflammation of the epithelium, too much absorption of bile acids from the bile, and too much absorption of water from the bile. A new surgical procedure called biliary lithotripsy offers distinct advantages over cholecystectomy. The advantages include no surgical incision, less pain, a shorter postoperative period, and a reduction in costs to the patient. Consequently, the patient has a 50% reduction in postoperative pulmonary complications because of this new procedure. Formerly, a cholecystectomy was performed, and that procedure was associated with a 50% reduction in the vital capacity on the first postoperative day. In fact, in the immediate postoperative period, the total lung capacity, vital capacity, and functional residual capacity all tend to decrease, thus causing a closure of the small airways and atelectasis. With the advent of biliary lithotripsy, the gallstones are broken into small fragments, and the patient receives either local anesthesia and sedation or general anesthesia. Complications of this procedure are associated with the type of anesthetic technique and its inherent complications and from the shock wave therapy used during the procedure. The most common problems from this procedure include nausea, vomiting, abdominal pain, hemoptysis, and diarrhea. Perianesthesia nursing care for a patient recovering from biliary lithotripsy should include the normal perianesthesia care of an upper abdominal surgical patient (see Chapter 37).

THE PANCREAS

The pancreas is situated in the upper abdomen behind the stomach. It is a slender organ that consists of a head, a body, and a tail (Fig. 14-4). Its main duct, through which pass the pancreatic enzymes, runs the entire length of the gland and opens into the duodenum along with the common bile duct. Scattered throughout the pancreas are small clusters of cells called the islets of Langerhans. They are responsible for the production and secretion of hormones that they empty directly into the blood stream; therefore the islets of Langerhans are considered an endocrine gland. Three types of cells are found in the islets of Langerhans: alpha, beta, and delta. The alpha cells are associated with the production of the hormone glucagon, and the beta cells are associated with insulin. The physiologic significance of the delta cells has not been determined.

Insulin is secreted in response to an increase in the concentration of glucose. The secretion of insulin is inhibited when a low concentration of glucose exists. Glucagon is frequently called hyperglycemic factor because it causes hyperglycemia by stimulating the breakdown of liver glycogen with consequent release of glucose into

the circulation. It also stimulates gluconeogenesis, which is the formation of glucose from noncarbohydrate sources.

The pancreas excretes juice for digesting all three major types of food: carbohydrates, fats, and proteins. The pancreatic juice also contains large amounts of bicarbonate ions, which help neutralize the acidic chyme as it passes into the duodenum from the stomach.

Pancreatitis

Acute pancreatitis is a serious complication of surgery on the biliary tract. It can occur as a result of common duct exploration during gallbladder surgery. Acute postoperative pancreatitis should be suspected if there is excessive pain, vomiting, fever, tachycardia, persistent ileus, or jaundice. The perianesthesia nurse should be aware of these symptoms, which, if detected, should be reported to the surgeon. Treatment of this disorder may include nasogastric suction, anticholinergic drugs, antibiotics, and replacement of fluids and electrolytes.

THE SPLEEN

Because of its anatomic location—not its physiologic functions—the spleen will be discussed here (see Chapter 37).

The spleen is an oval organ located in the upper left quadrant of the abdominal cavity. Its physiologic functions include the filtering of blood and foreign material, hematopoiesis, and, in some instances, the production of lymphocytes and antibodies.

The spleen is a highly vascular organ, and approximately 350 L of blood normally flows through it daily. The spleen acts as a reservoir of blood. It can store so many RBCs that splenic contraction can cause the hematocrit of the systemic blood to increase as much as 3% or 4%.

Normal health is possible after splenectomy because other tissues can assume the functions the spleen normally performs. Splenectomy is usually performed for the cure or alleviation of hematologic disease or because of its traumatic rupture. Because the spleen is friable and vascular, blood loss from a splenectomy can be high. It is therefore important for the perianesthesia nurse to assess the blood loss as well as the cardiovascular status of the patient during the recovery phase.

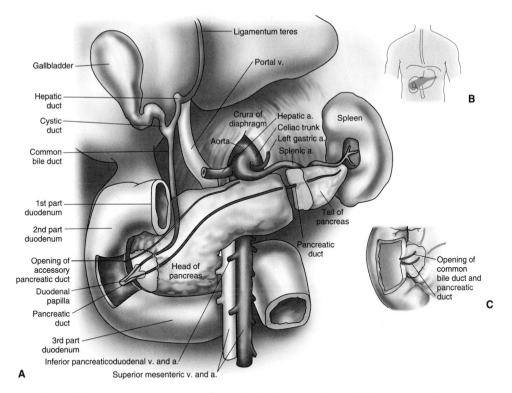

Fig. 14-4 **A,** Relationship of the pancreas to the duodenum, showing the pancreatic and bile ducts joining at the duodenal papilla. A section has been removed from the pancreas to expose the pancreatic duct. **B,** Anatomic position of the pancreas. **C,** Common variation. *(Redrawn from Jacob S, Francone C, Lossow WJ: Structure and function in man, ed 5, Philadelphia, 1982, WB Saunders.)*

BIBLIOGRAPHY

Alspach J: Core curriculum for critical care nursing, ed 5, Philadelphia, 1998, WB Saunders.

Atlee J: Complications in anesthesia, Philadelphia, 1999, WB Saunders.

Barash P, Cullen B, Stoelting R: Clinical anesthesia, ed 4, Philadelphia, 2000, Lippincott Williams & Wilkins.

Benumof J, Saidman L: Anesthesia & perioperative complications, ed 2, St Louis, 1999, Mosby.

Benumof J: Anesthesia and uncommon diseases, ed 4, Philadelphia, 1998, WB Saunders.

Bickley L, Hoekelman R: Bates' guide to physical examination and history taking, ed 7, Philadelphia, 1998, Lippincott Williams & Wilkins.

Bowdle T, Horita A, Kharasch E: The pharmacologic basis of anesthesiology, New York, 1994, Churchill Livingstone.

Conklin K: Maternal physiological adaptations during gestation, labor, and the puerperium, Semin Anesth 10(4):221-234, 1991.

DeFazio-Quinn D: Ambulatory surgical nursing core curriculum, Philadelphia, 1999, WB Saunders.

Ganong W: Review of medical physiology, ed 20, New York: McGraw-Hill Professional, 2001.

Guyton A, Hall J: Textbook of medical physiology, ed 10, Philadelphia, 2000, WB Saunders.

Hardman J, Limbird L: Goodman and Gilman's the pharmacological basis of therapeutics, ed 10, New York, McGraw-Hill, 2001.

Hiley M, Giesecke A: The patient with a full stomach, Semin Anesth 9(3):204-210, 1990.

Jacobs B, Swift C, Dubow H et al: Time required for oral ranitidine to decrease gastric fluid acidity, Anesth Analg 73:787-789, 1991.

Jacobsen W: Manual of post anesthesia care, 1992, Philadelphia, WB Saunders.

Katzung B, editor: Basic and clinical pharmacology, ed 8, Los Altos, Calif, 2000, Appleton & Lange.

Longnecker D, Murphy F: Dripps/Eckenhoff/Vandam introduction to anesthesia, ed 9, Philadelphia, 1997, WB Saunders.

Longnecker D, Tinker J, Morgan G: Principles and practice of anesthesiology, ed 2, St Louis, 1998, Mosby.

Martin J: Positioning in anesthesia and surgery, ed 3, St Louis, 1997, Mosby.

McIntosh L: Essentials of nurse anesthesia, New York, 1997, McGraw-Hill.

Miller R, editor: Anesthesia, ed 5, New York, 2000, Churchill Livingstone.

Nagelhout J, Zaglaniczny K: Nurse anesthesia, ed 2, Philadelphia, 2001, WB Saunders.

Palmer A, Waugaman W, Conklin K et al: Does the administration of oral bicitrate before elective cesarean section affect the incidence of nausea and vomiting in the parturient? Nurse Anesth 2(3):126-133, 1991.

Roberts A: Post anesthesia care of the biliary lithotripsy patient, J Post Anesth Nurs 56:392-396, 1990.

Stoelting, R: Pharmacology and physiology in anesthetic practice, ed 3, Philadelphia, Lippincott-Raven, 1999.

Stoelting R, Miller R: Basics of anesthesia, ed 4, New York, 2000, Churchill Livingstone.

Stone D: Perioperative Care: Anesthesia, medicine, and surgery, St Louis, 1998, Mosby.

Townsend C, editor: Sabiston textbook of surgery: the biological basis of modern surgical practice, ed 16, Philadelphia, 2001, WB Saunders.

Vila P: Acid aspiration prophylaxis in morbidly obese patients: famotidine versus ranitidine, Anesthesia 46:967-969, 1991.

Waugaman W, Foster S, Rigor B: Principles and practice of nurse anesthesia, ed 3, Norwalk, Conn, 1999, Appleton & Lange.

Weinberg G: Basic science review of anesthesiology, New York, 1997, McGraw-Hill.

The integumentary system performs many functions that influence the perianesthesia nursing interventions in the postanesthesia care unit (PACU). Aseptic technique, intravenous cannulation, and care of the burn patient are discussed in this chapter because of their involvement with the integumentary system.

DEFINITIONS

Chilblain: trauma caused by exposure to cold temperatures above freezing and associated with high humidity.

Desquamation: the process by which dead cells are shed at a fairly constant rate.

Frostbite: trauma caused by the crystallization of tissue fluids in the skin or subcutaneous tissue.

Immersion foot: trauma which occurs when the skin of the foot is exposed to water that is below 10°C (50°F) for a long period.

INTEGUMENTARY SYSTEM ANATOMY

The skin, or integument, provides a boundary between the internal and external environments of the body. The surface area covered by the skin is about $1.8\,m^2$ in the average male and $1.6\,m^2$ in the average female and accounts for 15% of the total body weight. It is divided into two major layers: the epidermis and the dermis, which includes the hypodermis.

The Epidermis

The epidermis consists of stratified squamous epithelium and has no blood vessels. The cells of the innermost—or basal—layer (stratum basale or stratum germinativum) of the epidermis are constantly dividing and producing cells of the outer layers. Basal cell cancer develops from this layer. The prickly layer—or stratum spinosum—which is located immediately above the basal layer, consists of cells that are connected by intercellular bridges. It is from this layer that squamous cell cancer arises (Fig. 15-1).

The granular layer, or stratum granulosum, contains three or four layers of cells. Squamous epithelial cells are converted in this layer into hard material by a process called cornification. The next layer, the stratum lucidum, develops only on the palms of the hands and the soles of the feet. The outermost epidermal layer—called the horny layer, or stratum corneum—comprises dead cells, keratin, surface lipids, and dirt. Dead cells are shed at a fairly constant rate by a process called desquamation. The epidermis also has keratinizing and glandular appendages. Keratinizing appendages comprise the hair and the nails, and glandular appendages include the sweat, scent, and sebaceous glands.

The Dermis

The dermis, or corium, lies below the epidermis and consists of collagenous, elastic, and reticular fibers. It also contains blood vessels, nerves, lymphatics, and smooth muscle.

The Hypodermis

The hypodermis functions as a shock absorber and heat insulator. Located under the dermis, it comprises fat, smooth muscle, and areolar tissue.

INTEGUMENTARY FUNCTIONS

The skin has many important functions, the most important of which is to act as a barrier between the internal and external environments. In addition, it plays an important part in body temperature and fluid regulation, excretion, secretion, vitamin D production, sensation, appearance, and many other functions that have yet to be identified.

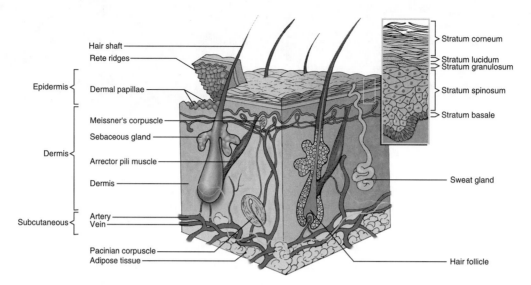

Fig. 15-1   Layers of the epidermis. *(From Monahan FD, Neighbors M: Medical-surgical nursing: foundations for clinical practice, Philadelphia, 1998, WB Saunders.)*

Thermoregulation

Skin, subcutaneous tissue, and fat in the subcutaneous tissue provide heat insulation for the body. Heat is lost from the body to the surroundings by radiation, conduction, convection, and evaporation (Fig. 15-2). Radiation of heat from the body accounts for about 60% of the total heat loss. In this mechanism, heat is lost in the form of infrared heat waves. Conduction of heat to objects represents about 3% of the total heat loss, whereas conduction of heat to the air represents about 15% of the total heat loss. When water is carried away from the skin by air currents, convection of heat occurs. Evaporation constitutes about 22% of the heat loss. Even when a person is not sweating, water still evaporates from the skin and the lungs. This insensible loss is about 600 ml per day.

The skin regulates body temperature by conserving heat in a cold environment. Sweating can lower the body temperature in hot environments. The sweat glands are innervated by the sympathetic and parasympathetic nervous systems. When the anterior hypothalamus in the preoptic area is stimulated by excess heat, impulses are sent from this area by way of the autonomic pathways to the spinal cord. From the spinal cord through the sympathetic outflow tracts, the

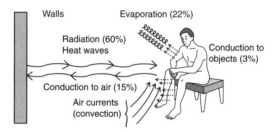

Fig. 15-2   Major mechanisms of heat loss from the body. *(From Guyton A, Hall J: Textbook of medical physiology, ed 10, Philadelphia, 2000, WB Saunders.)*

impulses go to the skin all over the body. The sweat glands are innervated by sympathetic nerve fibers. However, in these specific fibers, the neurotransmitter is acetylcholine. Consequently, these fibers are actually sympathetic cholinergic nerve fibers and are stimulated by epinephrine or norepinephrine.

The sweat gland consists of two portions: a deep subdermal coiled portion that secretes the sweat and a duct portion that conducts the sweat to the skin. Sweat has a pH of 3.8 to 6.5 and contains sodium, chloride, potassium, calcium, and lactic acid as well as urea. Therefore sweating is an act of excretion as well as secretion.

Protection

The skin protects the body from injurious physical, chemical, electrical, thermal, or biologic stimuli. Of particular importance to the perianesthesia nurse is the presence of bacteria on the skin that may cause sepsis when a patient's skin barrier is broken. Normal flora of the skin include gram-positive cocci and rods. Diphtheroids are also widely distributed on the skin, especially in moist areas. The normal pH of the skin is 4 to 6, from lactic acid and amino acid residues of keratinization.

When intact, the skin stops pathogenic organisms from entering the body and at the same time prevents the loss of water, electrolytes, and proteins to the external environment. Once the skin is broken, for example, by surgical incision or venipuncture, the barrier between the internal and external environments is broken. This is why aseptic technique is important whenever opening of the skin is anticipated or has occurred.

IMPORTANCE OF ASEPTIC TECHNIQUE

Because all skin has pathogenic organisms on it, skin can never be sterile. Precautions should be taken to reduce the number of pathogenic organisms that may be introduced into a wound. Handwashing technique is most important. This should be accomplished before care is given to the patient. A good mechanical scrub with a skin antiseptic, such as a soap containing iodine, should be done.

The surgical wound site should be kept clean, and the dressings should remain sterile. If any question about sterility because of excess bleeding, fluid, or physical contamination arises, the dressing should be changed. Special precautions to reduce the introduction of pathogenic organisms should be taken with patients who are prone to infection. This includes patients who are obese, anemic, or debilitated; those with vascular insufficiency, chronic obstructive pulmonary disease, and diabetes mellitus; and those with an immune deficiency, including patients who are on chemotherapy or chronic steroid therapy or who have acquired immunodeficiency syndrome (AIDS). Aseptic technique in wound care of these patients should include the wearing of a surgical mask and the use of sterile gloves and drapes.

Universal Precautions in the PACU

The Centers for Disease Control (CDC) developed the "Universal Precautions for Prevention of Transmission of the Human Immunodeficiency Virus (HIV) and Hepatitis B Virus (HBV) in Healthcare Settings," which is summarized in Box 15-1. The Occupational Health and Safety Administration's universal standards are presented in Box 15-2 and serve to supplement the CDC precautions.

Sterile Technique for Intravenous Therapy

Establishing an intravenous infusion should be accomplished with sterile technique. The site chosen for cannula (needle) placement should be prepared in a suitable fashion. An excellent method uses 1% iodine in 70% isopropyl alcohol. After at least 30 seconds of drying time, the iodine solution should be washed off with 70% isopropyl alcohol. Both agents should be applied with friction, applied from the center of the field to the periphery. An iodophor skin preparation may be substituted in patients with sensitive skin but should not be washed off with alcohol, because its antibacterial action may depend in part on the sustained release of free iodine. In the rare instance in which iodine preparations cannot be tolerated at all, vigorous, prolonged (more than 1 minute) washing with 70% isopropyl alcohol is acceptable.

After the intravenous administration route is established, the cannula (needle) should be securely anchored to prevent irritating to-and-fro motion and to avoid potential transport of cutaneous bacteria into the puncture wound. Although evidence is not conclusive, additional protection from infectious complications may follow topical antimicrobial applications to the infusion site. Because studies have demonstrated that antibiotic ointments may actually favor the selective growth of fungi, the use of topical antiseptic iodophor ointment should be considered. The intravenous site should be covered with a sterile dressing.

Burn Injuries

The care of the postoperative burn patient can be most challenging to the perianesthesia nurse. These patients usually present a complex array of pathophysiologic difficulties—from deranged fluid and electrolyte balance, respiratory complications, and disrupted temperature regulation to psychologic disturbances. A burn—no matter how small—represents a total body assault.

Infection is the most common and the most dreaded complication following a burn injury; therefore aseptic skin care is of primary importance. Nursing care of the patient with a burn injury is complex; the reader should refer to Chapter 42 for discussion of specific pathophysiologic processes, assessment, and nursing interventions for the burn patient in the PACU.

The four main types of burn injuries include cold, chemical, electrical, and thermal. A cold injury is trauma caused by exposure to cold. Conditions such as frostbite, chilblain, immersion foot, and trench foot are the result. Frostbite results from the crystallization of tissue fluids in the skin or subcutaneous tissue. Chilblain results from exposure to cold temperatures above freezing associated with high humidity. Immersion foot occurs when the skin of the foot is exposed to water that is below 10°C for a long period.

Chemical burns are produced by caustic agents—either acid or base. They are devastating because without appropriate emergency treatment, these agents continue to cause destruction of fascia, fat, muscle, and bone.

Electrical burns, which result from direct contact with electrical voltage, are deceiving in appearance. Although only the entrance and exit wounds may be visible, massive damage is often sustained as the high-energy sources follow conductive muscle and nerves. Damage may require amputation of extremities. Thermal injury often occurs in addition to the electrical burn from the heat of arcing currents or ignited clothing.

The most common type of burn injury is the thermal burn, which is caused by excessive heat. Metabolic derangement and problems in maintaining thermal control develop. Unless otherwise indicated, this discussion will cover thermal burns. The terms partial-thickness, deep-dermal, and full-thickness are commonly used to classify burn injuries. The terms first-degree, second-degree, third-degree, and sometimes fourth-degree burns are based on the characteristics and surface appearance of the burn wound.

A partial-thickness burn heals without grafting. This is when only part of the skin has been damaged or destroyed but enough epithelial cells remain in the skin to provide new epidermis, which includes hair follicles and sweat glands. The partial-thickness burn can also be referred to as a first- or second-degree burn. Partial-thickness burns can be divided into three categories: (1) superficial burns, in which there is partial skin loss but no dermal death and therefore no slough; (2) intermediate partial-thickness burn, typically characterized by healing from the level of the hair follicles; and (3) deep partial-thickness burn,

Box 15-2 OSHA Universal Standards Overview (Taken from 29 CFR Part 1910)

INFECTION CONTROL PLAN

Employers need to identify in writing all tasks, procedures, and role descriptions that carry the potential exposure.

Employers must develop a written Infection Control Plan that includes a schedule and method of implementation for each category of the standards.

An Infection Control Plan must be completed within 120 days of the effective date of the final standards.

The Infection Control Plan must be updated and reviewed as tasks and procedures are added or changed.

ENGINEERING AND WORK PRACTICE CONTROLS

Protective equipment must be available in appropriate sizes. It must be removed immediately after leaving the work area, or upon contamination, and placed in a designated receptacle for disposal, washing or disinfection.

Hands should be washed after contact with blood or other potential pathogens and after removal of protective gloves.

Contaminated needles should not be bent, broken, or otherwise manipulated.

Eating, drinking, applying cosmetics or handling of contact lenses should be prohibited in areas of potential exposure.

All laboratory specimens should be handled in a fashion that minimizes splashing or spraying.

PROTECTIVE EQUIPMENT

Personal protective clothing and equipment should be easily accessible, in the appropriate sizes, and replaced or repaired when necessary.

Gloves should be worn when handling blood or infectious materials or when handling items or surfaces soiled by blood or other pathogens.

Masks and eye protection should be worn whenever splashes, spray, or aerosols of blood may occur.

Gowns, warm-up jackets, or similar clothing should be worn if there is a potential for soiling clothes or skin contact.

The protective barrier selected should be appropriate for the procedure being performed and the anticipated occupational exposure.

The decision not to use protective clothing and equipment rests with the employee and not the employer.

HOUSEKEEPING

A written schedule for cleaning and disinfecting all anesthesia equipment and work surfaces is required as well as prompt cleaning and disinfecting at the end of a treatment or whenever contamination occurs.

Laboratory specimens to be transported should be placed in color-coded, leakproof bags with an appropriate label.

Disposal of infectious waste should be in accordance with all federal, state, and local regulations.

Sharps should be disposed of in impermeable, puncture-resistant containers that are accessible to the staff; sharps containers should be labeled and precautions taken to prevent overfilling of the receptacles.

Laundry contaminated with blood or other infectious materials must be placed in labeled or color-coded leakproof bags.

HEPATITIS B VACCINATION AND POSTEXPOSURE FOLLOW-UP

Employers must make the HBV vaccination available to all staff members who have occupational exposure to blood or other potential pathogens one or more times per month.

Postexposure follow-up and reporting of all staff with an occupational exposure to HBV are required.

HBV antibody testing should be made available to employees prior to deciding whether or not to receive the vaccination; if testing indicates that an employee has immunity to HBV, the employer is not required to offer the vaccine.

Following an occupational exposure, the employer should provide medical evaluation and follow-up care to the employee.

Permission for antigen or antibody testing of the source patient's blood should be obtained if possible to determine HBV and HIV infection status.

An employee with an occupational exposure should be tested as soon as possible for the determination of HIV and HBV status.

COMMUNICATION OF HAZARDS TO EMPLOYEES

Labels or other forms of warning should be placed on containers of infectious waste, refrigerators that are used to store blood, and containers used to transport laboratory specimens.

Employee training about the hazards associated with blood and other infectious materials

Continued

Box 15-2   OSHA Universal Standards Overview (Taken from 29 CFR Part 1910)–*cont'd*

and the protective measures required to minimize the risk of exposure should be accomplished within 150 days of the effective date of the final standards.

Employee training and inservice education are required for all new employees and annually thereafter.

Employee training should include epidemiology, symptomatology, modes of transmission of diseases, and work practice controls instituted to prevent contamination.

Employee training records should be maintained for 5 years.

Medical records should be maintained on each employee who receives the hepatitis B vaccine or who experiences an occupational exposure; medical records must be maintained for the duration of employment plus 30 years.

Reprinted with permission from Fay MF: Anesthesia: employee health safety, Anesth Today 2(4):6, 1991, CoMed Communications, Philadelphia, pubs.
HBV, Hepatitis B virus; *HIV*, human immunodeficiency virus.

which typically heals from the level of the sweat ducts.

A deep-dermal burn is a partial-thickness burn that can heal without grafting. However, if it is complicated by infection or mechanical trauma, it is likely to be converted into a full-thickness burn.

Full-thickness burns cause destruction of all the skin. No viable epithelial elements are present, and there may be destruction of the subcutaneous tissue, muscles, and bones. The wound must be grafted, as the skin does not regenerate. The full-thickness burn is equivalent to the third-degree burn. Destruction of the full-thickness burn extending to the structures underneath the skin to include the bone is called a fourth-degree burn.

BIBLIOGRAPHY

Alspach J: Core curriculum for critical care nursing, ed 5, Philadelphia, 1998, WB Saunders.

Atlee J: Complications in anesthesia, Philadelphia, 1999, WB Saunders.

Barash P, Cullen B, Stoetling R: Clinical anesthesia, ed 4, Philadelphia, 2000, Lippincott Williams & Wilkins.

Benumof J, Saidman L: Anesthesia & perioperative complications, ed 2, St Louis, 1999, Mosby.

Benumof J: Anesthesia and uncommon diseases, ed 4, Philadelphia, 1998, WB Saunders.

Bickley L, Hoekelman R: Bates' guide to physical examination and history taking, ed 7, Philadelphia, 1998, Lippincott Williams & Wilkins.

Bowdle T, Horita A, Kharasch E: The pharmacologic basis of anesthesiology, New York, 1994, Churchill Livingstone.

Centers for Disease Control: Universal precautions for prevention of transmission of the human immunodeficiency virus (HIV) and hepatitis B virus (HBV) in healthcare settings, Atlanta, 1989, Centers for Disease Control.

DeFazio-Quinn D: Ambulatory surgical nursing core curriculum, Philadelphia, 1999, WB Saunders.

Ganong W: Review of medical physiology, ed 20, New York, 2001, McGraw-Hill Professional.

Guyton A, Hall J: Textbook of medical physiology, ed 10, Philadelphia, 2000, WB Saunders.

Hardman J, Limbird L: Goodman and Gilman's the pharmacological basis of therapeutics, ed 10, New York, 2001, McGraw-Hill.

Jacobsen W: Manual of postanesthesia care, Philadelphia, 1992, WB Saunders.

Longnecker D, Murphy F: Dripps/Eckenhoff/Vandam introduction to anesthesia, ed 9, Philadelphia, 1997, WB Saunders.

Longnecker D, Tinker J, Morgan G: Principles and practice of anesthesiology, ed 2, St Louis, 1998, Mosby.

McIntosh L: Essentials of nurse anesthesia, New York, 1997, McGraw-Hill.

Miller R, editor: Anesthesia, ed 5, New York, 2000, Churchill Livingstone.

Nagelhout J, Zaglaniczny K: Nurse anesthesia, ed 2, Philadelphia, 2001, WB Saunders.

Sabiston D, editor: Textbook of surgery: the biological basis of modern surgical practice, ed 14, Philadelphia, 1990, WB Saunders.

Stoelting R: Pharmacology and physiology in anesthetic practice, ed 3, Philadelphia, 1999, Lippincott-Raven.

Stoelting R, Miller R: Basics of anesthesia, ed 4, New York, 2000, Churchill Livingstone.

Stone D: Perioperative care: anesthesia, medicine, and surgery, St Louis, 1998, Mosby.

Waugaman W, Foster S, Rigor B: Principles and practice of nurse anesthesia, ed 3, Norwalk, Conn, 1999, Appleton & Lange.

16

Over the past three decades, a virtual explosion of information about the immune system has occurred. Diseases once believed to be based in one of the other physiologic systems are now found, as a result of medical research, to have their bases in the immune system. For example, myasthenia gravis was once thought to be a neuromuscular disease; however, research has demonstrated the origin of the disease to be in the immune system. Today, in the postanesthesia care unit (PACU), perianesthesia nurses must treat patients who are immunosuppressed or are experiencing a hypersensitivity reaction or who have immune diseases such as acquired immunodeficiency syndrome (AIDS). An informed appreciation of the physiology and pathophysiology of the immune system is essential for the appropriate perianesthesia care of the surgical patient.

DEFINITIONS

Acquired immunity: the ability of the human body to develop an extremely powerful specific immunity against most invading agents.

Active acquired immunity: immunity that develops when a person comes into direct contact with a pathogen either by contracting the disease produced by the pathogen or by being vaccinated against the disease.

Antibody: a globulin molecule with the potential to attack agents that are foreign to the host.

Antigen: a protein, large polysaccharide, or large lipoprotein complex that stimulates the process of acquired immunity.

B lymphocytes or bursa-dependent cells: immunocompetent lymphocytes that are named for the preprocessing that occurs in the bursa of Fabricius of birds and is responsible for humoral immunity.

Cellular or cell-mediated immunity: a type of acquired immunity that uses sensitized lymphocytes as the primary defense.

Clone: a group of cells that originate from a single parent cell.

Hapten: a substance that has a low molecular weight and combines with an antigenic substance to elicit an immune response.

Humoral immunity: a type of acquired immunity that uses antibodies as the primary defense.

Immunodeficiency disease: immunosuppression that results from a deficiency of a single humoral antibody group or from a combined deficiency of both the T- and B-cell systems.

Immunity: the ability of the human body to resist almost all types of organisms or toxins that can damage tissues and organs.

Immunosuppression: a state of nonresponsiveness of the immune system to antigenic challenge.

Innate immunity: general processes in the human body–other than those of acquired immunity–that are responsible for protection against organisms and toxins.

Lymphopenia: decreased function of the lymphoid organs.

Passive acquired immunity: immunity that results when a person receives immune cells or immune serum produced by someone else.

Phagocytosis: the envelopment and digestion of bacteria or other foreign substances.

Sensitized lymphocytes: lymphocytes that are made competent by processing to facilitate their immunologic activity, such as their attachment to and destruction of a foreign agent.

Stem cells: an unspecialized cell that gives rise to specific specialized cells such as T and B lymphocytes.

T lymphocytes: sensitized lymphocytes that are responsible for cellular immunity.

PHYSICAL AND CHEMICAL BARRIERS

The body's first line of immunologic defense is the mechanical barrier provided by the epithelial surface. Some parts of the epithelium have extensions from their surface, such as the cilia and the mucus in the respiratory system. These extensions provide not only an additional physical barrier to the entrance of foreign substances but also an efficient removal system. In the stomach, hydrochloric acid, which is thought to have bactericidal action, is secreted. As an additional defense, the skin produces chemicals that inactivate bacteria. The surfaces of the boundary tissues also have specific defenses in the form of secretory antibodies. Consequently, surgical incisions, intravenous cannulation, and many other invasive procedures can cause major breaks in the first line of defense. Hence the perianesthesia nurse should use good aseptic or sterile technique to prevent an overwhelming bacterial invasion through the boundary tissues.

INNATE IMMUNITY

Innate or nonspecific immunity is the body's second line of immunologic defense against foreign material. In this type of immunity, activation occurs during each exposure to an invading substance. Recognition does occur at the level of distinguishing between self and nonself; however, the mechanisms of innate immunity cannot identify the specific invader.

Phagocytosis is the primary mechanism of innate immunity. The cells in the body that carry out the phagocytic functions of innate immunity are monocytes, which are macrophages, and neutrophils (polymorphonuclear leukocytes), which are microphages. The phagocytes' overall immunologic functions are to localize the antigen and to destroy, inactivate, or process it for handling by other components of the immune system. The process of phagocytosis can be enhanced by the combination of an antigen with a plasma protein called opsonin, a substance associated with the immune system. Finally, phagocytosis gives transitory protection to the body so that it will not be overwhelmed by foreign materials before the immune system (acquired immunity) is activated.

ACQUIRED IMMUNITY

Acquired or adaptive immunity is the body's third line of immunologic defense. It is mediated by the capability of specific antibodies or sensitized lymphocytes to recognize and to react to antigens from the offending agent. Two closely allied types of acquired immune mechanisms occur in the body: humoral immunity and cellular (cell-mediated) immunity.

Humoral Immunity

Humoral immunity is conferred by circulating antibodies found in the globulin fraction of blood proteins and are therefore called immunoglobulins (Ig). The processing that is involved to produce the immunoglobulin begins with the lymphocytic stem cells in the bone marrow. These stem cells, which are incapable of forming antibodies, make pre-B lymphocytes that are taken up by the lymph nodes and processed in the as yet unidentified "bursa-equivalent" tissue to become mature immunocompetent B lymphocytes. These processed B lymphocytes are then released into the blood, where they become entrapped in the lymphoid tissue. On stimulation by an antigen, the B lymphocyte specific for that antigen enlarges, divides, and differentiates into plasma cells that have specificity for that antigen. The plasma cells then produce and secrete an antibody or sensitized lymphocyte. During their first exposure to the antigen, lymphocytes from one specific type of lymphoid tissue form clones. The clones are responsive only to the antigen responsible for their initial development. On their second stimulation by the same antigen, the clones proliferate rapidly, thus leading to the formation of a large amount of antibody. Some cells in this clone mature to form plasma cells, whereas other cells of the clone become B lymphocyte memory cells. When the immune system responds to the first presentation of the antigen, the immune system will "remember" the antigen by means of the B lymphocyte memory cell. The immune system can remember the antigen for years. In other words, on the first stimulation by an antigen, the plasma cells produce antibodies (immunoglobulins) as their primary response. The primary response is usually evident about 4 to 10 days after the initial exposure to the antigen. On the second stimulation by the same antigen, a second response occurs. This secondary response, in which a massive amount of antibody specific to the antigen is produced within 1 or 2 days, lasts for months. The secondary response is more rapid, stronger, and more persistent than the primary response. This is because of the memory cells and clones that are produced by the initial exposure to the antigen. If the T lymphocytes are activated by the same antigen; the T-lymphocyte helper cells will enhance the response of the B lymphocytes. Therefore, because of this cooperative effort, the total number of lymphocytes in the lymphoid tissue increases markedly. On second exposure to an antigen, the same plasma cell can produce the particular antibody needed and can convert from one type of antibody secretion to another as needed. Once the specific antibodies from the plasma cells are no longer needed, further production of the antibodies is suppressed by the antibodies themselves or by T-lymphocyte suppressor cells (Fig. 16-1).

The immunoglobulins are large proteins with specific structural arrangements of polypeptide chains with specific amino acid sequences. The immunoglobulins are divided into five primary classes based on structural arrangements: IgA, IgD, IgE, IgG, and IgM.

IgA is a small molecule that constitutes about 15% of the total immunoglobulins and is present in most body secretions. This antibody activates complement through the alternate properidin pathway. Along with this, secretory immunity is mediated by IgA. The secretory antibodies are found on the mucosal surfaces of the oral cavity, the lungs, and the intestinal and urogenital tracts

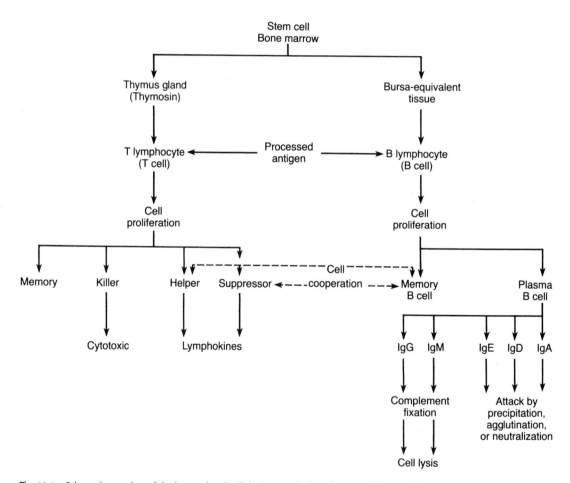

Fig. 16-1 Schematic overview of the humoral and cellular immunologic pathways and the resulting effector substances or mechanisms of activity.

as well as in mammary secretions. This secretory IgA differs from other antibodies in that it has a protein molecule—called a secretory piece—attached to it. Secretory IgA is effective against viruses and some bacteria.

IgD constitutes about 1% of the total immunoglobulins. The exact function of IgD is unknown. However, this immunoglobulin may be involved with the differentiation of the B lymphocytes, and a relationship has been suggested between IgD and antibody activity directed toward insulin, penicillin, milk proteins, diphtheria toxoid, thyroid antigens, and the products of abnormal tissue growth.

IgE is present in minute quantities (about 0.002% of total serum immunoglobulins) and is associated with type I immediate hypersensitivity reaction.

IgG is the smallest antibody, and it constitutes about 75% of the total plasma antibodies. It is the only antibody that can cross the placental barrier, thus conferring passive immunity to the fetus. IgG is the primary antibody involved in the secondary response. It is active against many bloodborne infectious agents such as bacteria, viruses, parasites, and some fungi.

IgM is the largest antibody, and it constitutes about 10% of plasma antibody. It is the main antibody involved in the primary antibody response, and IgM will fix complement.

Antibodies, once secreted by the plasma cells, protect the body against invading agents by three mechanisms of action: (1) attacking the antigen; (2) activating of the complement system, which results in cell lysis; and (3) activating the immediate hypersensitivity reaction, which localizes the invader and may negate its virulence. More specifically, antibodies can inactivate the invading antigen by precipitation, agglutination, neutralization, or complement fixation. Precipitation occurs when an insoluble antibody forms a complex with a soluble antigen (such as tetanus toxin), and the resulting antigen-antibody complex becomes insoluble and precipitates. When antigens are bound together and react with an antibody, agglutinated aggregates occur. Neutralization is achieved when antibodies cover the toxic sites of an antigenic agent or when antibodies counteract toxins released by bacteria. Rarely are the potent antibodies able to attack a cell membrane directly and cause lysis. However,

one of the powerful effects of the binding of the antigen-antibody complex is the activation of complement, which serves to amplify this interaction. More specifically, when IgG or IgM binds to an antigen, the complement system is activated, and a cascade system of nine different enzyme precursors (C1 through C9) reacts sequentially. The final result of the activation of the complement system is puncture of the antigen's cell membrane (cell lysis), thus rupturing of its cellular agents.

Cellular Immunity

Cellular immunity is the second type of specific immunity, and it uses T lymphocytes and macrophages. Some specific functions of the cellular immunity system are protection against most viruses, slow-acting bacteria, and fungal infections; mediation of cutaneous delayed hypersensitivity reactions; rejection of foreign grafts; and immunologic surveillance.

The T lymphocytes, like the B lymphocytes, originate from primitive stem cells and go through stages of maturation (see Fig. 16-1). Once the immature lymphocyte leaves the bone marrow, it migrates to the thymus gland, where it is acted on by the hormone thymosin. The T lymphocyte then becomes mature and immunocompetent. Thus they are thymus-dependent—or T—lymphocytes. These mature T lymphocytes can circulate in the blood and lymph, or they may come to rest in the inner cortex of the lymph nodes, where they may form subgroups of T lymphocytes.

These T lymphocytes function overall in the immune system by serving in regulatory, effector, and cytotoxic capacities. The regulatory T lymphocytes are the helper or suppressor T lymphocytes. These lymphocytes amplify or suppress responses of other T lymphocytes or responses of B lymphocytes. The helper T lymphocytes produce a soluble factor that is required, in some instances, for antibody formation by B lymphocytes. This helper action is most important for IgE and IgG production. The underproduction of helper cells is associated with AIDS. The suppressor T lymphocytes appear to regulate or to suppress the activity of B lymphocytes in the production of antibodies. Evidence indicates that the suppressor T lymphocytes can become pathologically active against helper T lymphocytes and other aspects of cellular immunity. For this reason, these suppressor T lymphocytes may have a role in immune tolerance and in the development of autoimmune disease, such as myasthenia gravis. Effector T lymphocytes are probably responsible for the delayed hypersensitivity reactions, the rejection of foreign tissue grafts and tumors, and the elimination of viral-infected cells. Effector T lymphocytes have antigen receptors on their surfaces that are significant in the initiation of cellular immunity. When an antigen enters the body, it undergoes processing by the phagocytes. The antigen then travels to the regional lymph node, which drains the area of antigen invasion. In this lymph node, the T lymphocyte recognizes the antigen, binds to the antigen, and proliferates. The T lymphocyte becomes sensitized when it comes into contact with the antigen. In addition, memory T lymphocytes result from this interaction. Hence on a second exposure to the antigen, a more intense, efficient, and rapid cellular immunity will result. This contact also results in the release of lymphokines by the T lymphocyte. Some of the lymphokines are (1) chemotactic factor, which recruits phagocytes into the area; (2) migration inhibitory factor, which prevents the migration of phagocytes away from the area; (3) transfer factor, which induces noncommitted T lymphocytes to form T lymphocytes of the same antigen-specific clone as the original cells; (4) lymphotoxin, which is a nonspecific cellular toxin; and (5) interferon, which inhibits the replication of viruses.

The direct cellular cytotoxicity that is mediated by cellular immunity involves cytotoxic lymphocytes—or killer cells—and macrophages. The role of these cytotoxic T lymphocytes is not well established; however, they are believed to be involved in nonspecific killing of viruses, rejection of allografts, and immune surveillance of malignant diseases.

HYPERSENSITIVITY REACTIONS

The immune system serves mainly to protect a person from harmful substances. However, in some instances, the activation of the immune system can cause many deleterious effects; this is termed allergic response or hypersensitivity reaction. Briefly, this response represents a magnified or inappropriate reaction by the host to an antigenic substance, and it can result in an immunologic disease. Hypersensitivity reactions are divided into four major categories and are called type I through type IV hypersensitivity reactions (Table 16-1).

Type I Hypersensitivity Reaction (Anaphylactic, Immediate)

Type I hypersensitivity reaction occurs in persons who were previously sensitized to a specific antigen. The antibodies formed against that antigen are of the IgE classification. The term reagins is used to describe these IgE antibodies. Reaginic antibodies bind to mast cells in tissues surrounding the blood vessels and to blood basophils. When the previously sensitized host is reexposed to the same antigen, the antigen reacts with the reaginic antibody that is attached to the cell, and an immediate swelling and then rupture of the basophil or mast cell results in a release of chemical mediators into the local environment. These chemical mediators include (1) histamine, which causes local vasodilatation and increased permeability of the capillaries; (2) slow-reacting substance of anaphylaxis, which causes prolonged contraction of some smooth muscle, such as that of the bronchi; (3) chemotactic factor, which draws neutrophils and macrophages into the area of the antigen-antibody reaction; and (4) lysosomal enzymes, which elicit a local inflammatory reaction. These chemical mediators act on the "shock organs," such as the mucosa, skin, bronchi, and heart. The resulting clinical manifestations of the type I reaction include urticaria, allergic rhinitis, allergic asthma, and, in severe cases, systemic anaphylaxis.

Type II Hypersensitivity Reaction (Cytotoxic)

In the type II hypersensitivity reaction, the antigen and the antibody complex react, thereby injuring the cell membrane or a surface tissue by direct destruction by antibody of cellular elements. The antibodies involved in the type II reaction are either IgG or IgM, and the reaction is enhanced by complement. Hemolytic anemia is an example of a type II reaction that affects the red blood cells (RBCs). For example, when penicillin is absorbed on the RBC membrane, the interaction of antipenicillin antibody, penicillin, and complement causes a reaction that results in the lysis of RBCs.

Table 16-1 **Categories of Hypersensitivity Reactions**

Type	Mechanism	Outcome	Reaction Time	Examples
I (anaphylactic)	Antigen-IgE reaction at surface of mast cells and basophils	Release of mediators	Immediate	Asthma Hay fever Systemic anaphylaxis
II (cytotoxic)	Binding of IgM or IgG with antigens on surface of cell; enhanced by complement fixation	Cell lysis and tissue damage	Variable	Hemolytic anemia Goodpasture's disease
III (arthus)	Microprecipitation of immune complex formed by antigen and IgM or IgG; enhanced by complement fixation	Tissue damage and release of vasoactive substances	4-18 hours	Serum sickness Farmer's lung Allergic alveolitis Glomerulonephritis SLE
IV (delayed)	Direct interaction of antigen with sensitized T lymphocytes	Release of mediators and tissue damage	24-48 hours	Contact dermatitis Tuberculosis

SLE, Systemic lupus erythematosus.

Type III Hypersensitivity Reaction (Arthus)

The type III hypersensitivity reaction involves the formation of immune complexes of antigen and antibody (IgG or IgM). These immune complexes precipitate in and around small vessels and damage the target tissue by activating complement. Also involved in this process is an inflammatory reaction that is initiated by the gathering of inflammatory cells and the release of vasoactive amines from platelets. As this process continues, polymorphonuclear leukocytes phagocytize the immune complexes and cause inflammation and necrosis of the blood vessels and surrounding tissue because of the release of lysosomal enzymes. Serum sickness and systemic lupus erythematosus are clinical examples of type III hypersensitivity reactions.

Type IV Hypersensitivity Reaction (Delayed or Cell Mediated)

Type IV hypersensitivity reaction is the only hypersensitivity reaction that does not involve antibodies. In the type IV reaction, the exposure to an antigen and the subsequent binding of the antigen with antigen-specific reactive T lymphocytes initiates the production of lymphokines from the T lymphocytes, with tissue damage as the end result. The antigen responsible for the type IV reaction can be bacterial, fungal, protozoan, or viral. Contact dermatitis, allograft rejection, and delayed response in tuberculin skin tests are examples of delayed hypersensitivity reactions.

LATEX ALLERGY

The prevalence of confirmed allergic reactions among healthcare workers ranges from 5% to 10%. Moreover, recent studies indicate that about 8% to 12% of the healthcare population become sensitized to latex. Since 1987—when universal precautions were instituted to prevent the spread of HIV, hepatitis viruses, and other infectious agents—healthcare workers have routinely worn latex gloves as a protective barrier.

Along with this, the Occupational Safety and Health Administration (OSHA) also instructed healthcare workers to wear protective material as a barrier. A great demand then occurred for surgical gloves and hence the accounts of the amount of latex proteins found in surgical gloves varied.

Many products contain latex, and at home they include rubber bands, some carpets, earphones, and mouse pads. In the hospital setting, tourniquets, pressure cuff tubing, and urinary catheters often contain latex. In the perianesthesia area, possible routes of exposure include contact with mucosa, direct contact of particles with an open surgical wound, and aerosolized particles that are bound to the powder in the latex article. Interestingly, these particles can stay suspended for up to 5 hours.

The degree of reactions to latex vary; irritant contact dermatitis is basically a nonallergic reaction. Symptoms such as dry, itchy, irritated areas that may be red and cracked usually occur within the first 6 to 24 hours after exposure. The reaction can be caused by exposure to powders added to the gloves, repeated hand washing and drying, and the use of cleaners and sanitizers. Because it is not a true allergy, it usually clears up after the irritant is removed.

Allergic contact dermatitis is also a nonallergic reaction. Symptoms, which usually occur within 24 to 48 hours, include erythema, vesicles, papules, pruritus, blisters, and crusting of the area that was touched by the latex. This type of response is caused by the chemical additives that are used in the manufacture of latex and are usually thiurams or carbamates.

Of major concern is the Type I immediate hypersensitivity, which is the IgE-mediated response. It usually occurs within minutes of exposure to the latex; however, it can occur within a few hours in some cases. A mild reaction is characterized by skin redness, urticaria, and itching. Severe reactions will produce reactions such as acute rhinorrhea, sneezing, angioedema, bronchospasm, and anaphylactic shock.

Many organizations are investigating latex allergies and the American Society of Anesthesiologists (ASA) has a task force that can be found on the Internet at www.asahq.org/ProfInfo/latexallergy.html. Also,

---

Box 16-1	**Patients Who Should be Strongly Considered at Risk for an Allergic Reaction to Latex**

- A complete medical history is the most reliable screening examination to predict a reaction to latex.
- History of atopic immunologic reactions.
- History of contact dermatitis.
- A history of documented immunologic reactions during a medical or surgical procedure of unknown etiology.
- A history of allergies to food products—including fruits, nuts, bananas, avocado, celery, fig, chestnut, and papaya.
- Neural tube defects—including spina bifida, myelomeningocele/meningocele, and lipomyelomeningocele.
- Patients who have had multiple operations.
- Patients who have had chronic bladder catheterizations.

---

the American Association of Nurse Anesthetists has an excellent web site on latex allergies at www.aana.com/crna/prof/latex.asp. Other helpful sites are the National Institute for Occupational Safety and Health at www.cdc.gov/niosh/latexalt.html, the Latex Allergy Home Page at WWW.netcom.com/~nam1/latex_allergy.html, and "how to manage a latex-allergic patient" at www.anes.com/lair/latex/manage.html.

The best treatment for a latex allergic response is avoidance. Patients that are at risk for a allergic reaction caused by latex are listed in Box 16-1. Healthcare personnel with known sensitivity should carry their own nonlatex—usually made of vinyl or neoprene. They also should use nonlatex tourniquets and latex-free or glass syringes and should use stopcocks to inject drugs. Intravenous line tubing should have no latex ports, or if the latex ports exist, they should be taped. Box 16-2 summarizes the various recommendations for patients with known or risk of latex allergic reactions.

Should the patient in the PACU develop a reaction to latex, the first intervention is to

---

Box 16-2 Summary of the Recommendations for Perianesthesia Care of Patients with Known or Risk of Latex Allergic Reactions

PREOPERATIVE AND INTRAOPERATIVE
- Remove all latex products from the operating room.
- Use a latex-free reservoir bag on anesthesia machine, oral airways, endotracheal tubes, and laryngeal mask airways.
- Use a latex-free breathing circuit with plastic mask and bag.
- Anesthesia ventilator must have a latex-free bellows.
- Place all monitoring devices, cords, and tubes (oximeter, blood pressure cuffs, electrocardiograph wires) in stockinet and secure with tape to prevent direct skin contact.
- Cover all rubber injection ports on IV bags with tape and label "do not inject fluid through ports."
- Use intravenous tubing without latex ports or cover with tape.
- Use nonlatex gloves.
- Use nonlatex tourniquets.

- Draw medication directly from opened multidose vials.
- Draw up medications immediately before the beginning of the case.
- Use latex-free or glass syringes.
- Use stopcocks to inject drugs.

POSTANESTHESIA PHASE OF CARE
- Place sign on the door and flag chart of the patient to alert personnel to the hypersensitivity.
- Make sure patient recovers in a private area.
- Use good handwashing techniques.
- Use only latex-free syringes and gloves.
- Use ampules or remove stoppers from vials before use.
- Cover injection ports on minibags and use latex-free tubings.
- Remain alert for signs and symptoms (hypotension, tachycardia, and bronchospasm) of a latex allergy response and have appropriate emergency drugs and equipment available.

---

remove the patient from ongoing exposure to the latex. The reactions can vary from mild respiratory reactions that can be treated on a symptomatic level, hives—which can occur immediately to several hours after exposure—to a type 1 hypersensitivity anaphylactic reaction.

Treatment for the type 1 reaction should consist of first carefully looking for the latex allergen such as rubber drains in the wound, inadvertent use of latex gloves, latex that contains urinary draining tubes, or IV tubing. Remove all latex from patients' bedsides; change gloves; discontinue antibiotics and blood administration; maintain the airway; administer 100% oxygen; intubate the trachea if necessary; and maintain intravascular volume support. Once the diagnosis of type 1 IgE mediated anaphylaxsis has been confirmed, epinephrine should be administered intravenously in doses of 0.1 mg/kg and titrate to effect. These small doses will stabilize the patient and avoid ventricular tachycardia and malignant arrhythmias.

IMMUNOSUPPRESSION

With the advent of organ transplantation, patients often arrive in the PACU in an immunosuppressed state. Consequently, it is important for the perianesthesia nurse to have a basic knowledge of the forms of immunosuppression and the appropriate nursing care measures that can be implemented for the immunosuppressed patient.

Forms of Immunosuppression

The nonresponsive state of the immune system may be caused by a natural tolerance to self-antigens, to a pathologic state, or to induced immunosuppression. Researchers are attempting to understand immunosuppression by artificially manipulating the immune system to produce a natural tolerance to self-antigens. Pathologic states such as lymphoma and leukemia are examples of the second form of immunosuppression, in which the immune system becomes unresponsive because of the pathologic changes in the immunocompetent cells. Induced immuno-suppression can be accomplished by the administration of an antigen, antisera or antibody; hormones and cytotoxic drugs; radiation; and surgery. For the most part, induced immunosuppression is used for tissue and organ transplants.

For patients who suffer from allergies, the administration of low-dose antigen provides relief in some instances from the antigen-antibody reaction. This desensitizing process produces antibodies that block the interaction between the antigen and the antibody-producing cells. Another method of providing tolerance to self-antigens is by the administration of antisera or antibody in an attempt to coat the antigenic sites. The object is to prevent immunocompetent cells from combining with the antigen. This method of immunosuppression is 100% effective in preventing Rh sensitization and ultimately erythroblastosis fetalis. Corticosteroids produce immunosuppression by reducing the amount of T and B lymphocytes circulating in the blood, blocking lymphokine release, and decreasing the number of monocytes. Cytotoxic drugs are used in the treatment of cancer and autoimmune diseases. The most popular drugs are azathioprine and cyclophosphamide. These drugs suppress immune system function by killing unstimulated lymphocytes. X-irradiation suppresses most of the immunocompetent cells by the induction of a profound lymphopenia. Surgical removal of the thymus gland, spleen, or lymph nodes may alter the immune response by removing tissue needed for the maturation of both the cellular and the humoral immune systems.

Perianesthesia Care of the Immunosuppressed Patient

The major responsibilities of the perianesthesia nurse caring for the immunosuppressed patient are prevention of and early diagnosis and treatment of infection. Opinions differ in regard to placement of the nonleukopenic patient in protective isolation. However, if the peripheral leukocyte count is less than 2000 cells per mm³, the patient probably will benefit from protective isolation. Before the patient is admitted to the PACU, sources of cross-contamination should be eliminated. Blood pressure cuffs and other equipment that are to be used directly on the

patient should be cleaned and disinfected with appropriate solutions. Aseptic technique should be followed at all times. In addition, needle puncture sites and surgical wounds should be cleaned and dressed with appropriate cleaners and ointments. If Foley catheters are used, open skin should be monitored closely for the beginning signs of infection. Immunosuppressed patients may not demonstrate the classic symptoms of infection. The temperature of the immunosuppressed patient should be closely monitored, and if it rises above 38° C, the attending physician should be notified immediately. The use of rectal thermometers should be avoided because they can cause mucosal injury and contamination.

BIBLIOGRAPHY

American Association of Nurse Anesthetists: Latex allergy protocol, J Am Assoc Nurse Anesthetists 61:223-224, 1993.

Atlee J: Complications in anesthesia, Philadelphia, 1999, WB Saunders.

Barash P, Cullen B, and Stoelting R: Clinical anesthesia, ed 3, Philadelphia, 1997, Lippincott-Raven.

Benumof J: Anesthesia and uncommon diseases, ed 4, Philadelphia, 1998, WB Saunders.

Benumof J, Saidman L: Anesthesia & perioperative complications, ed 2, St Louis, 1999, Mosby.

Floyd P: Latex allergy update, J Perianesth Nurs 15(1):26-30, 2000.

Gorringe-Moore R: Immunology and the lung. In Traver G, editor: Respiratory nursing: the science and the art, New York, 1982, John Wiley & Sons.

Grass J, Harris A: Postcesarean section analgesia, Wellcome Trends Anesthesiol 9(6):3-8, 1991.

Groenwald S: Physiology of the immune system, Heart Lung 9(4):645-650, 1980.

Guyton A, Hall J: Textbook of medical physiology, ed 10, Philadelphia, 2000, WB Saunders.

Hardman J, Limbird L: Goodman and Gilman's the pharmacological basis of therapeutics, ed 9, New York, 1996, McGraw-Hill.

Holzman R: Managing the latex-allergic and latex-sensitive patient, Audio-Digest Anesthesiology 42(11)1-2, 2000.

Jacobsen W: Manual of perianesthesia care, Philadelphia, 1992, WB Saunders.

Jocius M: Immunohematology and transfusion reaction, AANA J 50(1):42-48, 1982.

Katzung B, editor: Basic and clinical pharmacology, ed 2, Los Altos, Calif, 1984, Lange Medical Publications.

Longnecker D, Tinker J, Morgan G: Principles and practice of anesthesiology, ed 2, St Louis, 1998, Mosby.

McIntosh L: Essentials of nurse anesthesia, New York, 1997, McGraw-Hill.

Miller R, editor: Anesthesia, ed 3, New York, 1990, Churchill Livingstone.

Murray J: The normal lung, ed 2, Philadelphia, 1986, WB Saunders.

Nagelhout J, Zaglaniczny K: Nurse anesthesia, ed 2, Philadelphia, 2001, WB Saunders.

Paskawicz J, Chatwani A: Latex allergy: a concern for anesthesia personnel, The American Journal of Anesthesiology 28:435-441, 2001.

Rana A, Luskin A: Immunosuppression, autoimmunity, and hypersensitivity, Heart Lung 9(4):651-657, 1980.

Spindler J, Mehlisch D, Brown C: Intramuscular ketorolac and morphine in the treatment of moderate to severe pain after major surgery, Pharmacotherapy 10:51S-58S, 1990.

Stites D, Stobo J, Fudenberg A et al: Basic and clinical immunology, Los Altos, Calif, 1984, Lange.

Stoelting R: Pharmacology and physiology in anesthetic practice, ed 3, Philadelphia, 1999, Lippincott-Raven.

Stoelting R, Miller R: Basics of anesthesia, ed 4, New York, 2000, Churchill Livingstone.

Vance D: Interferon, J Post Anesth Nurs 2(1):43-44, 1987.

17

BASIC PRINCIPLES OF PHARMACOLOGY

The areas of pharmacokinetics and pharmacodynamics of the drugs used in perianesthesia care is ever changing. Consequently, a complete review of the principles and concepts of pharmacology is presented in this second section. The specific pharmacology of drugs related to perianesthesia care is discussed in the physiology chapters in section II along with the chapters dealing with anesthetic agents and adjuncts in this second section. It is believed that the pharmacology of the individual drugs can be best understood in relation to the functions of the physiologic system that is most impacted by the particular drug or classification of drugs.

The final portion of this chapter provides an overview of drug interactions between anesthetic and nonanesthetic drugs to include the herbal agents that can be purchased over the counter to include herbal preparations. These concepts are discussed in detail because they are increasingly relevant to the perianesthesia nurse. With the growth of interest in the fields of drug interaction, drug surveillance, and clinical pharmacology, knowledge of drug interactions in perianesthesia care should become an exceedingly meaningful and useful tool in the delivery of nursing care to the postanesthesiacare unit (PACU) patient.

DRUG RESPONSES

Drugs are administered by a certain route of administration at a certain dosage with the expectation of achieving a desired response. Many factors affect the time of onset, the intensity, and the duration of action of a particular drug. The perianesthesia nurse must become aware of the basic principles of drug interaction with the biologic system. Hence, a review of the basic concepts of drug responses is presented, with particular emphasis on the patient in the PACU.

DEFINITIONS

Additive effect: occurs when a second drug with properties similar to the first is added to produce an effect equal to the algebraic sum of effects of the two individual drugs.

Agonists: drugs such as dopamine that attach and activate specific receptors.

Antagonists: drugs such as Narcan that attach to a specific receptor and do not activate the receptor and prevents the agonist from stimulating the receptor.

Competitive antagonist: when the concentration of the antagonist is higher than the agonist concentration, which remains constant, with the result being antagonism of the agonist. This process is described in detail in regard to the pharmacology of the neuromuscular blocking drugs in Chapter 21.

Cross-tolerance: the result of two drugs with similar actions administered to a patient who has developed tolerance to that category of drugs (i.e., narcotics). The amount of each individual drug must be increased to achieve the desired effect. An example of cross-tolerance is a heroin addict receiving high-dose narcotics in the PACU to maintain minimal analgesia.

Efficacy of a drug: refers to the maximum effect that can be produced by a drug.

Hyperreactivity: an abnormal reaction to an unusually low dose of a drug. For example, patients with Addison's disease, myxedema, or dystrophia myotonica exhibit hyperreactivity to unusually low doses of barbiturates.

Hypersensitivity (anaphylaxis): refers to a drug-induced antigen-antibody reaction. The particular hypersensitivity reaction can be either a type I immediate (anaphylactic) or a type IV delayed reaction. Hypersensitivity reactions can occur with succinylcholine, antibiotics, and many other drugs that are administered in the PACU (see Chapter 16).

Hyporeactivity: an indication that a person requires excessively large doses of a drug to obtain a therapeutic or desired effect.

Idiosyncrasy: an unusual drug effect in a particularly susceptible patient, regardless of the dose. These susceptible patients usually have hypersensitivity or genetic dysfunction.

Metareactivity: unusual drug side effects unrelated to the dosage strength. Metareactivity is also referred to as an idiosyncratic reaction, such as the occurrence of skeletal muscle pain and increased intraocular pressure when succinylcholine is administered.

Pharmacodynamics: the study of the mechanisms of action of drugs and other biochemical and physiologic effects on the body.

Pharmacokinetics: the study of the movement of drugs throughout the body—including the process of absorption, distribution, localization in tissues, biotransformation, and excretion.

Potency of a drug: the dose required of a particular drug to produce a specific effect that is designated as the effective dose (ED). Similarly, that effect, when achieved in a particular percentage of patients, is called ED_{50} for 50% of the patients and ED_{95} in 95% of the patients who demonstrate that effect to the drug.

Receptors: that portion on a cell that drugs attach to which leads to a physiologic response. The receptors are selective in that they only recognize and bind to specific pharmacologic or physiologic agents.

Synergistic effect: addition of a second drug to a drug with properties similar to the first, thereby resulting in an effect greater than the algebraic sum of effects of the two individual drugs.

Tachyphylaxis: an acute drug tolerance—for example, succinylcholine administered by intravenous drip. Over time, a higher drip rate will be needed to achieve the required response.

Tolerance: a type of hyporeactivity that is acquired during chronic exposure to a drug in which unusually large doses are required to reach a desired effect. A prime example is a person who has become addicted to narcotics and who requires larger than normal doses to elicit the desired therapeutic response.

Dose-Response Relationships

The response of a drug in changing a physiologic state may be either quantal or graded. The quantal response is the final intended response, such as sleep, that is intended to be produced by the drug. The quantal data are usually plotted on a dose-response curve of log-dose distribution. The dose of the drug is plotted against the frequency of response to the drug. The median effective dose is the ED_{50} and represents the point on the slope of the curve when 50% of the subjects report a quantal response to the drug. The therapeutic index represents the relative safety of a drug and is the ratio between the toxic dose (TD_{50}) and the ED_{50}. The margin of safety is another way to measure the safety of a drug. It is the ratio between the time when 5% of the subjects experience toxic effects (TD_5) and the dose at which 95% experience the quantal or desired response (ED_{95}).

The graded response makes multiple evaluations of the response of the drug. A continuous scale that ranges from no response to maximum response is used. An example of graded response criteria is the train-of-four, which is used to measure the response to muscle relaxants (see Chapter 21). Usually, the percentage of skeletal muscle function represents the percentage of occupancy of the receptors by the drug being evaluated.

Pharmacokinetic Actions

Pharmacokinetics comprises the absorption, distribution, and elimination of a drug in the body. Consequently, pharmacokinetics can be viewed as what the body does to a drug.

The pharmacokinetic models for the distribution of drugs are based on either a physiologic or a compartmental model. The physiologic model for drug distribution quantifies a drug according to its distribution in various anatomic and physiologic compartments. For example, parameters such as tissue mass, blood volume and flow, partition coefficients, diffusion, and active transport mechanisms are considered in identifying the distribution of a drug. An example of the physiologic model is seen when distribution of the anesthetic drug thiopental is described. After thiopental is injected intravenously, it goes through various anatomic and physiologic organ systems. By redistribution from the brain, the drug is dissipated, and its anesthetic actions consequently are terminated. Because of the difficulty in obtaining human data for the physiologic model of drug distribution, this model is rarely used.

The compartmental model has replaced the physiologic model for determining drug distribution. This model mathematically predicts a drug's concentration in blood or plasma. A compartment represents a theoretical space. A mathematical model can be used to describe the pharmacokinetics of the disposition of a drug. A two-compartment model is usually used to depict a central compartment and a peripheral compartment. The central compartment includes plasma and blood cells and highly perfused tissues such as the heart, lungs, brain, liver, and kidneys. The peripheral compartment represents all other fluids and tissues in the body. With this two-compartment model, a drug can be introduced into the central compartment, move into the peripheral compartment, and then return to the central compartment where removal from the body occurs. The two-compartment model is constructed with the serum concentration versus time and is called the plasma concentration curve. From this curve, the distribution and elimination half-times of the drug can be determined with logarithms. The resulting curve (Fig. 17-1) can be divided into two phases: the distribution (alpha) phase and the elimination (beta) phase.

Elimination clearance quantifies the ability of the body to remove the drug. The major mechanisms for eliminating a drug from the body are hepatic clearance and renal clearance. The half-life ($T^1/_2$) of a drug is the time at which 50% of the total amount of the drug has been eliminated from the body. The elimination half-life ($T^1/_{2\beta}$) is the time when the plasma concentration is at 50% of the elimination phase; it is directly proportional to the volume distribution of the drug and inversely proportional to the drug clearance. Consequently, when the $T^1/_{2\beta}$ for a particular drug is known, a large initial dose called a loading dose of a drug can be given to achieve a therapeutic concentration. The drug can then be given by infusion or in multiple doses at calculated intervals, based on the $T^1/_{2\beta}$, to produce a steady-state plasma concentration. In addition, the time necessary for elimination of a particular dose of a drug can be predicted by the $T^1/_{2\beta}$. Usually, 95% of the drug can be eliminated in five half-lives.

Systemic Absorption by Routes of Administration
Oral Route of Administration.
When a drug is administered orally, it is absorbed in the small intestine, which has a large surface area. A drug must be lipid soluble to cross the gastrointestinal lining. After such absorption, the drug passes to the liver by way of the portal veins before it can enter the systemic circulation. The liver extracts and metabolizes some of the drug, a process termed the first-pass hepatic effect. The drugs that are particularly subject to this effect are lidocaine and propranolol, which is why these drugs

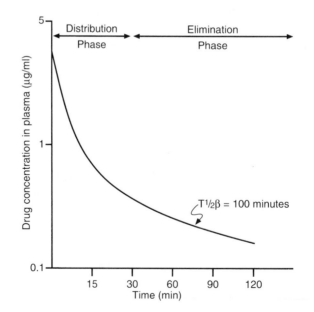

Fig. 17-1 Concentrations of a drug that is administered intravenously plotted on a logarithmic scale over time.

are administered in much higher doses orally than when they are given intravenously.

Oral administration of drugs in the PACU has some distinct disadvantages. For example, nausea and vomiting may occur, which reduces the amount of the drug available for absorption by the small intestine. Also, because the gastric volume and pH are altered either by preoperative drugs or anesthesia and surgery, the absorption process can be affected.

Sublingual Route of Administration. The sublingual route of administration has several important advantages over the oral route. This is because the sublingual route bypasses the first-pass hepatic effect. This route can be particularly favorable in the PACU for drugs such as nifedipine and nitroglycerin.

Subcutaneous and Intramuscular Routes of Administration. These routes of administration require simple diffusion from the site of injection into the systemic circulation. Consequently, they do not provide a reliable rate of systemic absorption. This is particularly true in the PACU when patients are hypothermic, hypotensive, and usually have some peripheral vasoconstriction. In addition, if a hypothermic patient in the PACU is administered a drug either subcutaneously or intramuscularly, the drug probably will not produce the desired effects. However, when the patient is rewarmed, a significant amount of the drug can be rapidly liberated from the injection site, thus causing a large concentration of the drug in the systemic circulation. This can be dangerous when narcotics are administered.

Intravenous Route of Administration. This route of administration facilitates the delivery of a desired concentration of a drug in a rapid and precise fashion. In the PACU, because patients generally experience a certain amount of hypothermia, hypotension, delirium, and unconsciousness, the intravenous route is most acceptable for administration of drugs.

Aerosolized Medications to the Respiratory Tract. This route of administration facilitates direct delivery from inhaled aerosols to a targeted organ which reduces the systematic drug exposure and side effects. Many aerosol delivery devices can be used to administer bronchoactive inhaled aerosols. The most commonly used method of administration in the PACU is the aerosolized nebulizer, in which a specific amount of drug is administered in a solution of normal saline is nebulized using a ventilator or oxygen delivery devices. Other devices to deliver the drug either orally or nasally by inhalation are the metered dose inhaler (MDI) with or without a holding chamber or spacer device, the small volume nebulizer (SVN), and the dry powder inhaler (DPI). The MDI, SVN, and the DPI devices deliver about the same percentage of the drug to the target organ, the lungs, with the MDI able to increase the patient flow rates better than the SVN and the DPI. Table 17-1 presents some of the drugs that activate the lung adrenergic and anticholinergic receptors in regard to onset, peak and duration. Table 17-2 summarizes the major drug groups and their intended outcome in respiratory care.

Removal of Drugs from the Systemic Circulation

The principal ways drugs are cleared from the systemic circulation are by the hepatic, biliary, and renal systems. The hepatic system has a high blood flow and can extract many lipid-soluble drugs from the systemic circulation. In the liver, drugs undergo biotransformation and become pharmacologically inactive. Enzyme induction or a decrease in protein binding enhances the hepatic clearance of some drugs (see Chapter 14). After they have been metabolized in the liver, drugs can be transported to the biliary system for excretion. Also, some drugs, such as the glucuronides, are actively transported to the bile and excreted in an inactive form.

The kidneys secrete many water-soluble drugs in their unchanged form. Renal excretion of drugs depends on the major physiologic processes that occur in the kidneys: glomerular filtration, active tubular secretion, and passive tubular reabsorption. Appropriate renal function is needed to facilitate many of the drugs administered in the perioperative period. Consequently, concern about renal function should merit a creatinine clearance or serum creatinine level because these laboratory tests correlate well with renal drug elimination.

Effects of Physiologic Dysfunction on Pharmacologic Action

Renal Disease. Kidney disease reduces the effectiveness of drug clearance. Indirectly, it also reduces hepatic clearance with a resultant production of exaggerated effects and a prolongation in the action of the drugs that experience a reduc-

Table 17-1 **Drugs Used in the PACU: Perianesthesia Drug List**					
Drug	Route	Onset	Peak	Duration Of Action	Classification
Adenosine (Adenocard)	IV	<20 Seconds	20-30 Seconds	1 Minute	Antiarrhythmic
Albuterol (Proventil, Ventolin)	INH	<5 Minutes	0.5-2 Hours	3-6 Hours	Bronchodilator
Alfentanil (Alfenta)	IV	1-2 Minutes	1-2 Minutes	10-60 Minutes	Opioid agonist
	Epidural	5-15 Minutes	30 Minutes	30 Minutes-1 Hour	
Aminocaproic acid (Amicar)	IV	1-2 Hours		8-12 Hours	Hemostatic agent
Aminophylline	IV	1-2 Minutes	30-60 Minutes	4-10 Hours	Bronchodilator
	PO	<30 Minutes	1-5 Hours	4-8 Hours	
Amrinone (Inocor)	IV	2-5 Minutes	10 Minutes	30 Minutes-2 Hours	Positive inotrope
Atenolol (Tenormin)	IV	5 Minutes	5 Minutes	12-24 Hours	β-Blocker
	PO	30-60 Minutes	2-4 Hours	24 Hours	
Atracurium (Tracrium)	IV	2-5 Minutes	3-5 Minutes	20-35 Minutes	Nondepolarizing neuromuscular blocker (NMB)
Atropine	IV-cardiac	30-60 Seconds	1-2 Minutes	15-30 Minutes	Anticholinergic
	IV-dry OS	30-60 Minutes	60-90 Minutes	4 Hours	
	ETT	10-20 Seconds			
	IM	5-40 Minutes	20-60 Minutes	2-4 Hours	
	INH	3-5 Minutes	15-90 Minutes	3-6 Hours	
Bretylium (Bretylol)	IV/IM	1-5 Minutes	20 Minutes-2 Hours	6-24 Hours	Antiarrhythmic
Bumetanide (Bumex)	IV	1-5 Minutes	15-30 Minutes	4 Hours	Loop diuretic
Bupivacaine (Marcaine)	Epidural	4-7 Minutes	30-45 Minutes	2-7 Hours	Local anesthetic
	Infiltration	2-10 Minutes	30-45 Minutes	3-7 Hours	
	Spinal	<1 Minute	15 Minutes	2-4 Hours	

Table 17-1	**Drugs Used in the PACU: Perianesthesia Drug List**–*cont'd*				
Drug	Route	Onset	Peak	Duration Of Action	Classification
Butorphanol (Stadol)	IV	1-2 Minutes	5-10 Minutes	3-4 Hours	Analgesic (agonist-antagonist combination)
	IM	10-15 Minutes	30-60 Minutes	3-4 Hours	
Captopril (Capoten)	PO	<15 Minutes	1-2 Hours	2-6 Hours	ACE inhibitor
Chloroprocaine (Nesacaine)	Epidural	6-12 Minutes	10-20 Minutes	30-60 Minutes	Local anesthetic; not to be used for spinal anesthesia
Chlorpropamide (Diabinese)	PO	1 Hour	3-6 Hours	60 Hours	Hypoglycemic
Cimetidine (Tagamet)	IV	30-45 Minutes	60-90 Minutes	4-5 Hours	H_2-receptor antagonist
	PO	15-45 Minutes	1-2 Hours	2-4 Hours	
Cisatracurium (Nimbex)	IV	1-4 Minutes	2-7 Minutes	22-65 Minutes	Nondepolarizing NMB
Clonidine (Catapres, Dixarit)	PO	30-60 Minutes	2-4 Hours	6-8 Hours	Antihypertensive
	IV	30-60 Minutes	2-4 Hours	6-10 Hours	
	Epidural	<15 Minutes	3-4 Hours		
	Spinal				
Cocaine HCl	Topical	<1 Minute	2-5 Minutes	30-120 Minutes	Topical anesthetic; vasoconstrictor
	PO	30-60 Minutes		2-4 Hours	Opioid agonist
	IM	20-60 Minutes		2-3 Hours	
Cyclosporine (Sandimmune)	PO	1-6 Hours	8-12 Hours	1-4 Days	Immunosuppressant
Dantrolene (Dantrium)	IV	<5 Minutes	60 Minutes	3 Hours	Skeletal muscle relaxant; treatment of malignant hyperthermia
	PO	1-2 Hours	4-6 Hours	8-12 Hours	
Desflurane (Suprane)	Inhalation	1-2 Minutes		Emergence in 8-9 Minutes	Inhalational anesthetic agent

Continued

Table 17-1 Drugs Used in the PACU: Perianesthesia Drug List—*cont'd*

Drug	Route	Onset	Peak	Duration Of Action	Classification
Desmopressin (DDAVP)	IV	30 Minutes	1.5-3 Hours	8-20 Hours	Synthetic vasopressin analogue
	Intranasal	<60 Minutes	1-5 Hours	8-20 Hours	
Dexamethasone (Decadron)	IV	<8 Hours	12-24 Hours	36-54 Hours	Long-acting corticosteroid
	IM	<8 Hours	1-2 Hours	72 Hours	
(Respihaler)	INH	<20 Minutes	2-4 Hours	12 Hours	
(Turbinaire)	Intranasal	<15 Minutes		12-24 Hours	
Diazepam (Valium)	IV	1-5 Minutes	4-8 Minutes	15-60 Minutes	Benzodiazepine
	IM	15-30 Minutes		3-6 Hours	
	PO	30-60 Minutes	1-2 Hours	3-6 Hours	
Digoxin (Lanoxin)	IV	5-30 Minutes	1-5 Hours	3-4 Days	Inotropic agent
	IM	30 Minutes	4-6 Hours	3-4 Days	
	PO	30 Minutes-2 Hours	6-8 hours	3-4 Days	
Diltiazem (Cardizem)	IV	1-3 Minutes	2-7 Minutes	1-3 Hours	Calcium channel blocker
	PO	30 Minutes	2-3 Hours	4-6 Hours	
	PO-extended	1-3 Hours	4-11 Hours	18-24 Hours	
Diphenhydramine (Benadryl)	IV	<3 Minutes	1-2 Hours	3-6 Hours	Antihistamine
	PO	1 hour	1-2 Hours	4-6 Hours	
Dobutamine (dobutamine)	IV	2 Minutes	1-10 Minutes	5-10 Minutes	Vasopressor (adrenergic agonist)
Dopamine (Intropin)	IV	2-4 Minutes	5 Minutes	<10 Minutes	Catecholamine
Doxacurium (Nuromax)	IV	>4 Minutes	6-10 Minutes	30-160 Minutes	Long-acting NMB
Doxapram (Dopram)	IV	20-40 Seconds	1-2 Minutes	5-12 Minutes	Respiratory and cerebral stimulant

Table 17-1   **Drugs Used in the PACU: Perianesthesia Drug List**—*cont'd*

Drug	Route	Onset	Peak	Duration Of Action	Classification
Droperidol (Inapsine)	IV/IM	3-10 Minutes	30 Minutes	8-16 Hours	Tranquilizer
Edrophonium (Enlon, Tensilon)	IV	30-60 Seconds	1-5 Minutes	5-20 Minutes	Anticholinesterase
	IM	2-10 Minutes	5-10 Minutes	10-40 Minutes	
Enalapril (Vasotec)	PO	1 Hour	4-6 Hours	12-24 Hours	ACE inhibitor
Enalaprilat (Vasotec IV)	IV	10-15 Minutes	1-4 Hours	6 Hours	ACE inhibitor
Enflurane (Ethrane)	INH	2-3 Minutes		15 Minutes	Inhalational general anesthetic
Enoxaparin (LMW Heparin)	SQ	20-60 Minutes	3-5 Hours	12 Hours	Anticoagulant
Ephedrine	IV	<30 Seconds	2-5 Minutes	10-60 Minutes	Sympathomimetic
	IM	1-3 Minutes	<10 Minutes	30-60 Minutes	
Epinephrine (Adrenalin)	IV	<30 Seconds	2-3 Minutes	5-10 Minutes	Catecholamine
	ETT	15-30 Seconds	15-25 Minutes		
	INH	1 Minute	1-5 Minutes	1-3 Hours	
	SQ	5-15 Minutes	20 Minutes	1-3 Hours	
Esmolol (Brevibloc)	IV	1-2 Minutes	5-6 Minutes	10-20 Minutes	Cardioselective blocker
Ethacrynic acid (Edecrin)	IV	5-15 Minutes	30 Minutes	2 Hours	Loop diuretic
Etidocaine (Duranest)	Infiltration	3-5 Minutes	5-15 Minutes	2-3 Hours	Local anesthetic
	Epidural	5-15 Minutes	15-20 Minutes	3-5 Hours	
Etomidate (Amidate)	IV	30-60 Seconds	1 Minute	5-14 Minutes	Nonbarbiturate hypnotic
Famotidine (Pepcid)	IV	<30 Minutes	30 Minutes	8-12 Hours	Histamine (H_2) antagonist
	PO	20-45 Minutes	1-3 Hours	8-12 Hours	

Continued

Table 17-1 Drugs Used in the PACU: Perianesthesia Drug List—*cont'd*

Drug	Route	Onset	Peak	Duration Of Action	Classification
Fenoldopam (Corlopam)	IV (Continuous infusion)	5 Minutes	15 Minutes	Rapidly metabolized after discontinued	Antihypertensive
Fentanyl (Sublimaze)	IV	<30 Seconds	3-7 Minutes	30-60 Minutes	Opioid agonist
	Epidural/ spinal	4-10 Minutes	<30 Minutes	3-8 Hours	
	IM	<8 Minutes	20-30 Minutes	1-2 Hours	
	Transderm	12-18 Hours	1-3 Days	3 Days	
Flumazenil (Romazicon)	IV	1-2 Minutes	6-10 Minutes	45-90 Minutes	Benzodiazepine-receptor antagonist
Furosemide (Lasix)	IV	2-5 Minutes	20-30 Minutes	2 Hours	Loop diuretic
	PO	30-60 Minutes	1-2 Hours	4-8 Hours	
Glucagon	IV/IM	5 Minutes	2-20 Minutes	10-30 Minutes	Antihypoglycemic
Glipizide (Glucotrol)	PO	60-90 Minutes	2-3 Hours	10-24 Hours	Hypoglycemic
Glycopyrrolate (Robinul)	IV	1-3 Minutes	3-5 Minutes	2-3 Hours	Anticholinergic
	IM	15-30 Minutes	30-45 Minutes	2-7 Hours	
Granisetron (Kytril)	IV	2-4 Minutes	5-8 Minutes	24 Hours	Serotonin receptor antagonist
Halothane (Fluothane)	INH	2-5 Minutes		Up to 1 hour after discontinued	Inhalation general anesthetic
Haloperidol (Haldol)	IV	5-30 Minutes	1 Hour	6-8 Hours	Long-acting tranquilizer
Heparin (Liquaemin, Panheparin)	IV	Immediate	Dose-dependent	Dose-dependent	Anticoagulant
	SQ	20-30 Minutes	2-4 Hours	12-16 Hours	
Hetastarch (Hespan)	IV	15-30 Minutes	1 Hour	24-48 Hours	Plasma expander
Hyaluronidase (Wydase)	SQ	Immediate		30-60 Minutes	Enzyme to increase absorption

| Table 17-1 | **Drugs Used in the PACU: Perianesthesia Drug List**—*cont'd* | | | | |

Drug	Route	Onset	Peak	Duration Of Action	Classification
Hydralazine (Apresoline)	IV	5-20 Minutes	10-60 Minutes	2-4 Hours	Direct-acting arterial vasodilator
	IM	10-30 Minutes	30-80 Minutes	2-8 Hours	
	PO	30-120 Minutes	2 Hours	2-8 Hours	
Hydrocortisone sodium succinate (Solu-Cortef)	IV/IM	5 Minutes		30-36 Hours	Corticosteroid
Hydromorphone (Dilaudid)	IV	<60 Seconds	5-20 Minutes	2-4 Hours	Opioid (mixed)
	IM/PO	15-30 Minutes	30-60 Minutes	4-6 Hours	
Ibutilide fumarate (Covert)	IV	Immediate	10 Minutes	10-30 Minutes	Antiarrhythmic
Insulin, Lente	SQ	1-4 Hours	7-15 Hours	18-26 Hours	Antidiabetic agent
Insulin, NPH	SQ	1-2 Hours	4-12 Hours	18-26 Hours	
Insulin, Regular	SQ	30-60 Minutes	1-5 Hours	5-8 Hours	
Insulin, Semilente	SQ	1-3 Hours	4-10 Hours	12-16 Hours	
Insulin, Ultralente	SQ	4-8 Hours	14-24 Hours	28-36 Hours	
Insulin, NPH 70/Reg30	SQ	30 Minutes	2-12 Hours	24 Hours	
Ipratropium (Atrovent, Itrop)	INH	15-30 Minutes	1-2 Hours	4-5 Hours	Cholinergic blocker for reactive airways disease
Isoflurane (Forane)	INH	1-2 Minutes		15 Minutes after discontinued	Inhalational general anesthetic
Isoproterenol (Isuprel)	IV	Immediate	1 Minute	1-5 Minutes	Sympathomimetic
Ketamine (Ketalar)	IV	30-60 Seconds	1 Minute	5-15 Minutes	Dissociative anesthetic
	IM	3-4 Minutes	5-8 Minutes	12-25 Minutes	
Ketorolac (Toradol)	IV	<1 Minute	30 Minutes	4-6 Hours	Nonsteroidal Antiinflammatory
	IM	<10 Minutes	45-60 Minutes	4-6 Hours	
	PO	30-60 Minutes	1-3 Hours	3-7 Hours	

Continued

Table 17-1	**Drugs Used in the PACU: Perianesthesia Drug List**–*cont'd*				
Drug	Route	Onset	Peak	Duration Of Action	Classification
Labetalol (Normodyne, Trandate)	IV	1-3 Minutes	5-15 Minutes	0.25-2 Hours	Adrenergic antagonist
	PO	20-40 Minutes	1-4 Hours	4-12 Hours	
Lansoprazole (Prevacid)	PO	1 hour	2 Hours	>24 Hours	Proton pump inhibitor
Levobupivacaine (Chirocaine)	SQ	2-10 Minutes	30-45 Minutes	200-400 Minutes	Local anesthetic
	Epidural	4-7 Minutes	30-45 Minutes	200-400 Minutes	
	Spinal	<1 Minute	15 Minutes	200-400 Minutes	
Lidocaine (Xylocaine)	IV	45-90 Seconds	1-2 Minutes	10-20 Minutes	Local anesthetic
	Epidural	5-15 Minutes	20-30 Minutes	60-120 Minutes	
	Infiltration	<60 Seconds	20-30 Minutes	30-120 Minutes	
	Spinal	<60 Seconds	<10 Minutes	60-90 Minutes	
Lorazapam (Ativan)	IV	1-5 Minutes	20-40 Minutes	4-6 hours	Benzodiazepine
	PO	20-30 Minutes	2 Hours	10-20 Hours	
Magnesium sulfate	IV	Immediate	2-3 Minutes	30 Minutes	Anticonvulsant
Mannitol (Osmitrol)	IV, diuresis	15-60 Minutes	1-3 Hours	3-8 Hours	Osmotic diuretic
	IV to lower: ICP	<15 Minutes	60 Minutes	3-8 Hours	
	IOP	30-60 Minutes	1-2 Hours	4-6 Hours	
Meperidine (Demerol)	IV	1-3 Minutes	5-20 Minutes	2-4 Hours	Synthetic opioid agonist
	IM	5-10 Minutes	30-50 Minutes	2-4 Hours	
	PO	10-45 Minutes	60 Minutes	2-4 Hours	

Table 17-1 Drugs Used in the PACU: Perianesthesia Drug List—*cont'd*

Drug	Route	Onset	Peak	Duration Of Action	Classification
Mephentermine (Wyamine)	IV	1-5 Minutes	5-15 Minutes	15-30 Minutes	Synthetic noncatecholamine that stimulates α-receptors
	IM	5-15 Minutes	15-30 Minutes	1-2 Hours	
Mepivacaine (Carbocaine)	Epidural	5-15 Minutes	15-45 Minutes	3-5 Hours	Local anesthetic
	Infiltration	3-5 Minutes	15-45 Minutes	45-90 Minutes	
Metaproterenol (Metaprel)	INH	<60 Seconds	60 Minutes	1-4 Minutes	Bronchodilator
Metaraminol (Aramine)	IV	1-5 Minutes	5 Minutes	10-15 Minutes	Synthetic noncatecholamine
	IM	5-15 Minutes	30 Minutes	1-2 Hours	
Methadone (Dolophine)	IV	1-3 Minutes	15 Minutes	6 Hours	Synthetic opioid
	IM	3-60 Minutes	30 Minutes	6 Hours	
	PO	30-60 Minutes	45 Minutes	6 Hours	
Methohexital (Brevital Sodium)	IV	<30 Seconds	30-120 Seconds	5-10 Minutes	Ultra ultra short-acting barbiturate
	Rectal	5-7 Minutes	5-10 Minutes	45-90 Minutes	
Methoxamine (Vasoxyl)	IV	<1 Minute	5 Minutes	15-60 Minutes	α-receptor agonist
	IM	15-20 Minutes	30 Minutes	60-90 Minutes	
Methylene Blue (Urolene Blue)	IV	<1 Minute	<1 Hour	Varies	Antidote for methemoglobinemia
Methylergonovine (Methergine)	IV	Immediate	5-10 Minutes	45 Minutes	Oxytocic
	IM	2-5 Minutes	30 Minutes	3 Hours	
Metoclopramide (Reglan)	IV	1-3 Minutes	30-60 Minutes	1-2 Hours	Dopamine-receptor antagonist-antiemetic
	IM	10-15 Minutes	30-60 Minutes	1-2 Hours	
	PO	30-60 Minutes	1-2 Hours	1-2 Hours	

Continued

Table 17-1 Drugs Used in the PACU: Perianesthesia Drug List—*cont'd*

Drug	Route	Onset	Peak	Duration Of Action	Classification
Metoprolol (Toprol)	IV	<5 Minutes	20 Minutes	5-8 Hours	β-Blocker
	PO	<15 Minutes	90 Minutes	12-19 Hours	
Midazolam (Versed)	IV	1-5 Minutes	2-5 Minutes	15-90 Minutes	Benzodiazepine
	IM	10-15 Minutes	30-60 Minutes	1-3 Hours	
	PO	10-15 Minutes	30-60 Minutes	2-6 Hours	
Milrinone (Primacor)	IV	2 Minutes	15 Minutes	2 Hours	Inotropic agent
Mivacurium (Mivacron)	IV	1.5-4 Minutes	2-5 Minutes	6-15 Minutes	Short-acting NMB agent
Morphine	IV	<1 Minute	20 Minutes	2-7 Hours	Opioid agonist
Morphine (Duramorph)	Epidural	60 Minutes	90 Minutes	6-18 Hours	Opioid agonist
	IM	1-5 Minutes	30-60 Minutes	3-7 Hours	
	PO	15-60 Minutes	30-60 Minutes	3-7 Hours	
	PO extended	60-90 Minutes	1-4 Hours	6-12 Hours	
	Spinal	<60 Minutes	1-2 Hours	12-24 Hours	
Nalmefene HCl (Revex)	IV	2 Minutes	5 Minutes	4-6 Hours	Opioid antagonist
	IV	2-3 Minutes	15-30 Minutes	3-6 Hours	
	IM	15 Minutes	30-60 Minutes	3-6 Hours	
Naloxone (Narcan)	IV	1-2 Minutes	5-15 Minutes	1-4 Hours	Opioid antagonist
	IM	2-5 Minutes	5-15 Minutes	1-4 Hours	
Naltrexone (ReVia, Trexan)	PO	5 Minutes	1 Hour	24-72 Hours	Opioid antagonist
Neostigmine (Prostigmin)	IV	<3 Minutes	7 Minutes	45-60 Minutes	Anticholinesterase

Table 17-1 Drugs Used in the PACU: Perianesthesia Drug List—*cont'd*

Drug	Route	Onset	Peak	Duration Of Action	Classification
Nicardipine (Cardene)	IV	1 Minute	15 Minutes	3 Hours	Calcium channel blocker
	PO	<30 Minutes	0.5-1 Hour	3 Hours	
Nifedipine (Procardia)	PO	15-20 Minutes	30-120 Minutes	4-12 Hours	Calcium channel blocker
	PO extended	20-30 Minutes	6 Hours	24 Hours	
	SL	5 Minutes	20-45 Minutes	4-12 Hours	
Nitroglycerin	IV	1-2 Minutes	1-5 Minutes	3-5 Minutes	Peripheral vasodilator
	Ointment	20-60 Minutes	3-6 Hours		
	SL	1-3 Minutes	30-60 Minutes		
	Transdermal	40-60 Minutes	18-24 Hours		
Nitroprusside (Nipride, Nitropress)	IV	30-60 Seconds		1-10 Minutes	Peripheral vasodilator
Nitrous oxide (N_2O)	INH	1-5 Minutes		5-10 Minutes after discontinued	General inhalation anesthetic
Nizatidine (Axid)	PO	30-60 Minutes	0.5-3 Hours	8-12 Hours	H_2-receptor antagonist
Norepinephrine (Levophed)	IV	<60 Seconds	1-2 Minutes	2-10 Minutes	Catecholamine
Omeprazole (Prilosec)	PO	1 Hour	2 Hours	72 Hours	Proton pump inhibitor
Ondansetron (Zofran)	IV	<30 Minutes	1-1.5 Hours	12-24 Hours	Serotonin (5-HT3) receptor antagonist
Oxazepam (Serax)	PO	30 Minutes	2 Hours	8-12 Hours	Benzodiazepine
Oxytocin (Pitocin)	IV	<30 Seconds	20-40 Minutes	60 Minutes	Oxytocic
	IM	3-5 Minutes	40 Minutes	2-3 Hours	
Pancuronium (Pavulon)	IV	1-3 Minutes	3-5 Minutes	40-90 Minutes	Nondepolarizing skeletal muscle relaxant

Continued

Table 17-1   Drugs Used in the PACU: Perianesthesia Drug List—*cont'd*

Drug	Route	Onset	Peak	Duration Of Action	Classification
Phentolamine (Regitine)	IV	1-2 Minutes		10-15 Minutes	α-adrenergic blocker
	IM	5-20 Minutes		30-45 Minutes	
Pentobarbital (Nembutal)	IV	Immediate	1-2 Minutes	15 Minutes	Barbiturate
Phenylephrine (Neo-Synephrine)	IV	<30 Seconds	1 Minute	15-20 Minutes	α-adrenergic agonist
	Nasal	0.5-4 hours			
Phenytoin (Dilantin)	IV	3-5 Minutes	1-2 Hours	22 Hours	Anticonvulsant
Physostigmine (Antilirium)	IV	3-8 Minutes	5-10 Minutes	0.5-5 Hours	Anticholinesterase
Pipecuronium (Arduran)	IV	2-3 Minutes	3-6 Minutes	45-120 Minutes	Long-acting NMB agent
Prilocaine (Citanest)	SQ	1-2 Minutes	<30 Minutes	0.5-1.5 Hours	Local anesthetic
	Epidural	5-15 Minutes	<30 Minutes	1-3 Hours	
Procainamide (Pronestyl)	IV	Immediate	5-15 Minutes	2.5-5 Hours	Antiarrhythmic
Procaine (Novocain)	SQ	2-5 Minutes	<30 Minutes	0.25-0.5 Hours	Local anesthetic
	Spinal	2-5 Minutes	<30 Minutes	0.5-1.5 Hours	
	Epidural	5-25 Minutes	<30 Minutes	0.5-1.5 Hours	
Prochlorperazine (Compazine)	IV	3-5 Minutes	15-30 Minutes	3-4 Hours	Antiemetic, antipsychotic
	IM	10-20 Minutes	15-30 Minutes	3-4 Hours	
	PO	30-40 Minutes	2-4 Hours	3-4 Hours	
	Rectal	60 Minutes	3-4 Hours		
Promethazine (Phenergan)	IV	3-5 Minutes	1-2 Hours	2-8 Hours	Phenothiazine, H_1-receptor antagonist
	IM	20 Minutes	1-2 Hours	2-8 Hours	

Table 17-1 Drugs Used in the PACU: Perianesthesia Drug List—*cont'd*

Drug	Route	Onset	Peak	Duration Of Action	Classification
Propofol (Diprivan)	IV	30-60 Seconds	1 Minute	5-20 Minutes	Nonbarbiturate anesthesia induction agent
Propanolol (Inderal)	IV	<2 Minutes	1 Minute	1-6 Hours	α-adrenergic receptor antagonist
	PO	30 Minutes	60-90 Minutes	8-12 Hours	
Protamine sulfate	IV	30-60 Seconds	<5 Minutes	2 Hours	Heparin antagonist
Pyridostigmine (Mestinon, Regonol)	IV	2-5 Minutes	10-13 Minutes	80-130 Minutes	Anticholinesterase
Ranitidine (Zantac)	IV	<15 Minutes	1-2 Hours	6-8 Hours	H₂-receptor antagonist
	PO	<30 Minutes	2-3 Hours	8-12 Hours	
Rapacuronium (Raplon)	IV	45-90 Seconds		15-30 Minutes	Short-acting NMB agent—*withdrawn from the market*
Remifentanil (Ultiva)	IV	1-5 Minutes		Opiate effect ceases 18 minutes after discontinued	Opioid
Ritodrine HCL (Yutopar)	IV	Immediate		3-6 Hours	α₂-adrenergic agonist—tocolytic agent
Rocuronium (Zemuron)	IV	45-90 Seconds	1-3 Minutes	30-120 Minutes	Nondepolarizing NMB agent
Ropivacaine HCl (Naropin)	SQ	1-5 Minutes		2-6 Hours	Amide local anesthetic
	Epidural	5-13 Minutes		3-5 Hours	
Salmeterol (Serevent)	INH	10-20 Minutes	30 Minutes	12 Hours	α₂-adrenergic agonist
Scopolamine (Transderm-Scop)	IV	Immediate		30-60 Minutes	Anticholinergic
	IM	30 Minutes		4-6 Hours	
	Transdermal	4 Hours		72 Hours	
Sodium citrate (Bicitra)	PO	2-10 Minutes	60 Minutes	60-90 Minutes	Nonparticulate neutralizing buffer
Somatostatin (Zecnil)	IV	5-10 Minutes	45 Minutes	1 Hour	Synthetic somatostatin

Continued

Table 17-1   Drugs Used in the PACU: Perianesthesia Drug List—*cont'd*

Drug	Route	Onset	Peak	Duration Of Action	Classification
Sotalol HCl (Betapace)	PO	1 hour	2.5-4 Hours	4-6 Hours	Antiarrhythmic
Sodium bicarbonate	IV	2-10 Minutes	10-30 Minutes	30-60 Minutes	Neutralizing buffer
Sodium citrate	PO	<60 Seconds	3-4 Minutes	2 Hours	Neutralizing buffer
Sodium nitroprusside	IV	30-60 Seconds	1-2 Minutes	1-10 Minutes	Antihypertensive
Succinylcholine (Anectine, Quelicin)	IV	30-60 Seconds	1 Minute	4-6 Minutes	Depolarizing skeletal muscle relaxant
	IM	2-3 Minutes	10-30 Minutes		
Sufentanil (Sufenta)	IV	1-3 Minutes	3-5 Minutes	20-45 Minutes	Opioid agonist
	Epidural/ spinal	4-10 Minutes	<30 Minutes	2-4 Hours	
Terbutaline (Brethine)	INH	5-30 Minutes	1-2 Hours	3-4 Hours	α_2-adrenergic agonist
	PO	30 Minutes	2-3 Hours	4-8 Hours	
	SQ	15 Minutes	30-60 Minutes	1.5-4 Hours	
Tetracaine (Pontocaine)	Spinal	<10 Minutes	15-60 Minutes	1.25-3 Hours	Local anesthetic
Thiamylal (Surital)	IV	Immediate		10-30 Minutes	Ultra short-acting barbiturate
Thiopental (Pentothal)	IV	30-60 Seconds	20-40 Seconds	5-15 Minutes	Ultra short-acting barbiturate
Torsemide (Demadex, Presaril)	IV	10 Minutes	1-2 Hours	6-8 Hours	Loop diuretic
Trimethaphan (Arfonad)	IV	Immediate		5-30 Minutes	Autonomic ganglion blocking agent, antihypertensive
Tubocurarine Chloride (Curare)	IV	<2 Minutes	4 Minutes	25-90 Minutes	Nondepolarizing NMB agent
Vancomycin (Vancocin)	IV	15-30 Minutes	4-6 Hours	8-12 Hours	Antimicrobial agent
Vasopressin (Pitressin)	IV	15-30 Minutes	30-60 Minutes	2-8 Hours	Antidiuretic hormone

Table 17-1	**Drugs Used in the PACU: Perianesthesia Drug List**–*cont'd*				
Drug	Route	Onset	Peak	Duration Of Action	Classification
Vecuronium (Norcuron)	IV	2-3 Minutes	3-5 Minutes	25-40 Minutes	Nondepolarizing NMB agent
Verapamil (Isoptin)	IV	2-5 Minutes	<10 Minutes	30-60 Minutes	Calcium channel blocker
	PO	30 Minutes	1-2 Hours	3-7 Hours	
	IM, IV, SQ	1-3 Hours		6-48 Hours	Water-soluble vitamin
	PO	Up to 5-7 days		2-5 days after therapeutic dose reached	Anticoagulant

Adapted from Nagelhout J, Zaglaniczny K, Haglund V: Handbook of nurse anesthesia, ed 2, Philadelphia, 2001, WB Saunders; and Waugaman W, Foster S, Rigor B: Principles and practice of nurse anesthesia, ed 3, Norwalk, Conn, 1999, Appleton & Lange.

tion in renal clearance. In renal drug clearance, the laboratory test of creatinine clearance, which measures glomerular filtration (see Chapter 11), can be used to predict the degree of a drug's renal clearance. Anesthetic drugs, such as d-tubocurarine (curare) and gallamine (Flaxedil), are excreted by the kidney mostly unchanged. In anephric patients or patients with severe kidney disease, the elimination clearance is decreased, and the $T^1/_{2\beta}$ is increased, thus prolonging the effects of the drugs, especially when they are administered at particular dosing intervals. However, a single dose of these nondepolarizing neuromuscular blocking agents is usually unaffected in the anephric patient.

Hepatic Disease.   Patients with hepatic diseases such as cirrhosis and ascites may have difficulty in clearing some anesthetic drugs from their bodies. Liver function testing is unreliable in predicting the level of impairment in hepatic clearance. Any patient with documented liver disease should be considered at risk for decreased clearance of drugs. Therefore in patients with documented hepatic disease, all drugs administered in the PACU should be titrated to desired effect to gain an appropriate pharmacologic outcome.

Cardiovascular Disease.   Cardiovascular diseases that cause a reduction in tissue perfusion have a significant impact on drug distribution and clearance. For example, when lidocaine is administered to patients with congestive heart failure, the dose should be reduced by one half because of changes in volume distribution and clearance. Postoperative cardiopulmonary bypass patients can experience a hemodilution of drugs. However, this change in the central compartment is transitory because the plasma drug concentration is compensated in the peripheral tissue compartment.

DRUG-DRUG INTERACTIONS

When a patient is simultaneously receiving two or more drugs, the drugs may or may not interact to cause a toxic reaction. Patients are often given drugs other than the ones associated with anesthesia and surgery. Thus in these patients, the potential for a drug-drug interaction is present (Table 17-3). These interactions are divided into two broad categories: pharmacokinetic and pharmacodynamic.

Pharmacokinetic Interactions

Interactions of a second drug that produces alterations in absorption, distribution, metabolism, or excretion of the first drug are known as pharmacokinetic interactions. Hence when one drug

Table 17-2 **The Major Drug Groups and Their Intended Outcome in Respiratory Care**		
Drug Group	**Intended Physiologic Response**	**Generic Agent (Trade Name)**
Adrenergic agents	α-adrenergic stimulation produces bronchial relaxation to reduce airways resistance and improve flow rates in patients who suffer from obstructive lung disease.	Epinephrine Isoproterenol (Isuprel) Isoetharine (Bronkosol) Terbutaline (Brethine) Metaproterenol (Metaprel) Albuterol (Ventolin) Pirbuterol (Maxair) Bitolterol (Tornalate) Salmeterol (Serevent) Procaterol (Mescalcin)
	α-adrenergic stimulation produces bronchial relaxation, peripheral vascular vasoconstriction and nasal decongestion.	Ephedrine Phenylephrine (Neo-Synephrine)
Anticholinergic agents	Relaxation of cholinergic (vagal)-induced bronchoconstriction to improve flow rates in patients who suffer from obstructive lung disease.	Ipratropium (Atrovent)
Mucoactive agents	Modification of the properties of the respiratory tract mucus to facilitate clearance of secretions.	Acetylcystine (Mucomist) Dornase alfa (Pulmozyme)
Corticosteroids	Reduce inflammation in the respiratory tract.	Dexamethasone (Decadron) Beclomethasone (Vanceril) Triamcinolone (Kenalog) Flunisolide (Aerobid) Fluticasone (Flonase/Flovent) Budesonide (Rhinocort)
Antiasthmatic agents	Inhibits the chemical mediators of inflammation to help prevent the onset of an asthma attack.	Cromolyn (Intal) Nedocromil (Tilade) Zafirlukast (Accolate) Zileuton (Zyflo) Montelukast (Singulair)
Antiinfective agents	Inhibits or stops specific infective agents, such as *P. carinii* (pentamidine), or respiratory syncyial virus (ribavirin), or for management of *P. aeruginosa* in cystic fibrosis (tobramycin).	Pentamidine Ribavirin (Rebetron) Tobramycin (TOBI)
Exogenous surfactants	Enhances lung compliance by reducing surface tension. Approved for direct intratracheal instillation.	Colfosceril (Exosurf) Beractant (Survanta)

Adapted from Rau J: Recent developments in respiratory care pharmacology, J Perianesth Nurs 13(6):362, 1998.

Table 17-3	**Drug-Drug or Drug-Induced Interactions in the PACU**		
Drug(s)	**Interactions**	**Result**	**Mechanism**
ANTIHYPERTENSIVE DRUGS			
Reserpine	Inhalation anesthetics	Hypotension	Inhibits the synthesis and storage of norepinephrine in the sympathetic nerve endings.
Propranolol	Inhalation anesthetics	Bradycardia, hypotension	Additive effect.
Verapamil	Halothane	Enhancement of A-V Block Potentiate all skeletal muscle relaxants	Additive inhibitor effect.
Clonidine	Inapsine	Rebound hypertension	Sudden inhibition of cardiovascular and vasoconstrictor centers.
Diuretics	Halothane	Hypotension	Reduced extracellular sodium and water, which is compensated for by vasoconstriction. Halothane dilates the constricted vascular beds.
Propranolol	Lidocaine	Enhanced negative inotropic effect	Propranolol reduces liver blood flow and lidocaine clearance.
Lidocaine Procainamide Bretylium Phenytoin Digitalis Quinidine Disopyramide Propranolol	d-Tubocurarine	Increased duration of neuromuscular blockade	Synergistic effect.
Digitalis	Succinylcholine	Arrhythmias	Direct effect or caused by the hyperkalemia that can be induced by succinylcholine.
Quinidine	Digitalis (digoxin)	Can produce digitalis intoxication	Decreases digitalis clearance and increases concentration of digitalis.
Propranolol	Heparin	Myocardial depression	Heparin increases free fatty acids, which displace propranolol from plasma protein binding sites leading to increased free propranolol.
Quinidine	Myasthenia gravis plus skeletal muscle relaxants	Postoperative respiratory depression	Blockade of acetylcholine receptors at neuromuscular postsynaptic membrane.
Digitalis	Thiazide diuretics	Increased potassium excretion by the kidneys	Combined effect of the two drugs on the kidneys promotes potassium excretion.

Continued

Table 17-3   Drug-Drug or Drug-Induced Interactions in the PACU—*cont'd*

Drug(s)	Interactions	Result	Mechanism
ANTIBIOTICS			
Neomycin Streptomycin Dihydrostreptomycin Polymyxin A Polymyxin B Colistin Viomycin Paromomycin Kanamycin Lincomycin Gentamicin Tetracycline	Nondepolarizing skeletal muscle relaxants	Potentiates nondepolarizing muscle relaxants, respiratory depression	Neuromuscular blockade caused by a reduction in the amplitude of the end-plate potential.
NARCOTICS			
Morphine Meperidine Sublimaze Sufentanil	Inhalation anesthetics	Potentiation, respiratory and cardiovascular depression	Depressant effects of inhalation anesthetics and the narcotics are additive.
Meperidine	Enovid Norinyl	Birth control pill potentiates meperidine	Excess female sex hormones with oral contraceptive therapy, which may slow the metabolism of meperidine.
SYMPATHOMIMETIC AMINES			
Epinephrine	Halothane Enflurane	Cardiac arrhythmias	Anesthetic agents sensitize the myocardium to endogenous and exogenous catecholamines.
ELECTROLYTES			
Increased extracellular potassium	Skeletal muscle relaxants	Increased resistance to depolarization and greater sensitivity to nondepolarizing muscle relaxants	Acute increase in extracellular potassium increases end-plate transmembrane potential, thus causing hyperpolarization.
Decreased extracellular potassium	Skeletal muscle relaxants	Increased effects of depolarizing muscle relaxants and increased resistance to nondepolarizing muscle relaxants	Acute decrease in extracellular potassium lowers resting end-plate transmembrane potential.
Increased calcium levels	Nondepolarizing skeletal muscle relaxants	Decreased response	Calcium increases the quantal release of acetylcholine and enhances the excitation-contraction coupling mechanism.

Table 17-3   Drug-Drug or Drug-Induced Interactions in the PACU—*cont'd*

Drug(s)	Interactions	Result	Mechanism
Magnesium ions	Muscle relaxants	Potentiation	Magnesium ions cause a partial muscle relaxation by blocking the release of acetylcholine.
Calcium chloride	Digitalis	Additive effect on the heart	High concentrations of calcium inhibit the positive inotropic actions of digitalis and potentiate digitalis toxicity.
MISCELLANEOUS			
Echothiophate iodide	Succinylcholine	Prolonged apnea	Echothiophate is a cholinesterase inhibitor, and succinylcholine is destroyed by pseudocholinesterase.
Tolbutamide	Dicumarol	Intensification of the effects of tolbutamide, leads to hypoglycemia	Dicumarol displaces tolbutamide from its binding site on plasma proteins and makes more tolbutamide available in the free form.
Succinylcholine	d-Tubocurarine	Prolonged apnea	Both drugs act at the acetylcholine receptor, thus causing a synergistic effect on the myoneural junction.
Procaine Nesacaine Pontocaine	Succinylcholine	Prolonged apnea	All these drugs are metabolized by the enzyme pseudocholinesterase. The concomitant use of these drugs may reduce the effective plasma concentration of the enzyme.
Furosemide Thiazide Ethacrynic acid	Nondepolarizing skeletal muscle relaxants	Intensified neuromuscular block	Electrolyte imbalance (hypokalemia).
Aminophylline	d-Tubocurarine Pancuronium	Antagonized neuromuscular blockade	End-plate effect is antagonized by the increase in neurotransmitter.
Procaine Lidocaine	Nondepolarizing and depolarizing skeletal muscle relaxants	Enhanced neuromuscular blockade	Decreased end-plate potential.
Lithium	Pancuronium Succinylcholine	Potentiated neuromuscular blockade	Lithium ions are substituted for sodium ions at a presynaptic level.
Chlorpromazine	Nondepolarizing skeletal muscle relaxants	Enhanced neuromuscular blockade	Potentiation of neuromuscular blockade.

Continued

Table 17-3	**Drug-Drug or Drug-Induced Interactions in the PACU**–*cont'd*		
Drug(s)	Interactions	Result	Mechanism
All inhalation anesthetics	Nondepolarizing skeletal muscle relaxants	Augment block in a dose-dependent manner in the following decreasing order of potency: isoflurane and enflurane, halothane, nitrous oxide	Central nervous system depression or presynaptic inhibition of acetylcholine.
Insulin	Corticosteroids, oral contraceptives, loop and thiazide diuretics	Reduction in effects	Insulin antagonizes the effects.
Diethylstilbestrol (Stilphostrol)	Succinylcholine	Prolonged neuromuscular blockade	Decreased plasma cholinesterase.
Hydrocortisone Dexamethasone Prednisolone	Phenobarbital	Decreased effects of the steroids	Increased metabolism.

alters any pharmacokinetic parameter of another, with a resultant alteration in the concentration of the drug at the receptor site, a pharmacokinetic interaction has taken place. In other words, the absorption, distribution, or elimination of the drug concentration at the receptor site is changed, which results in an altered pharmacologic response from the person.

Absorption. The absorption of one drug may be enhanced or inhibited by another drug. With the addition of epinephrine to solutions of local anesthetics, the absorption of the anesthetic is prolonged through the vasoconstrictive action of epinephrine. The local vasoconstriction produced by epinephrine delays the systemic absorption of the local anesthetic, and the effect of the local anesthetic ultimately is prolonged. When a patient has been administered a preoperative aluminum-containing antacid and then is administered tetracycline in the late postoperative period, absorption of the tetracycline will be reduced.

Distribution. Pharmaceutical incompatibility is one type of pharmacokinetic distribution interaction. This situation occurs, for example, when one drug reacts chemically with another. In this situation, when one drug (e.g., aspirin) displaces another drug (e.g., phenytoin) from plasma protein-binding sites, the blood concentration of the free drug will be increased, which may result in toxic blood levels. When a large dose of thiopental is administered to an obese patient who also receives halothane, the anesthetic action may be prolonged considerably and last well into the PACU phase. This is caused by the prolonged retention of thiopental in the adipose tissue because of the circulatory depressant action of halothane. Hence at the end of the period of anesthesia, the redistribution and subsequent elimination of thiopental are delayed, which causes a prolonged hypnotic effect.

Elimination

Biotransformation. When patients are administered enzyme-inducing agents, such as barbiturates and the antibiotic rifampin, the activity of the enzyme systems of the liver will be increased. This results in a more rapid metabolism and excretion of drugs that are metabolized by a particular liver enzyme system. For example, if a barbiturate were administered to a patient who is on a stabilized dose of the anticoagulant warfarin, the warfarin blood level might be reduced, which would result in a lowered prothrombin time. If this situation were to occur (stabilization by an anticoagulant and administration of an enzyme-inducing agent) and the barbiturate were to be discontinued, the nurse would have to monitor the patient for the potentially more serious problem of excessive anticoagulation and hemorrhage.

The drug cimetidine (Tagamet) is sometimes administered preoperatively to reduce the amount of gastric secretion and increase the gastric pH. Cimetidine is a potent inhibitor of drug metabolism and can slow the elimination of antipyrine, warfarin, diazepam, and propranolol. This effect results in an increased drug concentration and enhanced pharmacologic effect of the latter drugs.

Excretion. The pharmacokinetic parameters of concern in excretion relate to one drug facilitating or hindering the excretion of another. An example of this occurs when probenecid is administered together with penicillin. The outcome of this interaction is that the pharmacologic actions of penicillin are prolonged because of the slower $T_{1/2}$ produced by probenecid. Certainly, this can be considered a desirable drug-drug interaction.

Pharmacodynamic Interactions

Pharmacodynamic interactions occur when one drug alters the pharmacologic effects of another drug. For example, when a patient is being treated with an antibiotic such as an aminoglycoside or polymyxin and receives a skeletal muscle relaxant such as curare, a prolonged neuromuscular blockage may result. Another example is a patient who receives thiazide diuretic therapy who has resultant hypokalemia. If the patient is administered digitalis, digitalis toxicity may result. Also, if the patient on thiazide therapy is administered a nondepolarizing muscle relaxant, the neuromuscular blockade will be intensified.

DRUG-DRUG INTERACTIONS AND THE PACU

Antibiotics

Aminoglycoside and polymyxin antibiotics have been reported to interact with some anesthetic agents as well as skeletal muscle relaxants. Streptomycin and the other aminoglycoside antibiotics produce a partial neuromuscular blockade by inhibiting the release of acetylcholine from the presynaptic membrane and by stabilizing the postsynaptic membrane. The order of decreasing potency of aminoglycosides for causing a partial neuromuscular blockade is neomycin, kanamycin, amikacin, gentamicin, and tobramycin. When a nondepolarizing skeletal muscle relaxant such as curare or pancuronium, is administered to a patient who receives an aminoglycoside antibiotic, the neuromuscular blockade will be intensified and difficult to reverse pharmacologically. Studies indicate that the aminoglycoside neuromuscular blockade can sometimes be partially reversed by calcium and neostigmine, whereas the neuromuscular blockade produced by polymyxin B is enhanced by neostigmine and not reversed by calcium. The antibiotics that prolong the actions of the nondepolarizing skeletal muscle relaxants are neomycin, streptomycin, dihydrostreptomycin, kanamycin, gentamicin, polymyxin A, polymyxin B, colistin, lincomycin, and tetracycline. The antibiotics that enhance the pharmacologic actions of the depolarizing skeletal relaxant succinylcholine include neomycin, streptomycin, kanamycin, polymyxin B, and colistin. These drugs must usually be given for at least 2 weeks before any clinically significant depression in the neuromuscular transmission occurs; such a depression may produce only slight muscular weakness in the patient. Antibiotics that have no skeletal muscle relaxant properties are penicillin, chloramphenicol, and the cephalosporins.

Sympathomimetic Amines

The volatile inhalation anesthetics, particularly halothane, can sensitize the heart to sympathomimetic amines, such as epinephrine, thus producing cardiac arrhythmias. Patients who are recovering from halothane anesthesia in the PACU still have a significant amount of halothane in their bodies. Consequently, epinephrine or other sympathomimetic amines should not be administered to them. If epinephrine must be used for hemostasis or for vasoconstriction in a local anesthetic, the epinephrine concentration should not be greater than 1:100,000 to 200,000, and the total adult dose should not be greater than 10 ml of 1:100,000 solution in 10 minutes—that is, the total dose should not exceed 30 ml of 1:100,000 solution in 1 hour.

Antihypertensives

Estimates suggest that 1 to 2 million hypertensive patients are anesthetized each year in the United States. Anesthetic agents have been reported to produce changes in cardiac output, peripheral resistance, and regional blood flow patterns in normotensive and hypertensive patients.

Hypertension is treated by lowering systemic vascular resistance, by reducing cardiac output, or both. Antihypertensive drugs alter the circulatory hemostasis, strongly influence the activity of pressor amines, and may alter the response to muscle relaxants and narcotic analgesics. Antihypertensive drugs can produce systemic conditions that may result in a hypotensive crisis during anesthesia and in the immediate postoperative period. Therefore PACU patients who have been on long-term antihypertensive medication therapy and who have received a 100% potent inhalation anesthetic should be specifically monitored for cardiac dysrhythmias and hypotension. If a hypotensive crisis occurs in the PACU, the patient should have his or her legs elevated, and oxygen and—if necessary—vasopressors should be administered. The anesthesiologist and surgeon should be notified immediately so that specific treatment can be instituted.

Narcotics

Every perianesthesia nurse has probably observed the drug-drug interaction between narcotics administered in the PACU and the inhalation anesthetic agents administered in the operating room. If the patient has not completely eliminated the anesthetic agent and is administered a narcotic, a synergistic effect between the two drugs will occur. The outcome of this interaction is usually respiratory depression, because both drugs are respiratory depressants.

If the two drugs have interacted in this way, a narcotic (opioid) antagonist, such as naloxone (Narcan), can be administered to reverse the respiratory depression produced by the narcotic. However, naloxone will not reverse respiratory depression produced by the inhalation anesthetic agents such as halothane (Fluothane), enflurane (Ethrane), or isoflurane (Forane).

Naloxone reverses respiratory depression and analgesia produced by an opioid. In the PACU, reversing the respiratory depression and preserving some postoperative analgesia with nalbuphine (Nubain) are usually advantageous. The pharmacology of nalbuphine is discussed in detail in Chapter 20.

Steroids

Although exogenous steroids administered to a steroid-dependent patient is not actually an interaction of two drugs that alters one of the pharmacokinetic parameters, the problems resulting from this circumstance will be presented.

Patients experiencing adrenocortical insufficiency cannot withstand the stress of anesthesia and surgery. For example, if a patient with chronic obstructive pulmonary disease has been treated with long-term steroids, there will usually be some degree of adrenocortical insufficiency. Hence because of the alteration in the receptor site, the patient may react to surgery and anesthesia with hypotension, respiratory depression, or delayed recovery. To prevent a hypotensive crisis during the perioperative period, these patients are usually maintained on corticosteroids until, through, and after the surgical procedure.

Should these symptoms appear in a PACU patient who did not receive this steroid coverage, the preferred treatment would be hydrocortisone (see Chapter 13).

SPECIAL CONSIDERATIONS IN PHARMACOLOGY ASSOCIATED WITH PERIANESTHESIA CARE

Sedative Drugs for PACU Patients

Because of the stress response that is experienced by some patients in the PACU, sedative drugs are sometimes used to prevent the adverse physiologic effects of stress such as increased oxygen consumption, tachycardia, hypertension, and

Table 17-4	**Ramsay Sedation Scoring System**	
Ramsay Score	Clinical Parameters for Bedside Assessment of Sedation	Global Degree of Sedation
1	Anxious, restless, perhaps agitated	
2	Cooperative and oriented	Varying degrees of awake state
3	Easily arousable, responds appropriately	
4	Brisk response to light glabellar tap or loud auditory stimulus	
5	Sluggish response to glabellar tap or auditory stimulus	Varying degrees of asleep state
6	Asleep, does not respond to above stimuli	

From Prielipp R, Young C: Current drugs for sedation of critically ill patients, Seminars in Anesthesia, Perioperative Medicine, and Pain 20(2):85-94, 2001.

exacerbated hyperglycemia. The institution of drugs to promote sedation is a difficult task in the PACU because the patient may have residual effects of the intraoperative anesthetic agents still active in his or her body. Hence a bedside sedation scoring system is helpful in determining the degree of sedation and will help to predict when concerns about oversedation should be realized. Although many sedation scoring systems are available, the Ramsay Sedation Scoring System appears to be quite appropriate to assess drug-induced sedation. The Ramsay Scale consists of 6 scoring levels. The first three levels (Table 17-4) are usually administered while the patient is awake, and levels 4 through 6 are assessed during varying degrees of sleep. Drakulavic and associates in 1999 used univariate analysis to demonstrate that a Ramsay level of 4 or greater was associated with increased risk for nosocomial pneumonia. Because oversedation is associated with increased risk of edema, thromboemboli, gastric regurgitation, and aspiration—to name a few—patients in the PACU should have Ramsay Sedation levels in the range of 3 or less.

Herbal Medicinals

Over the past few years, the use of an herbal product has escalated to the point that over 24 million Americans use at least one herbal product. This industry has an annual sales of over $12 billion and is projected to only increase because of the ongoing dissatisfaction with conventional medicine and the healthcare system in general. What is most concerning to the healthcare practitioner is that of the Americans using alternative forms of therapy, including herbal products, over 60% of patients do not inform their family physicians of the drugs and/or therapies that they are using.

Because of the rapid onset in popularity in the use of herbal products, research in this area is lacking, particularly in the area of the impact on postoperative outcomes. In response to this, the American Society of Anesthesiologists (ASA) have issued a statement cautioning patients taking herbal products to refrain from those medications at least two weeks before surgery. Hence because of the possible negative perianesthesia outcome caused by herbal products, a brief overview of the more popular herbal products will be presented in Table 17-5.

Drugs Used in the PACU

Because of all the possible drugs used in the PACU, Table 17-1 presents most of the drugs that may be used in the perianesthesia care of the surgical patient.

Table 17-5 Herbal Drugs and Their Possible Interactions with Anesthesia

Herbal	Actions	Key Component	Untoward Effects
Aristolochia	Aphrodisiac and anticonvulsant	Aristolochic acid	Nephrotoxic and cardiogenic
Ephedra	Weight loss, stimulant, ergogenic	Ephedrine	Adrenergic stimulant—hypertension, bronchodilatation, diuresis, tachycardia
Feverfew	Temperature reduction Migraine prophylaxis, Treatment of rheumatoid arthritis	Parthenolide	Risk of bleeding, insomnia, anxiety (should discontinue this drug one week before surgery)
Garlic	Reduction in blood pressure, decrease in total cholesterol	Allicin	Risk of postoperative bleeding (should discontinue this drug one week before surgery)
Ginger	Decreases platelet aggregation, antiemetic, motion sickness	Oleoresins	Risk of postoperative bleeding (should discontinue this drug one week before surgery)
Ginkgo	Decreases RBC aggregation, memory loss, improved cognitive function, chronic venous insufficiency	Ginkgo biloba extract (GBE)	Significant risk of postoperative bleeding (should discontinue this drug one week before surgery)
Ginseng	Stress reduction; increased physical performance; improved cardiovascular function; anticancer properties; antioxidant	Ginsenosides	Insomnia, irritability, and mania; interactions with digoxin, warfarin and lithium (should discontinue this drug one week before surgery)
Golden Seal	Laxative antiinflammatory, antiemetic	Berberine; hydrastine	Seizures, respiratory depression, hypertension, electrolyte imbalance
Kava	Anxiolytic, analgesic, muscle relaxant, anticonvulsant, local anesthetic properties	Kavapyrones	MAO inhibition, platelet aggregation inhibition, potentiate anesthetics (should discontinue this drug one week before surgery)
St. John's Wort	Antidepressant, sedative/hypnotic	Hypericin, pseudohypericin	Should not be coadministered with other antidepressants. Potential to interact with amphetamines and adrenergic stimulants. Prolongs the effects of anesthesia. Because antidepressants may be used in the perioperative period, it should be discontinued one week before surgery.
Valerian	Sedative, muscle relaxant	Valerianic acid	Potentiate sedatives, including anesthetics

BIBLIOGRAPHY

Assemi M: Herbal preparations: concerns for operative patients, Anesthesia Today 10(3):17-23, 2000.

Atlee J: Complications in anesthesia, Philadelphia, 1999, WB Saunders.

Barash P, Cullen B, Stoelting R: Clinical anesthesia, ed 3, Philadelphia, 1997, Lippincott-Raven.

Benumof J, Saidman L: Anesthesia & perioperative complications, ed 2, St Louis, 1999, Mosby.

Bowdle T, Horita A, Kharasch E: The pharmacologic basis of anesthesiology, New York, 1994, Churchill Livingstone.

Cottrell J, Smith D: Anesthesia and neurosurgery, ed 4, St Louis, 2001, Mosby.

Drakulovic M, Torres A, Bauer T, et al: Supine body position as a risk factor for nosocomial pneumonia in mechanically ventilated patients: a randomized trial, Lancet 354:1851-1858, 1999.

Estafanous F: Opioids in anesthesia: II. Boston, 1991, Butterworth-Heinemann.

Farmer W, Silverman D: Potential effects of herbal medicinals on perioperative care, Seminars in Anesthesia, Perioperative Medicine, and Pain 20(2):110-117, 2001.

Ganong W: Review of medical physiology, ed 30, New York, 2001, McGraw-Hill Professional.

Guyton A, Hall J: Textbook of medical physiology, ed 9, Philadelphia, 1996, WB Saunders.

Hardman J, Limbird L: Goodman and Gilman's the pharmacological basis of therapeutics, ed 9, New York, 1996, McGraw-Hill.

Longnecker D, Murphy F: Dripps/Eckenhoff/Vandam introduction to anesthesia, ed 8, Philadelphia, 1992, WB Saunders.

McIntosh L, Essentials of nurse anesthesia, New York, 1997, McGraw-Hill.

Miller R, editor: Anesthesia, ed 5, New York, 2000, Churchill Livingstone.

Mueller R, Lundberg D: Manual of drug interactions for anesthesiology, ed 3, New York, 1996, Churchill Livingstone.

Nagelhout J: Drug interactions: introduction, Anesthesia Today 1(4):1-5, 1990.

Nagelhout J, Zaglaniczny K: Nurse anesthesia, ed 2, Philadelphia, 2001, WB Saunders.

Omoigui S: The anesthesia drugs handbook, ed 2, St Louis, 1995, Mosby.

Prielipp R, Young C: Current drugs for sedation of critically ill patients, Seminars in Anesthesia, Perioperative Medicine, and Pain 20(2):85-94, 2001.

Rau J: Recent developments in respiratory care pharmacology, J Perianesth Nurs 13(6):359-369, 1998.

Stoelting R: Pharmacology and physiology in anesthetic practice, ed 3, Philadelphia, 1999, Lippincott-Raven.

Stoelting R, Miller R: Basics of anesthesia, ed 4, New York, 2000, Churchill Livingstone.

Waugaman W, Foster S, Rigor B: Principles and practice of nurse anesthesia, ed 3, Norwalk, Conn, 1999, Appleton & Lange.

Wood M, Wood A: Drugs and anesthesia: pharmacology for the anesthesiologist, ed 2, Baltimore, 1990, Williams & Wilkins.

To anticipate how a patient will react when emerging from an inhalation anesthetic in the postanesthesia care unit (PACU), the perianesthesia nurse should have a thorough understanding of the pharmacologic concepts of inhalation anesthesia. Although the complexity of these agents, coupled with drug interactions and the various levels of physical health, makes it difficult to predict the exact nature of each patient's emergence from inhalation anesthesia, an understanding of some general principles will prepare the perianesthesia nurse for the most commonly expected outcomes.

BASIC CONCEPTS

Evolution of the Signs and Stages of Anesthesia

The five components of anesthesia are hypnosis, analgesia, muscle relaxation, sympatholysis, and amnesia. In the past, when diethyl ether was the primary general anesthetic administered, assessment of anesthetic depth with the signs and stages of anesthesia was quite simple—the patient could be monitored by assessment of the pupils, respiratory activity, muscle tone, and various reflexes. The ether signs and stages were devised to give some means of assessing the depth of anesthesia. The first three stages were described by Plomley in 1847, and a year later John Snow added a fourth stage—overdose. During World War I, Guedel more accurately defined and described the signs and stages of anesthesia. A graphic representation of these signs and stages is provided in Figure 18-1.

With the advent of modern anesthesia—which included the addition of fluorinated inhalation anesthetic agents, muscle relaxants, and various pharmacologic adjuncts—the usual predictable signs and stages as described by Guedel were abolished. However, in the PACU,

many of these pharmacologic adjuncts have been reversed or the effects have dissipated in the patient who is recovering from anesthesia. The classic signs and stages provide some help in the assessment and care of the postoperative patient. Consequently, a brief description—including the incorporation of some of the pharmacology of the modern anesthetics—will be given.

Stage I begins with the initiation of anesthesia and ends with the loss of consciousness. It is commonly called the stage of analgesia. This stage has been described as the lightest level of anesthesia and represents sensory and mental depression. Stage I is the level of anesthesia used when nitrous oxide is employed. Patients are able to open their eyes on command, breathe normally, maintain protective reflexes, and tolerate mild painful stimuli.

Stage II starts with the loss of consciousness and ends with the onset of a regular pattern of breathing and the disappearance of the lid reflex. This is also called the stage of delirium. It is characterized by excitement and, because of this, many untoward responses such as vomiting, laryngospasm, and even cardiac arrest may take place during this stage. With the use of anesthetic agents that act much more rapidly than ether, this stage is passed rather quickly. In addition, the induction of anesthesia is usually facilitated by short-acting barbiturates, which expedite a short duration of stage II.

Stage III is the stage of surgical anesthesia. Using ether anesthesia, it is defined as lasting from the onset of a regular pattern of breathing to the cessation of respiration. At this stage of anesthesia, response to surgical incision is absent. The modern concept of minimum alveolar concentration (MAC) is predicated in part by the signs and stages of surgical anesthesia. MAC is exceeded by a factor of 1.3 in stage

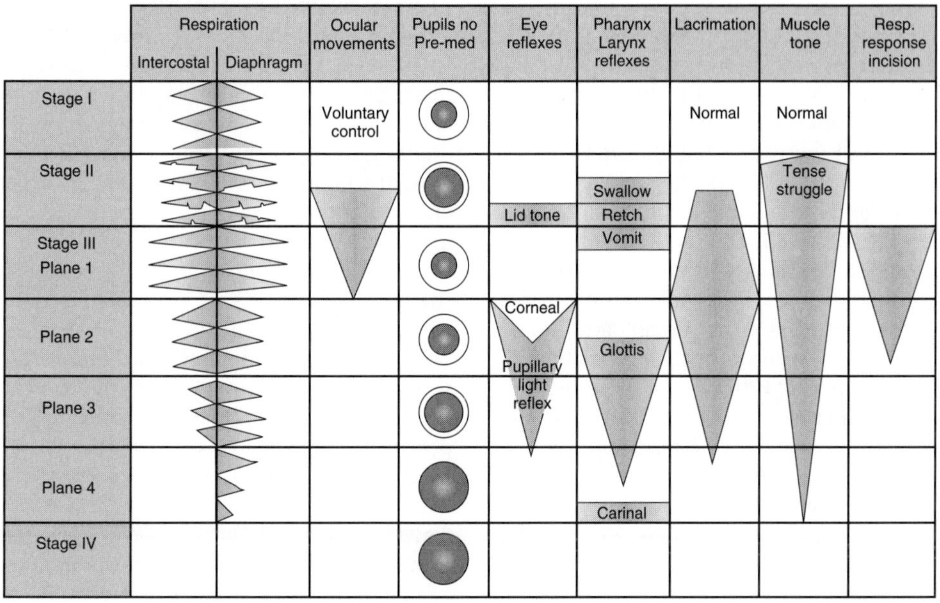

	Respiration		Ocular movements	Pupils no Pre-med	Eye reflexes	Pharynx Larynx reflexes	Lacrimation	Muscle tone	Resp. response incision
	Intercostal	Diaphragm							
Stage I			Voluntary control				Normal	Normal	
Stage II					Lid tone	Swallow / Retch			Tense struggle
Stage III Plane 1						Vomit			
Plane 2					Corneal / Pupillary light reflex	Glottis			
Plane 3									
Plane 4						Carinal			
Stage IV									

Fig. 18-1 The signs and reflex reactions of the stages of anesthesia. *(Adapted from Gillespie NA: Signs of anesthesia, Anesth Analg 22:275, 1943.)*

III because most patients do not respond to surgical incision at this level of anesthesia. Patients who receive 1.3 MAC anesthesia experience a depression in all elements of nervous system function—that is, sensory depression, loss of recall, reflex depression, and some skeletal muscle relaxation. From this point, with the modern anesthetics, increased MAC results in further respiratory, cardiovascular, and central nervous system (CNS) depression. The difficulty is that each of the newer agents affects the clinical signs, such as blood pressure, differently. Consequently, monitoring the level of anesthesia depends on the particular properties of each agent.

Most surgical procedures in which ether anesthesia was used were performed at this stage of anesthesia, which is divided into four planes. Plane 1 is entered when the lid reflex is abolished and respiration becomes regular. During this plane the vomiting reflex is gradually abolished. It is important for the nurse working in the PACU to know that swallowing, retching, and vomiting reflexes tend to disappear in that order during induction and reappear in the same order during emergence from anesthesia.

Plane 2 lasts from the time the eyeballs cease to move and become concentrically fixed to the beginning of a decrease of activity of the intercostal muscles, or thoracic respiration. The reflex of laryngospasm disappears during this plane. Plane 3 is entered when intercostal activity begins to decrease. Complete intercostal paralysis occurs in lower plane 3, and respiration is produced solely by the diaphragm. Plane 4 lasts from the time of paralysis of the intercostal muscles to the cessation of spontaneous respiration.

Tracheal tug often appears in association with deep anesthesia and intercostal paralysis. This represents an unopposed action of the diaphragm, displacing the hilum of the lung and thereby increasing traction on the trachea.

Stage IV lasts from the time of cessation of respiration to failure of the circulatory system. This level of anesthesia is considered the stage of overdose.

When ether is used as the sole inhalation agent, these signs and stages will be seen in reverse order on emergence from the anesthetic. No one clinical sign can be considered a reliable indicator of anesthetic depth by itself. All clinical signs must be viewed in the context of the patient's status along with the particular characteristics of the individual anesthetic agent used.

Some of the more reliable indicators of depth of anesthesia for the more modern inhalation anesthetics include changes in breathing pattern, eye movement, lacrimation, and muscle tone. Because the ventilation is under autonomic control, it is the most sensitive indicator of depth of anesthesia. In the PACU, a patient who is using diaphragmatic ventilation without the intercostal muscles should be considered to be in surgical anesthesia. As the ventilatory pattern returns to a more normal rate, rhythm, and pattern, the patient can be considered to be under light anesthesia and about to experience total emergence. Eye movement as opposed to pupillary size is a good indicator of anesthetic depth. Light anesthesia is present with eye movement. Deeper anesthesia is present when the eyes are close together in a cross-eyed position. Lacrimation does not occur during surgical anesthesia when a patient is receiving enflurane (Ethrane), isoflurane (Forane), or halothane (Fluothane). Conversely, if a patient received one of those drugs and is tearing, light anesthesia can be considered to be present. As the depth of anesthesia is increased, the amount of muscle tone decreases. Therefore if a patient in the PACU lacks muscle tone, especially in the jaw and abdomen, the patient should be considered to be in a surgical depth of anesthesia. When making the assessment of the degree of muscle tone, it is important that the perianesthesia nurse critically assess the degree of reversal of skeletal muscle relaxants (see Chapter 21) before determining the depth of anesthesia with the criterion of muscle tone. Finally, because the determinants of anesthesia depth have such a high degree of variability, all possible assessment tools should be incorporated into the care of the PACU patient. It goes without saying that the bottom line is constant vigilance of the patient's physiologic parameters during his or her emergence from anesthesia and the institution of appropriate nursing interventions based on an ongoing assessment.

Pharmacokinetics of Inhalation Anesthetics

The pharmacokinetics of inhalation anesthetics—as described by Stoelting—involves uptake, distribution, metabolism, and elimination. Basically, this involves a series of partial pressure gradients starting in the anesthesia machine, to the patient's brain for induction, and vice versa for emergence. The object of anesthesia is to achieve a constant and optimal partial pressure in the brain. The key to attaining anesthesia is having the alveolar partial pressure (PA) in equilibrium with the arterial (Pa) and brain partial pressure (Pbr) of the inhaled anesthetic. The partial pressure of an inhalation anesthetic in the brain determines the depth of anesthesia. The more potent the anesthetic, the lower the partial pressure of the agent required to produce a certain depth of anesthesia.

Movement of Inhalation Anesthetic from Anesthesia Machine to Alveoli.

The determinants of the PA are the inspired partial pressure of the inhalation anesthetic, the characteristics of the anesthesia machine's delivery system, and the patient's alveolar ventilation. The inhaled partial pressure (PI) is the concentration of the inhalation anesthetic that is delivered from the anesthesia machine. The impact of the PI on the rate of increase in the PA is called the concentration effect. The higher the inhaled concentration, the more rapid the induction of anesthesia. The anesthesia machine's delivery system has an impact on the depth of anesthesia and the speed of induction and emergence. For example, the rate of uptake of an anesthetic agent administered by inhalation can be reduced by the diffusion of the anesthetic agent into the rubber tubing of the anesthesia machine, the small losses of anesthetic agent from the body by diffusion across skin and mucous membranes, and—to a lesser extent—the metabolism of the agents by the body.

Alveolar ventilation plays the primary role in delivery of the anesthetic gas. It is determined in large part by the minute ventilation (V_E). If the V_E is high, the anesthetic concentration increases quickly in the alveoli, as does the concentration in the arterial blood. This is an important concept to understand because the reverse also is true. In the emergence phase of anesthesia, it is important to have a good V_E to ensure elimination of the anesthetic agent.

Movement of Inhalation Anesthetic from Alveoli to Arterial Blood. The movement of the inhalation anesthetic agent from the alveoli to the arterial blood depends on the blood-gas partition coefficient and the cardiac output. The rate at which the anesthetic is taken up by the blood and tissues is governed in part by the solubility of the agent in blood. This is expressed as the blood-gas partition coefficient, or the Oswald solubility coefficient. It is defined as the ratio of the concentration of an anesthetic in blood to that in a gas phase when the two are in equilibrium (Table 18-1). This is a difficult concept to understand because the more soluble the anesthetic agent is, the slower the agent is in producing anesthesia. This is because the blood serves as a reservoir, and a large volume of the agent must be introduced to attain an equilibrium between the blood partial pressure and the partial pressure in the lungs.

The blood conveys the anesthetic agent to the tissues. Consequently, a normal cardiac output is needed to facilitate the movement of the inhalation anesthetic through the tissues to the brain. The partial pressure increases most rapidly in the tissues with the highest rates of blood flow. Of interest is the great variation in blood perfusion of certain tissues in the body. The body tissue compartments can be divided into the following major groups:

1. The vessel-rich group, which consists of the heart, brain, kidneys, hepatoportal system, and endocrine glands.
2. The intermediate group of perfused tissues, which consists of muscle and skin.
3. The fat group, which includes marrow and adipose tissue.
4. The vessel-poor group, which has the poorest circulation per unit volume and comprises tendons, ligaments, connective tissue, teeth, bone, and other avascular tissue.

The vessel-rich group of tissues receives 75% of the cardiac output; thus the brain becomes saturated rapidly with an anesthetic agent administered by inhalation. On termination of the anesthetic, the reverse takes place, and the agent is rapidly removed from the brain.

The tissue tensions of the inhaled anesthetic increase and approach the arterial blood tension and ultimately the PA. One of the tissue groups that affects both the induction and emergence from anesthesia is the fat group. The oil-gas partition coefficient best exemplifies the process involved with the affinity of anesthesia agents to adipose tissue and ultimately the emergence from anesthesia. The oil-gas partition coefficient is defined as the ratio of the concentration of the anesthetic agent in oil (adipose tissue) to that in a gaseous phase when the two are in equilibrium (see Table 18-1). The oil-gas partition coefficients seem to parallel anesthetic requirements. In fact, one can calculate the MAC by knowing the oil-gas partition coefficient. With the constant of 150, the calculated MAC for an anesthetic with an oil-gas partition coefficient of 100 would be 1.5%.

Because some anesthetic agents are highly fat-soluble, they tend to be readily absorbed by the adipose tissue. This characteristic affects uptake

Table 18-1	**Properties of Inhalant Anesthetic Agents**			
	PARTITION COEFFICIENT			Minimum Alveolar Concentration (% in Oxygen)
Agent	Blood-Gas	Oil-Gas	Blood-Brain	
Methoxyflurane (Penthrane)	12.0	970.0	1.4	0.16
Halothane (Fluothane)	2.37	224.0	2.0	0.75
Enflurane (Ethrane)	1.9	98.5	1.4	1.68
Isoflurane (Forane)	0.97	93.7	1.6	1.15
Desflurane (Suprane)	0.42	18.7	1.3	6.58
Sevoflurane	0.69	53.4	1.7	1.71
Nitrous oxide	0.47	1.4	1.1	104.0

of the anesthetic agent, but of more importance is the prolonged recovery phase that usually ensues with a high oil-gas partition coefficient, such as in the case of halothane. Because adipose tissue is poorly perfused by blood, the adipose tissue releases the agent slowly to the blood at the termination of the anesthesia. Redistribution then takes place; some of the agent is eliminated by the lungs, which are vessel-rich, and some is distributed to the brain. The recovery period becomes significantly extended when—to allow for complete saturation of the adipose tissue—the administration time of the anesthetic agent is prolonged.

Halothane has an oil-gas partition coefficient that is about twice that of isoflurane or enflurane. Consequently, some authors question the use of halothane in the ambulatory surgical setting. However, clinical observation indicates that patients who receive halothane appear to emerge from anesthesia at about the same rate as they do from isoflurane. Therefore even with its relatively high oil-gas partition coefficient, halothane remains a popular inhalation anesthetic for use in the ambulatory surgical setting.

Movement of Inhalation Anesthetic from Arterial Blood to the Brain.
The transfer of the inhalation anesthetic from the arterial blood to the brain depends on the blood-brain partition coefficient of the agent and the cerebral blood flow. The blood-brain partition coefficient for most of the inhalation anesthetics is between 1.3 and 2 (see Table 18-1). The concentration gradient during induction of anesthesia is as follows:

$$PA > Pa > Pbr$$

During maintenance of surgical anesthesia, the brain tissue becomes saturated with the anesthetic agent, and the brain tissue is in equilibrium with the alveolar and arterial concentration. Consequently,

$$PA = Pa = Pbr$$

Emergence of Inhalation Anesthesia
When the administration of the anesthetic is terminated, a reverse gradient takes place. In this instance, the PA is almost zero, because only oxygen is administered during the emergence phase. The gradient that develops is as follows:

$$PA < Pa < Pbr$$

This gradient favors the removal of the anesthetic agent from the brain tissue. The partial pressure in the tissues declines first and is followed by that in the arterial blood. The agent returns to the lungs and is then eliminated into the atmosphere. The factors that affect the rate of elimination of the agent are the same ones that determine how rapidly an anesthetic agent takes a patient to surgical anesthesia. If a short procedure is performed (less than 1 hour), complete equilibrium among PA, Pa, and Pbr might not have occurred, and the recovery from anesthesia will be more rapid. The reverse is true; during long procedures in which equilibrium occurs, a prolonged emergence may be anticipated.

Potency of Inhalation Anesthetic Agents
Potency is determined by factors such as absorption, distribution, metabolism, excretion, and affinity for a receptor. The potency of the anesthetic agent refers to its ability to take the patient through all the stages of anesthesia to respiratory and circulatory arrest without the occurrence of hypoxia or the use of preanesthetic medication. Certainly, circulatory and respiratory arrests are not desired outcomes of the use of anesthetic agents; this feature is used merely to describe the potency of anesthetic agents that are used clinically. For example, halothane is 100% potent in comparison to nitrous oxide, which is 15% potent. Halothane, when administered with oxygen to meet the patient's metabolic needs and when given without premedication, takes the patient to circulatory and respiratory arrest, whereas nitrous oxide administered with oxygen takes the patient only to the first portion of surgical anesthesia and no further. Therefore, clinically speaking, potency of a drug makes little difference as long as the drug that is to be administered has an effective dose for a particular patient. This is why the concept of effective dose (ED) was developed. The ED is the dose of a drug necessary to produce certain effects in a certain percentage of patients. For example, an ED_{50} means that a drug produces a particular effect in 50% of the patients.

Another way of determining potency is with the use of the MAC. The MAC is found by determining the alveolar concentration (at 1 atm) required to prevent gross muscular movement in response to painful stimuli in 50% of anesthetized patients. The lower the MAC value, the more anesthetic potency of the inhalation anesthetic. The MAC of halothane in oxygen required to prevent patient movement in response to surgical incision is 0.75%. A geriatric patient may be administered 0.38% halothane in oxygen, which is commonly called half-MAC. "MAC hours" is the concentration in MAC units multiplied by the duration in hours of anesthetic administration. Consequently, the MAC hours for this patient is 0.76 (0.38 × 2). When 70% nitrous oxide is added to the halothane, the MAC decreases to 0.29%. Thus when halothane (or any 100% potent agent) is combined with a premedication and nitrous oxide, the MAC will decrease (see Table 18-1). "MAC awake" is the anesthetic dose at which patients respond to commands. It is also the dose of anesthetic at which most patients lose consciousness and recall. MAC awake usually corresponds with stage I of anesthesia. Another term used with MAC is MAC-BAR. This is the MAC required to block the adrenergic and cardiovascular responses to incision, and it corresponds to stage III, plane III anesthesia. The MAC is reduced in patients who are hypothermic, elderly, or pregnant. Narcotics, clonidine, diazepam, nitrous oxide, reserpine, and methyldopa also decrease the MAC. On the other hand, amphetamines, which release catecholamines, increase the MAC.

TECHNIQUES OF ADMINISTRATION
The inhalation anesthetics are usually administered by means of an anesthesia machine (Fig. 18-2). The anesthesia machine is essentially a breathing circuit that conveys the agent and oxygen to the patient. It consists of a mask, corrugated tubing, an absorber to remove expired carbon dioxide, a reservoir bag, unidirectional valves, a pop-off valve, and vaporizers (Fig. 18-3).

Circle Systems
A variety of techniques can be used to deliver gaseous agents with the anesthesia machine by adding or removing certain features. The most common technique used is the semiclosed circle method, in which some rebreathing of expired gases occurs by opening the pop-off valve to vent some of the gas to the atmosphere. The closed

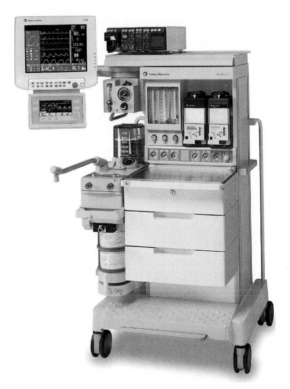

Fig. 18-2 Anesthesia machine apparatus. *(Used with permission from Datex-Ohmeda, Madison, Wis.)*

circle method is used when explosive gases are being administered or when low gas flows are desired for nonexplosive agents. In this technique, the pop-off valve is completely closed, and complete rebreathing of expired gases occurs. A carbon dioxide absorber is used in both the semiclosed and the closed techniques.

Insufflation Technique
The insufflation technique involves the delivery of large volumes of fresh gases administered continuously to the mouth by means of a hook made of hard plastic or metal. This technique permits the least rebreathing of expired gases, and, although it is not often used now, has the advantages of posing little resistance to breathing and not requiring complex equipment.

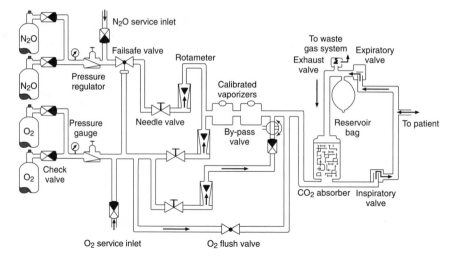

Fig. 18-3 Anesthesia machine circuit. Oxygen and nitrous oxide enter the machine from cylinders or from the hospital service supply. Pressure regulators reduce cylinder pressure to about 3 kg per cm^2. Check valves prevent transfilling of cylinders or gas flow from cylinders to the service line. The fail-safe valve prevents the flow of nitrous oxide if the oxygen supply fails. Needle valves in the flowmeters control flows to rotameters. Calibrated vaporizers provide a preselected concentration of volatile anesthetics. Gases are delivered to the circle absorber, where unidirectional valves ensure flow from the patient through the carbon dioxide absorber. Excess gas is vented through the exhaust valve into a waste gas scavenger system. The reservoir bag compensates for variations in respiratory demand. *(Adapted from Dripps RD, Eckenhoff JE, Vandam LD: Introduction to anesthesia: the principles of safe practice, ed 7, Philadelphia, 1988, WB Saunders.)*

Open Systems

The open, or nonrebreathing, technique ensures that the patient will inhale only the anesthetic mixture delivered by the anesthesia machine. Valves such as the Leigh, Fink, Rubin, or Stephen-Slater are used, and minimal rebreathing of the anesthetic gas occurs.

Semiopen Systems

The semiopen system allows exhaled gases to pass into the surrounding atmosphere, and some of the exhaled gases are rebreathed. Essentially, the semiopen method works without carbon dioxide absorption. The types of semiopen systems used are the open drop method, the Ayre T-piece, the Magill attachment, and the Bain anesthesia circuit.

The open drop method was one of the first anesthesia methods ever used, and it requires the least equipment. A volatile anesthetic agent is dripped over a wire mask covered with gauze. Oxygen is usually administered by the insufflation technique to supply the metabolic needs of the patient. The open drop technique is not used

in today's anesthesia practice because the anesthetic agents required in this technique are flammable and explosive.

The Ayre T-piece was devised to facilitate endotracheal anesthesia for infants and children (Fig. 18-4). One end of the T-piece is connected to the endotracheal tube, and the other end is open to the atmosphere. At the middle portion and at a right angle to the main limb a tube is attached, thus forming the T through which the delivery of the anesthetic agent is accomplished. The modified Ayre T-piece consists of a rebreathing bag connected by corrugated tubing to the escape end of the T-piece. This arrangement gives the system more versatility and provides a means of positive pressure to support ventilation. This method is simple and is used for children 4 years of age and younger.

The Magill attachment is similar to the modified Ayre T-piece, except that an expiratory valve is inserted into the circuit close to the face mask and is separated from the reservoir bag by corrugated tubing (Fig. 18-5).

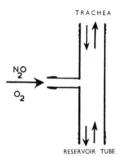

Fig. 18-4 The Ayre T-piece. Nitrous oxide-oxygen supplemented with ether enters through the side tube. The tracheal end of the T-piece is connected to the endotracheal tube. The end marked "reservoir tube" is open to the air. *(From Ayre P: The T-piece technique, Br J Anaesth 28:520, 1956.)* © The Board of Management and Trustees of the British Journal of Anaesthesia. Reproduced by permission of Oxford University Press/British Journal of Anaesthesia.

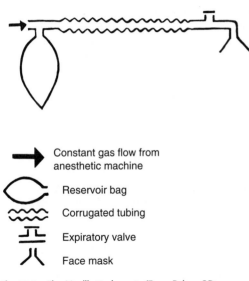

Constant gas flow from anesthetic machine

Reservoir bag

Corrugated tubing

Expiratory valve

Face mask

Fig. 18-5 The Magill attachment. *(From Dripps RD, Eckenhoff JE, Vandam LD: Introduction to anesthesia: the principles of safe practice, ed 6, Philadelphia, 1982, WB Saunders.)*

The Bain anesthesia circuit, introduced in 1972, consists of a tube within a tube. The inner noncorrugated tube, which provides fresh gases to the patient, is surrounded by a wider corrugated tube that conveys exhaled gases away from the patient. The circuit attaches to a bag mount that is attached to the anesthesia machine. The bag mount incorporates an exhaust valve and a bag port for attachment of an anesthesia bag or ventilator tubing (Fig. 18-6). The major advantage of this circuit is its versatility; it may be used for both children and adults; it has no directional valves; it is especially useful in surgical procedures involving the head and neck; and it does not require carbon dioxide absorption (no soda lime), yet patients may be maintained at a normal $PaCO_2$ and pH.

INHALATION AGENTS

Inhalant anesthetic substances may be divided into two groups: volatile and gaseous. Volatile anesthetic agents are chemicals in the liquid state at room temperature that have a boiling point above 20°C. Ethyl chloride, which has a boiling point of 12°C, is also included in this class of anesthetic agents. The volatile inhalation anesthetic agents are divided into two major categories: the halogenated hydrocarbons and the ethers. Examples of the halogenated hydrocarbons are halothane, chloroform, and trichloroethylene. Enflurane, methoxyflurane, isoflurane, and diethyl ether are examples of the ethers. The gaseous anesthetic agents, such as nitrous oxide and cyclopropane, are those in the gaseous state at room temperature. The anesthetic agents currently in use have evolved from the traditional inhalation anesthetics such as cyclopropane, chloroform, and diethyl ether. For that reason they will be described briefly before the current inhalation agents are presented in detail.

Traditional Inhalation Anesthetics
Chloroform (Trichlormethane). Chloroform was the most potent anesthetic agent available until the 1970s. It offered many advantages, such as excellent muscle relaxation, no irritation of the respiratory tract, rapid induction and emergence, and nonflammability. However, the disadvantages of chloroform are clinically significant. Because deep anesthesia can be achieved rapidly with small changes in concentration, it has a narrow margin of safety. The major problem with chloroform is that it is hepatotoxic and cardiotoxic and therefore is no longer administered to humans.

Because chloroform is a hydrocarbon, it has some excellent qualities that were preserved

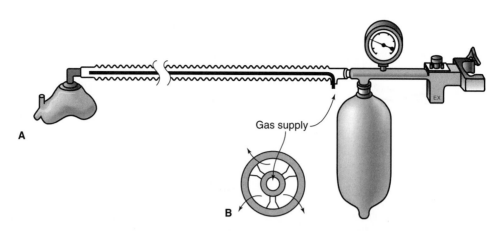

Fig. 18-6 Bain system breathing circuit. **A,** Tube-within-tube design. **B,** Cross-section of tubing. Arrows show air inflow and outflow. *(From Chu YK, Rah KH, Boyan CP: Is the Bain breathing circuit the future anesthesia system? Anesth Analg 56:84, 1977.)*

when researchers developed newer hydrocarbon inhalation anesthetic agents, such as halothane. In this way, chloroform served as a model for the modern inhalation anesthetics.

Cyclopropane. Cyclopropane was introduced into clinical anesthesia in 1934. It is a colorless gas with the characteristic odor of petroleum ether. It is stored in orange metal cylinders as a liquid under pressure. The most notable property of this drug is its speed of induction and emergence because of its blood-gas partition coefficient of 0.42. In fact, anesthesia can be induced in five or six deep tidal breaths in a premedicated patient.

The simplest of the cyclic hydrocarbons, cyclopropane is flammable and explosive in air and in oxygen. Like other explosive inhalation anesthetic agents, cyclopropane is no longer used in anesthesia practice.

Diethyl Ether. Ether, one of the first inhalation anesthetics administered in the United States, is rarely used today; therefore it is presented to the reader for its historical significance only. Ether has the relatively high blood-gas partition coefficient of 12.1. Consequently, when ether is administered alone, without any premedication, the induction time is long—usually 30 to 40 minutes. The same holds true for emergence. When the patient awakens, he or she usually has some degree of analgesia. Because of its rather high blood-gas partition coefficient, ether has a built-in safety factor that provides a wide margin

of safety for the patient. This consists of the fact that it is difficult to deepen the anesthesia rapidly; thus the anesthetist has a reasonable length of time to appraise the patient's status and make corrections before a deeper anesthetic plane is induced.

Ether has other advantages—it improves the blood pressure and causes excellent muscle relaxation; in addition, it can be used with all techniques and is inexpensive. The disadvantages of ether are that it is flammable and explosive and has been implicated in the occurrence of convulsions, nausea, and vomiting.

Ethylene. Ethylene, discovered in 1923, resembles nitrous oxide in its use in anesthesia practice. The gas is about 25% potent and takes the patient to the lower border of stage III, plane 1 of anesthesia while supplying the metabolic oxygen requirement. A unique property of this agent is that it is lighter than air and will rise. Ethylene is a very rapid-acting agent because of its blood-gas partition coefficient of 0.14. This agent has been eliminated from use in anesthesia departments solely because of its flammability and explosive properties.

Fluroxene (Trifluoroethyl Vinyl Ether, Fluoromar). Fluroxene was the first of the fluorine-containing hydrocarbons to be introduced into clinical practice. It is a mixed halogenated aliphatic ether that is flammable, although less so than the nonfluorinated ethers. Because fluroxene is a derivative of ether, postanesthetic nausea and vomiting are not uncommon with its use. Because it is explosive and has strong emetic properties, it is not used today.

Methoxyflurane (Penthrane). Methoxyflurane is a fluorinated alkyl ether that was introduced into anesthesia practice in 1959. It is nonflammable and nonexplosive in air, oxygen, or nitrous oxide mixtures at normal room temperature. Methoxyflurane can produce any desired depth of anesthesia in the absence of hypoxia and therefore meets the requirements for a 100% potent agent. The drug has a high blood-gas partition coefficient of 13 and thus features excellent controllability and analgesia, with good muscle relaxation.

Methoxyflurane was originally thought to be exhaled unchanged, but it is now known to be partially metabolized into several substances that contribute to renal dysfunction. The most important metabolite is free inorganic fluoride, which is nephrotoxic. The renal syndrome caused by methoxyflurane is called vasopressin-resistant high-output renal failure. Because methoxyflurane is nephrotoxic, it is no longer used in anesthesia practice.

Trichloroethylene (Trilene). Like chloroform and ether, trichloroethylene is not used today in anesthesia practice. The drug is related chemically to chloroform and ethylene. Because the drug decomposes to dichloroacetylene when it is exposed to soda lime, it was used only for its analgesic qualities in obstetrics, dentistry, and short surgical procedures. It was administered by techniques such as inhalers, insufflation, and blow-through vaporizers that did not have to incorporate soda lime in the circuit.

Modern Inhalation Anesthetics

Enflurane (Ethrane). Enflurane is a halogenated ether that is enjoying significant popularity in the practice of anesthesia. It is nonflammable, 100% potent, and very rapid-acting. Enflurane promotes a fair amount of muscle relaxation and strongly potentiates any nondepolarizing skeletal muscle relaxant, such as d-tubocurarine and pancuronium.

Enflurane, like halothane, causes cerebral vasodilatation, which results in an increase in cerebral blood flow if the patient is normotensive. When the patient is hypotensive, enflurane can reduce the cerebral blood flow. This agent may cause no change or small and inconsistent increases in intracranial pressure in neurosurgical patients who are hyperventilated. The hemodynamic effects of enflurane are similar to those of halothane; however, it depresses arterial blood pressure, stroke volume, and systemic vascular resistance. The cardiac depression that enflurane produces appears to be the result of direct negative inotropic effects on the heart, and it also produces a reduction in the peripheral vascular resistance. Enflurane tends to increase the heart rate—or it may keep it normal—and bradycardia does not usually occur. Enflurane sensitizes the myocardium to the effects of endogenous and exogenous catecholamines. However, a lower incidence of dysrhythmias has been associated with enflurane as compared with halothane. In comparison with halothane, enflurane is a more potent respiratory depressant and blunts a patient's response to hypercarbia.

Like methoxyflurane (another fluorinated ether), enflurane is metabolized to inorganic and organic fluoride. However, the maximum serum concentrations are not high enough to cause renal toxicity. However, a fluoride-induced nephrotoxicity is a potential hazard after the metabolism of enflurane. This topic is hotly debated because the amount of fluoride produced by enflurane needed to produce any clinical signs of nephrotoxicity is rather low. Some reports have suggested that enflurane causes slight hepatic dysfunction. These reports describe a mild, self-limited postoperative hepatic dysfunction that is most likely caused by inadequate hepatocyte oxygenation during enflurane anesthesia. Hence enflurane may not be the anesthetic of choice for a patient with compromised hepatic function.

The patient regains consciousness from enflurane quickly, partly because of its low blood-gas partition coefficient of 1.37. There usually is no residual analgesia; therefore when the patient regains consciousness, it is important to assess his or her pain and administer a narcotic analgesic if indicated. Some anesthetists administer a short-acting narcotic, such as fentanyl, at the end of the surgical procedure to reduce the amount of postoperative pain experienced by the patient in the PACU. Therefore the perianesthesia nurse should note at admission whether the patient has received any pain-relieving drugs during the intraoperative period.

The incidence of nausea and vomiting has been minimal with enflurane. Some patients have exhibited shivering that is unrelated to body temperature during emergence and recovery. Because enflurane is a halogenated agent, it continues to be studied as a possible cause of liver problems; however, it has yet to be linked with any hepatic syndrome.

Advantages of enflurane include marked cardiovascular stability, good operative analgesia, pleasant induction and emergence, and good patient acceptance. Enflurane is contraindicated in seizure disorders because it increases intracranial pressure and lowers the seizure threshold; in diabetes mellitus; with administration of catecholamines; in obstetric usage, especially in the first trimester of pregnancy; and in patients receiving enzyme inducers, particularly phenobarbital and phenytoin (Dilantin).

Halothane (Fluothane). Halothane is a saturated hydrocarbon. Unlike the traditional inhalation anesthetic agents, halothane was a product of planned research by chemists and pharmacologists whose aim was to synthesize a volatile compound that combined the properties of anesthetic potency with nontoxicity and nonflammability. Halothane is 100% potent and a very rapid-acting drug. It is also easily controlled, in that the depth of anesthesia can be changed quickly. Because it is such a potent agent, it is administered by finely calibrated vaporizers. Recovery to consciousness is rapid because of the small amounts absorbed by the brain tissue and the low blood-gas partition coefficient of 2.37.

Halothane has demonstrated a low incidence of postanesthesia nausea and vomiting. It does, however, sensitize the heart to catecholamines. Therefore, epinephrine should be administered cautiously to a patient in the PACU who has received halothane intraoperatively, because serious dysrhythmias may result. For the patient who is emerging from halothane (within 30 minutes of the termination of the intraoperative anesthetic), the following guidelines for the administration of epinephrine in the PACU will reduce the incidence of dysrhythmias. The epinephrine concentration should be no greater than 1:100,000 to 1:200,000, with a total adult dose not to exceed 10 ml of 1:100,000 solution in 10 minutes, or a total dose of 30 ml of 1:100,000 solution in 1 hour.

When the position of a patient is being changed during emergence from halothane, the maneuver should be carried out slowly and gently because compensatory vasoconstrictor mechanisms are depressed. Bronchial dilatation, myocardial depression, peripheral vasodilatation, and nonirritation of respiratory tissues are other features of this agent.

The use of halothane anesthesia as a possible cause of hepatitis continues to be the subject of research studies. It is well known that postoperative jaundice and liver failure may be caused by factors other than the anesthetic agent. However, because of the possibility that halothane may cause hepatitis in certain sensitized patients, it is usually not the anesthetic of choice when the patient has had recent exposure to halothane or has had any type of liver disease.

Halothane is widely used for all types of surgical procedures in patients of all age groups. The importance of maintaining the blood volume within reasonably normal limits should be stressed because of the peripheral-vasodilating action of halothane. Diminution of the blood volume by preoperative fluid restriction, diuretic therapy, and hemorrhage augment the hypotensive effect of halothane and should be corrected by intravenous infusions of the appropriate solutions.

Because the recovery phase of halothane is generally short, the postoperative analgesic phase is also short. Evaluation of postoperative pain should be thorough before a narcotic analgesic is administered to the patient, because the synergistic effect of halothane and a narcotic may result in marked respiratory depression.

Isoflurane (Forane). Isoflurane, an analogue of enflurane, is also a halogenated methyl ethyl ether. It produces a dose-related depression of the CNS. But, in contrast with enflurane, this anesthetic agent does not produce convulsive electroencephalographic abnormalities. Isoflurane reduces the systemic arterial blood pressure and total peripheral resistance. However, during isoflurane anesthesia, the heart rate is usually increased, and the cardiac output usually remains within normal limits. This agent produces respiratory depression as well as skeletal muscular relaxation in a dose-related fashion, because isoflurane markedly potentiates the actions of the nondepolarizing muscle relaxants. Of interest to the perianesthesia nurse is the fact that isoflurane does not sensitize the myocardium to cate-cholamines to the same extent as halothane does. Thus the chance of dysrhythmias is reduced when the patient has received isoflurane anesthesia.

The recovery phase is rapid because of isoflu-rane's low blood-gas partition coefficient of 0.97. The patient not only awakens promptly but is also quite lucid within 15 to 30 minutes after ter-mination of the anesthetic. However, clinical observation indicates that if the anesthesia time using isoflurane is longer than 45 to 60 minutes, the patient will probably experience a slower emergence phase than would be expected given that the drug has such a low blood-gas partition coefficient.

The lung volumes and capacities, as measured by the Wright respirometer, return to normal in less than 30 minutes along with the ability to raise the head, protrude the tongue, cough on command, and converse clearly. The blood pres-sure and pulse remain stable. Shivering is seen in 2% of patients, and nausea and vomiting occurs only occasionally.

Isoflurane possesses some excellent qualities—that is, a lack of sensitization of the heart to catecholamines, cardiovascular stability, limited biodegradation, good neuromuscular relaxation, and no CNS excitatory effects. Since its intro-duction into anesthesia practice, isoflurane has enjoyed continuing success among both anesthe-sia practitioners and perianesthesia nurses.

Sevoflurane.   Sevoflurane is a 100% potent inhalation anesthetic agent that has a blood-gas solubility coefficient of 0.69, which is near nitrous oxide, thus making it an extremely rapid-acting agent. Consequently, patients emerge from sevoflurane anesthesia in a matter of minutes when they have received this drug as the sole agent. It must be remembered that a rapid re-covery from an inhalation anesthetic usually mandates the need for analgesic drugs in the immediate postoperative period.

The drug is nonirritating to the respiratory tract, and the degree of patient acceptance is high. It can be used in place of halothane for the induction of anesthesia in children. Sevoflurane tends to decrease the blood pressure by decreas-ing the systemic vascular resistance. Like all other inhalation agents, this drug is a respiratory depressant and blunts the ventilatory response to

an increased $PaCO_2$. This drug does undergo some metabolism at about the same degree as does enflurane. The metabolites of sevoflurane include fluoride and hexafluoroisopropanol, and from a number of studies, no evidence of toxicity has been demonstrated in regard to the biodegra-dation of this agent. This is probably due to sevoflurane's rapid ventilatory excretion, in which the metabolic byproducts do not seem to be significantly detrimental to the patient.

Like the other ethers, sevoflurane does not sensitize the heart to catecholamines and hence does not predispose to arrhythmias. This inhala-tion agent does reduce cerebrovascular resistance and can increase intracranial pressure in a dose-related manner. In regard to its effect on skeletal muscle function, it enhances the action of the skeletal muscle relaxants. However, because of its rapid elimination, this characteristic does not have a significant impact on the care of a patient in the PACU who has received sevoflurane intraoperatively.

Sevoflurane possesses many outstanding qual-ities. It has great precision and control over anes-thetic depth, does not depress kidney or liver function, has little effect on heart rate, and—most of all—is extremely rapid, which will speed up the emergence of the patient in the PACU.

Desflurane (Suprane).   Desflurane is a fluorinated ether that is similar to isoflurane. This drug has a blood-gas partition coefficient that is the same as cyclopropane (0.42) and even less than nitrous oxide, which makes it extremely rapid-acting. As with sevoflurane, patient emergence is extremely rapid, and analgesia is needed in the immediate postoperative period. This drug produces a dose-related decrease in blood pressure and cardiac output that is slightly greater than the depression seen with equivalent doses of isoflurane. Because this drug is an ether-type inhalation agent, the incidence of cardiac dysrhythmias when epi-nephrine is administered is extremely low.

The pungency of desflurane irritates the respi-ratory tract and causes coughing, breathholding, and laryngospasm. Consequently, it is not rec-ommended as an inhalation induction agent, especially in the pediatric age group. This drug depresses respiration in the same fashion as does sevoflurane and thus blunts the response to an increased $PaCO_2$. Because this drug decreases cerebrovascular resistance, it will produce in a dose-related fashion. Desflurane also enhances the neuromuscular blockade produced by skeletal muscle relaxants. However, like sevoflurane, this action is not of consequence for the patient in the PACU, because of its extremely rapid ventilatory excretion during emergence. Finally, as opposed to sevoflurane, this drug resists biodegradation and is almost totally eliminated by the respiratory system and therefore does not have a negative effect on the kidney or liver.

Desflurane represents a new era in inhalation anesthesia in regard to its impact on the care of the patient in the PACU. More specifically, because of its low solubility, rapid emergence will become quite common, and a more rapid release from the PACU and a shorter length of stay in the hospital may be possible.

Nitrous Oxide. Nitrous oxide is the only inorganic gas used as an anesthetic agent. It is marketed in blue steel cylinders as a colorless liquid under a pressure of 30 atm. As the pressure is released, nitrous oxide returns to the gaseous state. It is readily soluble in water and heavier than air. Nitrous oxide was probably the first anesthetic agent to be used extensively. The fact that it is still being used indicates that, when used properly, it is a valuable and safe anesthetic agent.

Nitrous oxide supports combustion—that is, if a burning match is put into a jar containing nitrous oxide, it will continue to burn. However, this agent is not explosive. Although the nitrous oxide molecule contains oxygen, that oxygen is unavailable for respiration because nitrous oxide does not decompose in the body.

Nitrous oxide is a 15% potent agent; therefore, the maximum depth of anesthesia that can be produced while supplying the patient's metabolic need for oxygen is the middle of plane 1 of stage III anesthesia. This agent has no side effects unless hypoxia is present. It is nontoxic and nonirritating; however, nitrous oxide can cause postoperative nausea and vomiting. This is particularly true in the ambulatory surgical setting when the procedure lasts for 1—and quite probably for 2 or more—hours. Nitrous oxide is a rapid-acting agent in part because of its blood-gas partition coefficient of 0.47. This agent does not combine with hemoglobin but is carried in physical solution in the blood. It is excreted mostly unchanged by the lungs, although a small fraction is excreted through the skin. It does not sensitize the heart to epinephrine, and it provides a fair amount of analgesia. Even in subanesthetic concentrations it has an analgesic effect in humans, and 20% concentrations of the gas have been claimed to be as effective as 15 mg of morphine sulfate. If this agent were more potent, it would probably be considered an almost perfect anesthetic.

In current anesthesia practice, nitrous oxide serves an important role, because it is administered alone and in combination with various agents. Recently, the balanced technique of anesthesia has been favored because of the number of negative factors associated with some of the more potent volatile inhalation anesthetics. The balanced technique consists of the administration of narcotics that may or may not be in combination with a tranquilizer, a muscle relaxant, nitrous oxide, oxygen, and barbiturates. All the elements of anesthesia or nervous system depression are met: sensory block (analgesia), motor block (muscle relaxation), reflex block, and mental block (narcosis). For short procedures, when only light anesthesia is desired, a pent-nitrous technique is sometimes used. This consists of nitrous oxide, oxygen, and sodium thiopental. This technique provides narcosis and limited analgesia for brief, simple procedures.

When nitrous oxide is administered with a potent volatile inhalation anesthetic such as halothane, it acts as a carrier and also provides an additional analgesic effect. The second gas effect occurs because of nitrous oxide's rapid uptake, after which the potent volatile agent takes the patient to the desired surgical plane. The reverse takes place at termination of the anesthetic.

The solubilities of nitrogen and nitrous oxide differ greatly. Nitrous oxide is 30 times more soluble than nitrogen. An enclosed gas-filled space in the body expands if gas within it is more soluble than the gas respired. For this reason, any enclosed gas-filled cavity in the body expands because of the slow exchange of nitrogen from the cavity for the rapid exchange of large volumes of nitrous oxide from the blood. This is why the use of nitrous oxide is not recommended in surgical procedures for intestinal obstruction or pneumothorax. Nitrous oxide has been shown to dislodge a tympanoplasty graft because of the expansion of the air pocket in the middle ear. Consequently, in surgical procedures involving the middle ear, the administration of nitrous oxide is usually avoided. Of interest to the perianesthesia nurse is the possible role of nitrous oxide in altering the pressures in the middle ear; it has been suggested that nitrous oxide may cause nausea and vomiting caused by the resulting increased pressure in that area.

Diffusion hypoxia following nitrous oxide anesthesia is another area of concern for the perianesthesia nurse. This is sometimes called the Fink phenomenon. It occurs when not enough nitrous oxide is removed from the lungs at the end of the surgical procedure. Normally, 100% oxygen is administered at the end of the procedure to remove the nitrous oxide. This is called nitrous oxide washout. Diffusion hypoxia is directly related to the dilution of alveolar gas by the rapid diffusion of the nitrous oxide out of the blood. This outpouring of nitrous oxide into the alveoli occurs during the first 1 to 5 minutes after the nitrous oxide has been discontinued. Along with this, the rapid movement into the alveoli can cause a dilutional effect of the $PACO_2$ and ultimately a reduction in the stimulus to breathe. It is therefore highly advisable to administer oxygen by mask to all patients who are admitted to the PACU. This maneuver forestalls the development of severe hypoxia, should some unpredicted airway problem occur. Another measure for avoiding this complication is to provide adequate verbal and physical stimulation to the patient to promote good ventilatory effort. This approach should include encouraging the patient to sigh every 5 minutes to ensure adequate removal of the anesthetic gases.

ASSESSING THE EFFECTS OF INHALATION AGENTS IN THE PACU

When assessing the patient's degree of emergence from inhalation anesthesia, it is important for the nurse to understand the pharmacologic effects of each anesthetic agent and of the preoperative medications used. Along with this, the rate of recovery from inhalation anesthesia is predictable based on the solubility of the anesthetic agent, alveolar ventilation, and duration of the anesthetic. Each anesthetic agent is essentially a depressant drug. Certain volatile agents, such as halothane, enflurane, and isoflurane, possess a high degree of myocardial and respiratory depressant properties. One parameter for monitoring the emergence phase when these agents have been administered is the vital signs. Preanesthetic baseline vital sign readings are reliable postoperative indicators of the patient's cardiorespiratory status and can be used to assess the patient's stage of recovery. When this assessment is being made, however, all other factors of the patient's condition must also be considered. Total assessment of the patient recovering from anesthesia is discussed in Chapter 26. Most inhalation anesthetics cause some degree of depression of the respiratory system. Consequently, the $PaCO_2$ increases in a dose-related manner; frequency increases; and tidal volume is reduced. Because of the respiratory depression that all patients have after anesthesia and surgery, it is important that the perianesthesia nurse use the stir-up regimen that encourages the patient to perform the sustained maximal inspiration maneuver (see Chapter 26).

To understand the emergence phase of inhalation anesthesia, the nurse also needs a basic understanding of blood-gas and oil-gas partition coefficients. Anesthetic agents are usually administered in combinations, often with nitrous oxide as the carrier gas. The combination of agents usually consists of a 100% potent agent, a carrier agent, and oxygen to meet the metabolic needs of the patient. The agent with the highest blood-gas partition coefficient takes the longest time to be removed from the body. Therefore if a halothane–nitrous oxide–oxygen combination were administered to a patient, the halothane, which has the highest blood-gas partition coefficient, would be eliminated the most slowly.

Along with the factors attributed to the blood-gas partition coefficient, those attributed to the oil-gas partition coefficient should be considered in an evaluation of length of time of emergence from the anesthetic. When the intraoperative phase is of long duration, an agent that has a high oil-gas partition coefficient will redistribute into the adipose tissue. As mentioned previously, because the vascular supply to adipose tissue is sparse, the release of the agent to the blood is slow, and the emergence is prolonged. Both coefficients must be kept in mind when predicting the length of the emergence phase from an inhalation anesthetic agent. Halothane, for example, has the low blood-gas partition coefficient of 2.37, and one would expect a rapid recovery from its administration. However, halothane has a high oil-gas partition coefficient of 224, so when it is administered for longer than 1 hour, the adipose tissue will be saturated and emergence from the anesthetic agent prolonged. Nitrous oxide, enflurane, and isoflurane have low blood-gas and oil-gas partition coefficients.

Inhalation agents, because of their depressant effect on the hypothalamus, disrupt the regulation of body temperature that may be manifested by either a reduction or an elevation, depending on the environmental temperature. In the recovery phase, the emerging patient should be monitored for hypothermia or hyperthermia. Serious heat loss may occur in newborns, creating difficulties in the re-establishment of adequate ventilatory effort after surgery. Body temperature should be monitored in patients who were febrile before surgery and who received atropine before or during the operative procedure. Agents such as halothane, which have a direct vasodilatory effect on vascular smooth muscle, can cause a temperature drop of 1°C in esophageal temperature. Shivering and tremors have been reported during the postoperative period after halothane anesthesia, although this phenomenon has mostly been associated with a generalized loss of muscle tone during surgery and anesthesia.

Water and electrolyte balance is affected by inhalation anesthesia. Pituitary and adrenocortical systems appear to be affected in such a way that there is water and sodium retention and potassium loss after anesthesia. This balance is also affected, in part, by the stress of surgical trauma. Decreased glomerular filtration, increased tubular reabsorption, and varying degrees of oliguria exist in the recovery phase because of renal vasoconstriction. If renal blood flow is not impaired, glomerular function quickly returns to normal after the operation. The increased tubular reabsorption of water usually persists for 36 to 48 hours but may continue for several days in the elderly.

BIBLIOGRAPHY

Alspach J: Core curriculum for critical care nursing, ed 5, Philadelphia, 1998, WB Saunders.

Atlee J: Complications in anesthesia, Philadelphia, 1999, WB Saunders.

Barash P, Cullen B, Stoelting R: Clinical anesthesia, ed 4, Philadelphia, 2000, Lippincott Williams & Wilkins.

Benumof J: Anesthesia and uncommon diseases, ed 4, Philadelphia, 1998, WB Saunders.

Benumof J, Saidman L: Anesthesia & perioperative complications, ed 2, St Louis, 1999, Mosby.

Bickley L, Hoekelman R: Bates' guide to physical examination and history taking, ed 7, Philadelphia, 1998, Lippincott Williams & Wilkins.

Block R, Ghonem M, Ping S: Efficacy of therapeutic suggestions for improved postoperative recovery presented during general anesthesia, Anesthesiology 75:746-755, 1991.

Bowdle T, Horita A, Kharasch E: The pharmacologic basis of anesthesiology, New York, 1994, Churchill Livingstone.

Butterworth J: Atlas of procedures in anesthesia and critical care, Philadelphia, 1992, WB Saunders.

Chu Y, Rah K, Boyan C: Is the Bain breathing circuit the future anesthesia system? An evaluation, Anesth Analg 56:84-87, 1977.

DeFazio-Quinn D: Ambulatory surgical nursing core curriculum, Philadelphia, 1999, WB Saunders, 1999.

Dorsch J, Dorsch S: Understanding anesthesia equipment, ed 2, Baltimore, 1989, Williams & Wilkins.

Eger E: Clinical pharmacology of nitrous oxide: an argument for its continued use, Anesth Analg 71:575-585, 1990.

Eger E, Saidman L, Bradstater B: Minimum alveolar anesthetic concentration: a standard of anesthetic potency, Anesthesiology 26:756, 1965.

Ganong W: Review of medical physiology, ed 20, New York, 2001, McGraw-Hill Professional.

Guyton A, Hall J: Textbook of medical physiology, ed 10, Philadelphia, 2000, WB Saunders.

Hardman J, Limbird L: Goodman and Gilman's the pharmacological basis of therapeutics, ed 9, New York, 1996, McGraw-Hill.

Jacobsen W: Manual of post anesthesia care, Philadelphia, 1992, WB Saunders.

Jones R: Desflurane and sevoflurane: inhalation anaesthetics for this decade? Br J Anaesth 65:527-536, 1990.

Katoh T, Suguro Y, Nakajima R et al: Blood concentration of sevoflurane and isoflurane on recovery from anaesthesia, Br J Anaesth 69:259-262, 1992.

Katzung B, editor: Basic and clinical pharmacology, ed 8, Los Altos, Calif, 2000, Appleton & Lange.

Kulli J, Koch C: Does anesthesia cause loss of consciousness? Trends Neurosci 14(1):6-10, 1991.

Lake C, Hines R, Blitt C: Clinical monitoring: practical applications for anesthesia and critical care, St Louis, 2001, Mosby.

Litwack K: Core curriculum for post anesthesia nursing pactice, ed 3, Philadelphia, 1994, WB Saunders.

Longnecker D, Murphy F: Dripps/Eckenhoff/Vandam introduction to anesthesia, ed 9, Philadelphia, 1997, WB Saunders.

Longnecker D, Tinker J, Morgan G: Principles and practice of anesthesiology, ed 2, St Louis, 1998, Mosby.

Mazze R: The safety of sevoflurane in humans, Anesthesiology 77:1062-1063, 1992.

McIntosh L: Essentials of nurse anesthesia, New York, 1997, McGraw-Hill.

Miller R, editor: Anesthesia, ed 5, New York, 2000, Churchill Livingstone.

Nagelhout J, Zaglaniczny K: Nurse anesthesia, ed 2, Philadelphia, 2001, WB Saunders.

Redai I, Svyatets M, Mets B: Are volatile anesthetics cardioprotective agents? Seminars in Anesthesia, Perioperative Medicine and Pain 20(2):95-100, 2001.

Saidman L: The role of desflurane in the practice of anesthesia, Anesthesiology 74:399-401, 1991.

Stancer-Smiley B, Paradise N: Does the duration of N_2O administration affect postoperative nausea and vomiting? Nurse Anesth 2(1):13-18, 1991.

Stoelting R: Pharmacology and physiology in anesthetic practice, ed 3, Philadelphia, 1999, Lippincott-Raven.

Stoelting R, Miller R: Basics of anesthesia, ed 4, New York, 2000, Churchill Livingstone.

Stone D: Perioperative care: anesthesia, medicine, and surgery, St Louis, 1998, Mosby.

Tsai S, Lee C, Kwan W, Chen B: Recovery of cognitive functions after anaesthesia with desflurane or isoflurane and nitrous oxide, Br J Anaesth 69:255-258, 1992.

Waugaman W, Foster S, Rigor B: Principles and practice of nurse anesthesia, ed 3, Norwalk, Conn, 1999, Appleton & Lange.

Weinberg G: Basic science review of anesthesiology, New York, 1997, McGraw-Hill.

Wood M, Wood A: Drugs and anesthesia: pharmacology for the anesthesiologist, ed 2, Baltimore, 1990, Williams & Wilkins.

The time-tested use of the inhalation anesthetic agents has proved that they possess some definite disadvantages. Because of the biotransformation hazards that have been reported with the halogenated inhalation anesthetics, other techniques have been sought to provide general anesthesia. Intravenous anesthetics are now enjoying a wide range of use in the perioperative period. In fact, in current anesthesia practice, the use of intravenous drugs is now commonplace. Intravenous anesthetics are now grouped by primary pharmacologic action into nonopioid and opioid intravenous agents. The nonopioid agents are further grouped into the barbiturates, nonbarbiturates, and tranquilizers. These drugs can be injected in a rapid intravenous fashion to induce anesthesia, or they can be used via continuous infusion pump to facilitate maintenance of anesthesia. These drugs have certainly found their place in the practice of anesthesia to enhance patient outcomes.

MECHANISM OF ACTION OF THE NONOPIOID INTRAVENOUS ANESTHETICS

The nonopioid drugs appear to interact with gamma-aminobutyric acid (GABA) in the brain. GABA is an inhibitory neurotransmitter, and activation of the GABA receptors by GABA on the postsynaptic membrane causes inhibition of the postsynaptic neuron. The barbiturates appear to bind to the GABA postsynaptic receptor, with the net result of hyperpolarization of the postsynaptic neuron and inhibition of neuronal activity and, ultimately, loss of consciousness. Conversely, etomidate (Amidate), which is a nonbarbiturate induction agent, probably antagonizes the muscarinic receptors in the central nervous system (CNS) and also acts as an agonist to the opioid receptors. The resultant action of these drugs is a loss of wakefulness.

Tranquilizers such as the benzodiazepines bind to specific receptors in the limbic system. These benzodiazepine receptors use GABA as part of the neurotransmitter system. After the benzodiazepines have bound to the receptor, the action of GABA is enhanced, leading to the hyperpolarized state and ultimately to inhibition of neuronal activity. The drug flumazenil is a specific benzodiazepine receptor antagonist. Consequently, after the administration of a benzodiazepine agonist, flumazenil can be administered. The pharmacologic actions on the benzodiazepine receptor will be reversed, and neuronal activity will resume.

THE BARBITURATES

Intravenous anesthesia began with barbiturate anesthesia. The long-acting barbiturates were introduced clinically in 1927. It was not until 1934 that Tovell and Lundy began using thiopental in clinical anesthesia practice. Since then, barbiturate anesthesia has enjoyed great popularity and is still widely used in clinical anesthesia.

Thiopental (Sodium Pentothal)

Thiopental is most commonly injected intravenously to induce or sustain surgical anesthesia. It is usually used in conjunction with a potent inhalation anesthetic and nitrous oxide–oxygen combinations. The main reason for the use of other anesthetic agents with thiopental is that thiopental is a poor analgesic. For surgical procedures that are short and require minimal analgesia, thiopental and nitrous oxide–oxygen combinations can be used. This technique is commonly called the pent-nitrous technique. Thiopental is also used (1) to maintain light sleep during regional analgesia; (2) to control convulsions; and (3) to quiet a patient rapidly who is too lightly anesthetized during a surgical procedure.

The mode of action of thiopental involves a phenomenon of redistribution. Thiopental has the ability to penetrate all tissues of the body without delay. Because the brain, as part of the vessel-rich group, is highly perfused, it receives approximately 10% of the administered intravenous dose within 40 seconds after injection. The patient usually becomes unconscious at this time. The thiopental then redistributes to relatively poorly perfused areas of the body. In the brain, the level of thiopental decreases to half its peak in 5 minutes and to one tenth in 30 minutes. Recovery of consciousness usually occurs during this period. Recovery may be prolonged if the induction dose was excessive or if circulatory depression occurs that would slow the redistribution phenomenon. Thiopental is metabolized in the body at a rate of 10% to 15% per hour.

Thiopental is a respiratory depressant. The chief effect is on the medullary and pontine respiratory centers. This depressant effect depends on the amount of thiopental administered, the rate at which it is injected, and the amount and type of premedication given to the patient. The response to carbon dioxide is depressed at all levels of anesthesia and is abolished at deep levels of thiopental anesthesia. Therefore apnea can be an adverse outcome of high-dose thiopental.

Myocardial contractility is depressed and vascular resistance is increased after injection of thiopental, with the result that blood pressure is hardly affected, although it may be transiently reduced when the drug is first administered (when the vessel-rich group is highly saturated).

In addition to its being nonexplosive, the advantages of thiopental are (1) rapid and pleasant induction; (2) reduction of postanesthetic excitement and vomiting; (3) quiet respiration; (4) absence of salivation; and (5) speedy recovery after small doses. The disadvantages of the drug are adverse respiratory actions—including apnea, coughing, laryngospasm, and bronchospasm. Extravenous injection may result in tissue necrosis because of its highly alkaline pH (10.5 to 11).

Perianesthesia Care. Because thiopental may have an antianalgesic effect at low concentrations, some patients who have pain may be irrational, hyperactive, and restless during the initial recovery phase. The patient may exhibit some shivering related to lowered body temperature, which may result from a cold operating suite. Of concern to the perianesthesia nurse is the patient admitted with cold, clammy, cyanotic skin. This effect occasionally occurs with thiopental and is caused, in part, by the peripheral vasoconstrictive action of the drug.

If the anesthesia time exceeds 1 hour or if the total dose of thiopental exceeds 1 g, patients may have a delayed awakening time because of the redistribution of thiopental. This phenomenon is particularly common in obese patients, because the drug is highly fat-soluble. At present, no antagonist exists for the barbiturates. Therefore airway management and monitoring of cardiovascular status are important.

Methohexital (Brevital)

Methohexital is an ultra–short-acting barbiturate intravenous anesthetic agent. It is usually indicated for short procedures in which rapid, complete recovery of the patient is required. Methohexital is about three times as potent as thiopental, and the recovery time from anesthesia is extremely rapid (4 to 7 minutes) because the drug is redistributed from the CNS to the muscle and fat tissues and a significant portion of the drug is metabolized in the liver. Consequently, the clearance of methohexital is about four times faster than that of thiopental. Methohexital causes about the same degree of cardiovascular and respiratory depression as does thiopental. It should be mentioned, however, that this drug can cause coughing and hiccups and that, after injection, excitatory phenomena such as tremor and involuntary muscle movements may appear.

THE NONBARBITURATES

Etomidate (Amidate)

Etomidate, which is a derivative of imidazole, is a short-acting intravenous hypnotic that was synthesized in the laboratories of Janssen Pharmaceutica in Beerse, Belgium. It is not related chemically to the commonly used hypnotic agents. This drug is a mere hypnotic and does not possess any analgesic actions. Etomidate is quite safe to administer to patients, because it has a high therapeutic index. Metabolism of this drug is accomplished by hydrolysis in the liver and by plasma esterases, with the final metabolite being pharmacologically inactive. The cardiovascular effects of etomidate are minimal; when the drug is injected in therapeutic doses, only a small blood pressure decrease and a slight heart rate increase may be observed. Studies have also shown that etomidate causes a minimal reduction in the cardiac index and the peripheral resistance. This drug does not seem to produce arrhythmias. In regard to the respiratory system, etomidate causes a dose-related reduction in the tidal volume and respiratory frequency, which can lead to apnea. Laryngospasm, cough, and hiccups can occur during injection of this drug; however, the severity of these clinical phenomena can be reduced when the patient receives an opiate premedication.

Although this drug does cause some pain at the site of injection, it does not appear to cause a release of histamine. Spontaneous involuntary movements and tremor have been observed after the injection of etomidate. These involuntary movements can be reduced by an opiate premedication. Etomidate reduces both intracranial and intraocular pressure and therefore is considered safe to use in patients with intracranial pathologic conditions. This short-acting hypnotic is particularly well suited for the induction of neuroleptanalgesia and inhalation anesthesia. The induction dose ranges from 0.2 to 0.3 mg/kg, which produces sleep in 20 to 45 seconds after injection; the patient wakes within 7 to 15 minutes after induction.

Research has demonstrated that etomidate inhibits steroid synthesis and that patients who receive etomidate by continuous infusion have marked adrenocortical suppression for as long as 4 days. Even when etomidate is administered as a single dose, adrenal function is suppressed for 5 to 8 hours. Consequently, after the administration of etomidate there is a decrease in cortisol, 17-alpha-hydroxyprogesterone, aldosterone, and corticosterone levels. Because of this, etomidate is administered only to selected patients and is no longer administered by continuous intravenous infusion.

Propofol (Diprivan)

Propofol is a rapid-acting nonbarbiturate induction agent. It is administered intravenously as a 1% solution. The dosage for induction is 2 to 2.5 mg/kg. The dosage should be reduced in elderly patients and in patients with cardiac disease or hypovolemia. Along with this, propofol in combination with midazolam acts synergistically. In fact, the dosage of propofol can be reduced by 50% when it is administered in combination with midazolam. When propofol is used as the sole induction agent, it is usually administered over 15 seconds and produces unconsciousness within about 30 seconds. Emergence from this drug is more rapid than from thiopental or methohexital. This is because propofol has a half-life of 2 to 9 minutes. Hence the duration of anesthesia after a single induction dose is about 3 to 8 minutes, depending on the dose of the propofol. A major advantage of this drug is its ability to allow the patient a rapid return to consciousness with minimal residual CNS effects. Moreover, the drug's low incidence of nausea and vomiting is of particular importance to perianesthesia nursing care. In fact, propofol may possess antiemetic properties.

Propofol decreases the cerebral perfusion pressure, cerebral blood flow, and intracranial pressure. It does produce a reduction in the blood pressure similar in magnitude to or greater than thiopental in comparable doses. The decrease in blood pressure is also accompanied by a reduction in cardiac output or systemic vascular resistance. This reduction in blood pressure is more pronounced in elderly patients and in patients with compromised left-ventricular function. As opposed to the reduction in blood pressure, the pulse usually remains unchanged after the administration of propofol because of a sympatholytic or vagotonic effect of the drug. Therefore in some patients, bradycardia may be assessed after injection of propofol, and in this instance, an anticholinergic drug such as atropine or glycopyrrolate (Robinul) can be administered to reverse the bradycardia.

In regard to ventilation, propofol has a profound depressant effect on both the rate and depth of ventilation. In fact, after the induction dose is administered, apnea normally occurs. In fact, the incidence of apnea is greater after propofol than thiopental and may approach 100%. Consequently, if propofol is administered in the postanesthesia care unit (PACU), the perianesthesia nurse should be prepared to support the patient's ventilation and, if necessary, intubate the patient (see Chapter 27).

Clinically, this drug is useful for intravenous induction of anesthesia, especially for outpatient surgery. It is also an excellent choice for procedures requiring a short period of unconsciousness, such as cardioversion and electroconvulsive therapy. Also, propofol can be used for sedation during local standby procedures. This drug does not interfere with or alter the effects of succinylcholine because it has such a rapid plasma clearance. Propofol can be used intraoperatively in a continuous intravenous infusion, and the patients will still emerge from anesthesia in a rapid fashion without any CNS depression. This drug can be used in the PACU as a continuous infusion, and the level of sedation can be adjusted by titration to effect. The typical infusion rates for sedation with propofol are between 25 to 100 μg/kg/minute.

When administered within 12 hours of intravenous sedation, propofol is characterized by a more rapid recovery from its sedative effects than midazolam. Once propofol is discontinued, extubation can be performed in a short time; propofol is cleared very rapidly because of redistribution to fatty tissue and hepatic metabolism to inactive metabolites.

Long-term or high-dose infusions may result in hypertriglyceridemia, which is usually associated with elevated levels of pancreatic enzymes and possibly with pancreatitis. It should be noted that after very long infusions, plasma concentrations of propofol gradually increase unless the infusion rate is decreased over time. Current data seem to indicate that the recovery from propofol is less rapid after 12 hours of intravenous sedation. Propofol is contraindicated in patients sensitive to soybean oil, egg lecithin, or glycerol and is not recommended for PACU/ICU administration in children.

Perianesthesia Care. When a patient has received propofol for induction or even via continuous infusion, the perianesthesia nursing care should be based mainly on the other drugs that were used intraoperatively. This is because propofol is so rapid and has no cumulative effects; its effects are normally dissipated within 8 to 10 minutes. Consequently, the patient usually arrives in the PACU awake and in pain. Therefore analgesics should be titrated to effect. Titration is recommended in the immediate postoperative period because propofol and opioid analgesics can have a synergistic effect.

Propofol is an excellent addition to clinical anesthesia practice. It offers many advantages and few disadvantages. More specifically, propofol has one major advantage over all the other intravenous induction agents: early awakening. It can be used in the PACU if indicated. The major concern for the perianesthesia care of the patient who has received this drug is the level of postoperative pain. The nursing assessment and appropriate interventions for pain are the most important aspects of care of the patient who has received this drug (see Chapter 28).

THE TRANQUILIZERS

The Benzodiazepines

The benzodiazepines (BZs), which are tranquilizers, have enhanced the anesthetic outcomes of the surgical patient. They exert their activity by depressing the limbic system without causing cortical depression. More specifically, they interact with the inhibitory neurotransmitter GABA, thus resulting in reduced orientation (hypnotic effect), retrograde amnesia, anxiolysis, and relaxing of the skeletal muscle. Opiates and barbiturates enhance the hypnotic action of the benzodiazepines.

Diazepam (Valium). Diazepam is still a popular drug used in anesthesia practice. Because of its ability to allay apprehension, diazepam is indicated for use as a premedicant, as an adjunct to intravenous anesthesia, and as an induction agent. Recovery is usually not prolonged when diazepam is used for the induction of anesthesia. Diazepam can be used as the sole anesthetic agent for short diagnostic and surgical procedures and can also be used to provide sedation to make local anesthesia more acceptable to the patient.

Its principal action is to depress limbic system function. Important actions of diazepam are its ability to produce anterograde amnesia for as long as 48 hours postoperatively, to reduce anxiety, and to provide minimal cardiovascular depressant effects. Clinical doses of diazepam cause a slight degree of respiratory depression; however, when it is combined with an opiate, the chance of respiratory depression—including apnea—is greatly increased.

Diazepam may possess some muscle-relaxant properties. It has been reported that diazepam is antagonistic to depolarizing neuromuscular blocking agents such as succinylcholine and that the action of the nondepolarizing neuromuscular blocking agents (e.g., d-tubocurarine, pancuronium, and gallamine) are potentiated. Diazepam has been used clinically for psychomotor and *petit mal* seizures because of its anticonvulsant actions.

Because many patients who undergo cardioversion are debilitated, diazepam may be used to provide sedation for this procedure. Increments of 2.5 to 5 mg can be given at 30-second intervals until the speech of the patient is slurred or light sleep occurs. At the time of electrical discharge, the patient may experience brief muscle contraction and slight arousal. When this technique is employed, a significant number of the patients have complete amnesia regarding the event. Diazepam can also be used to provide anesthesia in endoscopic and dental procedures and to control behavior on emergence from ketamine. Finally, this drug also has strong anticonvulsant activity and can stop generalized seizure activity.

Intramuscularly administered diazepam can be quite painful to the patient. Along with this, the absorption is often poor. Also, when diazepam is administered intravenously, thrombophlebitis often occurs. When diazepam is administered intravenously, it should be injected slowly, directly into a large vein. The drug should not be mixed with other drugs or diluted. The onset of action of diazepam administered intravenously is immediate, and the duration of action varies from 20 minutes to 1 hour. When administered intramuscularly, its onset of action is about 10 minutes, and the duration of action may be as long as 4 hours. Adverse reactions to diazepam include hiccups, nausea, phlebitis at the site of injection, and occasional acute hyperexcited states.

Midazolam (Versed). Midazolam has become a popular drug in anesthesia practice and in the postanesthesia care of the surgical patient. Midazolam can be used for premedication, cardioversion, endoscopic procedures, and induction of anesthesia and as an intraoperative adjunct for inhalation anesthesia. It also is an excellent agent for sedation during regional anesthetic techniques. Midazolam's principal action is on the benzodiazepine receptors in the CNS, particularly on the limbic system, which results in a reduction in anxiety and profound anterograde amnesia. This drug also has excellent hypnotic, anticonvulsant, and muscle-relaxant properties.

The water-soluble midazolam may offer some advantages over diazepam. It causes depression of the CNS by inducing sedation, drowsiness, and—finally—sleep with increasing doses. Midazolam, in comparison to diazepam, is about three times as potent, has a shorter duration of action, and produces less incidence of injection pain and postinjection phlebitis and thrombosis. More specifically, this drug has a rapid onset of action, a peak in action between 10 and 30 minutes, and a duration of action between 1 and 4 hours. Midazolam administered at a dose of 0.2 mg/kg produces a decrease in blood pressure, an increase in heart rate, and a reduction in systemic vascular resistance. Midazolam should be used with caution in patients with myocardial ischemia and those with chronic obstructive pulmonary disease. Postoperative patients who have a substantial amount of hypovolemia should not receive midazolam. Along with this, midazolam does not affect intracranial pressure. Consequently, this drug can be used safely in neurosurgical patients in addition to patients with intracranial pathophysiology.

Because this drug can be administered in the PACU, it is of utmost importance to the postanesthesia nurse to monitor the patient for respiratory depression after injection. This is because midazolam causes a dose-dependent respiratory depression. Given that every patient in the PACU intraoperatively has received a plethora of depressant drugs, midazolam can be potentiated quite easily when administered in the PACU. Because of this potentiation factor, any dose of midazolam administered in the PACU should be considered effective enough to cause profound respiratory depression. Therefore oxygen and resuscitative equipment must be immediately available, and a person skilled in maintaining a patent airway and supporting ventilation should be present. Along with this, extra care should be observed in patients with limited pulmonary reserve and in the elderly and debilitated by reducing the dosage of midazolam by 25% to 30%.

Box 19-1   **Guidelines for the Use of Midazolam for the Treatment of Agitation in the PACU and Critical Care Setting**

Indications: For patients with respiratory or cardiac dysfunction. Promotes anxiolysis and amnesia.

Onset of action: 1-5 minutes

Peak of action: 2-5 minutes

Duration of action: 15-90 minutes

Dosages:

Load: 1-4 mg IV over 2-3 minutes

Max load: 5 mg in 1 hour (nonintubated patient)
10 mg in 1 hour (intubated patient)

Maint: 1-5 mg/hour (IVP)

Intravenous infusions: 1-50 mg/hour. No oral form available.

Tapering: Decrease infusion rate by 10% to 25% of maintenance rate every 24 hours. Should be discontinued by day 4.

Midazolam can be given by continuous infusion for patients who require sustained sedation. However, midazolam has a pH-dependent diazepine ring; and at physiologic pH the ring can close, causing CNS penetration; plus its metabolites are partially active, all of which make midazolam not the drug of choice for long-term sedation. Midazolam is sometimes used in the treatment of critically ill patients that are agitated. The guidelines for use can be found in Box 19-1.

Lorazepam (Ativan).   Lorazepam, a long-acting benzodiazepine, is used as a premedication in current clinical anesthesia practice and as a long-acting, slow-onset benzodiazepine for sedation in the PACU and ICU. This drug has actions similar to those of diazepam but has a slow onset of action from 20 to 40 minutes; the pharmacologic activity may last as long as 24 hours. Lorazepam produces profound anterograde amnesia, tranquilization, and a reduction of anxiety, and the drug provides good cardiovascular and respiratory stability. Therapeutic plasma concentrations are achieved in about 3 hours when the drug is given orally. The drug is well absorbed via the intramuscular route; however, the patient experiences a significant amount of

pain during the injection of the drug. Lorazepam can also be injected intravenously, and the patient may experience some burning on injection. Because of its slow onset and long duration, lorazepam is mainly used as a preanesthetic medication. If this drug has been administered in the preoperative period, the effects of lorazepam may last well into the postoperative period because of its prolonged action. If a narcotic is administered in the PACU to a patient who received lorazepam preoperatively, the nurse should monitor for increased narcotic sedation and respiratory depression because of the potentiation of the narcotic by lorazepam.

Caution should be taken with using lorazepam in the PACU for sedation. Lorazepam does not have any active metabolites. This long-acting but slow-onset benzodiazepine is often delivered by intermittent boluses but also may be administered as a continuous infusion. Peak effects are not observed for 30 minutes. However, the solvent for lorazepam contains polyethylene glycol 400 and propylene glycol, both of which have been implicated in the development of lactic acidosis, acute tubular necrosis, and hyperosmolar coma when lorazepam is used in prolonged, high-dose infusions. However, the toxic threshold for this effect has not been defined; hence high-dose infusions should be avoided, and monitoring for these side effects should be monitored.

Lorazepam is sometimes used in the treatment of critically ill patients that are agitated. The guidelines for use can be found in Box 19-2.

Flunitrazepam (Rohypnol).   Flunitrazepam is a long-acting benzodiazepine that is similar to diazepam. It is approximately 10 times more potent than diazepam when given intravenously. It is characterized by a high patient variability in regard to its effects. However, it produces pharmacologic actions similar to diazepam in regard to its cardiovascular, amnesic, and sedative-hypnotic properties. The major problems with this drug are its slow onset of action and prolonged recovery time. Its onset is within 30 minutes; it peaks in about 2 hours and has a duration of action of about 8 hours.

Flunitrazepam is manufactured worldwide and is neither manufactured nor approved for medical use in the United States. It has a "street" name of "rophy" and is usually smuggled into the United States through the mail or delivery serv-

---

Box 19-2 Guidelines for the Use of Lorazepam for the Treatment of Agitation in the PACU and Critical Care Setting

Indications: For patients with respiratory or cardiac dysfunction. Promotes anxiolysis and amnesia.

Onset of action: 1-5 minutes

Peak of action: 20-40 minutes

Duration of action: 4-6 hours

Dosages:

Load: 1-2 mg IV over 1-2 minutes

Max load: 4 mg in 1 hour (nonintubated patient)
6 mg in 1 hour (intubated patient)

Maint: 1-3 mg every 1-2 hours—IV push (IVP)

Intravenous infusions: 1-5 mg/hour

Precautions: Paradoxical effects can occur

Not dialyzed

Tapering: Decrease infusion rate by 10% to 25% of maintenance rate every 24 hours

---

ices. It is a highly abused drug that is usually taken by addicts with multiple addictions.

The Benzodiazepine Antagonists

Physostigmine (Antilirium). Physostigmine is an anticholinesterase that crosses the blood-brain barrier. Its action is to inhibit the enzyme acetylcholinesterase, which will result in an increase in the availability of acetylcholine at the receptors that are affected by the benzodiazepines in the CNS. The preponderance of acetylcholine counteracts the negative effects of glycine and GABA. Consequently, this drug provides a nonspecific reversal of the CNS side effects of the benzodiazepines scopolamine and ketamine. The dosage is 0.5 to 1 mg, and it should be administered slowly to prevent untoward cholinergic side effects. Because this drug is a nonspecific agent, a number of vagally mediated cholinergic side effects can occur after its administration. These effects include nausea, vomiting, salivation, bradycardia, bronchospasm, and seizures. Hence, because of its nonspecific properties, physostigmine is rarely used for the reversal of the untoward effects of the benzodiazepines.

Flumazenil (Romazicon). Flumazenil, a new benzodiazepine antagonist, has recently been intro-

duced into clinical practice in the United States. When introduced, the trade name was Mazicon; however, because the name was similar to the trade name Mavacron (mivacurium chloride), a neuromuscular-blocking agent, the name was changed to Romazicon. This drug antagonizes or reverses the effects of benzodiazepine-induced sedation at the benzodiazepine receptors. Consequently, it reverses the CNS effects of benzodiazepines such as the sedation and amnesia that are produced by diazepam and midazolam, for example. This drug also reverses the other effects produced by benzodiazepine agonists, including anxiolytic, muscle-relaxant, ataxic, and anticonvulsant actions. However, flumazenil may not be effective in the treatment for benzodiazepine-induced hypoventilation or respiratory failure. This drug is specific for the benzodiazepines and, more specifically, their receptors. Consequently, this drug does not reverse the effects of barbiturates, opiates, and ethanol. Flumazenil should be used with great caution in patients who have a history of epilepsy or chronic benzodiazepine usage because reversal with flumazenil in these patients can result in seizures. The incidence of postoperative nausea and vomiting is increased after flumazenil has been administered.

The usual reversal dose for flumazenil is 0.4 mg administered intravenously in 0.1 increments. Flumazenil should be administered very slowly to avoid the adverse consequences of abrupt wakening. A maximum dose for this drug is 1 mg. The onset of action is usually within 5 minutes, with a duration of action between 1 and 2 hours. Flumazenil has a shorter duration of action than most of the benzodiazepines, and consequently, the risk of resedation can occur after the initial reversal dose was administered. This is especially true when high doses of benzodiazepines were previously administered. Therefore after the administration of flumazenil, the patient should be monitored for resedation and other residual effects of benzodiazepines in the PACU and on the receiving unit. Should the patient develop signs of resedation, flumazenil should be given at 20-minute intervals as needed to reverse the sedation. In this situation, no more than 1 mg should be given at any one time, and no more than 3 mg should be given within a 1-hour period. This drug should prove to be a valuable asset in the care of the patient who has received an excessive dose of a benzodiazepine such as midazolam and diazepam. Consequently, flumazenil will be useful intraoperatively, postoperatively, and in the ICU.

The Butyrophenones

The butyrophenones are a class of tranquilizers that are characterized by producing a state of profound calm and immobility in which the patient appears to be pain-free and dissociated from his or her surroundings. They are a potent inhibitor of the chemoreceptor trigger zone–mediated nausea and vomiting. These drugs have some profound side effects but do seem to be useful in anesthesia and postanesthesia care of the surgical patient. The two major butyrophenones used in clinical practice are haloperidol and droperidol.

Haloperidol (Haldol). Haloperidol is a butyrophenone tranquilizer that has limited use in anesthesia practice because of its very long duration of action and its high incidence of extrapyramidal reactions. It is not approved for intravenous use and is usually administered intramuscularly at a dose from 2 to 5 mg. It is used in the treatment of psychoses and as an antiemetic. Haloperidol is sometimes used in the treatment of critically ill patients that are agitated. The guidelines for use can be found in Box 19-3.

Droperidol (Inapsine). Droperidol, which was originally investigated by Janssen Pharmaceutica, can be used alone or in combination with fentanyl (Sublimaze) as part of a neuroleptanalgesic technique. It produces a state of calm, disinclination to move, and disconnection from surroundings. It has an alpha-adrenergic blocking effect, which offers some protection against the vasoconstrictive components of shock; it leads to good peripheral perfusion; and it unmasks hypovolemia. More specifically, when a patient has compensated for a borderline hypovolemic state by activation of the alpha-vasoconstriction mechanisms, vital signs will be normal. When a drug such as droperidol is administered to this patient, by virtue of droperidol's alpha-blocking properties, the signs of hypovolemia will appear. Hence the patient's hypovolemia is "unmasked." Droperidol also protects against epinephrine-induced arrhythmias and has an antiemetic effect. In fact, because of its excellent antiemetic properties, droperidol is sometimes administered toward the end of the surgical procedure or in the

---

Box 19-3   Guidelines for the Use of Haloperidol for the Treatment of Agitation in the PACU and Critical Care Setting

Indications: For patients with respiratory or cardiac dysfunction. Promotes anxiolysis and amnesia.
Onset of action: 5-30 minutes
Peak of action: 1 hour
Duration of action: 6-8 hours
Dosages:
  Load: 2.5-5 mg IV over 1-2 minutes
  Max load: 20 mg in 1 hour (nonintubated and intubated patients)
  Maint: Once patient is controlled by loading dose, may decrease dose by 50% or by increasing dosing interval.
Precautions: Precipitates with heparin
  Decreases epinephrine and dopamine activity
  Contraindicated in Parkinson's disease
  Not dialyzed

PACU to reduce the risk of vomiting and aspiration in anxious patients. The antiemetic dose of droperidol is between 1 and 2.5 mg, which can be given intravenously. Also, by virtue of its alpha-blocking properties, this drug may be administered in the PACU on a short-term basis to reduce the afterload.

Droperidol is similar to chlorpromazine (Thorazine) in its CNS effects; however, its mechanism of action is different. Droperidol is more selective than chlorpromazine, because it provides more tranquility with less sedation and has less effect on the autonomic nervous system. Droperidol has been classified as a neuroleptic and is the main tranquilizing component of Innovar. (See following discussion in this section.) Among its negative effects, droperidol may cause hypotension by virtue of its alpha-adrenergic blocking effect and peripheral vasodilatation. It may cause extrapyramidal excitation, such as twitchiness, oculogyric seizures, stiff neck muscles, trembling hands, restlessness, and occasionally, psychologic disturbances (e.g., hallucinations). These can be reversed with atropine or antiparkinsonian drugs such as benztropine mesylate (Cogentin) and trihexyphenidyl hydrochloride (Artane). Clinically, patients who have received droperidol have reported the dichotomy of appearing outwardly calm while feeling terrified inside and unable to express how they feel. Hence the perianesthesia nurse should provide emotional support to all patients who have received droperidol.

Droperidol is known to potentiate the action of barbiturates and narcotics. It has a high therapeutic margin of safety with a rapid onset of 10 minutes, and its activity is lessened in 2 to 4 hours, although some effects last as long as 10 to 12 hours.

Droperidol is the prototype neuroleptic drug. A neuroleptic drug is one that reduces motor activity, lessens anxiety, and produces a state of indifference in which the person can still respond appropriately to commands. Neuroleptanalgesia is a state of profound tranquilization with little or no depressant effect on the cortical centers. Therefore neuroleptanalgesia is achieved by the combination of a neuroleptic such as droperidol and a potent narcotic analgesic such as fentanyl. A fixed-dose mixture of droperidol and fentanyl is called Innovar. Each milliliter of Innovar contains 0.05 mg of fentanyl and 2.5 mg of droperidol. When the fixed-dose approach is not desired, fentanyl (0.004 mg/kg) and droperidol (0.2 mg/kg) can be administered in slow intravenous doses. A step further is neuroleptanesthesia, the combination of a neuroleptanalgesic (droperidol plus fentanyl), a skeletal muscle relaxant, and nitrous oxide and oxygen. The main objective in developing neuroleptanesthesia is to provide for all types of operations a technique that does not depress the metabolic, circulatory, or central nervous systems as severely as do the inhalation anesthetics when used alone.

The United States Food and Drug Administration (FDA) has strengthened the warnings and precautions in the labeling for droperidol as the drug has been associated with fatal cardiac arrhythmias. More specifically, recent research has shown QT prolongations that indicate delayed recharging of the heart between beats within minutes after injection of droperidol at the upper end of the labeled dose range. Prolonged QT is dangerous because it can cause a potentially fatal heart arrhythmia known as torsades de pointes (TdP). The new warning is intended to facilitate the focus on the potential for cardiac arrhythmias during administration and to urge the practitioner to consider the use of alternative medications in patients at high risk for cardiac arrhythmias.

Perianesthesia Care. In the immediate postoperative period, the awakening from neuroleptanesthesia is usually rapid, extremely smooth, and uneventful. A striking feature is the extension of analgesia well into the postoperative period. It is difficult to explain the mechanism of such a prolonged pain-relieving effect with a drug such as fentanyl, in which the onset is so rapid and the duration of action is so short.

Nursing personnel in the PACU should constantly assess the patient for signs of respiratory depression. Narcotics should be avoided in patients who have received droperidol, or they should be given in minimal amounts. It is recommended that the dosage of narcotic agonists be reduced to as little as one fourth to one third the usual dose because of the additive potentiating effects of droperidol.

The patient should be encouraged to cough and perform the sustained maximal inspiration (SMI) maneuver in the PACU (see Chapters 10 and 26). Patients who have received droperidol or Innovar tend to drift back to sleep unless they are encouraged to move about their surroundings. The perianesthesia nurse will find that, because the analgesia extends into the postoperative period, the patient who has received neuroleptanesthesia is more willing to cough and perform the SMI. Innovar depresses both the respiratory rate and the tidal volume. The perianesthesia nurse should use verbal stimulation with these patients. This is because, if ordered, the patient will be able to take a deep breath; otherwise respiration may remain slow and shallow, or the patient may even become apneic. Consequently, the perianesthesia nurse must remain with the patient, provide verbal stimulation, and actively monitor for any signs of respiratory depression.

The perianesthesia nurse should monitor for extrapyramidal symptoms; although rare, they have been detected as long as 24 hours after a single administration of droperidol or Innovar. Most of the reported extrapyramidal reactions occurred in children younger than 12 years of age. Because of the length of action of droperidol, it is recommended that the perianesthesia nurse provide information about the drug to the nursing personnel on the surgical units via hospital in-service education programs.

Because of droperidol's long duration of action and tremendous potentiating effects, all PACU personnel should be alerted when a patient has received this drug either intraoperatively or postoperatively. Hence the patient's bed should have a tag on it to indicate that the patient has received either droperidol or Innovar and to serve as a visual reminder for the staff to reduce the dose of any narcotics or barbiturates given in the PACU.

THE DISSOCIATIVE ANESTHETICS

Ketamine

Traditionally, general anesthetic agents achieved control of pain by depression of the CNS. An anesthetic agent, ketamine, has been introduced that has a totally different mode of action. It selectively blocks pain conduction and perception, leaving those parts of the CNS that do not participate in pain transmission and perception free from the depressant effects of the drug. Ketamine is termed dissociative because patients who are totally analgesic usually do not appear to be asleep or anesthetized but rather disassociated from their surroundings. The drug is nonbarbiturate and nonnarcotic. It is administered parenterally and has a short duration. Early laboratory studies using ketamine suggested that most of the drug's activity is centered in the frontal lobe of the cerebral cortex.

The clinical characteristics of ketamine consist of a state of profound analgesia combined with a state of unconsciousness. The patient usually has marked horizontal and vertical nystagmus. The eyes are usually open and shortly become centered and appear in a fixed gaze. The pupils are moderately dilated and react to light. Respiratory function is usually unimpaired, except after rapid intravenous injection, when it may become depressed for a short time. Ketamine is sympathomimetic in action and is beneficial to asthmatic patients because of its bronchodilating effect. When patients receive ketamine, their pharyngeal and laryngeal reflexes remain intact. The tongue usually does not become relaxed, so the airway usually remains unobstructed. Ketamine accelerates the heart rate moderately and

increases both the systolic and the diastolic pressure for several minutes, after which the pulse and blood pressure return to preinjection levels. Finally, ketamine increases cerebral blood flow and, consequently, intracranial pressure. Therefore this drug definitely is contraindicated in patients who are at risk for increased intracranial pressure.

Ketamine can be administered intramuscularly or intravenously. The intramuscular dose is 4 to 6 mg/lb, and the anesthesia lasts from 20 to 40 minutes. The intravenous dose is usually 0.5 to 2 mg/lb with anesthesia lasting 6 to 10 minutes. Complete recovery from ketamine varies according to the duration of surgery and the amount of ketamine used throughout the procedure. When a single dose of intravenous ketamine is used, recovery time is usually rapid and does not exceed 30 minutes. When supplemental intravenous doses need to be administered, more particularly when supplemental intramuscular doses are required, recovery is often markedly prolonged, sometimes as long as 3 hours.

Perianesthesia Care. When patients are emerging from ketamine anesthesia, they may go through a phase of vivid dreaming—with or without psychomotor activity manifested by confusion, irrational behavior, and hallucinations. The perianesthesia nurse should be aware that such psychic aberrations are usually transient and appear to be preventable by avoiding early verbal or tactile stimulation of the patient, which helps prevent fear and anxiety reactions. Short-acting barbiturates administered intravenously can effectively control the psychic responses sometimes seen after the administration of ketamine. Pediatric patients seem to be less prone to these psychic disturbances. Results of a study revealed that droperidol, the tranquilizer component of Innovar, may be effective in eliminating some of the adverse psychic emergence phenomena of ketamine. Other tranquilizers such as diazepam have also been found effective in suppressing these phenomena. Thus when admitting a patient to the PACU, the nurse should be aware of any tranquilizers the patient may have received.

Once the patient has arrived in the PACU, he or she should be secluded from auditory, visual, and tactile stimuli and be observed for any signs of respiratory depression. Mechanical airway obstruction, particularly when caused by marked salivation, accounts for most of the instances of respiratory insufficiency after ketamine anesthesia. When the patient does not have adequate respiratory exchange, oxygen should be administered by mask until it is restored. Other important signs to watch for are persistent blood pressure elevation, tachycardia, bradycardia, dreaming, delirium, hallucinations, euphoria, and increased muscle tone. It should be stressed to all PACU personnel that attempts to rouse patients while they are still unable to see, hear, and orient themselves may set off a chain of anxiety reactions that may ultimately lead to severe psychomotor responses and even more irrational behavior.

The widespread use of ketamine requires an entirely new approach to perianesthesia nursing care. Certainly, the agent has many deficiencies, but commonly overlooked is the fact that it is one of the safest anesthetics. Its safety justifies its important place in the drugs used by the anesthesiologist. Ketamine appears to be an excellent anesthetic for pediatric patients, as the sole agent for short procedures, for inducing anesthesia in extremely poor-risk patients, and for patients with burns requiring surgical treatment. Certain adult orthopedic and diagnostic procedures have also been found suitable for the use of ketamine anesthesia.

Ketamine is the first of several drugs that will probably achieve clinical usage as dissociative agents. Its actions therefore should be well understood by the PACU staff to ensure effective, informed care of the patient.

OTHER AGENTS

Propanidid

Propanidid is a nonbarbiturate hypnoticanesthetic agent. The drug may be used as an induction agent or to produce transient anesthesia. It exerts a biphasic effect on respiration. After intravenous injection, an initial period of hyperventilation that is caused by stimulation of the carotid chemoreceptors ensues. This is followed by a short period of hypoventilation, periodic breathing, or apnea. When propanidid is administered, some degree of hypotension—usually due to cardiac depression—will be observed. Other side effects of propanidid are rigidity, coughing, hiccups, phonation, and uncontrollable movements.

The action of this drug is terminated by its being rapidly metabolized enzymatically by plasma pseudocholinesterase, whereas redistribution terminates the anesthetic action of the ultra–short-acting barbiturates. Recovery from propanidid is usually more complete, and accumulation does not occur with repeated administration in contrast with the barbiturates. Patients who receive propanidid usually have a smooth recovery with no "hangover" effect. During the emergence phase of this drug, headaches, nausea, and vomiting are more common than with thiopental. The patient may also complain postoperatively of an unpleasant taste. Propanidid has been in clinical use in Europe for many years; it is currently under investigation and therefore not available in the United States.

Steroid Anesthesia

Steroid anesthesia involves using steroids, administered intravenously, to produce an anesthetized state (loss of consciousness and immobility in response to stimuli). Currently, the major use of steroid anesthetics is as a substitute for the commonly used intravenous barbiturates.

Althesin. Althesin, which is currently enjoying wide popularity in Great Britain, is a combination of two steroids: alphaxalone and alphadolone acetate. At present, this drug is not available in the United States. Used mainly as an induction agent, althesin has a similar onset and about a 5- to 10-minute longer duration of action in comparison to thiopental. This drug does not seem to alter the cardiac output and often causes a short period of hyperventilation, which is sometimes followed by apnea. The major disadvantage of althesin is in the realm of hypersensitivity reactions. These reactions, which may be caused by histamine release, range from severe circulatory collapse, bronchospasm, and edema to a generalized erythematous reaction.

BIBLIOGRAPHY

Alspach J: Core curriculum for critical care nursing, ed 5, Philadelphia, 1998, WB Saunders.

Atlee J: Complications in anesthesia, Philadelphia, 1999, WB Saunders.

Barash P, Cullen B, Stoelting R: Clinical anesthesia, ed 4, Philadelphia, 2000, Lippincott Williams & Wilkins.

Benumof J, Saidman L: Anesthesia & perioperative complications, ed 2, St Louis, 1999, Mosby.

Benumof J: Anesthesia and uncommon diseases, ed 4, Philadelphia, 1998, WB Saunders.

Blouin R, Gross J: Ventilation and conscious sedation, Semin Anesth 15(4):335-342, 1996.

Borchardt M: Review of the clinical pharmacology and use of the benzodiazepines, J Perianesth Nurs 14(2):65-72, 1999.

DeFazio-Quinn D: Ambulatory surgical nursing core curriculum, Philadelphia, 1999, WB Saunders.

FDA strengthens warning for droperidol, FDA Talk Paper, Washington, DC, December, 2001.

Ganong W: Review of medical physiology, ed 20, New York, 2001, McGraw-Hill Professional.

Gold M, Sacks D, Grosnoff D et al: Comparison of propofol with thiopental and isoflurane for induction and maintenance of general anesthesia, J Clin Anesth 1(4):272-276, 1989.

Guyton A, Hall J: Textbook of medical physiology, ed 10, Philadelphia, 2000, WB Saunders.

Hardman J, Limbird L: Goodman and Gilman's the pharmacological basis of therapeutics, ed 9, New York, 1996, McGraw-Hill.

Katz R, editor: Propofol: a critical assessment, Semin Anesth 6(1, Suppl):1-54, 1992.

Katzung B, editor: Basic and clinical pharmacology, ed 8, Los Altos, Calif, 2000, Appleton & Lange.

Korttila K, Ostman P, Faure E et al: Randomized comparison of recovery after propofol-nitrous oxide versus thiopentone-isoflurane-nitrous oxide anaesthesia in patients undergoing ambulatory surgery, Acta Anaesthesiol Scand 34:400-403, 1990.

Longnecker D, Murphy F: Dripps/Eckenhoff/Vandam introduction to anesthesia, ed 9, Philadelphia, 1997, WB Saunders.

Longnecker D, Tinker J, Morgan G: Principles and practice of anesthesiology, ed 2, St Louis, 1998, Mosby.

McIntosh L: Essentials of nurse anesthesia, New York, 1997, McGraw-Hill.

Miller R, editor: Anesthesia, ed 5, New York, 2000, Churchill Livingstone.

Nagelhout J, Zaglaniczny K: Nurse anesthesia, ed 2, Philadelphia, 2001, WB Saunders.

Prielipp R, Young C: Current drugs for sedation of critically ill patients, Seminars in Anesthesia, Perioperative Medicine, and Pain 20(2):85-94, 2001

Reves J, Fragen RJ, Vinik HR et al: Midazolam: pharmacology and uses, Anesthesiology 62:310-324, 1985.

Sebel P, Larson J: Propofol: a new intravenous anesthetic, Anesthesiology 71:260-277, 1989.

Shepherd M: Multidisciplinary approach to developing guidelines for use of anesthetic agents in an intensive care unit, Anesthesia Today 6(1):15-18, 1995.

Short T, Chui P: Propofol and midazolam act synergistically in combination, Br J Anaesth 67:539-545, 1991.

Spiess B: Two new pharmacological agents for the 1990s: flumazenil and propofol, J Post Anesth Nurs 5(3):186-189, 1990.

Spindler J, Mehlisch D, Brown C: Intramuscular ketorolac and morphine in the treatment of moderate to severe pain after major surgery, Pharmacotherapy 10:51S-58S, 1990.

Stoelting R: Pharmacology and physiology in anesthetic practice, ed 3, Philadelphia, 1999, Lippincott-Raven.

Stoelting R, Miller R: Basics of anesthesia, ed 4, New York, 2000, Churchill Livingstone.

Stone D: Perioperative care: anesthesia, medicine, and surgery, St Louis, 1998, Mosby.

Vogelsang J, Hayes S: Butorphanol tartrate (Stadol): a review, J Post Anesth Nurs 6(2):129-135, 1991.

Waugaman W, Foster S, Rigor B: Principles and practice of nurse anesthesia, ed 3, Norwalk, Conn, 1999, Appleton & Lange.

White P: What's new in intravenous anesthesia. 1990 International Anesthesia Research Society Review Course Lectures. Cleveland, IARS, 105-114, 1990.

20

OPIOID INTRAVENOUS ANESTHETICS

Opioid intravenous anesthetics constitute a major portion of the clinical anesthesia process. These drugs enhance the effectiveness of the inhalation anesthetics. More specifically, the opioids meet much of the analgesic portion of the anesthesia process. Also, adding the opioids to the drugs used to provide general anesthesia can reduce the concentration of the inhalation anesthetic; as a result, a safer anesthetic can be administered to the patient. Because opioids are used to manage acute and chronic pain and are administered for general inhalation anesthesia and sedation and pain relief during regional anesthesia, their implications for the postanesthesia nursing care of the surgical patient are profound. The immediate postanesthesia phase is the time when the patient is most vulnerable to complications. Modern anesthesia care now uses many drugs that have residual anesthetic effects well into the postanesthesia period. These agents include the potent inhaled agents, muscle relaxants, benzodiazepines, and opioids. Respiratory depression is the most common adverse event in the postanesthesia care unit (PACU); hence the use and understanding of the various opioid agents will optimize patient outcomes.

THE CONCEPT OF OPIOIDS AND OPIOID RECEPTORS

Opioids are the substances, either natural or synthetic, that are administered into the body (exogenous) and bind to specific receptors and produce a morphine-like or opioid agonist effect. The endogenous opioids are the endorphins. The endorphins, which are produced in the body, attach to the opioid receptors in the central nervous system (CNS) to activate the body's pain modulating system. The term opioid is used because of the multitude of synthetic drugs with morphine-like actions, and with the advent of receptor physiology, it has replaced the term narcotic. Narcotic is derived from the Greek word for stupor and usually refers to both the production of the morphine-like effects and the physical dependence.

The naturally occurring alkaloids of opium are divided into two classes: phenanthrenes and benzylisoquinolines. The principal phenanthrene series of drugs includes morphine, codeine, and thebaine. Papaverine and noscapine, which lack opioid activity, represent the benzylisoquinoline alkaloids of opium.

The synthetic opioids have been produced by the modification of the chemical structure of the phenanthrene class of drugs. Drugs such as fentanyl (Sublimaze) and meperidine (Demerol) are examples of synthetic opioids.

The identification of specific opioid receptors has enhanced the understanding of the agonist and antagonist actions of this category of drugs. The opioid receptors are located in the CNS, principally in the brain stem and spinal cord. These receptors have been determined by the pharmacologic effect they produce when stimulated by a specific agonist along with how the effect is blocked by a specific antagonist. The four major categories of opioid receptors are the mu, delta, kappa, and sigma receptors.

The mu receptors are mainly responsible for the production of supraspinal analgesia effects when stimulated. These receptors are further divided into mu-1 and mu-2 types. Activation of the mu-1 receptors results in analgesia, and when the mu-2 receptors are stimulated, hypoventilation, bradycardia, physical dependence, euphoria, and ileus can result. The mu receptors are activated by morphine, fentanyl, and meperidine. The drug that is specific to the mu-1 receptor is meptazinol. The delta opioid receptors, when stimulated, serve to modulate the activity of the mu receptors. Stimulation of the kappa receptors results in spinal analgesia, sedation, and miosis with little effect on ventilation. The drugs that possess both opioid agonist and antagonist activities, such as nalbuphine (Nubain), have their principal action on the kappa opioid receptors. The last category of opioid receptors is the sigma receptors, and activation of these receptors results in dysphoria, hallucinations, hypertonia, tachycardia, tachypnea, and mydriasis. The drug naloxone (Narcan) attaches to all the opioid receptors and thus serves as an antagonist to all the opioid agonists.

THE OPIOIDS

Opioids, or narcotics, are becoming quite popular in anesthesia practice. They are usually used in the nitrous-narcotic (balanced) techniques, which involve the use of a narcotic, nitrous oxide, and oxygen, with or without a muscle relaxant, and thiopental for induction.

The effects of narcotics generally last well into the PACU phase, and every perianesthesia nurse should have a good knowledge of the pharmacologic actions of each narcotic that is administered to the patient in the perioperative phase of the surgical experience.

The administration of opioids in the perioperative period is not without the concern of overdosage. The major signs of overdosage of opioids are miosis, hypoventilation, and coma. If the patient becomes severely hypoxemic, mydriasis can occur. Airway obstruction is a strong possibility because the skeletal muscles become flaccid. Along with this, hypotension and seizures may occur. The treatment for an opioid overdosage is mechanical ventilation and the slow titration of naloxone. Consideration must always be given to the fact that some patients who become overdosed with an opioid may indeed be already physically dependent. Naloxone can precipitate an acute withdrawal syndrome.

Meperidine Hydrochloride (Demerol)

Meperidine was discovered in 1939 by Eisleb and Schauman. Because it is chemically similar to atropine, it was originally introduced as an antispasmodic agent and was not used as an opioid anesthetic agent until 1947. The main action of this drug is similar to morphine, and it stimulates the subcortical mu receptors, which results in an analgesic effect. Meperidine is about one tenth as potent as morphine and has a duration of action of about 2 to 4 hours. The onset of analgesia is prompt (10 minutes) after subcutaneous or intramuscular administration. All pain, especially visceral, gastrointestinal, and urinary tract, is satisfactorily relieved. This drug causes less biliary tract spasm than morphine; however, in comparison to codeine, meperidine causes greater biliary tract spasm. It produces some sleepiness but causes little euphoria or amnesia. Meperidine increases the sensitivity of the labyrinthine apparatus of the ear, which explains the dizziness, nausea, and vomiting that sometimes occur in ambulatory patients.

This narcotic may slow the rate of respiration, but the rate generally returns to normal within 15 minutes after intravenous injection. The tidal volume is not changed appreciably. In equivalent analgesic doses, meperidine depresses respiration to a greater extent than does morphine. Some authors have noted that meperidine may release histamine from the tissues. Occasionally, one may notice urticarial wheals that have formed over the veins where meperidine has been injected. The usual treatment is to discontinue the use of meperidine and, if the reaction is severe, to administer diphenhydramine (Benadryl). Diphenhydramine further sedates the patient, however, and should be administered only if truly warranted.

Meperidine in therapeutic doses does not cause any significant untoward effects on the cardiovascular system. When this drug is administered intravenously, it usually causes a transient increase in heart rate. When it is administered intramuscularly, no significant change in heart rate will be observed. One of the major concerns with this drug is that of orthostatic hypotension, probably caused by meperidine's interference with the compensatory sympathetic nervous system reflex. Hence after a patient has received meperidine, he or she should be repositioned slowly in a "staged" approach so as to avoid any possibility of hypotension.

Meperidine is generally metabolized in the liver; less than 5% is excreted unchanged by the kidneys.

Because of its spasmolytic effect, meperidine is the drug of choice for biliary duct, distal colon, and rectal surgery. It offers the advantages of little interference with the physiologic compensatory mechanisms, low toxicity, smooth and rapid recovery, prolonged postoperative analgesia, excellent cardiac stability in elderly and poor-risk patients, and ease of detoxification and excretion.

Morphine

Morphine, one of the oldest known drugs, has only recently been used as an opioid intravenous anesthetic agent. Alkaloid morphine is from the phenanthrene class of opium. The exact mechanism of action of morphine is unknown. In humans, it produces analgesia, drowsiness, changes in mood, and mental clouding. The analgesic effect can become profound before the other effects are severe and can persist after many of the side effects have almost disappeared. By direct effect on the respiratory center, morphine depresses respiratory rate, tidal volume, and minute volume. Maximal respiratory depression occurs within 7 minutes after intravenous injection of the drug and 30 minutes after intramuscular administration. Following therapeutic doses of morphine, the sensitivity of the respiratory center begins to return to normal in 2 or 3 hours, but the minute volume does not return to preinjection level until 4 or 5 hours have passed.

The greatest advantage of morphine is the remarkable cardiovascular stability that accompanies its use. It has no major effect on blood pressure, heart rate, or heart rhythm—even in toxic doses, when hypoxia is avoided. Morphine does, however, decrease the capacity of the cardiovascular system to adjust to gravitational shifts. This is important to remember because orthostatic hypotension and syncope may easily occur in a patient whose care requires a position change. This phenomenon is primarily the result of the peripheral vasodilator effect of morphine. Therefore, a position change for a patient who has received morphine should be accomplished slowly, with constant monitoring of the patient's vital signs.

Morphine may cause nausea and vomiting, especially in ambulatory patients, by virtue of direct stimulation of the chemoreceptor trigger zone. The emetic effect of morphine can be counteracted by narcotic antagonists and phenothiazine derivatives such as chlorpromazine (Thorazine), prochlorperazine (Compazine), and benzoquinamide (Emete-con) Histamine release

has been noted with morphine, and morphine also causes profound constriction of the pupils, stimulation of the visceral smooth muscles, and spasm of the sphincter of Oddi.

Morphine is detoxified by conjugation with glucuronic acid. Ninety percent is excreted by the kidneys, and 7% to 10% is excreted in the feces via the bile.

Morphine is used in the balanced, or nitrous-narcotic, technique with nitrous oxide, oxygen, and a muscle relaxant. This technique is useful for cardiovascular surgery, along with other types of surgery in which cardiovascular stability is required. The patient may arrive in the PACU still narcotized from morphine with an endotracheal tube in place. Mechanical ventilation for 24 to 48 hours is usually warranted. Morphine may or may not be supplemented during the time of ventilation. This type of recovery procedure facilitates a pain-free state and maximum ventilation of the patient during the critical phase of recovery. Morphine can also be used to provide basal narcosis when regional anesthesia is employed.

In the PACU, morphine is an excellent drug to use in the control of postoperative pain. When given intravenously, this drug has a peak analgesic effect in about 20 minutes, with a duration of about 2 hours. When it is administered intramuscularly, the onset of action is about 15 minutes, with a peak effect attained in about 45 to 90 minutes and a duration of action of about 4 hours.

Fentanyl (Sublimaze)

Janssen and associates introduced a series of highly potent meperidine derivatives that were found to render the patient free of pain without affecting certain areas in the CNS. Fentanyl appeared to be of special interest. In regard to analgesic properties, fentanyl is approximately 80 to 125 times as potent as morphine, and it has a rapid onset of action of 5 to 6 minutes and a peak effect within 5 to 15 minutes. The analgesia lasts 20 to 40 minutes when administered intravenously. Via the intramuscular route, the onset of action is 7 to 15 minutes; the analgesia usually lasts 1 to 2 hours. When fentanyl is administered as a single bolus, 75% of the drug will undergo "first-pass" pulmonary uptake. That is, the lungs serve as a large storage site, and this nonrespiratory function of the lung (see Chapter 10) limits the amount of fentanyl that actually reaches the systemic circulation. If the patient receives multiple doses of fentanyl by single injections or infusion, the first-pass pulmonary uptake mechanism will become saturated, and the patient will have a prolonged emergence because of increased duration of the drug. Consequently, during the admission of the patient to the PACU, the postanesthesia nurse must determine the frequency and amount of intraoperative fentanyl administration. Patients who have received a significant amount of fentanyl by infusion or by titration should be continuously monitored for persistent or recurrent respiratory depression. Along with this, fentanyl has been implicated in what is called a delayed-onset respiratory depression. In some patients, a secondary peak of the drug concentration in the plasma occurs about 45 minutes after the apparent recovery from the drug. This syndrome may occur because some of the fentanyl can become sequestered in the gastric fluid and then can become recycled into the plasma in about 45 minutes. Hence in the PACU, all patients who have received fentanyl should be continuously monitored for respiratory depression for at least 1 hour from the time of admission to the unit.

Fentanyl can be administered intraoperatively at three different dose ranges, depending on the type of surgery and the desired effect. For example, the low-dose range of 2 to 20 μg/kg attenuates moderately stressful stimuli. The moderate dose range is 20 to 50 μg/kg and strongly obtunds the stress response. The megadose range of as much as 150 μg/kg blocks the stress response and is particularly valuable when protection of the myocardium is critical.

Fentanyl shares with most other narcotics a profound respiratory depressant effect, even to the point of apnea. Rapid intravenous injection can provoke bronchial constriction as well as resistance to ventilation caused by rigidity of the diaphragmatic and intercostal muscles. This is commonly called the fixed chest syndrome and can occur when any potent narcotic analgesic is administered too rapidly via the intravenous route. Should this syndrome occur, intravenous succinylcholine (15 to 25 mg) will relieve the rigidity of the chest wall muscles. Once succinylcholine is administered for this purpose, the peri-anesthesia nurse should be prepared to ventilate the patient until the skeletal muscle relaxant properties of succinylcholine subside.

Fentanyl, unlike most narcotics, has little or no hypotensive effects and usually does not cause nausea and vomiting. Because of its vagotonic effect, it may cause bradycardia, which can be relieved by atropine or glycopyrrolate. Fentanyl can be reversed by the narcotic antagonist naloxone, which also reverses analgesia. Should fentanyl be reversed by naloxone in the PACU, the perianesthesia nurse should continue to monitor the patient for the possible return of respiratory depression, because the duration of the respiratory depression produced by the fentanyl may be longer than the duration of action of naloxone.

Fentanyl can be used alone in a nitrous-narcotic technique. It also is used in the PACU in the form of a low-dose intravenous drip for pain relief. Fentanyl is the narcotic portion of Innovar (see Chapter 19).

Sufentanil (Sufenta)

Sufentanil is an analogue of fentanyl and is approximately five to seven times as potent as fentanyl. Anesthesia with sufentanil can be induced more rapidly—with basically the same technique as that used for fentanyl—without increasing the incidence of chest wall rigidity. However, sufentanil can produce chest wall rigidity, so if it is administered in the PACU, equipment for administering oxygen by positive pressure and the skeletal muscle relaxant succinylcholine should be on hand. The incidence of hypertension with sufentanil is lower than with comparable doses of fentanyl. Bradycardia is infrequently seen in patients who receive sufentanil, and when high-dose sufentanil is used in combination with nitrous oxide-oxygen, the mean arterial pressure and cardiac output may be decreased. The recovery time from sufentanil from the time of injection is about the same as with fentanyl. This is because sufentanil is very rapidly eliminated from tissue storage sites, and consequently, the duration of action of sufentanil is about the same as with fentanyl. Also, initial studies indicate that the incidence of postoperative hypertension, the need for vasoactive agents, and the requirements for postoperative analgesics are generally reduced in patients who are administered moderate or high doses of sufentanil in comparison to patients given inhalation agents. Of particular interest to the perianesthesia nurse is that sufentanil has an additive effect that is exhibited in patients who receive barbiturates, tranquilizers, other opioids, general anesthetics, or other CNS depressants. This is especially true of benzodiazepines, because they can potentiate a profound hypotensive action. Hence when sufentanil is combined with any of these drugs, particular attention should be paid to any signs of decreased respiratory drive, increased airways resistance, and hypotension. Immediate countermeasures include maintaining a patent airway by proper positioning of the patient, by placement of an oral airway or endotracheal tube, and by the administration of oxygen. If indicated, naloxone should be employed as a specific antidote to manage the respiratory depression. The duration of respiratory depression after overdosage with sufentanil may be longer than the duration of action of the naloxone. Consequently, the patient should be constantly observed for the recurrence of respiratory depression, even after the initial successful treatment with naloxone. Hypotension can be treated with reversal with naloxone; however, fluids and vasopressors may be indicated (see Chapter 9).

Alfentanil (Alfenta)

Alfentanil is another analogue of fentanyl that is about one tenth as potent and has about one third the duration of action of fentanyl. The onset of action of this drug occurs in about 1 or 2 minutes, and the duration of action is 20 to 30 minutes. Alfentanil appears to have significant advantages over currently available opioid anesthetics. For example, it has no cumulative drug effects, and once the infusion of alfentanil is terminated, the emergence time is quite predictable. Alfentanil, like fentanyl, produces minimal hemodynamic effects and offers a high therapeutic index. In fact, the therapeutic index for alfentanil is higher than those of fentanyl and other opioids. A therapeutic index is the ratio of the lethal dose to the effective dose, and the higher the therapeutic index, the farther the lethal dose from the dose used to get the desired effect. More specifically, the therapeutic index of fentanyl is 270, which means that it is about four times safer

than morphine. Alfentanil's therapeutic index is about 2.5 times more favorable than that of fentanyl.

Alfentanil, in addition to having a place in the operating room, may also have important uses in the PACU. Its rapid onset and very brief duration of action make it advantageous for the immediate pain relief needs of PACU patients. As previously stated, the drug has about one third the potency of fentanyl, but its onset of action is at least three times faster; its duration is one third that of fentanyl, and it has a high therapeutic index, which makes alfentanil well suited for pain relief in the immediate postoperative period. The drug produces few cardiovascular effects and thus should be of great value in the prevention of dangerous reflexes, such as tachycardia during intubation. Clinical observation indicates that the recovery time for this drug is extremely rapid. Hence patients who receive this drug intraoperatively will most likely experience pain early in the immediate postoperative period, and the appropriate analgesic should be administered.

Remifentanil

Remifentanil is a very selective mu opioid agonist that has an analgesic potency about equal to fentanyl and 20 times as potent as alfentanil. This drug has some excellent pharmacologic properties in that it is brief in action, titratable, noncumulative, lacks histamine release, and has a rapid recovery after the discontinuation of the drug. The onset of this drug is within one minute. When the drug is discontinued, it will be metabolized quickly; its effects will disappear within 4 minutes. The remifentanil anesthetic technique is excellent for suppression of the stress response and allows for excellent depression of neurological responses. In regard to the immediate postanesthesia period, remifentanil is better than most all over intravenous opioid drugs in regard to residual effects because it has a very rapid recovery and less risk of postoperative respiratory depression.

This drug should probably not be used in the PACU; however if the drug is to be administered in the PACU, it should be administered *only* by a anesthesia clinician who is very experienced in the administration of the drug; some of the adverse effects of the drug may accompany its administration.

Remifentanil is given via intravenous infusion with an infusion pump and never should be administered by intravenous bolus. The drug can produce the "fixed chest" syndrome and can also cause nausea and vomiting, respiratory depression, and mild to moderate depression of the heart rate and blood pressure.

Pentazocine (Fortral, Talwin)

Pentazocine, an opioid agonist and antagonist analgesic, was first synthesized in 1959. The drug has significant activity and a low addiction potential. It is approximately one third as potent as morphine when given intramuscularly. Its advantage over morphine is that it can be given orally. It can be used preoperatively as well as postoperatively for the relief of pain from abdominal, cardiac, genitourinary, orthopedic, neurologic, and gynecologic surgery. The observed side effects of this drug include sedation, dizziness, nausea, and vomiting, but these occur infrequently.

Studies of the relative potency of this drug indicate that 30 mg of pentazocine is analgesically equivalent to 10 mg of morphine and 75 mg of meperidine. It has been established that pentazocine can relieve severe pain and is approximately two to four times less potent than morphine when administered parenterally.

Pentazocine can be used in the nitrous-narcotic technique. The respiratory depression produced by pentazocine is potentiated when general anesthetics are used concomitantly. Pentazocine produces an increase in systolic blood pressure and does not appear to have depressant effects on cardiac output. The drug should be used with caution in patients with renal or hepatic impairment. Pentazocine depresses the respiratory system in a manner comparable to morphine in equivalent analgesic doses. Tolerance to the analgesic effect of the drug does not appear to develop as it does with other narcotics. Because pentazocine is a narcotic antagonist at the mu receptors, administration of this drug to a patient who depends on opiates may induce abrupt withdrawal symptoms.

The onset of analgesic activity of pentazocine is approximately 2 or 3 minutes when it is given intravenously and 15 to 20 minutes when given intramuscularly. The duration of action is about 3 hours. When given orally, the drug is about one third as potent as when it is given intramuscularly.

Butorphanol (Stadol)

Butorphanol is a synthetic analgesic that is chemically related to the nalorphine-cyclazocine series with both narcotic and antagonist properties. More specifically, it serves as an agonist at the kappa and sigma opioid receptors. In regard to its analgesic potency, it is about 5 times more potent than morphine, 30 times more potent than meperidine, and 20 times more potent than pentazocine. Butorphanol can produce sedation, nausea, and respiratory depression. The respiratory depression is plateaulike in that 2 mg of butorphanol depresses respiration to a degree equal to 10 mg of morphine. The magnitude of respiratory depression with butorphanol is not appreciably increased at doses of 4 mg. The duration of the respiratory depression is dose-related and is reversible by naloxone. Intravenous administration of butorphanol can produce increased pulmonary artery pressure, pulmonary wedge pressure, left-ventricular end-diastolic pressure, systemic arterial pressure, and pulmonary vascular resistance. Consequently, this drug increases the workload of the heart, especially in the pulmonary circuit. Because of its antagonist properties, butorphanol is not recommended for patients who are physically dependent on narcotics, because butorphanol can precipitate withdrawal symptoms in those patients. See Table 20-1 for an overview of the clinical pharmacology of butorphanol.

Nalbuphine (Nubain)

Nalbuphine is a potent analgesic with narcotic agonist and antagonist actions. It is chemically related to oxymorphone and naloxone. This drug is an antagonist at the mu receptors, a partial agonist at the kappa receptors, and an agonist at the sigma receptors. Nalbuphine is as potent as morphine and about three times as potent as pentazocine on a milligram basis. At a dose of 10 mg/kg, nalbuphine causes the same degree of respiratory depression as does 10 mg of morphine. At higher doses, nalbuphine exhibits the same plateau effect as butorphanol (i.e., respiratory depression is not increased appreciably with higher doses). The respiratory depression produced by nalbuphine can be reversed by nalox-

Table 20-1	Comparison of Seven Analgesics						
	Morphine	Meperidine	Pentazocine	Butorphanol	Nalbuphine	Dezocine	Ketorolac
Indication	Moderate to severe pain	Moderate to severe pain	Moderate to severe pain	Moderate to severe pain	Moderate to severe pain	Moderate to severe pain	Moderate to severe pain
Recommended IM dose	10 mg	25-50 mg	30 mg	2 mg	10 mg	5-15 mg	15-30 mg
Recommended IV dose	4-10 mg	100 mg	30 mg	1 mg	10 mg	2.5-10 mg	Do not give IV
Time required for onset of analgesia	Rapid IV 30 min IM	Rapid IV 30 min IM	Rapid IV 20 min IM	Rapid IV 30 min IM	Rapid IV 15 min IM	5-15 min IV 15-30 min IM	30-60 min IM
Duration of analgesia	4 hr	2-4 hr	3-4 hr	3-4 hr	3-6 hr	2-3 hr	4-6 hr
Respiratory depression	High	High	Occurs, but less than morphine	Occurs, but less than morphine	Occurs, but less than morphine	Occurs, but less than morphine	None
Cardiovascular effect	Decreases cardiac workload	Decreases cardiac workload	Increases cardiac workload	Increases cardiac workload	Good cardiac stability	Good cardiac stability	Good cardiac stability
Abuse syndrome	High	High	Occurs; induces withdrawal syndrome	Occurs; induces withdrawal syndrome	Occurs; induces withdrawal syndrome	Occurs; induces withdrawal syndrome	None

Adapted from Wood M, Wood A: Drugs and anesthesia: pharmacology for the anesthesiologist, Baltimore, 1982, Williams & Wilkins.

one. Nalbuphine does not appear to increase the workload of the heart or to decrease cardiovascular stability. This drug has a lower abuse potential than does morphine; however, if it is given to a patient who is physically dependent on narcotics, withdrawal symptoms may appear. Signs of withdrawal include abdominal cramps, nausea and vomiting, lacrimation, rhinorrhea, anxiety, restlessness, elevation of temperature, and piloerection. Should these symptoms appear after the injection of nalbuphine, the administration of small amounts of morphine can relieve the objective effects of the syndrome. See Table 20-1 for an overview of the clinical pharmacology of nalbuphine.

Dezocine (Dalgan)

Dezocine is a strong analgesic drug that has both agonist and antagonist activities. Its potency, onset, and duration of action are similar to those of morphine, and its analgesic effects appear to be at the mu opioid receptors. Dezocine produces a degree of respiratory depression similar to that of morphine when given in similar analgesic doses. Respiratory depression does not increase progressively in doses higher than 30 mg/kg. The depression of respiration produced by dezocine can be reversed by naloxone. The effects of dezocine on the cardiovascular system appear to be minimal.

Dezocine is available in three concentrations (5, 10, and 15 mg/ml) for either intravenous or intramuscular administration. For relief of postoperative pain, an intravenous dose of 2.5 to 10 mg can be used, and for intramuscular administration, 5 to 15 mg is standard. The onset of analgesia is usually about 15 minutes for intravenous administration and 30 minutes for the intramuscular route. The peak analgesic effect and duration of action are about the same, regardless of the route of administration. Remedication with dezocine may be needed within 2 or 3 hours after its initial administration.

Dezocine should not be administered to patients who have developed a significant tolerance to opioid drugs from long-term use. This precaution is necessary because dezocine has some opioid antagonist properties, and if it is given to a patient who is physically dependent on narcotics, acute withdrawal symptoms can occur. Finally, because dezocine contains sodium metabisulfite, it should not be given to any patient who is allergic to this sulfite. In addition, asthmatics are more sensitive to sulfites than are nonasthmatics. Hence an asthmatic patient with a strong allergy history probably should not receive this drug.

Buprenorphine (Buprenex)

Buprenorphine is a parenteral opiate analgesic with agonist-antagonist properties that is 30 times as potent as morphine sulfate. This drug is a derivative of the opium alkaloid thebaine and has a low abuse potential. It is proposed that the mechanism of action of buprenorphine involves the binding of the drug to the opiate receptors in the CNS. More specifically, this drug is a partial agonist at the mu opiate receptors. Buprenorphine at a dose of 0.3 mg has about the same respiratory depressant effect as 10 mg of morphine. This drug may cause a decrease or, rarely, an increase in pulse and blood pressure. Given by the intramuscular route of administration, the onset of analgesia is within 15 minutes, with a peak analgesic effect in 1 hour and a duration of 6 hours. When administered intravenously, the onset and peak times are shortened.

Of importance to the perianesthesia nurse is the fact that the respiratory depressant effects of buprenorphine can be only partially reversed by naloxone. At present, no completely reliable specific antagonist is available to reverse the respiratory depressant effects produced by buprenorphine. Consequently, patients who have been administered this drug should be assessed for respiratory depression for the next 6 hours. When a PACU patient is transferred, the nursing staff on the surgical units must be advised of the administration of and ramifications of the use of this drug.

Ketorolac (Toradol)

Ketorolac is an analgesic that is classified as a nonsteroidal antiinflammatory drug (NSAID). Its mode of action is to inhibit the prostaglandin synthetase enzyme. Therefore it has analgesic, antiinflammatory, and antipyretic actions. On a dosage basis, 30 mg of this drug, given intramuscularly, is equal to about 12 mg of morphine or 100 mg of meperidine in degree of postoperative pain relief. This drug should not be administered intravenously and hence can be administered only by the intramuscular route. When it is used with supplemental opioids, ketorolac will afford excellent postoperative analgesia. For acute postoperative pain, an initial loading dose of 30 mg can be administered intramuscularly. Ketorolac can be administered every 6 hours thereafter at a dose of 15 mg. The duration of analgesia—but not the peak analgesic effect—is increased when the dose is increased beyond its recommended dosage range of 15 to 60 mg. Ketorolac should be given at a lower dose range for patients with renal disease, for the elderly (older than 70 years of age), and in patients weighing less than 50 kg. Because this drug is an NSAID and not an opioid, its lack of effect on psychomotor activities and on the respiratory system makes it an ideal analgesic for outpatient surgery.

Clinically, to take advantage of the peak effects of ketorolac, it is sometimes administered intramuscularly about 1 hour before the end of the surgical procedure. In this instance, the patient usually emerges from anesthesia in an analgesic state that lasts well into the immediate postoperative period. Hence to effectively design an analgesic plan in the PACU, the postanesthesia nurse must determine whether ketorolac was given intraoperatively so as to avoid analgesic overmedication.

The Narcotic Antagonists

Narcotic antagonists are used to reverse narcotic-induced respiratory depression. An opioid antagonist, such as naloxone, is a drug that completely antagonizes the effect of a narcotic. Drugs such as nalorphine (Nalline) and levallorphan (Lorfan) best typify the agonist-antagonists. These drugs partially reverse the effects of narcotics but also produce autonomic, endocrine, analgesic, and respiratory depressant effects similar to those of morphine.

Naloxone (Narcan). Naloxone, a pure antagonist, reverses the depressant effects of narcotics. More specifically, this drug antagonizes the opioid effects at the mu, kappa, and sigma receptors. This drug also reverses the analgesic effect of the narcotic, which is important to remember when assessing the patient's respiratory effort. Naloxone should be titrated according to the patient's response. Usually, 0.1 to 0.2 mg given slowly intravenously should be adequate for reversal. The onset of action of naloxone is 1 or 2 minutes, and if after 3 to 5 minutes inadequate reversal has been achieved, naloxone administration may be repeated until reversal is complete. If the patient shows no sign of reversal, assessment of other pharmacologic agents administered is indicated. Drugs such as halothane, barbiturates, and muscle relaxants are not reversed by naloxone.

The duration of action of naloxone is 1 to 4 hours, depending on the route and amount of drug used. If long-acting narcotics were used, the patient must be monitored for respiratory embarrassment after the administration of naloxone, because the depressant activity of the narcotic may return. If this phenomenon occurs, supplemental doses of naloxone can be used. The intramuscular route of administration has been shown to produce a longer-lasting effect.

An excessive dosage of naloxone may increase blood pressure, a finding that may be seen as a response to pain. Too-rapid reversal may induce nausea, vomiting, diaphoresis, or tachycardia. During the reversal procedure, the vital signs should be monitored, and naloxone should be used with caution in patients with cardiac irritability.

Naloxone does not produce respiratory depression as do other narcotic antagonists. It also does not produce any significant side effects or pupillary constriction. Naloxone reverses natural or synthetic narcotics, propoxyphene (Darvon), and the narcotic-antagonist analgesic pentazocine. Because reversal may precipitate an acute withdrawal syndrome, Naloxone should be administered with great caution in patients who are physically dependent on opioids.

Naltrexone. Naltrexone is a pure mu receptor antagonist; therefore its actions are similar to naloxone. This drug can be administered orally and can produce sustained opioid antagonist activity for as long as 48 to 72 hours. This drug can only be administered orally and is used in opioid detoxification as it can be used to facilitate withdrawal; once the patient has been completely detoxified, naltrexone can prevent relapses to opioids by blocking the euphoric effects of the opioid.

Levallorphan (Lorfan). Levallorphan is an agonist-antagonist of narcotic depression. It has essentially been replaced by naloxone. It acts as a narcotic antagonist in the presence of a strong narcotic effect. If used when no narcotic is present, respiratory depression may occur. It does not counteract mild respiratory depression and may in fact intensify it. Repeated doses decrease its effectiveness, and it eventually produces its own respiratory depression. Adverse reactions associated with levallorphan include dysphoria, miosis, drowsiness, nausea, and diaphoresis. It can also cause weird dreams, visual hallucinations, and disorientation.

SELECTED METHODS OF OPIOID ADMINISTRATION

Intrathecal and Epidural Routes of Administration

In an attempt to manage acute and chronic pain, the opioids can be administered via the subarachnoid or epidural space. The technique is called the neuraxial administration of opioids. This concept of pain relief is based on the fact that opioid receptors exist in the substantia gelatinosa on the dorsal horn of the spinal cord. More specifically, mu, kappa, and delta opioid receptors are located in the substantia gelatinosa. The pain relieved by the administration of neuraxial opioids is usually of the visceral as opposed to somatic type. When the opioid is administered via the epidural space, it crosses the epidural space to the opioid receptors in the spinal cord. Consequently, the dosage of the opioid, when administered into the epidural space, is usually 10 times the dosage of the opioid if it were to be administered via the subarachnoid space.

When 0.1 to 0.2 mg of preservative-free morphine (Duramorph) is administered into the subarachnoid space (intrathecal), the maximum concentration will be reached in about 5 to 10 minutes, with a duration of about 80 to 200 minutes. When morphine, 5 mg, is administered into the epidural space in the lumbar region, analgesia can last for as long as 24 hours. The patient should obtain pain relief in about 30 to 60 minutes after injection. If appropriate pain relief is not achieved, incremental doses of 1 to 2 mg can be administered. The maximum dose in a 24-hour period is 10 mg.

After spinal surgery, epidural morphine administered by the continuous epidural technique has both advantages and disadvantages. Its advantage is a profound degree of pain relief, especially for the first 12 to 18 postoperative hours. However, disadvantages of this technique are related to displacement of the epidural catheter and the length of action of the epidural morphine. If the epidural catheter becomes displaced and the morphine has been injected, only partial pain relief ensues. Because of the possibility of profound respiratory depression, opioids must be administered cautiously. In fact, a nonopioid drug such as ketorolac may be especially useful in this circumstance. Depending on the anticipated amount and length of pain, a patient-controlled analgesia (PCA) device can be started on the patient and have an immediate result of pain resolution. Along with this, the postanesthesia nurse can have a profound impact on reducing the pain threshold by repositioning and reassuring the patient. The new technology of apnea monitors can be quite useful to detect hypoventilation or apnea that can be created by the opioid in this technique. Hence the use of the apnea monitor on patients who are receiving epidural morphine will certainly aid the postanesthesia nurse in monitoring for respiratory dysfunction.

Other opioids that can be administered epidurally are fentanyl and sufentanil. These drugs offer some advantages over morphine because they are more suited for continuous infusion techniques because of their rapid onset and short duration of action. Also, because they have such a rapid clearance from the cerebrospinal fluid, less chance for these drugs to spread toward the head (rostral spread) exists. It has been demonstrated that rostral spread, which is associated more with

morphine, produces side effects such as nausea, pruritus, and the previously discussed delayed respiratory depression syndrome. Naloxone reverses this side effect; however, the analgesic effect also is reversed. In this instance, nalbuphine administration should be considered to reverse the respiratory depression and preserve some of the analgesia.

Patient-Controlled Analgesia

To aid in the reduction of pain, the intramuscular injection of opioids and nonopioids has long been the standard route of administration used by nursing personnel. This method of administration has the advantage of simplicity and no requirement for specialized equipment. Its disadvantages include variable uptake, pain on injection, and patient dissatisfaction with the level of pain relief. Patient dissatisfaction is based on the cyclic effect of pain. If a level of analgesia were produced, the adverse effects of pain could be controlled. Intravenous administration offers some advantages over the intramuscular approach. The administration of an opioid via the intravenous route offers the patient an immediate reduction in pain. However, this reduction is only temporary because no appropriate blood level of the opioid has been established.

To achieve an appropriate level of analgesia, a "loading dose"—followed by titration to effect—based on the pharmacokinetics of the opioid drug is used intraoperatively. The maintenance of an appropriate blood level of the opioid to achieve and maintain a level of analgesia is the goal of this technique. The blood level of the drug is called the minimum effective analgesic concentration (MEAC). Research has demonstrated that the MEAC varies among individuals. Through the use of technology, the principles of this intraoperative technique have been continued into the immediate postoperative period. Intravenous PCA is the method of choice for those patients who require continued analgesia. The peaks and valleys of analgesia can be avoided without the patient having to become totally dependent on the nurse's response for pain relief. PCA allows the patient more control of the situation by allowing him or her to "seek out" a particular level of analgesia—the MEAC.

In the PACU, the patient is administered a loading dose of the intravenous opioid to achieve the MEAC and then a PCA infusion pump is set up for the patient. The PCA pump is programmed for the administration of a particular opioid based on the patient's analgesic needs and the pharmacokinetics of the drug to be administered. The parameters to be programmed are the bolus dose, the lockout interval, and the low-dose continuous basal infusion rate. Consequently, by a "push of a button" on the PCA pump, the patient can attain immediate analgesia and receive the benefits of controlled pain relief by low-dose continuous infusion of the opioid.

The amount of the self-dose bolus should be low so as to avoid an acute increase in blood levels of the drug above the MEAC because, along with the concern about overdosage, blood levels above the MEAC have no analgesic value. The lockout interval, or "delay," is the setting used to block the use of the self-dose bolus button for a period of time. During this time, the PCA pump does not deliver the drug, even when the patient pushes the button. The lockout interval is usually short, so the patient can self-administer small incremental doses to maintain his or her MEAC, yet the interval should be long enough to prevent overdosage. The basal infusion rate is usually set at a rate necessary to provide analgesia when the patient is resting. See Table 20-2 for a suggested protocol for drug administration in PCA.

Patient-Controlled Epidural Analgesia

The concept of PCA has been adapted to epidural analgesia. In this instance, the PCA infusion pump can be attached to the epidural catheter. The opioid drugs that can be used in this technique are fentanyl and sufentanil. They can be used with great success for analgesia after cesarean section. The basal infusion rate keeps the patient analgesic and comfortable. The patient can self-administer a bolus of the opioid if the analgesia provided by the basal infusion rate is not sufficient. Also, the bolus opioid facilitates additional analgesia needed for turning and early ambulation. A suggested protocol for both fentanyl and sufentanil is provided in Tables 20-3 and 20-4. Because of the possibility of rostral spread, it is suggested that an apnea monitor be used on patients who are receiving patient-controlled epidural analgesia.

Monitoring the Patient Receiving Opioids in the PACU

In addition to the routine monitoring for the patient receiving opioids in the PACU, the respiratory rate (RR) should be monitored for not only the rate but also the trend. For example, if the RR decreases from 18 to 16 to 12 over a 45-minute interval, strong suspicion that excessive opioid effect has occurred and the modified stir-up regime should be instituted.

Table 20-2 Protocol for Opioid Administration in Intravenous PCA

	Loading	Dose	Interval	Dose
Drug	Adult	By weight	Adult	By weight
Morphine	0.5-4 mg every 10 minutes (total, 6-16 mg)	0.05 mg/kg (total, 0.05-0.2 mg/kg	0.5-2 mg	10-20 µg/kg
Meperidine (Demerol)	12.5-25 mg every 10 min (total, 50-125 mg)	0.5-1.5 mg/kg	5-10 mg	0.1-0.2 mg/kg
Fentanyl (Sublimaze)	25-50 µg every 5 min (total, 50-300 µg)	0.05-2.0 µg/kg (total, 0.5-4 µg/kg)	10-30 µg	0.25-0.5 µg/kg

Adapted from Bailey P: Respiratory effects of postoperative opioid analgesia, Semin Anesth 15(4):343-352, 1996.
PCA, Patient-controlled analgesia.
Basal rate or interval dose rate is optional as the demand-only mode of PCA is often prescribed. Lockout intervals range generally between 6 to 12 minutes.

Table 20-3	Protocol For Administration Of Fentanyl* By The PCEA System For Post-Cesarean Section Patients		
	PACU	Surgical Unit	For Complaint of Pain
Bolus	100 µg	—	50-100 µg
Dose	40 µg	40 µg	50-60 µg
Lockout	10 min	10 min	10 min
Basal rate	60 µg/hr	60 µg/hr	60-80 µg/hr
Limit	260 µg/hr	260 µg/hr	310-380 µg/hr

Adapted from Grass J, Harris A: Postcesarean section analgesia, Wellcome Trends Anesthesiol 9(6):3-8, 1991. Reproduced with permission of GlaxoSmithKline.
PCEA, Patient-controlled epidural analgesia.
*Mix fentanyl in 20 µg/ml solution.

Table 20-4	Protocol for Administration Of Sufentanil by The PCEA System For Post-Cesarean Section Patients		
	PACU	Surgical Unit	For Complaint of Pain
Bolus	30 µg	—	20 µg
Dose	8 µg	4 µg	8 µg
Lockout	10 min	10 min	10 min
Basal rate	6 µg/hr	6 µg/hr	6 µg/hr
Limit	46 µg/hr	26 µg/hr	26 µg/hr

Adapted from Grass J, Harris A: Postcesarean section analgesia, Wellcome Trends Anesthesiol 9(6):3-8, 1991. Reproduced with permission of GlaxoSmithKline.
PCEA, Patient-controlled epidural analgesia.

Along with monitoring the RR, peripheral pulse oximetry and, if required, detection of expired carbon dioxide or arterial blood gas monitoring can be used. The nervous system clinical indicators of significant opioid action should also be monitored. This would include observing for excess sedation, lethargy, apathy, dysphoria, nausea, vomiting, pruritus (especially facial), meiosis, and cough suppression.

If the patient is determined to be suffering from opioid-induced respiratory depression, pro-phylactic supplemental oxygen should be administered, and the modified stir-up regime should be instituted. If the patient is difficult to arouse, the airway should be supported and manually assisted ventilation by bag and mask may be required. Should the patient have excessive secretions and/or vomitus, a person skilled in airway management should be summoned, as tracheal intubation may be required. Pharmacologic treatment should include the use of naloxone. For the adult, it is suggested to start out with lower doses such as 0.1 mg and titrate to effect. This will lessen the adverse cardiovascular effects that can occur when the opioid is completely reversed with high dose naloxone.

OPIATE DETOXIFICATION IN THE PACU

With the advent of more people experiencing addiction to heroin, many methods of detoxification have been developed. The most common methods of opioid detoxification are methadone withdrawal, clonidine withdrawal, clonidine/naltrexone withdrawal, and the use of anesthesia-assisted rapid opiate detoxification (AAROD).

AAROD is in its experimental stages but has advantages over the other methods of detoxification in that it is rather rapid and less costly than the other forms of treatment. In this method, the patient is admitted to the psychiatric unit of the hospital to ensure nothing per mouth status, and a premedication is usually administered. The patient is usually administered multiple preprocedural oral medications—including clonidine (Catapres) to suppress the withdrawal symptoms, nizatidine (Axid) to prevent nausea and vomiting, and metoclopramide (Reglan) to decrease gastric acidity. The patient is then admitted to the PACU the next morning, and the procedure is initiated. Monitoring of this patient usually includes a continuous cardiac monitor, pulse oximeter, and a noninvasive blood pressure monitor. Oxygen is usually administered per nasal cannula, and emergency resuscitation equipment—including intubation equipment and cardiac arrest cart—is immediately available. Before the initiation of the procedure, midazolam and ondansetron are usually given. Then light sedation is produced by a propofol infusion, and the patient is dosed with intravenous naloxone. The patient will go through withdrawal signs and symptoms that usually include mydriasis, piloerection, and a mild increase in heart rate and blood pressure. After about 45 minutes the propofol is discontinued, and routine postanesthesia nursing care is provided. Emotional support and reassurance certainly are important to ensure an appropriate outcome. Once the patient is stabilized, a report should be given to the receiving nurse on the psychiatric unit, and the patient is discharged from the PACU and transported to the psychiatric unit.

BIBLIOGRAPHY

Alspach J: Core Curriculum for Critical Care Nursing, ed 5, Philadelphia, 1998, WB Saunders.

Atlee J: Complications in Anesthesia, Philadelphia, 1999, WB Saunders.

Bailey P: Respiratory effects of postoperative opioid analgesia, Semin Anesth 15(4):343-352, 1996.

Barash P, Cullen B, Stoelting R: Clinical Anesthesia, ed 4, Philadelphia, 2000, Lippincott Williams & Wilkins.

Benumof J: Anesthesia and uncommon diseases, ed 4, Philadelphia, 1998, WB Saunders.

Benumof J, Saidman L: Anesthesia & perioperative complications, ed 2, St Louis, 1999, Mosby.

Bowdle T, Horita A, Kharasch E: The pharmacologic basis of anesthesiology, New York, 1994, Churchill Livingstone.

Estafanous F: Opioids in anesthesia: II. Boston, 1991, Butterworth-Heinemann.

Ganong W: Review of medical physiology, ed 20, New York, 2001, McGraw-Hill Professional.

Guyton A, Hall J: Textbook of medical physiology, ed 10, Philadelphia, 2000, WB Saunders.

Hardman J, Limbird L: Goodman and Gilman's the pharmacological basis of therapeutics, ed 10, New York, 2001, McGraw-Hill.

Katzung B, editor: Basic and clinical pharmacology, ed 8, Los Altos, Calif, 2000, Appleton & Lange.

Longnecker D, Murphy F: Dripps/Eckenhoff/Vandam introduction to anesthesia, ed 9, Philadelphia, 1997, WB Saunders.

Longnecker D, Tinker J, Morgan G: Principles and practice of anesthesiology, ed 2, St Louis, 1998, Mosby.

McIntosh L: Essentials of nurse anesthesia, New York, 1997, McGraw-Hill.

Miller R, editor: Anesthesia, ed 5, New York, 2000, Churchill Livingstone.

Nagelhout J, Zaglaniczny K: Nurse anesthesia, ed 2, Philadelphia, 2001, WB Saunders.

Prielipp R, Young C: Current drugs for sedation of critically ill patients, Seminars in Anesthesia, Perioperative Medicine, and Pain 20(2):85-94, 2001.

Spindler J, Mehlisch D, Brown C: Intramuscular ketorolac and morphine in the treatment of moderate to severe pain after major surgery, Pharmacotherapy 10:51S-58S, 1990.

Stoelting R: Pharmacology and physiology in anesthetic practice, ed 3, Philadelphia, 1999, Lippincott-Raven.

Stoelting R, Miller R: Basics of anesthesia, ed 4, New York, 2000, Churchill Livingstone.

Vogelsang J, Hayes S: Butorphanol tartrate (Stadol): a review, J Post Anesth Nurs 6(2):129-135, 1991.

Waugaman W, Foster S, Rigor B: Principles and practice of nurse anesthesia, ed 3, Norwalk, Conn, 1999, Appleton & Lange.

Weinberg G: Basic science review of anesthesiology, New York, 1997, McGraw-Hill.

Wilson L, KeMaria P, Kane H et al: Anesthesia-assisted rapid opiate detoxification: a new procedure in the postanesthesia care unit, J Perianesth Nurs 14(4):207-216, 1999.

21

MUSCLE RELAXANTS

Neuromuscular blocking drugs (NMBDs), or muscle relaxants, have been used in clinical anesthesia since the early 1940s. Significant advances have been made in understanding the physiology of neuromuscular transmission and the pharmacology of muscle relaxants, which have contributed greatly to clinical anesthesia as it is now practiced. Muscle relaxants are not used exclusively in the field of anesthesia; in postanesthesia care units (PACUs) and intensive care units (ICUs) and in emergency department settings, these drugs may be required to enhance patient care.

Muscle relaxants are used (1) to facilitate endotracheal intubation; (2) for procedures requiring muscle relaxation, such as intraperitoneal and thoracic surgery; (3) in ophthalmic surgery to relax the extraocular muscles; (4) to terminate laryngospasm and eliminate chest wall rigidity, which may occur after rapid intravenous injection of a potent narcotic; and (5) to facilitate mechanical ventilation by producing total paralysis of the respiratory muscles.

PHYSIOLOGY OF NEUROMUSCULAR TRANSMISSION

Because of the frequent and routine intraoperative and postoperative use of drugs that alter the patient's neuromuscular function, it is important to review the anatomy and physiology of the neuromuscular system, with emphasis on the chemical changes that occur at the receptor sites. Activation of skeletal muscle is both an electrical and a biochemical event. The term conduction refers to the passage of an impulse along an axon to a muscle fiber. Transmission applies to passage of a neurotransmitter substance across a synaptic cleft (neuromuscular junction). The combined electrical and chemical event is called neurohumoral transmission.

As the fine terminal branch of a motor neuron approaches the muscle fiber, it loses its myelin sheath and forms an expanded terminal that lies close to a specialized area of muscle membrane called the end plate (Fig. 21-1). Between the end of the muscle fiber and the end plate is the synaptic cleft, or neuromuscular junction. This space between the nerve and muscle fibers is about 20 nm wide. Acetylcholine is the biochemical neurotransmitter involved in the initiation of muscle contraction. Acetylcholine or cholinergic receptors are classified as either nicotinic or muscarinic, respectively. The acetylcholine receptors are stimulated by acetylcholine. Anticholinesterase drugs such as neostigmine (Prostigmin), edrophonium chloride (Tensilon, Enlon), and pyridostigmine (Regonol) produce an increase in acetylcholine at the acetylcholine receptor. Therefore the pharmacologic effects of the anticholinesterase drugs are on both the nicotinic and muscarinic receptors. The nicotinic receptors are further classified as either N_1 or N_2 receptors. The N_1 receptors are located at the presynaptic cleft and influence the release of acetylcholine. The N_2 receptors are situated on the postsynaptic cleft in the neuromuscular junction and when occupied by acetylcholine will open their channels to allow the flow of ions down the cell membrane, thus resulting in the skeletal muscle contraction. It is the nondepolarizing neuromuscular blocking agents such as pancuronium (Pavulon) that produce a block of the N_2 receptor—thus causing an inability of the channel to conduct ions, which results in skeletal muscle paralysis. It should be noted that extrajunctional nicotinic receptors are located throughout the skeletal muscles. Their activity is normally suppressed by normal neural activity. However, when a patient is suffering from prolonged sepsis, inactivity, denervation, or burn trauma in the skeletal muscles, a proliferation of these extra-junctional nicotinic receptors will result. Hence these patients will usually demonstrate an exaggerated hyperkalemic response when succinylcholine is administered.

The muscarinic receptors are also subdivided into M_1 and M_2 receptors. M_1 receptors are located in the autonomic ganglia and the central nervous system, and the M_2 receptors are located in the heart and salivary glands. It should be noted that atropine and glycopyrrolate (Robinul) block both the M_1 and M_2 receptors.

Acetylcholine is formed in the body of the nerve cell and the cytoplasm of the nerve terminal and is stored in the small, membrane-enclosed vesicles for subsequent release. A quantum is the amount of acetylcholine stored in each vesicle and represents about 10,000 molecules of acetylcholine. The presynaptic membrane contains discrete areas of specialization that are thought to be sites of release of the transmitter. These presynaptic "active zones" lie directly opposite the N_2 cholinergic receptors, which are located on the postsynaptic membrane. This alignment ensures that the acetylcholine diffuses directly to the N_2 receptors on the postsynaptic membrane quickly and in a high concentration. The N_2 receptor, which responds to the neurotransmitter acetylcholine, is a glycoprotein that is an integral part of the postsynaptic membrane of the neuromuscular junction (see Fig. 21-1). New evidence indicates that a positive feedback mechanism also exists at the neuromuscular junction. Acetylcholine has a presynaptic action; hence acetylcholine receptors are located on the presynaptic membrane. This positive feedback mechanism enhances the mobilization and release of acetylcholine. Finally, the enzyme that hydrolyzes acetylcholine is acetylcholinesterase, which is located in the neuromuscular junction.

The initiation of skeletal muscle contraction occurs as a result of application of a threshold stimulus. An action potential traveling down the axon causes depolarization of the presynaptic membrane. As a result of this depolarization, the membrane permeability for calcium ions is increased, and the calcium enters, or influxes, into the presynaptic membrane. Calcium acts to unite the vesicle to the presynaptic membrane and causes the rupture of that coalesced mem-

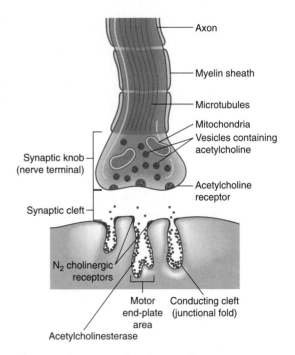

Fig. 21-1 The myoneural junction at resting state.

brane, thus releasing acetylcholine into the fluid of the synaptic cleft (Fig. 21-2).

The acetylcholine molecules released from the nerve terminal into the synaptic cleft are subject to two main processes: (1) attachment to N_2 cholinergic receptors located on the postsynaptic membrane, which leads to an opening of calcium channels that results in the movement of sodium into the region, which generates an end plate potential (EPP); and (2) attachment of acetylcholine to the presynaptic nicotinic receptor, which enhances the release of more acetylcholine. When enough EPPs are generated, an action potential will be propagated and will spread throughout the muscle and cause a change in the ionic permeability of the muscle sarcolemma. This process results in the release of calcium from the sarcoplasmic reticulum with a resultant increase in free calcium concentration in the muscle fiber. The process of excitation-contraction (E-C) coupling then takes place within that skeletal muscle cell. The physiologic outcome of E-C coupling is the contraction of the skeletal muscle. The increased concentration of

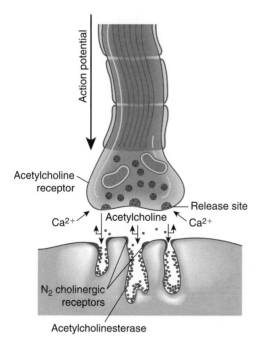

Fig. 21-2 The myoneural junction when a threshold stimulus is applied.

calcium in the muscle fiber leads to an interaction between troponin-tropomyosin and actin. This interaction causes the active sites on actin to be exposed and interact with myosin and slide together, thus resulting in muscle contraction. This sliding of actin and myosin is sometimes called the ratchet effect. The contraction of the muscle fibers is terminated when calcium is pumped back into the sarcoplasmic reticulum of the muscle fibers. The calcium is stored in the sarcoplasmic reticulum to be used when another action potential is generated.

Regulation and control of skeletal muscle contraction are also based on the enzymatic breakdown of acetylcholine. As previously discussed, the stimulus must be strong enough to release enough acetylcholine to bind to the postsynaptic N_2 cholinergic receptor. This process of competition between the postsynaptic N_2 receptor and acetylcholinesterase allows for some degree of regulation of the excitation process and for the recovery of the muscle cell membrane. The molecules of acetylcholine either diffuse in a random fashion to the N_2 receptor or are destroyed by

acetylcholinesterase. As the concentration gradient begins to decrease because of the destruction of acetylcholine by acetylcholinesterase, the N_2 receptor gives up its acetylcholine, which is then destroyed, and the skeletal muscle relaxes. A small portion of the acetylcholine can escape the acetylcholinesterase in the synaptic cleft and migrate into the extracellular fluid and from there into the plasma. Acetylcholine within the plasma is then destroyed by plasma acetylcholinesterase, or pseudocholinesterase, which is produced in the liver.

PHARMACOLOGIC OVERVIEW OF THE SKELETAL MUSCLE RELAXANTS

With the anatomy and physiology of neuromuscular transmission as a background, the principal pharmacologic actions of the nondepolarizing and depolarizing skeletal muscle relaxants will be discussed. Table 21-1 presents a pharmacologic overview of the commonly used skeletal muscle relaxants.

The prototypical nondepolarizing skeletal muscle relaxants are pancuronium and d-tubocurarine (curare). Pancuronium is an inhibitor of acetylcholine; is chemically viewed as two acetylcholine-like fragments; and has a bulky, inflexible nucleus. This drug attaches to the N_2 cholinergic receptors on the postsynaptic membrane and prevents depolarization. The skeletal muscle relaxant d-tubocurarine has the chemical structure of a monoquaternary compound. The principal pharmacologic action of this drug is to block the postsynaptic N_2 cholinergic receptor; in this way it stops acetylcholine from binding to the receptor, which results in a competitive neuromuscular blockade. The nondepolarizing skeletal muscle relaxants also block the presynaptic cholinergic receptor, thus resulting in binding of the acetylcholine and thereby preventing activation of the positive feedback mechanism.

The pharmacologic actions of the nondepolarizing skeletal muscle relaxants can be reversed by anticholinesterase drugs such as neostigmine. In effect, these drugs increase the quantum of acetylcholine at the postsynaptic membrane by preventing destruction of the acetylcholine by acetylcholinesterase. This promotes a more effective competition by the released acetylcholine with the nondepolarizing skeletal muscle relaxant that is occupying the N_2 receptor. Because of

Table 21-1 Pharmacologic Overview of the Commonly Used Neuromuscular Blocking Drugs

	Atracurium Besylate (Tracrium)	Pancuronium (Pavulon)	Vecuronium (Norcuron)	Doxacurium Chloride (Nuromax)	Pipecuronium Bromide (Arduran)	Mivacurium Chloride (Mivacron)	d-Tubocurarine	Metocurine (Metubine)	Succinylcholine (Anectine)
Nondepolarizing	Yes	Yes	Yes	Yes	Yes	Yes	Yes	Yes	No
Depolarizing	No	No	No	No	No	No	No	No	Yes
Intubation dose (IV mg/kg)	0.4-0.5	0.06-0.1	0.08-0.1	0.05-0.08	0.07-0.085	0.15	0.6	0.25-0.4	0.5-1.0
Intubation time (injection to relaxation in min)	2-2.5	4	2.5-3	4-5	2.5-3	2	6-8 (rarely used for intubation)	4	1
Muscle relaxation dose (IV mg/kg)	0.2-0.5	0.04-0.08	0.05-0.06	0.025-0.08	0.05	0.15-2	0.3	0.2-0.3	0.1-0.2 mg/kg (IV drip)
Recovery time (min)	30-45	84-114		60-160	50-150	12-15	74-87	94-117	4-6
Reversible?	Yes	Yes	Yes	Yes	Yes	Yes	Yes	Yes	No
When? (in min after initial dose)	20-35	40-60	25-30 (for 0.1 mg/kg) 40-80 (for 0.2 mg/kg)	2-30	10-20	8-11	40-60	45-60	
Cumulative effects?	No	Yes	Slight	Yes	Yes	Slight	Yes	Yes	No
Fasciculations and muscle soreness	No	No	No	No	No	No	No	No	Yes
Risk of histamine release	Minimal	Minimal	No	No	No	Yes	Significant	Moderate	Possible
Cardiovascular effects	Few	Slight ↑ in pulse and ↑ BP	None	None	None	Minimal	Hypotension	None	Slight ↓ in pulse

BP, Blood pressure; IV, intravenous.

the increased availability and mobilization of the acetylcholine, the concentration gradients favor acetylcholine and remove the nondepolarizing agents from the N_2 receptor, with the resultant return to normal contraction of the skeletal muscle.

The principal depolarizing skeletal muscle relaxant is succinylcholine (Anectine, Sucostrin). The molecular structure of this drug resembles two acetylcholine molecules back to back. Because of this structure, succinylcholine has the same effects as acetylcholine. Like acetylcholine, the succinylcholine molecule has a quaternary ammonium portion that is positively charged. This positively charged molecule is attracted by electrostatic action to the negatively charged N_2 receptor. Once the succinylcholine attaches to the receptor, a brief period of depolarization occurs that is manifested by transient muscular fasciculations. Succinylcholine also attaches to and activates the presynaptic acetylcholine receptor. This activation has an immediate effect of increased mobilization of acetylcholine in the motor nerve terminals. This explains why fasciculations are commonly observed after the administration of an intravenous bolus of succinylcholine. After the depolarization of the N_2 receptor takes place, succinylcholine promotes and maintains the receptor in a depolarized state and prevents repolarization. Succinylcholine has a brief duration of action because of its rapid hydrolysis of the succinylcholine by the enzyme pseudocholinesterase, which is contained in the liver and plasma. The actions of succinylcholine cannot be pharmacologically reversed.

NONDEPOLARIZING NEUROMUSCULAR BLOCKING AGENTS

Long-Acting Nondepolarizing Skeletal Muscle Relaxants

Tubocurarine Chloride (d-Tubocurarine Chloride, Curare). d-Tubocurarine chloride was first known as an arrow poison used by South American Indians. d-Tubocurarine blocks access of acetylcholine to the N_2 receptor at the neuromuscular junction of skeletal muscle. The action is a combination of electrical and chemical transmission; d-tubocurarine prevents depolarization by impeding leakage of the sodium ions necessary for depolarization.

The peak action of d-tubocurarine occurs 30 to 60 minutes after intravenous injection. Fifty percent to 70% of injected d-tubocurarine is excreted unchanged in the urine within 3 to 6 hours. In spite of this, the duration of action of d-tubocurarine is not unduly prolonged, even in the complete absence of renal function.

Side effects or variations in response to d-tubocurarine include histamine-like reaction, hypotension, increased airways resistance, and skin erythema. Consequently, asthmatic patients and those with a history of allergic reactions should receive a relaxant other than d-tubocurarine. d-Tubocurarine's ganglionic blocking action coupled with its histamine-like actions can cause hypotension in many patients.

Pancuronium Bromide (Pavulon). Pancuronium bromide was introduced into clinical anesthesia in 1972. This drug has demonstrated value—particularly in terms of its safety, cardiovascular stability, and skeletal muscle relaxant properties—and is receiving widespread clinical usage.

Chemically, pancuronium bromide is a biquaternary aminosteroid and is related to the androgens; however, it has no hormonal activities. Pancuronium's action is similar to but five times more potent than the action of d-tubocurarine. Also, like d-tubocurarine, pancuronium is reversible by an anticholinesterase agent, such as neostigmine, that is administered in combination with an anticholinergic such as glycopyrrolate or atropine. It has been demonstrated clinically that this particular skeletal muscle relaxant is extremely difficult to reverse pharmacologically within the first 20 to 30 minutes after injection. In the PACU, if a skeletal muscle relaxant is required for a short duration, another reversible skeletal muscle relaxant, such as d-tubocurarine or atracurium, should be chosen. About 30 to 40 minutes after injection, pancuronium is easily reversed by the combination of an anticholinesterase and anticholinergic drug preparation. Pancuronium is best suited for surgical procedures lasting more than 1 hour. It is well suited for patients who require complete muscle relaxation when receiving continuous mechanical ventilation. The dosage for adults is approximately 0.08 to 0.1 mg/kg of body weight. Relaxation lasts 60 to 85 minutes. If relaxation is required past this initial period, subsequent doses should be decreased to 0.02 to 0.04 mg/kg of body weight.

Pancuronium bromide does not produce ganglionic blockade, but it does block the M_2 cholinergic receptors in the heart. Consequently, when pancuronium bromide is administered, a slight 10% to 15% increase in heart rate will be observed. Pancuronium activates the sympathetic nervous system by promoting the release of norepinephrine and blocking its uptake at the adrenergic nerve endings. Hence after administration of this drug, a modest increase in mean arterial pressure and cardiac output will be produced. Although isolated cases of histamine release have been reported, pancuronium can probably be used in patients who have a marginal allergy history. Pancuronium bromide is compatible with anesthetic agents used clinically and is safe to use in most patients when a nondepolarizing skeletal muscle relaxant is indicated. However, pancuronium bromide is not indicated when a nondepolarizing muscle relaxant is to be used with caution. In addition, pancuronium should not be used in patients who are receiving chronic digitalis therapy because cardiac dysrhythmias have been reported. Finally, myocardial ischemia has been reported in patients with coronary artery disease when pancuronium is used. This ischemia is probably associated with the cardiac acceleration properties of the drug.

Pancuronium bromide should be avoided in patients with a history of myasthenia gravis. It is contraindicated in patients with true renal disease because a major portion of the drug is excreted unchanged in the urine. This agent is contraindicated in patients known to be hypersensitive to it or to the bromide ion.

Gallamine (Flaxedil).   Gallamine, the first synthetic skeletal muscle relaxant, was introduced into clinical anesthesia practice 6 years after d-tubocurarine was initially used. This nondepolarizing skeletal muscle relaxant has been shown to be one fifth as potent as d-tubocurarine, with a 25% shorter duration of action. In clinical doses, gallamine blocks the M_2 cholinergic receptors (much like the muscarinic cholinergic blocking effects of atropine), which results in tachycardia. This property has been used to advantage when the drug is combined with halothane (Fluothane), which is normally a vagal stimulant. However, gallamine activates the sympathetic

nervous system and also blocks the M_2 receptors. This leads to an imbalance in the autonomic nervous system in favor of the sympathetic nervous system. Ultimately, cardiac dysrhythmias can ensue after the administration of gallamine. Gallamine is excreted entirely unchanged by the kidneys, which explains reports of prolonged action of the drug in patients with poor renal function. Because of its effect on heart rate, gallamine occupies a very small component in clinical practice and is therefore only used in specific situations.

Metocurine Iodide (Metubine).   Metocurine, which was introduced into clinical anesthesia practice in 1948 as dimethyltubocurarine, is now regaining popularity. Metocurine is a nondepolarizing neuromuscular blocking agent that is a trimethylated derivative of d-tubocurarine and, like d-tubocurarine, is quite reversible by the drug combination of an anticholinesterase and an anticholinergic. The dosage for surgical relaxation is 0.2 mg/kg, and to facilitate endotracheal intubation, a dosage of 0.3 to 0.4 mg/kg is required. It is about one or two times as potent as d-tubocurarine in neuromuscular blocking potency and yet is less potent than d-tubocurarine in its ability to inhibit autonomic responses and to release histamine. Consequently, the clinical cardiovascular and hemodynamic effects of metocurine seem to be much less than those of d-tubocurarine. With the introduction of more potent long-acting drugs, which are free of cardiovascular effects, metocurine is used less often in today's clinical practice.

Doxacurium (Nuromax).   Doxacurium is a long-acting nondepolarizing neuromuscular blocking agent. It is similar to pancuronium in its length of action and dependence on appropriate renal function for clearance, but it is twice as potent as pancuronium. It is similar to atracurium in chemical structure. It has no histamine-releasing properties in its clinical dosage range, nor does it have any significant effect on the cardiovascular system; consequently, it offers excellent cardiovascular stability. The onset of action for the drug is about 4 to 9 minutes, with a duration of action of about 80 to 160 minutes that is potentiated by the inhalation anesthetics, particularly halothane. The dosage range for doxacurium is between 0.02 and 0.03 mg/kg for surgical relaxation and 0.05 to 0.08 mg/kg for facilitation of endotracheal intubation. Neostigmine 0.05 mg/kg as opposed to edrophonium should be used to reverse the neuromuscular blockade produced by doxacurium.

Doxacurium can be used in patients with liver failure with any change in onset and duration of action. In patients with renal failure, the time of onset is essentially the same; however, the duration is prolonged by about 30 minutes. Doxacurium can be used in the elderly patient because the time of onset and duration of action is about the same as in the younger population. Finally, doxacurium does not appear to be a trigger agent for malignant hyperthermia, and for patients on mechanical ventilation in the PACU who require a long-acting neuromuscular blocking agent, this drug would prove to be an excellent choice.

Because of the clinical trend towards the use of the intermediate and short-acting neuromuscular blocking agents, doxacurium is not used extensively in today's clinical practice.

Pipecuronium Bromide (Arduran). Pipecuronium is a long-acting nondepolarizing neuromuscular blocking agent with a chemical structure similar to pancuronium and vecuronium. The drug does not cause the release of histamine, nor does it have the circulatory side effects of tachycardia or hypotension. The dosage is 0.07 to 0.085 mg/kg. It has an onset of action of about 2 or 3 minutes, with a duration of action from 50 to 150 minutes. The neuromuscular blocking effects of the drug are prolonged more by isoflurane (Forane), followed by halothane, and lastly by nitrous-narcotic techniques. Pipecuronium can usually be reversed 10 minutes after it has been injected. For this particular drug, neostigmine is the preferred anticholinesterase-reversing drug. Because the kidney is its primary route of excretion, pipecuronium should not be used in patients with renal failure. This drug is more potent and shorter-acting in infants than in children and adults. Even though this drug is a nonvagolytic alternative to pancuronium, it does not enjoy wide clinical usage because of its long length of action.

Intermediate-Acting Nondepolarizing Skeletal Muscle Relaxants

Vecuronium Bromide (Norcuron). Vecuronium is a nondepolarizing skeletal muscle relaxant with a more rapid onset of action and shorter duration of action than pancuronium has. Actually, vecuronium is pancuronium without the quaternary methyl group in the steroid nucleus. Because of this structural difference, vecuronium has no effect on heart rate, arterial pressure, autonomic ganglia, or the alpha and beta adrenal receptors. The potency of vecuronium is equal to or slightly greater than that of pancuronium. Vecuronium has little or no cumulative effect. Although a portion of vecuronium is metabolized, most of the drug is excreted unchanged in the urine and bile. However, the neuromuscular blockade produced by vecuronium is not prolonged by renal failure. The duration of neuromuscular blockade produced by vecuronium is increased in patients with impaired hepatic function. It is of clinical interest that vecuronium, like atracurium, is less influenced by general inhalation anesthetics than are pancuronium and d-tubocurarine. The pharmacologic action of this drug is easily reversed by the combination of an anticholinesterase and an anticholinergic drug.

The onset of action of vecuronium is between 2.5 and 3 minutes, using the "normal" dosage of 0.08 mg/kg intravenously. Because of the rapid onset of action, vecuronium can be used for rapid-sequence intubation. In this instance, doubling the dosage of vecuronium to 0.2 mg/kg can achieve intubation conditions within 45 seconds to 2 minutes. Another method for using vecuronium for intubation is the "priming" technique. The object of this technique is to administer a small priming dose of vecuronium several minutes before the intubation dose is given to shorten the onset of neuromuscular blockade. The usual priming dose is 0.015 mg/kg, and after 3 minutes an intubation dose of 0.1 mg/kg is administered. The onset of neuromuscular blockade should be between 70 and 90 seconds. The main drawback of this technique is that some patients may develop symptoms of partial neuromuscular blockade. Sensations reported are heavy eyelids, blurred vision, and difficulty in swallowing. Therefore if this technique is used in the PACU, the nurse should warn patients of the possible symptoms, and ventilatory support should always be available.

Because of concerns about the priming technique, the "timing" technique was developed. In the timing technique, which is used mainly in the operating room, the patient is given vecuronium before sodium pentothal. Consequently, the induction of anesthesia is specifically timed to the onset of clinical muscular weakness. In this technique, the patient is given 0.1 to 0.2 mg/kg of vecuronium, and at the onset of weakness, as determined by the peripheral nerve simulator, a 4 mg/kg bolus dose of sodium pentothal is given. Intubating conditions occur within 1 minute.

Rocuronium Bromide (Zemuron). Rocuronium is a new nondepolarizing skeletal muscle relaxant with a chemical structure related to vecuronium. It has a rapid onset (1 to 1.5 minutes) and a short duration of action of 12 to 30 minutes. At a dose of 0.6 mg/kg, rocuronium provides excellent intubating conditions.

Rocuronium can be used in patients with renal failure and has a low potential for histamine release. Its actions are prolonged in patients with cirrhosis of the liver. Along with this, rocuronium's muscle relaxant actions are potentiated by the inhalation anesthetics.

Because rocuronium produces minimal cardiovascular effects and has such a fast onset and short duration of action, it is useful in intraoperative and postoperative periods.

Atracurium Besylate (Tracrium). Atracurium is a nondepolarizing skeletal muscle relaxant that offers an advantage over other skeletal muscle relaxants in that it does not depend on renal or hepatic mechanisms for its elimination. In fact, this quaternary ammonium compound breaks down in the absence of plasma enzymes through what is called Hofmann elimination and, to a lesser extent, through ester hydrolysis. Hofmann elimination is a nonbiologic method of degradation that occurs at a physiologic temperature and pH.

Atracurium is less potent than pancuronium and has a rapid onset of 1 to 3 minutes and a duration of action of about 30 to 45 minutes. To facilitate endotracheal intubation in the PACU setting, 0.3 to 0.5 mg/kg of atracurium should provide adequate skeletal muscle relaxation for intubation in about 2.5 minutes. To maintain mechanical ventilation in the PACU setting, an infusion rate of 10 µg/kg/min of atracurium may be used. Once the infusion has been discontinued, spontaneous ventilation by the patient will occur in about 30 minutes. The effects can be reversed with a combination of anticholinesterase and antimuscarinic in about 12 to 15 minutes after the discontinuation of the atracurium infusion.

Atracurium has many distinct advantages, such as not having its neuromuscular blockade prolonged by renal failure or impaired hepatic function. Also, it has little or no cumulative effect and is not influenced significantly by the specific general inhalation anesthetic dosage or concentration. Finally, this drug has little or no cardiovascular effect and is easily antagonized by the combination of an anticholinesterase and an anticholinergic.

Cisatracurium Besylate (Nimbex). Cisatracurium is a steroisomer of atracurium that is about three times as potent as atracurium with fewer side effects and is degraded by the same metabolic pathway as atracurium (i.e., the Hofmann elimination mechanism).

The average adult intubation dose of cisatracurium is 0.2 mg/kg and will have an onset of about 90 seconds, a peak in about 3 to 5 minutes, and a duration of action of about 40 to 50 minutes. A supplemental dose of 0.03 mg/kg will provide an additional 20 minutes of skeletal muscle relaxation. To maintain a stable state of skeletal muscle relaxation in the PACU, cisatracurium can be administered by infusion at a rate of 1 to 2 µg/kg/min.

This drug has all the assets of atracurium plus possesses a great advantage over atracurium of less histamine release. It does not have any particular effect on the cardiovascular system and because it undergoes an organ-independent clearance, it can be used in patients with hepatic or renal failure without a noticeable change in duration of action. It is well suited for many patients that undergo intermediate to long surgical procedures.

Short-Acting Nondepolarizing Skeletal Muscle Relaxants

Mivacurium Chloride (Mivacron). Mivacurium is a skeletal muscle relaxant that was introduced into clinical practice in 1992. Research has demonstrated that this drug has a shorter duration of action than any other currently approved nondepolarizing agent. Thus mivacurium may be suitable for providing skeletal muscle relaxation in surgical cases of short duration or for intubation when succinylcholine is not desirable. To facilitate good to excellent intubating conditions within 1.5 minutes, mivacurium can be given intravenously using the divided dose technique at a dose of 0.15 mg/kg; then, 30 seconds later, a second dose of 0.10 mg/kg should be given. Oxygen via bag-valve-mask system should be administered to the patient from the time of injection of mivacurium to the time of intubation. When mivacurium is administered in a bolus fashion, cutaneous flushing and arterial hypotension caused by systemic release of histamine have been reported. The average time of recovery from the drug is between 12 and 17 minutes after the last dose is given. Spontaneous recovery from mivacurium can occur without the use of reversal agents. However, if reversal agents are used, the recovery time is usually between 8 and 11 minutes.

Mivacurium is metabolized by pseudocholinesterase, which explains its short duration of action. Given in doses of 0.1 mg/kg or smaller, mivacurium does not cause facial flushing, hemodynamic changes, or histamine release. This skeletal muscle relaxant offers certain advantages over succinylcholine, such as its relative rapid rate of onset and short duration of action, its reversibility, and its approval for use in children and adolescents.

Rapacuronium Bromide (Raplon). Rapacuronium is a newly introduced nondepolarizing neuromuscular blocking drug that combines a rapid onset and a short duration. More specifically, at a dose of 1.5 mg/kg endotracheal intubation can be performed in one minute and it has a duration of action of approximately 15 minutes. It can be used for endotracheal intubation, and because of its clinical profile, it can be used in a variety of patients—including those with renal and hepatic dysfunction.

Because of recent safety issues regarding bronchospasm that arose in regard to rapacuronium, this drug has been voluntarily withdrawn from the market. Because this drug could be used in the PACU, it is extremely important that the perianesthesia nurse periodically examine the stock drugs to determine if any rapacuronium is in the inventory. If found, the drug should be immediately returned to the manufacturer.

Alcuronium Chloride (Alloferin). Alcuronium, which is chemically related to d-tubocurarine, is a new nondepolarizing skeletal muscle relaxant. It is about twice as potent as and much shorter in duration than d-tubocurarine. Administration of 0.2 mg/kg of alcuronium can produce muscular relaxation in 2 to 4 minutes that lasts about 20 minutes. Alcuronium is also reversible by combining an anticholinesterase and an anticholinergic drug. It produces about the same degree of hypotension as does d-tubocurarine and causes about the same amount of histamine release as does pancuronium. Because alcuronium is not metabolized and is excreted unchanged by the kidneys, it should be used with caution in patients with any type of renal dysfunction.

Reversal of Nondepolarizing Neuromuscular Blocking Agents

To restore neuromuscular transmission, the antagonist must displace the competitive neuromuscular blocking agent from the nicotinic receptor sites and open the way for depolarization of the postjunctional membrane. The antagonist is an antiacetylcholinesterase that blocks the enzymatic action of acetylcholinesterase located in the postsynaptic clefts so that acetylcholine is not hydrolyzed. The result is a buildup of acetylcholine at the end plate at the N_2 cholinergic receptor. The accumulated acetylcholine displaces the competitive neuromuscular blocking agent, which diffuses back into the plasma, thus reestablishing neuromuscular transmission.

Neostigmine and pyridostigmine are usually the anticholinesterase drugs of choice because of their long duration of action and reliability as compared with edrophonium chloride. However, research has demonstrated that edrophonium chloride is an effective reversal agent of neuromuscular blockades produced by vecuronium and atracurium. Atropine or glycopyrrolate, both antimuscarinic (anticholinergic) drugs, can be administered immediately before or in conjunction with the anticholinesterase to minimize the muscarinic effects of the anticholinesterase drug. The muscarinic effects include bradycardia, salivation, miosis, and hyperperistalsis. These effects are produced at lower concentrations of the anticholinesterase-type drug when administered (acetylcholine nicotinic effects are at the autonomic ganglia and the neuromuscular junction). Consequently, when an anticholinesterase drug is administered to reverse the nondepolarizing neuromuscular blocking agent at the N_2 receptor, an antimuscarinic drug is also given to prevent the adverse muscarinic cholinergic effects associated with the high dosage of anticholinesterase. Generally, 2.5 mg of neostigmine is the maximum dose required for reversal; however, the suggested limit is 5 mg. The method is to give atropine, 0.4 mg, or glycopyrrolate, 0.2 mg intravenously, over a 1-minute period, to observe for an increase in pulse rate, and then to administer 0.5 mg neostigmine intravenously and monitor the reversal. This procedure can be repeated until reversal has been achieved or until the limit of neostigmine that can be given is reached. If edrophonium chloride is indicated for reversal, the dosage is 0.5 mg/kg with 0.007 mg/kg of atropine.

Neostigmine should be administered cautiously. Cardiac monitoring is essential, especially in elderly or debilitated patients and in patients with cardiac disease. Atrioventricular dissociation and other dysrhythmias can be initiated by the anticholinesterases.

Pyridostigmine is an analogue of neostigmine. It facilitates the transmission of impulses across the myoneural junction by inhibiting the destruction of acetylcholine by acetylcholinesterase. Clinical data indicate a lower incidence of muscarinic side effects with this drug than with neostigmine. Like neostigmine, pyridostigmine should be administered with caution in patients with bronchial asthma or cardiac problems. Signs of overdosage are related to muscarinic and nicotinic receptor stimulation (Box 21-1). The muscarinic side effects are blocked with atropine or glycopyrrolate. Nicotinic responses can be blocked by drugs such as ganglionic or neuromuscular blocking agents. The recommended dosage for reversal is 0.15 mg/kg of intravenous pyridostigmine, in combination with 0.007 mg/kg of intravenous atropine. Full recovery occurs within 15 minutes in most patients; in others, it may require 30 minutes or more.

Another parasympatholytic agent, glycopyrrolate, has been substituted for atropine in the reversal technique. Its advantages over atropine are that it has a longer duration of action and a lower incidence of arrhythmias; it causes small, slow changes in the heart rate; and it does not cross the blood-brain barrier. The usual reversal dosage is 1 mg of neostigmine and 0.2 mg of glycopyrrolate in a 2-ml mixture. This dosage can be repeated if reversal is inadequate.

Box 21-1   Observable Responses to Stimulation of Receptors

Nicotinic

Stimulation of autonomic ganglia—both sympathetic and parasympathetic

Stimulation of adrenal medulla, resulting in the release of both epinephrine and norepinephrine

Stimulation of skeletal muscles at the motor end plate

Muscarinic

Stimulation or inhibition of smooth muscle in various organs or tissues

Stimulation of exocrine glands (i.e., salivary and sweat glands)

Slowing of cardiac conduction

Decrease in myocardial contractile force

DEPOLARIZING NEUROMUSCULAR BLOCKING AGENTS

Succinylcholine (Anectine, Quelicin, Sucostrin). Succinylcholine represents a valuable pharmacologic advance in modern anesthesia and in critical care, areas in which resuscitation of patients is required. This agent is usually included as one of the drugs available for emergencies, especially when endotracheal intubation is required. Outside the operating room, succinylcholine is used for electroshock therapy, to relieve pro-found laryngospasm, to control convulsions from tetanus, to manage ventilation of the flail chest, and during reduction of fractures or dislocations.

Although succinylcholine is widely used in the United States, it has side effects and complications that can be avoided through a basic understanding of the pharmacology of the drug.

Succinylcholine acts at the N_2 postsynaptic cholinergic receptor by causing a persistent depolarization of the end plate. It also acts on the presynaptic cholinergic receptor by causing an initial increase in acetylcholine at the motor end plate. This reaction is the reason that patients who receive succinylcholine have fasciculations when it is administered initially. It is a synthetic quaternary ammonium compound whose chemical structure closely resembles that of acetylcholine. The typical intravenous dose of succinylcholine to produce flaccid paralysis is 0.5 to 1.5 mg/kg and will have an onset of 30 to 60 seconds with a duration of about 5 to 10 minutes. The drug is hydrolyzed rapidly by plasma pseudocholinesterase, an enzyme produced by the liver, to succinylmonocholine and choline. Succinylmonocholine is further hydrolyzed by pseudocholinesterase and true cholinesterase, which found in the erythrocyte, to succinic acid and choline (see equations at bottom of page).

Advantages and Uses. Succinylcholine has certain advantages that, in most instances, justify its clinical use. Its very rapid onset of action, coupled with its short duration of action, has made this drug valuable when (1) rapid intubation is required; (2) laryngospasm is irreversible with positive pressure; (3) the skeletal muscles are rigid and prevent good ventilatory excursion; (4) procedures require a short duration of skeletal muscle relaxation, such as reduction of dislocations and fractures; and (5) electroconvulsive therapy is used to decrease the negative effects of seizures. Continued use over a 30-year period has shown succinylcholine to produce complications that can, in most instances, be prevented if the basic pharmacodynamics of the drug are understood.

In emergencies, succinylcholine remains the major muscle relaxant to facilitate endotracheal intubation. It should be stated that succinylcholine is contraindicated in children and adolescent patients except when used for emergency tracheal intubation or in instances in which immediate securing of the airway is necessary.

When this drug is used for a rapid-sequence intubation, the succinylcholine-induced fasciculations and the associated increase in gastric pressure should be reduced or eliminated by an intravenous injection of a small amount (3 mg per 70 kg of body weight) of d-tubocurarine. This "defasciculating" dose of d-tubocurarine should be administered about 1 or 2 minutes before the intravenous bolus injection of succinylcholine of 1.5 mg/kg.

Untoward Reactions. Because hydrolysis of succinylcholine depends on enzymatic activity, it is important to understand the atypical responses that may occur. Pseudocholinesterase activity in the plasma may be increased or decreased. Cases with increased activity are congenital and occur rarely. Patients with atypical pseudocholinesterase are resistant to succinylcholine and do not relax well. The reductions in pseudocholinesterase activity may be acquired or congenital. Acquired deficiencies are more important to understand because they are more common. They occur with liver disease, severe anemia, malnutrition, prolonged pyrexia, pregnancy, and recent renal dialysis. Drugs such as quinidine and propranolol (Inderal) inhibit pseudocholinesterase, as do echothiophate iodide eye drops (Phospholine). Patients with low pseudocholinesterase activity exhibit a prolonged response to these drugs.

Atypical pseudocholinesterase occurs alone in about one in 2800 people; this atypical form is inherited. Patients with genetically induced deficiencies of pseudocholinesterase have remained apneic for as long as 48 hours after a usual dose of succinylcholine. These patients require mechanical ventilation and constant nursing care. Patients with documented pseudocholinesterase deficiency should be advised to wear a Medic Alert bracelet. If anesthesia is required, these patients should be administered nondepolarizing skeletal muscle relaxants—such as pancuronium, d-tubocurarine, and gallamine—because these drugs can usually be reversed.

Disadvantages and Side Effects. Succinylcholine can be administered by single injection or continuous infusion. The single-injection method is used when neuromuscular relaxation is required for a short time, such as to facilitate endotracheal intubation. The usual intubation

---

Succinylcholine ⎯⎯⎯⎯⎯⎯⎯⎯⎯⎯→ Succinylmonocholine and choline
                 Pseudocholinesterase

Succinylmonocholine ⎯⎯⎯⎯⎯⎯⎯⎯⎯⎯⎯⎯⎯→ Succinic acid and choline
          True and pseudocholinesterase

dosage of succinylcholine is 1 mg/kg intravenously. During the first intravenous injection, cardiovascular status usually remains normal. If the injection must be repeated, the patient may exhibit profound bradycardia and various arrhythmias. Therefore monitoring the patient's cardiovascular status when succinylcholine is administered is important, especially if the dose is repeated.

Because children and adolescent patients are more likely than adults to have undiagnosed myopathies, a nondepolarizing skeletal muscle relaxant such as mivacurium (Mivacron) should be used for routine procedures in the PACU. More specifically, except when used for emergency tracheal intubation or in the instance in which immediate securing of the airway is necessary, succinylcholine is contraindicated in children and adolescent patients. This is because a patient with a myopathy in this age group who is administered succinylcholine can experience acute, fulminating destruction of skeletal muscle (rhabdomyolysis) that results in hyperkalemia and cardiac arrest.

If succinylcholine must be administered to an adolescent or child, the patient must be monitored completely because he or she is especially prone to bradycardia, even on the initial injection of succinylcholine. This complication can be easily overcome by prior administration of glycopyrrolate or atropine sulfate, either alone or mixed with succinylcholine. This appears to be the safest way of administering intravenous succinylcholine in this age group.

A disadvantage of the single-injection method with succinylcholine is that it causes fasciculations of the muscles. These "mini" contractions are a result of the initial depolarization of the skeletal muscle due to the positive feedback mechanism of initial stimulation of the presynaptic acetylcholine receptor. These contractions frequently lead to muscle pain, which is usually noted by the patient the day after surgery. This is particularly true in patients who are ambulatory soon after surgery. In ambulatory patients, muscle pains (myalgia) occur in 60% to 70% of cases. The incidence decreases to 10% in those patients confined to bed. Complaints of these patients include pain in their neck, back, and abdomen and when blinking their eyes, pain when smiling, and generalized pain when ambulatory. These objective symptoms are usually noticed first by the nurse in the PACU. It should be noted that the skeletal muscle pain around the neck area is sometimes described to the perianesthesia nurse as a "sore throat" caused by the endotracheal tube; in fact, the pain is caused by the myalgia from the succinylcholine. The pain usually does not require analgesics and subsides in a day or two. The fasciculations can be prevented by administering a nondepolarizing neuromuscular blocking drug at a pretreatment dose of between 5% and 10% of its normal intubation about 2 to 4 minutes before the injection of succinylcholine. It should be noted that if a pretreatment nondepolarizing drug was administered, the dose of succinylcholine should be increased by about 70%.

When succinylcholine is administered to patients in the presence of extensive burns, severe trauma, severe abdominal infections, tetanus, neuromuscular disease, or neurologic lesions such as paraplegia and quadriplegia, a release of potassium from the damaged muscle and nerve cells can result. The common denominator appears to be either massive tissue destruction or central nervous system injury with muscle wasting. This pathophysiologic process results when denervated muscle is stimulated by succinylcholine. This is because the extrajunctional nicotinic receptors proliferated during the skeletal muscle distruction. After activation of the nicotinic receptor by succinylcholine, response is enhanced in the ionic channels, with a resultant increase in the release of potassium into the circulation. Elevation of the serum potassium level, which can be as high as 10 to 15 mEq/L, has been reported. The result of this potassium elevation is cardiac dysrhythmias and cardiac arrest. The peak time for this reaction is 7 to 10 days after the injury. However, the critical period for these reactions is between posttraumatic days 1 and 180. Consequently, succinylcholine is contraindicated in patients who have injuries of major multiple traumas, extensive denervation of skeletal muscle, or upper motor neuron injury.

Succinylcholine has been implicated as one of the trigger agents of malignant hyperthermia (MH). Chapter 50 contains a complete description of the pathophysiology and treatment of MH.

In pediatric and adult patients anesthetized with halothane combined with succinylcholine as the muscle relaxant, an unusual incidence of plasma myoglobin has occurred. Myoglobin is an intracellular muscle protein and therefore should not be released into the plasma. If myoglobin is found in the plasma, it can only mean that the muscle membrane has been injured.

Succinylcholine can be administered in a drip infusion during a procedure that requires skeletal muscle relaxation for a longer period than a single injection can provide. It is usually administered in a 0.1% to 0.2% solution. If the infusion is administered for a prolonged period, the type of block can gradually change from a depolarizing block to a characteristic nondepolarizing block. The change is always from depolarization to nondepolarization, never in the reverse direction. This type of block is called a dual or phase II block (see p. 336). The exact time relationship and the mechanism of action are still uncertain. Treatment is by mechanical ventilation and by careful monitoring of the patient until the dual block disappears.

Succinylcholine increases intraocular pressure by about 7.5 mm Hg in both children and adults, in part because of the contraction of the extraocular muscles. When administered before succinylcholine to prevent contraction of the extraocular muscles, a nondepolarizing neuromuscular blocking drug does not completely extinguish the increase in intraocular pressure. Therefore even if succinylcholine is used with an NMBD, it is contraindicated in patients in whom an increase in intraocular pressure would be detrimental.

Hexafluorenium Bromide (Mylaxen)
Hexafluorenium bromide has both anticholinesterase and neuromuscular blocking effects. It is used clinically to potentiate the effects of succinylcholine and consequently to reduce the total amount of succinylcholine used during the surgical procedure. This approach averts the accumulation of breakdown products of succinylcholine and also reduces muscular fasciculations and twitching when succinylcholine is initially administered. Hexafluorenium bromide is not used much in clinical anesthesia practice because bronchospasm, tachycardia, hypotension, and cardiac dysrhythmias have been reported commonly after its use.

Decamethonium Bromide (Syncurine)
Decamethonium was first used clinically in 1949. This drug's action is similar to that of acetyl-choline in that it produces depolarization of the end plate of the neuromuscular junction. It liberates some histamine, but only about half as much as is released by use of d-tubocurarine. Decamethonium has no action on the myocardium, but it does produce fasciculations like succinylcholine does. This drug is not metabolized in the body and is excreted largely unchanged by the kidneys. The intravenous route of administration is the only satisfactory one for this drug. The onset of action for decamethonium is about 30 to 40 seconds after injection; its duration of action is about 15 to 20 minutes. Because of the difficulty in reversal and the problems of histamine release and fasciculations, decamethonium is rarely used in clinical anesthesia practice.

FACTORS INFLUENCING THE NEUROMUSCULAR BLOCKING AGENTS

Fluid Balance
Patients who are dehydrated are reported to be extremely sensitive to skeletal muscle relaxants. This finding is probably true because (1) dehydration decreases neuromuscular excitability; (2) the contracted extracellular fluid compartment permits an increase in the plasma concentration of the relaxant and thus intensifies the relaxant action; and (3) renal function is slowed, and the elimination time of the relaxant and its metabolites is prolonged.

Sodium
A deficit of sodium may prolong the neuromuscular block. Experimental evidence indicates that a sodium deficiency itself may result in a partial neuromuscular block.

Potassium
Potassium deficiency appears to increase the blocking action of d-tubocurarine and other nondepolarizing neuromuscular blocking agents. On the other hand, depolarizing neuromuscular blocking agents are required in larger amounts when potassium deficiency exists. Depolarization is prevented to some extent because a potassium deficiency appears to stabilize the muscle end plate. Potassium depletion can occur from decreased intake or excessive loss, such as in chronic pyelonephritis, primary aldosteronism, chlorothiazide therapy, and chronic diarrhea.

Magnesium

An increase in magnesium concentration causes a flaccid paralysis clinically similar to that caused by a nondepolarizing neuromuscular blocking agent. The principal action of magnesium is that it can enter the nerve terminal and replace or decrease the amount of calcium that enters, which stabilizes the postsynaptic membrane. Ultimately, depression of the release of acetylcholine occurs and reduces the EPP, which causes a partial neuromuscular block. Consequently, magnesium enhances a neuromuscular block produced by a nondepolarizing agent and, to a lesser extent, potentiates the block produced by succinylcholine.

Calcium

A deficiency in calcium prolongs the effects of nondepolarizing neuromuscular blocking agents by reducing the amount of acetylcholine released and by inhibiting neuromuscular transmission. The depolarizing neuromuscular blocking agents are also potentiated because a low calcium level aids depolarization. Conversely, the administration of calcium chloride solution in calcium deficiency states antagonizes the nondepolarizing effects of agents such as d-tubocurarine. Calcium chloride has a pronounced antagonism to the respiratory depressant effects of succinylcholine.

pH and Carbon Dioxide

The neuromuscular blocking effect of d-tubocurarine is intensified in acidosis and in states of elevated carbon dioxide tension. With drugs such as gallamine and succinylcholine, the neuromuscular blocking action is diminished. Alkalosis by itself decreases the effects of d-tubocurarine. Hyperventilation has been thought to augment the abdominal muscle relaxation produced by d-tubocurarine. One explanation of this phenomenon is that changes in pH or plasma concentrations of d-tubocurarine reflect a change in binding to the receptor substance.

Catecholamines

Epinephrine and ephedrine have an anticurare effect on skeletal muscle. Clinically, an antagonism to d-tubocurarine has been demonstrated. This effect is caused by an increase in acetylcholine release, the inhibition of acetyl-

---

Box 21-2 Neuromuscular Blocking Properties of Various Antibiotics

Antibiotics that increase the action of the nondepolarizing agents include the following:
Dihydrostreptomycin
Neomycin
Streptomycin
Kanamycin
Gentamicin
Polymyxin A
Polymyxin B
Lincomycin
Colistin
Tetracycline

Antibiotics that increase the action of succinylcholine include the following:
Neomycin
Streptomycin
Kanamycin
Polymyxin B
Colistin

Antibiotics that do not exert any neuromuscular blocking activity include:
Penicillin
Chloramphenicol
Cephalosporins

---

cholinesterase, a decreased excitability of muscle fibers, and the release of potassium when epinephrine and ephedrine are administered.

Mycins

Several antibiotics exhibit a nondepolarizing neuromuscular blocking property. This is because the aminoglycoside antibiotics potentiate the neuromuscular blockade by inhibiting the presynaptic release of acetylcholine. The resulting clinical difficulties are related to a combination of factors, including large doses of antibiotics, parenteral administration into body cavities that represent a large surface area for absorption, and concomitant use of a neuromuscular blocking agent. Neomycin and streptomycin have been most frequently implicated (Box 21-2).

Cardiac Antidysrhythmic Drugs

When administered intravenously, Lidocaine potentiates a preexisting neuromuscular blockade. This occurs because lidocaine stabilizes the postsynaptic membrane and depresses the skeletal muscle fibers. Quinidine interferes with the presynaptic release of acetylcholine at the neuromuscular junction. Consequently, it intensifies the neuromuscular blockade of both depolarizing and nondepolarizing skeletal muscle blocking agents. Finally, calcium channel blocking agents inhibit the calcium entry, with a resultant reduction in acetylcholine release followed by a reduction in neuromuscular function.

Temperature

Hypothermia antagonizes the action of d-tubocurarine and potentiates the action of succinylcholine or decamethonium. During the recovery phase of an anesthetic, when a neuromuscular blocking agent has been administered, young infants should be specifically monitored for return of skeletal muscle tone. This rule is especially in effect when a nondepolarizing relaxant is administered to infants, who are prone to have some hypothermia because of their immature heat-regulating systems.

Inhalation Anesthetics

The inhalation anesthetics produce a dose-dependent enhancement of the neuromuscular blockade of the nondepolarizing neuromuscular blocking agents. More specifically, this blockade is most pronounced when a patient has received either enflurane (Ethrane) or isoflurane. Halothane will produce a moderate amount of potentiation of nondepolarizing neuromuscular blocking agents, whereas nitrous oxide will only produce minimal potentiation of these agents. This potentiation of the neuromuscular blockade by the inhalation anesthetics results from depression of the central nervous system, and it ultimately reduces skeletal muscle tone. Consequently, patients in the PACU who have received nondepolarizing neuromuscular blocking agents intraoperatively and have not completely emerged from their inhalation anesthetic should be closely monitored by the use of a peripheral nerve stimulator for a reduction in skeletal muscle function. Also, an aggressive stir-up regimen should be instituted on these patients.

ASSESSMENT OF NEUROMUSCULAR BLOCKADE

Humans injected with d-tubocurarine at first have motor weakness; then their muscles become totally flaccid. The small, rapidly moving muscles—such as those of the fingers, toes, eyes, and ears—are involved before the long muscles of the limbs, neck, and trunk. The intercostal muscles and finally the diaphragm become paralyzed, and then respiration ceases.

The perianesthesia nurse should know the order of the return of muscle function after a patient has received a nondepolarizing muscle relaxant such as d-tubocurarine. The recovery of skeletal muscle function is usually in reverse order to that of paralysis; therefore the diaphragm is ordinarily first to regain function. The order of appearance of paralysis after injection with a nondepolarizing neuromuscular blocking agent can be assessed electromyographically as follows:

1. Small-sized muscle groups: Oculomotor muscles, muscles of the eyelids; muscles of the mouth and face; small extensor muscles of the fingers, followed by the flexor muscles of the fingers.
2. Medium-sized muscle groups: Muscles of the tongue and pharynx; muscles of mastication; extensor muscles of the limb, followed by flexor muscles of the limbs.
3. Large-sized muscle groups: Neck muscles, shoulder muscles, abdominal muscles, dorsal muscle mass.
4. Special muscle groups: Intercostal muscles, larynx, and diaphragm.

The order of paralysis is essentially the same after injection with a depolarizing neuromuscular agent, except that the flexor muscles are paralyzed before the extensor muscles. Patients who arrive in the PACU must be evaluated for residual effects from a neuromuscular blocking agent that was administered intraoperatively. In most instances, the action of the nondepolarizing neuromuscular blocking agent will be pharmacologically reversed at the end of the operation before the patient is admitted to the PACU; however, any patient who has received a neuromuscular blocking agent should be closely watched for signs of residual drug action. Box 21-3 describes the criteria for recovery from nondepolarizing neuromuscular blockade. The residual actions of the depolarizing muscle relaxants are similar to those of the nondepolarizing muscle relaxants, and the same nonrespiratory parameters and respiratory variables can be used to evaluate the neuromuscular blockade. The evoked (electrical stimulation) responses differ between the depolarizing and nondepolarizing neuromuscular blocking agents.

The peripheral nerve stimulator (PNS; Fig. 21-3) can be used in the PACU to assess the type and degree of a neuromuscular blockade. This electrical device can be used to stimulate the ulnar nerve at the wrist or elbow, and, on stimulation of the ulnar nerve, the nurse can observe the contraction of the fingers. The assessment of the depth of neuromuscular blockade using electrical stimulation is useful when more than 70% of the N_2 receptors are blocked by a skeletal muscle relaxant. However, in most instances, if the patient has a normal tidal volume, vital capacity, and maximal inspiratory force and can lift his or her head for 5 seconds, the use of the

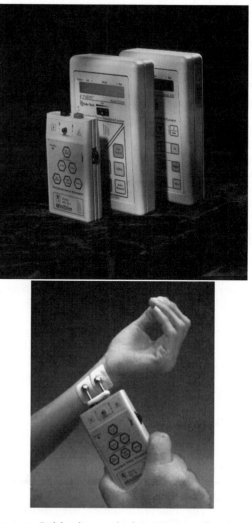

Fig. 21-3 Peripheral nerve stimulator. *(Courtesy Life-Tech, Inc., Stafford, Texas.)*

PNS is not warranted. If identification of the type of neuromuscular blockade used (depolarizing or nondepolarizing) is needed, or if some of the aforementioned parameters are marginal, the train-of-four or sustained tetanus using the PNS can be used to provide the objective data for assessment.

Although the mechanisms producing the nondepolarizing block differ from the depolarizing block, the diagnostic criteria using a PNS for assessing a nondepolarizing and phase II dual block are basically the same. Miller points out

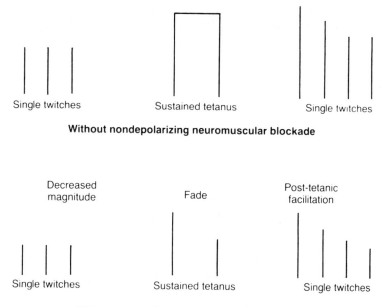

Without nondepolarizing neuromuscular blockade

With nondepolarizing neuromuscular blockade

Fig. 21-4 Magnitude of posttetanic facilitation without and with nondepolarizing neuromuscular blockade. *(Adapted from Donati F: Monitoring neuromuscular blockade. In Saidman L, Smith NT: Monitoring in anesthesia, ed 3, Woburn, Mass, 1993, Butterworth-Heinemann.)*

that the hallmark of a nondepolarizing neuromuscular blockade is an inability to sustain contraction in response to a tetanic stimulus and posttetanic facilitation. A tetanic stimulus is the usual 50 Hz of current for 5 seconds (sustained tetanus) produced by a PNS. Posttetanic facilitation is a twitch after the response to tetanic stimuli higher than the twitch immediately before tetanus. If a patient has a partial nondepolarizing neuromuscular block, an unsustained contraction called fade is seen after the initial tetanic stimulus (Fig. 21-4). Fade is caused by the decreased mobilization of acetylcholine in the nerve terminal because the presynaptic acetylcholine receptor is blocked by the nondepolarizing muscle relaxant. The responses to electrical stimulation result from the interaction of acetylcholine released and the number of N_2 cholinergic receptors occupied by the relaxant. In patients with a partial nondepolarizing neuromuscular block, the first three single electrical stimuli are of enough intensity to produce a twitch, but the twitch produced is not of the same

magnitude as a twitch produced in a subject who has not received a nondepolarizing skeletal muscle relaxant (see Fig. 21-4). The three electrical stimuli cause the normal quantum of acetylcholine to be released at the synaptic cleft; however, in this instance, the reduction in twitch magnitude is the result of the number of acetylcholine receptors being occupied by the nondepolarizing relaxant. Consequently, if the patient has had a complete nondepolarizing neuromuscular block in which all the N_2 cholinergic receptors were occupied, no twitch would be elicited from the three electrical stimuli.

In a normal subject, when a tetanic stimulus is applied for 5 seconds, the quantum of acetylcholine that is released decreases during the stimulus period. Along with this, only a fraction of nicotinic cholinergic receptors are activated at any one time to trigger an action potential. The excess in nicotinic cholinergic receptors is the safety margin of neuromuscular transmission. Consequently, in the normal subject who receives a tetanic stimulus, the magnitude of the twitch response is maintained because of the large nicotinic cholinergic receptor pool; however, if 75% of the nicotinic receptors are occupied by a nondepolarizing neuromuscular relaxant, for example, the twitch response will not be maintained, and fade (unsustained contraction) will occur because the usual margin of safety of excess acetylcholine receptors has been abolished. Between the termination of a tetanic stimulus and the first single-twitch stimulus, a buildup of acetylcholine occurs in the presynaptic knob. Thus after sustained tetanus, when the first electrical stimulus is administered, the height of the first twitch will be greater than the pretetanic twitches. These large posttetanic twitches (posttetanic facilitation) return to the pretetanic height as the acetylcholine mobilization also returns to the pretetanic level. Finally, more than 70% of the nicotinic cholinergic receptors must be occupied before this tetanic stimulation test will be sensitive enough to detect neuromuscular blockade.

The major drawback to the delivery of a 50-Hz tetanic stimulus to an awakened patient in the PACU is pain and general discomfort. For the patient who is awake and reactive, it is better to use the train-of-four stimulation to assess the degree of neuromuscular blockade caused by nondepolarizing skeletal muscle relaxants. In this test, the ulnar nerve is used, and four supramaximal electrical stimuli—2 Hz 0.05 seconds apart—are administered by a PNS. This test, which produces minimal discomfort to the awakened patient, is sensitive only when more than 70% of the nicotinic cholinergic receptors are occupied. The index of neuromuscular blockade in this test is the ratio of the fourth to the first twitch amplitude. More specifically, when the fourth response is abolished, a 75% block exists (Fig. 21-5). When the third and second responses to stimulation are abolished, the respective reductions in neuromuscular blockade are 80% and 90%. Finally, when all four twitch responses are absent, a 100%, or complete, block exists.

The depolarizing neuromuscular blockade is characterized by an absence of posttetanic facilitation, a decreased response to a single impulse, a decreased amplitude (but sustained response to a tetanic stimulus), and, if present, a train-of-four ratio between the first and fourth stimulus that is greater than 70%.

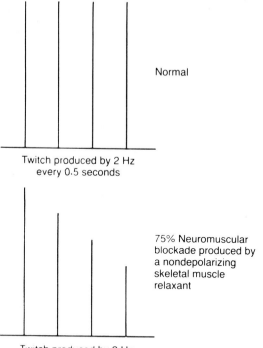

Normal

Twitch produced by 2 Hz every 0.5 seconds

75% Neuromuscular blockade produced by a nondepolarizing skeletal muscle relaxant

Twitch produced by 2 Hz every 0.5 seconds

Fig. 21-5 Diagrammatic illustration of the train-of-four in normal response and 75% neuromuscular blockade produced by a nondepolarizing skeletal muscle relaxant.

SPECIAL PROBLEMS IN THE PACU

A prolonged response to succinylcholine sometimes occurs because a patient does not possess the proper blood level of pseudocholinesterase. Other causes of a prolonged response include (1) overdosage; (2) temperature changes; (3) acid-base imbalance; (4) carcinoma; (5) antitumor agents; (6) antibiotics; (7) myasthenia gravis; and (8) liver disease.

If a patient who arrives in the PACU is apneic, controlled respiration must be initiated and maintained as long as necessary. Careful monitoring of vital signs and evaluation of renal function are important. The neuromuscular block can be identified with the PNS. If electrical stimulation results in vigorous contractions, it is unlikely that the apnea is the result of residual neuromuscular block. Consideration must then be given to other agents that may have caused the apneic state. The response of patients with

Table 21-2 Summary of the Response of Patients with Neuromuscular Disorders to Muscle Relaxants

Disorder	Pathophysiology	Response to Nondepolarizing Muscle Relaxant	Response to Depolarizing Muscle Relaxant
Hemiplegia	Sequelae of CVA; caused by an upper motor neuron in the cerebral motor cortex	Resistance	Hyperkalemia can occur as early as 1 week and as late as 6 months after stroke
Parkinson's disease	Extrapyramidal disorder	Normal	Hyperkalemia may occur
Multiple sclerosis	Demyelinating disorder of the CNS	Normal	Hyperkalemia may occur
Diffuse intracranial lesions	No focal neurologic deficits or muscular denervation or paralysis (i.e., ruptured cerebral aneurysm)	Normal	Hyperkalemia and possible cardiac arrest
Tetanus	Acute infectious disease of the CNS caused by the endotoxin released by *Clostridium tetani*	Normal	Hyperkalemia and possible cardiac arrest
Paraplegia and quadriplegia	Traumatic or pathologic transection of the spinal cord and interruption of pyramidal tracts	Increased response	Hyperkalemia as early as 3 weeks and as late as 85 days after spinal cord injury
Amyotrophic lateral sclerosis (ALS)	Degenerative disease of motor ganglia in the anterior horn of the spinal cord and of the spinal pyramidal tracts	Increased response	No reports of hyperkalemia in ALS; however, myotonia-like contracture may occur in ALS patients; avoid succinylcholine in patients with significant muscular denervation
Muscular denervation	Result of traumatic peripheral nerve damage—muscles undergo atrophy	Normal response	Muscular contracture and hyperkalemia
Myasthenia gravis (MG)	Postsynaptic reduction in the number of ACh receptors caused by autoimmune disease	Increased response and prolongation of effects	Resistance and early appearance of phase II (dual) block
Myasthenic syndrome	Differs clinically and electromyographically from MG; associated with small cell carcinoma of the lung and results in presynaptic lesion at the neuromuscular junction	Exaggerated response	Exaggerated response
Myotonias	Lesion in the muscle fiber distal to the neuromuscular junction; common symptom is delayed relaxation of skeletal muscles after voluntary contractions	Increased and prolonged; some report normal response	Unpredictable; many reports of increased rigidity
Muscular dystrophies (MD)	Disorder of the muscle fiber proper that may be secondary to a neurogenic disorder	Normal to prolonged response; ocular MD has a very high sensitivity to d-tubocurarine	Unpredictable; best to avoid use of succinylcholine

CVA, Cerebrovascular accident; *CNS*, central nervous system; *ACh*, acetylcholine.

neuromuscular disorders to muscle relaxants may include resistance, increased response, hyperkalemia, and even cardiac arrest. Table 21-2 is presented as a summary of the possible untoward responses in the clinical setting.

Phase II Block

Various terms are used to describe the different types of blocks that succinylcholine is able to produce. The phase I block is synonymous with the depolarizing block the drug ordinarily produces. It is characterized by a dose-dependent reduction in a single twitch without fade after a well-sustained tetanus and no posttetanic facilitation when the PNS is used.

Phase II block is also known as a dual block, desensitization, or open channel block. This block is caused by a conformational change in the presynaptic and postsynaptic cholinergic receptors. This anatomic change results in desensitization to the stimulation of acetylcholine. The characteristics of this block as demonstrated by the PNS are fade during the train-of-four and poorly sustained tetanus and posttetanic facilitation. The same clinical features are seen when d-tubocurarine is used; however, this does not mean that the two blocks are the same, because good evidence suggests that the d-tubocurarine and succinylcholine phase II blocks differ in several respects. Some clinicians believe that the phase II block produced by succinylcholine can be reversed with anticholinesterases such as edrophonium, which has a shorter duration of action than neostigmine. Edrophonium is used in this situation because it either reverses or potentiates the block. If potentiation occurs, it will be of a shorter duration than if neostigmine were used. Most experts believe that routine reversal to antagonize the dual block is unwarranted. It is more advisable to ventilate the patient and wait for return of the normal neuromuscular transmission.

Recurarization

Recurarization is the reappearance postoperatively of the pharmacologic actions of a nondepolarizing skeletal muscle relaxant that was administered intraoperatively. The hazard of recurarization after the use of gallamine (Flaxedil) represents a significant problem that may be encountered in the PACU. This compli-

cation arises when renal insufficiency exists. The interesting facet of this complication is that even when the gallamine is reversed sufficiently at the end of the anesthetic, recurarization may still occur for as long as 8 hours. This reappearance may be partly caused by the fading of the effect of the neostigmine. Gallamine is normally excreted after 2 hours, but in renal insufficiency the excretion of the drug is poor and may take as long as 30 hours. Therefore in patients with renal insufficiency in whom gallamine was used, signs of delayed excretion (weakness of the ocular muscles, difficulty in swallowing, or decrease in ventilation) should warrant attention. If symptoms appear, the required level of the reversal agent (neostigmine) must be maintained until that portion of the gallamine has been eliminated so that symptoms do not reappear. If recurarization occurs, the postoperative use of morphine and similar narcotics should be avoided because these agents will enhance a residual neuromuscular block sufficiently to make it clinically significant.

Recurarization from d-tubocurarine does not usually occur because only 20% to 40% of the drug is excreted through the kidneys. In some reported cases, recurarization due to d-tubocurarine was caused by an increased sensitivity of the myoneural junction associated with a decrease in the plasma potassium concentration.

Bradycardia

Another problem that occurs in the PACU is the appearance of bradycardia when a patient has received an atropine-neostigmine combination at the end of the anesthetic. The bradycardia is usually the result of the longer duration of action of neostigmine in comparison to that of atropine. The treatment for this problem is glycopyrrolate. Glycopyrrolate should not be administered, however, until other causes of bradycardia are eliminated, such as pain, hypoventilation, and a full bladder.

BIBLIOGRAPHY

Alspach J: Core curriculum for critical care nursing, ed 5, Philadelphia, 1998, WB Saunders.

Atlee J: Complications in anesthesia, Philadelphia, 1999, WB Saunders.

Barash P, Cullen B, Stoelting R: Clinical anesthesia, ed 4, Philadelphia, 2000, Lippincott Williams & Wilkins.

Basta S, Savarese K, Ali H et al: Clinical pharmacology of doxacurium chloride: a new long-acting nondepolarizing muscle relaxant, Anesthesiology 69:478-486, 1988.

Bevan D, Smith C, Donati F: Postoperative neuromuscular blockade: a comparison between atracurium, vecuronium, and pancuronium, Anesthesiology 69(2):272-276, 1988.

Benumof J: Anesthesia and uncommon diseases, ed 4, Philadelphia, 1998, WB Saunders.

Benumof J, Saidman L: Anesthesia & perioperative complications, ed 2, St Louis, 1999, Mosby.

Bickley L, Hoekelman R: Bates' guide to physical examination and history taking, ed 7, Philadelphia, 1998, Lippincott Williams & Wilkins.

Bowdle T, Horita A, Kharasch E: The pharmacologic basis of anesthesiology, New York, 1994, Churchill Livingstone.

Brown J, Foster S, Anderson C et al: The literature and perspectives on muscle relaxants for rapid-sequence induction, Nurse Anesth 2(2):72-88, 1991.

DeFazio-Quinn D: Ambulatory surgical nursing core curriculum, Philadelphia, 1999, WB Saunders.

Emmott R, Bracey B, Goldhill D et al: Cardiovascular effects of doxacurium, pancuronium, and vecuronium in anaesthetized patients presenting for coronary artery bypass surgery, Br J Anesth 65:480-486, 1990.

Erkola O, Karhunen U, Sandelin-Hellqvist E: Spontaneous recovery of residual neuromuscular blockade after atracurium or vecuronium during isoflurane anaesthesia, Acta Anaesthesiol Scand 33:290-294, 1991.

Ganong W: Review of medical physiology, ed 20, New York, 2001, McGraw-Hill Professional.

Goldhill D, Whitehead J, Emmott R et al: Neuromuscular and clinical effects of mivacurium chloride in healthy adult patients during nitrous oxide-enflurane anaesthesia, Br J Anaesth 67(3):289-295, 1991.

Guyton A, Hall J: Textbook of medical physiology, ed 10, Philadelphia, 2000, WB Saunders.

Hardman J, Limbird L: Goodman and Gilman's the pharmacological basis of therapeutics, ed 10, New York, 2001, McGraw-Hill.

Jacobsen W: Manual of post anesthesia care, Philadelphia, 1992, WB Saunders.

Katzung B, editor: Basic and clinical pharmacology, ed 8, Los Altos, Calif, 2000, Appleton & Lange.

Lambalk L, De Wit A, Wierda J et al: Dose-response relationship and time course of action of Org 9426: a new muscle relaxant of intermediate duration evaluated under various anesthetic techniques, Anaesthesia 46:907-911, 1991.

Larijani G, Bartkowski RR, Azad SS: Clinical pharmacology of pipecuronium bromide, Anesth Analg, 68:734-739, 1989.

Longnecker D, Murphy F: Dripps/Eckenhoff/Vandam introduction to anesthesia, ed 9, Philadelphia, 1997, WB Saunders.

Longnecker D, Tinker J, Morgan G: Principles and practice of anesthesiology, ed 2, St Louis, Mosby, 1998.

McIntosh L: Essentials of nurse anesthesia, New York, 1997, McGraw-Hill.

Miller R, Rupp S, Fisher D et al: Clinical pharmacology of vecuronium and atracurium, Anesthesiology 61(4):444-453, 1984.

Miller R, editor: Anesthesia, ed 5, New York, 2000, Churchill Livingstone.

Nagelhout J, Zaglaniczny K: Nurse anesthesia, ed 2, Philadelphia, 2001, WB Saunders.

Oduro K: Glycopyrrolate methobromide: comparison with atropine sulfate in anaesthesia, Can Anaesth Soc J 22(4):466-473, 1975.

Ostheimer G: A comparison of glycopyrrolate and atropine during reversal of nondepolarizing neuromuscular block with neostigmine, Anesth Analg 56:182-186, 1977.

Pittet J: Neuromuscular effect of pipecuronium bromide in infants and children during nitrous oxide-alfentanil anesthesia, Anesthesiology 73(2):432-436, 1991.

Reep B: Complications associated with the administration of succinylcholine, AANA J 40(3):193-203, 1972.

Savarese J, Hassan H, Antonio R: The clinical pharmacology of metocurine: dimethyltubocurarine revisited, Anesthesiology 47(3):277-284, 1977.

Schweinefus R, Schick L: Succinylcholine: "good guy, bad guy," J Post Anesth Nurs 6(6):410-419, 1991.

Stoelting R: Pharmacology and physiology in anesthetic practice, ed 3, Philadelphia, 1999, Lippincott-Raven.

Stoelting R, Miller R: Basics of anesthesia, ed 4, New York, 2000, Churchill Livingstone.

Stone D: Perioperative Care: anesthesia, medicine, and surgery, St Louis, 1998, Mosby.

Waugaman W, Foster S, Rigor B: Principles and practice of nurse anesthesia, ed 3, Norwalk, Conn, 1999, Appleton & Lange.

Weinberg G: Basic science review of anesthesiology, New York, 1997, McGraw-Hill.

Wicks T: Mivacurium chloride, Nurse Anesth 3(4):173-182, 1992.

Zarr G: Pharmacology of neuromuscular blockade and antagonism. In Waugaman W, Foster S, Rigor B: Principles and practice of nurse anesthesia, ed 3, Stamford, Conn, 1999, Appleton & Lange.

Zuurmond W, van Leeuwen L: Atracurium versus vecuronium: a comparison of recovery in outpatient arthroscopy, Can J Anaesth 35(2):139-142, 1988.

22

LOCAL ANESTHETICS

Charles H. Moore, PhD, CRNA

Local anesthetic agents are defined as pharmacologic agents capable of producing a loss of sensation in an area of the body. They were first used in 1884, when cocaine was employed as a topical anesthetic agent by Freud and Köller, and in 1885, when Halsted used cocaine to prevent nerve conduction in the lower extremities. The actual advent of the use of local anesthetics in anesthetic practice was not until 1943, when Lofgren synthesized procaine. Local anesthetics are used in all forms of regional anesthesia. The term regional anesthesia refers to the various anesthetic techniques that use local anesthetic agents to block nerve conduction in an extremity or a region of the body (see Chapter 23). Among the types of regional anesthesia are topical, infiltration, field block, and conduction. Topical anesthesia is produced when an anesthetic agent is applied to a surface, such as the skin, mucus membrane, urethra, nose, and pharynx. A new topical anesthetic that can be used on the skin to provide analgesia during venipuncture is called EMLA (eutectic mixture of local anesthetics). This drug is a mixture of 2.5% lidocaine and 2.5% prilocaine. Infiltration anesthesia is produced by injecting a local anesthetic into the tissue to be cut. Field block anesthesia is produced by injecting a local anesthetic agent into the surrounding tissues of an area being prepared for operation. Conduction anesthesia is produced by injecting a local anesthetic agent into a nerve or nerves that supply a region of the body to eliminate sensation or motor control or both. Epidural and subarachnoid blocks are conduction blocks.

The use of regional anesthesia has become popular in modern anesthesia practice because,

when indicated, it offers many advantages over general inhalation anesthesia. To facilitate optimal recovery of the surgical patient from this type of anesthetic, the postanesthesia care unit (PACU) nurse must first have a complete knowledge of the physiology of nerve conduction as well as the pharmacology of local anesthetic agents, including their mechanism of action, effects, and toxicity.

PHYSIOLOGY OF NERVES, NERVE CONDUCTION, AND LOCAL ANESTHETICS

Nerves conduct impulses, or action potentials, that provide information to the central nervous system (CNS) about the type, degree, and magnitude of pain. Inside the nerve cell (including the axon) is cytoplasm that contains positively charged potassium ions and negatively charged proteins. The potassium ions can freely move in and out of the cytoplasm, whereas the proteins are not freely diffusible. The fluid outside the nerve cell and axon contains positively charged sodium ions and negatively charged chloride ions. These ions are freely diffusible into the cytoplasm. However, via a sodium pump, the sodium is quickly pushed out of the nerve cell. Outside the nerve cell, the concentration of the negatively charged ion chloride is large and the concentration of the positively charged potassium is low. Inside the nerve cell, this ratio is reversed; the concentration of potassium is high and the concentration of the negatively charged chloride ions is low. The freely diffusible potassium ions are held inside the nerve cell by an excess of negatively charged ions. Because of the excess of negatively charged ions, an electrical potential of about −70 to −90 mV exists.

When the nerve impulse is conducted down the nerve fiber, the nerve membranes become permeable (because of depolarization) to the positively charged sodium ions. These sodium ions are conducted through pores, or sodium channels, in which a "gate" regulates their passage to the inside of the nerve cell. As the sodium ions reach the inside of the nerve cell, the electrical potential changes to +40 mV. This change from negative to positive is about 110 mV and represents the movement of an action potential down a nerve fiber or, in neurophysiologic terms, propagation of an action potential. Once the sodium has reached a certain ionic concentration, the gate closes in the sodium channels. The membrane permeability to potassium increases, thus allowing potassium back into the cytoplasm, and sodium is pumped out of the nerve cell, which will slowly return the ionic potential to its resting level of −70 to −90 mV.

Local anesthetics are quite lipid soluble and, consequently, can diffuse through the cell membrane into the axoplasm. They ionize and occupy a receptor near the gate of the sodium channel. Thus the local anesthetic prevents the opening of the gate, and sodium cannot enter the inside of the nerve, which results in a slowing of the rate of depolarization. Consequently, a nerve action potential cannot be reached, and blockage of the nerve's electrical conduction system ensues.

The afferent nerve fibers that conduct impulses to the spinal cord are classified as A, B, and C, based on fiber diameter and conduction velocity. The A fibers are further divided into A-alpha, A-beta, A-gamma, and A-delta fibers. The large-diameter A fibers are myelinated and have the fastest conduction velocity. The A-alpha fibers have the largest diameter and the fastest conduction velocity. They provide innervation of motor function to the skeletal muscles. The moderately myelinated A-beta fibers are the next largest in diameter and speed, and they are responsible for touch and pressure. The sensation of proprioception and skeletal muscle tone are maintained by the A-gamma fibers, which are smaller in diameter and are slower than the preceding A-beta fibers. The A-delta fibers are lightly myelinated and are the smallest and slowest of the A fibers. They are responsible for

---

Box 22-1 Emergence Sequence of a Nerve Block

1. Motor paralysis
2. Proprioception (awareness of body or extremity position) lost
3. Pressure sense abolished
4. Tactile sense lost
5. Slow and fast pain
6. Temperature discrimination lost
7. Sensation of warmth by patient
8. Block of cold temperature fibers
9. Vasomotor block-dilatation of skin vessels and increased cutaneous blood flow

---

conducting sensations of fast pain, touch, and temperature. The lightly myelinated B fibers are smaller than the A fibers and are the preganglionic autonomic fibers. The smallest fibers are the unmyelinated C fibers. They function as postganglionic sympathetic fibers and also conduct sensations such as slow pain and temperature.

Local anesthetics can penetrate and prevent nerve conduction in the smallest nerve fibers first and the large A-alpha fibers last. Consequently, during the emergence from conduction anesthesia, a particular order of return is seen that is based solely on the reduced concentration gradient of the local anesthetic and the fiber size (Box 22-1). For example, after epidural and peripheral nerve or plexus blocks, the large A-alpha fibers will return first, and the patient will have a return of motor function. The next fibers to return are the A-beta and A-gamma, and the patient will have a return of proprioception, touch, and pressure. Finally, a return of pain and a loss of a sensation of warmth occurs as a result of low concentration of local anesthetic in the A-delta, B, and C fibers.

Pain, which is called nociception, is a protective mechanism that occurs when tissues are damaged. There are two major types of pain: fast and slow. Fast pain is a well defined, stabbing sensation that is rather short in duration. Causes of fast pain include surgical incision and pin pricks. Fast pain is conducted via the small afferent, myelinated A-delta nerve fibers. Slow pain is not well defined and is characterized as a burning or aching sensation. In this type of pain, even after the pain stimulus is removed, the pain may continue. The efferent conducting nerves in this instance are the unmyelinated C fibers.

THE LOCAL ANESTHETICS

The ideal local anesthetic should have the following properties: selectivity of action, low toxicity, complete reversibility, nonirritation, short latency, good penetration, sufficient duration, solubility in saline and water, stability, and compatibility with vasoconstrictors. Not all local anesthetic agents possess all these attributes. As new agents are discovered, they are measured against these criteria.

In regard to their analgesic activity, local anesthetic agents can be divided into three groups according to potency. Procaine and chloroprocaine are the least potent of the commonly employed agents, whereas lidocaine, cocaine, mepivacaine, and prilocaine are compounds of intermediate potency—that is, they are twice as potent as procaine. Tetracaine, bupivacaine (and its isomers ropivacaine and chirocaine), and etidocaine are drugs of high potency that are approximately six to eight times more active than procaine.

The local anesthetic agents are grouped pharmacologically into two categories: the amides and the esters (Table 22-1). The amides are metabolized in the liver, have no real history of documented allergic reactions, have good penetration, and are stable. Drugs in this category are lidocaine, mepivacaine, prilocaine, etidocaine, and bupivacaine. The esters, except for cocaine, are hydrolyzed primarily in the plasma by plasma pseudocholinesterase and are metabolized more rapidly than the amides. Because the esters are metabolized to para-aminobenzoic acid, they are associated with an increased incidence of allergic reactions. In general, the esters have poor penetrance, rare allergic reactions, and fair to poor stability. Epinephrine is added to some local anesthetic agents because it is a vasoconstrictor and therefore prolongs the activity of the local agent and decreases its toxicity by slowing its uptake.

The Short-Duration Local Anesthetics

Procaine (Novocain). Procaine was one of the first ester local anesthetics, first synthesized by Einhorn in 1905. Because it ionizes so quickly, it has poor spreading and penetrating properties. Because it can produce vasodilatation, epinephrine is usually added to procaine to delay systemic absorption. The use of procaine is usually for infiltration anesthesia in a 1% or 2% solution or spinal anesthesia in a 5% solution. Allergic reactions have been reported after repeated doses of procaine.

Chloroprocaine (Nesacaine). Chloroprocaine is an analogue of procaine with low toxicity, a rapid onset of 10 minutes, and a short duration of action of about 45 minutes. Chloroprocaine can be used for most types of regional anesthesia. However, chloroprocaine with preservatives is rarely administered epidurally because of the risk of neurotoxicity caused by accidental injection into the subarachnoid space. Along with this, chloroprocaine is not used for spinal anesthesia because of its potential of neurotoxicity. Preservative-free chloroprocaine can still be used for epidural anesthesia without risk of neurotoxicity. The multiple-dose vial of chloroprocaine with preservatives (sodium bisulfite and methylparaben) should be used only for infiltration anesthesia. Rapid, inadvertent intrathecal injection of a low pH and bisulfite-containing solution can cause motor and sensory deficits.

The Intermediate-Duration Local Anesthetics

Cocaine. Cocaine has three distinctive actions: (1) it can block nerve conduction; (2) it can produce euphoria and sympathetic and CNS stimulation; and (3) it is highly addictive. Cocaine is used primarily for topical anesthesia and probably should not be administered parenterally. This is because it is addictive and has many toxic side effects when administered in any form other than topical. The major cardiovascular effect of cocaine is that it interferes with the reuptake mechanism of catecholamines and consequently can potentiate all vasopressors and cause cardiac dysrhythmias and seizures when administered in high doses.

Lidocaine (Xylocaine). Lidocaine is one of the most widely used local anesthetics in the world. It can be used for topical, infiltration, field block, spinal, epidural, and caudal anesthesia. For topical anesthesia, a 4% solution is usually used, and in this form its onset of action is about 5 minutes, and its effects last for about 20 minutes. When lidocaine is administered for local

Table 22-1   Local Anesthetic Agents: Esters and Amides

Agent	Use	Discussion
ESTERS		
Cocaine	Topical: 4%-20% for use in nose and throat procedures; duration, 10-55 minutes; maximum dose, 3 mg/kg	Topical use only; vasoconstrictor; CNS stimulant in abuse
Procaine (Novocain)	Topical: 10%-20% required; infiltration: 0.25%-0.5%; nerve block: 1%-2%; duration, 20-30 minutes plain, 45 minutes with epinephrine; maximum dose, 10 mg/kg plain and 14 mg/kg with epinephrine	Low potency, rapid hydrolysis in plasma, mild acetylcholine inhibition, poor stability
Chloroprocaine (Nesacaine)	Infiltration: 10 mg/ml solution; peripheral nerve block: 10 and 20 mg/ml solution; epidural block: 20-30 mg/ml solution	Not topically active; more potent but shorter duration of action than procaine. The safest local anesthetic in regard to systemic toxicity. The onset of action is 6-12 minutes, and the duration of anesthesia is 30-60 minutes. Total dose should not exceed 1 g with epinephrine and 800 mg without epinephrine; 12 times more potent than procaine
Tetracaine (Pontocaine)	Topical: 0.5%-1%, duration, 55 minutes; infiltration: 0.1%-0.25%; nerve block: 0.25%, duration, 3-4 hr plain, 5-7 hours with epinephrine; maximum dose, 1.5-2 mg/kg plain and 2-3 mg/kg with epinephrine	
AMIDES		
Lidocaine (Xylocaine)	Topical: 2%-4% onset, 2-4 minutes, maximum dose, 3 mg/kg; nerve block: 1%-2%, maximum dose, 4-5 mg/kg plain or 7 mg/kg with epinephrine; duration, 1 hour plain, 2 hours with epinephrine; antiarrhythmic, 1 mg/kg bolus, then 1-2 mg/min intravenous drip	Rapid onset, intense analgesia, good penetration, stable. As antiarrhythmic, it depresses the automaticity of the Purkinje fibers and decreases their effective refractory period
Mepivacaine (Carbocaine)	Infiltration: 0.5-1%; nerve block: 1-2%, maximum dose, 5-6 mg/kg plain, and 7 mg/kg with epinephrine; duration, 1.5 hr plain, 2 hr with epinephrine	Derivative of lidocaine; less penetrance, slower metabolism; ineffective topically
Bupivacaine (Marcaine)	Infiltration: 0.1%-0.25%; nerve block: 0.25%-0.5%; long-acting, up to 12 hours	Less penetrance than other amides
Ropivacaine	Labor: 0.1%-0.2% less motor block	Less cardiotoxicity than Bupivacaine
Levobupivacaine	Infiltration: 0.25%; epidural 0.75%, onset 15 minutes, duration 5-7 hours	Similar to bupivacaine; similar efficacy but enhanced safety profile compared to bupivacaine
Dibucaine (Nupercaine)	Topical: 2 mg/ml ointment, up to 15 ml; spinal: 2.5-5 mg/ml	Mainly used as topical anesthesia; because of high systemic toxicity, rarely used for spinal anesthesia
Etidocaine (Duranest)	Infiltration: 2.5-5 mg/ml solution; peripheral nerve block: 5 and 10 mg/ml solution; epidural block: 5 and 10 mg/ml solution	Greater potency and longer duration of action than lidocaine. Maximum dose of a single injection should not exceed 400 mg in the adult

infiltration in a 0.5% to 1% solution, the onset of anesthesia is from 2 to 5 minutes, with a duration of action of about 75 minutes. For brachial plexus (axillary) blocks, the drug has an onset of about 5 to 10 minutes and a duration of about 60 minutes without epinephrine and 120 minutes with epinephrine. A caudal block requires a 1% or 2% solution of lidocaine. The onset of anesthesia is between 5 and 15 minutes, with a duration of about 100 minutes with epinephrine and 60 minutes without epinephrine.

Over the past decade the use of 5% lidocaine for spinal anesthesia has come into question. Case reports and other studies have implicated 5% lidocaine as the cause of neurologic symptoms following spinal anesthesia. In an attempt to limit the potential for neurologic sequelae after spinal anesthesia with lidocaine it is now recommended that lidocaine be used in a 1.5% solution rather than the traditional 5% concentration.

The onset of spinal anesthesia is between 5 and 10 minutes, and the duration is about 60 minutes without epinephrine and 90 minutes with epinephrine.

Lidocaine can be used as an antidysrhythmic agent at an intravenous dose of 1 mg per kg. Infusion rates for this drug range from 20 to 50 µg/kg per minute. Lidocaine can be used for postoperative analgesia when it is administered in a slow, continuous intravenous infusion. When this technique is used, the plasma level of lidocaine should be between 1 and 2 µg/ml. Lidocaine can also be used to prevent increases in intracranial pressure and hypertension associated with endotracheal intubation, a bolus dose of 1.5 mg/kg of lidocaine given intravenously is helpful. The upper limits of safe dosage for this drug are between 200 and 400 mg without epinephrine and 500 mg with epinephrine. Toxic symptoms develop when the blood level of lidocaine increases about 5 µg/ml. Seizures and respiratory and cardiac depression have been reported when the blood level of lidocaine is higher than 8 µg/ml.

Mepivacaine (Carbocaine).   Mepivacaine, an amide local anesthetic, is similar to lidocaine in its uses and onset of action; however, its duration of action is longer than lidocaine. Mepivacaine does not produce vasodilatation and consequently is an attractive alternative to other local anesthetics that require epinephrine. Mepivacaine should not be used for topical anesthesia.

The upper limits of safe dosage for the drug are 400 mg without epinephrine and 500 mg with epinephrine. At high doses, mepivacaine can depress both respiratory and cardiac functions.

Prilocaine (Citanest).   Prilocaine is quite similar to lidocaine in its uses and potency. However, it has a lower toxicity and shorter duration of action than lidocaine. The major reason that prilocaine is not as widely used as lidocaine is that it can cause significant complications. One complication associated with prilocaine is methemoglobinemia, especially when the dosage exceeds 500 mg. The treatment for this problem is usually methylene blue given over 5 minutes intravenously at a dosage of 1 to 2 mg/kg.

The Long-Duration Local Anesthetics

Bupivacaine (Marcaine; Sensorcaine).   Bupivacaine is an amide local anesthetic that is about four times as potent as lidocaine. Like lidocaine, it is widely used in clinical practice. For infiltration anesthesia, it can be used in a 0.125% to 0.25% solution without epinephrine. For this type of anesthesia, it has an onset of 5 to 15 minutes and a duration of about 200 minutes. The duration of action of bupivacaine can be doubled by the addition of epinephrine. For axillary block and other nerve block techniques, including epidural anesthesia, bupivacaine is administered in a 0.25% to 0.5% solution. In this instance, the onset of action is about 15 minutes, and the duration is about 2 to 4 hours. For spinal anesthesia, 0.75% bupivacaine is in a solution with dextrose. The dose range is between 5 and 20 mg, and the onset is between 8 and 15 minutes, with a duration of action between 2 and 4 hours. Bupivacaine is the drug of choice for lower extremity surgery when a tourniquet is used. Tourniquet pain is transmitted by the very small C fibers. Bupivacaine is able to better block the C fibers than is tetracaine.

A 0.75%, or 7.5 mg/ml, concentration of bupivacaine is not recommended for obstetric (except spinal) or intravenous regional anesthesia. The upper limits for safe dosage with this drug are 150 mg without epinephrine and 200 mg with epinephrine. In patients who receive diazepam (Valium), bupivacaine can be potentiated because diazepam increases the bioavailability of bupivacaine. If bupivacaine is accidentally administered intravenously, acute cardiovascular collapse can ensue.

Ropivacaine. Ropivacaine is a new local anesthetic that resembles bupivacaine in potency and length of action. It may have certain advantages over bupivacaine when used in obstetrics. This is because it produces less motor blockage while it keeps the patient analgesic. Ropivacaine can be used for epidural anesthesia because it produces a rapid onset of sensory loss and has a relatively long duration.

Levobupivacaine (Chirocaine). Levobupivacaine is a newly released amide local anesthetic that contains only the pure S-enantiomer of bupivacaine. Studies indicate that levobupivacaine may be less toxic than bupivacaine at similar analgesic concentrations. Currently, however, levobupivacaine does not enjoy widespread use.

Etidocaine (Duranest). Etidocaine resembles lidocaine in time of onset; however, its duration of action is considerably longer than lidocaine. It is effective in infiltration, spinal, epidural, and caudal anesthesia. It can cause a profound motor blockade and, consequently, should not be administered to obstetric patients. The safe dosage limit for etidocaine is 300 mg without epinephrine and 400 mg with epinephrine.

Tetracaine (Pontocaine). Tetracaine is an ester local anesthetic that resembles procaine and chloroprocaine. It is metabolized by plasma pseudocholinesterase at a slower rate than other ester local anesthetics.

It is used predominately for spinal anesthesia in a 1% solution. The dosage range for spinal anesthesia is usually between 5 and 20 mg, with an onset of about 7 to 10 minutes and a duration of about 60 to 90 minutes. The addition of a vasoconstrictor increases the duration of the spinal block to about 120 to 180 minutes. Tetracaine can be potentiated by cimetidine (Tagamet). When the blood concentration of tetracaine exceeds 8 μg/ml, serious problems can occur, including seizures and severe depression of the respiratory and cardiovascular systems.

Complications of Use of Local Anesthetics

Allergic Reactions. Allergic reactions to local anesthetic drugs can be divided into four types: (1) contact dermatitis; (2) serum sickness, which includes fever, lymphadenopathy, and urticaria 2 to 12 days after injection; (3) anaphylactic reaction, characterized by dyspnea, cyanosis, and death; and (4) atopic response, which includes

---

Box 22-2	**Signs of Overdosage of Local Anesthetic Agents**

CENTRAL NERVOUS SYSTEM
Stimulation of:
Cortex: excitement, disorientation, euphoria, dizziness, hallucinations, muscle twitching, numbness of fingers or lips, and convulsions
Medulla:
    Cardiovascular center: hypertension, tachycardia
    Respiratory center: increased respiratory rate and variations in rhythm
    Vomiting center: nausea and vomiting
Depression of:
Cortex: unconsciousness
Medulla:
    Vasomotor center: hypotension
    Respiratory center: apnea

PERIPHERAL NERVOUS SYSTEM
Heart: bradycardia due to direct depression
Blood vessels: vasodilatation from direct action

---

bronchospasm, urticaria, and angioneurotic edema.

When the allergy is being evaluated, the first consideration is whether or not the reaction is caused by added epinephrine. Symptoms such as tachycardia, palpitations, restlessness, and anxiety indicate epinephrine as the causative agent.

Overdosage. Overdosage of local anesthetic agents can occur because of inadvertent intravenous injection of the local anesthetic, variation in patient response, or injection of the local anesthetic into a highly vascular area. Box 22-2 summarizes the signs of overdosage of the local anesthetic agents.

The treatment and nursing care of a patient who has had an overdosage of a local anesthetic agent begin with the administration of 100% oxygen. Oxygen should be administered to the patient at the first sign of local anesthetic toxicity. This should be followed by preparation for the management of convulsions, hypotension, and respiratory depression. Diazepam should be administered to suppress local anesthetic-induced seizures. Intubation and mechanical ventilation may be indicated. Vasopressors such as epinephrine may also be indicated.

BIBLIOGRAPHY

Barash P, Cullen B, Stoelting R: Clinical anesthesia, ed 3, Philadelphia, 1997, JB Lippincott.

Cousins M, Bridenbaugh P: Neural blockade. In Clinical anesthesia and management of pain, ed 3, Philadelphia, 1998, Lippincott-Raven.

De Jong R: Local anesthetics, St Louis, 1994, Mosby.

Guyton A: Textbook of medical physiology, ed 8, Philadelphia, 1991, WB Saunders.

Hardman J, Limbird L: Goodman and Gilman's the pharmacological basis of therapeutics, ed 9, New York, 1996, McGraw-Hill.

Macintyre P, Ready B: Acute pain management: a practical guide, ed 2, New York, 2001, WB Saunders.

Mcleod G, Burke D: Levobupivacaine, Anaesthesia 56:331-341, 2001.

Miller R, editor: Anesthesia, ed 5, Philadelphia, 2000, Churchill Livingstone.

Saleh K: Practical points in understanding local anesthetics, J Post Anesth Nurs 7(1):45-47, 1992.

Schneider M, Ettlin T, Kaufmann M et al: Transient neurologic toxicity after hyperbaric subarachnoid anesthesia with 5% lidocaine, Anesth Analg 76(5): 1154-1157, 1993.

Waugaman W, Foster S, Rigor B: Principles and practice of nurse anesthesia, ed 3, Norwalk, Conn, 1999, Appleton & Lange.

Wood M, Wood A: Drugs and anesthesia: pharmacology for the anesthesiologist, ed 2, Baltimore, 1990, Williams & Wilkins.

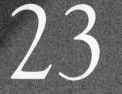

REGIONAL ANESTHESIA

Charles H. Moore, PhD, CRNA

The term regional anesthesia refers to the various anesthetic techniques that use local anesthetic agents to block nerve conduction in an extremity or a region of the body. The use of regional anesthesia has become popular in modern anesthesia practice because, when indicated, it offers many advantages over general inhalation anesthesia. To facilitate optimal recovery of the surgical patient from this type of anesthetic, the postanesthesia care unit (PACU) nurse should have a complete knowledge of all the particular regional anesthetic techniques employed.

SPINAL AND EPIDURAL ANESTHESIA

Anatomy of the Spine

The vertebral column comprises 33 vertebrae (7 cervical, 12 thoracic, 5 lumbar, 5 sacral, and 4 coccygeal). The ligaments of the vertebral column, which bind it together and protect the spinal cord, are the supraspinous ligament, intraspinous ligament, ligamentum flavum, posterior longitudinal ligament, and anterior longitudinal ligament (Fig. 23-1). When a midline spinal puncture is made, the needle will traverse the first three ligaments.

The spinal cord, which is a continuation of the medulla oblongata, occupies the upper two thirds of the vertebral canal. It is approximately 18 inches long, and it ends at the lower border of L1. The lower portion of the spinal cord then becomes the filum terminale, which connects to the bone of the coccyx vertebra and holds the spinal cord in place. The spinal cord is encased by three membranes: the dura mater, the arachnoid, and the pia mater. The outermost membrane is the dura mater, which consists of two

layers (periosteal and dural) and ends at S2. Between the dura and the ligamentum flavum is the epidural space, which is a potential space filled with loose fatty tissue and blood vessels. It is in this space that local anesthetic solutions are introduced when the epidural regional anesthetic technique is used. The arachnoid layer consists of a thin membranous sheath. The innermost layer is called the pia mater, and it is separated from the arachnoid layer by a subarachnoid space filled with cerebrospinal fluid (CSF). This space is where local anesthetic solutions are deposited when the spinal technique of producing regional anesthesia is used.

There are 31 pairs of spinal nerves that travel from the spinal column through the layers of the cord and exit at the intervertebral foramina. There are 8 cervical, 12 thoracic, 5 lumbar, 5 sacral, and 1 coccygeal pairs of spinal nerves. It is these nerves that are blocked by the local anesthetic drug to produce anesthesia.

Spinal Anesthetics
Techniques of Administration.   Because a lumbar puncture may be performed in the PACU, a brief description of the procedure of lumbar puncture will be presented. Before the procedure is started, the PACU nurse should ensure that the spinal (or epidural) procedure is not contraindicated. The absolute contraindications are anatomic abnormalities, coagulation abnormalities, patient refusal, infection at the site of the needle insertion, and uncorrected hypovolemia. The relative contraindications are chronic back pain, bacteremia, neurologic disorders such as multiple sclerosis, and patients who are receiving minidose heparin.

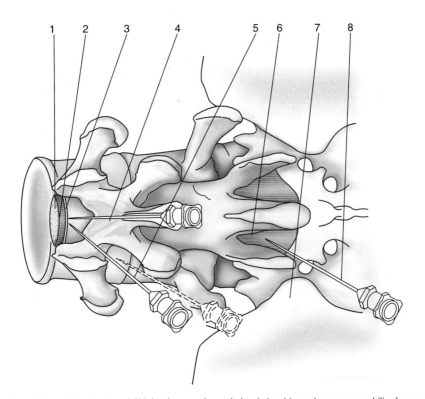

Fig. 23-1 The dorsal view of the fourth and fifth lumbar vertebrae, their relationship to the sacrum and iliac bones, and the most frequently used approaches for needle puncture in subarachnoid and lumbar peridural techniques. Numerals represent the following: (1) the cauda equina; (2) the dura mater; (3) the ligamentum flavum at the L3–L4 interspace; (4) the midline approach for spinal and epidural techniques, in which the needle is introduced between the spines of L3 and L4 vertebrae, traversing the supraspinous and interspinous ligaments before piercing the ligamentum flavum; (5) the paramedian approach at this level where the needle puncture site is 1 to 2 cm lateral to the above midline approach; if the initial approach results in contacting the lamina of the vertebrae as shown in the dotted needle silhouette, the needle is walked cephalad and medially until it slips off the lamina and contacts the ligamentum flavum as shown; (6) the large interspace between S5 and L1, which is situated 2 cm medial and cephalad from (7) the posterior superior iliac spine; (8) the needle can be introduced at this site in the Taylor approach for either subarachnoid or epidural puncture. *(From Miller R: Anesthesia, ed 2, New York, 2000, Churchill Livingstone.)*

Once it has been determined that the spinal procedure is not contraindicated, the PACU nurse should obtain the patient's baseline vital signs. These should include the blood pressure, pulse, respiratory rate, and oxygen saturation. The blood pressure cuff and pulse oximeter should remain in place throughout the procedure. Also, the nurse should describe the procedure to the patient and answer any questions he or she might have. Verbal contact with the patient throughout the procedure is important in reducing fear and anxiety.

Proper positioning of the patient is important in facilitating the success of this procedure. The lateral decubitus position or sitting position can be used. To place the patient in the lateral decubitus position, the patient is turned on his or her side, the knees are then bent and drawn up near the patient's chin, and his or her back is arched out toward the person who is performing the lumbar puncture. A pillow may be placed under the patient's head to help align the spine and to add comfort during the procedure. The assistant should stand near the patient's stomach to secure his or her knees and provide for safety throughout the procedure. At this time the patient's back should be inspected for signs of any dermatologic infectious process that may be present. If an infectious process near the lumbar puncture site is found, the procedure should be canceled. Once the patient is properly positioned, the person performing the procedure should first wash his or her hands and then open the lumbar puncture tray so that the sterile components are available and—using sterile technique—don the sterile gloves. The drugs are then drawn into the syringes and the needles and equipment examined for any signs of damage. The back is then washed (prepped) with antiseptic solution, after which the sterile drapes are placed over the patient's back. Throughout the procedure, the PACU nurse should continue to explain each maneuver to the patient. An imaginary line, called Tuffier's line, is then drawn between the iliac crests. This line crosses the spine between the third or fourth lumbar interspace. Because the spinal cord terminates at the L2 interspace, from L3 and below are used when the lumbar puncture is performed. Once the interspace has been identified, a local anesthetic (usually procaine) is deposited subcutaneously and into the supraspinous ligament with a 25-gauge needle. A needle introducer is then placed through the skin, the supraspinous ligament, and interspinous ligaments. The spinal needle is inserted through the introducer and is passed through the ligamentum flavum and the dura and enters the subarachnoid space. The stylet is removed, and CSF can be seen at the hub of the needle. Blood-tinged CSF or lack of free flow is a contraindication to the injection of the anesthetic solution. If the blood-tinged CSF becomes clear, the anesthetic solution can be administered. Before the syringe is connected to the hub of the needle, the patient should be secured and told not to move or cough by the PACU nurse. The patient should also be told that his or her legs will feel warm after the anesthetic solution is injected. The syringe is then secured to the hub of the needle, and after aspiration to ensure that CSF is still present, the anesthetic solution is injected. After the solution is injected, the syringe is aspirated to verify the presence of CSF, thus confirming the introduction of the medications into the subarachnoid space. After confirmation, the syringe, needle, and introducer

are removed simultaneously. Next, the PACU nurse and the person who performed the lumbar puncture place the patient in the supine position. Before the patient is moved, he or she should be told not to try to move or cough because that would increase the spread of the anesthetics.

Once the patient is supine, his or her blood pressure, pulse, respiratory rate, and oxygen saturation should be assessed at 1-minute intervals for the first 5 to 10 minutes and then every 5 minutes during the next half hour. If the oxygen saturation drops below 94% or the blood pressure decreases by 20% of the baseline reading, the anesthesia practitioner should be notified immediately.

If a local anesthetic was administered into the subarachnoid space, the dermatome level (Fig. 23-2) should be closely monitored using a supersaturated alcohol sponge or a pin. With either method, patients should be informed fully about the procedure to ascertain the dermatome level. In this procedure, the nurse touches the patient's shoulders with either the alcohol sponge or the pin. The patient is instructed to tell the nurse when he or she feels the same sensation. The nurse then touches the skin with the sponge or pin at about the sacral area and moves up slowly at intervals of about 1 inch, corresponding with the dermatomes. When the patient says the sensation is the same as the one felt on the shoulder, that dermatome is so noted (see Fig. 23-2) as the level of the anesthetic.

Mechanism of Action. After the local anesthetic drug is injected into the subarachnoid space, a level of anesthesia will be achieved that depends on the dosage of the agent used, the rate of injection, the specific gravity of the fluid injected, and the position of the patient following injection. The level of anesthesia is called the dermatome level (see Fig. 23-2). A dermatome is that area of the skin that is supplied by a single spinal nerve. The face is supplied by the trigeminal nerve, and the remaining portions of the body's cutaneous areas are supplied in sequence by dermatomes C2 through S5. Some of the major topographic landmarks that can be depicted by a pinprick to detect sensory loss are L1 to T12, the inguinal ligament and iliac crest; T10, the umbilicus; T6, the xiphoid; T4, the nipples; T1, the clavicle; and C7, the middle finger. The order of blockage of the various nerve modalities is shown in Table 22-1 in Chapter 22.

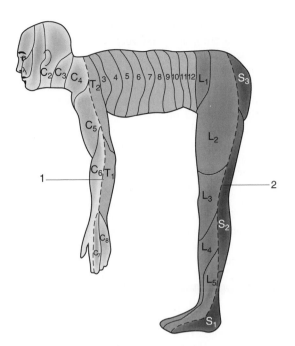

Fig. 23-2 The dermatomes of the body show an orderly craniad to caudad sequence. Positioning the body as shown allows the complex arrangement of dermatomes on the limbs to be more readily understood. On the upper extremity, the limb dermatomes are distributed symmetrically about the axial line *(1)*. Note that dermatomes C5 and C6 are distributed on the preaxial border of the limb, and the postaxial dermatomes—C8, T1, and T2—are distributed on the postaxial part of the limb. C7, which is the central dermatome of the limb, is distributed more distally (i.e., over the middle finger). There is an orderly sequence on the trunk from T3 to L1. The dermatome distribution of the lower extremity is also arranged around the axial line *(2)*. Large areas of skin— that is, L2 and L3—have been borrowed from the trunk to supplement the true leg dermatomes of L4 through S3. Note that as in the upper extremity, the craniad dermatomes, L4 and L5, are distributed on the preaxial border of the limb, and the caudad dermatomes, S2 and S3, are distributed on the postaxial border of the limb. The central dermatome S1 is distributed over the lateral aspect of the plantar surface and lateral border of the foot. *(Adapted from Foerster O: The dermatomes in man, Brain 56:1, 1933, Oxford University Press.)*

During the recovery from a spinal anesthetic, the anesthesia works its way back from the extremities toward the site where the anesthetic was administered. Therefore the areas near the site of injection are the last to recover.

Complications. The complications of spinal anesthesia are high spinal block, hypotension, nausea and vomiting, backache, palsies and paralysis, urinary retention, postspinal headache, and meningitis.

High Spinal Block. When the local anesthetic rises in the CSF, the major nerves exiting the spinal cord can be effectively blocked. The effects of the spread of the anesthetic into the cervical region are usually short lived, because dilution of the anesthetic produces a lower concentration of the drug. Some objective symptoms associated with a high spinal anesthetic are agitation, hypotension, nausea, diaphragmatic breathing (absence of intercostal muscle function), and an inability to speak audibly. The treatment of a high spinal block is initiated in the operating room and consists of efficient ventilation and oxygenation and the maintenance of the blood pressure by vasopressors. This block is a reversible complication; when the local anesthetic drug wears off, the patient will recover. PACU care consists of maintaining the treatment initiated in the operating room. The patient may be intubated and possibly placed on a ventilator. As the local anesthetic agent wears off, the patient may be unable to maintain tidal volume because of partial paralysis of the respiratory muscles. Ventilation of the patient should be assisted until an adequate tidal volume can be maintained. It is inadvisable to place the patient in a head-up position in an effort to limit the spread of the anesthetic—the anesthetic is already "fixed" at a level in the CSF, and raising the head can reduce cerebral blood flow, thus resulting in medullary ischemia.

The perianesthesia nurse should establish verbal contact with the patient to decrease the anxiety and apprehension he or she may feel because of being partially sedated, having difficulty in breathing, and being unable to move about.

To enhance the cardiac output, the patient's legs may be elevated to promote the return of venous blood from the lower extremities to the heart. If the vital signs still indicate neurogenic shock after this maneuver has been performed, vasopressor therapy will usually be instituted. Vasopressors used to treat this complication are usually of the alpha-adrenergic variety, because total spinal block produces a type of neurogenic shock. The alpha-adrenergic vasopressors produce peripheral vasoconstriction, which aids in returning the blood to the heart, thereby improving the cardiac output. Alpha-adrenergic vasopressors that may be used in this situation are phenylephrine (Neo-Synephrine) or norepinephrine (Levophed) and are discussed in Chapter 5.

Because of the height of the spinal block, the patient may also experience some bradycardia, which can be treated with atropine or glycopyrrolate (Robinul). Nausea and vomiting may also occur. Suction should be available, and antiemetics may have to be administered to the patient.

Hypotension. Postoperative hypotension caused by a sympathetic blockade from a spinal anesthetic leads to venous dilation, which results in a decreased venous return and reduces the cardiac output. This problem is most likely to occur during the first 30 minutes in the PACU, and, if the patient is hypotensive, assessing for bleeding—which may be causing the hypotension—is important. If bleeding is not the cause, treatment should be instituted and the anesthesiologist should be notified. If bleeding is the cause, the attending physician should be notified. The first line of treatment is to ensure that hydration is adequate. Often, the infusion of 500 ml of crystalloid along with the elevation of the legs corrects the postoperative spinal hypotension. If the hypotension continues, it can best be treated by vasopressors.

Nausea and Vomiting. Nausea and vomiting can be a result of hypotension, hypertension caused by the vasopressors, motion during change in position, or apprehension. If hypotension or hypertension is present, the anesthetist should be notified. It is important for the PACU nurse to assess the cause of the nausea and vomiting. Blood pressure should be taken and oxygen administered to the patient. Should vomiting occur, the patient should be placed in a Trendelenburg position with his or her head to the side, and a clear airway should be established and maintained. The anesthetist should be summoned if the patient experiences nausea or vomiting (see Chapter 10).

Palsies and Paralysis. Palsies and paralysis usually occur postoperatively in the peripheral nerves. Of the cranial nerves, the sixth cranial nerve is most often involved. In the PACU phase of the spinal anesthetic, the nurse should assess neurologic function of the extremities as the anesthetic wears off. If the patient has double vision or any other decrease in peripheral nerve function, the anesthetist and the surgeon should be notified.

Urinary Retention. Urinary retention is usually caused by trauma to the bladder during surgery or decreased bladder tone due to the anesthesia. The patient complains of severe pain and may become hypertensive or bradycardic. If the condition is not diagnosed and corrected, the patient may become incoherent and thrash about in bed. The PACU nurse should assess the patient for a distended bladder or hypoxia because the symptoms are almost identical. If urinary retention is the problem, the patient should be encouraged to void. If the patient cannot void, the surgeon should be notified and an order for catheterization of the bladder obtained.

Postspinal Headache. The true postspinal headache is caused by a persistent leak of CSF through the needle hole in the dura mater. Postspinal headache is usually transient but annoying to the patient. The pain usually becomes severe when the patient is upright and lessens when he or she is in a supine position. The location of the pain is usually occipital or frontal. The patient may also complain of tinnitus and diplopia.

As a prophylactic measure, most patients who have received a spinal anesthetic are encouraged to remain in the supine position for at least 6 to 8 hours following surgery. Some research indicates that the supine-bedrest prophylaxis is unnecessary and of no value in preventing postspinal headache. The advent of smaller-gauge needles has reduced the incidence of postspinal headache. Conservative treatment of the patient with this complication involves optimal hydration, analgesics, and reduction in environmental noise. However, if the postspinal headache becomes incapacitating or does not respond to conservative treatment within the first 2 days after the administration of the spinal anesthetic, an epidural blood patch procedure may be performed. This procedure involves administering 10 to 20 ml of the patient's own blood into the epidural space at the site of the previous lumbar puncture. This procedure seals the hole in the dura mater; prompt pain relief usually follows.

Epidural Anesthetics

Mechanism of Action. Epidural (peridural) block is produced by depositing an anesthetic agent in the epidural space. The location on the vertebral column or the segment where the epidural block is performed determines the type of epidural anesthesia the patient will receive. Thoracic epidural block, lumbar epidural block, and caudal epidural block or caudal anesthesia are the possible types of epidural anesthetic.

Techniques of Administration. Epidural block is usually performed in the same manner as the spinal block. The patient is placed into the sitting or lateral decubitus position, his or her back is prepped, and the needle is inserted into the epidural space. After it has been determined that the needle is in the epidural space, a test dose of the anesthetic solution is injected. Blood pressure, pulse, respiratory rate, and oxygen saturation are then determined. If vital signs are unchanged, the remainder of the anesthetic is incrementally administered. The needle may be removed, or a catheter may be placed through the needle into the epidural space for the continuous (serial) epidural technique. Monitoring the patient after epidural block is similar to monitoring after the spinal technique.

The morphine epidural technique is becoming popular as a way to reduce postoperative pain. Epidural morphine may be administered intraoperatively or in the immediate postoperative period. The pharmacology of epidural morphine is discussed in detail in Chapter 20. The major risk with epidural morphine is respiratory depression. Epidural morphine can depress respiration from 2.5 to 16.5 hours or longer. Consequently, monitoring for respiratory depression requires close surveillance of the patient's respiratory rate and oxygen saturation. To enhance the monitoring parameters, an apnea monitor should provide another alarm system to alert PACU personnel to the patient's respiratory depression. Fentanyl in a continuous infusion or in a patient-controlled modality also is used for postoperative pain management. Fentanyl may have a lower incidence of side effects such as pruritus and respiratory depression. This drug is discussed in Chapter 20.

The epidural block is the anesthetic technique of choice for cesarean section and is indicated in poor-risk patients and in those with cardiac, pulmonary, and metabolic diseases. It is also well suited for patients who have had thoracic or upper abdominal surgical procedures. In this instance, the epidural is usually placed preoperatively, and the patient may receive both general and epidural anesthesia. This combination of two anesthesia techniques has been quite successful in reducing postoperative pulmonary complications and enhancing pain relief.

The epidural block is contraindicated in patients being given anticoagulants, when hemorrhage or shock is present, when the patient has had previous back surgery, and when local inflammation exists.

Combined Spinal-Epidural Technique (CSE)

The combined spinal-epidural technique is a combination spinal and epidural technique that is performed by first inserting an epidural needle into the epidural space. A spinal needle is then passed through the epidural needle into the subarachnoid space, and spinal medication is injected. The spinal needle is then withdrawn, and a catheter is placed in the epidural space for future use. Because of the versatility of this combined technique, CSE is increasing in popularity. The CSE technique minimizes or eliminates some of the disadvantages of both spinal and epidural yet maintains their advantages. Specifically, CSE offers the rapid onset, profound analgesia, and reduced toxicity of spinal block combined with the potential for improving an inadequate block or lengthening the duration of anesthesia with epidural supplementation via epidural catheter. Preparation for anesthesia, side effects, precautions, contraindications, and postoperative care are essentially the same as those for spinal and epidural block. The CSE technique is most commonly used in obstetrics and for orthopedic, general, urological, and gynecological surgery.

PACU Care After Spinal, Epidural, or CSE Anesthesia

After the patient's arrival in the PACU, care must be exercised when moving him or her because the block's residual effects, such as lack of motor and sensory function, are still present. Care should be taken in positioning the patient, because good body alignment is needed to reduce muscle soreness or injury. The patient's joints should not be hyperextended, and the bedclothes should not press on his or her toes.

If a patient has any residual spinal anesthesia while in the PACU, care should be taken to avoid rapid position change, which causes severe decreases in blood pressure. This is because the circulatory system cannot compensate adequately for rapid position change when anesthesia is present.

If intravenous sedation was given during the operation, respiratory function should be monitored closely by the use of a pulse oximeter. Oxygen should be administered to all block patients until their motor and sensory functions return adequately. The patient should be encouraged to cough and breathe deeply every 15 minutes to reduce the incidence of atelectasis.

The patient should be checked for any signs of bladder distention. Catheterization may be required, especially in patients who have had pelvic or perineal surgery.

AXILLARY OR BRACHIAL PLEXUS BLOCK

Nerve blocks are employed to produce anesthesia in specific areas of the body. They are usually used for orthopedic, obstetric, and vascular surgical procedures. They are relatively safe and usually have good patient acceptance.

The axillary or brachial plexus block is used to anesthetize the arm to facilitate surgery below the elbow. When this block is performed, either the axillary or the supraclavicular approach is used.

PACU Care After Axillary or Brachial Plexus Block

PACU care of the patient who has received an axillary block centers on patient education and observation for complications. The patient should be taught that motor function will be lost and that no attempts should be made to move his or her arm. Injuries to the face and to the surgical site have been reported because the patient arm with reduced motor control managed to "flop" on his or her face or hit on the side rail.

If the supraclavicular approach was used, pneumothorax is a possible complication. The first sign is a complaint by the patient of pain in the chest that is accentuated by deep breathing. Other signs of pneumothorax are increased reso-

nance to percussion, absence of or decreased breath sounds, lag in expansion on the affected side in comparison with the unaffected side, and difficulty in "getting breath."

PACU care involves administering oxygen and advising the anesthetist of the complication. Analgesics are usually administered, and after a chest radiograph is made, more definitive treatment may be instituted.

When the supraclavicular approach is used to perform the brachial plexus block, Horner's syndrome can result. This occurs when the anesthetic solution spreads so that it involves the stellate ganglion. Symptoms of this syndrome, which appear on the side where the block is performed, are flushing of the face, constricted pupils, ptosis, and stuffiness of the nose. Horner's syndrome clears as the block wears off.

Another complication caused by the supraclavicular approach is blockage of the phrenic nerve. The incidence of this complication is related to the spread of anesthetic solution and is usually unilateral. Generally, no signs and symptoms occurs, and the complication clears as the block dissipates itself.

Obliteration of the radial pulse is a possible complication of the axillary approach to the brachial plexus. It is caused by bleeding or the use of too large a volume of anesthetic solution. The radial pulse usually returns in 2 to 4 hours.

INTRAVENOUS REGIONAL ANESTHESIA

The intravenous regional—or Bier—block was named for August K. Bier, who originated it in 1908. It is useful for emergency procedures on the forearm and hand, especially for a procedure such as Colles' fracture reduction, and is simple to administer. The Bier block involves starting an intravenous infusion in the hand, exsanguinating the arm with an Esmarch latex bandage, inflating a double pneumatic tourniquet above the elbow, and then removing the Esmarch bandage and injecting the local anesthetic agent (bupivacaine or lidocaine) while the tourniquet remains inflated. At the end of the surgical procedure, the tourniquet is released and the analgesia will cease within 5 to 10 minutes. Usually, no sequelae from the anesthetic agent occur; by the time the venous blood from the limb has passed through the lungs and has mixed with the rest of the venous return, the systemic arterial blood levels are not clinically significant because of the dilution effect. Should the blood levels of the local anesthetic remain high, the patient will experience cardiovascular depression, which is usually manifested by bradycardia. This cardiovascular depression is usually quite transient. If this situation arises, vigilant monitoring coupled with appropriate interventions such as oxygen and glycopyrrolate (Robinul) or atropine will usually correct the problem.

The intravenous regional technique can also be used for surgery on the lower leg and foot. Although it requires a larger tourniquet and more local anesthetic agent, it is an effective technique for this type of surgery.

PACU Care After Intravenous Regional Anesthesia

When the patient arrives in the PACU, all analgesia provided by the local anesthetic agent used in the intravenous regional anesthesia has usually dissipated. Medication for the relief of pain can be given soon after the patient's arrival. The PACU nurse should assess the patient's level of sedation—including the amount of premedication and sedation during the surgical procedure—before administering the pain medication.

BIBLIOGRAPHY

Barash P, Cullen B, Stoelting R: Clinical anesthesia, ed 3, Philadelphia, JB Lippincott.

Cousins M, Bridenbaugh P: Neural blockade. In clinical anesthesia and management of pain, ed 3, Philadelphia, 1998, Lippincott-Raven.

Cramer C: Postanesthetic management of regional anesthesia, J Post Anesth Nurs, 1(4):236-243, 1986.

Hardman J, Limbird L: Goodman and Gilman's the pharmacological basis of therapeutics, ed 9, New York, 1996, McGraw-Hill.

Kingsley C: Epidural analgesia: your role, RN 64(3): 53-57, 2001.

Macintyre P, Ready B: Acute pain management. a practical guide, ed 2, New York, 2001, WB Saunders.

Miller R, editor: Anesthesia, ed 5, Philadelphia, 2000, Churchill Livingstone.

Rawal N, Van Zundert A, Holmstrom B et al: Combined spinal-epidural technique, Regional Anesthesia 22(5):406-423, 1997.

Wood M, Wood A: Drugs and anesthesia: pharmacology for the anesthesiologist, ed 2, Baltimore, 1990, Williams & Wilkins.

24

TRANSITION FROM THE OPERATING ROOM TO THE PACU

Kay Ball, RN, MSA, CNOR, FAAN

The practice of nursing is directed toward the patient by helping to promote and maintain health through various interventions. Nursing care of the surgical patient is quite intricate; it continues to change daily as new technology, advanced techniques, complex patient conditions, and evolving nursing practices impact patient outcomes. Surgical patient care is administered by perioperative and perianesthesia registered nurses; therefore, continual and clear communication between these specific professionals is vital.

PERIOPERATIVE NURSING

Perioperative nursing care involves the "nursing activities that address the needs of patients, their families, and significant others that occur preoperatively, intraoperatively, and postoperatively."[1] Perioperative nursing services can be delivered in a variety of environments, from the preoperative area to the postanesthesia care unit. A perioperative nurse is defined "as the registered nurse who, using the nursing process, designs, coordinates, and delivers care to meet the identified needs of patients whose protective reflexes or self-care abilities are potentially compromised because they are having operative or other invasive procedures."[2]

PERIANESTHESIA NURSING

The scope of perianesthesia nursing practice involves the "assessment, diagnosis of, intervention for, and evaluation of perceived, actual or potential, physical or psychosocial problems that may result from the administration of sedation/analgesia or anesthetic agents and techniques."[3] Perianesthesia nursing is multidimensional and ranges from the preanesthesia phase (patient assessment and preparation) through postanesthesia phase I (transition from a totally anesthetized state to one that requires less acute interventions), postanesthesia phase II (helping to prepare patient/family/significant other for care of the patient in the home or in an extended care facility),[4] and postanesthesia phase III (providing ongoing care for those surgical patients who require extended observation or intervention after discharge).[5]

COMMUNICATION BETWEEN PERIOPERATIVE AND PERIANESTHESIA NURSES

No matter how nurses describe their practices or roles (perioperative or perianesthesia), the basic foundation of nursing practice remains the same: high-quality care for the surgical patient. Therefore nurses who provide care during surgical procedures that involve sedation, analgesia, or anesthetics must work very closely with nurses who provide care after the procedure to foster continuity of care, quality services, and desired patient outcomes.

Care of the surgical patient involves planning, collaboration, and communication between the perioperative and perianesthesia registered nurses, who must always demonstrate effective verbal, written, and listening skills. As the care of the surgical patient is transferred from the perioperative nurse in one area to the perianesthesia nurse in another area, effective and complete communication is vital. This communication can be in the form of written documentation or verbal reports.

Written and Verbal Communication

Written documentation provides a basis for verbal reports and is usually in the form of standardized operative and/or anesthesia records. AORN's recommended practice for "Documentation of Perioperative Nursing Care" notes that the "patient's record should reflect the perioperative patient's plan of care, including assessment, diagnosis, outcome identification, planning, implementation, and evaluation."[6] Documentation should include information about the patient's status, assessment notes, plan of care, nursing interventions, and a continuous evaluation of nursing care and patient responses. The written patient operative record facilitates communication and provides continuity of care while also serving as a legal record of the care provided. A verbal report is the vehicle used when giving a "snapshot" or abbreviated symposia of the patient status and care delivered.

To examine the issues of communication and documentation between the perioperative nurse and the perianesthesia nurse, the basic questions of why, when, where, who, how, and what must be explored.

WHY: Verbal reports highlight written documentation on the patient record. A written report records the details of the patient care, whereas a verbal report is a quick description or overview used when the patient's care is being transferred to another nurse.

WHEN: A formal written report begins with the admission of the patient for the surgical procedure and extends through discharge. Written reports documenting patient information before admission or after discharge may be added to the patient's chart. A verbal report from the perioperative nurse to the perianesthesia nurse begins when the call is made to the PACU to announce the completion of the surgical procedure and request to transfer the patient to the PACU. At this time, any special needs must be communicated (i.e., ventilator needed). The verbal report continues when the patient is actually admitted to the PACU.

WHERE: Ideally the written patient record is kept with the patient during transfer from the operating room into the PACU. The verbal report is given when the patient's care is being transferred from the perioperative nurse to the perianesthesia nurse in the PACU.

WHO: Written patient reports are completed by the perioperative nurse, anesthesia provider, and the surgeon (or his or her designee). Usually the verbal report is given by the anesthesia provider and the perioperative registered nurse. In a few surgical environments, the perioperative nurse may call the perianesthesia nurse on the phone to give a report while the anesthesia provider and an orderly (patient care assistant) transfer the patient to the PACU. Ideally the perioperative nurse and anesthesia provider should accompany the patient to the PACU. Sometimes the surgeon or his or her assistant also participate in the patient transportation and verbal report.

HOW: The written patient record is documented on a healthcare facility–approved standardized form. The verbal report is usually given in person from one professional to another, but verbal reports have also been given via telephone or computer, depending on the patient acuity and facility protocols.

WHAT IS REPORTED: The American Society of PeriAnesthesia Nurses (ASPAN) recommends that patient reporting should contain[7]:

Relevant preoperative status, such as vital signs, radiology findings, laboratory values, oxygen saturation, allergies, effects of preoperative medications, disabilities, substance abuse, physical or mental impairments, mobility limitations, prostheses, etc.

Anesthesia technique and agents

Length of time anesthesia administered, time reversal agents given

Type of procedure

Estimated fluid/blood loss and replacement

Complications occurring during anesthesia course, treatment initiated, response

Emotional status on arrival to the operating or procedure room

Numerical score, if used

Different healthcare providers, including the anesthesia provider, perioperative nurse, and surgeon, are involved with giving the report during the transference of care to the PACU nurse. Box 24-1 includes suggestions on topics to report from each professional.[8]

An Example: Reporting Patient Positioning. The importance of reporting specific and appropriate information about the patient's surgical

Box 24-1	Suggestions on Topics to Report from Each Professional

ANESTHESIA PROVIDER MAY REPORT:

Patient name, gender, age, procedure, physician
History of present illness
History of chronic illness
Relevant preop lab tests
Type of anesthesia administered
Patient response to anesthesia agents
Duration of anesthesia
Reversal agents
Narcotics
Antibiotics
Fluid replacement and type (I & O)
Invasive monitoring lines
Vital signs
Allergies
Other conditions
Medications given
Complications related to the procedure
Orders

PERIOPERATIVE NURSE MAY REPORT:

Baseline patient assessment
Positioning during procedure
Skin prep
ESU pad placement and removal assessment
Use of special equipment (laser, endoscope)
Intraoperative irrigation fluids
Administration of medications or dyes from surgical field
Implants, transplants, explants
Dressing
Drains, stents, catheters
Sensory or motor limitations
Prosthesis presence
Other pertinent patient information
Information about the family or others waiting for the patient

SURGEON MAY REPORT:

Immediate orders
Diagnostic tests for PACU
Interventions needed in PACU

From Fortunato N: Berry & Kohn's operating room technique, ed 9, St Louis, 2000, Mosby.

experience can be critical. The perianesthesia nurse must receive the full details of the patient's condition, interventions, and plan of care. In the hustle and bustle of today's surgical environment, seemingly minor details that may have major effects on the patient's recovery can be disregarded in the documentation and reporting.

For example, reporting the positioning used during a surgical procedure may seem trivial and insignificant to the perioperative nurse and may often be overlooked. However, patient injuries from prolonged or improper positioning during the surgical procedure have been assessed and documented by astute PACU nurses. AORN recommended practices note that perioperative documentation should include "patient positioning and/or repositioning devices and supports, including immobilization devices used during the surgical procedure."[9]

The impact of improper positioning is not immediately recognized in the OR; therefore positioning must be documented and reported to allow the perianesthesia nurse to look for symptoms of potential problems. The results of improper positioning can be discovered during the assessment of various body systems—including the cardiac and vascular, skin, musculoskeletal, nervous, and respiratory systems. Positioning during a surgical procedure can influence breathing patterns, gas exchange, cardiac output, tactile sensory perception, mobility, and skin integrity. The perianesthesia nurse should assess the patient carefully understanding that different systems may be compromised from faulty positioning during surgery.

Cardiovascular. Cardiac output can indicate intraoperative positioning injuries and can easily be assessed by measuring the patient's blood pressure. The following list provides some examples:

- Hypotension or hypertension can be caused by the type of anesthesia administered but can be intensified by specific positioning during a surgical procedure.
- Regional or general anesthesia may cause peripheral blood vessels to dilate (from the relaxation of the muscle lining of the blood vessels) and lead to venous pooling, a decrease in circulating blood volume, and a fall in blood

pressure if the extremities are in a dependent position.

- Reverse Trendelenburg, lithotomy, or jack-knife positions can contribute to venous pooling because of the dependent position of the lower extremities.
- Pooling of the blood in the trunk may be caused from unusual pressure on the abdomen from the thighs during lithotomy position, which compresses the external iliac artery that distributes blood to the abdominal wall, external genitalia, and lower limbs.
- Lowered blood pressure may be from unusual pressure or tension to the major blood vessels (such as the inferior vena cava) from improper positioning or through the inappropriate positioning of deep retractors.
- Hyperabduction of the arm (>90 degrees) can cause axillary and subclavian vessels to be stretched and compressed between the first rib and the clavicle. This can cause the radial pulse to be undetectable and could result in arterial thrombosis.

Skin. The skin is the largest organ of the body and the first line of defense against infection; therefore the skin must be inspected thoroughly by the perianesthesia nurse to determine whether any positioning injury has resulted.

Four potential positioning injuries can cause skin problems. They are described in the following discussions.

Pressure. Pressure injuries are the most common skin injuries caused by inappropriate positioning. A lower pressure on the skin surface sustained for a prolonged time cannot be tolerated as easily as a greater pressure for a shorter time period. The PACU nurse should note what time surgery began to determine the possibility of the formation of pressure ulcers from lengthy surgical procedures.

If the patient's skin is thin, tissue can be easily compromised. With prolonged pressure, blood vessels may constrict and occlude, thus leading to possible ischemia, which is the first step to pressure ulcer formation. Years ago research demonstrated that pressures over 32 mg Hg cause arterioles to constrict and occlude, thus leading to decreased nourishment and oxygenation of the

capillary beds. Ischemia and microscopic necrosis can then result and cause pressure ulcerations.[10] Injuries from prolonged pressure may not be evident for hours or even days and may even be missed by the perianesthesia nurse. Because a pressure ulcer starts at a bony prominence and extends to the skin, it takes a while to manifest itself at the skin level; therefore a pressure ulcer may not be readily identified. Research has noted that 1 in every 12 patients who has surgery over 3 hours can develop at least one pressure ulcer within 4 days of surgery.[11]

Head injuries also may not be immediately evident in the PACU. With prolonged pressure on the scalp, localized postoperative alopecia may result. This condition may present with a reddened area or may not be evident until days or weeks after the surgery. Pain and swelling may occur where the pressure has been applied intraoperatively. Repositioning the head every 30 minutes during a procedure and in the PACU can minimize this problem.

Shearing. Shearing injuries occur when the skin stays stationary while the underlying tissue moves during patient positioning. The tissue layers moving on each other cause the tissue and vessels to be stretched and damaged. The perianesthesia nurse may note that the skin integrity has been broken, or a redness or discoloration may occur when shearing injuries are sustained.

Friction. Friction injuries occur when the skin is moved across a rough surface during positioning or when the skin is rubbed with operating-room devices such as a safety strap or face mask. The perianesthesia nurse may note that the skin has become abraded during a potential friction injury that may lead to inflammation, infection, and pain. Friction injuries may involve deeper levels of skin and tissues, which may not be immediately evident during the PACU experience.

Maceration. Maceration injuries are caused from prolonged contact of the patient's skin with fluids (e.g., pooling of prep solutions, incontinence, sweat, or irrigants) during a surgical procedure. This contact with fluids causes the skin to weaken and become more vulnerable to pressure, shearing, or friction injuries. The perianesthesia nurse should consider maceration injuries if the skin integrity has been compromised.

Musculoskeletal System. The structural framework of the body skeleton consists of over 200 bones that provide support and allow movement to occur. Unusual pressure or overextension of a joint or extreme positioning coupled with anesthesia agents that lead to relaxation can cause musculoskeletal injuries. Stretching of a joint or ligament can lead to increased pressure on an area, thus compromising the bone by decreasing the blood supply. The perianesthesia nurse may notice discoloration or redness over a bony prominence or joint that could indicate an injury. Moreover, the patient's subjective complaints of pain in a specific joint may suggest a musculoskeletal problem.

Nervous System. The two components of the nervous system are the central nervous system and the peripheral nervous system. The peripheral nervous system is more vulnerable to positioning injuries with pressure and stretching of structures that leads to pain. These injuries can be temporary or permanent which may result in a disability. Neural injuries from positioning usually are delayed in discovery in the PACU, thus making tracing the original injury back to the surgical experience more difficult.

The most frequently injured nerves from positioning problems are the following:

- Ulnar nerve that extends from the upper arm to the lower arm. When the compression of the ulnar nerve is near the elbow, a clawing effect of the fingers may be present.
- Lower extremity nerves in the legs that may be injured by improper stirrup use or by positioning devices not used properly.
- Brachial plexus that consists of a network of nerves from the clavicle down the upper arm. When the arm is overextended, a numbness or palsy of the hand, arm, or wrist may result.
- Lumbosacral nerves that are located in the lower back region. When a patient is placed in the lithotomy position for a long procedure, the lumbosacral nerves can be stretched, thus leading to weakness of the quadriceps muscle or a sensory deficit in the anterior thigh area.

Respiratory System. If the lungs are not allowed to expand well because of positioning problems during a surgical procedure, the alveoli can begin to close, thus decreasing the exchange of respiratory gases. A pulse oximeter applied to the recovering patient in the PACU will note any changes or respiratory problems that may have resulted from prolonged or improper positioning.

SUMMARY

Thorough communication from the perioperative professionals to the perianesthesia nurse is imperative and will directly impact the outcomes in the care of the surgical patient. Whether in written or verbal format, continuity of patient care and attention to the details of the surgical event and the patient's responses to the interventions is vital to ensure a smooth transition from the intraoperative surgical suite into the PACU. The perioperative nurse must be diligent in observing what details to document and verbalize, and the perianesthesia nurse must be unfailing in listening and observing patient details that could indicate untoward responses to the surgical event. Never should the importance of this critical part of communication within nursing be overlooked.

Florence Nightingale wrote in *Notes on Nursing* in 1860, "In dwelling upon the vital importance of sound observation, it must never be lost sight of what observation is for. It is not for the sake of piling up miscellaneous information or curious facts, but for the sake of saving life and increasing health and comfort."[12]

REFERENCES

1. AORN: Standards, recommended practices, and guidelines, Denver, 2001, AORN.
2. AORN: Standards, recommended practices, and guidelines, Denver, 2001, AORN.
3. ASPAN: Standards of perianesthesia nursing practice, Cherry Hill, NJ, 2000, ASPAN.
4. ASPAN: Standards of perianesthesia nursing practice, Cherry Hill, NJ, 2000, ASPAN.
5. AORN: Standards, recommended practices, and guidelines, Denver, 2001, AORN.
6. ASPAN: Standards of perianesthesia nursing practice, Cherry Hill, NJ, 2000, ASPAN.

7. Fortunato N: Berry & Kohn's operating room technique, ed 9, St Louis, 2000, Mosby.
8. AORN: Standards, recommended practices, and guidelines, Denver, 2001, AORN.
9. Kosiak M: Etiology and pathology of ischemic ulcers, Physiological Medical Rehabilitation 40:60-69, 1959.
10. American Health Consultants: Are you overlooking your OR in the battle against pressure ulcers? Wound Care 3(6), 1998.
11. Nightingale F: Notes on nursing (an unabridged republication of the first American edition published by D. Appleton and Company in 1860), Toronto, 1969, Dover Publications.

ASSESSMENT AND MONITORING
OF THE PERIANESTHESIA PATIENT

The primary purpose of the postanesthesia care unit (PACU) is the critical evaluation and stabilization of postoperative patients, with emphasis on anticipation and prevention of complications that result from anesthesia or the operative procedure. It is therefore imperative that a knowledgeable, skillful perianesthesia nurse fully assesses the condition of each patient not only at admission and at discharge but also at frequent intervals throughout the postanesthesia period. Assessment must be a continuous and complete process that leads to sound nursing judgments and the implementation of therapeutic care. Assessment includes gathering information from direct observation of the patient (the primary source), from the physician and other healthcare personnel, and from the medical record and the care plan.

Traditionally, perianesthesia nurses have, with only limited information, performed the role of caring for the surgical patient in the vulnerable postanesthesia state. However, to assess the perianesthesia patient and plan and implement appropriate care, it is imperative that preoperative information be available as a basis for comparison with postoperative data. The perianesthesia nurse has a professional obligation to consider the patient's history, clinical status, and psychosocial state. The necessary data may be gathered by chart review, personal preoperative visit, and consultation with other healthcare members who are providing care to the patient. The collection of such information should be a coordinated effort with all involved members of the healthcare team.

This chapter discusses the assessment of postoperative patients and their common needs. Specific assessments related to patient age, the type of surgical procedure, and problems that result from complicated diagnoses are dealt with in the following chapters. The assessment and management of postoperative pain is presented in Chapter 28.

PREOPERATIVE ASSESSMENTS

Preoperative evaluation of both the physical and the emotional status of the surgical patient is extremely important, and nursing brings a unique perspective to this assessment. Nurses in a number of subspecialties—including perianesthesia nurses, operative room nurses, and general unit nurses—have advocated this assessment. Having each nurse who will care for the patient make a preoperative visit seems redundant and may be overwhelming for the patient. More appropriately, nurses should treat each other as colleagues who communicate needs for specific information, coordinate the collection of such information, and document data to be used for planning care. Multidisciplinary care conferences can be instrumental in educating all those who will care for the surgical patient and in developing communication patterns.

Because many PACU departments now include preoperative holding areas, it may be necessary for the perianesthesia nurse to participate in the patient's preoperative interview and assessment. A complete preoperative nursing assessment should include relevant preoperative physical and psychosocial status, past medical history (including anesthesia history), length of fasting, understanding of the surgery and postoperative course, and the need for follow-up services. The preoperative physical assessment should include documentation of temperature, pulse, blood pressure, respirations, oxygen saturation, height, and weight and a review of systems. Nursing diagnoses are established based on analysis of data collected during the assessment phase, and an appropriate plan of care is generated.

ADMISSION OBSERVATIONS

Physical assessment of the perianesthesia patient must begin immediately on admission to the PACU. The patient is accompanied from the operating room to the PACU by the anesthesiologist (or nurse anesthetist), who reports to the receiving nurse on the patient's general condition, the operation performed, and the type of anesthesia used for the surgery. In addition, the nurse should be informed of any problems or complications encountered during the surgery and anesthesia.

Because all anesthetics are depressants, postoperative assessment and care generally are the same, regardless of the specific agent used. For special precautions required for certain agents, review the chapters on anesthesia (see Chapters 17 through 23).

Rapid assessment of the life-sustaining cardiorespiratory system is of initial concern. Ensure that the airway is patent and that respirations are free and easy. Check and record the patient's blood pressure, pulse, rate of respiration, and oxygen saturation level. Quickly inspect all dressings and drains for gross bleeding. These baseline observations, which are made immediately on admission, should be reported to the anesthesiologist in attendance and recorded in the admission note.

Once these initial observations are made, it is essential to systematically assess the patient's total condition. This assessment may be made from head to toe or by systems, whichever the individual nurse prefers; the observations are essentially identical. Because the authors' preference is for a systems approach, the following outline of postanesthesia assessment is presented. It should be noted that each system of the body has an integral function, and therefore all observations are interrelated.

RESPIRATORY FUNCTION

Because the postanesthesia patient has experienced some interference with his or her respiratory system, maintenance of adequate gas exchange is a crucial aspect of care in the PACU. Any change in respiratory function must be detected early so that appropriate measures can be taken to ensure adequate oxygenation and ventilation. The most significant respiratory problems encountered in the immediate postoperative period include hypoventilation, airway obstruction, aspiration, and atelectasis.

Respiratory assessment is coupled with the related responses of the cardiovascular and neurologic systems to provide for total evaluation of the adequacy of gas exchange and ventilatory efficiency. Respiratory function is evaluated by clinical assessment. Additionally, pulse oximetry is used to assess arterial oxygenation, and capnography is used to evaluate the adequacy of ventilation. Arterial blood gas measurements may also be a part of the respiratory assessment (see Chapters 10 and 27).

Clinical Assessment

Inspection. The resting respiratory rate of a normal adult is approximately 16 to 20 breaths per minute. Infants and children have a higher respiratory rate and a lower tidal volume than adults (see Chapter 46). Respirations should be quiet and easy and have a regular rate and rhythm. The chest should move freely as a unit, and expansion should be equal bilaterally. Alterations in symmetry may be caused by many factors, including pain that may cause splinting at the incision site, consolidation, and pneumothorax. Note the character of the respirations; intercostal retractions, bulging, nasal flaring, or use of the accessory respiratory muscles are signs of respiratory distress. The depth of respiration is as important as the rate. Shallow respiration is the cardinal sign of continuing depression from anesthesia or preoperative medications, but it may be caused by many other factors, including incisional pain, obesity, tight binders, and dressings that restrict movements of the thoracic cage or abdomen. Shallow respirations and use of the neck and diaphragmatic muscles may also indicate recurarization from the use of skeletal muscle relaxants such as succinylcholine, atracurium, pancuronium, and vecuronium. The presence of chest movements alone, however, does not provide evidence that adequate gas exchange is occurring.

Airway obstruction may be present when the normal duration of inspiration versus exhalation is altered. Restlessness, confusion or anxiety, and apprehension are the earliest signs of hypoxemia and carbon dioxide (CO_2) retention and should receive immediate attention to determine their cause. The patient's color should also be regularly evaluated. Although this assessment is difficult, it provides important information about the respiratory function. However, it is crucial to remember that cyanosis is a late sign of severe tissue hypoxia; when it appears, immediate and vigorous efforts must be instituted to determine and correct the cause of hypoxia. The noninvasive monitors that are increasingly used in the PACU provide an effective means of continuously and objectively assessing gas exchange; pulse oximeters monitor hemoglobin oxygen saturation, and capnographs evaluate the adequacy of ventilation. These monitors will be discussed later in this chapter.

Note the presence of an artificial airway; airways are used primarily to maintain a patent air passage so that respiratory exchange is not hampered. Four types of airways commonly used are (1) the balloon-cuffed endotracheal tube (extends from the mouth through the glottis to a point above the bifurcation of the trachea); (2) the balloon-cuffed nasotracheal tube (extends from the nose to the trachea); (3) the oropharyngeal airway (extends from the mouth to the pharynx and prevents the tongue from falling back and obstructing the trachea); and (4) the nasopharyngeal airway (extends from the nose to the pharynx). The airway must be kept clear of secretions for adequate gas exchange to occur, and it may need to be suctioned if gurgling develops. The airway should not be removed until the laryngeal and pharyngeal reflexes return; these reflexes enable the patient to control the tongue, to cough, and to swallow. If the patient "reacts on the airway" (attempts to eject it), gagging—which progresses to retching and vomiting—may occur. The airway should be removed as soon as clinically possible in this instance to avoid aspiration.

An endotracheal tube can be removed as soon as the patient is adequately reversed and able to maintain the airway without it and when the danger of aspiration is over. This point may be difficult to determine; it is usually much easier to determine when a patient needs an airway than to decide when such an adjunct is not needed. Therefore if PACU policy permits removal of an airway, it should definitely include insertion of an airway. Both procedures should, of course, be accompanied by appropriate education and skill training for the nurses who will perform them.

Palpation.   Palpation and inspection of the chest may be carried out simultaneously to validate observations such as symmetry of expansion. In addition, crepitation may be heard or fremitus may be felt. The temperature, the level of moisture and general turgor of the skin, and the presence of any edema should be noted.

Percussion.   The normal sound over the lungs is resonance. Dullness heard where there should normally be resonance indicates consolidation or filling of the alveolar or pleural spaces by fluid.

Listening and Auscultation.   First, listen to the patient's respirations unaided. Normal respiration should be quiet; noisy breathing indicates a problem. Extraneous sounds always indicate some kind of obstruction; however, quiet breathing does not always indicate the absence of problems. An accumulation of mucus or other secretions evidenced by gurgling in any of the respiratory passages may cause airway obstruction and should be removed immediately. Purposeful coughing with good expiratory airflow is the most effective way of clearing secretions. If the patient is not yet reactive enough to do this alone, the secretions must be suctioned out orally and nasally. Nasotracheal suctioning may be useful to clear secretions and to stimulate cough, but the catheter is ineffective for reaching secretions distal to the carina. Obstruction may also occur from poor oropharyngeal muscle tone caused by the muscle-relaxant effect of general anesthesia plus the rolling back of the tongue. To relieve this obstruction, provide anterior pressure support on the angle of the jaw to open the air passages.

Crowing may indicate laryngospasm—a sudden, violent contraction of the vocal cords that may result in complete or partial closure of the trachea. If spasms continue, the airway must be maintained by the insertion of an endotracheal tube. Total blockage of the airway caused by laryngospasm produces no sound because of the absence of moving air. Equipment and medications for emergency tracheostomy should be readily available in the PACU.

Wheezing may indicate bronchospasm caused by a reflex reaction to an irritating mechanism. Bronchospasm occurs most often in patients with preexisting pulmonary disease—such as severe emphysema, reactive airway disease, pulmonary fibrosis, and radiation pneumonitis. Laryngeal edema after endotracheal intubation is not uncommon and can contribute significantly to airway obstruction. Acute changes in the patient's skin condition, cardiovascular status, and bronchospasm after regional anesthesia must alert the nurse to a possible allergic reaction, but this event is rare.

Listen to the patient's chest with a stethoscope for quality and intensity of breath sounds. Locate and identify any abnormality, and describe it in the patient's medical record. Total absence of breath sounds on one side may signal the presence of pneumothorax (collapsed lung), obstruction, or fluid or blood within the pleural space. Auscultation of breath sounds in the PACU is often difficult, because the patient often cannot sit up or respond to commands to breathe deeply with the mouth open. Positioning the patient on alternating sides during the stir-up regimen provides an opportunity to examine the posterior lung field.

Monitoring Oxygenation by Pulse Oximetry

A pulse oximeter noninvasively measures the arterial oxygen saturation (SaO_2) in the blood (called SpO_2 when measured by pulse oximetry). Therefore it is a valuable adjunct to the clinical assessment of oxygenation. Many clinical indicators, such as the patient's color and the characteristics of the respirations, are subjective, and

the physical signs of cyanosis are not evident until hypoxia is severe. Pulse oximetry monitoring is objective and continuous, and it provides an early warning of developing hypoxemia, thus allowing intervention before signs of hypoxia appear. Consequently, pulse oximetry has been widely adopted in the PACU as a tool for both safety monitoring and patient management. As a confirmation of its importance, the American Society of PeriAnesthesia Nurses (ASPAN) Standards of Postanesthesia Nursing Practice (1991) requires evaluation of all PACU patients with pulse oximetry at admission and discharge, and ASPAN recommends a pulse oximeter for every patient care unit in a Phase I PACU.

A pulse oximeter consists of a microprocessor-based monitor and a sensor (Fig. 25-1). In addition to an SpO_2 display, most oximeters display the pulse rate and have an adjustable alarm system that sounds when values register outside a designated range. A variety of sensors is available, each intended for application to specific sites and for use on patients of various sizes (the manufacturer's instructions describe these requirements). The sensor is applied to a site with a good arterial supply. The most common application site is a finger or toe (hand or foot in neonates); other sites include the nose, the forehead, or the temple. Both reusable sensors and disposable adhesive sensors are available, and disposable sensors allow for patient-dedicated monitoring when infection control concerns are present.

Technology Overview. A pulse oximeter uses plethysmography to detect the arterial pulse and spectrophotometry to determine SpO_2. The pulse oximetry sensor incorporates a red and an infrared light-emitting diode (also known as an LED) as light sources and a photodiode as a light

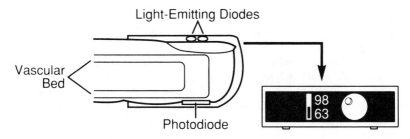

Fig. 25-1 A pulse oximeter uses two light-emitting diodes and a photodiode to determine the arterial hemoglobin saturation.

detector. In the most common type of sensor—a transmission sensor—the light sources and detector are positioned on opposite sides of an arterial bed, such as around the finger. In a reflectance oximetry sensor, they are positioned on the same surface, such as on the forehead.

With both transmission and reflectance sensors, red and infrared light passes into the tissue, and the detector measures the amount of light absorbed. Because oxyhemoglobin and deoxyhemoglobin differ in their absorption of red and infrared light, the detector can determine the percentage of oxyhemoglobin in the arterial pulse.

Applications.   Pulse oximetry is used in many clinical settings for safety monitoring and as a patient management tool. As a safety monitor, a pulse oximeter detects hypoxemia caused by unanticipated events such as severe atelectasis, bronchospasm, airway displacement, disconnections or kinks in the breathing circuit, and cardiac arrest. As a patient management tool, it is valuable in titrating oxygen therapy, weaning a patient from mechanical ventilation, and evaluating response to medications or other interventions that are intended to improve oxygenation.

In addition to these broad applications, certain uses of pulse oximetry are of particular value in the PACU. For example, postoperative patients can become significantly hypoxemic during transport to or from the PACU. Pulse oximetry during transport can diagnose undetected hypoxemia and identify a need for supplemental oxygen. Also, as indicated by the ASPAN standards, it is a valuable adjunct to clinical assessments in determining readiness for PACU discharge. When evaluated by pulse oximetry, some patients judged to be stable and ready for transfer based on clinical evaluation alone have been found to be hypoxemic.

Interpretation of SpO$_2$ Measurements.   To adequately interpret SpO$_2$, considering the mechanisms of oxygen transport is essential. Approximately 98% of the oxygen in blood is bound to hemoglobin; SaO$_2$ and SpO$_2$ reflect this blood oxygen. The remaining blood oxygen is dissolved in plasma; blood gas analysis measures the partial pressure exerted by this oxygen dissolved in plasma (PaO$_2$). It is the dissolved oxygen that is used to meet immediate metabolic needs. The oxygen bound to hemoglobin serves as the reservoir that replenishes the pool of dissolved oxygen (see Chapter 10).

The rate at which oxygen binds to hemoglobin is primarily controlled by two factors: the PaO$_2$ and the affinity of hemoglobin for oxygen. This relationship between SaO$_2$ and PaO$_2$ is represented by the oxyhemoglobin dissociation curve. The curve is sigmoid in shape, and its position is affected by a number of physiologic variables that change the affinity of hemoglobin for oxygen (Fig. 25-2).

Many factors that shift the oxyhemoglobin dissociation curve are commonly seen in PACU patients. For example, a hypothermic patient may have a left-shifted curve. In such a patient, a given SpO$_2$ as measured by pulse oximetry may correspond to a lower than normal PaO$_2$. Although oxygen saturation may be adequate, hemoglobin will have a greater affinity for oxygen and be less willing to release oxygen to meet tissue needs. Warming the patient to a normothermic range facilitates oxygen unloading from the hemoglobin molecule and helps maintain adequate tissue oxygenation.

Clinical Issues.   As with any technology, important clinical issues must be considered to use pulse oximetry appropriately. As just discussed, shifts in the oxyhemoglobin dissociation curve that are caused by abnormal values of pH, temperature, PCO$_2$, and 2,3-diphosphoglycerate must be considered. It is also important to consider the patient's hemoglobin level because a pulse oximeter cannot detect depletion in the total amount of hemoglobin. When pulse oximetry is used on a postoperative patient with a low hemoglobin level, a high SpO$_2$ value may not reflect adequate oxygenation. The amount of hemoglobin, although it is well saturated with oxygen, may be inadequate to meet tissue needs because fewer carriers are available to transport oxygen.

Adequate oxygenation is a factor of not only adequate oxygen saturation and hemoglobin values but also adequate oxygen delivery (which necessitates appropriate cardiac output) and the ability of the tissues to effectively use oxygen. When oxygen demand exceeds oxygen supply, tissue hypoxia results. Pulse oximetry readings therefore should be assessed in conjunction with all other indices of oxygenation.

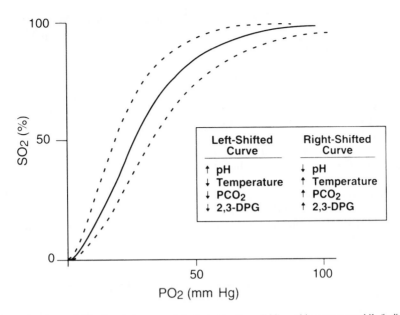

Fig. 25-2 The normal oxyhemoglobin dissociation curve is indicated by the solid line. This curve may shift (indicated by the broken lines) whenever pH, temperature, PCO_2, or 2,3-DPG values are increased or decreased. *SO_2,* Oxygen saturation; *PO_2,* partial pressure of oxygen; *PCO_2,* partial pressure of carbon dioxide; *2,3-DPG,* 2,3-diphosphoglycerate.

Dysfunctional hemoglobins, variants of the hemoglobin molecule that are unable to transport oxygen, present a similar problem. Despite the high SpO_2 level, hemoglobin may be insufficient to carry oxygen. Carboxyhemoglobin is hemoglobin that is bound with carbon monoxide and therefore is unavailable for carrying oxygen. Its effect must be considered in patients with burns or carbon monoxide poisoning and in those who smoke. In methemoglobinemia, the iron molecule on the hemoglobin is oxidized from the ferrous to the ferric state. This form of iron is unable to transport oxygen. Methemoglobinemia, although rare, may occur in patients who receive nitrate-based and other drugs and in those who are exposed to a variety of toxins. When dysfunctional hemoglobins are suspected, assessment of oxygenation by pulse oximetry must be supplemented with arterial blood gas saturations measured by a laboratory cooximeter to determine whether dyshemoglobins are present and oxygenation is adequate.

Perfusion at the sensor application site must be sufficient for the pulse oximeter to detect pulsatile flow. This is an important consideration for some PACU patients, such as those treated with vasoconstrictors, those who are markedly hypothermic, and those who have significantly reduced cardiac output. When applying the sensor, select a well-perfused site. If in doubt, check the pulse and adjacent capillary refill. If the monitor is unable to track the pulse, first evaluate the patient for adverse physiologic changes. Next, ensure that blood flow is not being restricted, such as by a flexed extremity, a blood pressure cuff, an arterial line, any restraints, or a sensor that is applied too tightly. Local perfusion to the sensor site can be improved by covering the site with a warm towel or by use of a convective warming device such as the Bair Hugger. Certain sensors, such as nasal sensors, are designed for application to areas where perfusion is preserved even when peripheral perfusion is relatively poor. Finally, some pulse oximeters use an electrocardiogram (ECG) signal as an aid in identifying the pulse, thus enhancing the instrument's ability to detect a weak pulse.

The patient movement seen in the PACU can produce false signals that interfere with the pulse oximeter's ability to identify the true pulse, thus leading to unreliable SpO_2 and pulse rate readings. When movement presents a problem, check whether the sensor is properly and securely applied; a sensor that is loosely attached or incorrectly positioned can magnify the effect of motion. If the problem persists, consider moving the sensor to a less active site. Also, pulse oximeters that use the ECG signal as an aid in identifying the pulse can have an enhanced ability to distinguish between the true pulse and artifacts produced by motion. The result is more reliable SpO_2 readings.

Normally, venous blood is nonpulsatile and is not detected by a pulse oximeter. In the presence of venous pulsations, the SpO_2 value provided by the pulse oximeter may be a composite of both arterial and venous saturations. Venous pulsations may occur in patients with severe right-sided heart failure or other pathophysiologic states that create venous congestion and in patients receiving high levels of positive end-expiratory pressure. They may also occur when the sensor is placed distal to a blood pressure cuff or occlusive dressing and when additional tape is wrapped tightly around the sensor. When venous pulsations are present, the perianesthesia nurse should take care in interpreting the SpO_2 readings and, if possible, attempt to eliminate their cause.

Because pulse oximeters are optical measuring devices, the perianesthesia nurse must be aware of additional factors that can influence the reliability of SpO_2 readings. To ensure good light reception, the sensor's light sources and detector must always be positioned according to the manufacturer's specifications. In the presence of bright lights, such as infrared warming devices, fluorescent lights, direct sunlight, and surgical lights, the sensor must be covered with an opaque material to prevent incorrect SpO_2 readings. Also, agents that significantly change the optical-absorbing properties of blood, such as recently administered intravascular dyes, can interfere with reliable SpO_2 measurements. The use of pulse oximetry with certain nail polishes, especially those that are blue, green, and reddish-brown in color, may result in inaccurate readings. If nail polish in these shades cannot be removed, the sensor should be applied to an alternate unpolished site.

Monitoring Ventilation by Capnography

Monitoring CO_2 in respiratory gases provides an early warning of physiologic and mechanical events that interfere with normal ventilation. Capnography, which measures CO_2 at the patient's airway, is increasingly used in the PACU. It allows continuous assessment of the adequacy of alveolar ventilation, the function of the cardiopulmonary system, ventilator function, and the integrity of the airway and the breathing circuit. Consequently, it enables early detection of many potentially catastrophic events, including the onset of malignant hyperthermia, esophageal intubation, hypoventilation, partial or complete airway obstruction, breathing circuit leaks or disconnects, a large pulmonary embolus, and cardiac arrest.

Two variants of the instrument are available. A capnometer provides numeric measurement of exhaled CO_2 levels. A capnograph provides the same numeric information, and it also displays a CO_2 waveform. Both types of instruments usually incorporate an adjustable alarm system and often have trending and printing capabilities. The following discussion focuses on the use of capnographs, because they allow more complete and effective patient assessment than do capnometers. As discussed later, changes in the shape of the CO_2 waveform can provide crucial diagnostic information about ventilation, similar to the way in which the waveform provided by an ECG can provide crucial diagnostic information about the heart.

Technology Overview. To measure exhaled CO_2, the most common type of capnograph passes infrared light at a wavelength that is absorbed by CO_2 through a sample of the patient's respiratory gas. The amount of light that is absorbed by the patient's gas reflects the amount of CO_2 in the sample.

Capnographs differ in the manner in which they obtain respiratory gas samples for analysis. Sidestream (or diverting) capnographs transport the sample through narrow-gauge tubing to a measuring chamber. Mainstream (or nondiverting) capnographs position a flow-through measurement chamber directly on the patient's airway. Special adapters are available to allow sidestream capnographs to be used on nonintubated patients. The sample adapter should be placed as close to the patient's endotracheal tube or airway as possible.

Sidestream capnographs incorporate moisture-control features that are designed to minimize clogging of the sample tube, protect the measurement chamber from moisture-induced damage, and minimize the risk of cross-contamination. The design of these moisture-control systems significantly impacts a monitor's ease of use. Most rely on water traps, which must be emptied routinely. A new technology uses a special system of filters and tubing to dehumidify the sample, thus eliminating the need for water traps.

Capnographs also differ in their calibration requirements. Many require removal of the patient from the respiratory circuit and adjustment of the instrument with special mixtures of calibration gases. Advanced capnographic technology includes automatic calibration and does not require any user calibration skills or time.

The Normal Capnogram. To effectively use capnography, it is important to understand the components of the normal CO_2 waveform (capnogram), which are illustrated in Figure 25-3. Early in exhalation, air from the anatomic dead space, which is virtually CO_2 free, is measured by the instrument. As exhalation continues, alveolar gas reaches the sampling site, and the CO_2 level increases rapidly. The CO_2 concentration continues to increase throughout exhalation and reaches the alveolar plateau because alveolar gas dominates the sample. At the end of exhalation, the peak (end-tidal) CO_2 ($ETCO_2$) occurs, which in the normal lung is the best approximation of alveolar CO_2 levels. The CO_2 concentration then drops rapidly as the next inhalation of CO_2-free gas begins.

End-Tidal Versus Arterial CO_2. Under normal conditions, when ventilation and perfusion are well matched, $ETCO_2$ closely approximates arterial CO_2 ($PaCO_2$). The difference between the $PaCO_2$ and the $ETCO_2$ levels is referred to as the alveolar-arterial CO2 difference (a-$ADCO_2$). $ETCO_2$ is usually as much as 5 mm Hg lower than $PaCO_2$. When the two measurements differ significantly, an anomaly in the patient's physiology, the breathing circuit, or the capnograph is usually present. Significant divergence between $ETCO_2$ and $PaCO_2$ is often attributable to increased alveolar dead space. CO_2-free gas from nonperfused alveoli mixes with gas from perfused regions, thus decreasing the $ETCO_2$ measurement. Clinical conditions that cause increased dead space—such as pulmonary hypoperfusion, cardiac arrest, and pulmonary embolus—can increase the a-$ADCO_2$. Changes in the a-$ADCO_2$ can be used to assess the efficacy of the treatment; as the patient's dead space improves, the PAO_2-PaO_2 narrows. Alternatively, a significant PAO_2-PaO_2 can indicate incomplete alveolar emptying (such as with reactive airway disease), a leak in the gas-sampling system that allows loss of respiratory gas, and contamination of respiratory gas with fresh gas.

Interpretation of Changes in the Capnogram. An abnormal capnogram provides an initial warning of many events that warrant immediate intervention. Abnormalities may be seen on a breath-by-breath basis or when the CO_2 trend is examined. For this reason, it is preferable to visualize both the real-time waveform and the CO_2

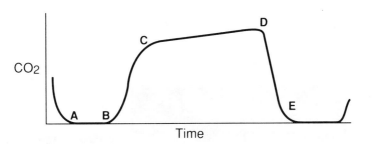

Fig. 25-3 The normal capnogram. *AB,* Beginning exhalation, dead space; *BC,* initial alveolar emptying; *CD,* end-alveolar emptying; *D,* end-tidal CO_2; *E,* inspiration (CO_2-free gas).

trend on the monitor display. This discussion will provide a few examples of changes produced by significant events that commonly occur in the PACU.

A sudden decrease in $ETCO_2$ to a near-zero level indicates that the monitor is no longer detecting CO_2 in exhaled gases (Fig. 25-4). Immediate action is crucial to detect and correct the cause of this loss of ventilation. Possible causes include a completely blocked endotracheal tube, esophageal intubation, a disconnection in the breathing circuit, and inadvertent extubation. The latter three possibilities are particularly likely if the decrease in $ETCO_2$ coincides with movement of the patient's head. Only after eliminating possible clinical causes for this decrease in $ETCO_2$, investigate whether a clogged sampling tube or instrument malfunction may be causing the problem.

An exponential decrease in $ETCO_2$ over a small number of breaths usually signals a life-threatening cardiopulmonary event that has dramatically increased dead space ventilation (Fig. 25-5). Sudden hypotension, pulmonary embolism, and circulatory arrest with continued ventilation must be considered.

A gradual increase in the $ETCO_2$ level while the capnogram retains its normal shape usually indicates that ventilation is inadequate to eliminate the CO_2 that is being produced (Fig. 25-6). This situation can be the result of a small ventilator leak or a partial airway obstruction that reduces minute ventilation. It can also reflect increased CO_2 production associated with increased body temperature, the onset of sepsis, or shivering. Of particular importance, a large increase in $ETCO_2$ can be one of the earliest signs of malignant hyperthermia, which may not begin until after emergence from anesthesia.

A gradual decrease in the $ETCO_2$ level commonly occurs in the patient who is anesthetized, narcotized, hyperventilated, or hypothermic (Fig. 25-7).

Assessment of the capnogram can reveal information about the quality of alveolar emptying. For example, the patient with bronchospasm is unable to completely empty his or her alveoli, and the resulting capnogram will not have an alveolar plateau (Fig. 25-8). The $ETCO_2$ reported by the capnograph in this instance is not a good estimate of alveolar CO_2. Effective administration of bronchodilator therapy commonly improves alveolar emptying and results in a more normal capnogram.

Clinical Issues. In addition to the diagnostic usefulness of changes in the capnogram, some

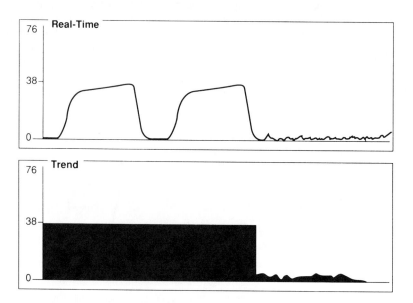

Fig. 25-4 Sudden decrease in end-tidal CO_2 to near-zero level.

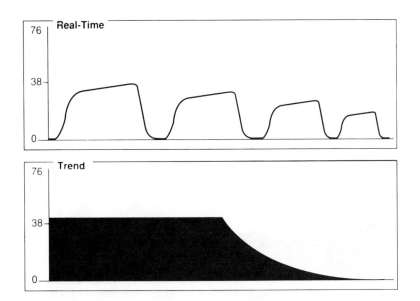

Fig. 25-5   Exponential decrease in end-tidal CO_2.

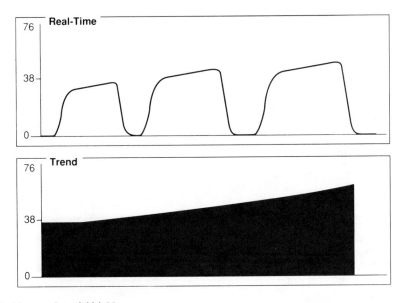

Fig. 25-6   Gradual increase in end-tidal CO_2.

specific applications of capnography are particularly valuable in the PACU. Of primary importance is its ability to provide early warning of hypoventilation that, in the PACU, may be secondary to anesthesia, sedation, analgesia, or pain.

A falling $ETCO_2$ may indicate pulmonary hypoperfusion due to blood loss or hypotension. During rewarming, $ETCO_2$ values are likely to increase as metabolic activity increases. Capnography can signal when shivering is producing an

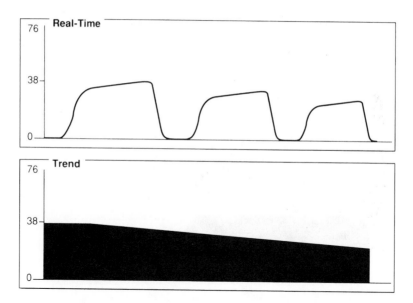

Fig. 25-7 Gradual decrease in end-tidal CO_2.

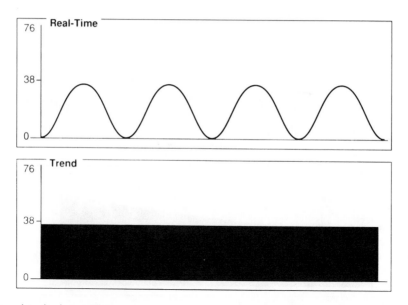

Fig. 25-8 Incomplete alveolar emptying.

unacceptable increase in oxygen consumption and metabolic rate. During ventilator weaning, capnography is valuable in assessing the adequacy of ventilation.

Recent studies have demonstrated the value of capnography in monitoring the course and efficacy of cardiopulmonary resuscitation (CPR). $ETCO_2$ measurements, which decrease during cardiac arrest, typically reach about 50% of normal levels during effective CPR. When spontaneous circulation is restored, $ETCO_2$ values increase dramatically.

The presence and persistence of normal $ETCO_2$ values are also useful determinants in confirming tracheal intubation, because CO_2 is not normally found in the esophagus. However, capnography cannot be substituted for chest auscultation and radiograph in eliminating the possibility of bronchial intubation.

CARDIOVASCULAR FUNCTION AND PERFUSION

The three basic components of the circulatory system that must be evaluated are (1) the heart as a pump; (2) the blood; and (3) the arteriovenous system. The maintenance of good tissue perfusion depends on a satisfactory cardiac output. Therefore most assessment is aimed at evaluating cardiac output.

Clinical Assessment

Observe the overall condition of the patient, especially skin color and turgor. Peripheral cyanosis, edema, dilatation of the neck veins, shortness of breath, and many other findings may be indicative of cardiovascular problems. In addition to checking all operative sites for blood loss, note the amount of blood lost during surgery and the patient's most recent hemoglobin level.

Blood Pressure Monitoring

Arterial blood pressure must be assessed in the preoperative physical assessment, on admission to and discharge from the PACU, and at frequent, regular intervals during the PACU stay. Arterial blood pressure is currently measured either noninvasively (indirectly) or invasively (directly). Noninvasive methods include manual cuff measurement with either an aneroid or mercury sphygmomanometer and automatic measurements with an electronic blood pressure monitor. Invasive measurement may be accomplished via a transduced arterial line. A clear understanding of proper technique is essential to ensure accurate and reliable readings with all the blood pressure measurement methods.

Noninvasive Measurement

Manual Method. An aneroid or mercury-type sphygmomanometer with inflatable cuff and stethoscope is required for the standard auscultatory blood pressure measurement technique. It is essential to use the correct cuff size. The width of

the inflatable bladder that is encased inside the cuff should be 40% to 50% of upper arm circumference. A bladder that is too wide underestimates blood pressure, whereas a bladder that is too narrow overestimates blood pressure. The length of the bladder should be at least 80% of the arm circumference.

The cuff is placed on the extremity, with the inflatable bladder positioned directly over the artery at the level of the heart. The brachial artery is the site most commonly used for blood pressure measurement. If the upper extremities are unavailable for cuff placement because of operative issues or other problems, the lower extremities may be used. The bladder of the cuff should be centered over the posterior surface of the lower third of the thigh, and pressure may be auscultated over the popliteal artery or at the ankle over the posterior tibial artery (just posterior to the medial malleolus). Systolic pressure in the legs is usually 20 to 30 mm Hg higher than in the brachial artery.

The cuff is inflated, and when cuff pressure exceeds the arterial pressure, arterial blood flow will cease and the pulse will no longer be palpated. As pressure is released by turning the valve of the inflation bulb, blood flow will resume, and audible (Korotkoff) sounds will be noted with the stethoscope. These sounds change in quality and intensity throughout further cuff deflation and generally disappear. The American Heart Association recommends that the systolic pressure be noted as the first audible sound in the cuff-deflating process. The diastolic pressure is marked by the disappearance of sounds in the adult patient and the muffling of sounds in the pediatric patient.

A common cause of error in blood pressure measurement is an auscultatory gap that may be present, especially in hypertensive patients. This gap is a silent interval between the systolic and diastolic pressures. During this gap, the pulse is palpable. Therefore to avoid mistakenly low systolic readings, the cuff should be inflated until the pulse is obliterated. Blood pressure readings should be recorded completely, including the systolic pressure, the point at which the sounds become muffled and when they cease, and, if present, the range of the auscultatory gap.

Auscultatory blood pressure measurements may be completed quickly and easily under many circumstances. The accuracy and reliability of the readings may be affected by low flow states (including decreased cardiac output and vasoconstriction) or decreased sound transmission caused by factors related to the patient (edema and obesity) or the environment (noise). Cuff size and placement, user error, and improperly calibrated manometers may also contribute to unreliable readings. Because measurements are intermittent and must be initiated by the user, blood pressure changes may go unnoticed in the postoperative patient with labile hemodynamics or sudden blood loss. The use of automatic blood pressure monitors that can be set to measure blood pressure at regular, frequent intervals can minimize some of this risk.

Automatic Method. Automatic blood pressure monitoring with electronic devices has become increasingly prevalent in the PACU. The devices are commonly used to provide frequent blood pressure measurements over relatively brief periods, when the need for arterial sampling is minimal to absent, and when the risks of arterial lines cannot be justified.

One of the most commonly used automatic noninvasive blood pressure methods is based on oscillometric technology. The cuff is chosen and applied according to conventional technique. Oscillations of the arterial wall are occluded as the cuff is inflated and are detected during cuff deflation. Systolic pressure is indicated at the onset of oscillations. As cuff pressure decreases, oscillations increase in amplitude and peak at the mean arterial pressure. The point at which oscillations disappear is the diastolic pressure (Fig. 25-9). All three pressures are normally reported on oscillometric monitoring devices.

Automatic noninvasive blood pressure monitors may be set to cycle at various measurement periods. The instruments alarm when systolic and diastolic pressures register outside of a preset range. Equipment should be calibrated on a regular basis, and preventive maintenance should include assessment for leaks. The use of automatic devices may be limited in patients with low-flow states or high peripheral vascular resistance and in those who are severely obese or edematous. These devices provide only intermittent measurements and are less desirable for assessment of the labile patient.

Newer advances in noninvasive blood pressure technology, currently available for

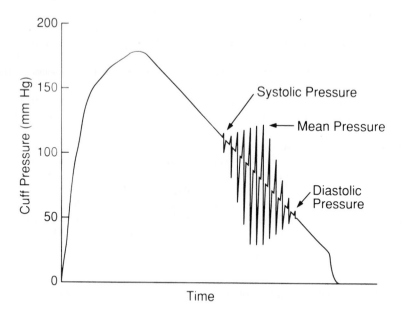

Fig. 25-9 Oscillometric blood pressure measurement. Systolic pressure is indicated at the onset of oscillations. Mean arterial pressure occurs when oscillations peak in amplitude. The point at which oscillations disappear is the diastolic pressure.

intraoperative monitoring of the anesthetized patient, include continuous monitoring capabilities that ensure detection in sudden blood pressure variations. The only other method of continuous blood pressure monitoring currently available is invasive arterial blood pressure technology.

Invasive Measurement. Invasive arterial pressure measurements are most commonly obtained via cannulation of the radial artery but may be obtained at other arterial sites as well. A continuous flush solution is connected to the intraarterial catheter and is slowly infused into the arterial vessel under pressure. The pressure within the artery is transmitted through the column of fluid to the transducer. The transducer then converts this pressure to an electrical signal that can be converted to millimeters of mercury and displayed on the monitor. A corresponding arterial waveform, or pressure pulse, is also displayed on the monitor.

Arterial blood pressure measurements are continuous and are indicated for hemodynamically high-risk patients. Changes in patients' pressures can be observed on an ongoing basis. This technology may also be chosen in patients for whom indirect measurements fail, because of diminished or absent Korotkoff sounds (as in obese or edematous patients), and with high peripheral vascular resistance. The direct arterial access is also beneficial if the patient requires frequent blood samples for laboratory analysis.

To ensure more reliable arterial blood pressure readings, the clinician should balance and calibrate the system according to the manufacturer's specifications. The transducer must always be balanced and positioned at the fourth intercostal level at the midaxillary line. Aseptic technique must always be used during placement and maintenance of the arterial line and transducer.

Damping of the arterial waveform with subsequent unreliable readings may occur for a variety of reasons, including clotting and kinking of the arterial catheter, positioning of the catheter against the arterial wall, and the presence of air bubbles within the arterial line system. Loose connections, calibration error, and equipment failure may also contribute to unreliable readings.

An Allen test should be performed before radial artery cannulation to minimize the risk of hand ischemia (see Chapter 9). If arterial lines are discontinued in the PACU, constant pressure should be applied to the site for 10 to 15 minutes or until bleeding has ceased. A pressure dressing should be applied, and the site should be checked frequently for any bleeding.

Complications and risks of invasive arterial blood pressure monitoring include infection, thrombosis, emboli, tissue ischemia, hemorrhage, and vessel perforation. Arterial blood pressure monitoring is generally contraindicated in patients with septicemia, coagulopathies, irradiated arterial sites, anatomic anomalies, inadequate collateral blood flow, or thrombosis.

Clinical Issues. To assess their significance, blood pressure readings in the postoperative period must be compared with preoperative baseline measurements. A low postoperative blood pressure may be the result of a number of factors—including the effects of muscle relaxants, spinal anesthesia, preoperative medication, changes in the patient's position, blood loss, poor lung ventilation, and peripheral pooling of blood. The administration of oxygen to help eliminate anesthetic gases and to assist the patient in awakening causes an increase in blood pressure. Deep breathing, leg exercises, verbal stimulation, and conversation can be instituted to raise the blood pressure. A low fluid volume may be augmented by increasing the rate of intravenous fluids, which helps maintain the arterial pressure. Any method designed to raise the pressure must be instituted with consideration for the patient's overall condition.

An increase in blood pressure postoperatively is not uncommon because of the effects of anesthesia, respiratory insufficiency, or decreased respiratory rate and depth causing CO_2 retention. The surgical procedure, with its accompanying discomfort, also causes increased blood pressure. Emergence delirium, with its excitement, struggling, and pain, may also be a causative factor in a transient increase in blood pressure. Obviously, it is important to determine the cause before treatment is instituted. In patients with uncontrolled hypertension, continuous intravenous antihypertensive medications may be required. However, it is extremely important to diagnose the cause of the hypertension so that effective therapy may be employed rapidly.

Pulse Pressure Monitoring

Pulse pressure is an important determinant in the evaluation of perfusion. Because of the pulsatile nature of the heart, blood enters the arteries intermittently, thus causing pressure increases and decreases. The difference between the systolic and diastolic pressures equals the pulse pressure. The pulse pressure is affected by two major factors: the stroke volume output of the heart and the compliance (total distensibility) of the arterial tree. The pulse pressure is determined approximately by the ratio of stroke output to compliance. Therefore any condition that affects either of these factors also affects the pulse pressure.

To evaluate the patient's cardiovascular status accurately, all signs and symptoms must be evaluated individually as well as within the body system as a whole. For example, cool extremities, decreased urine output, and narrowed pulse pressure may be indicative of decreased cardiac output, even in the presence of normal blood pressure.

Pulses. The rate and character of all pulses should be assessed bilaterally. Examine the pulses simultaneously to determine their equality and time of arrival. Peripheral arterial occlusion is not uncommon; if it is suspected, a Doppler instrument can be of great value in detecting the presence or absence of blood flow. Occlusion is an emergency and must be reported to the surgeon at once.

Irregularities in pulse are most commonly caused by premature beats, generally premature ventricular contractions (PVCs) or premature atrial contractions (PACs). These irregular rhythms should be thoroughly investigated before therapy is initiated.

ELECTROCARDIOGRAPHIC MONITORING

The perianesthesia nurse must have a basic understanding of cardiac monitoring and should be able to interpret the basic cardiac rhythms and dysrhythmias and correlate them with expected cardiac output and its effects on the patient's condition. According to the most recent ASPAN standards, ECG monitoring should be available for each patient in a Phase I PACU and should be readily available for patients in Phase II units. Arrhythmias of any type may occur at any time and in any patient during the postoperative period. Therefore accurate ECG monitoring and interpretation are mandatory skills for

the perianesthesia nurse (see Chapter 9). This section is designed to provide an introduction to specific problems of cardiac monitoring in the PACU.

Any type of cardiac arrhythmia may be seen in the PACU. The causes of specific arrhythmias must be carefully differentiated before any treatment is instituted. Some commonly encountered problems are reviewed here, but the list is by no means complete.

All abnormal rhythms should be documented with a rhythm strip and recorded in the patient's progress record. Any questionable rhythms should be documented by a complete 12-lead ECG.

Electrical monitoring of the patient's heart is only one assessment parameter and must be interpreted in conjunction with other salient parameters before therapy is initiated. Cardiac monitors generally depict only a single lead. They do not detect all rhythm disturbances and alterations, and a 12-lead ECG is essential to define a conduction problem accurately.

Lead Placement

The skin where the electrode will be placed should be clean, dry, and smooth. Excessive hair should be removed; moisture or skin oils should be removed with alcohol or acetone and the skin mildly abraded to obtain good adherence of the electrode.

Site selection on the chest is based on a triangular arrangement of positive, negative, and ground electrodes. Avoid placing electrodes directly over the diaphragm, areas of auscultation, heavy bones, or large muscles. Allow adequate space for application of defibrillator paddles in the event that defibrillation should become necessary. Figure 25-10 depicts the most commonly used electrode leads. The modified lead II is the most commonly used because it is the most versatile; it is useful in assessing P waves, PR intervals, and atrial arrhythmias. The modified chest lead I is useful for assessing bundle branch block and differentiating between ventricular arrhythmias and aberrations. This lead is useful when the patient is known to have preexisting cardiac disease. The Lewis lead is useful when P waves are difficult to distinguish using other leads.

Sinus Arrhythmias

Sinus Bradycardia. Figure 25-11 shows a slow heart rate—less than 60 beats per min. Its rhythm may be irregular owing to accompanying sinus arrhythmias. All other complex features are normal.

Sinus bradycardia is commonly encountered in the PACU because of the depressant effects of anesthesia. Young, healthy adults, especially those who are normally physically active, often have bradycardia. Usually no treatment is necessary except to continue the stir-up regimen. Excessive parasympathetic stimulation from pain may cause bradycardia, in which case appropriate analgesics should be administered and other pain-relieving measures initiated. If the patient shows symptoms of low cardiac output, the physician should be notified and treatment instituted using atropine to block vagal effects or isoproterenol to stimulate the cardiac pacemaker. If temporary pacing wires are available, either atrial or ventricular pacing can be attempted.

Sinus Tachycardia. Figure 25-12 shows a fast heart rate—more than 100 beats per minute. The rhythm may be slightly irregular, and all other complex features are normal.

Sinus tachycardia results from any stress and may be encountered in the PACU because of numerous causes, including the stress of surgery, anoxia, fever, overhydration, hypovolemia, pain, anxiety, or apprehension, or any combination of these factors. Tachycardia is an important postoperative sign and should be fully evaluated before treatment is instituted. Increasing tachycardia is an early sign of shock and must be thoroughly investigated. Treatment must be specific and based on removal of the underlying cause (see Chapter 51). The patient should be assessed carefully for his or her ability to tolerate the rapid rate. The deleterious effects of tachycardias are generally related to diminished stroke volume and cardiac output. In general, the patient with previously normal cardiac function can tolerate tachycardias as high as 160 beats per minute without manifesting symptoms. Poor tolerance with a resultant decrease in cardiac output occurs when the diastolic interval—and thus the ventricular filling time—is significantly compromised.

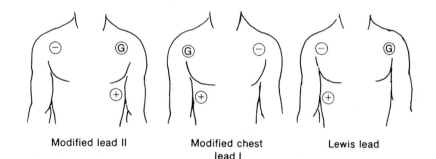

Modified lead II   Modified chest lead I   Lewis lead

Fig. 25-10 Basic electrode placement.

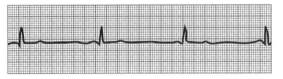

Fig. 25-11 Sinus bradycardia (lead III).

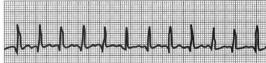

Fig. 25-12 Sinus tachycardia (lead I).

Sinus Arrest (Atrial Standstill). Sinus arrest is failure of the sinoatrial (SA) node to discharge, with resulting loss of atrial contraction. The rate remains within normal ranges. The rhythm is regular except when the SA node fails to discharge. P waves and QRS complexes are normal when the SA node is firing and absent when it fails to discharge.

Common causes of sinus arrest in the PACU are the depressant effects of anesthesia or analgesics and electrolyte disturbances. Treatment is aimed at eliminating depressant drugs from the body and correcting electrolyte imbalances. This arrhythmia must be brought to the attention of the physician immediately, because persistent sinus arrest constitutes an emergency, and CPR must be initiated.

Supraventricular Arrhythmias

Supraventricular arrhythmias consist of supraventricular extrasystole (PAC), atrial tachycardia, atrial flutter, and atrial fibrillation. Supraventricular arrhythmias occur in about 10% to 40% of patients after coronary artery bypass graft surgery. These rhythms should be documented with a 12-lead ECG. Their cause has been related to a number of possible factors, such as an inflammatory reaction to surgical trauma, insufficient "protection" of the atria during surgery, atrioventricular (AV) node ischemia, and sudden withdrawal of beta blockers. A correlation exists between persistent atrial activity during cardioplegic arrest and postoperative supraventricular arrhythmias.

Premature Atrial Contraction. PAC, or atrial premature beat, occurs earlier than expected, resulting from an irritable focus in the atrium (Fig. 25-13). Cardiac rate and rhythm are normal except for their prematurity. The P wave configuration of the premature beat usually differs from that of the normal beat. The PAC is followed by a pause that is not fully compensatory.

This arrhythmia results from anxiety and is commonly encountered in the PACU. No treatment is necessary unless the PACs become frequent or the patient becomes symptomatic. If pharmacologic therapy becomes necessary, agents such as propranolol and verapamil can be administered.

Atrial Tachycardia. Atrial tachycardia is a rhythm disturbance that is a rapid, regular supraventricular heart rate that results from an irritable focus of five or more PACs in succession (Fig. 25-14). The rate is 150 to 200 beats per minute with a regular rhythm.

This rhythm should be documented with a full 12-lead ECG. The physician should be notified to institute therapy. Maneuvers that enhance vagal tone—such as the Valsalva maneuver and carotid sinus massage—may be successful in terminating this arrhythmia. Antiarrhythmic agents such as digitalis, quinidine, and verapamil may cause the patient to revert to normal sinus rhythm. If these measures are unsuccessful, cardioversion with countershock will be necessary.

Atrial Flutter. Atrial flutter consists of rapid supraventricular contractions resulting from an ectopic focus with varying degrees of ventricular blocking (Fig. 25-15). Its cause is the same as that of PACs and atrial tachycardia. The rhythm is

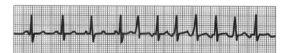

Fig. 25-14 Atrial paroxysmal tachycardia—onset in middle of record (lead I).

Premature beat

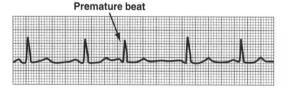

Fig. 25-13 Atrial premature beat (lead I).

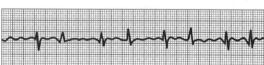

Fig. 25-15 Atrial flutter—2:1 and 3:1 rhythm (lead I).

usually regular; the atrial rate is 250 to 350 beats per minute. Treatment is the same as for atrial tachycardia.

Atrial Fibrillation. In atrial fibrillation, one or more irritable atrial foci discharge at an extremely rapid rate that lacks coordinated activity (Fig. 25-16).

Atrial fibrillation occurs commonly in patients with atrial enlargement from mitral valve disease or from long-standing coronary artery disease and is often preceded by PACs, tachycardia, or flutter. Clinically, the patient has an irregular heartbeat, pulse rate, and, usually, a noticeable pulse deficit. Cardiac output decreases in varying degrees. Normally, atrial filling and contraction account for 30% of ventricular filling. Without this atrial filling, or "atrial kick," of volume into the ventricle, stroke volumes and thus cardiac outputs are diminished. Treatment involves digitalis, quinidine, verapamil, atrial pacing, or cardioversion.

Ventricular Arrhythmias

Myocardial ischemia and perioperative myocardial infarction remain the two major causes of ventricular arrhythmias; however, bradycardia, hypokalemia, hypoxemia, acidosis, and hypothermia are also potential causes.

Premature Ventricular Contraction. PVC is a rhythm disturbance involving an earlier-than-expected ventricular contraction from an irritable focus in the ventricle (Fig. 25-17). The rhythm is regular except for the premature beat, and the rate is normal.

The P wave is absent from the premature beat. A wide, bizarre, notched QRS complex that may be of greater-than-normal amplitude is present. A widened T wave of greater-than-normal amplitude is present after the premature beat and is of opposite deflection to that of the QRS complex.

The PVC is followed by a pause that is fully compensatory (i.e., the time of the PVC plus the pause time equals the time of two normal beats).

PVCs are commonly encountered in the PACU and can occur in any patient. Occasional PVCs occur normally and need no treatment. Multiple PVCs may indicate inadequate oxygenation, and when they occur, the patient's respiratory status should be thoroughly assessed. Other causative factors of PVCs include electrolyte disturbances, acid-base imbalance, drug toxicity, and hypoxemia of the myocardium.

Treatment of PVCs is based on the underlying cause and obliteration of the irritable focus. Occasional, isolated PVCs need not be treated. If PVCs occur more frequently than five per minute, if a successive run of two or more occurs, if they are multifocal, or if they occur during the vulnerable period on the ECG complex, they must be treated, because they are the precursors of the more lethal ventricular arrhythmias.

Ventricular arrhythmias present in the setting

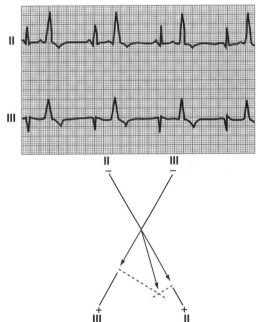

Fig. 25-17 Premature ventricular contractions (leads II and III). *(From Guyton A, Hall J: Textbook of medical physiology, ed 10, Philadelphia, 2000, WB Saunders.)*

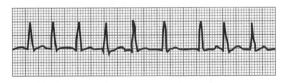

Fig. 25-16 Atrial fibrillation (lead I).

of bradycardia should be treated with atropine or with overdrive pacing to eliminate ventricular escape rhythms. Otherwise, lidocaine should be the first drug of choice to treat ventricular arrhythmias.

Ventricular Tachycardia. Three or more consecutive PVCs constitute ventricular tachycardia (Fig. 25-18). The rhythm is fairly regular, and P waves are not seen. Occasionally, patients may have ventricular tachycardia and be asymptomatic, but usually they experience anxiety, palpitations, fluttering, pounding in the chest, dizziness, faintness, and precordial pain. If ventricular tachycardia is prolonged, cyanosis, mental confusion, convulsions, and unconsciousness develop as a result of decreased blood and oxygen supply to the brain.

The causative factors of ventricular tachycardia are essentially the same as those for PVCs. Most commonly, ventricular tachycardia in the PACU is the result of hypoxia, drug toxicity, or underlying heart disease.

Ventricular tachycardia must be treated immediately. If the patient initially tolerates the arrhythmia, treatment should be instituted with lidocaine. If the patient has cardiac decompensation and circulatory insufficiency, cardioversion with direct-current (DC) electrical countershock should be immediately instituted. Immediate notification of the physician is essential.

Ventricular Fibrillation. A rapid, irregular quivering of the ventricles that is uncoordinated and incapable of pumping blood characterizes ventricular fibrillation (Fig. 25-19). This rhythm disturbance is the major death-producing cardiac arrhythmia. The immediate initial treatment is external DC countershock (Fig. 25-20). Ventricular fibrillation may occur spontaneously without any forewarning, or it may be preceded by evidence of ventricular irritability. Patients likely to develop ventricular fibrillation include those with underlying heart disease, those who evidenced ventricular irritability in the operating room during surgery, and those with symptoms of shock. All of these patients should be monitored continuously throughout their recovery periods.

If ventricular fibrillation is not immediately terminated with countershock, CPR is instituted without delay. The anesthesiologist should be summoned immediately (see Chapter 53).

HEMODYNAMIC MONITORING

Although more prominent in cardiac surgery, additional hemodynamic monitoring is commonly used with patients of higher acuity who do

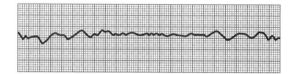

Fig. 25-19 Ventricular fibrillation (lead II).

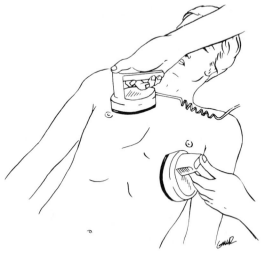

Fig. 25-20 The emergency administration of external direct-current countershock. *(From Sanderson RC: The cardiac patient, Philadelphia, 1972, WB Saunders.)*

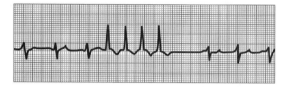

Fig. 25-18 Ventricular paroxysmal tachycardia (lead III).

not receive care in many PACUs. Hemodynamic monitoring can be accomplished via the following invasive lines: a flow-directed pulmonary artery catheter, a central venous pressure catheter, a left-atrial or right-atrial catheter, a pulmonary artery thermistor catheter, or a peripheral arterial catheter (A-line). The parameters obtained from these various lines, the catheter insertion sites, and the placement and monitoring methods are presented in Table 25-1

Table 25-1	**Methods for Invasive Monitoring of Hemodynamic Parameters**			
Parameters	Catheter Placement	Insertion Sites	Monitoring Method	Special Considerations
RAP	Proximal port of FDPAC lies in the right atrium	Brachial Jugular Subclavian	Water manometer	Intermittent readings at lowest fluctuation*
	Distal end of RAC or CVP lies in the right atrium	Direct insertion through RA wall[†]	Transducer[‡]	Intermittent or continuous readings on mean[§]
PAP	Distal end of FDPAC lies in right or left branch of pulmonary artery Distal end of PATC lies in main pulmonary artery	Brachial Jugular Subclavian Direct insertion through PA wall[†]	Transducer	Readings on systole and diastole
PCWP	Inflation of balloon on tip of FDPAC allows it to float into a wedged position in a smaller branch of the pulmonary artery	Brachial Jugular Subclavian	Transducer	Intermittent readings on mean[§]
LAP	Distal end of the LAC lies in left atrium	Direct insertion through LA wall[†]	Water manometer	Intermittent reading recorded at lowest fluctuation*
MAP	Distal end of catheter lies in a peripheral artery	Radial Brachial Femoral	Anaeroid manometer	Midpoint of needle fluctuation
			Transducer	Continuous readings on mean[§]

Adapted from Whitman GR: Bedside hemodynamic monitoring. In Horvath PT, editor: Care of the adult cardiac surgery patient, New York, 1984, John Wiley & Sons.

RAP, Right-atrial pressure; *PAP,* pulmonary artery pressure; *PCWP,* pulmonary capillary wedge pressure; *LAP,* left-atrial pressure; *MAP,* mean arterial pressure; *FDPAC,* flow-directed pulmonary artery catheter; *RAC,* right-atrial catheter; *LAC,* left-atrial catheter; *CVP,* central venous pressure; *PATC,* pulmonary artery thermistor catheter.

*Fluctuation indicates a patent catheter and good position in the thorax.

[†]Direct insertion is achieved during an open chest procedure via a median sternotomy incision. The exit site is via a stab wound at the distal portion of the median sternotomy. The catheter is attached to skin with suture. Removal is achieved by removing the suture and applying gentle traction to the catheter to free it from the chamber wall. The catheter is sutured to chamber wall with absorbable suture so that it releases easily. Chest tubes remain in place until such lines are removed, owing to the possibility of bleeding.

[‡]To convert mm Hg to cm H_2O, multiply mm Hg reading times 1.36.

[§]Biphasic waves are measured on mean.

and depicted in Figure 25-21. Problems associated with maintaining these lines are summarized in Table 25-2.

Right-Atrial Pressure

The normal right-atrial pressure ranges from 0 to 7 mm Hg. Pressures exceeding that level can be the result of fluid overload, right-ventricular failure, tricuspid valve abnormalities, pulmonary hypertension, constrictive pericarditis, or cardiac tamponade. Values in the lower range are usually indicative of hypovolemia.

Pulmonary Artery Pressure

Pulmonary artery systolic pressures normally range from 15 to 25 mm Hg, whereas a normal pulmonary artery diastolic pressure is 8 to 15 mm Hg. Hypovolemia contributes to low pressure readings. Increased volume loads that can develop with an atrial or ventricular septal defect or left-ventricular failure can create elevations in pressure. Additionally, obstructions to forward flow that can be caused by mitral stenosis or pulmonary hypertension can lead to an elevation in pulmonary artery pressures.

Pulmonary Capillary Wedge Pressure

Normal pulmonary capillary wedge pressure (PCWP) recordings are between 6 and 15 mm Hg. Values in this range can be caused by an increased volume load, as is seen in left-ventricular failure, or they can be created by an obstruction to forward flow. Such obstructions may be caused by mitral stenosis or regurgitation or by a pulmonary embolism. Lower values may result from hypovolemia or indicate an obstruction to left-ventricular filling, which could occur with a pulmonary embolism, pulmonary stenosis, or right-ventricular failure.

Left-Atrial Pressure

Normal left-atrial pressures range from 4 to 12 mm Hg. As is seen with the PCWP, elevations in left-atrial pressure are associated with volume overloads or obstructions to forward flow, the latter of which may consist of left-ventricular failure states, mitral or aortic valve dysfunctions, or constrictive pericarditis. Lower recordings are generally a consequence of hypovolemia from inadequate volume or related to an obstruction to forward flow. Such an obstruction may

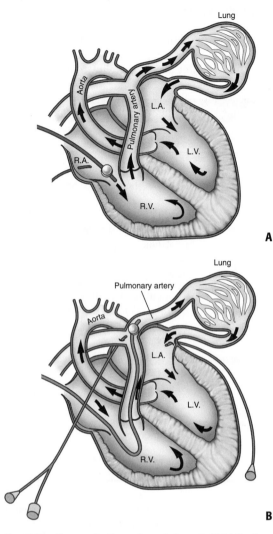

Fig. 25-21 Placement of hemodynamic lines. **A,** Distal tip of a flow-directed pulmonary artery catheter (FDPAC) lying in the right atrium as it floats toward the pulmonary artery, and the distal tip of a right atrial catheter directly inserted through the right atrial wall lying in the right atrium. **B,** Distal tip of an FDPAC advancing into a wedged position. Also illustrated is the distal tip of a pulmonary artery thermistor catheter lying in the pulmonary artery after direct insertion through the pulmonary artery wall and the distal tip of a left atrial catheter lying in the left atrium after direct insertion through the left atrial wall near or in a pulmonary vein. *R.A.,* Right atrium; *L.A.,* left atrium; *R.V.,* right ventricle; *L.V.,* left ventricle. *(From Whitman GR: Bedside cardiovascular monitoring. In Horvath PT: Care of the adult cardiac surgery patient, New York, 1984, John Wiley & Sons.)*

Table 25-2 **Potential Problems Associated with Invasive Hemodynamic Monitoring**

Potential Problems	Etiology	Precautions/Treatment

ALTERATIONS IN PRESSURE WAVE CONFIGURATIONS

Dampened tracings	*Technical*	
	Air in system	Check system for bubbles; flush bubbles out of system.
	Disconnection in system	Inspect and tighten all connections.
	Blood on transducer head	Flush until transducer dome clears of blood; change dome if necessary.
	Kinked catheter	Remove dressing to ascertain whether catheter is kinked externally
	Catheter tip against wall	Turn patient's head or reposition extremity in which that catheter is inserted; watch for improvement in tracing. Gently aspirate catheter from various angles to determine at which angle the best flow is achieved; tape and redress the catheter at the angle at which the best flow is achieved. Gently flush catheter in an attempt to push tip away from vessel wall. NEVER flush a catheter in which a clot is suspected.
	Physiologic	
	Clot on catheter tip	Attempt to aspirate blood from catheter. If possible, keep aspirating until clot is retrieved or blood no longer seems thickened. Flush system until the line is cleared and a readable tracing reappears. If blood cannot be aspirated, notify the physician.
	With an FDPAC this may also indicate the catheter has advanced forward and is in a wedged position*	Make sure balloon is deflated. Recheck system and line. If no improvement, obtain a chest radiograph and notify physician.
Abrupt exaggeration of pressure tracings	*Technical*	
	Loss of calibration of level of transducer	Recalibrate and relevel transducer.
	Physiologic	
	Slippage of catheter out of chamber or vessel	Avoid traction on intravascular lines; tape catheter to skin or secure with suture.
	FDPAC slipping from pulmonary artery to right ventricle. This is characterized by a systolic pressure that remains the same while the diastolic pressure falls into the range of the right-ventricular end-diastolic pressure	Inflate balloon in attempt to let catheter float back into pulmonary artery. If catheter does not migrate back into pulmonary artery, obtain a chest radiograph and notify a physician.

Continued

Table 25-2	**Potential Problems Associated with Invasive Hemodynamic Monitoring**—*cont'd*	
Potential Problems	**Etiology**	**Precautions/Treatment**
	RAC, PAC, or PATC has slipped out of vessel wall into thoracic cavity	Attempt to aspirate to see whether catheter is still in the vessel. If blood returns, flush system and attempt to obtain readable pressure tracings. If no blood return is achieved, notify physician and remove catheter, per protocol.
ALTERATIONS IN VASCULAR INTEGRITY		
Venous and arterial spasms	Irritation to vessels during prolonged insertion attempts	Apply local anesthetic to catheter surface or administer anesthetic by intravenous route. Use a guidewire to facilitate insertion. Cool catheter to make it less flexible and easier to insert.
Thrombophlebitis	Irritation to vessels from prolonged insertion attempts or from constant motion of catheter against vessel	See "venous and arterial spasms," discussed earlier. Secure catheter in place with either tape or suture. Avoid prolonged infusions of chemically irritating medications. Maintain adequate dilutions. Observe for signs and symptoms of phlebitis, and notify physician for possible withdrawal of catheter. Distal placement of stopcocks, connecting catheters, and tubing permits atraumatic blood sampling and flushing.
Embolization	Clot embolization from thrombophlebitis or from clot on catheter tip	Always aspirate catheter first if clot is suspected. NEVER FLUSH.
	Pulmonary embolism with infarct from FDPAC	Observe for changes in chest radiograph that indicate pulmonary embolization.
	Cerebral embolization from LAC catheter	Observe for neurologic changes that may indicate embolization from LAC.
	Peripheral embolization with extremity ischemia from peripheral arterial lines	Observe for ischemic changes of the extremity in which the catheter is located.
Air embolization	Loose connections	Secure and tighten all connections. Vigilantly observe LAC catheter because even minute amounts of air in this system can lead to serious neurologic complications.
	Rupture of balloon on FDPAC caused by overinflation or after normal use because the latex layer on the balloon absorbs lipoproteins from the blood and slowly loses elasticity, thus increasing its incidence of rupture	Inflate balloon slowly, and do not overinflate. Limit inflations. Allow balloon to empty air passively back into syringe. Avoid aspirating air back, because this weakens integrity of balloon. Aspirate only if air fails to return passively. If air does not return and rupture is questioned, sterile saline can be injected into balloon and attempts made to aspirate it back. Failure to aspirate fluid back indicates a leak, and the physician should be notified.

Table 25-2	**Potential Problems Associated with Invasive Hemodynamic Monitoring**—*cont'd*	
Potential Problems	**Etiology**	**Precautions/Treatment**
Vessel erosion or hemorrhage	Inadequate hemostasis after insertion	Apply firm pressure for 15 to 20 minutes.
Bleeding from insertion site: Rupture of a branch of the pulmonary artery	Overinflation of the balloon in a normal-sized vessel	Do not attempt to inflate the balloon if tracing already appears wedged. Inject only prescribed amount of air into balloon.
	Normal inflation of balloon in a too-small vessel	Inject air slowly, and stop injecting if resistance is felt. Inject only amount of air required to obtain a wedge tracing.
	Repeated normal inflations in a brittle or susceptible vessel	Limit wedge intervals in high-risk patients, such as patients with pulmonary hypertension or long-standing mitral valve disease.
Atrial dysrhythmias	Irritation of RA from RAC or during insertion of FDPAC	Withdraw CVP catheter to level of superior vena cava, and obtain readings from that area. Continue with insertion of FDPAC, because dysrhythmias are usually self-limiting and stop once catheter tip exits the right atrium.
Ventricular dysrhythmias	Irritation of right ventricle from tip of FDPAC during insertion procedure or from catheter tip slipping out of the pulmonary artery and back into the right ventricle	Continue with insertion of FDPAC, because dysrhythmias are usually self-limiting and stop once the catheter passes into the pulmonary artery. If catheter tip falls back into the right ventricle from the pulmonary artery, inflate the balloon, because this will cushion the tip of the catheter and may alleviate the dysrhythmias. Administer lidocaine if ventricular dysrhythmias continue. Notify physician, obtain a chest radiograph, and manipulate catheter, per hospital policy.
INFECTIONS		
Local infection	Faulty aseptic techniques during insertion or during subsequent dressing changes	Maintain sterility during insertion. Change dressings with sterile technique and tubings, per hospital policy.
Systemic infection	Faulty aseptic technique during insertion	Avoid spasms during insertion. Avoid development of thrombophlebitis along vessel. Change indwelling catheters and insertion sites every 48-72 hours. This may be impossible in patients with difficult vascular access sites. In these situations, rethreading a new catheter over a guidewire at the previous insertion site can be done every 48 to 72 hours. However, once the

Continued

Table 25-2	**Potential Problems Associated with Invasive Hemodynamic Monitoring**—*cont'd*	
Potential Problems	Etiology	Precautions/Treatment
		site is questionable or the patient develops symptoms of sepsis, such as elevated temperatures and white blood cell count, a new line at a new site is required.
Endocarditis	Extension of a local insertion site. Infection along the catheter and into the circulation	Culture per hospital policy. Observe for the development of new murmurs.

Adapted from Whitman GR: Bedside hemodynamic monitoring. In Horvath PT, editor: *Care of the adult cardiac surgery patient,* New York, 1984, John Wiley and Sons.
See Table 25-1 for abbreviations.
*Note: Wedging of the catheter in a postoperative patient may be a common occurrence for two reasons: (1) the catheter may have advanced forward during operative procedure when the chest was open and the lungs were not fully inflated, because there was less resistance to forward advancement; and (2) as hypothermia is reversed and the patient and catheter rewarm, its increased flexibility may allow it to float forward.

be a pulmonary embolism or pulmonic valve stenosis, or it may result from right-ventricular failure.

Mean Arterial Pressure

Normal mean arterial pressures generally range between 80 and 120 mm Hg. In a postoperative cardiac surgical patient, pressures lower than 60 mm Hg are generally avoided, because coronary artery filling may be limited or impeded when parameters reach this level and may contribute to an ischemic or infarction state. Conversely, pressures higher than 120 mm Hg are avoided because they place too much stress on newly created suture lines that could readily rupture under sustained pressures.

Cardiac Output and Cardiac Index

Cardiac output is the amount of blood ejected by the ventricle in 1 minute. Normal cardiac output is 5 to 6 L per min; it is calculated by the following formula:

$$SV \times HR = CO$$

in which SV = stroke volume, HR = heart rate, and CO = cardiac output.

Cardiac index is calculated by the following formula:

$$CO/BSA = CI$$

in which BSA = body surface area in m^2 and CI = cardiac index. Normal CI ranges from 2.5 to 3.5 L/min/m^2. Because CI takes body size into consideration, it is a better indicator of the patient's perfusion status.

Systemic Vascular Resistance

Systemic vascular resistance (SVR) is the resistance the left ventricle must work against to eject its volume of blood. Normal SVR is 900 to 1300 dynes/second/cm^{-5}. An elevated SVR can create enough resistance to left-ventricular ejection that cardiac output and cardiac index will decrease, which will lead to a state of hypoperfusion or shock. Infusion of vasodilators and afterload-reducing agents can counteract this elevation. SVR is calculated using the following formula:

$$SVR = (MAP - CVP) \times 80/CO$$

in which MAP = mean arterial pressure and CVP = central venous pressure.

Pulmonary Vascular Resistance

Pulmonary vascular resistance (PVR) is the resistance the right ventricle must work against to eject blood into the pulmonary bed. Normal PVR is 80 to 240 dynes/second/cm^{-5}. An elevated PVR can create enough resistance to right-ventricular ejection that right-sided failure or infarction can develop. Infusion of vasodilators or pulmonary artery dilators such as aminophylline can counteract these elevations. PVR is calculated using the following formula:

$$PVR = [PAM - (PCWP \text{ or } LAP)] \times 80/CO$$

in which PAM = pulmonary artery mean pressure and LAP = left-atrial pressure.

CENTRAL NERVOUS SYSTEM FUNCTION

All anesthetics affect the central nervous system (CNS), and it can be assumed for the present—even though we do not know exactly how narcosis occurs—that anesthetics are general, nonselective depressants. The complexity of the CNS, coupled with our incomplete knowledge of how it functions, makes it a most difficult system to evaluate.

Assessment of the CNS in the PACU generally involves only gross evaluation of behavior, level of consciousness, intellectual performance, and emotional status. A more detailed assessment of CNS function is necessary for patients who have undergone CNS surgery, and that discussion occurs in Chapters 8 and 35.

Emergence from Anesthesia

Patients arrive in the PACU at all levels of consciousness, from fully awake to completely anesthetized. With modern anesthesia techniques, however, most patients respond appropriately by the time they are established in the PACU and become oriented quickly when the stir-up regimen is begun (see Chapter 26). With the use of fluorinated and narcotic anesthetics, emergence is generally quiet and uneventful. Occasionally, a patient will become agitated and thrash about; this seems to occur more often in adolescents and young adults than in patients of other age groups. Emergence delirium also tends to occur more frequently in patients who have undergone intraabdominal and intrathoracic procedures (see Emergence Excitement in Chapter 26). Additional information on emergence can be obtained by reviewing the chapters on specific anesthetic agents (see Chapters 17 through 23).

The perianesthesia nurse can facilitate patient orientation by telling the patient where he or she is, that the surgery is over, and what time it is as

---

Box 25-1	**Factors Influencing Body Temperature of the PACU Patient**

Anesthesia
Preoperative medications
Age of patient
Site and temperature of intravenous fluids
Vasoconstriction (secondary to blood loss or anesthetic agent)
Vasodilation (secondary to regional anesthesia or use of halothane)
Body surface exposure
Temperature of irrigations
Temperature of ambient air

---

a part of the stir-up regimen. Reorientation occurs in reverse order from anesthesia: the patient first becomes oriented to person, then place, then time. This order, of course, may not hold true for the patient who was somewhat confused or disoriented before surgery, which emphasizes the importance of recording accurate information about the mental status of the patient before anesthesia.

Alterations in cerebral function are often the first signs of impaired oxygen delivery to the tissues. Therefore an orderly and periodic assessment of mental function is necessary to detect early evidence of abnormal cerebral function. Restlessness, agitation, and disorientation in the PACU may be ascribed to a number of other causes and are often difficult to evaluate. The use of continuous pulse oximetry can assist the perianesthesia nurse in determining whether symptoms may be related to hypoxemia.

THERMAL BALANCE

The measurement of the patient's body temperature in the PACU is particularly important. The most recent ASPAN standards state that, at minimum, the preoperative assessment, initial postoperative physical assessment, and discharge evaluation of the patient in Phases I and II PACUs should include documentation of temperature. Normal body temperature may vary from 35.9°C to 38°C. In the normal healthy adult, body temperature remains fairly constant because of the balance between heat production and heat loss. Alterations in body temperature

Box 25-2 Physiologic Alterations Associated with Hypothermia and Hyperthermia	
HYPOTHERMIA	**HYPERTHERMIA**
Bluish tint to skin (cyanosis)	Pale skin (mottled)
Increased metabolic rate with shivering, then decreased metabolic rate	Increased metabolic rate
Decreased oxygen consumption	Increased oxygen consumption
Decreased muscle tone	Decreased muscle tone
Decreased heart rate	Increased heart rate (rapid and bounding)
Dysrhythmias	Dysrhythmias
Decreased level of consciousness	Alterations in CNS (patient may be agitated)

occur often in the postoperative patient. Factors that affect the body temperature in the PACU patient are listed in Box 25-1.

Premedications, anesthesia, and the stress of surgery all interact in a complex fashion to disrupt normal thermoregulation. Both hypothermia (temperature below 36°C) and hyperthermia (temperature above 39°C) are associated with physiologic alterations that may interfere with recovery (Box 25-2).

Patients at the age extremes and those who are extremely debilitated are at even greater risk for postoperative development of temperature abnormalities.

The accuracy of axillary, rectal, or oral measurement is often debated. Core temperature (approximate value of temperature of blood perfusing the major metabolically active organs) is only estimated by oral and rectal temperature readings. Invasive techniques that use the thermistor on a pulmonary artery catheter, the tympanic membrane, or the bladder as a site for monitoring temperature are more accurate. Unless required during surgery or because of a specific problem, these temperature-monitoring modalities are seldom used in the PACU.

Shell (skin) temperature may be measured at the axilla or forehead with conventional thermometers or liquid crystal temperature strips. Shell temperature does not accurately reflect core temperature, although it may at least indicate gross trends.

Infrared tympanic membrane thermometry is increasingly used in the PACU. It is noninvasive and nontraumatic and may be used with patients of all sizes. When placed over the outer third of the auditory canal, the sensor on this otoscope-like thermometer gathers emitted infrared energy from the ear and translates this energy into a temperature reading within seconds. The infrared tympanic thermometer has been found to accurately track core temperature as measured by the thermistor tip of a pulmonary artery catheter.

Management of the hypothermic patient is directed toward the restoration of normothermia and the avoidance of shivering. Warm blankets may be placed over the patient as specific hospital protocol allows. Convective warming devices, such as the Bair Hugger, provide a safe and effective means of gradually rewarming the patient. Hypothermia and hyperthermia are discussed in greater detail in Chapters 26, 42, and 50.

FLUID AND ELECTROLYTE BALANCE

Evaluation of a patient's fluid and electrolyte status involves total body assessment. Imbalances readily occur in the postoperative patient for a number of reasons, including the restriction of food and fluids preoperatively, fluid loss during surgery, and stress (Table 25-3). The normal body response to stress of surgery is renal retention of water and sodium. In addition, patients often have abnormal avenues of postoperative fluid loss.

Fluid Intake

Each patient must be evaluated to determine his or her baseline requirements and the fluid needed to replace abnormal losses. The normal adult who is deprived of oral intake requires 2000 to 2200 ml of water per day to make up for urinary output and insensible loss.

Table 25-3	**Common Clinical States Affecting Fluid and Electrolyte Balance in the PACU**
Clinical State	**Effect on Fluid and Electrolyte Balance**
Pain	Heightened response
Anesthesia	to stress
Fear	Water and sodium
Trauma	retention
Acute renal failure	Impaired acid-base regulatory mechanism
Blood loss	Impaired fluid
Immobilization	circulation
"–ostomies"	Excessive loss of fluid
Nasogastric suction	by abnormal routes
Bleeding	Potassium and sodium
Vomiting	deficit
Thyroidectomy	Calcium deficit
Treatment of acidosis	
Excessive administration of citrated blood	

Intravenous Fluids.   Most patients admitted to the PACU from the operating room will be receiving intravenous fluids. The anesthetist must have an open intravenous line for the administration of necessary medications and replacement fluids intraoperatively, and an open line is needed postoperatively to supply necessary fluids, electrolytes, and medications. Because all efforts to substitute for normal oral intake of electrolytes and adequate volumes of fluid are at best temporary and inadequate, the first objective is to return the patient to adequate oral intake as soon as possible. Until this objective can be attained, an intravenous line must be maintained. The nurse should be aware of the type and amount of any fluid being administered and any medications that may have been added to it.

The intravenous site should be checked to ensure that the needle or cannula is still in the vein and that no extravasation has occurred. Watch for kinks or disconnected tubing, and

ensure that the rate of infusion is accurate. The intravenous site should be positioned comfortably; a board may be helpful to maintain the intravenous site if the patient should become restless.

Pediatric patients may require a protective device over the site or soft restraints to prevent dislodging of the needle or cannula. A simple paper cup device can be helpful in preventing dislodgment of the intravenous line from the scalp veins of small infants. Snip the bottom out of the cup; thread the cup over the tubing; place the large opening over the intravenous site; and secure the cup to the baby's head with tape crisscrossed over the entire cup. In addition to providing protection for the intravenous site, this method allows the nurse to check the insertion site frequently.

After ensuring that the intravenous fluids are infusing correctly, check to see what fluids, if any, are to follow or if the infusion is to be discontinued.

If the patient is receiving total parenteral nutrition and intralipids, only feeding solutions should go through this line; another intravenous pathway must be secured for other uses. Multilumen catheters allow for the administration of multiple fluids and medications and can be transduced to provide continuous hemodynamic monitoring, if indicated.

The flow of intravenous fluids in the patient receiving hyperalimentation, the patient who is fluid-restricted, the infant and small child, and the patient who is receiving intravenous analgesia or vasopressors should always be regulated by electronic fluid administration devices.

Oral Fluids

Oral intake must be prohibited after anesthesia until the laryngeal and pharyngeal reflexes are fully regained, as evidenced by the patient's ability to gag and swallow effectively. If the patient is permitted oral intake, it is best to start with small amounts of ice chips, because these are less likely to cause nausea and vomiting. Some PACUs use isotonic ice chips that are made from a balanced electrolyte solution, such as Lytren. If ice chips are well tolerated, the patient can progressively increase oral intake to include water and other clear liquids. Kool-Aid and fruit-flavored popsicles are well tolerated and accepted by both children and adults. In addition, carbonated beverages may be soothing to a patient who feels slightly nauseated. The management of postoperative nausea and vomiting is discussed in Chapters 14 and 26.

Fluid Output

Normal output in the average adult results from obligatory urinary output and insensible avenues of loss, including evaporation of water from the skin and exhalation during respiration. The amount of urine necessary for the normal renal system to excrete waste products of a day's metabolism is approximately 600 ml. Optimally, 30 ml/hour or more of urine should be obtained from a catheterized adult to ensure proper hydration and kidney function. Urinary output should be closely monitored in the recovery phase; measurement of urinary output and urine specific gravity yields important clues to the overall status of the patient and may alert the nurse to overhydration or dehydration or the development of shock.

A lower than normal urinary output can be expected in the postoperative patient as a result of the body's normal reaction to stress; however, an unduly small volume of urine (less than 500 ml in 24 hours) may indicate the presence of renal insufficiency, and the physician should be notified.

If a Foley catheter is in place, a more accurate observation of hourly output is available. If urine volume is low and specific gravity remains fixed at a low level, renal insufficiency is indicated. A small urine volume plus a high specific gravity indicates dehydration. In addition to the volume and specific gravity of urinary output being noted, the urine should be examined for the presence of pus, blood, or casts.

The perianesthesia nurse must evaluate abnormal as well as normal avenues of output. Abnormal ways include external losses from vomiting, nasogastric tubes, T-tubes, and fistula or wound drainage and temporary functional losses from fluid shifting within the body, such as hemorrhage into soft tissues and the edema of surgical wounds.

The surgical site should be noted on admission to the PACU, and the dressing should be checked for drainage. The perianesthesia nurse must be aware of the presence of any drains and the expected amount of drainage. Drainage tubes should be checked to ensure patency, and the amount, color, and odor of any drainage should be observed and documented. All tubes should be secure and either clamped shut or connected to drainage apparatus as ordered by the physician. A summary of imbalances that may occur with abnormal avenues of output is presented in Table 25-4. Any deviations from the normally expected drainage in a specific route should be reported promptly to the surgeon.

Obviously, the accurate measurement and recording of all intake and output is vital to the assessment of each patient's fluid and electrolyte status. Keeping a running total on the postoperative flow sheet is essential for quick assessment of fluid status.

In addition to observing and assessing avenues of intake and output, the perianesthesia nurse should be alert to symptoms of fluid and electrolyte imbalance, which are summarized in Table 25-5.

PSYCHOSOCIAL ASSESSMENT

Assessment of the patient's psychological and emotional well-being is an important component of perianesthesia nursing. As with any other assessment, this must be made in the context of the whole patient. Illness, hospitalization, surgery, and pain all take on a variety of values, depending on the person who experiences them. The meaning of the surgery to the person must be explored preoperatively and will probably have been obtained by other healthcare providers; this information should be communicated to the perianesthesia nurse who will care for the patient. Likewise, the perianesthesia nurse must ensure that additional assessment information and psychosocial care in the PACU are shared with those who will care for the patient after his or her discharge from the unit.

Almost all surgical patients experience a degree of anxiety about anesthesia and the surgical procedure and a fear of postoperative pain. The physical signs and symptoms of anxiety are the same as those produced by any stressor. Reactions are mediated by the sympathetic nervous system and are listed in Box 25-3.

Symptoms of anxiety must be carefully differentiated from those of other causes. Differentiation is particularly difficult while the effects of anesthesia are still present.

Table 25-4	**Imbalances that May Occur with Abnormal Avenues of Output**		
Fluid	**pH**	**Content (mEq/L)**	**Likely Imbalances with Significant Losses**
Gastric juice (fasting) (nasogastric suction)	1-3	Na^+ 60 K^+ 10 Cl^- 85 HCO^{-3} 0-15	Metabolic alkalosis Potassium deficit Sodium deficit Fluid volume deficit
Small intestine (suction) Jejunum	7-8	Na^+ 111 K^+ 4.6 Cl^- 104 HCO^{-3} 31	Metabolic acidosis Potassium deficit Sodium deficit
Ileum		Na^+ 117 K^+ 5.0 Cl^- 105	Fluid volume deficit
New ileostomy		Na^+ 129 K^+ 11 Cl^- 116	Potassium deficit Sodium deficit Fluid volume deficit Metabolic acidosis
Biliary tract fistula	7.8	Na^+ 148 K^+ 5.0 Cl^- 101 HCO^{-3} 40	Metabolic acidosis Sodium deficit Fluid volume deficit
Pancreatic fistula	8.0-8.3	Na^+ 141 K^+ 4.6 Cl^- 76 HCO^{-3} 121	Metabolic acidosis Sodium deficit Fluid volume deficit

Adapted from Bland J: Clinical metabolism of body water and electrolytes, Philadelphia, 1963, WB Saunders; and Guyton AC: Textbook of medical physiology, ed 7, Philadelphia, 1986, WB Saunders.

Box 25-3	**Signs and Symptoms of Anxiety**

Tachycardia
Increased blood pressure
Pale cool skin
Increased respiratory rate
Hyperventilation
Increased muscle tone
Restlessness/agitation
Dilated pupils

A quiet, calm environment is important to the postanesthesia recovery of the surgical patient. A calm, confident nurse can do much to allay anxiety for the postoperative patient through both verbal reassurance and touch. Hearing is the first sense to return after anesthesia. It is not necessary to yell at patients; they may not respond even if they can hear. In fact, yelling at patients may increase their anxiety early in the PACU period because they may believe they are not recovering as quickly as they should.

Attention to comfort—including minimal environmental noise and stimuli—and the reassuring presence of the nurse are calming. Once the patients have fully regained consciousness, simply talking to them may help allay anxiety. Simple, factual statements repeated often are best. At this point, the nurse may be able to explore the cause of the distress with the patients.

Table 25-5 Signs and Symptoms of Acute Fluid and Electrolyte Imbalance	
Imbalance	**Symptoms and Findings**

Hyperosmolarity
  Water excess
  Sodium deficit
	Polyuria (if kidneys are healthy), twitching, hyperirritability, disorientation, nausea, vomiting, weakness, serum Na$^+$ ↑ 120 mEq/L

Isotonic disturbances
  Dehydration
  Circulatory collapse
  Volume excess
	Weakness, nausea, vomiting, oliguria, postural drop in systolic blood pressure, elevated hematocrit, normal serum Na$^+$ →
	SHOCK
	Dyspnea, cough, sweating, edema

Hydrogen ion imbalances Metabolic acidosis	Apathy, disorientation, increased rate and depth of respiration → Kussmaul's respiration, symptoms of K$^+$ excess, ABG pH ↓ 7.35, HCO^{-3} ↓ 25, acid urine with pH ↓ 6.0
Metabolic alkalosis	Increased irritability, disorientation, shallow, slow respirations, periods of apnea, irregular pulse, muscle twitch, ABG pH ↑ 7.45, HCO^{-3} ↑ 29, alkaline urine with pH ↑ 7.0
Respiratory acidosis (CO$_2$ retention)	Increased rate and depth of breathing, tachycardia and other arrhythmias, drowsiness, ABG pH ↓ 7.4, PCO$_2$ ↑ 40, HCO^{-3} 25-35
Potassium imbalances Deficit (hypokalemia)	Weakness, mental confusion, shallow respirations, hypotension, arrhythmias, serum K$^+$ ↓ 3.5 (this is a measurement of extracellular K$^+$ and only gives a vague reflection of intracellular balance)
Excess (hyperkalemia)	Intestinal colic, oliguria, bradycardia, cardiac arrest, serum K$^+$ ↑ 5 mEq/L
Calcium imbalances Deficit (hypocalcemia)	Tingling of the fingers, laryngospasm, facial spasms, painful muscle spasms, positive Trousseau's sign, positive Chvostek's sign, convulsions, palpitations, cardiac arrhythmias, serum Ca^{2+} ↓ 4.5 mEq/L
Excess (hypercalcemia)	Not usually seen in the PACU. Usually caused by pathology involving the parathyroid glands

ABG, Arterial blood gas.

For the patient in acute distress due to anxiety, a mild tranquilizer, such as diazepam (Valium), midazolam (Versed), and lorazepam (Ativan), may be indicated; however, these benzodiazepines should be used judiciously. One advantage of their use is that they potentiate narcotics and often allow a reduction of the narcotic analgesia dosage necessary to control pain. Because apnea is a common side effect when benzodiazepines are given to patients receiving narcotics, continuous respiratory monitoring with pulse oximetry and capnography is indicated.

Attention to the psychosocial ramifications of specific surgical interventions is provided in each of the following chapters on postanesthesia care. These comments are incorporated into the overall text whenever deemed appropriate. For further discussion of the relationship between pain and anxiety, see Chapter 28.

SUMMARY

Obviously, the perianesthesia nurse must be an expert in assessment. The perianesthesia nurse must not only understand the normal physiologic functioning of the human body but also be able to differentiate and evaluate the variety of pathologic symptoms that may arise in the postanesthesia patient. The perianesthesia nurse must be aware of the interrelationships between mind and body and must be sensitive to the psychosocial factors influencing the patient's reactions. Knowledgeable assessment of the postanesthesia patient is essential for the provision of safe and effective medical treatment and nursing care.

BIBLIOGRAPHY

Alspach J: Core curriculum for critical care nursing, ed 5, Philadelphia, 1998, WB Saunders.

Altsberger D, Shrewsbury P: Postoperative pain management: the PACU nurse's challenge, J Post Anesth Nurs 3(6):399-403, 1988.

American Society of PeriAnesthesia Nurses: Standards of postanesthesia nursing practice, Thorofare, NJ, 2002, ASPAN.

Atlee J: Complications in anesthesia, Philadelphia, 1999, WB Saunders.

Barash P, Cullen B, Stoetling R: Clinical anesthesia, ed 4, Philadelphia, 2000, Lippincott Williams & Wilkins.

Benumof J: Anesthesia and uncommon diseases, ed 4, Philadelphia, 1998, WB Saunders.

Benumof J, Saidman L: Anesthesia & perioperative complications, ed 2, St Louis, 1999, Mosby.

Bickley L, Hoekelman R: Bates' guide to physical examination and history taking, ed 7, Philadelphia, 1998, Lippincott Williams & Wilkins.

Bowdle T, Horita A, Kharasch E: The pharmacologic basis of anesthesiology, New York, 1994, Churchill Livingstone.

Cook KG: Assessment and management of anxiety in recovery room patients, Curr Rev Recov Room Nurses 7(5):51-55, 1983.

Coté C, Todres I, Goudsouzian N, Ryan J: A practice of anesthesia for infants and children, ed 3, Philadelphia, 2001, WB Saunders.

DeFazio-Quinn D: Ambulatory surgical nursing core curriculum, Philadelphia, 1999, WB Saunders.

Drain C: Physiology of the respiratory system related to anesthesia, CRNA: The Clinical Forum for Nurse Anesthetists 7(4):163-180, 1996.

Drain C: Pathophysiology of the respiratory system related to anesthesia, CRNA: The Clinical Forum for Nurse Anesthetists 7(4):181-192, 1996.

Drain C: Anesthesia care of the patient with reactive airways disease, CRNA: The Clinical Forum for Nurse Anesthetists 7(4):207-212, 1996.

Durbin N: The application of Doppler techniques in critical care, Focus Crit Care 10(3):44-46, 1984.

Estafanous F: Opioids in anesthesia: II. Boston, 1991, Butterworth-Heinemann.

Estafanous F, Barash P, Reves J: Cardiac Anesthesia, ed 2, Philadelphia, 2001, Lippincott Williams & Wilkins.

Fraulini KE: Coping mechanisms and recovery from surgery, Assoc Operating Room Nurses J 37(6):1198-1208, 1983.

Ganong W: Review of medical physiology, ed 20, New York, 2001, McGraw-Hill Professional.

Guyton A, Hall J: Textbook of medical physiology, ed 10, Philadelphia, 2000, WB Saunders.

Hardman J, Limbird L: Goodman and Gilman's the pharmacological basis of therapeutics, ed 10, New York, 2001, McGraw-Hill Professional.

Henneman EA, Henneman PL: Intricacies of blood pressure measurement: reexamining the rituals, Heart Lung 18(3):263-273, 1989.

Holtzclaw BJ: Shivering: a clinical nursing problem, Nurs Clin North Am 25(4):977-986, 1990.

Kataria BK, Harnik EV, Mitchard R et al: Postoperative arterial oxygen saturation in the pediatric population during transportation, Anesth Analg 67:280-282, 1988.

Katzung B, editor: Basic and clinical pharmacology, ed 8, Los Altos, Calif, 2000, Appleton & Lange.

Kaye A: Essential neurosurgery, ed 2, St Louis, 1997, Mosby.

Kruse DH: Postoperative hypothermia, Focus Crit Care 10(2):48-50, 1983.

Jacobsen W: Manual of postanesthesia care, Philadelphia, 1992, WB Saunders.

Lake C, Hines R, Blitt C: Clinical monitoring: practical applications for anesthesia and critical care, St Louis, 2001, Mosby.

Longnecker D, Murphy F: Dripps/Eckenhoff/Vandam introduction to anesthesia, ed 9, Philadelphia, 1997, WB Saunders.

Longnecker D, Tinker J, Morgan G: Principles and practice of anesthesiology, ed 2, St Louis, 1998, Mosby.

Martin J: Positioning in anesthesia and surgery, ed 3, St Louis, 1997, Mosby.

McCarthy EJ: Ventilation-perfusion relationships, AANA J 55(5):437-440, 1987.

Miller KM, Taylor BT: Standard care plans for the postanesthesia care unit, J Post Anesth Nurs 6(1):26-32, 1991.

Miller R, editor: Anesthesia, ed 5, New York, 2000, Churchill Livingstone.

Motoyama E: Smith's anesthesia for infants and children, ed 6, St Louis, 1996, Mosby.

Murray J, Nadel J: Textbook of respiratory medicine, ed 3, Philadelphia, 2001, WB Saunders.

Nagelhout J, Zaglaniczny K: Nurse anesthesia, ed 2, Philadelphia, 2001, WB Saunders.

New W: Pulse oximetry, J Clin Monit 1(2):126-129, 1985.

Pesci B: Neuromuscular blockage and reversal agents: a primer for postanesthesia nurses, J Post Anesth Nurs 1(1):42-47, 1986.

Sanders A: End-tidal carbon dioxide monitoring during cardiopulmonary resuscitation: a prognostic indicator for survival, JAMA 262(10):1347-1351, 1989.

Shields JR: A comparison of physostigmine and meperidine in treating emergence excitement, MCN 5:(3)170-175, 1980.

Shinozaki T, Deane R, Perkins FM: Infrared tympanic thermometer: evaluation of a new clinical thermometer, Crit Care Med 16(2):148-150, 1988.

Skoog RE: Capnography in the postanesthesia care unit, J Post Anesth Nurs 4(3):147-155, 1989.

Spindler J, Mehlisch D, Brown C: Intramuscular ketorolac and morphine in the treatment of moderate to severe pain after major surgery, Pharmacotherapy 10:51S-58S, 1990.

Stoelting R: Pharmacology and physiology in anesthetic practice, ed 3, Philadelphia, 1999, Lippincott Raven.

Stoelting R, Miller R: Basics of anesthesia, ed 4, New York, 2000, Churchill Livingstone.

Stone D: Perioperative care: anesthesia, medicine, and surgery, St Louis, 1998, Mosby.

Swedlow DB: Capnometry and capnography: the anesthesia disaster early warning system, Semin Anesth 5(3):194-205, 1986.

Toledo LW: Pulse oximetry: clinical implications in the PACU, J Post Anesth Nurs 2(1):12-17, 1987.

Traver G, Tremper Mitchell J, Glodquist-Priestley G: Respiratory care: a clinical approach, Gaithersburg, Md, 1991, Aspen Publishers.

Vaughn MS: Shivering in the recovery room, Curr Rev Recov Room Nurses 6(1):3-7, 1984.

Vogelsang J, Hayes S: Butorphanol tartrate (Stadol): a review, J Post Anesth Nurs 6(2):129-135, 1991.

Waugaman W, Foster S, Rigor B: Principles and practice of nurse anesthesia, ed 3, Norwalk, Conn, 1999, Appleton & Lange.

Waxman SJ, Waxman SG: Correlative neuroanatomy, ed 24, Norwalk, Conn, 1999, Lange Medical Publishers.

Weinberg G: Basic science review of anesthesiology, New York, 1997, McGraw-Hill.

26

CARE OF THE PERIANESTHESIA PATIENT

Denise O'Brien, MSN(c), RN, CPAN, CAPA

Nursing care of postanesthesia patients who are emerging from anesthesia is reviewed in this chapter. Postanesthesia care includes the stir-up regimen, intravenous and transfusion therapy, maintenance of respiratory function, infection control, and general comfort measures. Emergence excitement and delayed emergence, which may alter the postanesthesia patient's recovery, are also reviewed.

THE STIR-UP REGIMEN

The stir-up regimen is probably the most important aspect of postanesthesia nursing care. Patients transition to an awake state more quickly than in the past or even arrive in the PACU awake and alert; however, preventing complications remains important. Like most other postanesthesia care unit (PACU) activities, the basics of the stir-up regimen are aimed at preventing complications, primarily atelectasis, and venous stasis. Five major activities—deep-breathing exercises, coughing, positioning, mobilization, and pain management—constitute the stir-up regimen.

Deep-Breathing Exercises

The primary factor that contributes to postoperative pulmonary complications is decreased lung volumes. The major factor that contributes to low lung volumes in the PACU patient is a shallow, monotonous, sighless breathing pattern caused by general anesthesia, pain, and opioids. Full inflation of the lungs prevents small areas of patchy atelectasis from developing and assists in the elimination of inhalation anesthetics, thus hastening the awakening process. Intravenous anesthesia differs from inhalation anesthesia in that, one injected, little can be done to expedite

removal of the drug; however, the prevention of atelectasis by deep breathing remains just as important.

The patient must be stimulated to take three or four deep breaths every 5 to 10 minutes. Full expansion is important. This may be impeded by a number of factors that are discussed in Chapter 25. Every effort must be made to enhance the patient's ability to expand the lungs. Patients who are emerging from anesthesia may have difficulty participating in the activity because of their reduced levels of consciousness and awareness.

The sustained maximal inspiratory (SMI) maneuver is a method to enhance the lung volumes of postoperative patients. The SMI maneuver consists of the patient inhaling as close to total lung capacity as possible and—at the peak of inspiration—holding that volume of air in the lungs for 3 to 5 seconds before exhaling it. Ideally, the patient will have received instruction and coaching in the postoperative use of this maneuver. The patient may use an incentive spirometer that provides visual or auditory feedback and observation of inspiratory volume.

Incentive spirometry is used to prevent or assist in reversing atelectasis, promote normal lung expansion, and improve oxygenation. Instruction and practice before surgery provide patients the opportunity to master the device and establish a baseline for themselves before anesthetic and surgical interventions. Devices currently available include disposable flow-oriented and volume-oriented incentive spirometers that are inexpensive and can be used by the patient at home. Incentive spirometry may have greater use after the immediate postanesthesia period because patients are more awake and capable of manipulating the devices than they are in the PACU.

Coughing

The patient must be instructed to cough in addition to the SMI maneuvers. The best way to clear the air passages of obstructive secretions is a purposeful cough. Cough effectiveness depends on the inspired tidal volume and the velocity of expired airflow. For the patient who is recovering from anesthesia, the cascade cough is the most effective cough maneuver. The patient should be taught to take a rapid, deep inspiration to increase the volume of air in the lungs, which will in turn dilate the airways, thus allowing air to pass beyond the retained secretions. On exhalation, the patient should perform multiple coughs at subsequently lower lung volumes. With each cough during exhalation, the length of the airways that undergo dynamic compression will increase, thus enhancing cough effectiveness.

Coughing is most effective when the patient is sitting up. Splinting of incisions and adequate analgesia facilitate a good cough. If the patient is unable to sit upright, positioning the patient in a side-lying position with hips and knees flexed or in a semi-Fowler's position with head and arms supported with pillows and with knees flexed will decrease abdominal tension and allow maximal movement of the diaphragm, thereby improving the effectiveness of the cough.

Between cascade cough maneuvers, the patient should be encouraged to inhale and close the glottis. This dilates the airways and, by increasing the pleural pressure, further compresses the airways to "milk" the secretions toward the larger airways, where they can be removed in successive cough maneuvers.

If an effective cough cannot be produced, secretions from the respiratory passages must be suctioned manually. If the patient cannot or will not cough effectively, it may be necessary to stimulate cough by means of tracheal suctioning or manual pressure to the trachea. A cough is stimulated by finger pressure against the trachea just above the manubrial notch; the maneuver is also known as tracheal tickle. Because this maneuver may also produce retching and vomiting, it should be used cautiously.

Preoperative teaching of postoperative breathing exercises and coughs and their importance is effective and should be included in the preoperative regimen whenever possible. Patients scheduled for surgery may attend formal teaching sessions before surgery or may receive instructions for coughing, deep breathing, and incentive spirometry through educational booklets, video programs, and visits to preoperative testing departments.

Positioning

When possible, patients in the PACU should be maintained in a semi-prone, side-lying position. The semi-prone position promotes maintenance of a patent airway, prevents aspiration of vomitus into the trachea, and permits optimal ventilation of the lower lung lobes. Frequent repositioning of patients (at least every hour) is essential to prevent atelectasis and peripheral stasis. The patient's position should be changed from side to side. Care must be taken to ensure that all drainage tubes and intravenous catheters remain in place and patent and that no tension on any of these lines is created. As soon as they are able, patients should be encouraged to turn and change positions alone.

Mobilization

To prevent venous stasis, patients must be encouraged to move their legs and arms rhythmically. Patients should flex and extend their extremities. Mobilization and flexion of the muscles aid venous return, automatically cause deep breathing, and improve cardiac function.

Pain Management

Achievement of the stir-up regimen's first four activities is difficult if adequate pain relief is not provided. Opioids depress the cough reflex and ciliary action and may lower alveolar ventilation by direct depression of the respiratory center. If breathing is painful and splinting occurs or if the patient refuses to cough or move because of pain, respiratory or embolic complications may occur. Pain relief is discussed in detail in Chapter 28.

Modifications of the Stir-Up Regimen

Modifications of the stir-up regimen may be needed depending on the type of anesthesia used and the operative procedure performed. When ketamine is used, a rigorous stir-up regimen is eliminated from routine PACU care, and verbal and tactile stimulation of the patient are minimized as much as possible. Cough must be eliminated after eye surgery and other delicate plastic surgery procedures. Stimulation of the patient with increased or potentially increased intracranial pressure must be undertaken carefully to avoid dangerous and potentially life-threatening pressure changes.

Positioning is probably the activity most often modified in the stir-up regimen. Positioning of the patient and modifications of the stir-up regimen after specific surgical procedures and anesthetics are discussed in related chapters.

EMERGENCE EXCITEMENT

Most patients emerge from general anesthesia in a calm, tranquil manner. Some patients, however, emerge in a state of "excitement," a condition characterized by restlessness, disorientation, crying, moaning, irrational talking, and inappropriate behavior. In the extreme form of excitement, which is called emergence delirium, the patient screams, shouts, and wildly thrashes.

The incidence of emergence excitement is higher among children, the elderly, and in those with a history of drug dependency or psychiatric disorders. Medications administered preoperatively or intraoperatively—including ketamine, droperidol, opioids, benzodiazepines, large doses of metoclopramide, and atropine—may precipitate delirium. Patients who are emotional or anxious before induction of anesthesia or who awaken restrained are at increased risk of emergence excitement or delirium.

The PACU nurse should assess the patient's status if emergence excitement is encountered. Check the patient's respiratory function, airway patency, and oxygen saturation first because restlessness and agitation are well-known manifestations of hypoxia. Other causes include a full bladder, cramped or sore muscles and joints from prolonged abnormal positioning on the operating table, the presence of pain, incomplete reversal of neuromuscular blockade, withdrawal from alcohol and other drugs, central anticholinergic syndrome, acid-base disturbances, and electrolyte abnormalities.

The restless patient requires constant careful observation. Gentle physical restraint may be required to prevent injury. Several nurses or attendants may be needed. Treatment is symptomatic. If hypoxia, pain, and full bladder are ruled out, a change in position may have a quieting effect. Physostigmine may be used to reverse central anticholinergic drug effects. Anxiolytics, such as midazolam, usually calm the patient. If sedative treatment is instituted, the patient should be monitored for respiratory depression. Nurses should be alert to increased agitation after benzodiazepine administration. These agents may contribute to restlessness rather than decreasing it; this is a paradoxical reaction to benzodiazepines.

DELAYED EMERGENCE

Occasionally patients awaken from anesthesia more slowly than expected. Causes include prolonged action of anesthetic and other drugs; metabolic problems such as hypoglycemia, hypocalcemia, hyponatremia, and hypermagnesemia; hypovolemia; hypothermia; and neurologic injury. Respiratory inadequacy with resultant hypercarbia and hypoxemia may result from opioids, sedatives, other anesthetic agents and adjuncts, or neurologic causes.

Treatment consists of thorough assessment and identification of the cause or causes of the delayed arousal. Oxygenation and ventilation along with adequate cardiac output must be maintained. Residual anesthetic agents may be treated with maintenance of ventilation. Residual opioids, sedatives, neuromuscular blocking agents, and anticholinergics may be reversed with the appropriate antagonists. Metabolic disturbances should be corrected. If hypothermia is the suspected cause, warming measures are instituted with appropriate temperature monitoring. Neurologic evaluation may be needed if other causes of delayed arousal have been excluded.

INTRAVENOUS THERAPY

Postoperative parenteral fluid requirements vary with the patient's preoperative status and with the surgical procedure. For a discussion of fluid and electrolyte imbalance, see Chapter 12.

TRANSFUSION THERAPY

The administration of whole blood or blood components (serum, plasma, red blood cells [RBCs], platelets) is less common, although it is often a life-saving treatment modality for the postoperative patient. However, the inherent dangers are numerous, and perianesthesia nurses must be well aware of the principles of safe administration of blood and blood components.

Whole Blood

The only indication for whole blood transfusion in the PACU is hypovolemic shock to restore and maintain circulating blood volume that has been depleted from hemorrhage or trauma. The nurse may anticipate this need in patients who have required emergency surgery and in patients who have been subjected to extensive dissection. The only other indications for whole blood transfusions are exchange transfusions to remove toxic substances from the blood or to prime the oxygenating pump for cardiac surgery. These are rare occurrences in the PACU. Most other clinical situations that require replacement therapy can be handled with blood components, plasma volume expanders, and crystalloids.

Patients who are anticipating blood loss that requires replacement during elective operative procedures may donate autologous blood before the scheduled procedure. As many as six units may be obtained through collections as frequently as every week. This preoperative autologous donation, acute normovolemic hemodilution (in which blood is removed immediately before the procedure and the patient infused with intravenous fluids; at the end of the procedure, the stored blood is reinfused), and autotransfusion of blood (scavenged either intraoperatively or postoperatively) commonly are used for replacement instead of homologous blood transfusions. Patients may also name designated donors to give blood for their operations, although the blood of these donors may be no safer than the blood of volunteer donors.

Every possible safeguard must be exercised to prevent the administration of incompatible blood to the patient who needs replacement. Before any blood or blood component is administered, including autologous donor units, typing and cross-matching of the donor and the recipient blood must be done. Whether it is known in advance that the patient will need blood replacement for major surgery or only that the patient might need blood replacement based on possible planned operative procedures, this typing and cross-matching should be completed before the start of surgery, and compatible blood should be available for administration.

Great care must be taken in the identification of the recipients and the unit of blood prepared for them. An information form that lists the donor's and recipient's types, cross-matches and identification number, the recipient's name, and the date must be cross-checked with the label on the unit of blood to be administered and with the patient's identification bracelet. At least two persons should be involved in the identification of the recipient, preferably two nurses or a physician and a nurse. Because postanesthesia patients are often not well known by the nurse and often only partially conscious because of anesthesia, scrupulous attention must be directed toward positive identification of the recipient. If any discrepancy exists, do not give the blood until clarification is obtained. Once positive identification of the recipient and the unit of blood to be transfused is established, the blood must be inspected for hemolysis and abnormal cloudiness or color. RBCs settle to the bottom of whole blood, and plasma rises to the top. Before the transfusion is begun and from time to time during the transfusion, whole blood should be gently and thoroughly mixed by tilting the bag back and forth.

Blood and blood components should be administered via large-bore intravenous catheters in a large vein of the forearm or through a central venous catheter. Blood administration sets should be used for transfusions. The drip chamber must be filled to cover the filter before the infusion is started. If the filter becomes clogged during the infusion, it may be cleared by squeezing the flexible drip chamber above the filter after the clamp has been completely closed. Squeezing the chamber resets the level. Squeezing the plastic drip chamber above the filter ensures that particulate matter will not be forced into the filter and that the filter will not be bent. Multiple transfusions and some blood components require special filters or administration sets, or both.

The recommended solution to infuse with blood and blood components is 0.9% sodium chloride injection (USP). It is completely compatible with blood. Small clumps or globules of RBCs may form when blood is administered with dextrose in water and many of the balanced solutions (e.g., Ringer's injection, USP; lactated Ringer's injection, USP) contain calcium, which may cause citrated blood to clot. Solutions that contain calcium or a potent drug (e.g., any anesthetic or neuromuscular blocking agent) should never be used in the primary infusion line when blood is administered by secondary or piggyback hookup.

Before beginning the blood administration, obtain baseline vital signs, including temperature, and note the status of the infusion site. Untoward reactions to blood generally occur with the first 50 ml of the transfusion; start the transfusion slowly (20 to 40 drops/min) for the first 15 minutes. If no symptoms of reaction develop, the rate of administration may be increased to 80 to 100 drops/min or the rate ordered by the physician.

A unit of blood is usually administered over a period of 1 to 2 hours; however, in emergency situations, such as shock or hemorrhage, a unit of blood can be infused within 10 minutes under pressure. A pressure cuff similar to a blood pressure cuff is slipped over the collapsible plastic blood container and pumped to compress the bag and literally push the blood into the patient's veins. When pressure transfusion equipment is used, every precaution must be exercised to prevent air from entering the system and causing an air embolus. All tubing and the blood container itself must be checked for leaks. The infusion site must be monitored carefully for signs of infiltration to prevent the infusion of blood into subcutaneous tissue.

Blood may need to be warmed, especially in emergencies and when large volumes are infused or when the patient is hypothermic or has cold agglutinin disease or sickle cell disease. Rapid infusion of refrigerated blood can cause cardiac arrhythmias or cardiac arrest, especially when given through a central venous catheter, and hypothermia. Warming devices available include dry-heating and water-bath types.

Once the blood infusion is started, the flow rate should be checked frequently. Changing the height of the intravenous stand or the bed may alter the rate of the infusion, as will repositioning of the patient, changes in location of the catheter in the vein, or alterations in the tone of the vein.

Transfusion Reactions

The exact incidence of transfusion reactions is unknown. Reports of their incidence vary from 0.2% to 10%, and some reactions are undoubtedly unrecognized and unreported.

Nurses in the PACU must be especially adept at assessing the patient receiving blood because many of the signs and symptoms of an adverse reaction to blood may be difficult to separate from those caused by other variables such as the patient's illness, surgery, or medications (including anesthesia). In addition, the patient who is not fully conscious may not complain of symptoms. Blood transfusion reactions or complications may be either immediate or delayed. Immediate reactions include hemolytic, febrile nonhemolytic, and allergic reactions. Nonimmunologic complications include transmission of infectious disease and bacterial contamination.

Hemolytic Reactions. Fifty to 75 ml of ABO-incompatible blood can precipitate a hemolytic reaction that results in agglutination—or clumping—of RBCs, which blocks the patient's capillaries, thus obstructing the flow of blood and oxygen to vital organs. In time, hemolysis of the RBCs occurs, thus releasing free hemoglobin into the plasma. Free hemoglobin may plug the renal tubules and disrupt the work of the nephrons, thus resulting in renal failure. Improper storage, overheating, or freezing of blood may also cause hemolysis of the cells and release of free hemoglobin.

The clinical signs of the hemolytic reaction occur quickly and include sudden hypotension; tachycardia; substernal chest pain; abdominal, leg, and back pain; dyspnea; and sensorium changes, most often anxiety. Headache may be one of the awakened patient's first complaints. Pain may occur along the vein path. Fever and chills develop later, along with hemoglobinuria, which leads to oliguria. Many of these symptoms may be significantly masked under the influence of anesthesia. Bleeding from the wound strongly suggests that the patient has received incompatible blood; it is also a poor prognostic sign.

Febrile Reactions. Febrile reactions are most often caused by sensitivity to leukocytes and platelets and are seen most often in patients who have received multiple transfusions. A febrile reaction may also be attributed to bacterial contamination. In febrile or bacterial contamination reactions the patient may complain of headache and chills, followed by a rapid rise in temperature. Backache, nausea, vomiting, diarrhea, and abdominal pain follow. Hypotension and tachycardia develop quickly. Pyrogenic reactions caused by the polysaccharide products of bacterial metabolism are manifested by the same symptoms, except that blood pressure does not drop, and the temperature usually returns to normal within 12 hours.

Allergic Reactions. Allergic reactions occur in about 1% of all transfusions and are most often seen in patients who have a history of allergy. Symptoms include mild edema and urticaria, sometimes accompanied by pruritus, occasionally by fever and chills, and bronchial wheezing. More severe reactions include symptoms of asthma, bronchospasm, severe dyspnea, laryngeal edema, and finally, anaphylactic shock.

Treatment of Immediate Reactions. At the first sign of a reaction, the transfusion must be stopped and the physician notified. The donor blood unit and administration set, along with a sample of the recipient's blood (drawn from a site other than the intravenous catheter where the blood was administered), should be sent to the blood bank for transfusion reaction investigation. The first voided specimen should be sent to the laboratory and tested for hemoglobin and urobilinogen. Urine output must be monitored carefully. Ideally, a Foley catheter should be inserted and hourly output recorded. Vital signs must be monitored and the patient treated according to his or her symptoms. The intravenous line should be kept open with normal saline. Blood transfusion with properly matched blood may be needed to correct blood volume deficits and control shock. Vasopressors may be required to control blood pressure but must be used with caution because they may contribute to renal damage, especially if blood volume has not been restored. Oxygen and epinephrine may be used to treat dyspnea and wheezing. Steroids and broad-spectrum antibiotics may be necessary to treat reactions caused by bacterial contamination. Antihistamines and antipyretics are given to the patient who experiences an allergic reaction. Diuretic therapy (e.g., furosemide) and the infusion of 0.9% sodium chloride or 5% dextrose in 0.45% sodium chloride may be prescribed to maintain hydration and urine flow of more than 100 ml/hr.

Delayed Reactions

Delayed reactions include the transmission of disease (hepatitis, cytomegalovirus, human immunodeficiency virus-$^1/_2$, human T-cell lymphotropic virus-I/II), transfusion siderosis, graft-versus-host disease, circulatory overload, citrate intoxication, cardiac dysrhythmias, and bleeding caused by depleted coagulation factors.

Circulatory overload results when fluid is infused into the circulatory system either too rapidly or in too great a quantity. Elderly patients and those with minimal cardiac reserve are particularly susceptible. The use of packed RBCs in these patients should be considered carefully. Symptoms of circulatory overload include cough; dyspnea; edema; tachycardia; hemoptysis; and frothy, pink-tinged sputum. If the patient is conscious, he or she may complain of a pounding headache, a feeling of constriction around the chest, back pain, and chills. If these symptoms develop, the transfusion should be stopped and the physician notified.

When large amounts of banked blood are transfused, citrate intoxication may occur. If the blood is infused rapidly, the liver cannot metabolize the citrate ions, which combine with the calcium in the blood, thus causing calcium deficit symptoms such as tingling of the fingers, muscular cramps, and nervousness. If the calcium deficit is not corrected, cardiac dysrhythmias, including ventricular fibrillation, may occur. Treatment consists of slow intravenous administration of calcium gluconate, 1 g for every 1000 ml of blood the patient received. If calcium gluconate is unavailable, calcium chloride may be used, but this is more irritating to the veins.

The rapid infusion of cold blood may result in cardiac dysrhythmias or cardiac arrest. Blood should be warmed to room temperature or passed through a warming coil, taking care not to overheat it, which would cause hemolysis of the RBCs.

In cases of massive blood replacement, bleeding from dilution of coagulation factors and platelets can occur. If massive transfusions are required, it is suggested that several fresh blood infusions (<4 hours old) be used along with banked blood.

Blood must be properly stored and refrigerated at 5°C—except for platelets. In most instances, blood should be stored in the blood bank until required. If blood is to be kept in the PACU, proper storage requirements must be met. When units of blood prepared for a given recipient are not used, they should be promptly returned to the blood bank.

Blood Component Transfusions

Packed Red Blood Cells. The use of packed RBCs can eliminate many of the problems associated with whole blood transfusion. Packed cells are prepared by drawing off about two thirds of the plasma, either through the natural settling-out process or by centrifugation. Patients who require RBCs to improve the oxygen-carrying capacity of the blood should be treated with packed cells to minimize volume increase and the risks of circulatory overload or cardiovascular failure. In addition, a better balance of sodium, potassium, and ammonium ions is maintained, and citrate intoxication is prevented. When plasma is removed, the antibody content of blood is markedly reduced and hence minimizes reactions to plasma factors.

Platelets and Plasma Proteins. Other blood components that may be used in the PACU include platelets and the plasma proteins. Transfusion of platelets is the treatment of choice when bleeding occurs and the platelet count is less than 10,000/μl. Spontaneous bleeding may occur if the platelet count is less than 10,000/μl. For a surgical patient who is bleeding, platelet counts of 50,000 to 100,000 μl in the perioperative period may justify transfusion of platelets. Platelets may be administered through a standard blood administration set or a special component administration set.

Plasma proteins may be used to treat specific deficits. Albumin may be used to treat shock caused by hemorrhage, trauma, or infection. It is prepared in concentrations of 5% in buffered saline and of 25% in salt-poor diluent. It is administered with a large-bore catheter and may be infused through standard intravenous tubing. Plasma protein fraction (PPF) is heat treated like albumin; it destroys antibodies and thereby eliminates compatibility problems. Hepatitis and HIV cannot be transmitted by PPF or albumin because the pasteurization process destroys the viruses.

PPF consists of 83% albumin and 17% globulins extracted from plasma. It is less pure than albumin and can cause hypotension from vasoactive contaminants.

Fresh-frozen plasma thawed slowly forms a precipitate that is separated and refrozen. This cryoprecipitate consists of factor VIII and fibrinogen and is used to control bleeding caused by factor VIII deficiency. It is also indicated for the treatment of von Willebrand's disease and for fibrinogen or factor XIII replacement.

Nonblood Volume Substitutes

Dextran is a synthetic plasma substitute that may be used in acute hemorrhage as a volume expander until more specific blood components can be given. It is inexpensive, readily available, and carries no risk of disease transmission. Dextran may interfere, to some extent, with platelet function and may be associated with a transient prolongation of bleeding time. Hypersensitivity reactions can occur; therefore patients should be closely monitored during the first 30 minutes of infusion. Certain blood typing and cross-matching methods are affected by dextran. Dextran is administered through standard intravenous tubing.

Hetastarch is an artificial colloid. It is a synthetic starch molecule derived from corn that closely resembles human glycogen. Available in a 6% hetastarch in 0.9% sodium chloride solution, hetastarch is claimed to be less likely to produce allergic reactions and to have minimal effects on coagulation when infused in moderate amounts (<1500 ml total volume). It is also used for volume replacement and expansion following acute blood loss from trauma, burns, and surgery.

MAINTENANCE OF RESPIRATORY FUNCTION

Oxygen Therapy

The optimal use of the oxygen-carrying capacity of arterial blood is the goal of oxygen therapy. All anesthetized patients have experienced some interference with their respiratory processes, and for this reason most experts suggest routine oxygen administration to all postanesthesia patients. However, oxygen is a drug and should be treated as such, with full prescription information provided by the anesthesia care provider.

This information may be contained in standard orders that are individualized for each patient. Low-flow oxygen administration assists the patient in maintaining adequate oxygenation of all tissues. Optimal arterial oxygen tension should be between 70 and 100 mm Hg. Patients with chronic lung disease may be maintained with low-flow oxygen administration, which keeps the oxygen tension in the range of 50 to 70 mm Hg. Pulmonary processes should be monitored carefully in the PACU. Pulse oximetry monitoring of all patients who have received an anesthetic is recommended in the initial postanesthesia period.

Pulse oximetry, a noninvasive technique, measures arterial oxygen saturation of functional hemoglobin. In the postanesthesia setting, continuous monitoring of a patient's oxygen saturation assists in manipulating the fraction of delivered oxygen (F_DO_2) levels and in identifying episodes of desaturation and hypoxia. Normal pulse oximetry values are 97% to 99%. Oxygen saturation as measured by pulse oximetry (SpO_2) values of 95% or greater are acceptable. Preanesthetic baseline SpO_2 values should be noted; patients may normally fall below the normal range on room air. Attempting to maintain higher oxygen saturation levels than the patient's baseline level may result in prolonged oxygen therapy and PACU stays.

Sensor site selection and application, ambient light, motion, electrical interference, and impaired blood flow (low perfusion states, excessive edema) may influence SpO_2 levels. Temperature, pH, $PaCO_2$, hemodynamic status, and anemia affect accurate measurement. These factors alter the oxyhemoglobin dissociation curve and oxygen delivery. Additionally, dysfunctional hemoglobins (carboxyhemoglobin, a byproduct of smoking and smoke; methemoglobin, formed from drugs such as lidocaine and nitroglycerin) may result in false elevation of oximetry values.

Nurses should never be reluctant to draw arterial blood gases to aid in the assessment of a patient's status. For discussion of arterial blood gases and the method for obtaining their measurement, see Chapter 10.

Complications of oxygen therapy can occur, and nurses should be aware of them. Oxygen-induced hypoventilation, atelectasis, substernal chest pain, and toxicity may occur when high concentrations are administered over prolonged periods ($FIO_2 > 0.5$ for >24 hours). Decreased SpO_2 is difficult to detect clinically. For more detailed discussions of these complications, the reader should refer to the respiratory references at the end of this chapter.

Methods of Administration

Routine oxygen administration in the PACU can be accomplished with nasal cannula (prongs) or face masks. Table 26-1 lists commonly used oxygen delivery methods. Nasal cannulas are advantageous for routine short-term oxygen administration in the PACU. The cannula is made of plastic tubing with two soft plastic tips that insert into the nostrils about 1.5 cm. The prongs deliver 100% oxygen, thus yielding a final inspired oxygen concentration of 30% to 40% when a 4 to 6 L per minute flow is used. The prongs are easily inserted, comfortable, inexpensive, and disposable. Simple, clear plastic disposable face masks may be used for oxygen administration in the PACU. They are also easy to apply and comfortable. The oxygen concentration inspired depends on the mask fit and the patient's inspiratory flow rate; however, an oxygen flow rate of 5 to 8 L per minute yields an FIO_2 of approximately 40% to 60%. Face masks in the PACU must be clear to provide adequate observation of the patient's nose and mouth. The mask should be removed intermittently to dry the face.

Humidity

Surgery and anesthesia often interrupt the normal functioning of the nose in heating and humidification of inspired air. When oxygen is administered by nasal cannula at flow rates of less than 4 l per minute or by Venturi mask, humidification is generally unnecessary because adequate amounts of humidified room air are inspired. At higher flow rates, humidification or nebulization may be needed in the PACU.

Humidifiers convert water from the liquid to the gaseous state, whereas nebulizers produce tiny water particles. Humidifiers are used to add water vapor to the airway, whereas a nebulizer can provide both water vapor and particulate water or medication or saline aerosols to the airway. Aerosol therapy can be used to administer antibiotics, bronchodilators, and corticosteroids.

Table 26-1 **Methods of Oxygen Administration**			
Method	FIO_2	Flow (l/min)	Comments
LOW-FLOW METHODS			
Nasal cannula (prongs)	0.24-0.4	5-6	Comfortable to wear; patient can breathe orally or nasally and still raise FIO_2; humidification unnecessary
Simple face mask	0.4-0.6	5-8	Adjustable to fit face; may be hot and uncomfortable for patients. Poorly tolerated; potential for skin irritation from tight fit and oxygen contact
Face tent	0.3-0.55	4-10	Less confining; useful when extra humidity needed
Partial rebreathing mask	0.35-0.6	6-10	Mask with attached reservoir bag; no valves on mask (exhalation ports open)
HIGH-FLOW METHODS			
Nonrebreathing mask	0.4-1	6-15	Mask with reservoir bag; one-way valves on exhalation side ports of mask; one-way valve between mask and bag for inhalation
"Venturi" mask	0.24-0.55	2-14	Believed accurate delivery of desired FIO_2; may be less if patient is hyperpneic or unable to keep mask in position on face
T-piece or Brigg's	0.21-1	2-10	Used with endotracheal or tracheostomy tube; provides accurate delivery of desired FIO_2 and humidification; most often used when weaning patients from ventilator assistance before endotracheal tube removed
Mechanical ventilator	0.21-1	Direct from supply	Pressure, volume, flow, and oxygen percentage all adjustable

FIO_2, Fraction of inspired oxygen concentration.

Mechanical Ventilation

Rarely, some patients who are recovering from anesthesia may require some form of mechanical ventilation in the PACU. Various techniques such as positive end-expiratory pressure (PEEP), continuous positive airway pressure (CPAP), and intermittent mandatory ventilation (IMV) are used to improve the respiratory status of the patient. Table 26-2 gives the terminology of the common ventilatory modes.

Positive End-Expiratory Pressure. PEEP is a technique that can be used to help prevent collapse of the alveoli during the expiratory phase of ventilation, to increase the lung's functional residual capacity (FRC), and to reduce the amount of physiologic shunting. PEEP also increases the PaO_2, which will usually enable the FIO_2 to be reduced, thus lessening the chances of oxygen toxicity. In patients with preexisting obstructive lung disease, PEEP should probably be used cautiously, because it may overexpand relatively normal alveoli. When it is used under such circumstances, the dead space increases and occasionally causes a decrease in the PaO_2 and an increase in the $PaCO_2$.

When a patient is placed on PEEP, hemodynamic status should be monitored because this ventilatory technique retards venous return and may cause a decrease in cardiac output, especially in the hypovolemic patient. In some instances, the reduced cardiac output can cause a decrease in systolic blood pressure. Other parameters to be monitored are vital signs, skin perfusion, and urine output.

Table 26-2	**Terminology: Common Ventilatory Modes**
Abbreviation	**Term**

MECHANICAL VENTILATION WITH POSITIVE AIRWAY PRESSURE

A/C	Assist–control ventilation
CMV	Continuous mandatory ventilation
IMV	Intermittent mandatory ventilation
SIMV	Synchronized intermittent mandatory ventilation
PSV	Pressure support ventilation
PEEP	Positive end-expiratory pressure
APRV	Airway pressure-release ventilation

SPONTANEOUS BREATHING (SB) WITH POSITIVE AIRWAY PRESSURE

CPAP	Continuous positive airway pressure
BiPAP	Bilevel positive airway pressure

Continuous Positive Airway Pressure. CPAP helps keep the lungs expanded. The patient breathes out against increased pressure as high as 10 to 20 cm H_2O, but the mechanics of ventilation do not change. The lung performs at a larger, more inflated volume, thereby increasing the FRC and decreasing the tendency to atelectasis. CPAP is a technique that can be used for weaning a patient from a ventilator. When CPAP is being used, the patient should be monitored for tachypnea, tachycardia, increase in blood pressure, arrhythmias, or generalized distress, which should be reported to the physician, if detected.

Intermittent Mandatory Ventilation. IMV was originally devised to facilitate the weaning process from mechanical ventilation. It is currently used when a patient is first given mechanical ventilation. This technique allows patients to breathe on their own as often and as deeply as they would like; it also ensures that every minute a set tidal volume is delivered at a predetermined back-up rate. IMV allows gradual progression from complete ventilatory support by the ventilator to spontaneous provision of ventilation by the patient.

Nursing Responsibilities. All PACU nurses must be familiar with the specific types and modes of operation of ventilators used in their

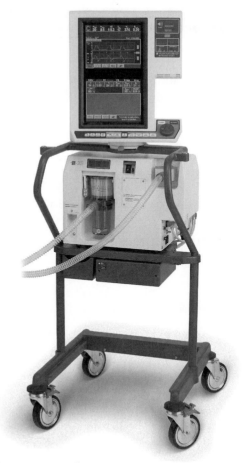

Fig. 26-1 840 Ventilator System. A volume ventilator used either to assist or to control a patient's respirations. *(Reprinted by permission of Nellcor Puritan Bennett Inc., Pleasanton, Calif.)*

area (Fig. 26-1; see Table 26-2). However, some nursing responsibilities remain the same regardless of mechanical ventilator. The following list discusses these responsibilities.

1. Ascertain that the patient is being ventilated by frequently observing the chest for bilateral synchronous and equal expansion and by listening for bilaterally present and equal breath sounds.
2. Check the airway frequently for complete patency. See that the patient ventilator system is free of significant leaks by listening for air gurgling in the upper airway during

ventilation and by comparing the exhaled volume with the tidal volume set on the ventilator.

3. Ensure that the cuff is never overinflated. Inflate the cuff until there is no leak on tidal ventilation and a small, barely audible leak on sigh volume.

4. Empty the ventilatory hoses frequently of excess water from condensation.

5. Be sure that proper humidification is being delivered to the patient by noting the presence of water droplets in the ventilator hoses.

6. The humidifier should be checked and filled frequently to ensure proper humidification.

7. The temperature gauge should be between 32.2°C and 36.6°C, and the ventilator hoses and the humidifier should be warm to the touch, never cold or hot.

8. There must never be any pull on the patient's endotracheal or tracheostomy tube.

9. Tracheostomy wound care should be performed as needed during the postanesthesia phase.

10. Ascertain frequently that all alarms on the ventilator are on and functioning properly.

The observations and checks of mechanical devices often seem simple and routine but are an important part of nursing the mechanically ventilated patient. Ideally, all these checks, along with measured parameters of the patient's respiratory status, should be recorded on a flow sheet attached to the patient's bed or to the ventilator.

Suctioning

When large amounts of secretions accumulate that cannot be handled effectively by coughing, suctioning must be instituted to assist the patient in clearing air passages.

Oral and Nasal Suctioning. Suctioning the nose and mouth is simple and safe. This procedure is commonly used to assist patients in eliminating secretions before they have regained full consciousness and cannot spit out secretions. The catheter used should be soft and pliable. The technique should be clean but need not be strictly sterile. A Yankauer or tonsil suction tip may be used to remove oral secretions from the mouth and over the tongue; however, care must

be exercised to avoid breaking or chipping the teeth.

Tracheal Suctioning. Tracheal suctioning may be performed through the mouth or nose, via endotracheal tube, or through a tracheostomy tube (Fig. 26-2). Tracheal suctioning must be accomplished atraumatically using aseptic technique. A selection of sterile suctioning catheters in a variety of sizes should be kept at the bedside of every patient in the PACU along with sterile gloves and sterile water or normal saline. The catheter chosen for suctioning should not have an external diameter that exceeds by one third the internal diameter of the tube to be suctioned. Most commonly, a 14 or 16 French size is used for adult patients. The catheter must not completely occlude the trachea or endotracheal tube.

The procedure should be explained to the patients even if they are apparently totally unconscious. Explaining the procedure alleviates fear and also helps gain cooperation from the patients to the extent that they are able.

Before suctioning the patient, ensure proper ventilation. In most patients, suctioning lowers the arterial pressure of oxygen 30 to 35 mm Hg. Because suctioning removes oxygen, which may in turn initiate cardiac dysrhythmias, the nurse should assess the total physiologic condition of the patient before beginning the procedure. Are they restless, agitated, or disoriented? Although these conditions can be caused by other factors, they often indicate inadequate oxygenation. Conscious patients can be asked to take four or five deep breaths. The patient who cannot cooperate must be preoxygenated with an air-mask-bag unit (Ambu) or anesthesia bag. Ambus deliver variable oxygen concentrations (FIO_2 between 30% to 95%) and volumes. Flow rates should be at least 10 to 15 L/min to achieve higher FIO_2. Higher volumes can be obtained by using two hands to compress the bag. If the patient has an endotracheal airway in place and is on a ventilator, several sigh volumes can be delivered at 1.0 FIO_2 before suctioning.

To suction patients with no airway adjunct, the nurse should instruct them to stick out their tongues. Grasp the tongue with a gauze pad, and apply gentle traction to make the glottis open and move in line with the trachea. Lubricate the catheter tip with a small amount of water-soluble jelly. Gently insert the catheter into the nostril.

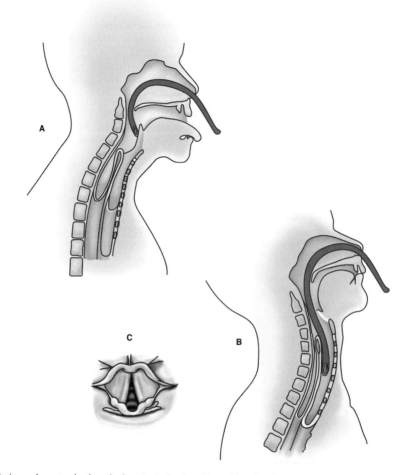

Fig. 26-2 Technique of nasotracheal suctioning. **A,** Optimal position of head to direct the catheter tip anteriorly into the trachea. The neck is flexed, and the head is extended. The tongue is protruded (and held in place with a 4 × 4 gauze). **B,** After the catheter has been advanced into the trachea, the tongue is released, and the patient's head may be more comfortably positioned. **C,** View of the vocal cords from above. The cords are most widely separated during inspiration. *(Redrawn from Sanderson RG, editor: The cardiac patient, Philadelphia, 1972, WB Saunders.)*

A slight curvature in the tubing may facilitate intubation of the larynx. Advance the catheter until intubation of the trachea is accomplished. Listen through the catheter or feel for air movement against your cheek through the proximal end of the catheter. An increasing intensity of breath sounds or more air against the cheek indicates nearness to the larynx. If the breath sounds decrease or the patient begins to gag, the catheter is in the hypopharynx. Draw back and advance again. A sudden cough indicates the presence of the catheter in the larynx; advance quickly with the next breath.

Once the catheter is positioned in the trachea, apply intermittent suction by alternately occluding and opening the vent of the Y-connector with the thumb and withdraw the catheter in a spiral motion. If an airway adjunct is present, suctioning may be accomplished through it.

Never apply suction until the catheter is in the trachea, and never apply suction longer than 15 seconds. One useful trick is for the nurse to hold his or her breath while suctioning the patient as a reminder of the time limits. Monitor the patient carefully during all suctioning procedures. Any form of suctioning can lead to dysrhythmias, and prolonged suctioning may produce hypoxia, asphyxia, and cardiac arrest. Remember that suctioning removes oxygen as well as secretions; therefore the patient should be oxygenated before and after the procedure.

Suctioning is not without risk of complication, nor should it be done routinely. Appropriate indications for suctioning are the presence of bronchial secretions, identified visually by auscultation or—in the mechanically ventilated patient—by rising airway pressures from retained secretions. Hypoxemia is the most common complication that can lead to atelectasis and dysrhythmias. Other complications include mucosal trauma, infection, paroxysmal coughing, and increased systemic and intracranial pressures.

Tracheostomy care is discussed in Chapter 29.

INFECTION CONTROL

Infection control in the PACU is always a problem. All postoperative patients are exceedingly vulnerable to infection because their body defenses are depressed. Prevention of the spread of infection involves blocking infectious agents from the three major avenues of transmission in the PACU: air, human carriers, and inanimate objects used in the care of patients—particularly instruments.

When a patient is received in the PACU for whom air may reasonably be expected to act as a vector, he or she should be isolated in a single room and the hospital's standard isolation techniques carried out. Ideally, a separate isolation room with glass partitions should be planned for the PACU to allow for separation of isolation cases. Ease of observation of a patient placed in the isolation room is essential. If patients in isolation cannot be fully observed, they should be attended until complete recovery from anesthesia. The Centers for Disease Control and Prevention recommendations for isolation precautions and the institution's own system for isolation precautions should be reviewed regularly.

The Occupational Safety and Health Administration (OSHA) mandates that standard precautions (the treating of blood and certain body fluids as if infectious), engineering controls, work practice controls, personal protective equipment, and housekeeping protocols be complied with in the healthcare environment. Pertinent references can be found in the list at the end of the chapter.

Primary to infection control and prevention of disease transmission is handwashing. All personnel should wash their hands thoroughly after caring for each patient; no deviation from this practice should occur. Handwashing facilities must be easily accessible to the observation area. In an emergency or if handwashing facilities are not readily available, antiseptic hand cleaners must be provided.

Disposable patient care items such as drinking glasses, catheter sets, and irrigation sets have contributed immensely to infection control programs. Many of these products are used in the PACU; they must be used as specified and then discarded and must not be resterilized for reuse. All items that are not disposable should be cleaned and sterilized appropriately after use before contact with a new patient. OSHA standards address the disposal of regulated waste and cleaning of reusable items.

Personnel must be scrupulous in their personal hygiene. Personnel should never work in the PACU if they know or suspect that they have any infectious disease, especially an upper respiratory infection. Open cuts or sores should disqualify a person from working with postoperative patients.

The wearing of scrub attire in the PACU has been questioned. Although recommendations for its use continue, no definitive studies exist to indicate that scrub suits should be mandatory. The proximity and access to the operating suite may determine the dress code for staff and visitors.

Every hospital has its own physical limitations, and modifications in isolation techniques must be made to fit the circumstances. Good practice dictates using scientific principles and knowledge when making plans to prevent the spread of infection.

GENERAL COMFORT AND SAFETY MEASURES

General comfort and safety measures are important parts of postanesthesia care. For safety, at least two nurses (one of whom is a registered nurse) should always be present whenever patients are recovering. An unconscious patient should never be left alone, and side rails should be raised on the bed whenever direct patient care is not being provided. The wheels of the bed should be locked to prevent sliding when care is being rendered.

General physical measures such as cleanliness should not be overlooked in the PACU. Comfort measures, important to the total well-being of the patient, are often forgotten in the hustle of caring for postanesthesia patients. As soon as the patient is settled into the unit and assessment has been accomplished, all excess skin preparations and electrodes should be removed; in addition to providing comfort, washing off excess skin preparations gives the nurse an excellent opportunity to further assess the patient's general condition. A backrub at this time may prevent later complaints of discomfort from positioning for long periods in the operating room. This is also a good time to change the patient's position, assist with range-of-motion exercises, and encourage deep breathing. Frequent position changes help prevent atelectasis, promote circulation, and prevent pressure from developing on the skin surfaces.

Mouth care with lemon-glycerin swabs may be comforting to the patient who has not only had nothing by mouth but also has been medicated with an anticholinergic or glycopyrrolate to reduce secretions. When patients are fully conscious and their laryngeal reflexes have returned, they can rinse their mouths with mouthwash and water. Ice chips and small sips of water or juice may be offered to the patient who can tolerate fluids. A petrolatum-based ointment should be applied to the lips after mouth care to prevent drying and consequent cracking.

Patients often complain of being cold when they return from the operating suite. This is caused in part by the effects of anesthesia and premedications and in part to the cool atmosphere of the operating suite and the PACU. This must be explained to the patient. Warming measures should be instituted on arrival to the PACU if the patient is hypothermic. Warmed cotton blankets, thermal foil drapes, radiant lamps, and convective warming devices are available.

Devices should be used according to the manufacturers' recommendations to avoid patient injury.

The normothermic patient may shiver or complain of feeling cold; warm blankets may provide psychological comfort, and pharmacologic and active warming interventions may be needed to reduce or eliminate shaking. Blankets of any type should not, however, obscure the intravenous lines, arterial lines, or other monitoring apparatuses from the direct view of the attending nurse. The patient's temperature must be monitored closely to avoid overheating.

In addition to physical comfort measures, remember to provide psychological comfort. Reorientation, especially to time and place, is important to the postanesthesia patient, as is constant reassurance that the surgery is completed and that all went well. The nurse's presence at the bedside or gentle touch may also be comforting to the patient.

TRANSFER OF THE PATIENT FROM THE PACU

When the patient has recovered from the effects of anesthesia, vital signs will have stabilized; if no surgical complications have arisen, the patient is ready for transfer to the nursing unit or discharge area. The patient's postanesthesia recovery score, if a scoring system is used, should meet preestablished minimums, unless criteria for exception are noted. The patient should have regained a satisfactory level of consciousness to the point of being oriented and able to call for assistance, if necessary, and should be clean, dry, and dressed in appropriate hospital garb. All dressings should be dry and intact, and all drainage receptacles should be emptied. The patient should be seen by a licensed practitioner before discharge, or the name of the responsible physician should be documented in the patient's record. The PACU nurse should discharge the patient when the patient meets medically approved discharge criteria.

No patient should be discharged immediately after receiving an initial dose of a opioid medication. Discharge should be delayed to assess the patient for pain relief and adverse side effects of the medication. Pain assessment and management should be documented in the patient's record for ongoing evaluation of pain intensity and treatment effectiveness.

A summarizing PACU discharge note should be written on the patient's progress record to indicate condition and time of transfer. The nurse should alert the receiving unit that the patient is being transferred and request the preparation of any specialized equipment for care and the assignment of a receiving nurse.

Patients may be transferred on a stretcher or bed as required by their condition and the operative procedure. Ensure that the patient is adequately covered with bed linens, including a warmed blanket if hallways are kept cool. Lock the side rails of the stretcher in place. Ideally, two persons should be used to wheel the stretcher to the receiving unit. The person in back pushes; the person in front steers; both move at a reasonable speed. Transport personnel vary by institution, and decisions regarding who transports may vary based on the patient's condition, staffing, and unit needs.

A receiving nurse should meet the patient on arrival to the unit and direct the transfer to the patient's room. The patient is transferred to the bed along with all apparatuses. Safety precautions must be strictly followed. Always use at least two people to transfer the patient. A third person may be necessary to assist with the patient transfer if extra equipment or multiple drainage tubes are present. Stabilize both the bed and the stretcher by locking the wheels when transferring the patient from one to the other. Ensure that all drainage tubes and catheters are safely transferred, that no kinking occurs, and that they do not become tangled underneath the patient. All drainage receptacles should remain below the level of the patient. Intravenous tubing and solution must be carefully transferred from the portable stand attached to the stretcher to the bedside stand or holder. Drainage tubes should be connected to suction or gravity drainage as indicated, and their proper functioning checked. Ensure that the patient's call light is positioned within the patient's reach along with any other items that may be needed. Check the intravenous infusion rate, and adjust as necessary. Side rails on the bed should be raised.

The report may be written, telephoned, faxed or given in person to the receiving nurse. The PACU nurse should give a complete report to the receiving nurse, including pertinent facts about the following:

1. The operative procedure performed.
2. The anesthesia used and any reversal agents given.
3. The patient's general condition and postanesthesia course.
4. The incision, any drains placed, and the dressing.
5. Any drainage tubes or catheters.
6. Intake and output, including intravenous fluids (colloid and crystalloid) given, estimated blood loss, and time of void or catheterization. The flow sheet should be reviewed.
7. Any medications given in the PACU, especially analgesics, and the patient's response and level of comfort.

BIBLIOGRAPHY

American Society of Anesthesiologists: Questions and answers about transfusion practices, ed 3, Park Ridge, Ill, 1997, American Society of Anesthesiologists.

American Association of Blood Banks, America's Blood Centers, and the American Red Cross: Circular of information for the use of human blood and blood components. Aug 2000 (revised). American Association of Blood Banks. Retrieved online Feb 5, 2002, from *http://www.aabb.org/all_about_blood/coi/aabb_coi.htm*

American Society of PeriAnesthesia Nurses: Clinical guideline for the prevention of unplanned perioperative hypothermia, J Perianesth Nurs 16(5):305-314, 2001.

American Society of PeriAnesthesia Nurses: Standards of perianesthesia nursing practice 2000, Cherry Hill, NJ, 2000, American Society of PeriAnesthesia Nurses.

Black JM, Hawks JH, Keene AM: Medical-surgical nursing: clinical management for positive outcomes, ed 6, Philadelphia, 2001, WB Saunders.

Finucane BT, Santora AH: Principles of airway management, ed 2, Philadelphia, 1996, WB Saunders.

Greensmith JE, Aker JG: Ventilatory management in the postanesthesia care unit, J Perianesth Nurs 13(6):370-381, 1998.

Longnecker DE, Murphy FL: Dripps/Eckenhoff/Vandam introduction to anesthesia, ed 9, Philadelphia, 1997, WB Saunders.

Lynn-McHale DJ, Carlson KK: AACN procedure manual for critical care, ed 4, Philadelphia, 2001, WB Saunders.

Marley RA: Postoperative oxygen therapy, J Perianesth Nurs 13(6):394-412, 1998.

Stoller JK, Kester L: Respiratory care protocols in postanesthesia care, J Perianesth Nurs 13(6):349-358, 1998.

27

ASSESSMENT AND MANAGEMENT OF THE AIRWAY

Melissa A. Hotchkiss, MSNA, CRNA
Cecil B. Drain, PhD, RN, CRNA, FAAN

Airway assessment and management are principal skills required of all personnel in the postanesthesia care unit (PACU). Intubation of the trachea is a skill that should be reserved for nursing personnel who are specifically trained to perform this maneuver. The perianesthesia nurse should be familiar with the intubation technique and capable of performing it quickly and efficiently. Airway management skills, including endotracheal intubation, can be developed in the operating room setting under the mentorship of a nurse anesthetist or an anesthesiologist. Using the same mentor, the perianesthesia nurse should continue to practice the intubation skills on a monthly basis in the operating room.

ORAL AIRWAY MANAGEMENT

Patients may arrive in the PACU still experiencing the depressant effects of the anesthetic, and because they are obtunded, airway obstruction can occur. Some of the indications of airway obstruction include increased respiratory effort, retraction of the various muscles of respiration, a rocking chest motion, abnormal breath sounds, and evidence of hypoxemia and hypercarbia. In some instances, the obtunded patient's tongue and epiglottis may fall back on the posterior pharyngeal wall, thus occluding the airway. When this happens, the nurse should place the patient in a supine position with the head tilted backward and the neck hyperextended. The nurse should then lift the angle of the lower jaw upward using moderate pressure (Fig. 27-1). Often, this maneuver is all that is required for spontaneous respirations to return. If spontaneous respirations do not return, the oral cavity should be inspected for foreign material and the oral pharynx suctioned if necessary. If large particles are present,

the nurse should turn the patient's head to the side and remove the particles manually.

If spontaneous ventilation does not occur, positive-pressure breathing must be instituted. If possible, a bag-valve-mask unit that is connected to an oxygen source should be used. The requirements for a bag-valve-mask unit are addressed in Box 27-1. The perianesthesia nurse should be positioned behind the patient's head—not at his or her side. The mask should be fitted over the patient's mouth and nose with his or her neck hyperextended. The lower jaw should be lifted at its angle with the other fingers of the hand holding the mask. The thumb of that hand should be placed at the top of the mask, and pushing down will provide compression over the bridge of the nose to reduce air leaks (Fig. 27-2).

After the mask is properly applied, the patient should be ventilated. While the perianesthesia nurse is ventilating the patient, an assistant should assess the adequacy of the positive-pressure breathing by auscultating the chest. If an assistant is not present, the perianesthesia nurse should check to see if the chest rises and falls or if air escapes during expiration. These are rough estimates of ventilation, and they may not be completely accurate about adequacy of ventilation. If breath sounds are not heard during auscultation or if the rough estimates are inconclusive, an oropharyngeal airway should be inserted (Fig. 27-3). This airway can be extremely stimulating to patients in the PACU who are awake or lightly anesthetized. The results of stimulation of reflexes include bradycardia, retching, vomiting, and laryngospasm.

The oropharyngeal airway may relieve the airway obstruction by providing a mechanical conduit for air to pass between the base of the

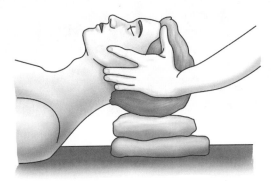

Fig. 27-1 Technique of lifting the jaw by placing the fingers behind the mandible to overcome soft-tissue obstruction of the upper airway. *(From Dripps R, Eckenhoff J, Vandam L: Introduction to anesthesia: the principles of safe practice, ed 6, Philadelphia, 1982, WB Saunders.)*

Box 27-1	**Requirements for Bag-Valve-Mask Unit**

Self-refilling but without sponge rubber inside (because of the difficulty in cleaning and disinfecting and in eliminating ethylene oxide and because of fragmentation)
Nonjam valve system at 15 L/min oxygen inlet flow
Transparent, plastic face mask with an air-filled or contoured, resilient cuff
Standard 15 mm/22 mm fittings
No pop-off valve, except in pediatric models
System for delivery of high concentrations of oxygen through an ancillary oxygen outlet at the back of the bag or by an oxygen reservoir
True nonrebreathing valve
Oropharyngeal airway
Satisfactory practice on mannequins
Available in adult and pediatric sizes

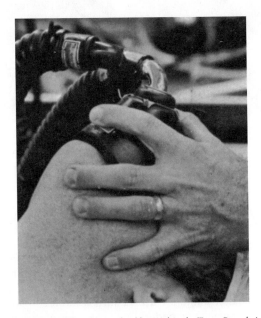

Fig. 27-2 Holding the mask with one hand. *(From Dorsch J, Dorsch S: Understanding anesthesia equipment, Baltimore, 1975, Williams & Wilkins.)*

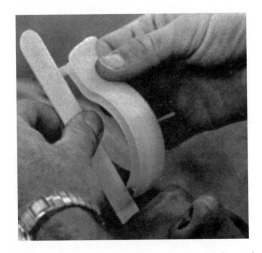

Fig. 27-3 Insertion of an oral airway. The airway is inserted with the use of a tongue blade to displace the tongue forward. *(From Dorsch J, Dorsch S: Understanding anesthesia equipment, Baltimore, 1975, Williams & Wilkins.)*

tongue and the posterior oropharynx. To place an oropharyngeal airway, the perianesthesia nurse should first open the patient's mouth with the right hand and, using the left hand, place a tongue blade toward the posterior aspect of the tongue. Slight pressure should then be applied to draw the tongue forward. Holding the oropharyngeal airway in the right hand, the nurse should slip it in over the tongue blade into the orophar-

ynx. The airway should not be twisted or forced into place, and the airway insertion procedure should be accomplished quickly and carefully so as to avoid trauma to the soft tissue and teeth.

In comparison to the oropharyngeal airway, the nasopharyngeal airway is less stimulating to the irritant receptors in the upper airway, especially in awake or lightly anesthetized patients. The nasopharyngeal airway should be lubricated with a local anesthetic water-soluble lubricant, such as 1% lidocaine, and gently passed with the right hand through the nares along the curvature of the nasopharynx to the oropharynx. The nasopharyngeal airway should not be forced. If resistance is encountered, the other naris should be used. When positioned properly, the nasopharyngeal airway should rest between the base of the tongue and the posterior pharyngeal wall. This airway should not be used in a patient with a nasal septal deformity, a leakage of cerebrospinal fluid from the nose, or a coagulation disorder.

Once the oropharyngeal or the nasopharyngeal airway has been placed properly, ventilation should be continued. Then assessment of adequacy of ventilation should be repeated. With insertion of the oropharyngeal airway, the patient will often resume ventilation. In this instance, the patient should be given a breath via the bag-valve-mask unit to assist his or her breathing effort and to help remove excess carbon dioxide. If the patient continues to be apneic, positive-pressure breathing should be continued by using large tidal volumes (10 to 12 ml/kg) at a rate of 14 to 16 breaths/min.

INTUBATION OF THE TRACHEA

If the perianesthesia nurse cannot ventilate the patient, even after placement of an oropharyngeal or nasopharyngeal airway, endotracheal intubation should be performed. Endotracheal intubation and intratracheal intubation are synonymous terms that indicate the placement of a tube directly into the trachea. When the endotracheal tube is placed through the mouth, the method is called orotracheal intubation. Other indications for endotracheal intubation in the PACU are inability of the patient to protect his or her airway, prolonged mechanical ventilation, cardiac arrest, and respiratory arrest.

The perianesthesia nurse should be familiar with the technique of tracheal intubation and be capable of performing it quickly and efficiently, knowing that the conditions under which intubation is performed in the PACU are less than

ideal. The patient's position in the bed, excess upper airway secretions, and intact reflexes all increase the difficulty in performing this maneuver in the PACU.

Equipment for Tracheal Intubation

Adult and pediatric intubation equipment should be kept in the PACU at all times. This equipment should be inspected daily and after each use. For a list of the suggested items to be kept in the PACU, see Box 27-2. Table 27-1 shows the recommended sizes for endotracheal tubes. Because of their importance, the laryngoscope and tracheal tubes will be discussed in detail.

Laryngoscope. The laryngoscope is used to visualize the larynx and the anatomic structures in close proximity to the larynx (Fig. 27-4). The laryngoscope has two main parts: the handle and the blade. The handle holds the laryngoscope and houses batteries that provide electricity for the light on the side of the blade. The blade consists of three sections: the spatula, the flange, and the tip. The spatula can be straight or curved; it is the long main shaft of the blade. It compresses and moves the soft tissue of the lower jaw to facilitate direct vision of the larynx. The flange, which is on the side of the spatula, deflects tissue that may obstruct the direct vision of the larynx. The tip, at the distal end of the spatula, is either curved or straight and serves to elevate the epiglottis, either directly or indirectly. The blade is attached to the handle at a connection called the hook-on fitting. The perianesthesia nurse is strongly encouraged to practice connecting the blade to the handle before using the laryngoscope in an emergency.

The Macintosh and Miller blades are the most popular types in clinical use. The Macintosh is a curved blade with the flange on the left side to aid in moving the tongue so as to enhance visual exposure of the larynx. The Macintosh blade (Fig. 27-5) comes in four sizes: no. 1 for the infant, no. 2 for the child, no. 3 for the medium adult, and no. 4 for the large adult. For most adults, the no. 3 medium adult is the blade of choice. The Miller blade (see Fig. 27-5) is a straight spatula with a curved tip. This blade has five sizes: no. 0 for the premature infant, no. 1 for the infant, no. 2 for the child, no. 3 for the medium adult, and no. 4 for the large adult. The Miller nos. 0 and 1 are the blades of choice for

Box 27-2	**Suggested Equipment for PACU Pediatric and Adult Airway Management Carts**

PEDIATRIC ENDOTRACHEAL EQUIPMENT
Small laryngoscope handle
No. 2 Macintosh curved blade
No. 1 Miller straight blade
Pediatric oral airways
Assorted pediatric masks
   Child's anatomic masks
   Randell-Baker-Soucek masks
Assorted tracheal tubes
   Reverse-angle endotracheal tubes
   Cole tubes
   Reinforced latex tube with stylet
   Plastic thin-walled tube

PEDIATRIC LMA EQUIPMENT
LMA-Classic: Sizes 1, 1½, 2, 2½, and 3
LMA-Unique: Sizes 3 and 4
20 cc syringes to inflate LMA
Pediatric oral airways

ADULT ENDOTRACHEAL EQUIPMENT
Laryngoscope handle
Laryngoscope blades
   Nos. 2 and 4 Miller
   No. 3 Macintosh
Stylet
Sterile gauze with topical water-soluble anesthetic
   lubricant
Sizes 6- through 9-mm cuffed tracheal tubes
10 ml syringe to inflate the cuff
Small hemostat
Tongue blades for airway insertion
Assorted-sized oropharyngeal airways

ADULT LMA EQUIPMENT
LMA-Classic: Sizes 3, 4, 5, and 6
LMA-Unique: Sizes 3, 4, and 5
60 cc syringes to inflate LMA
Adult oral airways

Table 27-1	**Recommended Sizes For Endotracheal Tubes**

Age/Sex	Internal Diameter (mm)
Premature	2.0
Newborn	2.5
6 months	3.5
1 year	4.0
2 years	5.0
4 years	5.5
6 years	6.0
8 years	6.5
10 years	6.5-7.0
12 years	7.0-7.5
14 years	7.5-8.0
Adults	
Female	8.0-8.5
Male	9.0-9.5

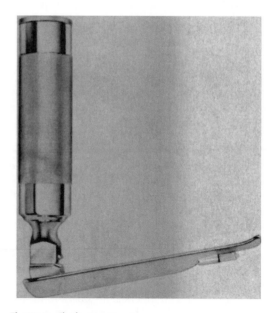

Fig. 27-4 The laryngoscope.

premature and fullterm infants, whose anatomic structures are more receptive to the use of a straight blade. Many anesthesia practitioners use the no. 2 Miller to intubate adults. The perianesthesia nurse is encouraged to use both the straight and the curved blades and then to decide on the blade of preference. In most instances, the curved blade is easier to use than the straight blade; however, the exposure of the vocal cords is not as good as with the straight blade.

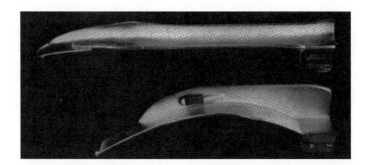

Fig. 27-5 The most frequently used laryngoscope blades: Miller *(top)* and Macintosh *(bottom)*. *(From Miller R, editor: Anesthesia, New York, 1981, Churchill Livingstone.)*

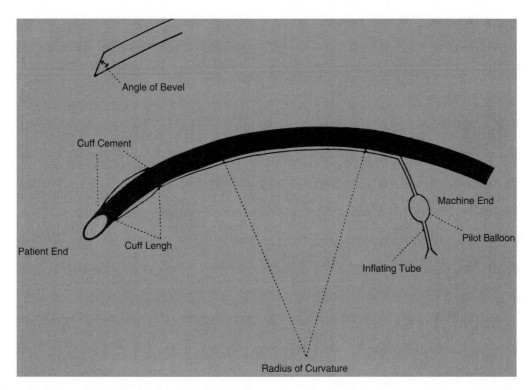

Fig. 27-6 The curved tracheal tube. *(From Dorsch J, Dorsch S: Understanding anesthesia equipment, Baltimore, 1975, Williams & Wilkins.)*

Tracheal Tube. The tracheal tube is also called the endotracheal tube, intratracheal tube, or catheter (Fig. 27-6). It is usually made from natural or synthetic rubber or plastic. The proximal, or machine, end protrudes from the patient's mouth and receives the adaptor. The distal, or patient end, has a slanted portion called the bevel. An uncuffed tracheal tube should be used on patients who are 8 years of age or younger. Endotracheal tubes are numbered according to their internal diameter in millimeters. Near the distal end of the tracheal tube is a cuff. Also leading away from the cuff is an inflating tube with a pilot balloon at its proximal end to indicate whether the cuff is inflated. Above the pilot balloon is a plug or one-way valve to which the inflation syringe is attached.

The cuff is an inflatable sleeve that provides a leak-resistant fit between the tube and the trachea when inflated. It also prevents aspiration and allows positive-pressure ventilation of the lungs. The cuff is permanently attached to the tracheal tube at the distal end. Concerning inflation volume, there are high- or low-residual-volume cuffs, which refer to the amount of air that can be withdrawn from the cuff after it has been inflated and allowed to deflate spontaneously with the tube patent and open to the air. The high-residual-volume cuff is also referred to as a low-pressure cuff. The low-residual-volume cuff is also called a high-pressure cuff. The arterial pressure in the tracheal wall is about 30 torr, and the venous pressure in that area is about 20 torr. Most clinicians agree that a low-pressure (high-residual-volume), thin-walled cuff should be inflated to a pressure of about 17 to 23 torr. Local tracheal complications are associated with the cuff, especially after longer periods of intubation. Excessive cuff pressure is the primary factor to cause ulceration, necrosis, and tracheal stenosis. These complications occur because high cuff pressure reduces the blood supply in the tracheal mucosa. For long-term ventilation, the cuffs should be long, with a large residual volume.

In an emergency, the perianesthesia nurse should choose an endotracheal tube that is one size smaller than the size normally recommended for the patient. When making this choice, many clinicians look at the little finger of the patient because a small-sized little finger indicates that the patient has an opening at the vocal cords that is smaller than normal. Also, a stylet made of malleable metal or plastic should be inserted inside the endotracheal tube to improve its curvature and maintain its shape. Before the stylet is placed inside the tracheal tube, it must be covered with a water-soluble lubricant to ease its withdrawal from the tube after placement. The end of the stylet should be about 3 cm from the distal end of the tracheal tube and should not protrude beyond the bevel because damage to the vocal cords can occur.

Oral Endotracheal Intubation

Before oral endotracheal intubation is attempted, additional equipment should be immediately available and ready for use. Such equipment includes a tonsil suction connected to a working suction device, McGill forceps, 1-inch tape, a 10-ml empty syringe, and an anesthesia bag system or bag-valve unit. Also, throughout the procedure, the patient's oxygen saturation should be monitored continuously with a pulse oximeter.

The essential steps in the technique of oral endotracheal intubation are positioning the patient, positioning his or her head, inserting the blade of the laryngoscope, raising the epiglottis, visualizing the vocal cords, placing the tracheal tube, and assessing the patient. The methods for accomplishing these steps are discussed in the following sections.

Positioning the Patient. Move the patient up so that his or her head is at the top of the bed. Raise the head of the bed (or the entire bed, if possible) so that the patient's face is approximately at the level of the standing perianesthesia nurse's xiphoid process.

Positioning the Head. Place a firm 4-inch pillow or ring under the head. Flex the patient's head at the neck. This position is called the sniffing position (Fig. 27-7) because of the flexion of the head at the neck and extension of the head. The nurse places his or her right hand on the patient's forehead to extend the head.

Inserting the Blade. With the fingers of the right hand, open the jaw wide, making sure that the lips are spread away from the teeth. With the laryngoscope in the left hand, insert the moistened or lubricated blade between the teeth at the right side of the patient's mouth. Advance the blade slowly inward, past the tonsillar pillars and toward the midline of the oral cavity, sweeping the tongue toward the left side of the mouth. A major key to a successful intubation is moving the tongue to the left, out of the visual path to the vocal cords. At this point, the right hand can be placed under the patient's occiput to extend the head. The epiglottis should now be visualized; it is a red, leaf-shaped structure that will appear behind the tip of the blade as the laryngoscope is advanced down the oral cavity.

Raising the Epiglottis and Visualizing the Vocal Cords. With the epiglottis under direct vision, slip the straight blade just beneath the tip of the epiglot-

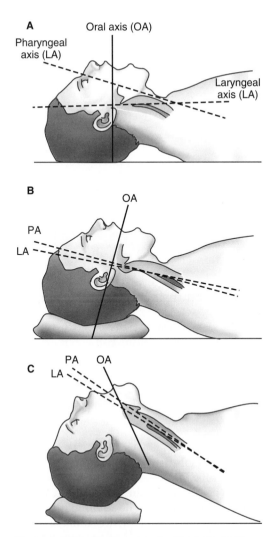

A
Oral axis (OA)
Pharyngeal axis (LA)
Laryngeal axis (LA)

B
OA
PA
LA

C
PA OA
LA

Fig. 27-7 Positioning for endotracheal intubation. **A,** The patient is in the supine position, with alignment of the oral, pharyngeal, and laryngeal axes. **B,** Placement of pad or ring under the patient's occiput (sniffing position) aligns the pharyngeal and laryngeal axes. **C,** Extending the patient's head at the atlanto-occipital joint now aligns all three axes, which provides the shortest distance and most nearly straight line from the mouth to the larynx. *(Redrawn from Miller R, editor: Anesthesia, ed 5, New York, 2000, Churchill Livingstone.)*

tis, gently lift the blade forward and upward at a 45-degree angle, and hold the wrist rigid (Fig. 27-8). If a curved blade, such as the Macintosh, is used, slip the tip of the blade between the epiglottis and the base of the tongue (see Fig. 27-

8). With the left hand, lift forward and upward on the handle at a 45-degree angle. The epiglottis will fold onto the blade, and the vocal cords should then be visible.

Regardless of whether a curved or straight blade is used, the handle should not be used as a lever with the upper teeth as a fulcrum because the tip of the blade will push the larynx up and out of sight and the teeth can become chipped or broken.

At this point, if the vocal cords cannot be visualized, an assistant should apply gentle external downward pressure on the larynx (the Sellick maneuver); the vocal cords should come into view. If the blade is passed too far, it will enter the esophagus. If this happens, withdraw the blade, ventilate the patient with 100% oxygen, and perform the procedure again. While ventilating the patient, think about what went wrong, and design an alternative strategy to facilitate a successful intubation of the trachea.

Placing the Tracheal Tube. When the vocal cords are visualized, an assistant should place the tracheal tube—with a stylet properly inserted to maintain a curve and the cuff deflated—in the right hand. Pass the tracheal tube with the right hand to the right of the tongue and blade through the vocal cords until the cuff disappears behind the vocal cords or until the tip of the tracheal tube protrudes 2 or 3 cm into the trachea.

Assessing the Patient. Once the tracheal tube is in place, remove the blade with the left hand while holding on to the tube with the right hand. Place the laryngoscope on the patient's bed or on a table, and slowly remove the stylet without dislodging the tracheal tube. The patient end to the tracheal tube should then be connected to a bag-valve unit or an anesthesia bag system and ventilated while an assistant auscultates the chest for breath sounds. The breath sounds should be assessed in all four quadrants, and the stomach also should be auscultated. If no breath sounds are heard or if a "gurgling" sound is heard over the stomach, deflate the cuff, remove the tracheal tube, and ventilate the patient with a mask, using 100% oxygen. While ventilating the patient, think about why the attempt was unsuccessful, review the procedure, and reintubate the patient. If breath sounds are heard on only one side of the chest (usually the right side, not the left), withdraw the tube at 1-cm intervals until the breath

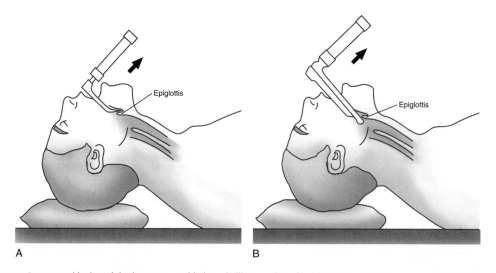

A   B

Fig. 27-8 Proper positioning of the laryngoscope blade to facilitate endotracheal intubation. **A**, With a curved blade (e.g., Macintosh), the tip is placed into the space between the base of the tongue and the pharyngeal surface of the epiglottis, which is called the vallecula. **B**, With a straight blade (e.g., Miller), the tip is placed on the laryngeal surface of the epiglottis. Regardless of the type of blade used, once the blade is in position, the forward and upward movements on the handle (arrows) exert pressure on the long axis of the blade, which serves to elevate the epiglottis and expose the vocal cords. *(Redrawn from Miller R, editor: Anesthesia, ed 5, New York, 2000, Churchill Livingstone.)*

sounds are bilateral. Using a 10-ml syringe full of air, inject a volume of air (about 4 to 6 ml) into the pilot balloon until leakage around the cuff is minimal or stops. The cuff leak is assessed by placing the bell of the stethoscope over the larynx. Once tube placement and cuff pressure are correct, insert an oral airway and secure the tube with adhesive tape.

Documentation of the procedure should include the number of attempts, the degree of visualization of the vocal cords, whether the intubation was traumatic or atraumatic, the quality of breath sounds, the amount of air injected into the cuff, the cuff pressure, the tracheal tube size, and the laryngoscope blade type and size.

Ventilating the Patient.   The adult patient should be ventilated approximately 14 to 18 times/min at a tidal volume of 8 to 10 ml/kg. Infants should be ventilated at approximately 26 to 30 times/min at a volume large enough to raise their chest on inspiration. However, when time permits, a tidal volume of 7 ml/kg should be used. Children should be ventilated at a rate of 18 to 24 breaths/min. The tidal volume to be delivered

can be determined in the same manner for infants.

Nasotracheal Intubation
When the tube is inserted through the nose, the method is called nasotracheal intubation. When nasotracheal intubation is done without the use of a laryngoscope, the method is called a blind nasotracheal intubation. Direct-vision intubation is the insertion of an endotracheal tube with the aid of a laryngoscope. When using the direct-vision method to perform a nasotracheal intubation, the perianesthesia nurse may use Magill forceps (Fig. 27-9). A description of the nasal intubation technique can be found in many anesthesia textbooks.

Intubation has many advantages. It provides a route for mechanical ventilation, reduces the amount of anatomic dead space, and protects the patient from aspiration of blood, mucus, or foreign material into the tracheobronchial tree. It also relieves upper airway obstruction and provides an access route for removing excess secretions in the airways.

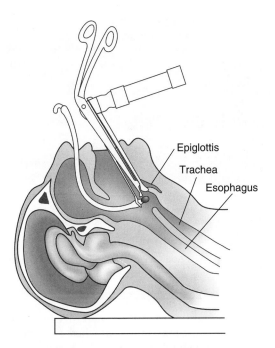

Fig. 27-9 Use of Magill forceps for nasal intubation. *(From Collins VJ: Principles of anesthesiology, ed 2, Philadelphia, 1976, Lea & Febiger.)*

Epiglottis

Trachea

Esophagus

The disadvantage of intubation is that it may produce trauma to the teeth, lips, soft palate, epiglottis, vocal cords, and other tissues in that region.

Perianesthesia Care of the Intubated Patient

Nursing care of the intubated patient involves (1) frequent auscultation of the chest for bilateral breath sounds to ensure correct placement of the endotracheal tube; (2) frequent suctioning of the oral cavity and, if clinically required, suctioning down inside the endotracheal tube to remove secretions; and (3) maintenance of verbal communication with the intubated patient to reduce anxiety. The perianesthesia nurse must reassure the patient that the attendants are constantly observing him or her. In addition, the nurse should provide the patient with a means of communication. Warning: when suctioning down an endotracheal tube, always administer at least five maximal ventilations of 100% oxygen before performing the suctioning procedure.

Extubation of the Intubated Patient

When it is determined that the patient can be extubated, the perianesthesia nurse should first ensure that all intubation, suction, and ventilation equipment is at the patient's bedside and is operational. Then the entire procedure should be explained to the patient. Depending on the amount and location of secretions, the trachea, the nasopharynx, or both, should be suctioned. All secretions must be aspirated from the upper airway to reduce the incidence of coughing and laryngospasm. Next, the patient should be ventilated with 100% oxygen for about 2 minutes. A syringe is then placed into the side valve, and the tracheal tube cuff is deflated. The patient should be asked to take a deep breath, and at the end of the inspiration, the tube should be gently removed. If the patient is completely awake and responding, the oral airway should also be removed. Then 100% oxygen should be administered by mask and the patient assessed for dyspnea, stridor, and airway obstruction. Oxygenation should be assessed continually by the pulse oximeter.

Adverse Sequelae After Tracheal Intubation

Hoarseness and Sore Throat. On emergence from anesthesia, some patients who have been intubated intraoperatively will complain of a very sore throat. Although the incidence of a sore throat after intubation is low, it is a significant discomfort to the patient. The incidence of sore throat increases dramatically when the patient's head is turned frequently or is placed intraoperatively in an abnormal position.

Assessment of the patient who complains of sore throat should include visual assessment of the oropharynx and auscultation of the chest. Abnormal findings should be reported to the anesthesiologist. Counseling the patient is probably the most important nursing intervention. The nurse should review the anesthesia record to determine whether the patient was intubated and whether the procedure was traumatic (such as multiple attempts and difficult intubation). Sore throats usually result from traumatic intubations.

Interventions consist of telling the patient that he or she had a tube in the throat during surgery to help with breathing and that throat discomfort may occur for 1 to 3 days. When the patient understands the reason for the discomfort and learns that it is not life-threatening, the discomfort often will become less severe. If treatment is required, dexamethasone (Decadron) may be given to reduce the inflammation; also, an ice bag or chips of ice may be given to the patient to relieve the symptoms.

Laryngospasm. Partial or complete closure of the vocal cords can occur because of increased secretions or as a reflex caused by stimulation of the irritant receptors. Assessment reveals reduced or no breath sounds. If partial laryngospasm is present, the patient will make crowing sounds, especially on inspiration. Interventions include the administration of 100% oxygen under positive pressure with a bag-valve-mask unit, and if the patient cannot be ventilated, intravenous administration of succinylcholine and reintubation are mandated (see Chapter 21).

Aspiration of Gastrointestinal Contents. Aspiration of gastrointestinal contents is a complication that may be seen in weak and debilitated patients and in those with neurologic disease or intestinal obstruction. See Chapter 14 for a complete discussion of this syndrome.

Laryngeal Mask Airway (LMA). The laryngeal mask airway was developed in the 1980's by a British anesthesiologist, Dr. Archie Brain. The product first became available in the United States in 1992. Over the last 10 years, modifications have been made to the design of the original LMA, known as the LMA-Classic, that have resulted in numerous LMA products that are useful for a variety of patient airway needs.

LMA-Classic. The LMA-Classic was designed to provide an alternative method of airway management that was intermediate in intensity between the facemask and the endotracheal tube (ETT) (Fig. 27-10). The reusable, latex-free device consists of three basic components. The first component is the soft, inflatable cuff that, when inserted correctly, conforms to the hypopharynx with its opening facing the patient's laryngeal opening. At the proximal end on the inside of the cuff is a set of aperture bars located at the junction of the cuff and airway tube that allows passage of air into the cuff yet prevents airway anatomy, such as the epiglottis, from entering the tube and blocking the airway passage. The cuff is connected to the second component, an airway tube, which is a large-bore tube with a 15 mm standard connector on the end.

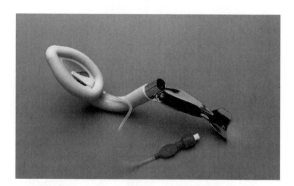

Fig. 27-10 LMA Classic™. *(Used with permission of The Laryngeal Mask Company Limited, United Kingdom.)*

The tube acts as a gas conduit for ventilation, and if needed, an endotracheal tube can be passed through the LMA into the vocal cords for intubation. The size of the ETT passed through the LMA depends on the size of the LMA inserted. Lastly, an inflation line is attached to a pilot balloon that permits inflation and deflation of the LMA cuff.

The LMA-Classic is used for a variety of patient circumstances during general anesthesia and is commonly used for patients who will be spontaneously breathing during the anesthetic. The LMA is often well-tolerated in the lightly anesthetized, semi-conscious patient. The LMA is available in eight sizes and can be used in patients ranging in size from neonates to over 100 kg. More importantly, the LMA has been used routinely in managing difficult and emergent airway situations. The device has proven successful in providing a bridge or temporary airway in patients in whom a permanent airway has not been obtained. Recently, the LMA has been included in two nationally recognized association protocols—the ASA Difficult Airway Algorithm and the American Heart Association Guidelines for 2000 for Cardiopulmonary Resuscitation and Emergency Cardiovascular Care for Advanced Cardiac Life Support (ACLS).

Insertion of the LMA is simple, and most providers find the learning curve to be gentle. After the cuff is deflated so that it is flat and free of wrinkles, the anterior portion of the cuff is lubricated with a water-soluble product. The patient is then placed in the preferred position—the sniffing position—although a neutral position can be used in patients with actual or suspected cervical spine injury. The provider places his or her dominant index finger at the junction between the cuff and the airway tube while ensuring the solid black line on the tube faces the patient's upper lip. The cuff is placed against the patient's hard palate, and it is moved back and forth against the palate to effectively lubricate the airway and prevent the cuff from folding over on insertion. Without forcing, the LMA is advanced as far down into the pharynx as possible. The nondominant hand holds the tube, and the dominant finger is withdrawn from the LMA device. Without the nurse holding onto the device, the LMA is now inflated following the maximum cuff inflation volume recommended in the product literature. Correct placement of the LMA may be observed during inflation; a slight and upward movement of the LMA in the airway as well as notable swelling in the neck may occur after cuff inflation. It may be necessary to insert an oral airway next to the LMA tube to prevent occlusion of the airway tube as patients regain consciousness. Auscultating bilateral breath sounds as well as checking for the presence of end-tidal carbon dioxide confirms placement of the LMA device.

Additional LMA products are available for management of the patient's airway. The LMA-Unique is the disposable version of the LMA-Classic. This product is often found in pre-hospital settings and in code carts and other airway management carts. The LMA-Flexible is a wire-reinforced device used primarily in patients who undergo procedures that involve the head or neck area. The flexible airway tube permits the airway product to be positioned away from the surgical field while an adequate seal is maintained. The LMA-Fastrach is designed to facilitate tracheal intubation (Fig. 27-11). The reusable device differs from the classic LMA design primarily in its rigid, anatomically curved airway tube that is connected to a metal handle. The handle is used to facilitate one-handed insertion and removal as well as to adjust the LMA cuffs position and the glottis alignment placement of the ETT. The aperture bars of the classic LMA have been replaced in the Fastrach by an epiglottic elevating bar. The elevating bar is designed to lift the epiglottis as the ETT passes through the LMA device, which may decrease

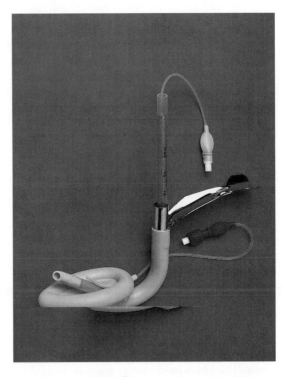

Fig. 27-11 LMA Fastrach™. *(Used with permission of The Laryngeal Mask Company Limited, United Kingdom.)*

the risk of arytenoids trauma or esophageal placement. The newest LMA product, introduced in 2000, is the LMA-ProSeal.

The LMA ProSeal is designed specifically to separate the alimentary and respiratory tracts while improving the laryngeal seal. The newly improved seal offers higher airway seal pressure during positive pressure ventilation and may be used in either the spontaneously breathing patient or the paralyzed patient. A built-in bite block provides protection from occlusion by the patient, and a removable introducer allows insertion of the product without the need to place fingers directly in the patient's mouth. Another unique feature of this product is the ability to blindly pass a gastric tube through the device, thus allowing for stomach decompression and drainage.

The following are guidelines for the perianesthesia nurse for care of patients in the PACU who presently have or had an LMA inserted for anesthesia. If an LMA is present in the PACU patient, a few important points should be remembered. The LMA is designed to be removed in either an awake patient or deeply anesthetized patient. Awake removal of the LMA is the most common and preferred technique, especially in the adult patients. Most patients are able to open their mouths on command for removal of the LMA. Because cuff deflation before the return of effective swallowing and coughing reflexes may allow secretions in the upper airway to enter the larynx and cause laryngospasm, do not deflate the LMA cuff until the LMA is being removed. Also, it is important to not remove the bite block or oral airway before removing the LMA device; this consideration prevents the patient from occluding his or her airway by biting down on the LMA tube. For patients who still have an LMA present in the PACU, no need to manually support the airway exists. In fact, lifting the jaw may actually displace the LMA cuff and cause laryngospasm or malposition.

Although LMA products may differ regarding indications for use in patient airway management, important similarities for product usage exist. The LMA products are contraindicated in patients at risk for aspiration and regurgitation because the devices do not protect the airway from gastric secretions.

LMA products are also contraindicated in patients with upper airway pathology or obstruction. LMA devices are advantageous for use in patients who are professional speakers who require a general anesthetic. Because LMA devices do not come in contact with the vocal cords, voice changes caused by vocal cord trauma are less likely. The devices are especially useful in patients who have a difficult mask airway because of distorted facial anatomy or presence of a beard. LMA products have gained access in many areas of health care and the ease of insertion combined with the variety of different products to choose from has allowed healthcare professionals to provide a greater degree of airway management and safety for their patients.

BIBLIOGRAPHY

Alspach J: Core curriculum for critical care nursing, ed 5, Philadelphia, 1998, WB Saunders.

Atlee J: Complications in anesthesia, Philadelphia, 1999, WB Saunders.

Austin R: Respiratory problems in emergence from anesthesia, Int Anesthesiol Clin 29(2):25-36, 1991.

Barash P, Cullen B, Stoelting R: Clinical anesthesia, ed 4, Philadelphia, 2000, Lippincott Williams & Wilkins.

Benumof J: Anesthesia and uncommon diseases, ed 4, Philadelphia, 1998, WB Saunders.

Benumof J, Saidman L: Anesthesia & perioperative complications, ed 2, St Louis, 1999, Mosby.

Bickley L, Hoekelman R: Bates' guide to physical examination and history taking, ed 7, Philadelphia, 1998, Lippincott Williams & Wilkins.

Bowdle T, Horita A, Kharasch E: The pharmacologic basis of anesthesiology, New York, 1994, Churchill Livingstone.

Brimacombe JR, Brain AIJ: The Laryngeal mask airway: a review and practical guide, London, 1997, WB Saunders.

Butterworth J: Atlas of procedures in anesthesia and critical care, Philadelphia, 1992, WB Saunders.

Class P: Nursing considerations for airway management in the PACU, Curr Rev Post Anesth Care Nurses 14(1):3-7, 1992.

Coté C, Todres I, Goudsouzian N, Ryan J: A practice of anesthesia for infants and children, ed 3, Philadelphia, 2001, WB Saunders.

DeFazio-Quinn D: Ambulatory surgical nursing core curriculum, Philadelphia, 1999, WB Saunders.

Ganong W: Review of medical physiology, ed 20, New York, 2001, McGraw-Hill Professional.

Guyton A, Hall J: Textbook of medical physiology, ed 10, Philadelphia, 2000, WB Saunders.

Hardman J, Limbird L: Goodman and Gilman's the pharmacological basis of therapeutics, ed 10, New York, 2001, McGraw-Hill.

Jacobsen W: Manual of post anesthesia care, Philadelphia, 1992, WB Saunders.

King T, Adams A: Failed tracheal intubation, Br J Anaesth 65:400-414, 1990.

Lake C, Hines R, Blitt C: Clinical monitoring: practical applications for anesthesia and critical care, St Louis, 2001, Mosby.

Longnecker D, Murphy F: Dripps/Eckenhoff/Vandam introduction to anesthesia, ed 9, Philadelphia, 1997, WB Saunders.

Longnecker D, Tinker J, Morgan G: Principles and practice of anesthesiology, ed 2, St Louis, 1998, Mosby.

Martin J: Positioning in anesthesia and surgery, ed 3, St Louis, 1997, Mosby.

McIntosh L: Essentials of nurse anesthesia, New York, 1997, McGraw-Hill.

Miller R, editor: Anesthesia, ed 5, New York, 2000, Churchill Livingstone.

Motoyama E: Smith's anesthesia for infants and children, ed 6, St Louis, 1996, Mosby.

Nagelhout J, Zaglaniczny K: Nurse anesthesia, ed 2, Philadelphia, 2001, WB Saunders.

Pesola G, Kvetan V: Ventilatory and pulmonary problem management, Anesthesiol Clin North Am 8(2):287-309, 1990.

Stoelting R: Pharmacology and physiology in anesthetic practice, ed 3, Philadelphia, 1999, Lippincott-Raven.

Stoelting R, Miller R: Basics of anesthesia, ed 4, New York, 2000, Churchill Livingstone.

Stone D: Perioperative care: anesthesia, medicine, and surgery, St Louis, 1998, Mosby.

Waugaman W, Foster S, Rigor B: Principles and practice of nurse anesthesia, ed 3, Norwalk, Conn, 1999, Appleton & Lange.

Weinberg G: Basic science review of anesthesiology, New York, 1997, McGraw-Hill.

Whitten C: Anyone can intubate, ed 2, San Diego, 1990, Medical Arts Publications.

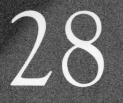

PAIN MANAGEMENT IN THE PACU

Philip Hughston Ewing, MD
Stephen P. Long, MD

Pain has evolved as a protective mechanism in response to tissue damage. It is defined as an unpleasant sensation and emotional experience that is associated with a damaging or noxious stimulus. Although pin pricks, paper cuts, and sore muscles are consequences of our everyday activities, neither the clinician nor the patient should view pain as an acceptable consequence of an operative procedure. Pain has no value in this setting, and the undertreatment of pain results in negative physiologic, psychologic, and economic effects. Inadequate management of pain increasingly has become a legal issue as patients have sought legal advice after poor treatment of pain in the hospital setting.

As its science and practice mature, the responsibility for pain management in surgical patients will be shared among all of caregivers from admission to follow-up after discharge. However, the role of PACU personnel will not diminish with this team-oriented approach because effective interventions begin from the moment the patient arrives from the operating room. Despite these advances the overall challenge of pain management remains unchanged—to provide analgesia in the narrow window between the undesirable states of pain and sedation. Optimal pain control permits breathing exercises with the incentive spirometer, coughing, repositioning, and earlier mobilization to decrease the occurrence of deep vein thrombosis and pulmonary embolus. These activities allow earlier discharge and more rapid recovery.

UNDERSTANDING PAIN:
A BASIC FUND OF KNOWLEDGE

The perianesthesia nurse has a solid understanding of anesthesia, the stress response, the inflammatory response, and hemodynamics. To effectively treat pain, the PACU staff also needs a working knowledge of pain management to augment their knowledge of postoperative patients. This introduction includes the physiology of pain, analgesic pharmacology and delivery (including common side effects and adverse effects), and noninvasive interventions. Obviously, the PACU staff should also have hands-on knowledge about the use and troubleshooting of IV PCA and epidural catheter pumps.

The modern model of pain identifies the four requirements for the production of pain: transduction, transmission, modulation, and perception. Transduction occurs when mediators such as substance P, serotonin, histamine, and bradykinin are released at the site of tissue injury. These mediators stimulate peripheral sensory afferent nerves that extend to the dorsal horn of the spinal cord. Transmission of this stimulus occurs when ascending nerves running from the dorsal horn to the brain are stimulated by the peripheral sensory afferents. Descending pathways to the dorsal horn modulate the activity of the peripheral nerves by the release of enkephalins and endorphins. Perception of pain occurs in the brain and reflects the modulation of the transduction of the pain stimulus, which ranges from amplification to suppression.

Analgesic pharmacology encompasses a wide range of drug classes, each of which can be categorized by the four components of the pain experience as described above. Three drug classes in particular are the most important in the PACU setting: local anesthetics, antiinflammatories, and opioids. Both local anesthetics and antiinflammatories act at the site of tissue injury to prevent the transduction of pain to the spinal cord. Local anesthetics such as lidocaine stabilize cell membranes to prevent excitation of nerves that detect painful stimuli. Antiinflammatory drugs can reduce the effects of the inflammatory mediators produced by the arachidonic acid cascade at the site of injury. It is important to stress the importance of prostaglandins in this process; not only do they produce pain but also sensitize the nerves to other pain-producing substances. Nonsteroidal antiinflammatory drugs (NSAIDs) have recently become increasingly important in the operative setting with the introduction of ketorolac tromethamine, the first NSAID to be indicated for parenteral use. Newer COX-2 NSAIDs—both orally administered and parenterally delivered—are even more significantly affecting the attenuation of the pain experience.

Opioids are the gold standard of the various postoperative analgesics; this drug class acts primarily at the level of the spinal cord where they influence both transmission and modulation at the level of the mu receptor.

Various delivery mechanisms are available for opioid analgesia. Intramuscular (IM) delivery traditionally was dominant; however, not only is that modality painful in and of itself, it also produces erratic analgesic because of varied absorption. In the past, the use of IM meperidine was even considered the standard of care for pain relief. This practice has fallen out of favor for a number or reasons. IM administration of meperidine in particular has not only inconsistent pharmacodynamics but has a number of undesirable physiologic side effects as well. These side effects include the potential for the induction of seizures caused by the epileptogenic metabolite normeperidine and strong anticholinergic effects. Elderly patients in particular may suffer from the anticholinergic side effects of the drug, which can cause long-lasting sedation that is particularly problematic in the Alzheimer's patient. It is also important to note that the recommendation of meperidine (at the exclusion of other more desirable narcotics such as morphine or hydromorphone or fentanyl) for pancreatitis and cholecystectomy is based on data that have not been borne out in the clinical setting and currently probably has minimal validity.

Intravenous bolus administration of opioids is the best and most efficient delivery system in the PACU patient environment. It affords not only quicker onset of drug and desired analgesic effect but also more ability to control effects via proper dose selection and titration for effectively meeting a patient's unique pain control requirements during the ever-constant change in individual physiology throughout the postoperative period.

The epidural (EPI) and intrathecal (IT) delivery of analgesics in the early 1980s revolutionized the way in which postoperative patients recovered as well. Not only do EPI and IT provide preemptive analgesia, they also provide more consistent levels of analgesia with more stable and smaller amounts of drugs required and delivered. Of particular interest with this delivery modality is the ability for smaller amounts of narcotic to provide significantly longer duration of analgesia because of the placement of the narcotic analgesic in close proximity to the site of action—the mu receptor in the spinal cord.

Of course, with the development of long-acting oral preparations of opioids as well as the transdermal delivery systems of opioids, patients may be effectively transitioned from parenteral delivery, which is not normally compatible with home use, to more user-friendly systems easily adaptable to the home environment and outpatient system.

In terms of particular opioid agents, we rely primarily upon pure μ-agonists such as morphine as our first line for analgesia. The μ-agonists reduce the release of excitatory neurotransmitters by the primary afferent neuron at its synapse in the spinal cord. Patients may experience pruritis and sedation, as well as nausea and vomiting when taking morphine, but the most feared side effect of this drug class is respiratory depression. Postoperative patients who are emerging from anesthesia require careful monitoring while initially being treated with opioids, especially after the first dose, when some—although admittedly very few patients—might experience anaphylaxis (most commonly confused with histamine release) or rapid respiratory decompensation. Hydromorphone is somewhat less sedating than morphine and significantly decreases the release of itch-producing histamine. Therefore patients who experience pruritis after receiving morphine are often switched to an equianalgesic dose of hydromorphone. Furthermore, hydromorphone may cause less nausea and vomiting while providing a more intense analgesic experience. One must remember that hydromorphone is 5 to 8 times more potent than morphine, so the dose must be adjusted accordingly. For instance, the patient who receives 1 mg of morphine would require only 0.2 mg of hydromorphone, the equianalgesic dose.

Other commonly used opioids include fentanyl and its derivatives. The synthetic drug fentanyl is a highly lipophilic drug that can be used in the operating room, the PACU, and the inpatient setting and for chronic pain treatment. In the operative and PACU settings, this drug is used to balance analgesia with the sedating effects of anesthetic agents. It is important to note that fentanyl and its cousins are both more potent and shorter-acting than the historic comparator, morphine; therefore effective analgesic doses in the operating room may wear off rapidly in the PACU, thus necessitating more frequent and earlier titration in the PACU patient. Fentanyl—like morphine and hydromorphone—is a particularly effective choice of analgesic for IV or EPI administration.

A few side effects are common to the opioids. Respiratory depression was mentioned previously; however, its danger cannot be understated because it is not an idiosyncratic or uncommon reaction. Respiratory depression can occur in all patients if a large enough opioid dose is given or if the medication is given too quickly or too frequently. Caution should be exercised in the patients suffering from hepatic and renal failure caused by potential drug accumulation secondary to inadequate clearance or metabolism. It must be noted that although opiates may not be solely responsible for postoperative ileus—particularly in patients undergoing abdominal surgery (length of surgery and amount of bowel physically handled predispose to ileus even more)—they share the common and universal effect of constipation. Although this is not the primary responsibility of the PACU nurse, it is worth recognizing that the thorough caregiver ensures that the patient receives, at the time of discharge, a stool softener or promotility agent to prevent stool impaction and uncomfortable and problem-

atic constipation. This is an important step in discharge planning and instruction.

A number of other medications can augment the pain relief provided by narcotics and NSAIDs. These adjunctive medications include anxiolytics and sedative/hypnotics like the barbiturates and benzodiazepines, muscle relaxers, tricyclic antidepressants, and cell membrane stabilizers also used to treat seizure disorders. Other adjuncts may be used to treat the side effects of pain medications, including antihistamines, antiemetics (Zofran, promethazine, compazine), stool softeners, and promotility agents. Another important class of drugs is the antagonists. Intravenous naloxone can be used to rapidly reverse the mental sedation and respiratory depression caused by narcotics, although it may cause precipitous opioid withdrawal if not carefully and diligently titrated in all but cases of respiratory arrest. Naloxone should be readily available in the PACU and on all patient medication carts on the floor when opioid agonists are being administered. Flumazenil is the benzodiazepine antagonist that is used to reverse sedation due to overreaction to benzodiazepines. It too may be used in a case with profound respiratory depression. It should be noted that rapid administration of flumazenil has been shown to precipitate seizures. Therefore careful dose adjustments and titration must be ensured.

As noted, analgesia may be provided in a number of different routes—including oral, intravenous, transdermal, and via the epidural or spinal injection. Intramuscular injections are avoided for the pharmacologic reasons mentioned previously but also because the injections can cause patient discomfort. Oral analgesia is typically avoided after major surgeries in which general analgesia is used and a postoperative ileus is expected. However, oral analgesia may be appropriate in ambulatory settings.

Injectable analgesics are often preferred in the postoperative patient for the reasons already mentioned. Intramuscular injection is an ineffective approach caused by complicated pharmacodynamic factors. The delivery and absorption is inconsistent among patients; therefore peak concentration and analgesic effect are not predictable. An added problem is the discomfort associated with this method of delivery. Intravenous access allows the provider to give rapid relief of pain and offers the patient the ability to titrate individually the need for pain medication when patient-controlled analgesia (PCA) pumps are available. IV PCA has become the standard of care after inpatient operative procedures.

Currently, transdermal fentanyl is the only transdermal system available for widespread analgesic use. Fentanyl patches have the advantage of easy dosing with one patch lasting for up to three days; unfortunately, the system takes a full 12 hours to reach full analgesic effect. Similarly, the pharmacologic effects of the patches remain for up to 12 hours after removal. Therefore patients who suffer from respiratory depression may require repeated doses of opiate antagonists as the drug, which is readily absorbed by fat, becomes available for systemic absorption. Although clinical studies that examine the efficacy of these transdermal delivery systems are limited, their general use in postoperative pain management is quite limited and requires cautious planning.

Patients who have been using opioids for chronic/cancer pain, however, will require significantly more analgesia than other, opioid-naïve patients. Likewise, the side effects profile of opioids in these patients will be lessened acutely. It is not uncommon for patients who have developed a tolerance to opioids to require 20% to 30% more medication than a patient who is opioid-naïve.

Epidural opioids represent a nearly direct delivery system of analgesics to the substantia gelatinosa in the dorsal horn. This specific area of delivery provides the optimal ratio of analgesic effect to safety of delivery. Opioids and/or local anesthetics are generally administered via a catheter placed either at the beginning of the surgery or at the conclusion, before emergence from general anesthesia. Normally, the epidural catheter is used as an anesthetic adjunct during the surgical procedure and is continued post-operatively as the primary method of analgesic delivery. Combining a very dilute concentration of local anesthetic agent with opioid agent results in sensory blockade without major motor blockade. This combination technique optimizes the basic physiologic principles discussed earlier by covering all of the pain sites and blocking them. Because combination therapy is used, better anal-

gesia with fewer side effects occurs, primarily because the amount of any one single agent that would normally be used is lessened.

Sometimes, the anesthetist chooses to deliver "single-shot" analgesics via the epidural catheter, and the catheter is either removed or intermittently bolused. Although more effective than IV or IM bolus, this technique is not as effective at maintaining consistent levels of analgesia as continuous delivery or epidural PCA. In best-case scenarios—with morphine as the agent for single delivery—analgesia lasts about 12 hours in the epidural space. Because delivery via the intrathecal (spinal) space deposits the medication even closer to the mu receptors within the dorsal horn of the spinal cord, analgesia with morphine administered this way may last up to 24 hours. One must remember that the side effects of spinally administered opioids in comparison to epidural opioids may be more intense and severe—especially pruritis, nausea, urinary retention, and respiratory depression. In both cases of EPI and IT delivery, one must be extraordinarily judicious in providing supplemental opioid analgesia for breakthrough pain via the oral or IV route because dangerous side effects can occur. Hence vigilant monitoring is a requirement in these circumstances. Still, the benefits of superb analgesia with the concomitant reduction in both morbidity and mortality far outweigh the reported but infrequent risks.

The optimal combination of EPI medications for postoperative pain management is a mixture of dilute local anesthetic agent (blocking the sensory/sympathetic, A-delta, and C-polymodal fibers) with low concentration of opioid. Using epidurally administered opioids, one is able to reduce tenfold the amount of agent that would normally be administered via IV or IM routes. Thus when a patient may require 100 mg of morphine IV in a 24 hour period, that same patient would normally require only 10 mg of epidurally administered morphine. Adding a local anesthetic such as 0.0625% bupivacaine may reduce the opioid amount even more.

Two drugs are historically most often used for epidural delivery and the choice of drug depends upon the type of analgesia required. Morphine, the first and most commonly used opioid in the epidural space, is less lipophilic than fentanyl and thus spreads easily in the epidural space and provides for more diffuse spinal mediated analgesia. Morphine may be delivered in the lumbar space and provide analgesia to surgical dermatomes far from the injection site. On the other hand, lipophilic fentanyl has a limited distribution and offers a more local analgesic effect in a classically dermatomal distribution. Intrathecal dosing allows even more direct delivery of the opioid to the site of action in the spinal cord. Intrathecal doses of morphine and fentanyl are reduced by a factor of ten compared to epidurally administered opioids because the drugs do not need to cross the dura to reach their target. Some authors support the use of hydromorphone for epidural and intrathecal analgesia; however, at this point, this is an off-label indication. However, because it has properties somewhere between the very hydrophilic morphine and very lipophilic fentanyl, it may provide better analgesia with less rostral spread and CNS depression (associated with morphine) or with less systemic update (associated with fentanyl).

Epidural patient-controlled analgesia is a newer and more commonly applied delivery modality used for patients undergoing major extremity, abdominal, vascular, or thoracic surgery. Using the same principles as IV PCA (less nursing time, less total drug required, patient sense of control, fewer side effects) but with even more profound analgesia and even fewer side effects (in comparative studies of EPI PCA versus IV PCA), EPI PCA has gained significant popularity and acceptance across the country. In the last 10 years an abundance of "acute pain services" have stressed the "team concept" of physician, nurse, pharmacist, and others to more optimally manage patients with state-of-the-art analgesia delivery systems. The primary instrument of analgesia delivery for these services has been epidurally administered analgesics.

Nonpharmacologic adjuncts—including psychologic approaches and transcutaneous electric nerve stimulation (TENS)—are often overlooked. The psychologic approaches change the way in which the patients perceive pain and allow some central modulation with endogenous opioids such as endorphins and enkephalins. Psychologic approaches include but are not limited to biofeedback, meditation, visualization, and hypnosis. TENS is an underused technique in which

pads that allow gentle electrical stimulation are placed periincisionally. Studies have shown that TENS reduces postoperative pain by 25% to 30%. TENS is noninvasive and causes little, if any, discomfort for the patient. In addition, the use of splinting, ice therapy, and other historic techniques used by nursing specialists remain quite effective in reducing postoperative pain.

OPERATIVE PAIN MANAGEMENT: THE MODERN APPROACH

Appropriate and aggressive postoperative pain management is an ideal that has been supported by nurses for decades. Regrettably, physician providers and others (including insurers and hospital administrators) did not place equal emphasis on this matter until the federal government, through the United States Department of Health and Human Services (HHS), published the first clinical practice guidelines on this topic in the early 1990s. The Agency for Health Care Policy and Research published the guide geared to all healthcare providers who participate in the care of patients who undergo procedures or surgeries which produce pain. This literally revolutionized the ways in which patients were viewed during recovery.

Effective pain management begins before the first skin incision; in fact, the initial surgical assessment provides information that is vital to pain control. Note that the thoroughness of the preoperative assessment reflects the nature of the procedure to be performed; patients admitted for emergency procedures are likely to have a minimal evaluation before surgery. The preoperative interview includes an assessment of the patient's surgical needs, pain history, and history of analgesic use as well as the patient's cognitive approach to coping with pain. The interview also offers an opportunity to introduce the patient to the staff and educate the patient about the procedure. This is the perfect time for the patient to learn about pain control options in the context of other postoperative interventions such as splinting and incentive spirometry. These interventions are best taught before surgery, when the patient can provide full attention and is not suffering the effects of postanesthesia sedation. It is the ideal time to discuss the role of the PCA pump—or "pain button"—which some patients find to be confusing. This discussion also gives the patient the assurance that his or her pain will be controlled. The patient should also have a basic physical exam during the interview that consists of vital signs, examination of posture and positioning, assessment of affect, and evaluation of the patient's level of activity.

Cues for which to look during the preoperative interview are previous or current use of narcotics, coping mechanisms, or anxious personality traits. A patient who has used high doses of narcotics, either legal or illegal, may have developed tolerance to opioids. These patients will require larger doses of analgesics that cover the "maintenance" dose required to prevent withdrawal as well as additional analgesic to provide pain relief. Coping mechanisms may also be evident during the preoperative assessment. Just as patient may prepare for surgery by donating blood for autologous transfusion, patients may prepare themselves by learning relaxation techniques. This approach certainly is not universal but it emphasizes the fact that pain is a physical and psychological experience. Anxious patients may make this point resoundingly clear. These patients may have a recovery period that is complicated by pain; careful, detailed explanation of the surgery and the postoperative period should help most patients.

Intraoperative management is critical to the patient's experience of pain. Both inhalation and intravenous anesthetics provide poor analgesia; therefore narcotic analgesics are administered to balance the anesthetic effect. Anesthesia alone allows transmission and transduction to occur in the absence of perception and, perhaps, modulation. Opioids are administered to decrease transmission and down-regulate the activity of ascending and descending neurons. Local anesthetics dampen the transduction of pain signals that are produced at the site of the incision. It is also important to note that perioperative NSAIDs have been used for their antiinflammatory and analgesic properties. Furthermore, the inflammatory response to surgical intervention allows inflammatory mediators to be released long after the procedure is completed. The new COX-2 NSAIDs may prove to be particularly efficacious in decreasing pain and decreasing opioid use but not predisposing to bleeding problems.

For multiple reasons, the immediate postoperative setting is perhaps the most difficult and challenging arena in which to manage pain. The PACU nurse faces many challenges and must address the components of the stress response after an invasive procedure, psychological duress associated with emergence from anesthesia, other bothersome concomitants of surgery (catheters, restraints, etc.), and the other effects of anesthesia. The PACU should be prepared to be a soothing place for the patient to recover; every attempt should be made to minimize unpleasant environmental stimuli—such as bright lights, loud noises, or extremes of temperature. To optimize pain control in the PACU—and after transfer to the floor—it is essential that the verbal report to the PACU nurse include information about the type of anesthesia and about any analgesics that were used. As mentioned before, analgesia with fentanyl may wear off rapidly because of its short half-life. On the other hand, regional analgesia may persist until the patient has left the PACU to go to the floor. It is also critical to determine what type of incision was used for the surgery. Incisions of the upper abdomen, chest, back, anorectal region, joints, and vertical abdominal incisions are noted to be the most painful.

Objective assessment begins as soon as the patient hits the PACU because the patient has monitoring systems in place to record blood pressure, heart rate, urinary output, etc. Nevertheless, it is equally important to collect subjective data from the patients as their level of sedation permits. Sedated patients may not be able to verbalize their feelings very well; also, stoic patients may not complain in spite of intense pain and suffering. The basic questions focus on the onset of pain and its location, intensity, quality, timing, and modifying factors. The onset of pain may reflect the decreasing effect of analgesia and anesthesia. However, a new onset of pain in the PACU should alert the nurse to patient positioning problems; pathologic pain caused by myocardial infarction, pulmonary embolus, and so on should be considered. Such issues are often clarified by asking the patient to identify the location of their pain.

Much work has been done to develop a system to quantify the intensity of pain. Numerous pain scales are available including the verbal rating scale, the visual analog scale, and the descriptive pain intensity scale. Providers may find their favorite among this group but also may use one scale for certain subsets of patients. An available illustrated version is appropriate for use in children and others that may have difficulty expressing their pain in words. With a pain scale, it is often helpful to ask the patient to identify their worst imaginable pain (Fig. 28-1). This helps serve as an anchor for the scale that can be used to understand the context of the patient's pain and to evaluate the success of any interventions.

The quality of the pain can help identify its source. Pain from superficial structures is often described as pricking or burning; deeper sources cause aching, throbbing, or radiating pain. Sometimes one can infer that pain is intense when the patient uses the words "gnawing" or "tiring." Similarly, the timing of pain is related to its source. Both the timing and the modifying factors of pain (such as position and activity) can help reveal the source of the pain.

The perianesthesia nursing assessment should then focus on examining the patient. This exam should begin with assessment of the vital signs. Common sources of pain in the postoperative patient are the incision, pressure points, and IV access sites or surgical drains. The initial exam

should focus on these problem areas to reduce or prevent their impact on the patient's pain experience. Other problems such as dry mouth and a distended bladder can cause discomfort. The exam may reveal physical findings that suggest that the patient is in pain. Physiologic changes related to sympathetic activation include hypertension, tachycardia, tachypnea, pallor, dilated pupils, and increased muscle tension; nausea, vomiting, bradycardia and hypotension are parasympathetically mediated changes caused by pain in the hollow organs. Cold perspiration and restlessness are also common. Van Poznak (see bibliography at end of chapter) suggests that irregular respiratory patterns that lack an expiratory pause are a good indicator of pain. He recommends using these patterns to titrate analgesics with a method that is described. Behavioral changes may also contribute to the assessment of pain; a patient may display excitement, irritability, depression, unusual quietness, withdrawal, and behavioral reverses. One must exercise caution when identifying pain as the source of these changes; some patients display these changes when anxious. Drain and Cain

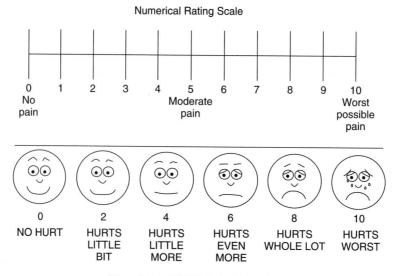

Fig. 28-1 Pain Rating Scales. The Numerical Rating Scale or visual analog scale is useful for evaluating adults' pain status, and the Wong-Baker FACES Pain Rating Scale is useful in rating pain in the pediatric population. *(From Wong DL: Wong's Nursing care of infants and children, ed 7, St Louis, 2003, Mosby.)*

recommend differentiating between state and trait anxiety. They define state anxiety as that which is related to the fright, uncertainty, and helplessness that patients experience as a result of their admission for surgery. On the other hand, trait anxiety describes the feelings that a patient has without the stress of surgery.

Withdrawal syndromes are an important aspect of perianesthesia nursing assessment that often goes unrecognized. Identifying these syndromes can help clarify the clinical picture and prevent potentially life-threatening complications such as delirium tremens. The opiate withdrawal syndrome includes anxiety, jittery behavior, rhinorrhea, hypotension, muscle twitching, sweating, pupillary dilation, gooseflesh, nausea, and vomiting. Obviously, this syndrome shares many symptoms with others that may indicate postoperative pain; rhinorrhea and gooseflesh may be subtle indicators that the patient is not merely in pain. The alcohol withdrawal syndrome includes headaches, malaise, and irritability that can progress to seizures, autonomic instability, and delirium with auditory and tactile hallucinations. The generalized seizures that accompany frank delirium tremens may be lethal.

After the nursing assessment of the patient, analgesics should be administered if the patient is in pain. Outdated guidelines historically suggested that patients at the extremes of age should be given less pain medications because supposedly they tolerated more pain. However, recent studies conclusively show that pediatric and geriatric populations do not have higher tolerances to pain and that these patients should receive adequate analgesia similar to any other age group. In fact, inadequate analgesia in the elderly patient may predispose to autonomic hyperactivity and associated comorbidity factors such as tachycardia, myocardial ischemia, myocardial infarction, cerebral ischemia, hypertension, and possible CVA. The pediatric population in particular should be dosed on a milligram per kilogram basis, but older patients, including teenagers, can be started on one of several textbook "standard dosages." Patients who have orders for IV PCA pumps often require a loading bolus, and attention should be paid to getting adequate analgesia via this modality before establishing the patient delivery component of the device—certainly before discharge from the PACU (Table 28-1). Under no circumstances should a patient who is capable of using a PCA device in the PACU have that device disconnected during transport from the PACU to the floor. This process may take long periods of time and cause the patient to go without analgesia during a prolonged transport time to the unit as well as during report to the accepting unit.

The patient should be monitored carefully after the first dose of a narcotic analgesic because of the risks of respiratory depression and anaphylaxis. If respiratory depression occurs, it will usually be seen within the first five to seven minutes of administration. After this time, the patient may be reassessed for the response to the medication. According to Van Poznak, continued assessment of the patient's respiratory status may allow the caregiver to titrate the analgesia to the appropriate dose. He notes that patients who are in pain have irregular respiratory patterns that have short or nonexistent pauses between breaths.

Patients who are admitted for ambulatory surgery are often discharged to home from the

Table 28-1	**Dosing for the Drugs Morphine and Hydromorphone**					
Drug	IV Dose	Pediatric Dose	PCA Bolus	PCA Dose	PCA Basal	PCA Limit
Morphine	10 mg q4h	0.1-0.2 mg/kg q2-4h	PRN	0.5-2 ml	0-0.5 ml	≤20 ml
Hydromorphone	1-4 mg q4-6h	0.01-0.02 mg/kg q4h	PRN	0.2-1.0 ml	0 ml	≤6 ml

Adapted from Ballantyne J, Fishman SM, Abdi S: The Massachusetts general hospital handbook of pain management, ed 2, Philadelphia, 2002, Lippincott Williams & Wilkins.

Box 28-1 ASPAN Position Statement on Pain Management

ASPAN has the responsibility for defining the practice of perianesthesia nursing. An integral part of this responsibility involves identifying the educational requirements and competencies essential to perianesthesia nursing practice and the educational needs of the patients and family regarding pain assessment and management.

ASPAN sets forth this position statement to promote the optimal level of practice and to present a consistent standard of care that documents sound clinical judgment in the management of postoperative pain.

BACKGROUND

ASPAN has defined a standard for pain management (Standard XI) with the intent of providing guidelines, which represent what is believed to be an optimal level of practice. To assist members in achieving this standard, ASPAN published pain management competency material in the Competency Based Orientation and Credentialing Program. In response to continued concerns from perianesthesia nurses, ASPAN's Standards and Guidelines Committee conducted a review of literature to identify current issues related to pain assessment and management. The following issues were identified:

1. As many as 50% of postoperative patients in both hospitals and outpatient surgical centers are undermedicated and suffer unrelieved pain.[1-4]
2. The practice of undermedicating for pain occurs regardless of the patient's age.[5,6]
3. Frequently the patient's self-report of pain is not taken into consideration when choosing the dosage of medication to give for pain relief.[7,8]
4. Inadequate pain management affects postoperative recovery and behaviors associated with that recovery.[5,6,9]
5. A prevalent cause of ineffective pain management is the professional's lack of knowledge related to pain physiology, medications, and protocols.[4,10]
6. There is still an overriding concern that the use of opioids in the treatment of acute postoperative pain control will contribute to psychological dependence.[11]

7. Patient and family education addressing postsurgical pain management remains inconsistent.[12]
8. Pain management should begin preoperatively with patient and family education addressing use of a pain scale as well as methods of postoperative pain control.
9. The Agency for Health Care Policy and Research (AHCPR) suggests that practitioners are too rigid when managing acute postoperative pain and should set goals to reduce its incidence and severity. Guidelines have been published by this agency for acute pain management.[13]

POSITION

It is therefore the position of ASPAN that a collaborative plan should be developed between the anesthesia department and the perianesthesia nurses to address pain management within the perianesthesia setting. The following points of action should be addressed:

1. The goal should be to relieve as much pain as possible to allow for activity, relaxation, prevention of complications, and promotion of optimal health and healing.
2. Areas of education in pain management for health care professionals should include the following:
   a. Physiology of pain management
   b. Assessment techniques
   c. Methods of intervention (pharmacological and nonpharmacological)
   d. Management of side effects and complications related to each intervention
   e. Evaluation of successful management
   f. Ethical considerations
   g. Age and cultural considerations
   h. Patient and family education issues
3. Whenever possible, the patient's plan of care for pain management should begin during the preoperative interview.
4. The patient's self-report of pain is the best measurement tool to use when assessing pain.
5. The use of reliable and valid pain scales should be a standard part of the pain assessment.
6. Measurement of outcomes should reflect timely, appropriate interventions and achievement of desired effects.

Continued

Box 28-1   ASPAN Position Statement on Pain Management—*cont'd*

EXPECTED OUTCOMES

Perianesthesia nurses need to familiarize themselves with this position statement and inform and educate peers, nurse managers, hospital administrators, and physicians.

Anesthesiologists and perianesthesia nurses need to collaborate in the development of a multidisciplinary plan of care (protocol, critical pathway, care map, etc.) to provide safe, appropriate, and effective pain management.

ASPAN, as the voice of perianesthesia nursing practice, must externalize this information by sharing this position statement with regulatory agencies and professional organizations that interface with perianesthesia nursing areas.

APPROVAL OF STATEMENT

This statement was recommended by a vote of the ASPAN Board of Directors on April 16, 1999 and approved by a vote of the ASPAN Representative Assembly on April 18, 1999 in Honolulu, Hawaii.

ANA: Code for nurses with interpretative statements, Washington, DC, 1995, American Nurses Association.

Anonymous: Surgical patient's no. 1 fear: pain, Today's Surgical Nurse 18:7, 1996.

ASPAN: Competency-Based Orientation and Credentialing Program, Cherry Hill, NJ, 1997, American Society of PeriAnesthesia Nurses.

Bishop A, Scudder J: Nursing ethics: therapeutic caring presence, Boston, 1996, Jones and Bartlett Publishers.

Heiser R, Chiles K, Fudge M et al: The use of music during the immediate postoperative recovery period, AORN J 65:777-778, 781-785, 1997.

Miaskowski C, Jacox A, Hester N et al: Interdisciplinary guidelines for the management of acute pain: Implications for quality improvement. Journal of Nursing Care Quality (Education of) 7:1-6, 1992.

Schwartz-Barcott C, Fortin J, Kim-Hesook S: Client-nurse interaction: testing for its impact in preoperative instruction, International Journal of Nursing Studies 31:23-35, 1994.

By the American Society of PeriAnesthesia Nurses, 10 Melrose Avenue, Suite 110, Cherry Hill, NJ 080037-3696; toll-free (877) 737-9696, fax: (856) 616-9601. E-mail: aspan@aspan.org. Copyright 1997-2001, American Society of PeriAnesthesia Nurses.

PACU with oral analgesics. Combinations of oxycodone, hydrocodone, or codeine and acetaminophen are very commonly used in this scenario. The combination of narcotic and NSAID has a synergistic effect that allows much better analgesia than with either drug on its own. It is imperative that the patient is informed about the risks of high levels of acetaminophen. Patients should be cautioned about taking more than four grams of the acetaminophen component per day, especially those who already have impaired liver function. Considerable research has focused on long-acting, sustained release opioid analgesics both as preoperative analgesics and for postoperative pain control. These agents allow some preemptive analgesia as well as continuous release of opioid in the recovery period. Likewise, the postoperative use of NSAIDs is now widely accepted as state-of-the-art analgesia due to the different site of action of these agents (both COX-1 and COX-2). They also act synergistically with opioids and local anesthetics to improve pain control and reduce the total amount of any one agent otherwise administered by itself. One must weigh the benefits with the possible risks of NSAID use in patients, particularly when bleeding or ulceration is anticipated.

SUMMARY

The role of the perianesthesia nurse has changed as the understanding of pain has improved. Aggressive interventions that are available today allow for optimal pain control and rapid recovery. The key to understanding these interventions lies in the physiologic basis for pain, analgesic pharmacology, and methods for delivery of analgesics. A working clinical and basic science knowledge of these topics is essential to the mastery of pain management in the postoperative setting.

Implementation of basic pain management principles coupled with newer state-of-the-art and standard-of-care techniques can reduce postoperative morbidity and mortality. In the practical sense, aggressive postoperative analgesia by a caring staff makes the hospital stay not only safer but more cost-effective and pleasant for all those involved. The most important person is, of course, the patient for whom we are entrusted to care. The current ASPAN position statement on Pain Management can be found in Box 28-1.

REFERENCES

1. Anonymous: Most patients face pain, often unrelieved, after surgery, Am J Nurs 96:68, 1996.
2. Campese C: Development and implementation of a pain management program, AORN J 64: 931-940, 1996.
3. Bormarm D, Hansen K: Improving pain management through staff education, Nursing Management 28:55-57, 1997.
4. Thornborough J: Developing a pain management protocol in the PACU, Today's Surgical Nurse 20:23-27, 1998.
5. Fortin J, Schwartz-Barcott D, Rossi S: The postoperative pain experience: a description based on the McGill Pain Questionnaire, Clinical Nursing Research 1:292-304, 1992.
6. Pasero C, McCaffrey M: Managing postoperative pain in the elderly, Am J Nurs 96:38-46, 1996.
7. Reid D, Evans M, Topiko J et al: Postoperative pain, Canadian Nurse 88:55, 1992.
8. Malek C, Olivieri R: Pain management: documenting the decision making process, Nursing Case Management 1:64-76, 1996.
9. Getker-Black S, Hart F, Hoffman J et al: Preoperative self-efficacy and postoperative behaviors, Applied Nursing Research 5:134-139, 1992.
10. Carr E: Overcoming barriers of effective pain control, Professional Nurse 12:412-416, 1997.
11. Aiher J, Coghlan A, Martin K et al: Children win with improved pain management, Canadian Nurse 88:19-21, 1992.
12. Jones S, Villalobos J: Incorporating clinical research findings into practice, Journal of Nursing Staff Development 12:46, 1996.

13. Agency For Health Care Policy and Research: Acute pain management in infants, children, and adolescents: operative and medical procedures, Rockville, Md, 1992, Department of Health and Human Services.

BIBLIOGRAPHY

Abram S: Preemptive analgesia, Seminars in Anesthesia 16(4):263-270, 1997.

Allen H: Difficult cases in postoperative pain management, Seminars in Anesthesia 16(4):271-279, 1997.

Atsberger DB, Shrewsbury P: Postoperative pain management: the PACU nurse's challenge, J Post Anesth Nurs 3(6):399-403, 1988.

Berry PH, Dahl JL: Making pain assessment and management a healthcare priority through the new JCAHO pain standard, Journal of Pharmaceutical Care in Pain and Symptom Control 8(2):5-20, 2000.

Drain CB, Cain RS: The nursing implications of postoperative pain, Military Medicine 146:127-130, 1981.

Edwards WT, Breed RJ: The treatment of acute postoperative pain in the postanesthesia care unit, Anesthesiology Clinics of North America 8(2): 235-265, 1990.

Long SP: The management of postoperative pain and the rationale for preemptive anesthesia, Journal of Back and Musculoskeletal Rehabilitation 9:279-297, 1997.

Sinatra RS, Levin S, Ocampo CA: Neuroaxial hydromorphone for control of postsurgical, obstetric, and chronic pain, Seminars in Anesthesia, Perioperative Medicine and Pain 19(2):108-131, 2000.

U.S. Department of Health and Human Services, Agency for Health Care Policy and Research, Clinical practice guideline for acute pain management: operative or medical procedures and trauma, AHCPR Publication Number 92-0032, Rockville, Md, 1992.

Van Poznak A: The role of respiratory patterns in the treatment of pain and anxiety, J Post Anesth Nurs 3(3):189-191, 1987.

Wetchler BV: Managing pain in the postanesthesia care unit, J Post Anesth Nurs 1(1):52-56, 1986.

CARE OF THE EAR, NOSE, THROAT, NECK, AND MAXILLOFACIAL SURGICAL PATIENT

DEFINITIONS

Ankyloglossia ("tongue tied"): a short lingual frenulum that may cause difficult suckling in the infant and subsequent speech impairment. It is treated surgically by clipping of the frenulum.

Cochlear implant: a prosthesis with internal electrode is surgically implanted into the cochlea so that an external microphone later can be applied to stimulate the eighth cranial nerve and provide sound for a deaf person.

Endoscopy: nasal surgery performed using direct vision with endoscopic equipment.

Ethmoidectomy: removal of ethmoid bone.

Fenestration: reconstruction of the outer and middle parts of the ear by means of a new drum or skin flap; creation of a new window into the internal ear mechanism with a newly established drum or skin flap.

Glossectomy: removal of the tongue.

Intranasal antrostomy (antral window): creation of an opening in the lateral wall of the nose under the middle turbinate and the removal of the anterior end of the inferior turbinate.

Labyrinthectomy: opening of the labyrinth to destroy the inner ear in an attempt to relieve medically uncontrollable symptoms of unilateral Meniere's syndrome.

Laryngectomy: removal of the larynx; total laryngectomy is the complete removal of the cartilaginous larynx, the hyoid bone, and the strap muscles connected to the larynx, and possible removal of the preepiglottic space along with the lesion.

Laryngofissure: opening of the larynx for exploratory, excisional, or reconstructive procedures.

Laryngoscopy: direct examination of the interior of the larynx with a laryngoscope.

Mastoidectomy: removal of mastoid air cells and of the tympanic membrane. Radical mastoidectomy also involves removing the malleus, incus, chorda tympani, and mucoperiosteal lining.

Myringotomy: incision of the tympanic membrane under direct vision and insertion of tubes to facilitate drainage.

Ossiculoplasty: reconstruction of the ossicular chain.

Paletouvuloplasty: the reconstruction of the posterior section of the palate and the uvula.

Radical antrostomy (Caldwell-Luc operation): use of an incision into the canine fossa of the upper jaw and exposure of the antrum for removal of bony, diseased portions of the antral wall and contents of the sinus; establishment of drainage by means of a counteropening into the nose through the inferior meatus to establish a large opening in the nasoantral wall of the inferior meatus, which will ensure adequate gravity drainage and aeration and will permit removal of all diseased tissue in the sinus under direct vision.

Stapedectomy: removal of the stapes, followed by the placement of a prosthesis.

Submucosal resection: removal of either cartilaginous or osseous portions of the septum that lie between the flaps of the mucous membrane and the perichondrium to establish an adequate partition between the left and right nasal cavities, thereby providing a clear airway for both the internal and external cavities and the parts of the nose.

Tonsillectomy and adenoidectomy (T&A): surgical removal of the tonsils and adenoids.

Tracheostomy: opening of the trachea and insertion of a cannula through a midline incision in the neck below the cricoid cartilage.

Tympanoplasty (myringoplasty): reconstruction of the tympanic membrane.

SURGERY ON THE EAR

Otologic surgery has been revolutionized by

433

antibiotics, the operating microscope, new and more delicate instruments, and an increased understanding of the anatomic structures involved (Figs. 29-1 and 29-2). New methods have been devised to treat hearing loss surgically by correcting conduction apparatus abnormalities, and selected patients can now be surgically relieved of the disabling symptoms of sensorineural hearing loss.

Most otologic procedures are now performed in the day surgery arena. The immediate postanesthesia care for patients who have undergone surgery on the ear is generally the same, regardless of the procedure. Immediate postoperative complications are rare. Occasionally, excessive bleeding may occur, especially if a large blood vessel has been entered during the operation. If bleeding has occurred, it should be reported to the postanesthesia care unit (PACU) nurse who will provide care for the patient upon admission. Immediate postanesthesia assessment should follow the same format as for any patient who is undergoing general anesthesia. In addition, postanesthesia assessment should include testing for function of the facial nerve. The patient should be instructed to frown, smile, wrinkle the forehead, close the eyes, bare the teeth, and pucker the lips. Inability to perform these actions indicates injury to the facial nerve and should be appropriately indicated in the patient's medical record and reported to the surgeon.

If surgery has been performed near the brain (inner ear), check for clear fluid in the ear or on the dressings that may indicate cerebrospinal fluid leakage. Aseptic technique for all dressings and protection from infection are especially important elements in the care of the patient who has undergone surgery on the ears, because infection can easily be transmitted to the meninges and the brain. The outer ear is highly vascular and susceptible to circulatory damage and excoriation. The outer ear may even become necrotic if circulation is impaired by excessive pressure from or malpositioning of a dressing. Assessment of the dressing should therefore include proper positioning.

Postanesthesia positioning of the patient who has undergone ear surgery should be indicated by the surgeon. If position is unimportant, the patient should be allowed to assume a position of comfort, usually with the head of the bed elevated to facilitate drainage. This position also

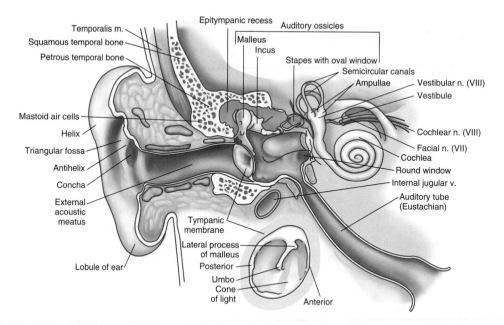

Fig. 29-1 Frontal section through the outer, middle, and internal ear. *(Redrawn from Jacob SW, Francone CA: Elements of anatomy and physiology, ed 2, Philadelphia, 1989, WB Saunders.)*

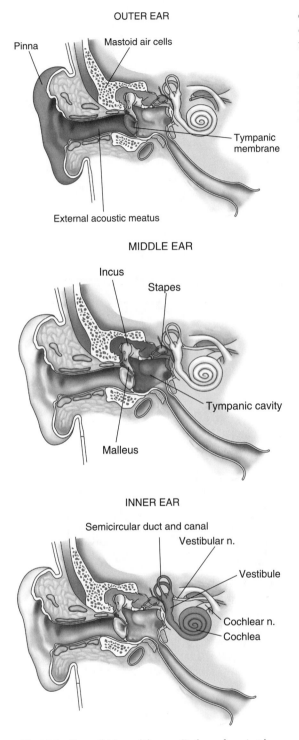

OUTER EAR

Pinna

Mastoid air cells

Tympanic membrane

External acoustic meatus

MIDDLE EAR

Incus

Stapes

Tympanic cavity

Malleus

INNER EAR

Semicircular duct and canal

Vestibular n.

Vestibule

Cochlear n.

Cochlea

Fig. 29-2 Three divisions of the ear. *(Redrawn from Jacob SW, Francone CA: Elements of anatomy and physiology, ed 2, Philadelphia, 1989, WB Saunders.)*

decreases the need to move the head to see. Generally, lying on the unoperated side is most comfortable for the patient.

Nausea, vertigo, and nystagmus commonly occur in patients after ear surgery. The patient may minimize discomfort by remaining in the position ordered, moving slowly, and avoiding quick, jerky movements. Advise the patient to take slow, deep breaths through the mouth to minimize nausea. Antiemetic drugs and sedatives such as dimenhydrinate (Dramamine), diazepam (Valium), droperidol (Inapsine), and chlorpromazine (Thorazine) may be ordered to prevent or treat nausea and vertigo. Avoid jarring the bed. When approaching the patient, place your hand on top of the patient's head as a reminder not to turn toward you suddenly when you speak. Avoid sudden turns and move slowly when transporting the patient. Particular attention must be paid to maintaining the integrity of the airway should nausea and vomiting occur.

Special Considerations

Myringotomy. This is the most common procedure performed on infants and small children. Special pediatric considerations must be given in the immediate postanesthesia phase to airway management, safety, parental involvement, and outpatient teaching. Position the patient so as to promote drainage from the ear. A small piece of sterile cotton may be placed loosely in the external ear to absorb the drainage that commonly occurs. The cotton should be changed often to avoid contamination.

Mastoidectomy. A firm, bulky dressing is placed over the ear and held in place with a circular head bandage after mastoidectomy. This dressing may be reinforced, if necessary, but should be changed only by the physician. Minimal serosanguineous drainage may be expected, but bright bloody drainage should be reported to the surgeon.

The patient should be placed in a position of comfort, usually on the unoperated side. Grafts are often taken from the arm or leg for radical mastoidectomy, and the donor sites should be assessed for drainage and treated according to local policy. Dizziness and vertigo are common following mastoidectomy and may be treated with the previously mentioned measures.

Tympanoplasty. Patients are usually positioned on the unoperated side after tympanoplasty. Care must be taken to keep bandages and grafts in place. Patients should be instructed not to blow their noses or cough and to avoid sneezing to prevent disruption of the grafts.

Fenestration. Fenestration is not commonly performed; however, it may occasionally be the procedure of choice for patients who have lost effective hearing in both ears. It is a major surgical procedure and is usually performed under general anesthesia. Nausea, vertigo, and pain on moving the jaws can be expected following fenestration. The patient is usually placed on the operated side to keep drainage from the operative site from entering the ear. The patient may be allowed to change position from the operated side to the back for nursing care and comfort.

Stapedectomy. Patients who have undergone stapedectomy are usually admitted to the PACU with ear packing in place, and this packing should not be disturbed (Fig. 29-3). Occasionally, patients postoperatively complain of vertigo. Patients should be advised to avoid blowing their noses, coughing, and sneezing.

Cochlear Implant. Patients who have undergone a cochlear implant require the same postanesthesia care as any other ear surgery patient. It is important to verify the integrity of the facial nerve. These patients do not have hearing immediately postoperatively and require emotional support and a means of communication.

SURGERY ON THE NOSE AND SINUSES

Nasal and sinus surgery may be accomplished under local or general anesthesia. The disposition of the patient is determined by the nature and type of surgery and anesthesia as well as the postanesthesia course related to complications and sedation required in the PACU. It may be necessary to observe the patients in an inpatient setting overnight before their discharge from the hospital.

The anatomy of the nasal cavity is shown in Figure 29-4.

Nasal Surgery

Conscious patients admitted to the PACU after nasal surgery should be placed in a semi-Fowler's position to promote drainage, reduce local edema, minimize discomfort, and facilitate respi-

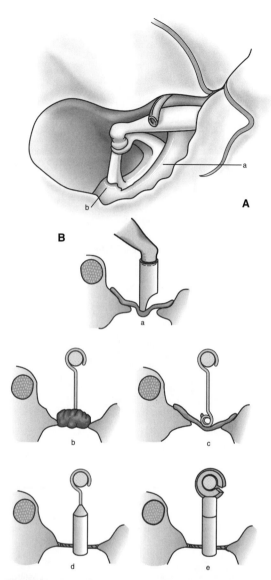

Fig. 29-3 A, Stapedectomy. Adequate footplate exposure is achieved when the facial canal *(a)* and the pyramidal process *(b)* are seen. **B,** Stapedectomy prostheses: *(a)* vein/polyethylene strut (Shea); *(b)* wire/fat (Schuknecht); *(c)* wire on compressed Gelfoam (House); *(d)* wire/Teflon piston; *(e)* Teflon piston (Shea). *(A and B from Paparella MM, Shumrick DA: Otolaryngology, Vol 2, Philadelphia, 1973, WB Saunders.)*

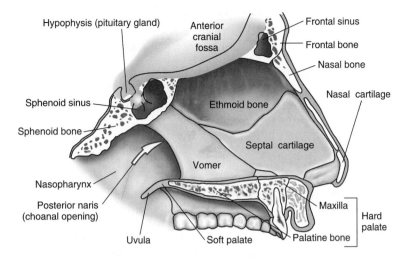

Fig. 29-4 Sagittal section through the nose showing components of the nasal septum. *(Redrawn from Jacob SW, Francone CA: Elements of anatomy and physiology, ed 2, Philadelphia, 1989, WB Saunders.)*

ration. Some postoperative serosanguineous drainage is expected; however, the nurse should observe closely for gross bleeding. The patient is usually admitted with one or both nostrils packed and a "mustache dressing" in place to catch any drainage from the packing. The position of the nasal packs and the amount of drainage should be checked frequently. The mustache dressing may be changed as necessary; it is not unusual for it to be changed two or three times within a 4-hour period. Another method commonly used to facilitate postoperative drainage is the insertion of nasal stents. This approach affords more comfort and permits nasal breathing.

The back of the patient's throat should be checked frequently for blood. Frequent belching (from the accumulation of blood in the stomach) and frequent swallowing as well as the classic signs of hemorrhage, such as tachycardia, are additional signs of unusual bleeding. The patient should be instructed not to blow his or her nose and not to swallow secretions but rather to spit them into a basin. An ample supply of disposable tissues along with an emesis basin should be placed within easy reach of the patient.

Airway obstruction or laryngeal spasm may occur if a postnasal pack accidentally slips out of place. A flashlight, scissors, and a hemostat for emergency removal of nasal packing and emergency airway equipment must be kept readily available at the patient's bedside.

Fluids are withheld until bleeding is controlled, vomiting and nausea have subsided, and independent airway management has been established. Occasionally, an antiemetic may be ordered to alleviate nausea and vomiting.

Mouth breathing, bleeding, and postnasal drainage create a dryness and an offensive taste and odor in the patient's mouth, so once the gag reflex has returned, oral hygiene is a priority. Lemon-glycerine swabs or mouthwash may be used for mouth care and to make the patient more comfortable. A petrolatum-based ointment may be applied to the lips to prevent drying and cracking.

Ice packs across the nose may be ordered to minimize pain, edema, discoloration, and bleeding. These ice packs should be small and lightweight.

Oxygen should be delivered via cool mist mask through a face tent because dry mucus membranes often produce coughing, dyspnea, and decreased respiratory exchange. Ice chips may be a comfort measure if intake is warranted.

Sinus Surgery

Following surgery on the sinuses, the patient is usually admitted to the PACU with packing in place. It is not unusual for the patient to report feelings of numbness in the upper lip and teeth. Following general anesthesia, the patient should be positioned well on one side to prevent aspiration of drainage. The conscious patient should be placed in a semi-Fowler's position, with the head elevated 45 degrees to promote drainage and minimize edema. The same general care, including oral hygiene and instructions to the patient not to blow his or her nose, should be followed as for the patient with nasal surgery.

SURGERY ON THE TONGUE

The tongue occupies a large portion of the floor of the mouth. Surgery on the tongue generally involves excision of benign or malignant lesions, correction of congenital anomalies, or repair of traumatic lacerations. Lesions may be excised without associated neck dissection; however, when the lesion is malignant, surgical treatment usually involves a combined operation that may include radical neck dissection and resection of both the mandible and the tongue.

Local anesthesia is used for minor surgical procedures such as incision and longitudinal closure of the frenulum in ankyloglossia. Local infiltration is also used to repair lacerations caused by trauma. More extensive surgical procedures on the tongue require endotracheal anesthesia.

Postoperatively, the patient must be placed in a side-lying position with the head slightly dependent to allow for the drainage of secretions out of the mouth. When protective reflexes have returned, the patient should be placed in a sitting position to promote venous and lymphatic drainage.

Maintenance of the airway is the most crucial nursing concern. Suctioning equipment with soft-tipped catheters must be immediately available at the bedside. The patient should be instructed to allow saliva to run out of the mouth. A wick of gauze may be placed in the patient's mouth to assist in the elimination of secretions. Swelling of the tongue may occur and thus obstruct the airway. Therefore an intubation tray should be readily available.

Because of the vascular nature of the tongue and oral cavity, postoperative bleeding may be a problem. If excessive bleeding occurs, local pressure should be applied until the surgeon can be notified and repair effected in the operating room.

THROAT SURGERY

Surgery on the throat and neck is generally accomplished under general anesthesia. Aside from routine care and assessment, specific postanesthesia care for the patient who has undergone surgery on the throat involves (1) close observation for bleeding from the surgical site; (2) maintenance of a patent airway; (3) prevention of aspiration of secretions; and (4) awareness of possible cerebral neurologic complications that may develop.

The most common procedures are tonsillectomy, either alone or in combination with adenoidectomy, and tracheostomy.

Tonsillectomy and Adenoidectomy

Most patients who undergo tonsillectomy (Fig. 29-5) and adenoidectomy (T&A) are children and young adults. Patients who have undergone T&A with local anesthesia or are admitted to the PACU fully conscious may be positioned on their backs with their heads elevated 45 degrees. Patients who return following general anesthesia and who are unconscious or semiconscious must be placed in the tonsillar position—well over on the side with the face partially down. The Trendelenburg position may be used to facilitate drainage. The patient's airway and chest expansion must be in full view of the nurse to ensure maximum respiratory integrity at all times. In this position, secretions are easily drained from the mouth. An oral airway should be left in place until the swallowing reflex has returned and the patient can handle secretions. The patient should be advised to spit out secretions as much as possible and to try not to cough, clear the throat, blow the nose, or talk excessively. An ice collar may be applied to minimize pain and postoperative bleeding. The administration of cool, humidified air to the T&A patient provides comfort, helps minimize swelling, and supplies oxygen.

The most common complication of T&A is postoperative bleeding. Frequent swallowing, clearing of the throat, and vomiting of dark blood are indications of possible bleeding. The nurse

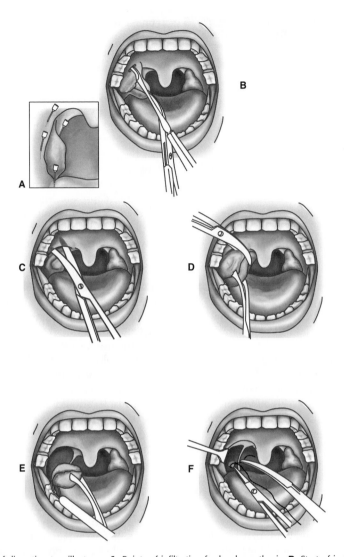

Fig. 29-5 A method of dissection tonsillectomy. **A,** Points of infiltration for local anesthesia. **B,** Start of incision with tonsil knife at attachment of anterior pillar to the tonsil superiorly. **C,** Separation by scissor dissection of the superior pole of the tonsil. **D,** Continuation of dissection of tonsil from its attachment to pillars and bed of tonsillar fossa. **E,** Separation of the tonsil by snare at the lower pole, including the plica triangularis. **F,** Hemostasis. *(A through F from Boies LR, Hilger JA, Priest RE: Fundamentals of otolaryngology: a textbook of ear, nose, and throat diseases, ed 4, Philadelphia, 1964, WB Saunders.)*

should frequently check the back of the throat with a flashlight for trickling blood. If any of the cardinal symptoms of hemorrhage—such as decreased blood pressure, tachycardia, pallor, and restlessness—occur, the surgeon should be notified. Because the surgeon may wish to treat a bleeding episode in the PACU, a tonsil tray should be available (Box 29-1). An electrocautery unit and appropriate illumination with a headlight should be available, along with suction equipment. Postoperative bleeding after T&A can often be controlled by the application of

Box 29-1	**Contents of Tonsil Tray**

Tongue depressors
1 Hurd retractor
2 Mouth gags
1 Allis clamp
2 Tonsil hemostats
1 Short sponge forceps
1 Pair scissors
Sterile towels
Epinephrine hydrochloride (Adrenalin) 1:1000
1 Set tonsil suture needles
1 Needle holder
1 Glass medicine cup
1 Sterile basin
Cotton balls
Tonsil tampons
1 Soft rubber catheter
Petrolatum

vasoconstrictors via nasal packing with pressure. If significant bleeding occurs, however, the patient may have to return to the operating room for suturing or cauterizing of blood vessels.

With the advent of laser dissection of tonsils and adenoids, swelling of the tissue in the hypopharyngeal area is increased. Close observation as well as measures to alleviate swelling are crucial. The advantage of laser dissection is that the potential for bleeding is significantly decreased.

Once the patient is conscious and the reflexes have returned, ice chips and fluids may be offered. Large swallows of lukewarm fluids seem to cause the least discomfort to these patients. Sucking may precipitate bleeding, so a straw should not be offered to the patient. Oral hygiene, including alkaline mouthwash, may provide comfort. Apply petrolatum ointment to the lips to prevent drying and cracking.

Patients who have undergone T&A are especially prone to laryngospasms and must be observed closely for patency of the airway. Airway obstruction may be created by swelling of the palate or nasopharynx, swelling in the retropharyngeal space, or swelling of the tongue and nose. If laryngospasm does occur, positive pressure via Ambu bag and 100% fraction of inspired oxygen

(FIO_2) is administered. If this is not effective in breaking the spasm, it may be necessary to reintubate the patient and administer succinylcholine and narcotics as prescribed.

Laryngoscopy

Laryngoscopy may be accomplished with local or general anesthesia. If the patient's gag and cough reflexes have been obliterated, the patient should not be given anything orally until these reflexes have fully returned. The conscious patient may be placed in a semi-Fowler's position on either side. If unconscious, the patient should be placed in the side-lying position to avoid aspiration. Cool mist, sips of water and intravenous narcotics may help relieve coughing that often occurs.

These patients are especially susceptible to the development of laryngospasm, and the most important observations in the postlaryngoscopy patient are aimed at ascertaining the patency of the airway. Laryngeal stridor, dyspnea, decreased oxygen saturation, or shortness of breath should alert the nurse to respiratory impairment, and the anesthesiologist should be notified. Equipment for endotracheal intubation and emergency tracheostomy should be immediately available at the bedside should laryngeal edema or laryngospasm develop (Box 29-2).

A certain amount of throat discomfort can be expected and may be relieved by the use of an ice collar. The administration of high-humidity oxygen by face tent or mask decreases throat irritation. After the cough and gag reflexes have returned, the patient may be allowed sips of warm normal saline, which is soothing to irritated tissues. If severe pain occurs in either the throat or the chest, the physician should be notified. Watch for signs of hemorrhage—including coughing or regurgitation of blood, apprehension, and the classic signs of tachycardia and lowered blood pressure.

In patients who have had a laryngoscopy (with biopsy) or removal of polyps, vocal rest is important. Coughing should be avoided if possible, and paper and pencil or a "Magic Slate" should be made available so the patient can communicate without talking. If intractable coughing does occur, it may be necessary to consult the anesthesiologist for further measures of control, including pharmacotherapeutics such as codeine and lidocaine to suppress the cough reflex.

Box 29-2   Contents of Tracheostomy Tray

1 Adson or Poole suction (without guard)
1 No. 3 knife handle with No. 15 blade
1 No. 11 blade
1 Metzenbaum scissors
1 One-point sharp scissors
1 Curved tenotomy scissors
1 Collier needle holder
1 6-inch needle holder
2 Adson forceps
1 Tissue forceps
1 Dressing forceps
4 Curved mosquito forceps
2 Straight mosquito forceps
2 Allis clamps
4 Small towel clips
1 Sponge stick (or forceps)
1 Probe
1 Grooved director
1 Goiter right-angle retractor
1 Tracheostomy hook
2 Vein retractors
2 Army-Navy retractors
1 Tonsil suction with tip screwed on
1 10-ml, 3-ring syringe
1 25-gauge 5/8-inch needle
1 Prep cup
1 Medicine glass
Tracheostomy tubes, 1 each, sizes 00-8
4 Hand towels
1 Trousseau tracheal dilator

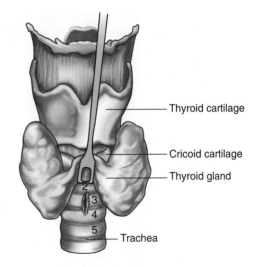

Fig. 29-6   Incision for a tracheostomy. *(Redrawn from Jacob SW, Francone CA: Elements of anatomy and physiology, ed 2, Philadelphia, 1989, WB Saunders.)*

- Thyroid cartilage
- Cricoid cartilage
- Thyroid gland
- Trachea

Box 29-3   Bedside Equipment Needed for a Patient With Tracheostomy

Suction equipment
Respirator
Ambu or anesthesia bag
Extra sterile tracheostomy tray, including tracheostomy tubes of proper size, sterile forceps, tracheal hook, and Trousseau tracheal dilator (see Box 29-2)
Sterile gauze squares
Sterile scissors
Tracheostomy ties
Cleaning solutions for the tracheostomy tube and the incision
Syringe
Hemostat (for inflating the tracheostomy tube cuff)

Tracheostomy

A tracheostomy—an incision into the trachea and the insertion of a cannula—may be done as either an emergency or an elective procedure (Fig. 29-6). Ideally, a tracheostomy is performed in the operating suite under controlled conditions. Tracheostomies are done to improve the airway and to provide access for suctioning of secretions from the trachea and bronchi. The PACU nurse should know what condition necessitated the tracheostomy.

PACU personnel should anticipate the arrival of a tracheostomized patient and have the necessary items at the bedside (Box 29-3).

A variety of tracheostomy tubes are available,

and the nurse should be familiar with those used in the particular institution. Several common types are shown in Figure 29-7.

Immediate postanesthesia care of the newly tracheostomized patient includes a complete assessment of the patient's general condition

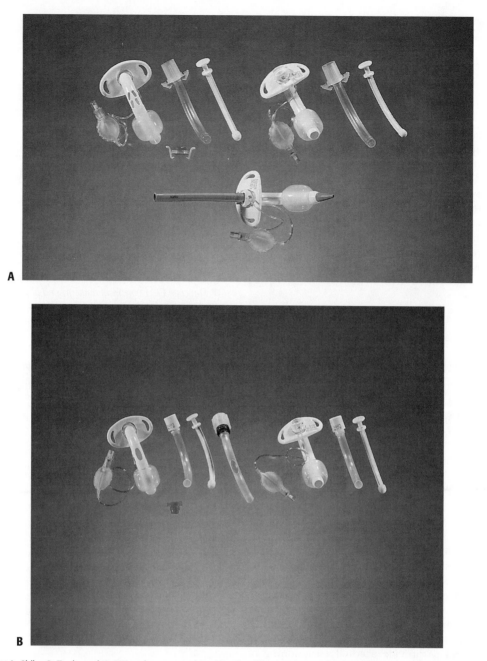

Fig. 29-7 A, Shiley® Tracheosoft® XLT tracheostomy tubes. (*Reprinted by permission of Nellcor Puritan Bennett Inc., Pleasanton, Calif.*) **B,** Shiley® fenestrated low-pressure cuffed tracheostomy tube, showing *(a)* the outer cannula with a fenestration above the cuff; *(b)* decannulation cannula used to plug the tracheostomy tube; *(c)* inner cannula; and (d) obturator. (*From Kersten LD: Comprehensive respiratory nursing: a decision-making approach, Philadelphia, 1989, WB Saunders.*)

as well as detailed attention to respiratory status and tracheostomy wound care. Because of the many nursing needs and the necessity of intensive, ongoing respiratory assessment, the newly tracheostomized patient requires constant attendance.

Assessment of respiratory function should include all parameters mentioned in previous chapters. The nurse should auscultate the patient's chest frequently for normal bilateral breath sounds and report any adventitious sounds or indications of pulmonary congestion. Pulse oximetry should be used to assist in assessment.

Suctioning and Tracheostomy Care. Patency of the newly created airway is vital, and frequent suctioning is necessary because of increased secretions from the tracheobronchial tree caused by trauma. Suctioning the tracheostomy must be sterile and atraumatic; a sterile disposable catheter and glove should be used for each procedure. A suction catheter in a plastic sleeve provides a means of suctioning without the use of gloves and is most convenient for use in the PACU. Catheters should be smooth and small enough to pass easily into the lumen of the tracheostomy tube without obstructing it.

As with any suctioning technique, the patient should be hyperventilated with increased FIO_2 both before and after the procedure. To suction, insert the catheter 6 to 8 inches into the tracheostomy tube. Do not apply suction during insertion. Apply suction intermittently by occluding the air valve with the thumb and at the same time slowly withdrawing the catheter in a twisting motion. Suctioning should not continue for longer than 5 seconds. Time should be allotted between each suctioning for adequate oxygenation of the patient. Suctioning often stimulates forceful coughing, which is effective in bringing up secretions, so the nurse should be prepared to wipe expelled secretions away from the tracheostomy tube orifice with plain gauze squares. To determine the effectiveness of the suctioning, the chest should be auscultated immediately afterward.

If deep suctioning is indicated, a coudé-tip catheter should be used. Insert the catheter with the tip pointing in the direction of the main stem bronchus to be suctioned. Recent evidence indicates that positioning the patient's head to the

left or the right has little effect, if any, on which bronchus will be entered.

If the patient's secretions are exceptionally thick, the physician may order instillation of 3 to 5 ml of sterile normal saline into the tracheostomy tube to help loosen secretions and promote coughing. Although this is a common procedure, whether it is actually effective is questionable, and if the normal saline is not immediately removed by suctioning, it may produce the effects of any inhaled fluid as well as acting as a contaminant. More effective measures to ensure liquefaction of secretions include providing inspired air that is well humidified and ensuring that the patient is well hydrated.

Immediate postanesthesia care of the newly tracheostomized patient also includes care and cleaning of the tracheostomy tube, which may be necessary as often as every hour. A variety of methods may be used to clean the inner cannula of the tracheostomy tube, including normal saline and hydrogen peroxide or 2% sodium bicarbonate solution. A small test tube brush or pipe cleaners may be used to scrub off sticky crusts of mucus. Regardless of the method, it must be a sterile procedure, and no supplies should be used that may leave on the cannula any lint or other debris that may be inhaled by the patient.

Wound drainage from the tracheostomy is generally minimal; however, soiling of the tracheostomy dressing occurs from secretions and sweating. The dressings should be changed as often as necessary, and the skin should be kept clean and dry to prevent maceration and infection. The skin around the stoma should be cleansed with hydrogen peroxide and normal saline and dried with sterile gauze pads, and an antibiotic ointment such as bacitracin should be applied. The tracheostomy dressing should be plain gauze with the edges bound and should have no cotton filling or loose strings. Special tracheostomy "pants" that fit over the tracheostomy tube and have all edges sewn make the best dressing. Sterile gauze may be cut halfway to the center and fitted over the tube (Fig. 29-8); however, this approach has the disadvantage of cut edges that may fray and allow bits of gauze to enter the wound or the trachea.

Fabric tapes or ties or Velcro devices are used to secure the tracheostomy tube in place. These

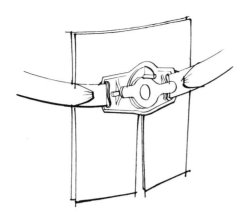

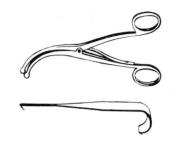

Fig. 29-9 Tracheal dilator and hook. *(Adapted from Sutton, AL: Bedside nursing techniques in medicine and surgery, ed 2, Philadelphia, 1969, WB Saunders.)*

Fig. 29-8 Gauze square cut to use as tracheostomy dressing. *(From Sutton, AL: Bedside nursing techniques in medicine and surgery, ed 2, Philadelphia, 1969, WB Saunders.)*

should be checked frequently to ensure the proper tension. If they are too tight, they will be uncomfortable for the patient and may compress the external jugular veins. If they are too loose, the cannula will slide up and down in the trachea or even be expelled. When the tapes are tied so that one finger can easily slip underneath, the tension is right.

Complications. When complications of a tracheostomy occur, PACU nurses should be especially astute in observing for signs of danger. The most common complication is respiratory obstruction caused by external pressure, foreign bodies, tracheal edema, or excessive secretions. If suctioning does not relieve airway obstruction, the tracheostomy tube may be removed immediately, the tracheal stoma held open with a tracheal dilator and hook or forceps (Fig. 29-9), and the surgeon or anesthesiologist summoned.

Occasionally, a tube is coughed out either because the ties are not sufficiently tight or because the tube is too short. If a tube is accidentally expelled, it must be reinserted by persons qualified to do so. In some institutions, nurses practice changing tracheostomy tubes under the supervision of physicians so that if accidental expulsion should occur in the PACU, the nurse will be skilled in replacement. If the tube cannot be inserted easily, the stoma should be held open and the surgeon called. Misplacement or displacement of the tube is a common complication and must be corrected immediately (Fig. 29-10).

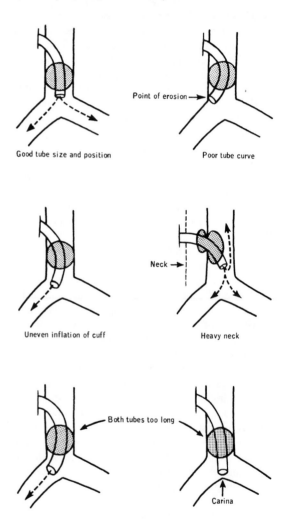

Fig. 29-10 Tracheostomy tube positions and factors that affect them. *(From Murphy ER: Intensive nursing care in a respiratory unit, Nurs Clin North Am 3:433, 1968.)*

Obstruction below the tracheostomy tube may create respiratory insufficiency. Respiratory adventitious sounds, unequal lung expansion, and marked respiratory efforts—including supraclavicular, intercostal, and substernal retractions—should alert the nurse to this problem, and the physician should be notified.

Some bloody secretions from the tracheal stoma may be expected in the immediate postoperative period, but frank bleeding is abnormal, and the surgeon should be notified. Sometimes, bleeding from a thyroid vein or other neck vessel next to the tube occurs, and blood—which runs down into the trachea—is sprayed about with every cough. This is usually not serious and can often be controlled with local packing with petrolatum gauze. Occasionally, however, serious bleeding does occur, and the patient must be taken back to the operating room, where the wound is reopened and the bleeding vessel ligated.

Subcutaneous emphysema may occur as a complication of tracheostomy if the wound is sutured too tightly about the tracheostomy tube, thus allowing air to enter the subcutaneous tissues, or it may result from an overly large incision or a partially obstructed tube. Although subcutaneous emphysema is annoying, it is usually not serious and generally clears after several days. If the nurse notices a crackling sensation under the skin of the neck, chest, or face of the patient, it should be reported to the surgeon because removal of a suture or two may readily correct this problem.

The complications of tracheostomy in infants and children are almost always more serious, because the relative size of the airway is smaller, and tolerance for any obstruction is lessened.

Emotional support of the patient with a new tracheostomy is important and begins immediately upon the patient regaining consciousness. Although the patient may have been well prepared with regard to the loss of ability to speak, awakening in that state is still a traumatic event. A pad and pencil should be readily available to allow the patient to communicate.

Laryngectomy

Partial laryngectomy (Table 29-1) is the surgical treatment of choice for patients with a limited

malignant process of the vocal cords. It is commonly performed through a laryngofissure, and tracheostomy is usually performed concomitantly to ensure a good airway during the immediate postoperative period. Postanesthesia nursing care is essentially the same as that for a posttracheostomy patient.

Postoperative subcutaneous emphysema is not uncommon and should be reported to the surgeon. Laryngectomy patients have trouble swallowing and need frequent suctioning and reassurance.

Supraglottic laryngectomy is performed for carcinoma of the epiglottis and adjacent structures above the level of the true vocal cords. A tracheostomy is mandatory for these patients; they also have a great deal of difficulty swallowing and require close observation and assistance with elimination of saliva and other secretions.

Total laryngectomy is reserved for patients with advanced carcinoma of the true cords (Fig. 29-11). Tracheostomy is always performed. Some means of communication should be established preoperatively for postoperative use.

The primary nursing concern after laryngectomy is maintenance of an adequate airway. Tracheostomy care, as previously discussed, should be deftly carried out and the air well humidified. In the immediate postanesthesia period, the patients need frequent suctioning not only of the tracheostomy but also of the nose and mouth, because they cannot blow their noses and may have difficulty spitting. Frequent mouth care provides additional comfort, and a petrolatum ointment should be applied to the lips to prevent drying and cracking.

Postoperatively, the patient should be positioned on the side until full consciousness is regained. When conscious, the patient may be positioned in a low semi-Fowler's position with the head elevated about 30 degrees. This position promotes drainage, minimizes edema, prevents uncomfortable pressure on suture lines, and facilitates respirations.

Dressings should be checked frequently for excessive drainage and reinforced or changed as necessary. Sometimes, drainage catheters are placed under the wound flaps to remove fluid from the potential dead space left after removal of the larynx and related structures. Drainage

Table 29-1 **Laryngectomy**		
Structures Removed	Structures Remaining	Postoperative Conditions
TOTAL LARYNGECTOMY		
Hyoid bone	Tongue	Loses voice; breathes through tracheostomy;
Entire larynx (epiglottis, false cords, true cords)	Pharyngeal walls Lower trachea	no problem swallowing
Cricoid cartilage		
Two or three rings of trachea		
SUPRAGLOTTIC OR HORIZONTAL LARYNGECTOMY		
Hyoid bone	True vocal cords	Normal voice; may aspirate occasionally,
Epiglottis	Cricoid cartilage	especially liquids; normal airway
False vocal cords	Trachea	
VERTICAL (OR HEMI-) LARYNGECTOMY		
One true vocal cord	Epiglottis	Hoarse but serviceable voice; normal airway;
False cord	One false cord	no problem swallowing
Arytenoid	One true vocal cord	
One half thyroid cartilage	Cricoid	
LARYNGOFISSURE AND PARTIAL LARYNGECTOMY		
One vocal cord	All other structures	Hoarse but serviceable voice; occasionally almost normal voice; no airway problem; no swallowing problem
ENDOSCOPIC REMOVAL OF EARLY CARCINOMA		
Part of one vocal cord	All other structures	May have a normal voice; no other problems

catheters must be connected to a constant vacuum source at 40 to 60 mm Hg, and free drainage must be maintained within the system. This may be accomplished by use of a Hemovac drainage device (Fig. 29-12). Excessive bloody drainage should be reported to the surgeon. The most common site of hemorrhage is the base of the tongue.

Laryngectomy patients are frequently very apprehensive upon awakening and should have someone in close attendance at all times. Although patients may be prepared for postoperative loss of voice, their first experiences of being voiceless and unable to call for help are always extremely frightening. A bell to ring or other noisemaker is more reassuring in this instance than the routine pencil-and-paper communication system.

RADICAL NECK SURGERY

The radical neck procedure itself is relatively simple; it involves removal of all the subcutaneous fat, lymphatic channels, and some of the superficial muscles within a prescribed area of the neck (Fig. 29-13). Generally, the procedure involves the removal of the sternocleidomastoid muscle, omohyoid muscle, internal and external jugular veins, and all lymphatic tissue on one side of the neck. It is the purposeful resection of the 11th cranial (spinal accessory) nerve that causes atrophy of the large trapezius muscle. In the modified neck dissection, the accessory nerve and the internal jugular vein are spared.

Postanesthesia nursing care of the patient after radical neck surgery is somewhat less demanding than that after laryngectomy because these patients do not have a tracheostomy and can talk

Before laryngectomy

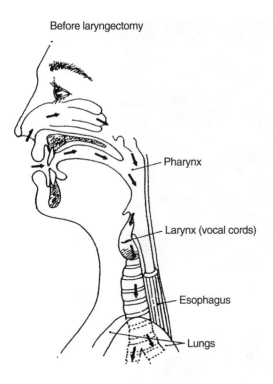

Pharynx

Larynx (vocal cords)

Esophagus

Lungs

After laryngectomy

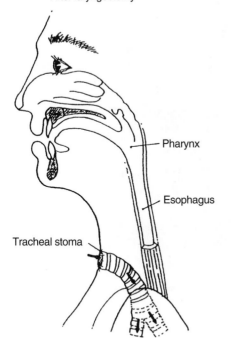

Pharynx

Esophagus

Tracheal stoma

and eat normally. The patient should be placed in a low semi-Fowler's position with the head elevated 30 to 45 degrees to improve venous return. Pillows must be used cautiously when patients are positioned to avoid restricting venous return or compressing the bases of pedicle flaps. Venous congestion, when present, gives the patient's face a purplish hue. This hue can be differentiated from cyanosis caused by inadequate ventilation by observing the color of the extremities to confirm good circulation and close monitoring of oxygen saturation. Postoperative pain is usually minimal after radical neck dissection and can be managed with the usual analgesics.

Dressings are minimal. Skin flaps are secured over drainage tubes, which should be connected to constant suction at 40 to 60 mm Hg. The suction catheters constantly working under the skin flaps suck them firmly against the neck. Approximately 70 to 120 ml of serosanguineous drainage can be expected the day of operation. This amount drastically decreases the second day and becomes minimal (less than 30 ml) the third day. If the dressing soaks through with blood, the surgeon should be notified immediately.

Edema of the recurrent laryngeal nerve and of the nerves to the pharynx may cause difficulty in swallowing and in expectorating secretions; therefore frequent, gentle suctioning of oral secretions may be needed. Extreme care must be taken to avoid any trauma to the internal suture lines. A gauze wick placed in the corner of the patient's mouth can alleviate the annoyance of constant dribbling of mucus and saliva. Mouth care is important for the comfort of this patient and can be accomplished by any of the conventional methods.

Complications
Edema of the lower part of the face on the same side as the surgery is to be expected. Lower facial paralysis may occur because of injury of the facial nerve during dissection. The most common com-

Fig. 29-11 Total laryngectomy. *(From Keith RL: Looking forward . . . a guidebook for the laryngectomy, ed 3, 1995, Rochester, MN, Mayo Foundation. By permission of Mayo Foundation for Medical Education and Research.)*

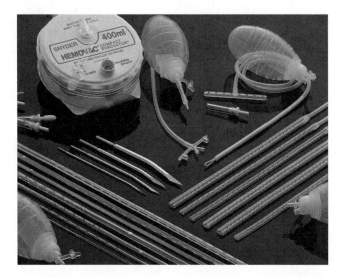

Fig. 29-12 Silicone evacuator (Snyder Hemovac drainage) device is a closed suction apparatus and blood receptacle for facial and neck surgery. (*Courtesy of Zimmer Inc., Warsaw, Ind.*)

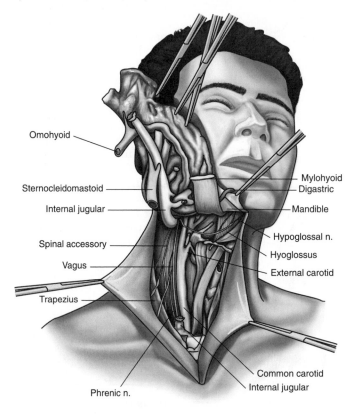

Fig. 29-13 Drawing showing the extent of the usual radical neck dissection. The specimen is retracted superiorly. As is shown, resection of the posterior belly of the digastric muscle permits high ligation of the internal jugular vein and also facilitates dissection around the hypoglossal nerve. (*Redrawn from Converse JM: Reconstructive plastic surgery, Vol 3, Philadelphia, 1964, WB Saunders.*)

plication after radical neck dissection is hemorrhage, which is most often the result of inadequate hemostasis in the immediate postoperative period. The most serious complication is rupture of the carotid artery ("carotid blowout"). This is an uncommon event and occurs almost exclusively when radical neck dissection is combined with total laryngectomy. It is more likely to occur in a patient who preoperatively has had a course of radiation therapy or who has a fistula that bathes the carotid artery in secretions. If the danger of a blowout of the carotid artery is present, all personnel should be aware of it and know what to do if it occurs.

If a carotid blowout occurs, digital pressure with gauze pads, bath towels, or anything available should be applied immediately and help summoned. Intravenous fluids must be started immediately if they are not already infusing. Fluids should be administered at an increased rate to replace loss and combat shock. Inflate the cuff on the tracheostomy tube, and perform tracheal suctioning to prevent aspiration of blood. Most importantly, maintain a patent airway and administer oxygen. Patients on "carotid precautions"—that is, those who may experience this complication—should be typed and crossmatched for whole blood, and appropriate emergency equipment—including gauze pads, vascular clips, and suture ties—should be immediately available at the bedside.

Reconstruction Surgery in Head and Neck Cancer

Any of a large variety of reconstructive procedures may be employed to reestablish both contour and function after the removal of large areas of the head and neck for malignant disease. Skin grafts have largely been replaced with skin flaps or muscle-skin combined flaps that can cover extensive areas both inside and outside the neck. These flaps provide a lining of the throat or mouth and can also replace excised skin on the external surfaces. The commonly used flaps are the pectoralis major muscle-skin unit and the deltopectoral flap, both from the anterior chest area. In rare instances, a free flap may be used. This flap is usually a muscle-skin flap that is moved a long distance from one area of the body to another. To be successful, this type of flap requires the microsurgical repair of its tiny artery and vein with an artery and vein in its new location. In general, these reconstructive flaps must be free of any pressure or dressings. A light coat of antibacterial ointment is usually applied along the suture lines, and the area is frequently observed for color, warmth, and bleeding. Because these flaps depend on a single small artery and vein, any kinking or external pressure may result in the death of the flap.

MAXILLOFACIAL SURGERY

The care of patients with extensive maxillofacial surgery follows the principles outlined earlier for tracheostomy care and care after laryngectomy or radical neck dissection. The care of these patients is extremely demanding, and attention to detail is the basis for the prevention of complications.

Maxillofacial surgery may be required to correct trauma and fractures or to correct congenital skeletal deformities. Following this type of surgery, the patient will be in intermaxillary fixation (IMF) with his or her jaws wired shut. Care revolves around protection of the airway.

Some additional emergency equipment is required at the bedside of patients who are admitted with IMF—including wire cutters, a suture set, additional nasal airways, small suction catheters, and gauze pads. On admission of the patient, the surgeon should review placement of the IMF wires with the nurse. A line drawing of these wires indicating which to cut in case of extreme emergency (e.g., cardiac or respiratory arrest) should be posted at the head of the bed.

Preoperative preparation of the patient who is undergoing IMF is particularly important and should include instructions on how to clear secretions or remove vomitus while remaining in IMF. The patient should also be taught how to use the suction catheter. These instructions will have to be repeated frequently in the PACU as the patient recovers. Having the jaws wired closed is a frightening experience for any patient, no matter how well prepared that patient is. Blood, emesis, lingual and pharyngeal edema, hematoma formation, or laryngospasm may further compromise the oral airway, which is already obstructed as much as 90% by fixation of the jaws. Reassurance is provided by maintaining proximity to the patient, ensuring a means to attract attention, and explaining fully all treatments and procedures.

The patient will arrive in the PACU with a nasotracheal tube in place. Extubation should not be considered until the patient is fully awake and reflexes have returned sufficiently to allow handling of secretions. A soft nasal airway may be inserted following extubation to assist in maintaining a patent airway.

Observe closely for bleeding. Some oozing of blood is normal, but excessive amounts should be reported to the surgeon. Frequent, gentle suctioning with a small catheter assists in keeping the airway clear by removing blood and saliva. The patient may be more comfortable doing this independently when able. It is reassuring to these patients to have a suction catheter in hand for use as necessary.

Vomiting and subsequent aspiration is a significant risk for this patient. A nasogastric tube is frequently used to reduce the likelihood of nausea and vomiting. Ensure that it is correctly positioned and patent. Antiemetics should be administered as necessary, and pain should be treated promptly to prevent the development of nausea and vomiting.

Despite all efforts to prevent it, vomiting may occur. If still drowsy, the patient should be turned immediately to the lateral or semiprone position and the emesis suctioned out via the nose or mouth. If the patient is awake, assist him or her to sit up, lean over, and allow emesis to flow out of the mouth and nose. Retract the cheeks by holding them out with the fingers. Most importantly, repeat instructions and reassurances quietly but confidently to keep the patient calm. It is rarely necessary to cut the wires.

The patient should be positioned with the head of the bed elevated 30 degrees to assist in maintaining the airway by controlling edema. Ice packs are usually ordered postoperatively to assist in controlling edema and promote comfort. A surgical glove partially filled with cracked ice can be used, or ice collars can be molded to the jaws, chin, or nose. Iced saline gauze pads may be applied to the eyes.

Petrolatum ointment or other emollient cream should be applied to the lips and corners of the mouth to relieve tenderness and prevent drying and cracking. Dental wax can be molded and applied to protruding wires, which are quite irritating to the oral mucosa.

When the patient is fully awake and protective reflexes have sufficiently returned, rinsing the mouth with warm saline will provide additional comfort. The patient may then also have small sips of liquids.

BIBLIOGRAPHY

Alspach J: Core curriculum for critical care nursing, ed 5, Philadelphia, 1998, WB Saunders.

Arnet G, Basehore LM: Dentofacial reconstruction, Am J Nurs 84(12):1488-1490, 1984.

Atlee J: Complications in anesthesia, Philadelphia, 1999, WB Saunders.

Balkany TJ: The Cochlear implant, Otolaryngol Clin North Am 19:217-449, 1986.

Ball KA: Lasers: the perioperative challenge, St Louis, 1990, Mosby.

Barash P, Cullen B, Stoelting R: Clinical anesthesia, ed 4, Philadelphia, 2000, Lippincott Williams & Wilkins.

Benumof J: Anesthesia and uncommon diseases, ed 4, Philadelphia, 1998, WB Saunders.

Benumof J, Saidman L: Anesthesia & perioperative complications, ed 2, St Louis, 1999, Mosby.

Bickley L, Hoekelman R: Bates' guide to physical examination and history taking, ed 7, Philadelphia, 1998, Lippincott Williams & Wilkins.

Darvich-Kodjouri C: Nursing care of the patient with a new tracheostomy, Curr Rev Recov Room Nurses 3(7):18-23, 1985.

DeFazio-Quinn D: Ambulatory surgical nursing core curriculum, Philadelphia, 1999, WB Saunders.

Frost CM, Frost DE: Nursing care of patients in intermaxillary fixation, Heart Lung 12(5):524-528, 1983.

Ganong W: Review of medical physiology, ed 20, New York, 2001, McGraw-Hill Professional.

Gotta A: Airway management for maxillofacial trauma, Curr Rev Post Anesth Nurses 10(5):34-39, 1988.

Guyton A, Hall J: Textbook of medical physiology, ed 10, Philadelphia, 2000, WB Saunders.

Hardman J, Limbird L: Goodman and Gilman's the pharmacological basis of therapeutics, ed 10, New York, 2001, McGraw-Hill Professional.

Lake C, Hines R, Blitt C: Clinical monitoring: practical applications for anesthesia and critical care, St Louis, 2001, Mosby.

Litwack K, Zeplin K: Practical points in the management of laryngospasm, J Post Anesth Nurs 4(1):36-39, 1989.

Longnecker D, Murphy F: Dripps/Eckenhoff/Vandam introduction to anesthesia, ed 9, Philadelphia, 1997, WB Saunders.

Longnecker D, Tinker J, Morgan G: Principles and practice of anesthesiology, ed 2, St Louis, 1998, Mosby.

Lyons RJ, Coren DA: The head and neck patient, AORN J 40(5):751-760, 1984.

Mapp C: Trach care: are you aware of all the dangers? Nursing 18(7):34-43, 1988.

Miller R, editor: Anesthesia, ed 5, New York, 2000, Churchill Livingstone.

Murray J, Nadel, J: Textbook of respiratory medicine, ed 3, Philadelphia, 2001, WB Saunders.

Nagelhout J, Zaglaniczny K: Nurse anesthesia, ed 2, Philadelphia, 2001, WB Saunders.

Patton C: The critical airway, Curr Rev Post Anesth Nurses 13(5):35-39, 1991.

Rook JL, Rook M: Head and neck cancer, J Post Anesth Nurs 4(6):263-277, 1989.

Saunders WH, Havener WH, Keith CF et al: Nursing care in eye, ear, nose, and throat disorders, St Louis, 1979, Mosby.

Smalley PJ: Lasers in otolaryngology, Nurs Clin North Am 25(3):645-655, 1990.

Stoelting R: Pharmacology and physiology in anesthetic practice, ed 3, Philadelphia, 1999, Lippincott-Raven.

Stoelting R, Miller R: Basics of anesthesia, ed 4, New York, 2000, Churchill Livingstone.

Stone D: Perioperative care: anesthesia, medicine, and surgery, St Louis, 1998, Mosby.

Townsend C, Beauchamp R, Evers B et al: Sabiston textbook of surgery: the biological basis of modern surgical practice, ed 16, Philadelphia, 2001, WB Saunders.

Traver G, Tremper Mitchell J, Glodquist-Priestley G: Respiratory care: a clinical approach, Gaithersburg, Md, 1991, Aspen Publishers.

Waugaman W, Foster S, Rigor B: Principles and practice of nurse anesthesia, ed 3, Norwalk, Conn, 1999, Appleton & Lange.

30 CARE OF THE OPHTHALMIC SURGICAL PATIENT

Carole Muto, RN, BSN, CPAN

There are unique rewards and challenges in the assessment and care of people who are undergoing eye surgery in the postanesthesia care unit (PACU). Often the perianesthesia nurse shares in the joy and excitement as a patient experiences dramatically improved vision minutes after cataract surgery. Conversely, the same nurse may carry a recovered toddler to the arms of weeping parents after the distressing loss of their child's eye because of retinoblastoma. The primary goals of the plan of care following eye surgery should be safe and successful postanesthetic recovery and comfort in keeping with ASPAN guidelines, but the special cognitive and advocacy needs of eye patients are also identified in the PACU. These needs must be met through education, discharge planning and postdischarge assessment beginning in the preanesthesia phase and continuing on to the Phase II or ambulatory surgery setting.[1]

Ophthalmologic advances have proceeded at an incredible pace during the past decade. Eye surgery is performed safely on fragile premature infants and neonates as well as on the very elderly. The special concerns that apply to specific age groups must be considered. In caring for infants and children, a thorough understanding of normal growth and development is essential. The perianesthesia nurse should be certified in Pediatric Advanced Life Support (PALS) as well as in ACLS. Elderly ophthalmic patients may have complex medical histories, sensory deficits, and senile dementia. Diabetes mellitus—a leading cause of blindness in adults between the ages of 21 and 60—leads to eye surgery for many in this age group.[2] Meticulous attention to details of the patient's ocular and medical history and type and course of anesthesia is vital to providing optimal perioperative care.

Most eye surgical procedures today are performed as same day or ambulatory outpatient surgery. Cataract surgery, after which few restrictions are necessary, is often performed with topical anesthesia and almost exclusively on an outpatient basis. Patients—including those who have had an eye removed—may be discharged to home the same day of general anesthesia. Discharge criteria are in keeping with other nonophthalmic types of surgery. In all cases postoperative care instructions should be discussed both preoperatively and postoperatively with the patient and a significant other. Instructions should also be written, preferably in large type, so that they may be reviewed as necessary after discharge. Special postoperative instructions that pertain to ophthalmic patients may include how to self-administer eye drops, proper application of the protective eye shield, face down or other positioning techniques after retina surgery, and emphasis on stringent hand-washing to prevent infection. For enucleated patients with a hydroxyapatite orbital implant, interdisciplinary involvement may include referral to an ocularist. Care of the patient undergoing day surgery is outlined in Chapter 43.

Ophthalmic surgical procedures for which patients may be admitted to the hospital for inpatient care include retinal detachment repair with instillation of a gas bubble, which requires special positioning; repair of ruptured globe caused by trauma, which requires intravenous antibiotics; application of radioactive plaque for eye tumors; glaucoma surgery that requires postoperative measurement of intraocular pressure, especially if the patient is monocular; enuclea-tion in children. The anatomy of the normal eye is shown in Figure 30-1.

DEFINITIONS

Anterior segment: the intraocular segment of the eyeball occupied by the aqueous that lies in front of and is separated from the vitreous-filled posterior segment by the lens and zonule; it is subdivided by the iris into anterior and posterior chambers.

Blepharoplasty: surgical repair of an eyelid. Often per-formed for ptosis or blepharophimosis of the eyelid (Fig. 30-2).

Cataract: opacity of the lens. Surgical treatment con-sists of removal of the lens.

Chalazion: a chronic granulomatous inflammation of one or more of the meibomian glands in the tarsal

plate of the eyelid. Surgical treatment consists of inci-sion and curettage.

Dacryocystitis: infection of the lacrimal sac.

Dacryocystorhinostomy: creation of a new pathway from the lacrimal sac to the nasal cavity.

Dermatochalasis: relaxation of the skin of the eyelid because of atrophy. Surgical treatment is blepharoplasty.

Ectropion: eversion of the margin of the eyelid. Surgi-cal treatment is to shorten the lower lid in a horizontal direction.

Entropion: inversion of the margin of the eyelid; it usually affects the lower lid but may affect the upper lid. Surgical treatment involves either removing a base triangle of skin, muscle, and tarsus and suturing the edges together to evert the lid margin or exposing the orbicular muscle, dividing it, and suturing it to the lower border of the tarsus.

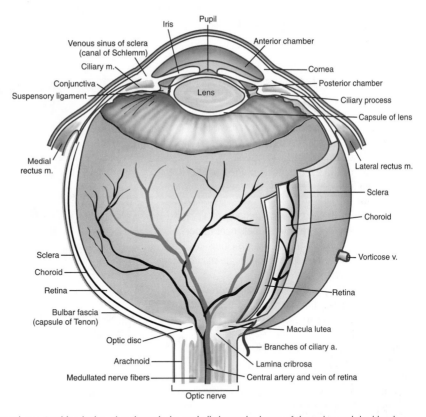

Fig. 30-1 Anatomy of the normal eye. A midsagittal section through the eyeball shows the layers of the retina and the blood supply. *(Redrawn from Jacob SW, Francone CA, Lossow WJ: Structure and function in man, ed 5, Philadelphia, 1982, WB Saunders.)*

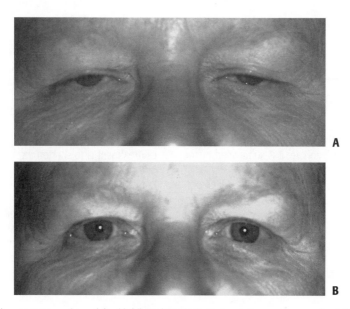

Fig. 30-2 **A**, Preoperative appearance of an adult with bilateral ptosis. **B**, Postoperative appearance after bilateral ptosis repair. *(Courtesy of Dr. Robert B. Penne; Wills Eye Hospital, Philadelphia.)*

Enucleation: removal of the entire eyeball after the eye muscles and optic nerve have been severed.

Epiphora: excess tearing; it may be caused by blocked lacrimal drainage system. Surgical treatment for epiphora and dacryocystitis caused by blockage is probing of the lacrimal duct.

Evisceration of the eye: removal of the contents of the eye, leaving the sclera intact and the muscles attached to the sclera.

Exenteration of the eye: radical removal of all orbital contents usually for unresectable malignant tumors of the eyelids, conjunctiva, intraocular structures and orbit. In many cases an eyelid-sparing technique may be used to expedite healing.[3]

Glaucoma: a disease of the eye characterized by increased intraocular pressure. Surgical treatment is aimed at establishing an evacuation route for outflow of aqueous fluid.

Goniotomy: surgery for congenital glaucoma in which the trabecular meshwork is incised.

Hydroxyapatite implant: an orbital implant made of natural material derived from ocean coral that resembles human bone in chemical and porous structure. After enucleation the eye muscles can be attached directly to this implant, thus allowing it to move within the orbit just like the natural eye.

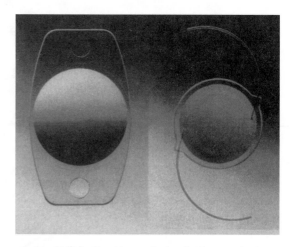

Fig. 30-3 Examples of intraocular lens implants used today. *(Courtesy of Wills Eye Hospital, Philadelphia.)*

Intraocular lens (IOL) implant: synthetic lens used to replace the crystalline lens after cataract surgery. The latest versions include a soft, foldable lens that can fit through an even smaller incision and the bifocal intraocular lens (Fig. 30-3).

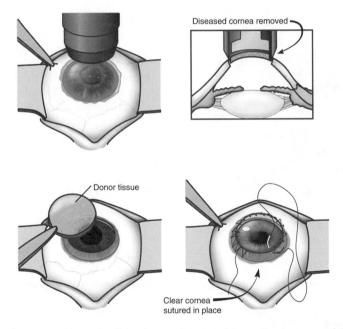

Diseased cornea removed

Donor tissue

Clear cornea
sutured in place

Fig. 30-4 Corneal transplant surgery. Upper, the diseased cornea is removed. Lower, the donor corneal tissue is placed in the opening and is sewn in place with a very fine suture. *(Courtesy of the Department of Medical Illustration and Audio Visual Education, Baylor College of Medicine, Houston.)*

Keratoplasty: transplantation of or a portion or the entire thickness of the cornea (Fig. 30-4).

LASIK (Laser-Assisted in Situ Keratomileusis): a corneal procedure in which the eximer laser is used to reshape the cornea, thus correcting farsightedness (hyperopia), nearsightedness (myopia), and astigmatism.

Ocularist: a carefully trained technician skilled in the arts of fitting, shaping, and painting ocular prostheses.

Oculcardiac reflex: a decrease in pulse rate associated with traction on extraocular muscles or compression of the eyeball; especially sensitive in children; may produce systolic cardiac arrest.

Phacoemulsification: the procedure of fragmentation of the lens with ultrasound combined with aspiration for cataract surgery (Fig. 30-5).

Plaque: a radioactive device (usually containing iodine-125) that is surgically applied to the sclera over an intraocular neoplasm. It is used to treat retinoblastoma and uveal malignant melanoma.[4]

Proptosis: protrusion of the eyeball.

Pterygium: a fleshy triangular growth extending from the conjunctiva and encroaching on the cornea. Surgical treatment is by excision.

Ptosis: drooping of the upper eyelid. Surgical treatment involves either elevating the lid with a sling or shortening the levator muscle of the lid (levator resection).

Retinoblastoma: malignant retinal tumor of infancy.

Retinopexy: surgical correction of retinal detachment (Fig. 30-6) by sealing the hole. Sealing is accomplished by causing scar formation with heat, electrical current, or cryotherapy.

Scleral buckle: surgical correction of a retinal detachment by compression of the sclera to rejoin the underlying retinal pigment epithelium to the detached sensory retina; used in conjunction with retinopexy.

Strabismus: condition in which the eyes are not simultaneously directed toward the same object. Esotropia is inward deviation of the eyes, and exotropia is outward deviation. Surgical treatment involves changing the relative strength of individual muscles either by resection (the shortening of a muscle by removal of part of the tendon) or by recession (the surgical transfer of a muscle insertion backward from the original attachment on the eye).

Tonometer: a hand-held noncontact instrument used to measure intraocular pressure in postoperative eyes.

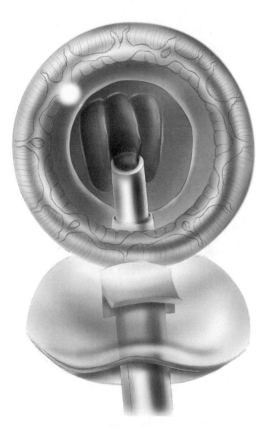

Fig. 30-5 The phacoemulsifier passes through the keratome incision at the apex of the scleral flap. Phacoemulsification of the nucleus is completed followed by aspiration of the cortex through the same incision. *(From Johnstone MA: Combined single incision cataract/trabeculectomy, Operative Techniques in Cataract and Refractive Surgery, 2(2):49, 1999.)*

Topical anesthesia: the topical application of local anesthetic that dispenses with akinesia as part of the operating conditions for cataract extraction. It avoids all the complications of needles in the orbit.

Trabeculectomy: creation of a drainage channel from the anterior chamber to the subconjunctival space; used to treat intractable glaucoma.

Vitrectomy: surgical removal of vitreous gel from the eye, usually to clear blood or opacified vitreous that blocks sight or to sever vitreous traction bands that pull on the retina and detach it. The clouded gel is replaced with specialized gas or silicone oil (Fig. 30-7).

ANESTHESIA

Ophthalmic procedures are often performed with monitored anesthesia care (MAC) with the administration of intravenous sedation in conjunction with a local anesthetic block.[5] Midazolam, fentanyl, and propofol are administered in the preoperative area before the block injection. Commonly used local anesthetics for eye surgery are bupivicaine, mepivacaine, lidocaine, and procaine. The type of block—retrobulbar, peribulbar, parabulbar, subconjunctival, lid, or facial—will depend on the type of surgery (Fig. 30-8). Ophthalmic surgery can be classified as intraocular or extraocular. Cataract, glaucoma, corneal, and vitrectomy procedures are intraocular; eye muscle surgeries, scleral buckling, enucleation, and oculoplastic surgeries are extraocular[6] (see Fig. 30-6). For cooperative adults local anesthesia is preferred to general anesthesia to avert the restlessness and nausea or vomiting associated with general anesthesia. Risks of local anesthesia are injection into the optic nerve, globe perforation, or retrobulbar hemorrhage with peribulbar and retrobulbar blocks.[5] The perianesthesia nurse should be alert to the potential of these complications, although they are rare. Facial drooping on the side of the operated eye after a facial block is sometimes present on the patient's arrival to the PACU. Usually this resolves as the anesthetic wears off.

Topical anesthesia is not a new technique, but it has recently gained popularity, primarily in cataract surgery.[5] Tetracaine 4% ophthalmic solution is used for its rapid onset and moderate duration of action. The patient may also receive intravenous sedation during the procedure. Benefits of topical anesthesia outweigh the risks associated with general, retrobulbar, and peribulbar anesthesia. With topical anesthesia, cataract surgery patients have better visual acuity immediately postoperatively and less pain.[7] In some practice settings, short eyesurgical procedures such as nasolacrimal duct probing may be performed on children with topical anesthesia in conjunction with propofol sedation.[8]

Infants, children, uncooperative or particularly anxious patients, and psychotic persons usually require general anesthesia. General anesthesia is also indicated when a local anesthetic

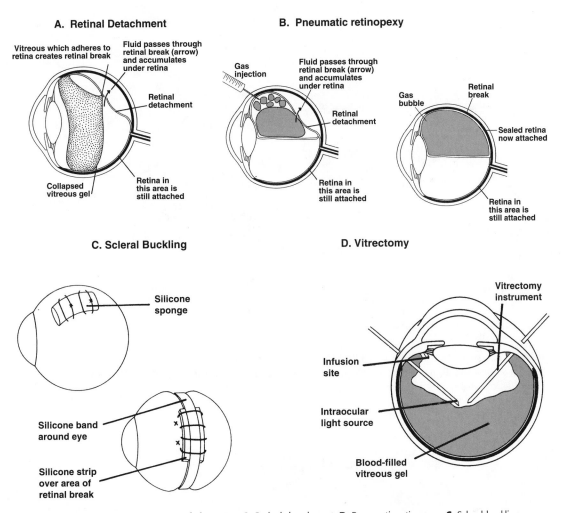

Fig. 30-6 Retinal detachment surgery and vitrectomy. **A,** Retinal detachment; **B,** Pneumatic retinopexy; **C,** Scleral buckling; **D,** Vitrectomy. *(Courtesy of Wills Eye Hospital, Philadelphia.)*

might exacerbate an eye problem; when surgery is to be performed on a lacerated cornea, ruptured globe, or optic nerve decompression; or when the surgery planned is extensive, as in enucleation or evisceration. The ophthalmic patient who has undergone general anesthesia must be assessed and receive care as previously described for patients who are undergoing general anesthesia. The special precaution for these patients is that

modifications in care must be made to prevent stress on the eyes and surrounding musculature (see Fig. 30-1).

PERIANESTHESIA CARE

Cardiorespiratory Assessment and Care

The patient usually arrives in the PACU awake. Immediate postoperative assessment of

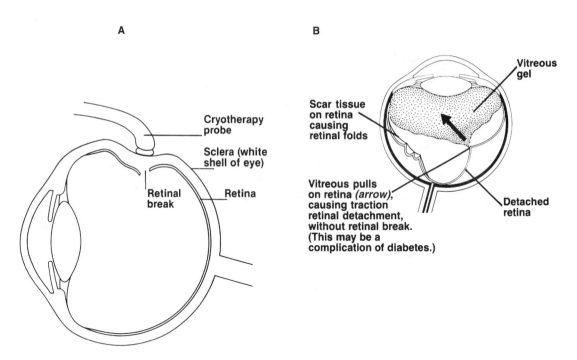

Fig. 30-7   **A,** Cryotherapy is a process in which a freezing probe is applied briefly to the outside of the eyewall to promote sealing of a retinal hole. **B,** Traction retinal detachment for which the patient may undergo vitrectomy. *(Courtesy of Wills Eye Hospital, Philadelphia.)*

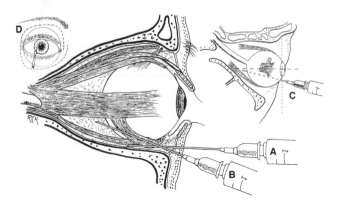

Fig. 30-8   Traditional retrobulbar block. *(Hamilton RC: Retrobulbar anesthesia, Operative Techniques in Cataract and Refractive Surgery 3(3):116, 2000.)*

the cardiorespiratory system should proceed as described in Chapter 26. Vital signs are monitored, and the stir-up regimen is started. One challenge is keeping the patient's lungs clear without increasing intraocular pressure. Cough-ing may increase intraocular pressure, thus potentially damaging the affected eye. Deep rhythmic breaths at frequent intervals assist in the prevention of atelectasis. The nurse should coach the patient in deep inspirations and concentration on breathing to help avoid coughing. Sucking on ice chips or throat lozenges may soothe the throat and prevent coughing. In some instances, lidocaine 1 mg/kg given intravenously may be ordered to ease coughing. If coughing persists and cannot be controlled, the surgeon must be notified.

Special cardiorespiratory situations may arise related to the patient's eye condition or surgery (Table 30-1). It is not uncommon for vasovagal syncope to occur in the PACU after eye surgery. The patient becomes lightheaded, nauseated, flushed, feels warm, and may even lose consciousness for several seconds. Immediate therapy includes intravenous fluids, oxygen, lowering the head of the stretcher and raising the feet. If the patient has symptomatic bradycardia and hypotension that does not respond to these interventions, atropine, glycopyrrolate, or ephedrine may be ordered.

The use of intravenous mannitol for its ocular hypotensive effect during eye surgery increases the potential for congestive heart failure in elderly patients or patients with poor cardiac output. The flat position of eye surgery tends to compound this potential.[9] In glaucoma patients being treated with topical beta-blockers, serious systemic effects from their eye drops—such as bradycardia, heart failure, hypotension, arrhythmias, and myocardial infarction—may develop.[10]

These patients may require a medical doctor's evaluation and transfer to a tertiary facility for continued monitoring.

The oculocardiac reflex is a response to manipulation of eye muscles and tissue during surgery. A child's strabismus repair, retinal surgery, or direct pressure on the orbital contents after enucleation can also evoke this reflex response. It is associated with bradycardia and may cause hypotension and ventricular dysrhythmias, which can continue into the postoperative period.[9]

In addition, incidence of malignant hyperthermia in patients with strabismus and blepharoptosis may be increased.[5,11] In these situations, early recognition and efficient appropriate response is critical.

Nausea and Vomiting

In ophthalmic surgery patients, nausea and vomiting can cause increased intraocular pressure, eye wound dehiscence, iris prolapse, and intraocular bleeding[11] and therefore should be avoided as much as possible.[11] Strabismus and retinal detachment surgeries have a higher incidence of postoperative nausea and vomiting than other eye surgeries. As a precaution, oral fluids and diet are delayed for a brief period after general anes-

Table 30-1 **PACU Issues Relating to Ophthalmic Surgery**

Postoperative Problems	Considerations
Pain	Routine vs. corneal abrasion, acute angle-closure glaucoma
Nausea/vomiting	Type of surgery, pain, anxiety, oculocardiac reflex
Dysrhythmias	Systemic and eye medications, hypoventilation, OCR
Mental status	Iatrogenic problems, preexisting disease
Hypotension	Diuretics, anesthesia, cardiovascular toxicity of local anesthetics
Hypertension	Eye medications, history of hypertension, bladder distension
Oculocardiac reflex	Ocular traction, orbital pressure, pain
Malignant hyperthermia	1:15,000 pediatric population, 1:50,000 adult population, increased index of suspicion with associated musculoskeletal disorders, strabismus
Bladder distension	After diuretics
Apnea and bradycardia	In premature infants, overnight monitoring for apnea and bradycardia

From Acquadro MA: Recovery room care and problems following ophthalmic and otolaryngologic surgery. In KE McGoldrick, editor: Anesthesia for ophthalmic and otolaryngologic surgery, Philadelphia, 1992, WB Saunders.

thesia. The anesthesia team often administers a prophylactic antiemetic regimen of ondansetron (Zofran), ranitidine (Zantac), and metoclopramide (Reglan) alone or in combination. In the PACU, patient movement should be minimized and hypotension avoided. If the patient complains of thirst, he or she may moisten the mouth with oral swabs dipped in ice water (taking care to minimize stimulation of the oropharynx). Despite preventative measures, nausea and vomiting may still occur, and prompt recognition is important so that treatment can begin without delay. Usual therapy is the administration of oxygen by nasal prongs or by, encouraging the patient to breathe slowly and deeply to avoid retching, appropriate fluid volume replacement to treat hypovolemic hypotension, and antiemetics. In addition to ondansetron, antiemetics commonly used in the PACU for ophthalmic surgery patients are prochloperazine (Compazine), droperidol (Inapsine), or trimethobenzamide (Tigan). Pediatric patients who experience nausea and vomiting in the PACU may receive ondansetron usually at a dose of 0.15 mg/kg intravenously.

The perianesthesia nurse must determine whether pain is contributing to the nausea and vomiting. Although narcotics can precipitate nausea, nausea caused by eye pain and headache may actually require narcotic administration to relieve the nausea.[11] This can be especially effective if given in conjunction with antiemetics. Persistent nausea and vomiting accompanied by pain may indicate intraocular hemorrhage, which necessitates immediate intervention by the ophthalmologist.

Pain Management

Many patients report no pain in the PACU after eye surgery. The eye is usually quite comfortable because of the effects of the local block, the intraoperative use of topical anesthesia, topical nonsteroidal antiinflammatory agents, and cholinergic blockers, such as atropine, which paralyze the ciliary muscle. Ophthalmic ointments that contain antiinflammatory or antibiotic agents are often applied to the eye before patching. These ointments soothe the eye and promote comfort but may blur patients' vision.

When localized pain in the eye does occur, it can be related to the use of surgical retractors

(Fig. 30-9), surgical wounds, and pressure dressings.[11] Complaints of itching, scratchy or grating feelings, or a "pins and needles" sensation should be interpreted as pain and treated as such. Reassurance and acetaminophen (Tylenol) are usually quite effective with these discomforts. Headache, which often follows anterior segment surgery, is also usually relieved with acetaminophen.[11]

Trauma to the eyes and the surrounding tissue is quite common among all age groups and often results in emergency eye surgery.[12] Pain from corneal abrasion, eyelid lacerations, and sharp injuries to the globe may be quite intense.[11,13] The administration of narcotic analgesia may be required to control the pain. If fentanyl, morphine sulfate, or other opiates are necessary for pain relief, they should be used in conjunction with an antiemetic to decrease the chance of nausea and vomiting. Eye pain in some same-day adult patients may be treated with intravenous or intramuscular ketorolac (Toradol). However, ketorlac is generally not used for patients with oculoplastic procedures or procedures in which bleeding may be a postoperative concern. Infants and children should be assessed for pain and medicated depending on their age, surgical procedure performed, and severity of pain.

Moist, cold, or iced compresses are routinely ordered for patients who are recovering from

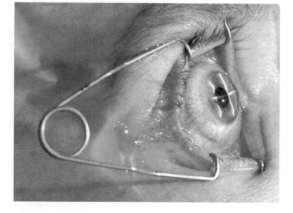

Fig. 30-9 The speculum used for the LASIK procedure separates the eyelids widely. *(Copyright 2001. Ray Swords Photography [swordsra@mindspring.com]. In McLeod SD, McDonnell PJ: Refractive surgery, Ophthalmology Clinics of North America 14(2):288, 2001.)*

oculoplastic procedures and eye muscle surgery. They help prevent swelling and promote comfort. Compresses should be lightweight and may be applied to the surgical eye in awake patients as early as possible for 15 to 20 minutes. The peri-anesthesia nurse should be alert to the possibility of the oculocardiac reflex being elicited by pressure on the eye and should remove the compresses at once if symptoms occur. Diffuse periorbital pain may indicate acute glaucoma, a serious postoperative complication of eye surgery.[11] Acute glaucoma may occur after glaucoma surgery, cataract extraction, corneal transplantation, and vitreoretinal surgery.[14] For significant pain that is not relieved with the prescribed analgesics, an ophthalmologist must be consulted immediately.

Intraocular Pressure

The potential for increased intraocular pressure is an important consideration in the postoperative care of ophthalmic patients.[15] As described above, prompt management of pain, nausea, and vomiting are indispensable. Other factors associated with increased intraocular pressure that should be avoided are systolic hypertension; ketamine used in anesthesia; and straining, as in Valsalva's maneuver.[14] The exertion of hard crying—often a problem with children and infants—should be minimized as much as possible. Some children respond well to being held by the nurse, or—if feasible—a parent may be called

to the PACU to hold the child. Because exertion against the restraints increases intraocular pressure, patients should not be restrained. In both children and adults, tranquilizers may be required to ensure patient cooperation and a smooth recovery course.

Excessive lid swelling, periorbital swelling, or evidence of proptosis as well as abnormally severe complaints of eye pain should be promptly reported to the patient's surgeon.[11] In cases of suspected ocular hypertension, the ophthalmologist may measure the intraocular pressure in the PACU with a pneumatic tonometer (Fig. 30-10).

Positioning

The nurse should begin to orient the patient as soon as he or she enters the PACU. To avoid any startle reflexes, it is particularly important to warn the ophthalmic patient when he or she is about to be moved and touched. Every caution is observed when the patient is transferred from stretcher to bed to avoid bumping and jarring. Movement should be slow and smooth and kept to a minimum. The patient's head should be positioned comfortably so that straining of the neck does not occur.

Specific instructions on head positioning are provided by the surgeon and will vary according to the type of eye surgery. For retinal reattachment surgery, a face-down position commonly is ordered to promote continuing reattachment. The patient assumes this position only when fully

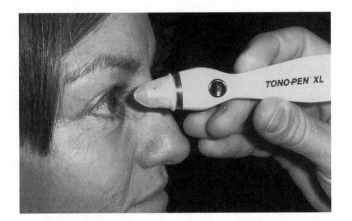

Fig. 30-10 Technique of tonometry with the pneumotonometer. *(Courtesy of Wills Eye Hospital, Philadelphia, 2002.)*

recovered from the anesthetic. The head of the stretcher generally is elevated to at least 30 degrees for patients with oculoplastic, eye muscle, and enucleation surgeries. Care should be taken to prevent pressure on the operated eye.

If the patient has had an operation on only one eye or has only one eye bandaged, it is important to determine just how much sight exists in the unaffected eye. It is not safe to assume that the patient can see with the unoperated eye. The patient may agree to wear a patch on the unaffected eye, which serves to remind the nursing personnel that the patient is sightless and requires additional care. The nurse should tell the patient exactly what is expected of him or her.

Dressings

Dressings are often not required, especially after relatively minor procedures, topical anesthesia, or plastic ophthalmic surgery. Hemorrhage or excessive discharge is uncommon. A slight, blood-tinged, watery discharge from the eyes is not unusual and may be gently wiped from the face, taking care not to apply pressure to the eye. Although infrequent, hemorrhage may be a problem after enucleation, exenteration, or orbital surgery. If bleeding occurs in the PACU, the surgeon may be able to control it with pressure, but in some instances, the patient may need to return to the operating room.

Often one or both of the eyes are bandaged with sterile eye patches. If bandages are present, these should not be disturbed. The patient must be prevented from disturbing the bandage or inadvertently rubbing the eyes.

After enucleation, a firm pressure dressing is applied for 24 hours. An alternative to enucleation for treatment of ocular tumors is the use of iodine plaque irradiation. The iodine plaque is sutured over the base of the tumor under local anesthesia. The plaque remains in place for a calculated amount of time, depending on the strength of the iodine plaque and the size of the tumor. A lead shield is placed over the operative eye to protect the health care personnel and visitors from radiation exposure (Fig. 30-11). Whenever both eyes are bandaged, extra care must be taken to orient the patient and to provide reassurance. Eye shields made of clear plastic or perforated metal may be placed alone

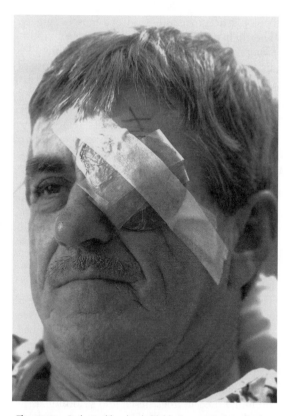

Fig. 30-11 Patient with a lead shield after surgical application of iodine plaque. *(Courtesy of Wills Eye Hospital, Philadelphia.)*

or over the dressing as an additional protection for the eye. Dressings should not be changed unless ordered by the surgeon, and if they are accidentally dislodged, they should be replaced and the physician notified. The tape used to hold eye patches or shields in place should not extend to the maxilla, because movement of the jaw may cause disruption of the dressing. The perianesthesia nurse should reinforce the shield as necessary.

Psychologic Aspects of Care

Perianesthesia care of ophthalmic surgery patients calls not only for keen physical assessment skills but also a serious sensitivity to the meaning of sight and a proactive, creative approach to promoting comfort and preventing complications. The perianesthesia nurse must be

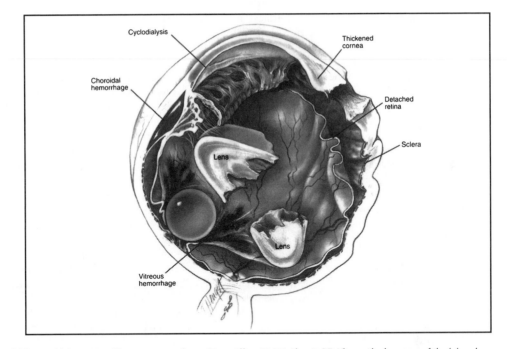

Fig. 30-12 Child's eye hit by a BB, with severe contusions. *(From Alfaro III DV, Liggett PE: Vitreoretinal surgery of the injured eye, Philadelphia, 1999, Lippincott-Raven.)*

prepared to provide significant support through both verbal communication and gentle touch. Unnecessary noise can be especially annoying to visually impaired patients and can heighten feelings of stress and pain. Promotion of a quiet, peaceful PACU environment will help to soothe patients who may be worried or nervous about the outcome regarding their vision.

Some patients may leave the PACU fully recovered from their anesthetic and elated with the immediate result of improved vision. Chen points out that for many patients with facial nerve paralysis who have corrective ptosis and brow ptosis surgery, results are very gratifying: "[p]atients' general appearance and psychologic well-being are all greatly improved, and their vision is preserved and protected as well."[16] Most patients, however, experience some degree of emotional distress and may require a great deal of empathy and reassurance.[17,18] Our eyes and the sense of sight are precious, and when sight is threatened by disease or surgery, we are understandably anxious and apprehensive. Injuries—

particularly those produced by imbedded foreign bodies—may provoke even greater anxiety for the patient who goes to surgery with the prognosis for visual acuity completely unknown (Fig. 30-12). It is important that the perianesthesia nurse be armed with factual information from the surgeon about expectations for the patient so that his or her reassurances are realistic. As eye surgery moves from the traditional hospital recovery room to more diverse practice settings, the PACU nurse's role is expanding; advocacy and interpersonal understanding are as important as hemodynamic monitoring and pain management.[13] A collaborative approach with other members of the perianesthesia team and a holistic picture of patients needs are crucial to optimal outcomes for ophthalmic surgical patients.

REFERENCES

1. Niehbuhr BS, Muenzen P: A study of perianesthesia nursing practice: the foundation for

newly revised CPAN and CAPA certification examinations, J Perianesth Nurs 16(3):163-173, 2001.

2. Elfervig LS, Elfervig JL: Proliferative diabetic retinopathy, Insight: The Journal of the American Society of Ophthalmic Registered Nurses 26(3), 88-91, 2001.

3. Shields JA, Shields CL, Demirci H et al: Experience with eyelid-sparing orbital exenteration: the 2000 Tullos O. Coston Lecture (electric version), J American Society of Ophthal Plast Reconstr Surg 17(5):355-361, 2001.

4. Boyd-Monk H, Augsburger JJ: Treatment of primary intraocular cancers: retinoblastoma and uveal malignant melanoma, J Ophthalmic Nurs Technol 16(4), 183-187, 1997.

5. Greenbaum S: Ocular anesthesia, Philadelphia, 1997, WB Saunders.

6. Mason G, Gacka-Hubler C: The surgical specialties—part 1: ophthalmic otolaryngologic, dental, and plastic reconstructive procedures. In N Burden: Ambulatory surgical nursing, Philadelphia, 1993, WB Saunders.

7. Hutchisson B, Nicoladis CB: Topical anesthesia: a new approach to cataract surgery, AORN J 74(3):340-350, 2001.

8. Movaghar M, Kodsi S, Merola C et al: Probing for nasolacrimal duct obstruction with intravenous propofol sedation, J AAPOS 4(3): 179-182, 2000.

9. Carlson K: Certification review for perianesthesia nursing, Philadelphia, 1996, WB Saunders.

10. Netlant PA: Cardiovascular effects of topical caretolol hydrochloride and timolol maleate in patients with ocular hypertension and primary open-angle glaucoma, American Journal of Ophthalmology 123(4):465-466, 1997.

11. Acquadro MA: Recovery room care and problems following ophthalmic and otolaryngologic surgery. In KE McGoldrick, editor: Anesthesia for opthalmic and otolaryngologic surgery, Philadelphia, 1992, WB Saunders.

12. Cioffi GA: Ophthalmology for the health care professional, Baltimore, 1997, Williams & Wilkins.

13. Wright KW: Textbook of ophthalmology, Baltimore, 1997, Williams & Wilkins.

14. Shields MB: Textbook of glaucoma, ed 4, Baltimore, 1998, Williams & Wilkins.

15. Spaeth GL: The use of antimetabolites with trabeculectomy: a critical appraisal, Journal of Glaucoma 10(3), 145-150, 2001.

16. Chen, WP: Occuloplastic surgery: the essentials, New York, 2001, Thieme Medical Publishers Inc.

17. Newell FW: Ophthalmology principles and concepts, St Louis, 1996, Mosby.

18. Scott IU, Schein OD, Feuer WJ et al: Emotional distress in patients with retinal disease, American Journal of Ophthalmology 131(5): 584-589, 2001.

31

CARE OF THE THORACIC SURGICAL PATIENT

Kim Litwack, PhD, RN, FAAN, CPAN, CAPA, CFNP

Thoracic surgery involves procedures in the structures within the chest cavity, including the lungs, heart, great vessels, and esophagus. In this chapter, discussion will center on procedures of the lungs and respiratory system. Specific postanesthesia care after cardiac surgery is discussed in Chapter 32; care after surgery of the great vessels is discussed in Chapter 33; and care after surgery of the esophagus is discussed in Chapter 37.

Lung surgery may be recommended for the diagnosis and treatment of:

Persistent cough
Hemoptysis
Wheezing
Obstruction
Abnormal chest x-ray
Cancer
Tumors (solitary pulmonary nodules)
Small areas of long-term infection (highly localized tuberculosis or mycobacterium)
Pockets of infection (abscess)
Permanently enlarged (dilated) bronchus (bronchiectasis)
Permanently enlarged (dilated) section of lung (lobar emphysema)
Permanently collapsed lung tissue (atelectasis)
Injuries with collapsed lung tissue (atelectasis, pneumothorax, hemothorax)
Correction of congenital or acquired chest wall deformities

DEFINITIONS

Atelectasis: collapse of the alveoli, caused primarily by obstruction of lower airways. Most commonly caused by accumulation of respiratory secretions but may also be caused by diminished lung volumes, tumors, prolonged bronchospasm, and foreign bodies.

Bronchoscopy: direct visualization of the tracheobronchial tree by use of a lighted scope (Fig. 31-1). It is used for diagnostic and therapeutic interventions to visualize structures of the tracheobronchial tree; to remove secretions, washings, mucus plugs or foreign bodies; and to perform a tissue biopsy or to apply medication. May be combined with laser (YAG) therapy for ablation of tracheal and bronchial obstructions. May be performed in the operating room, special procedures unit, or at the patient's bedside, depending upon the degree of urgency and the patient's status.

Chest tube: placement of a drainage tube into the intrapleural space to remove air and blood with the goal of restoring normal negative pressure and to allow re-expansion of the lung. Placed on the operative side following open chest procedures.

Chest wall reconstruction: repair of chest wall defects caused by trauma or tumor, by use of muscle or omentum (underlying abdominal tissue). Provides for protection of underlying structures and organs and provides support for respiration.

Decortication of the lung: removal of fibrous deposits or restrictive membranes on the visceral or parietal pleura that interfere with ventilatory action. Goal is to restore normal lung function.

Hemothorax: accumulation of blood or serosanguineous fluid or both within the pleural cavity, compromising lung expansion.

Lobectomy: removal of one or more lobes of the lung. Preferred procedure when cancerous lesion involves a single lobe of the lung. Used primarily in treatment of bronchial cancer. Also used in treatment of bronchiectasis, emphysematous blebs, large benign tumors, fungal infections, and congenital anomalies.

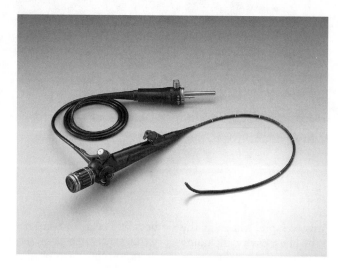

Fig. 31-1 Flexible fiber-optic bronchoscope. *(Courtesy Olympus America., Inc., Melville, NY.)*

Mediastinoscopy: direct visualization of lymph nodes or tumors at the tracheobronchial junction, subcarina, or upper lobe bronchi via a lighted scope. This is done by passing the mediastinoscope through a small incision at the suprasternal area and then down along the anterior course of the trachea. Diagnostic procedure for patients with identified changes on chest x-ray.

Needle biopsy: insertion of a needle with subsequent aspiration of lung tissue or fluid for diagnostic purposes. Generally performed under local anesthesia via a percutaneous approach.

Pneumonectomy: removal of an entire lung, most commonly for lung cancer when lobectomy cannot be performed for total removal of bronchial cancer.

Pneumothorax: accumulation of air or gas within the pleural cavity, thus compromising lung expansion. May occur as direct result of a thoracotomy incision or after chest wall trauma such as a stab wound.

Segmentectomy (segmental resection): excision of individual bronchovascular segments of the lobe of the lung with ligation of segmental branches of the pulmonary artery and vein and division of the segmental bronchus. Conserves healthy tissue while allowing for removal of localized lesion.

Sleeve resection: surgical removal of part of the bronchi, leaving healthy tissue for reanastomosis, thus preserving some tissue and lung function. Used primarily for metastatic disease in either the right or left upper bronchus.

Sternotomy: incision through the sternum.

Thoracentesis: insertion of a needle through the chest wall into the pleural space to remove either air or fluid to relieve lung compression or for diagnostic purposes. Removed fluid is evaluated for chemical, bacteriologic, and cellular composition. This procedure may be performed at the bedside, generally under local anesthesia.

Thoracoplasty/thoracostomy: removal of ribs or portions of the ribs to reduce the size of the thoracic space and to collapse a diseased lung.

Thoracotomy: incision into the chest cavity. May be used as a diagnostic tool to diagnose or stage cancer. Provides a definitive diagnosis in more than 90% of cases. Closed thoracotomy is used to place chest tubes or catheters for drainage of air or fluid to restore normal negative pressure within pleural space. It also may be used to create surgical access port for video-assisted lobectomy and other endoscopic procedures.

Transplantation: removal of diseased recipient lung(s) with immediate replacement of cadaveric donor lung(s).

Volume reduction surgery: incision and removal of those parts of the lung that are the most destroyed—most commonly from emphysema—to allow for full function of remaining lung structures.

Wedge resection: excision of a small, wedge-shaped section from the peripheral portion of the lobe of a lung. Commonly used to remove cancerous growths in the outer section of the lung to spare lung tissue and function.

ANESTHESIA

Invasive surgery involving the chest cavity is generally performed under general anesthesia, although diagnostic procedures such as bronchoscopy, needle biopsy, and thoracentesis are commonly performed under local (topical) anesthesia, often with small, titrated amounts of intravenous sedation. Epidural catheters may also be placed preoperatively for use during surgery and for extended postoperative pain control after pneumonectomy or lobectomy. Because these procedures all involve the airway in addition to anesthesia, patients will be asked to be NPO before any procedure.

Topical anesthesia involves the instillation or spray of a local anesthetic, commonly 4% lidocaine hydrochloride (Xylocaine), onto the laryngeal and pharyngeal surfaces. Although uncommon, toxic reactions and/or bronchospasm can occur; therefore emergency equipment should be readily available. Recovery of the patient after topical anesthesia requires airway assessment, ready availability of emergency resuscitation equipment, and the administration of humidified oxygen after the procedure. The patient must be given nothing by mouth until the pharyngeal and laryngeal reflexes have returned (2 to 4 hours). Patients should be advised to rest their voices following the procedure; in fact, the surgeon may prescribe a time interval for voice rest. Once the gag reflex has returned, throat lozenges and warm drinks may help to relieve the sore throat that inevitably follows bronchoscopy.

Epidural anesthesia involves placement of a catheter into the epidural space of the thoracic vertebrae with subsequent instillation of an infusion combination of narcotic and local anesthetic to achieve sensory blockade of pain without compromising motor function required for coughing, deep breathing, and ambulating. The catheter may be left in place for up to three days postoperatively for pain control, which may be regulated solely by medical personnel or may be patient-controlled. Epidural anesthesia is commonly used as an adjunct to general anesthesia.

General anesthesia involves the administration of some combination of inhalational anesthetics, intravenous anesthetics, benzodiazepines, narcotic analgesics, muscle relaxants, and reversal agents and aims to render the patient amnestic and pain-free. Somatic, autonomic, and endocrine reflexes are eliminated, and skeletal muscle relaxation is achieved. Because of the effects of general anesthesia on respiratory function and effort, in conjunction with a preexisting compromise in the respiratory system necessitating surgery, it is imperative that nursing care emphasize respiratory assessment, monitoring, and application of prompt intervention if evidence of compromise is noted postoperatively.

PERIANESTHESIA NURSING CARE AFTER THORACIC PROCEDURES

Positioning

Positioning after thoracic procedures varies; therefore it is important to check medical orders. The patient may be kept in a side-lying position until awake, and then the head of the bed is elevated 30 to 45 degrees to facilitate ventilation. This position allows the diaphragm to drop into normal position, thus enhancing lung expansion and, if present, facilitating chest tube drainage. After lobectomy, segmentectomy, and wedge resection, the patient can be turned freely from side-to-side to allow full expansion of lung tissue on both the operative and nonoperative side. After pneumonectomy, the patient may be placed on the back or on the operative side. The patient is *not* positioned side-lying on the nonoperative side, because the mediastinum is no longer confined by lung tissue and may move freely, thereby compressing the remaining lung or creating traction or torsion of the vena cava. Additionally, if the bronchial stump were to rupture and bleed profusely, the unaffected lung would be compressed by secretions from the pneumonectomy site.

Position changes are important following thoracic surgery. If the patient has an outpatient procedure, such as bronchoscopy, position changes will be made independently. If the patient has a chest tube in place, the perianesthesia nurse will need to assist with position changes to ensure system patency and patient comfort. Position changes also include early return to ambulation, with the goal of promoting patient comfort, drainage of secretions, and prevention of venous stasis and atelectasis.

Respiratory Assessment and Care

On arrival, the patient will be placed on oxygen via the delivery system required per the extent of the patient's surgery, preexisting medical conditions, and need for continued assistance. This may include a nasal cannula after bronchoscopy, face-mask or face-tent, or mechanical ventilation. Delivered oxygen should be given with humidification to help thin tracheobronchial secretions, thus permitting the ciliary mechanism and coughing to clear the airway.

The perianesthesia nurse should assess respiratory function on arrival, beginning with inspection of the patient's respiratory effort and ease of effort. Respiratory rate is noted; 10 to 20 breaths per minute is considered normal. A rate of greater than 20 is considered to be tachypnea and may be caused by pain, hypoxemia, hypoventilation, or secretions. The use of pulse oximetry will help to quickly assess for hypoxemia. A rate of less than 10 is considered bradypnea, which may occur secondarily to anesthetic and narcotic administration. The patient may also arrive in the postanesthesia care unit (PACU) intubated, either on a T-piece—if respiratory effort is sufficiently present but loss of airway patency is a concern—or intubated on mechanical ventilation—if airway and ventilation are concerns.

Breath sounds should be assessed for depth, clarity, and the presence of adventitious sounds—including crackles, rhonchi, or a pleural friction rub. The use of accessory muscles should be noted. Accessory muscle actions include nasal flaring, suprasternal retractions, diaphragmatic breathing, and intercostal retractions.

The regularity of breathing is assessed as regular, irregular, or ventilated. Ventilator settings are confirmed, and if arterial blood gases are drawn, adjustments are made—if necessary—after assessment of results. Ongoing pulse oximetry monitoring is necessary for any patient who has undergone a thoracic surgical procedure.

If the patient is intubated, it may be to protect the airway, to assist ventilation or to provide a means for management of secretions through suctioning. Tracheal suctioning of the postthoracic surgical patient may be necessary to assist in removing accumulated secretions.

Respiratory Management

The modified stir-up regimen—including positioning, mobilization, SMI, cascade coughing, and pain relief—is especially important for a patient recovering from a thoracic surgical procedure. Positioning and mobilization have already been discussed. The SMI and cascade coughing exercises are the easiest ways to maintain a patent airway after the patient is reactive to verbal commands. Preoperative teaching is extremely important; the patient who has been well educated and knows what is expected of him or her postoperatively can cooperate by taking a deep breath, holding it for 3 seconds and then exhaling (the SMI), and then taking a deep breath and coughing throughout exhalation (the cascade cough). Effective preoperative teaching will enhance the effectiveness of the modified stir-up regimen even if the patient is not fully reactive.

Once the patient is fully conscious, rigorous SMIs and cascade coughing are continued every hour. This regimen is most effective with the patient sitting up to allow full lung expansion. If the patient cannot sit up, raise the head of the bed and have him or her bend the knees to relax the abdominal muscles. The patient is instructed to inspire deeply and hold the breath for 3 seconds to expand the lungs and relax the abdominal muscles so that the belly pouches out. Four to five SMIs are taken, and then the patient is instructed to perform the cascade cough to clear the tracheobronchial tree of accumulated secretions. After the patient performs about three cascade coughs, a "forceful" cough will then usually be produced spontaneously, thus clearing the airways of secretions. Endotracheal secretions are usually excessive after thoracic surgery because of the tracheobronchial tree during the operation and intubation, decreased lung ventilation, and a decreased cough reflex. Pain or fear—or both—may interfere with the patient's ability to perform the SMI and cascade cough.

Pain Management

Although pain following bronchoscopy will usually be limited to a sore throat, the thoracic surgical patient should be told preoperatively to expect a fair amount of postoperative incisional pain. The patient should also be told that pain relief measures will be available and may include epidural analgesia, patient-controlled analgesia, and nurse-administered narcotics. Pain medications should be given in adequate doses and in a timely manner because pain interferes with the needed activities required postoperatively—including deep breathing, coughing and progressive mobilization. As narcotics can diminish respiratory function, care must be taken in their administration, especially after general anesthesia.

In addition to analgesics, pain relief measures can include using a pillow to splint the incision while coughing. Because coughing is the most effective way to clear secretions, pain medication should be offered and given regularly.

Fluid Management

Optimal hydration after thoracic surgery is important to prevent the increased viscosity of mucus to facilitate the removal of secretions. Oral fluids may be started as soon as the patient recovers from anesthesia and the danger of nausea and vomiting has passed. Intravenous fluids are also used after more extensive surgery, to ensure hydration and to continue fluid replacement for losses in the operating room. Removal of large segments or of a total lung (pneumonectomy) significantly reduces the size of the pulmonary circulation, thus predisposing the patient to the development of pulmonary edema if fluids are administered too rapidly or in too large a volume. The surgeon will write postoperative fluid orders. Accurate intake and output records are particularly important.

Chest Tube Management

Surgery on the structures of the chest that involves entry into the thoracic cavity will result in air entry and the development of a pneumothorax (atmospheric pressure admitted into the pleural cavity and collapse of the lung). Placement of a pleural chest tube after open-chest procedures allows for drainage of air and blood, restoration of normal negative pressure, and re-expansion of the collapsed lung. As blood is heavier than air, blood will pool in the lower portion of the pleural space, whereas air will accumulate in the upper portion. Therefore two chest tubes usually will be placed through the chest wall via a stab wound or via incision. An upper or anterior chest tube is placed in the second intercostal space to allow for air removal. A lower or posterior chest tube is placed in the sixth to eighth intercostal space to allow for drainage from the pleural space (Fig. 31-2). The chest tubes will be sutured in place with purse-string sutures, and covered with a dressing. The chest tube insertion site should be palpated for the presence of crepitus (also known as subcuta-

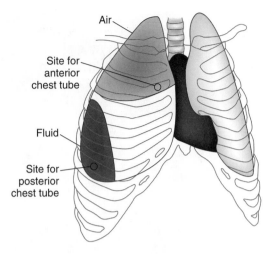

Fig. 31-2 Because air rises to the top of the cavity, chest tube placement for treatment of a pneumothorax is at the second intercostal space, close to the sternum. Chest tube placement for fluid removal is generally at the level of the 6 to 8 lateral intercostal space because this is where fluid will collect.

neous emphysema) caused by air trapping in subcutaneous tissue. Crepitus feels like crunchy cereal under the skin. If noted, the surgeon should be notified for probable resecuring of the chest tube.

The chest tubes will be connected to a drainage system that uses positive pressure, gravity, and suction to facilitate evacuation of air and fluid to re-expand the collapsed lung. The air trapped in the chest creates the positive pressure. Gravity assists primarily in fluid evacuation, and suction, when applied, facilitates removal of both air and fluid. Suction is generally established at 20 cm negative pressure unless specifically ordered differently. Wall units will have a manometer in place to allow for correct setting of suction pressure. Once the air and fluid are removed, the visceral and parietal pleura are brought back together again, and the pressure in the interpleural space becomes negative once again, thus re-expanding the lung.

In the past, drainage systems ranged from one-bottle to two-bottle to three-bottle systems, all with water seal to draw out air and fluid, thus allowing for re-expansion of the lung. These systems had to be set up by nursing personnel,

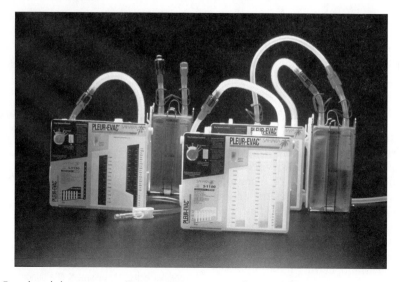

Fig. 31-3 Pleur-Evac chest drainage systems. *(Courtesy Genzyme Corporation, Cambridge, Mass.)*

which included gathering the required number of bottles, establishing a system for measurement, and maintaining sterility. Cumbersome in nature and subject to breakage, they have been replaced in most systems with disposable, prefabricated chest drainage units such as the Pleur-Evac or Atrium system (Fig. 31-3).

The principles of positive pressure, gravity, and suction still apply to these systems, yet they are simpler to use and transport and are associated with a lower rate of infection and system disruption. The pleural drainage system has three basic compartments, each with its own specific function. The first compartment, the collection chamber, receives air and fluid from the chest cavity. This compartment is vented to the second chamber, known as the water-seal chamber. This chamber acts as a one-way valve so that air can enter from—but not back into—the collection chamber. If bubbling is noted in this chamber, the lung has not re-expanded. The third chamber is the suction control chamber, which is used to apply controlled suction to the system to facilitate evacuation of air and fluid and to promote re-expansion of the lung. Some of these units have even been designed to allow for reinfusion of collected drained blood for autotransfusion.

As the goal of chest tube placement is evaluation of air and fluid, the system must remain patent. The perianesthesia nurse must ensure patency of the chest tubes, drainage tubing, and the system through periodic, regular assessments. A chest x-ray is often performed on admission to the PACU to ensure placement and lung function. Proper functioning of the system is evidenced by fluctuation or bubbling of the fluid in the water seal tubing in response to the patient's respiration. If no fluctuation is noted, the system should be evaluated for proper functioning. The tubing must not kink and should form a straight line from patient to collection unit to allow for unobstructed gravitational flow. "Milking" or "stripping" the chest tube may dislodge clots of blood blocking the tubing. This should be done in the direction away from the patient, toward the drainage system to prevent forcing clots back into the pleural space. If the system shows no fluctuation/bubbling with respiration and the tubing has been deemed clear, the physician should be notified, especially in the immediate postoperative period. In the latter days of recovery, the absence of fluctuation/bubbling signals re-expansion of the lung, with further evidence provided by full return of breath sounds and chest x-ray. However, in the PACU, failure of the system will prevent lung re-expansion. Any acute respiratory difficulty or pain should be referred immediately to the surgeon.

Complications

Risks of General Anesthesia. The risks of general anesthesia for any patient—regardless of the underlying medical condition and surgical procedure—include the potential for respiratory and cardiovascular compromise. In the presence of underlying pulmonary disease and surgery that involves the thoracic cavity, the potential for respiratory compromise—including hypoxemia, hypoventilation and atelectasis—increases greatly. The perianesthesia nurse should be prepared to evaluate for respiratory and ventilatory adequacy and to intervene with appropriate interventions if compromise is noted. This may include the need to simply stimulate the patient to take deep breaths, to increase the concentration of oxygen being delivered, or to anticipate and assist with reintubation if necessary.

Wound Infection. As with any surgical procedure, the risk of infection is possible. Prophylactic antibiotics may be given for major thoracic surgical procedures, including lobectomy and pneumonectomy, and will be used if prolonged postoperative mechanical ventilation is anticipated.

Bleeding. After bronchoscopy, bleeding should be limited to no more than lightly pink-tinged or slightly blood-streaked sputum. Grossly bloody sputum and coughing up frank blood should be reported to the surgeon and anesthesia provider immediately. After a more invasive procedure such as lobectomy or pneumonectomy, the surgical site must be inspected for bleeding and the chest tube for the presence of bloody drainage. If chest tube drainage seems excessive (greater than 100 cc/hour) or does not decrease in volume over time or if fresh bleeding is noted, the physician should be notified to evaluate for hemorrhage. Even if drainage is excessive, the chest tube should never be clamped unless specifically ordered. Clamping of the chest tube may result in the development of a tension pneumothorax, which is considerably more dangerous than an open pneumothorax.

Pneumonia. Although pneumonia is unlikely to develop in the immediate postoperative period, diminished ventilatory effort and prolonged bedrest are strong predictors of pneumonia potential. The patient should be encouraged on arrival to the PACU to take deep breaths, to cascade cough, and, if ordered, to use the incentive spirometer to prevent atelectasis and pneumonia. The use of sterile technique when suctioning is essential.

Worsening of Existing Heart Problems. Underlying cardiac disease should be carefully evaluated and documented before surgery. Any patient with preexisting cardiac disease should have continuous ECG monitoring in the PACU because these patients commonly develop cardiac dysrhythmias. These dysrhythmias may range from benign to life-threatening. Sinus tachycardia and atrial fibrillation are the most commonly seen dysrhythmias in the early recovery phases.

BIBLIOGRAPHY

Barash P, Cullen B, Stoelting R: Clinical Anesthesia, ed 4, Philadelphia, 2000, Lippincott Williams & Wilkins.

Benumof J, Saidman L: Anesthesia & perioperative complications, ed 2, St Louis, 1999, Mosby.

Bernard L: The pulmonary surgical patient. In K Litwack, editor: Core curriculum for postanesthesia nursing practice, ed 3, Philadelphia, 1995, WB Saunders.

Carroll P: Nursing the thoracotomy patient, RN 55(6): 34-43, 1995.

Carroll P: Chest tubes made easy, RN 55(3): 46-55, 1995.

Drain C: Pathophysiology of the respiratory system related to anesthesia, CRNA: The Clinical Forum for Nurse Anesthetists 7(4):181-192, 1996.

Gordon P, Norton J, Merrell R: Refining chest tube management: analysis of the state of practice, Dimens Crit Care Nurs 14(1):1:6-12, 1995.

Kozier B, Erb G: Monitoring a patient with chest drainage, techniques in clinical nursing ed 2, Menlo Park, Calif, 1993, Addison-Wesley.

Litwack K: Postanesthesia care nursing, ed 2, St Louis, 1995, Mosby.

Longnecker D, Tinker J, Morgan G: Principles and practice of anesthesiology, ed 2, St Louis, 1998, Mosby.

Martin J: Positioning in anesthesia and surgery, ed 3, St Louis, 1997, Mosby.

Miller R, editor: Anesthesia, ed 5, New York, 2000, Churchill Livingstone.

Murray J, Nadel J: Textbook of respiratory medicine, ed 3, Philadelphia, 2001, WB Saunders.

Nagelhout J, Zaglaniczny K: Nurse anesthesia, ed 2, Philadelphia, 2001, WB Saunders.

Norman M et al: Improved lung function and quality of life following increased elastic recoil after lung volume reduction surgery in emphysema, Respiratory Medicine 92:653-658, 1998.

O'Hanlon N. Clinical savvy: commonly asked questions about chest tubes, Am J Nurs 5:60-64, 1996.

Thys D, Schwartz A, Hillel Z: Textbook of cardiothoracic anesthesiology, New York, 2001, McGraw-Hill Professional.

Wolfe W: Complications of thoracic surgery: recognition and management, St. Louis, 1992, Mosby.

WEB RESOURCES

www.ahealthyme.com
www. cts.usc.edu
www.hopkinsmedicine.org/jhtop/Surgery/Surgical_Approaches/surgical_approaches.html
www. drkoop.com/conditions/ency/article
www.nhlbi.nih.gov
www.lungusa.org
www.cancer.org

32

CARE OF THE CARDIAC SURGICAL PATIENT

Karen "Toby" Haghenbeck, PhD, RN, C, CCRN
Karen D. Keeler, RN, BSN, CCRN, CEN

The concept of cardiac surgery as a viable option for patients with heart disease or trauma did not develop until the late 1800s, largely because of the emotional as well as technical difficulties inherent in the concepts of the heart itself. The perceived seat of the soul and a vital hemodynamic structure, the heart was viewed as untouchable on both fronts. The first surgical manipulation occurred in 1896, when Rehn successfully closed a stab wound in the ventricle of an unconscious man. Since then, success in the treatment of cardiac trauma has continued, and major developments have occurred in many aspects of treatment. In the 1950s, the development of the cardiopulmonary bypass machine and techniques made open heart surgery a viable option. Today, procedures ranging from valve and myocardial structure repair and replacement and direct manipulation of the coronary arteries to transplantation, implantation of assist devices, and total mechanical replacement of the heart are common.

In many institutions, patients are transferred directly from surgery to a special cardiac surgical intensive care unit (CSICU), where they remain for 1 to 3 days before transfer to a regular nursing unit. During this period these patients require intensive hemodynamic monitoring and rapid intervention to prevent many of their normal postoperative states (e.g., hypothermia and hypertension) from progressing to postoperative complications (e.g., myocardial infarction and hemorrhage). Discharge from the hospital usually occurs within 7 to 10 days after the surgical intervention.

The length of the preoperative period and thus patient preparation time can vary greatly.

The postanesthesia care unit (PACU) nurse should be aware of the level of knowledge, understanding demonstrated, and anxieties that both the patient and the family are experiencing. It is helpful—although not always practical—for the PACU nurse to provide the preoperative instruction for the patient and family or to make an introductory visit to them before surgery.

This chapter is designed to familiarize the PACU nurse with postoperative care for the cardiac patient. Additional study is a necessity, and the reader is directed to the reference list at the end of this chapter for sources that discuss the continuum of care needed by the patient hospitalized for cardiac surgery.

DEFINITIONS

Annuloplasty: a surgical technique in which the annulus of the valve is manipulated to decrease the size of the valvular orifice and thus limit valvular regurgitation; this can be accomplished by suturing portions of the valvular annulus. More recently, this has been done by using a plication ring, which is a cloth-covered flexible metal ring that is placed over the valve orifice, with the annulus of the valve attached to the ring (Fig. 32-1). This procedure is most commonly performed on tricuspid and mitral valves.

Aortic regurgitation: a condition that occurs when the aortic valve does not totally close because the cusps do not completely approximate with each other during diastole. This can occur as a result of congenital or rheumatic heart disease, infective endocarditis, trauma, aortic dissection, or Marfan's syndrome. This lesion is also known as aortic insufficiency.

Aortic stenosis: a narrowing of the orifice of the aortic valve itself or of the areas adjacent to the aortic valve.

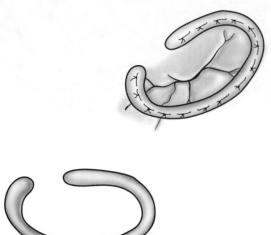

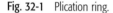

Fig. 32-1 Plication ring.

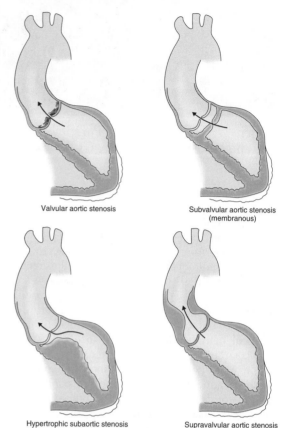

Valvular aortic stenosis

Subvalvular aortic stenosis
(membranous)

Hypertrophic subaortic stenosis

Supravalvular aortic stenosis

Fig. 32-2 Schematic representation of various types of left-ventricular outflow tract obstructions.

These narrowings create an obstruction to left-ventricular outflow and can be generally classified as three different types: valvular, subvalvular, and supravalvular. In the most common type, the valvular, there is a fusion of the commissures of the valve leaflets that leaves only a small opening. This lesion can occur as a congenital process, as in the bicuspid valve, or as an acquired disease process, such as in rheumatic heart disease. The second most common type is a subvalvular aortic stenosis. This lesion is usually caused by a fibrinous diaphragm located a few millimeters below the valvular leaflets. Another type of subvalvular stenosis occurs when the intraventricular septum becomes hypertrophied and creates an obstruction to left-ventricular outflow. This lesion is known as idiopathic hypertrophic subaortic stenosis or hypertrophic obstructive cardiomyopathy. The most infrequently seen form of aortic stenosis is the supravalvular type, in which the aorta is constricted just above the ostia of the coronary arteries. This lesion may be considered a coarctation of the ascending aorta. Figure 32-2 illustrates the different types of left-ventricular outflow tract obstructions.

Aortic valve disease: a disease that is usually caused by rheumatic involvement of the aortic valve in which the valve cusps become thick and fibrotic or that is the result of a congenital bicuspid valve. Aortic valve disease places increased amounts of work on the left ventricles, thus resulting in increased afterload, left-ventricular hypertrophy, and decreased compliance.

The left-ventricular cavity becomes reduced, and the atrial contribution to cardiac output becomes important to maintain adequate preload and forward flow of blood and to contribute to a more forceful ventricular contraction. Loss of this atrial contribution, or "kick," through the development of atrial arrhythmias can result in a marked decrease in cardiac output with resultant pulmonary edema.

Aortocoronary bypass grafts: see myocardial revascularization.

Atrial septal defect (ASD): a hole through the atrial septum. An ostium secundum defect is a defect high in the atrial septum for which no etiologic factors are known. Some secundum defects are associated with anomalous pulmonary veins returning oxygenated blood into the superior vena cava or into the right atrium. An ostium primum lesion is a defect low in the atrial septum and may involve the tricuspid and mitral valves and the upper portion of the intraventricular septum. Ostium primum defects develop after arrested embryonic development of the endocardial cushions that normally meet with the ventricular and atrial septa to form the four chambers of the heart. Atrioventricularis communis is a severe lesion that is caused by extensive nondevelopment of the endocardial cushions. In this lesion there is an ostium primum defect; portions of the mitral and tricuspid leaflets form a common valve; and a ventricular septal defect exists. Both ostium primum defects and atrioventricularis communis are also known as endocardial cushion defects or atrioventricular canal defects because of their similar embryonic origins. Closure of septal defects is accomplished by suturing or patching the defect with a graft of pericardium or prosthetic material. Appropriate manipulation and reconstruction of the involved valves are also performed if necessary. Anomalous pulmonary veins are diverted to the left atrium. Figure 32-3 illustrates the areas affected by these lesions.

Balloon valvotomy/valvuloplasty: an invasive, nonsurgical procedure that consists of dilatation of a cardiac valve by inflation of a balloon passed by catheter technique across the valve. It is an important component of therapy for children, young adults and for patients who are too elderly or medically compromised to withstand an operation.[1] Balloon valvotomy (i.e., dilatation of a cardiac valve by inflation of a balloon) is most often performed on the mitral valve. Complications of valvotomy include development of mitral regurgitation, cardiac perforation, and cerebral embolus.

Cardiac catheterization: a technique in which a radiopaque plastic catheter is inserted into the right or left heart via a percutaneous puncture or a cutdown into the femoral or brachial artery or vein to obtain pressure, volume, and oxygen saturation determinations from the intracardiac chambers and the great blood vessels (i.e., superior and inferior vena cava, pulmonary artery, and aorta). In addition, injection of a contrast medium can be used to assist in identifying intracardiac and intracoronary artery structural alterations as well as in obtaining cardiac output and ejection fraction values and wall motion studies. Generally, a "right-heart" catheterization yields data concerning the inferior and superior vena cava, the right atrium and ventricle, and the pulmonary artery. A "left-heart" catheterization yields information concerning the left atrium and ventricle, the aorta, and the coronary arteries if a selective coronary arteriography study is performed.

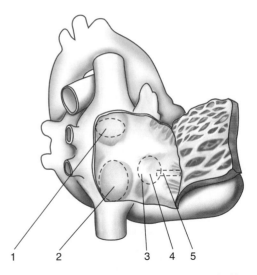

Fig. 32-3 Schematic representation of areas involved with various atrial septal defects: (*1*) anomalous pulmonary vein; (*2*) ostium secundum defects; (*3*) ostium primum defects; (*4*) ventricular septal defect; and (*5*) leaflet of mitral valve.

Cardioplegia: a paralysis of the heart or cardiac arrest. The purpose of cardioplegia is protection against ischemic injury during the aortic cross-clamp period during cardiac surgery. Although different methods can be used to induce this arrest, the term cardioplegia is most commonly used to refer to hyperkalemic solutions that produce this arrest effect. The solutions may be administered with antegrade infusion, retrograde infusion, or a combination of both techniques. Infused into the aortic root, these solutions enter the ostia of the coronary arteries and perfuse the myocardium. In addition to potassium, these solutions can have numerous additives, such as other electrolytes, blood, and antiarrhythmic agents. The purpose of these other agents is to provide a physiologically balanced environment, to provide energy substrates, and to decrease ventricular irritability.

Cardiopulmonary bypass (CPB): a temporary substitution for the heart and lungs by an oxygenator pump. With CPB, direct visualization and manipulation of a noncontracting heart are achieved. At the same time, blood is oxygenated; carbon dioxide is removed; and systemic blood flow is sustained. Venous access is achieved by placing cannulas in the venae cavae and the right atrium. Blood is then circulated through the CPB circuit where it becomes oxygenated. It is then

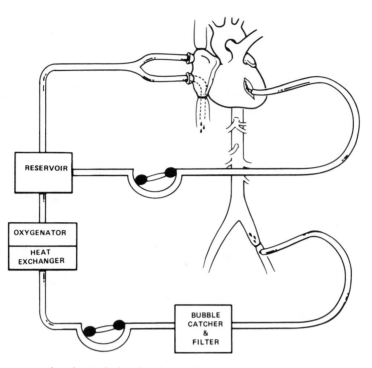

Fig. 32-4   Schematic representation of a standard cardiopulmonary bypass circuit.

returned to the patient via arterial cannulas that are located in the aorta or femoral or iliac arteries. Commonly used types of oxygenators are the rotating disk, the bubble, and the membrane (Fig. 32-4).

Coarctation of the aorta: a narrowing of the aorta that can occur anywhere between the aortic arch and the femoral bifurcation. There are generally two types of coarctations: preductal and postductal (Fig. 32-5). In the preductal type, the pulmonary artery communicates with the distal aorta through a ductus. In this situation, blood flow from the right ventricle and the pulmonary artery supplies the lower half of the body, whereas flow from the left ventricle and the aorta supplies the upper torso. With this anomaly other concurrent intracardiac defects, such as ventricular septal defects and transposition of the great arteries, are usually present. In the postductal type, there is a localized constriction, usually just distal to the left subclavian artery. This narrowing is usually followed by poststenotic dilatation. Correction is accomplished by excising the coarctation and then performing an end-to-end anastomosis, with or without a graft, to establish continuity. In the preductal type, appropriate correction of the associated intracardiac defects is also performed.

Commissurotomy: the opening or separation of fused valvular commissures. Either closed or open commissurotomy may be performed. In mitral stenosis, closed commissurotomy with a transventricular dilator can be performed. In this procedure a dilator is inserted through the left-atrial appendage and then through the mitral valve. The valve is then dilated to the appropriate degree. If the patient is suspected of having a left-atrial thrombus that could be easily embolized, an open procedure is performed with both a dilator and digital pressure.

Hypothermia: the elective cooling of the patient during cardiac surgery. Two general methods are used: systemic and local. Systemic cooling is accomplished by lowering the patient's temperature to 25°C to 30°C with the use of the CPB circuit. Local cooling refers to cooling the myocardium to levels of 0°C to 10°C. This can be accomplished by placing an ice slush solution in the pericardial area as well as by administering a cold cardioplegic solution. The purpose of both the local and the systemic use of hypothermia is to diminish cellular demands and limit ischemic injury.

Implantable cardioverter-defibrillator (ICD): a device, first introduced in 1980, developed to provide a shock

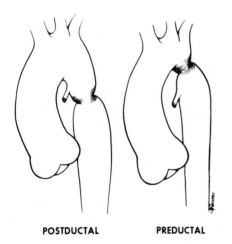

POSTDUCTAL   **PREDUCTAL**

Fig. 32-5 Postductal and preductal types of coarctation of the aorta.

to the heart for tachycardia above a predetermined rate, has the capability of providing bradycardia and tachycardia therapy.

Class I indications according to the American College of Cardiology and the American Heart Association for ICD implantation include (1) spontaneous sustained ventricular tachycardia (VT); (2) cardiac arrest not due to a reversible cause; (3) nonsustained VT or ventricular fibrillation (VF) with coronary artery disease, previous myocardial infarction, left ventricular dysfunction and inducible VF or sustained VT at EP study that is not suppressed by a class I antiarrhythmic drug, and syncope of undetermined origin with clinically relevant, hemodynamically significant sustained VT or VF induced at EP study when drug therapy is ineffective, not tolerated, or not preferred.[2] The system consists of a pulse generator and lead system with shocking electrodes for cardioversion and defibrillation and electrodes for sensing and pacing the heart. Before 1993, a two-patch technique was used; the patches were placed over the diaphragmatic surface and over the posterobasal portion of the left ventricle via anterior thoracotomy. Some patients may still have this system in place.

Transvenous implantation of the ICU may be done in the operating room or the cardiac catheterization laboratory. External defibrillation pads are usually placed on the patient's chest and all connections verified before draping. Testing of the sensing and cardioversion/defibrillation thresholds is performed by inducing VT and VF. If sufficient, the generator is turned on and tested for adequate sensing and cardioversion-defibrillation. If defibrillation is adequate, the generator is turned off and placed in a pocket in the left upper chest area and the incision is closed.

The ICD is activated when the patient is transferred out of the PACU, ICU, or cardiac catheterization laboratory. Complications are rare, and studies have shown 98% freedom from sudden death at 1 year and 94% at 5 years.

Mechanical assist devices: these devices can be divided into two general types: temporary assist and permanent assist. The purpose of temporary assist devices is to provide the failing heart with support over a short period, such as hours or days. Examples of temporary assist devices include the intraaortic balloon pump (IABP) and the external left-ventricular and right-ventricular assist devices (LVAD, RVAD).

The intraaortic balloon is a sausage-shaped balloon mounted on a catheter that is inserted most often through the femoral artery and is then placed distal to the left subclavian artery in the descending thoracic aorta. The action of the balloon is to inflate during diastole and deflate during systole. Inflation allows the blood to be pushed cephalad into the aortic root, which increases coronary artery blood supply. Deflation of the balloon just before systolic ejection creates a negative intraaortic pressure and therefore decreases afterload. Afterload is the impedance against which the ventricle must work to open the aortic valve. By increasing coronary blood flow and decreasing afterload, the total work of the heart is reduced, thereby providing an environment that supports the recovery of a failing myocardium.

Another variety of temporary cardiac assist devices, the external ventricular assist device, is indicated for use in patients with markedly impaired ventricular function who, following cardiac surgery, develop ventricular failure unresponsive to pharmacologic and IABP support. Although these devices vary in their specific design, their technique generally consists of removing blood via cannulas from the left atrium or ventricle and reinfusing it into the aortic root. This technique bypasses the ventricle and therefore requires no ventricular contraction. Blood flow in these systems can be either pulsatile or nonpulsatile and can be propelled by roller, centrifugal, or pneumatically powered drive systems. In these temporary systems, the cannulas and pumps are most often situated outside the chest cavity.

Research on a permanently implantable mechanical heart assist device is advancing in two directions. The totally artificial heart, developed by Jarvik at the University of Utah, has arrived at the stage of clinical use. This system consists of two pneumatically driven, elliptic, artificial ventricular chambers. Blood flows through these chambers in a manner similar to that in the natural heart, going from the right side through the lungs and then into the left chamber. At this point the blood is ejected into the systemic circulation. The pumping action in the chambers is supplied by a pusher-plate system that is controlled by a console external to the patient. The chambers are attached to the console via drive lines that exit from the patient in the abdominal region. This system requires complete excision of the natural myocardium. The other thrust in the development of a permanent artificial device is toward a permanently implantable LVAD in which the natural heart would remain in place while cannulas and a pump system divert blood flow from the left atrium or ventricle into the aorta. Implanted in the chest cavity, this device would also require external drive lines and a drive system. The advantage to this system is that if there were a catastrophic failure of the artificial pump, the natural pump—the heart—could maintain the patient until arrival at a medical facility. This device currently has numerous successes in animal models. For both of these systems, technology to eliminate the cumbersome drive systems is less than half a decade away.

Minimally invasive coronary artery bypass grafting: an operation that uses a smaller incision than usual and sometimes without cardiopulmonary bypass. Minimally invasive CABG reduces operative trauma, speeds patient recovery, allows the patient faster return to normal activities, and reduces costs. Two categories of minimally invasive CABG are (1) beating heart CABG (performed without CPB); and (2) port-access CABG performed with CPB and the use of femoral access for arterial and venous cannulation. The procedure is still evolving, and long-term data are not yet available.

Mitral regurgitation: a condition that occurs when the mitral valve does not totally close because the leaflets do not completely approximate with each other during diastole. This lesion can occur as a result of a rheumatic process in which the leaflets and the chordae tendineae are progressively shortened. The ischemia or infarction that is associated with coronary artery disease can cause a rupture or elongation of the papillary muscles or the chordae tendineae and also create a regurgitant state. In addition, connective tissue disorders, syphilis, Marfan's syndrome, and systemic lupus erythematosus can produce this state by their effect on the papillary muscles and on the chordae.

Mitral stenosis: a narrowing of the normal aperture of the mitral valve due to one or a combination of the following: a growth of rheumatic nodules on the valve where the leaflets meet, a thickening of the valves, a fusion of the commissures, or a shortening and thickening of the chordae tendineae. It is most commonly seen as a consequence of rheumatic heart disease.

Myocardial protection techniques: techniques or procedures designed to expedite the surgical procedure and to limit the amount of ischemic tissue injury that can occur. These techniques and procedures consist of the following:

1. Electrical arrest of the myocardium with alternating current during diastole. This allows a quiet operative field, which expedites surgical repair and hence limits ischemic time.
2. Anoxic arrest, produced by crossclamping the aorta. The effect of this technique is similar to that of electrical arrest of the myocardium with alternating current during diastole.
3. Hypothermia, both local and systemic, which serves to decrease cellular metabolism and thus limits ischemic damage (see Hypothermia).
4. Chemical cardioplegia, the infusion into the aortic root of electrolyte, pharmacologic, or blood solutions that assist in chemically arresting the myocardium. This also limits the amount of cellular damage (see Cardioplegia). In addition to these techniques, care is taken to prevent VF because this arrhythmia increases wall tension and oxygen consumption.

Myocardial revascularization: surgical intervention in which blood flow is diverted past significant obstructions in the coronary arteries to inadequately perfused myocardium distal to the obstruction. This allows adequate oxygenation of these ischemic sections. Most often, portions of the saphenous vein harvested from the patient's leg are used as the conduits for blood flow. One portion of the vein is anastomosed in an end-to-side fashion to the aorta, and the other end is similarly anastomosed to the coronary artery distal to the obstruction (Fig. 32-6). In addition to the saphenous vein, the right and left internal mammary arteries are well suited for myocardial revascularization. Arising from the aorta, these vessels extend along the inside of the chest wall. For revascularization purposes, they are distally dissected off the chest wall and are left attached proximally to the aorta. Their distal ends are then attached to vessels on their respective sides. Other conduit vessels that are attached in the same manner

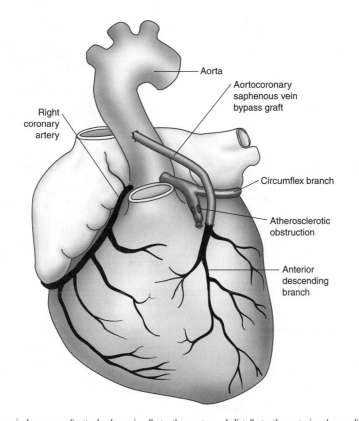

Aorta

Aortocoronary saphenous vein bypass graft

Right coronary artery

Circumflex branch

Atherosclerotic obstruction

Anterior descending branch

Fig. 32-6 Saphenous vein bypass graft attached proximally to the aorta and distally to the anterior descending coronary artery past the atherosclerotic obstruction.

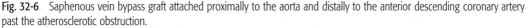

as the saphenous vein include portions of the cephalic vein and of a specially processed human umbilical vein. Bypass grafts are usually performed on the major coronary arteries, such as the right coronary artery, the two major branches of the left coronary artery, the left anterior descending artery, or the circumflex artery. However, grafts can be attached to any vessel that has a 1-mm diameter. Because of this, other vessels—such as the diagonal artery or other branches of the major arteries (e.g., the posterior descending artery of the right coronary artery)—also can be revascularized. Myocardial revascularization is also known as coronary artery bypass or aortocoronary grafting.

Patent ductus arteriosus (PDA): a duct between the pulmonary artery and the aorta. This structure, which is normally present in fetal life, usually closes within 1 or 2 weeks after birth. Failure to close can predispose the patient to the development of pulmonary hypertension or cardiac failure. Closure can be surgically achieved by ligation of the ductus or by division of the ductus followed by oversewing of the ends.

Percutaneous transluminal coronary angioplasty (PTCA): a widely accepted nonsurgical treatment modality for acute or chronically obstructed coronary arteries. The exact mechanism in which angioplasty improves vessel patency is still debatable, but it appears to restore patency by compression and rupture of the atherosclerotic plaque by creating a crack or fracture down to the internal elastic membrane. These "cracks" that extend from the lumen appear to improve vessel patency by creating new channels for coronary blood flow. Healing at the angioplasty site may, in itself, mimic the original atherosclerotic plaque, thus causing a restenosis of the vessel. Restenosis occurs in 25% to 35% of patients and usually recurs within 3 to 6 months after the angioplasty procedure.

PTCA is performed in a cardiac catheterization laboratory using fluoroscopy to guide catheter placement.

Local anesthetics and mild sedation are employed to help relax the patient and reduce discomfort. The patient needs to be awake; alert; and able to verbalize the occurrence of chest discomfort, shortness of breath, or other adverse reactions. The patient is monitored for arrhythmias and the presence of ischemia and injury. The guide catheter is inserted through a cutdown over the right femoral artery. The balloon is inflated in a stepwise manner; the amount of pressure applied to inflate the balloon and the duration of the inflation are determined by the physician based on the patient's symptoms, the presence of ischemia, and the percentage of dilatation achieved with each inflation. Complications from the PTCA procedure include prolonged chest pain, myocardial infarction, coronary artery dissection, or spasm and often necessitate an emergency CABG. Other techniques have been developed with rotoblation and the transluminal extraction catheter (TEC) device, in which the catheter "drills" through the lesion, with the former pulverizing the lesion into minuscule particles to be absorbed by the body and the latter pulverizing the lesion with the TEC device "sucking out" the particles into an attached vacuum bottle. Laser angioplasty is also being used with the insertion of stents to maintain vessel patency. Care of the patient after PTCA includes monitoring of vital signs and cardiac rhythm to detect early signs of ischemia and impending infarction, assessing for bleeding at the site of the right femoral artery, and palpating pulses in the extremities for possible arterial thrombosis. Sheaths may be left in place overnight, and once removed, direct pressure—most often by the use of 5-lb sandbags—is applied to the site for approximately 6 hours. The patient is maintained on bed rest for about 8 hours after the procedure to prevent any potential bleeding from the cannulation site. Patients generally are discharged home the following day.

Pericardiectomy: the partial excision of an adhered, thickened, fibrotic pericardium to relieve constriction of a compressed heart and great blood vessels. In patients with chronic cardiac effusions, the creation of a pericardial window between the pericardial sac and the pleural space can also be accomplished. The opening to the pleural space allows chronically accumulating fluid to be reabsorbed.

Pulmonary artery banding: a procedure in which the pulmonary artery is constricted with tape to reduce its diameter and to decrease the pulmonary blood flow. This is usually performed as one of several stages before a complete surgical correction. The goal of this

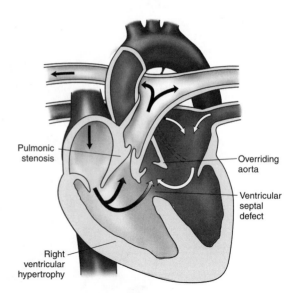

Fig. 32-7   Four features of tetralogy of Fallot: pulmonary stenosis; ventricular septal defect; overriding aorta; and right-ventricular hypertrophy. *(From Kenner CA, Lott JW: Comprehensive neonatal nursing: a physiologic perspective, ed 3, St Louis, 2003, WB Saunders.)*

technique is to prevent the development of pulmonary hypertension.

Pulmonary stenosis: fusion of the valve cusps at the commissures, which creates an obstruction to the right-ventricular outflow tract. In infundibular stenosis, fibromuscular obstruction occurs proximal to the valve. Most commonly, repair is accomplished via an open procedure under direct visualization. The stenotic valve is opened wide, and the fused commissures are sharply excised back to the annulus. Correction can also be performed by a closed procedure, in which a valvulotome is inserted via a right ventriculotomy and the stenotic leaflets are separated when it is withdrawn.

Tetralogy of fallot: a congenital entity with four distinctive features (Fig. 32-7): (1) a high ventricular septal defect; (2) pulmonary stenosis; (3) overriding of the ventricular septal defect by the aorta; and (4) hypertrophy of the right ventricle. The current trend is to proceed with an elective procedure for correction, generally when the patient is 3 to 5 years old. If the child is severely symptomatic before this age, a corrective or a palliative procedure is performed, according to the surgeon's preference. Currently, the most commonly performed palliative procedure is the Blalock-Taussig, or systemic-pulmonary anastomosed, technique. In this procedure, the subclavian artery is anastomosed to the pulmonary artery, thereby producing an increase in blood flow to the lungs. In a corrective procedure, a complete resection of the infundibular or pulmonary valve stenosis and closure of the ventricular septal defect are performed. If previously constructed palliative shunts are present, they are closed before the initiation of the corrective procedure.

Transplantation: with the improvement in pharmacologic management and infection prophylaxis, cardiac transplantation 1-year survival rates are approaching 90%. Potential candidates are patients who are considered to be in the New York Heart Association's functional class IV and who have less than a 10% chance of surviving for 6 months. Contraindications for transplantation include significant pulmonary hypertension, the presence of systemic disease, a recent pulmonary infarction, or active systemic infection. Heart donors are persons with irreversible, catastrophic brain injury who are younger than 30 years of age and do not have atherosclerotic heart disease. Removal of the donor heart is accomplished by transection of the vena cava, the pulmonary artery and veins, and the aorta. The donor heart is then transported to the recipient's institution in an iced saline bath with ischemic times of less than 4 hours. The recipient's heart is surgically removed once the donor heart has arrived in the operating room. The posterior and lateral atrial walls, the vena caval inflow tracts, the pulmonary vein orifices, and the atrial septum remain intact while the remainder of the heart is excised. The donor heart is then attached at the atria, the pulmonary artery, and the aorta. Except for the addition of infection and rejection monitoring, these patients receive the same postoperative care given other general cardiac surgery patients. If no complications ensue, they are generally discharged from the hospital in 3 weeks.

Transposition of the great arteries (TGA): a congenital anomaly in which the pulmonary artery arises from the left ventricle and carries oxygenated blood back to the lungs and the aorta arises from the right ventricle and carries unoxygenated blood into the systemic circulation. An uncommon anomaly, this condition is fatal unless a concomitant anomalous shunt, such as a septal defect or PDA between the systemic and pulmonary circulations, is also present. These lesions allow adequate mixing of the blood between the two circulations. To maintain the patency of the atrial septal defect, a balloon atrial septostomy is usually performed. In addition, prostaglandin E is administered to maintain the patency of the PDA. A variety of corrective procedures can be used to achieve a repair, with the selection of the procedure being dictated by the patient's anatomic structure and the surgeon's preference. Arterial, ventricular, and intraatrial repairs can be performed. The two intraarterial repairs are the Senning and the Mustard procedures. In both types, the atrial chambers are reconstructed so that pulmonary venous blood returns to the right atrium and systemic venous blood returns to the left atrium. Surgical correction of this anomaly is undertaken as early as possible.

Tricuspid regurgitation: a condition that occurs when the tricuspid valve does not totally close because the leaflets do not completely approximate in diastole. This lesion is more common than tricuspid stenosis and can develop because of rheumatic changes, after a right-ventricular infarction, or transiently from annular dilatation that results from right-ventricular failure.

Tricuspid stenosis: a narrowing of the orifice of the tricuspid valve. Although this condition occurs infrequently, it can be associated with rheumatic heart disease or bacterial endocarditis.

Valve replacement: a surgical procedure in which the natural valve is replaced with an artificial valve. Whatever the cause, repair consists of excising the natural valve and its attached apparatus, such as the chordae tendineae of the mitral valve, and inserting a prosthetic valve. Prosthetic valves can be classified into two groups: mechanical and biologic. Types of mechanical valves currently used are the caged-ball, the tilting-disk, and the bileaflet valves (Fig. 32-8). The caged-ball valve consists of a metallic cage attached to a sewing ring. In the center of the cage is a hollow metal or plastic ball that moves forward in the cage, thus allowing blood to flow through the valve. When the ball rests on the sewing ring, it impedes flow. An example of the caged-ball type is the Starr-Edwards valve.

The tilting-disk valve consists of a free-floating, thin, lens-shaped disk occluder made of pyrolytic carbon mounted on a semicircular sewing ring. The disk tilts or pivots upward when the valve is open, which allows blood flow. When the valve is closed, the disk lies on the sewing ring. Examples of the tilting disk valve are the Björk-Shiley and the Lillehei-Kaster valves. The St. Jude Medical® valve, a bileaflet valve, consists of a sewing ring in which reside two semicircular leaflets that open centrally. SJM is a registered trademark of St. Jude Medical Inc. This valve is well suited

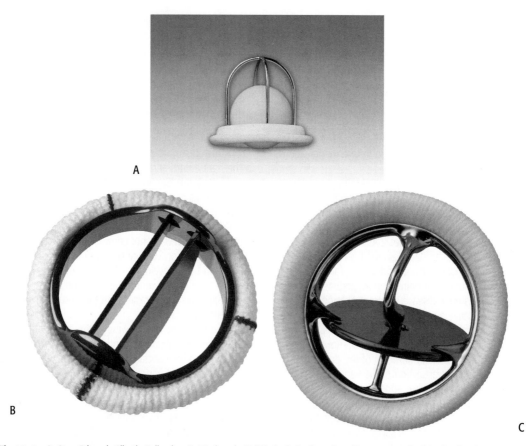

Fig. 32-8   **A,** Starr-Edwards Silastic Ball valve. **B,** Medtronic Hall™ single leaflet valve. (*A, courtesy of Edwards Lifesciences, Irvine, Calif. B, Copyright Medtronic, Inc., Minneapolis. C, Copyright St. Jude Medical Inc., 2002. All rights reserved.*)

for use in children and adults with small aortic roots because of its size and design.

Mechanical valves are extremely durable and withstand wear over a long period. One disadvantage associated with their use is the high incidence of thromboembolic events. For this reason, patients with these valves need lifelong anticoagulation therapy. This is usually initiated 3 to 5 days after surgery, when all their intracardiac lines and chest tubes are discontinued and immediate postoperative hemorrhage is no longer a concern. Oral coumarin therapy is then started and titrated appropriately to achieve prothrombin times of two-and-a-half times normal.

Biologic valves can be classified as xenograft (from animal cadaver tissues) or homograft (from human cadaver donor tissue). Xenografts can be made from porcine aorta or bovine pericardium. The Hancock and Carpentier-Edwards valves are porcine valves. The

Ionescu-Shiley valve is an example of a bovine pericardial valve. The advantage of biologic valves resides largely in the decreased incidence of thromboembolic events associated with their use. Despite this, some physicians maintain their patients on prophylactic anticoagulation drugs for 6 months after biologic valve replacement, particularly if the patient has had a history of a mural thrombus, atrial fibrillation, or an enlarged left atrium. Disadvantages of biologic valves are that they are not as durable as mechanical valves; they are prone to tissue degeneration and calcification of their leaflets and may therefore require reoperation and replacement earlier than mechanical valves.

An occasional postoperative problem after valve replacement for aortic stenosis is the hyperdynamic left-ventricle syndrome, which may also occur in patients with long-standing hypertension. This syndrome is characterized by extreme hypertension that occurs in the immediate postoperative period and is not responsive to increasingly larger dosages of vasodilators. Widening pulse pressure secondary to a diastolic decrease in blood pressure from effects of the vasodilators is seen with a consequential decrease in myocardial oxygen supply. Simultaneously, oxygen demand increases as a result of systemic hypertension and tachycardia. If left untreated, left-ventricular failure occurs with decreased cardiac output, increased pulmonary artery wedge pressure (PAWP) with eventual hypotension, and cardiac arrest. Medical management includes lowering the rate of vasodilators, adding a director peripheral vasodilator to treat hypertension, and using beta-blockers if tachycardia coexists.

Conversely, patients with aortic insufficiency (AI) have a volume-overloaded ventricle with increased compliance. Irreversible left-ventricular dysfunction may result from chronic volume overload in patients with AI. Some of these patients may not benefit from having the aortic valve replaced. Massive AI with dilated chambers and large changes in volume are associated with minimal changes in pressure. This factor limits the usefulness of postoperative left-atrial or PAWP pressures. After valve replacement for acute or chronic AI, a state of peripheral vasodilatation with low diastolic pressure sometimes occurs. If ventricular performance is hampered and no contraindications are present, an alpha-adrenergic agonist may be used. This approach is often used in septic patients with acute AI from infectious endocarditis.

Patients who are undergoing mitral valve replacement need to be observed for both right-ventricular and left-ventricular failure. Right-ventricular failure may occur intraoperatively at the time CPB is discontinued or in the early postanesthesia period. Low cardiac output despite adequate preload, increased central venous pressure, normal or low PAWP, and right-ventricular distention should alert the nurse to the onset of right-ventricular failure.

Patients with chronic mitral insufficiency have an enlarged left ventricle that is accustomed to low-pressure "pop-off" of the incompetent valve. Implantation of a prosthesis or repair of a dysfunctional valve results in a competent mechanism that creates a postoperative afterload mismatch. Sodium nitroprusside (Nipride) is often used postoperatively to decrease the afterload caused by the new competent valve.

Acute mitral insufficiency is better tolerated than acute AI. The most common causes of acute mitral insufficiency are papillary muscle rupture or dysfunction secondary to ischemia or injury and ruptured chordae tendineae. The left-atrial pressure increases because it cannot accommodate the regurgitant volume. This high left-atrial pressure is transmitted to the pulmonary veins. Large **V** waves can be seen on PAWP tracings. Forward output decreases and results in pulmonary edema. Management of these patients includes digoxin, diuretics, inotropic support with dopamine or dobutamine, and afterload reduction with sodium nitroprusside or nitroglycerin.

Ventricular aneurysm repair: a surgical technique used to correct a ventricular aneurysm. Ventricular aneurysms most often result from a large myocardial infarction or numerous smaller adjacent infarctions in which a portion of the myocardial wall becomes necrotic, thin, and weak. This portion then does not contract during systole but instead bulges outward, which decreases the patient's cardiac output. Additionally, the endothelial layers of the aneurysm become roughened, which promotes the development of large mural thrombi, thus leaving the patient at high risk for an embolic event. Also, the perimeter around the necrotic area can alter conduction pathways and create reentrant ventricular arrhythmias because it consists largely of varying amounts of fibrous tissue. The surgical technique consists of excising the aneurysm at its perimeter and carefully removing the thrombus inside to avoid embolization. Then the edges of the ventricle are joined with sutures. If the patient has been experiencing recurrent VT, an endomyocardial mapping might also be performed. With this technique, the aneurysm is first removed; next, a small electrode probe is attached to the surgeon's fingers and passed over the edges of the endothelial portion of the remaining ventricle; finally, activation potentials are observed. This procedure assists in differentiating fibrous tissue from viable tissue. The endothelium is then peeled back, and all fibrous tissue is removed. This eliminates tissues that are a source of reentrant rhythms. The edges of the ventricle are then closed as previously described (Fig. 32-9).

Ventricular septal defect: a defect that consists of a hole through the ventricular septum. This defect is usually located in the upper portion of the septum just anterior to the membranous septum. A ventricular septal defect can be congenital or acquired; those of congenital origin sometimes close spontaneously. In an adult, these are most commonly acquired from myocardial ischemia following an infarction of the septal wall (Fig. 32-10). In both types, closure of the defect can be accomplished either with the use of a synthetic patch or by oversewing the edges, depending on the size of the defect.

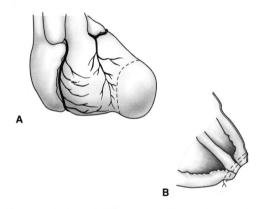

A

B

Fig. 32-9 **A**, A ventricular aneurysm is illustrated. **B**, Repair consists of excision of the aneurysm and approximation of the edges of the left ventricle.

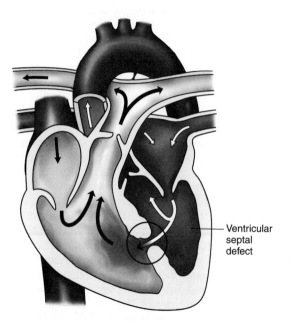

Ventricular septal defect

Fig. 32-10 Schematic representation of a ventricular septal defect. The size and location of the defect vary from patient to patient. *(From Kenner CA, Lott JW: Comprehensive neonatal nursing: a physiologic perspective, ed 3, St Louis, 2003, WB Saunders.)*

INTRAOPERATIVE CONSIDERATIONS

The most commonly used approach in cardiac surgery is the median sternotomy. However, anterolateral or posterolateral thoracotomy incisions or a transverse sternotomy with a bilateral thoracotomy can also be used. The median ster-notomy approach allows exposure of the anterior mediastinum without entry into the pleural cavities. With this approach, the sternum is split with a saw. At the conclusion of the procedure, the sternum is closed with stainless steel wires, and the skin is approximated subcutaneously with suture. The pericardium that was incised during the surgery is left open at the end of the procedure. Pericardial chest tubes are placed anteriorly and posteriorly in the pericardium to facilitate drainage. They exit via stab wounds at the distal portion of the mediastinal incision. If either of the pleurae was opened during the procedure, then pleural chest tubes are also inserted.

Once the sternum is opened, the patient is placed on CPB, and hypothermia and cardioplegic infusions are initiated. Although CPB is an essential component of cardiac surgery, it is not without potential problems. With prolonged use of an oxygenator pump (usually 4 hours or longer), various coagulation, volume, respiratory, and neurologic dysfunctions may develop.

Physiologic Changes Associated with Cardiopulmonary Bypass

Patients who undergo surgery requiring CPB are subject to several physiologic changes. Personnel involved with the care of these patients should be familiar with the physiologic changes that occur during the initial perianesthesia period. Epinephrine and norepinephrine levels are markedly elevated during CPB. Hyperglycemia and impaired insulin responses are present and result in use of fat stores for energy until carbohydrate metabolism returns to normal levels. Secretion of antidiuretic hormone and aldosterone is also increased, stimulated by different mechanisms associated with the physiologic components of stress. Serum complement that is activated in combination with the crystalloid solutions employed to prime the CPB pump cause a marked increase in total body water and interstitial edema.

With an understanding of these mechanisms, one can expect to see excess fluid in the interstitial spaces. Postoperative fluid requirements should be minimal, especially when rewarming has been instituted. Rewarming itself also causes fluid shifts. This excess fluid usually redistributes itself by the second or third day postoperatively and will be excreted spontaneously or from the use of diuretic therapy. CPB and hypothermia also alter coagulation factors and platelet formation. When exposed to the foreign surfaces of the CPB pump, platelets clump together. A decrease in the remaining number of platelets occurs along with a decrease in the aggregative and adhesive functions of remaining platelets. Release of vasoactive substances occurs as platelets are destroyed. In addition, exposure to the CPB pump causes a breakdown of plasma proteins, including gamma globulin, which in turn may cause fat microemboli release, microcoagulation, and clotting factor consumption and increased vascular permeability. The stresses of CPB also cause destruction of erythrocytes and leukocytes.

Also of importance is hypothermia-related hypocarbia. The body temperature usually remains lower than normal during the early postoperative hours. Slowly, the body temperature returns to normal, and occasionally rebound hyperthermia occurs. However, as rewarming takes place, carbon dioxide is produced; consequently, hypercarbia can develop, and ventilator settings should be adjusted to produce a minute volume necessary to facilitate normocarbia. In addition, if rebound hyperthermia occurs or if rewarming devices are not regulated and monitored appropriately, a hyperthermic overshoot will occur. Again, this reaction is undesirable, because hyperthermia increases myocardial oxygen demand and consumption.

Anesthesia

Anesthesia for cardiac surgery varies from hospital to hospital and also can vary depending on the type of cardiac repair undertaken. For example, in the repair of a mitral valve in which no evidence of significant pulmonary involvement exists, agents that increase pulmonary vascular resistance should be avoided. Commonly employed inhalation agents include halothane, enflurane, methoxyflurane, and nitrous oxide. Barbiturates, such as thiopental and methohexital, are used to accomplish the rapid sequence of induction and intubation. Other induction agents, such as etomidate and ketamine, can be used depending on the physiologic status of the patient. Morphine sulfate, sufentanil, and fentanyl are the narcotic analgesics that are most commonly used. Morphine can assist in increas-

ing the cardiac index, because it decreases systemic vascular resistance. Also, because fentanyl has a negligible myocardial effect, it is also a commonly used analgesic. Antianxiety agents such as diazepam and midazolam—in addition to narcotic analgesics—are employed in the early postoperative period.

PACU CARE

After cardiac surgery, most patients require monitoring of their heart rate, arterial blood pressure, and oxygen saturation during transport from the surgical suite to the PACU or cardiac ICU. This is because these patients can develop acute circulatory instability either because of their normally recovering physiologic state or to inadvertent movement or displacement of the numerous invasive lines and tubes they require. On admission to the PACU, the nurse should assess these parameters immediately. If either of these parameters indicates circulatory or ventilatory dysfunction, immediate resuscitative measures should be instituted.

If, at a quick glance, circulatory and ventilatory status appear adequate, then admission routines should be begun. The respiratory therapist or anesthesiologist usually attaches the patient to the ventilator, establishes the initial ventilator settings, and sets the alarms. Once the patient is attached to the ventilator, the nurse auscultates both lung fields and repeats that assessment often until the patient's discharge from the PACU. Arterial blood gas values are determined on admission and as needed thereafter. Patients remain intubated until the effects of anesthesia subside and hemodynamic stability is achieved and maintained. Controlled ventilation is used initially. As patients begin to generate their own respirations, they are switched to intermittent mandatory ventilation modes, in which they gradually increase their spontaneous respirations to maintain adequate minute ventilations. Once patients are maintaining an adequate respiratory rate, they are switched to continuous positive airway pressure (CPAP) systems. With CPAP, the patient determines the respiratory rate, and the ventilator provides the positive pressure to the airway that the glottis normally provides when the patient is not intubated. The use of CPAP prevents microatelectasis and increases the functional residual capacity of the lung. Once the patient maintains adequate arterial blood gas levels on CPAP, extubation usually follows quickly. After extubation, face masks or nasal cannulas are used to deliver supplemental oxygen.

A continuous ECG recording is established, alarm limits are set, and a strip recording is obtained. A 12-lead ECG is obtained as soon as possible and is repeated daily for the first 3 days. Rhythm strips are then obtained and documented; cardiac rhythm is assessed frequently and documented at least every 2 hours. Lead selection varies, but MCL_1—in which the left-atrial and right-atrial leads are in their respective places and the third lead is placed on the fourth right intercostal space—is commonly used. Electrode placement with this lead does not interfere with defibrillation procedures or with mediastinal or chest tube dressing placement. The apical pulse is auscultated and validated with the ECG recording. If the patient has a temporary external pacer in place, the nurse should check and record the type of pacer, the mode, the rate, and the milliamperage and determine whether the pacer is functioning adequately. If the patient is not being paced, then the nurse needs to ensure that the unused pacemaker wires are covered with gauze or electrical tape, placed in a plastic covering (a finger cot), and securely dressed and attached to the chest to protect the patient from electrical hazard. Usually, two ventricular and two atrial pacing wires are attached to the epicardium with absorbable suture before the chest is closed. These wires then exit the chest via stab wounds on either side of the sternal incision. The atrial wires are usually on the right and the ventricular wires on the left. They are most often left in place for a few days after surgery and may be used to assist in cardiac rhythm control. Before the patient is discharged from the hospital, the wires are totally removed by gentle traction or they are clipped off at the skin level, thus leaving a portion of them attached to the epicardium and residing in the subcutaneous tissues.

All intravascular lines are attached to transducers or manometers. Their patency is ascertained and their values or wave tracings, or both, are continuously displayed and recorded. Commonly measured intravascular parameters include the following pressures: mean arterial, right atrial, mean pulmonary artery, pulmonary artery systolic, pulmonary artery diastolic, pulmonary capillary wedge, and left atrial. In addition to providing these directly measured parameters, these values assist in calculating indirect or derived hemodynamic parameters, such as cardiac output and cardiac index, systemic vascular resistance, and pulmonary vascular resistance. All of these parameters assist in assessing both left-ventricular and right-ventricular status and are invaluable in determining pharmacologic, fluid, and mechanical therapies for the postoperative cardiac surgery patient. Once these intravascular lines are appropriately monitored, the nurse reviews and assesses with the anesthesiologist all intravascular lines and solutions with regard to type, drugs being infused, flow rates, patency, and expiration times, if applicable. Intake and output recordings with running totals are made and documented hourly. Volume administration and replacement treatments are largely determined by the individual patient's hemodynamic parameters, and responses can vary greatly from hour to hour.

The patient's neurologic status is assessed on admission and every 30 to 60 minutes thereafter until arousal from anesthesia. Once the patient has been aroused, neurologic assessments are decreased to every 2 hours. The Glasgow Coma Scale can be used for these checks (see Chapter 35).

Chest tube drainage systems are established. Water-seal drainage or autotransfusion systems with 15 to 20 cm of negative suction are most commonly used. The amount and type of chest tube drainage are frequently assessed and recorded on an hourly basis. Drainage that exceeds 100 ml/hr should be brought to the attention of the physician. Chest tubes are usually removed on the first or second postoperative day—so long as intracardiac lines have been removed, no evidence of fluid accumulation is present on the chest radiograph, and drainage has been less than 200 ml in the last 6 hours. Most patients will have one or two mediastinal chest tubes that facilitate pericardial drainage after surgery. If the pleural spaces were opened during the procedure or the internal mammary arteries were dissected off the chest wall, or both, then pleural chest tubes will also be present to facilitate drainage and to prevent a pneumothorax.

An admission temperature is obtained, and rewarming therapies are instituted, if necessary.

During rewarming, temperatures are recorded hourly, and rewarming devices are discontinued just before the patient reaches normothermia. This slightly premature discontinuation is performed to avoid a hyperthermic overshoot, which is common. In this situation, temperatures may overshoot the 37°C (98.6°F) level and elevate to levels of 38°C to 40°C (100.4°F to 104°F).

An abdominal assessment is performed on admission and every 2 hours thereafter until bowel sounds return. A nasogastric tube is in place to relieve gastric distention and facilitate removal of gastric contents. It is usually attached to low intermittent suction or gravity drainage and removed at the time of extubation. Analysis of pH and tests for the presence of occult blood may be performed on gastric secretions if they begin to resemble coffee grounds. Once the nasogastric tube is removed, the patient is given ice chips and resumes a clear liquid diet within the first 24 hours.

A retention catheter is in place, and urinary outputs are recorded on admission to the PACU and then hourly. The appearance of the urine is also monitored closely. During the first few hours after surgery, massive diuresis of 2 to 3 L of pale, dilute urine is usually common. This is a result of use of diuretics that are generally administered during the discontinuation of CPB pumping to facilitate the removal of fluid that has sequestered during surgery in the interstitial space. Once this initial diuresis resolves, urine color and consistency return to normal. At that time, it is desirable to keep urinary output at levels higher than 0.5 ml/kg/hr.

Peripheral pulses as well as skin color and temperature are assessed and recorded hourly. All incisions and intravascular and tube insertion sites are observed. The patient is placed in a semi-Fowler position with his or her legs supported at the knees and calves slightly elevated. This facilitates venous return from the legs and limits swelling, particularly in patients with saphenous vein incisions. Legs are wrapped from toes to hips with elastic leg wraps or antiembolism stockings.

Following these admission routines, a written assessment is performed. The frequency of assessing and documenting the hemodynamic parameters discussed earlier and routines is dictated by the patient's response to and recovery from surgery. Recovery time varies from patient to patient but generally occurs within 12 to 48 hours. During that time—largely because of the techniques of CPB, hypothermia, anesthesia, and surgical manipulation of the myocardium—numerous normal postoperative physiologic alterations occur. With correct interventions, these normal physiologic responses are short-lived and reversible. However, two problems do exist. First, although these alterations are reversible, if they are not identified early and quickly reversed, they can lead to complications. Such is the case with uncontrolled hypertension that can develop into hemorrhage if fresh suture lines are disrupted. Second, these normal alterations often resemble complications and thus may be missed in their early stages. For example, the initial absence of a pedal pulse may be attributed to hypothermia and vasoconstriction only to be traced later to a vascular embolism. For these reasons, it is incumbent on the PACU nurse to be knowledgeable about the causes, assessment factors, and interventions for both normal physiologic alterations and complications that can occur after cardiac surgery. In the following section, these alterations and potential complications will be briefly reviewed.

COMPLICATIONS

Cardiovascular System

A number of predisposing factors are known to increase the incidence of postoperative complications and early mortality. These include preoperative cardiac conditions such as myocardial dysfunction; recent myocardial infarction; and previous CABG surgery or systemic conditions such as advanced age, obesity, diabetes mellitus, and chronic obstructive pulmonary disease.

The surgical risks of CABG can be assessed quite accurately preoperatively, and complications can be anticipated by taking preoperative risk factors into consideration.

Complications related to CABG and valvular surgery can generally be classified as either cardiac or noncardiac. Cardiac complications include myocardial infarction, congestive heart failure, tamponade, decreased cardiac output, arrhythmias, and postoperative hypertension. Noncardiac complications include hemorrhage; wound dehiscence and infection; and neurologic, renal, pulmonary, and gastrointestinal problems. Each complication will be addressed individually.

Cardiac Complications of CABG and Valvular Surgery

Myocardial Infarction. Despite better myocardial protection with hypothermia, cardioplegic arrest, and topical hypothermia during surgery, myocardial infarction still remains the most common and serious postoperative complication and the main cause of early death after surgery. Suboptimal myocardial protection may result secondary to uneven distribution of cardioplegic solutions in the coronary arteries. Subendocardial ischemia may occur secondary to a distended left ventricle and incomplete revascularization. All serve as common causes of new infarction.

Hemorrhagic infarction may occur 1 to 4 hours postoperatively as a result of reperfusion injury. It is often manifested as a malignant reperfusion arrhythmia such as VT that is unresponsive to antiarrhythmic therapy, and cardiogenic shock develops quickly. Sudden reperfusion of an ischemic area is thought to cause hemorrhagic necrosis because of a rapid influx of calcium ions into the ischemic myocardial cells. The appearance of new Q waves postoperatively has been shown to adversely affect early and late survival. A number of other predictors of perioperative myocardial infarction include left main stenosis, multivessel disease, absence of collateral circulation, the number of grafts, and the duration of CPB.

Ischemic changes sometimes occur within the first 48 hours after surgery as a result of spasm of bypassed or unbypassed coronary arteries. Treatment with intravenous nitroglycerin or calcium channel blockers is usually effective in relieving the spasm.

Congestive Heart Failure (Alterations in Myocardial Contractility). Although relatively uncommon after CABG surgery, congestive heart failure remains a serious complication and is the second most common cause of early mortality.

Alteration in myocardial contractility with resultant low cardiac outputs and shocklike states can also develop postoperatively. The causes include a perioperative myocardial infarction or an ischemic state, faulty surgical repair, myocardial edema from surgical manipulation, metabolic disturbances, and depression from hypothermia and anesthesia. The patient clinically demonstrates a decrease in cardiac output and cardiac index, hypotension, elevated systemic vascular resistance, elevated filling pressures, acidosis, tachycardia, and decreased urine output. If the condition is the result of faulty surgical repair, the patient should immediately be returned to the surgical suite for correction.

The treatment includes a balance of pharmacologic and mechanical circulatory support throughout the period of recuperation, which may last from 1 to 5 days. Depending on the hemodynamic status of the patient, different combinations of inotropic and vasopressor agents are used as initial therapy, with the addition of mechanical support if cardiac output remains low despite inotropic stimulation and optimal filling pressures, as indicated by a pulmonary capillary wedge pressure higher than 22 to 25 mm Hg.

In most instances, decreased cardiac output occurs as a result of terminating CPB, and immediate attention is required. Temporary support by resuming CPB for about 30 minutes may be enough to relieve myocardial ischemia and improve ventricular contractility to a level that will allow smooth weaning with low dosages of inotropic support.

Cardiac Tamponade. Cardiac tamponade develops when blood or fluid accumulates in the pericardial cavity sufficient to compress the heart. This compression of the heart results in ineffective filling and ejection. Signs therefore consist of low cardiac output and cardiac index, hypotension, tachycardia, equalization of the right-atrial and left-atrial pressures, development of pulsus paradoxus, narrowed pulse pressure, muffled heart sounds, widening of the mediastinum on chest radiograph, and alteration in neurologic status. Observation of the quality of chest tube drainage is critical in this situation. Normally, chest tube drainage in cardiac surgical patients is thin, red, and nonclotted. This is because blood resides in the chest cavity for a brief period before it exits via the chest tubes. Because of this residence time, it is exposed to the mechanical effects of the contracting heart and the motion of the lungs. This allows the blood that normally begins to clot once it leaves its vessel to lyse the clot it forms and thus become thin, nonclotted drainage by the time it exits the chest tube. If clots begin to appear in the chest tubes, this indicates that relatively fresh bleeding is occurring, because blood has no residence time in the chest cavity.

In this situation, the incidence of tamponade is higher, because the chest tubes become clotted off easily. Therefore sudden cessation of previously heavily clotted drainage is a primary indicator for the nurse at the bedside that a tamponade may be developing. Tamponade occurs most commonly in the first 6 hours after surgery. The specific cause can be either rapid, active bleeding from a suture line or continuous, slow oozing from a coagulopathy that exceeds the ability of the chest tube to drain it. A tamponade may also develop after the removal of intracardiac lines, as a result of which bleeding occurred. Treatment consists of reoperation. If the patient becomes acutely unstable, the chest will be reopened in the PACU. Opening of the chest cavity frequently relieves the compression enough that relatively stable vital signs immediately ensue. The patient can then be taken to the surgical suite for complete repair on a less emergent basis. A reoperation to relieve a tamponade does not usually delay the patient's recovery or prolong hospitalization.

Dysrhythmias. Rhythm disturbance can occur postoperatively in as many as 30% of patients who undergo cardiac surgery. Caused by ischemic, pharmacologic, metabolic, or iatrogenic effects, these disturbances can range from atrial to ventricular in nature. Ischemia due to infarction, hypoxemia, or hypotension may serve as the precipitant drive for dysrhythmia. Inotropic drugs, with their contractile and chronotropic effects, or acid-base imbalances and electrolyte abnormalities may also cause dysrhythmias. Iatrogenically, mechanical irritation from some intracardiac lines and from the patient's endogenous catecholamine release may create irregularities. The high incidence of dysrhythmias demands that continuous monitoring be performed for the first 48 hours on these patients, even if they are discharged to a regular nursing unit in that period. Aggressive treatment of electrolyte imbalances and correction of hypoxic states are the first priorities. The massive diuresis some patients experience frequently precipitates hypokalemia and thus numerous arrhythmias. Therefore potassium replacement is aggressive, and efforts are made to maintain serum potassium concentrations at levels higher than 4 mEq/L. If correction of these imbalances fails to eliminate the dysrhythmia, pacing may be

undertaken via the temporary external pacing wires inserted during the surgical procedure.

Peripheral Vasoconstriction (Postoperative Hypertension). Factors that contribute to the development of peripheral vasoconstriction include the patient's own sympathetic drive triggered by anxiety and the surgical manipulation of the heart and the great vessels with their attached pressor receptors. Additionally, CPB, systemic hypothermia, and vasoactive drugs contribute to this vasoconstriction. The patient physically presents with pale, cold extremities; temperature lower than 37°C (98.6°F); increased systemic vascular resistance; absent pulses; tachycardia; and varying degrees of hypertension. If left unattended, the hypertension can disrupt new surgical anastomoses, and the increased systemic vascular resistance can assist in creating a state of myocardial depression because of the high afterload effect it creates. Treatment approaches consist of immediate rewarming and administration of vasodilating agents—including intravenous sodium nitroprusside, nitroglycerin, and phentolamine. These agents have relatively immediate effects and can be easily reversed once their use is discontinued. The PACU nurse usually titrates the dosage of these agents to maintain the mean arterial blood pressure at 60 to 120 mm Hg and to bring systemic vascular resistance back to normal levels.

Noncardiac Complications of CABG and Valvular Surgery

Hemorrhage. Coagulation difficulties and hemorrhage pose a potential threat to the postanesthesia CABG surgical patient. Coagulation dysfunction often occurs as a result of using the oxygenator pump 4 hours or longer. Bleeding difficulties may occur as a result of direct trauma to the blood components from solid synthetic surfaces and systemic heparinization associated with CPB.

Preoperative evaluation should detect most coagulation disturbances and dictate treatment for correction before surgery. Previous health problems should also be taken into account as possible causes of coagulation disturbances, such as in patients with uremic and hepatic diseases.

The main causes of postoperative mediastinal bleeding include inadequate surgical hemostasis and coagulation disorders. Surgical hemostasis at the end of CPB is the best prophylactic measure against postoperative bleeding. Particular attention to the internal mammary artery sites is required because of the extensive dissection from the chest wall. Risk of bleeding often is the result of pericardial adhesions that have formed. Adequate heparin reversal with confirmation by a whole-blood activated coagulation time (ACT) or activated partial thromboplastin time (APTT) should be performed (see Chapter 9). Even if the results of these studies are normal, heparin may still be released from body stores and cause a heparin rebound phenomenon. Therefore an initially normal ACT or APTT result does not guarantee that subsequent bleeding is unrelated to the effects of heparin. Another prophylactic measure to reduce intraoperative and postoperative bleeding is the drug aprotinin. This antiinflammatory agent has been used traditionally to manage pancreatitis. Aprotinin may be indicated for patients who are undergoing repeat or complicated CABG procedures and for patients who have taken aspirin in the perioperative period and who have had a CABG procedure.

Mediastinal exploration is indicated when signs of cardiac tamponade develop with bleeding of more than 500 ml/hr or less or more than 300 ml/hr for 6 hours or longer. The decision to reoperate should be made before the patient becomes hemodynamically unstable. On reexploration for bleeding, oozing from the mediastinal wound is more commonly found as opposed to active bleeding. After evacuation of clots and hematomas, bleeding can usually be controlled.

Sternal Wound Dehiscence and Infection. Three to four percent of the postoperative CABG patients have difficulty with sternal wound healing. Although sterile dehiscence of the sternal bone is possible, superficial wound infection, sternal osteitis, and mediastinitis are more common. Predisposing factors include advanced age, obesity, diabetes mellitus, and chronic obstructive pulmonary disease. Postoperative bleeding that necessitates reexploration significantly contributes to sternal wound infection. Infection may occur at any time, but it is usually diagnosed 6 to 12 days postoperatively. Treatment consists of intravenous antibiotics, opening of the wound, debridement, and removal of all foreign objects, including sutures. Once the sternal wound is clean, reconstruction can take place about 1 or 2 weeks after debridement. Intra-

venous antibiotics are continued for at least 1 week after wound closure.

Inadequate Volume Status. Inadequate volume status can easily develop in postoperative patients. Hypovolemia can be induced by inadequate volume management in conjunction with or following rewarming in which there is rapid vasodilatation. Hypovolemia can also be associated with diuretic and vasodilator therapies, hemorrhage from active or slow-oozing bleeders in the chest or from coagulopathies associated with CPB, or inadequate reversal of the effects of the heparin used during CPB. Hypervolemia develops as interstitial fluid moves back into the intravascular space or if overaggressive volume replacement occurs. Assessment of these states requires extensive hemodynamic monitoring and understanding of the numerous processes involved. Signs and symptoms specific to hypovolemia or hypervolemia should be sought. Interventions for hypovolemia consist first of replacement with crystalloid agents. If the patient is suspected of having a moderate capillary leak syndrome caused by prolonged bypass times or if the patient had significant peripheral edema, then colloidal solutions are more appropriate. If persistent hemorrhage from coagulopathies exists, transfusion with replacement factors such as fresh-frozen plasma, platelet concentrates, and other factors may be indicated. If hemorrhage is related to technical factors, reoperation is required, and replacement solutions in the interim can be autotransfused blood, whole blood, or packed cells.

Respiratory System

The effects of anesthesia, sedation, and CPB commonly create moderate episodes of impaired gas exchange with concurrent moderate alterations in the arterial blood gas values. These episodes, largely atelectatic in nature, are usually self-limiting or easily resolved with the sustained maximal inspiration (see Chapter 25), chest physiotherapy, and the administration of supplemental oxygen. A hemothorax or a pneumothorax may develop. In these situations, more negative pressure may be added to the drainage systems, or placement of additional chest tubes may be required. A volume overload from overaggressive replacement or mobilization of fluid from the third spaces may exist and can hamper gas exchange. In this situation, diuretic therapy would be instituted. In rare instances, a noncardiac permeability pulmonary edema can develop. Because this entity is associated with a high mortality rate, mechanical ventilatory assistance and pharmacologic and fluid therapies are quite intensive.

Nervous System

Temporary and permanent sensory, motor, perceptual, and cognitive deficits can occur during the perioperative period.

Permanent deficits can usually be attributed to a low cerebral perfusion state from inadequate cardiac output or to an embolic phenomenon from intracardiac thrombi, calcified valve fragments, plaque embolization from the aortic cross-clamp, or air embolization from intracardiac lines. The magnitude of the deficit is determined by the degree of neurologic involvement. These are usually identified early in the postoperative period when the effects of anesthesia have resolved. Some of these deficits may not be identified until after extubation. Transient deficits that can last from hours to days can occur in as many as one fourth of cardiac surgical patients. These transient deficits can range from a slowness to arouse to confusion and delirium.

Renal System

Prerenal and acute renal failure states can develop after cardiac surgery. Inadequate cardiac output from myocardial depression or inadequate volume replacement can lead to prerenal oliguria. In this situation, blood urea nitrogen and serum sodium levels increase and serum creatinine levels remain the same. There is low sodium content in the urine as the body attempts to save sodium and thus increase its intravascular volume; the urine plasma osmolality ratio remains 1:1.5. If these states continue for prolonged periods, acute renal failure can ensue. Treatment focuses on maintaining an adequate volume replacement and on increasing cardiac output, perhaps with an inotropic agent. In addition, renal emboli from intracardiac thrombi or hemolysis from blood transfusions can also lead to the development of acute renal failure. In the event of acute renal failure, serum creatinine and urea levels elevate and remain in a 10:1 ratio, urine sodium levels increase, and the plasma urine osmolality ratio falls to a 1:1 ratio.

Transient hematuria can occur after discontinuation of CPB or after autotransfusion of shed mediastinal blood. These events are usually short-lived and either clear up themselves or resolve following infusion of an osmotic diuretic such as mannitol.

Gastrointestinal System

Gastric complications that can develop include mesenteric or splenic ischemia or infarction from intracardiac thrombi or air emboli. Immediate surgical intervention may be necessary in these situations. Gastric distention can occur if the patient swallows air. This distention can cause cardiac problems as well as pulmonary complications. Stress ulceration can also develop; however, in recent years its incidence has decreased with the more frequent use of cimetidine, ranitidine, or famotidine.

Peripheral Vascular System

Vascular complications can include both venous and arterial thrombus formation and embolism development. Venous thrombus can develop because of stasis from immobilization and inactivity in the immediate postoperative period. Arterial complications are largely associated with various intravascular devices such as intraarterial lines and intraaortic balloon catheters. Assessment of pulses should be ongoing, but particular attention should be given to the performance of the Allen test after radial artery line removal. The Allen test assesses for the patency of the radial and ulnar arteries. In addition, the status of lower extremity pulses, skin color and temperature, and motor activity should be monitored closely in the presence of an intraaortic balloon catheter, particularly during insertion and removal. Passive and active range-of-motion exercises and early ambulation are advocated and encouraged in these patients to prevent some of the foregoing complications. In the recovery areas, the patient is instructed and assisted in performing active dorsiflexion and extension of the feet and ankles. These maneuvers facilitate venous return and decrease stasis.

REFERENCES

1. Finkelmeier BA: Cardiothoracic surgical nursing, ed 2, Philadelphia, 2000, Lippincott.
2. Gregoratos G, Cheitlin MD, Connill A et al:

ACC/AHA guidelines for implantation of cardiac pacemakers and antiarrhythmia devices: a report of the American College of Cardiology/American Heart Association Task Force on Practice Guidelines (Committee on Pacemaker Implantation), J Am Coll Cardiol 31:1175, 1998.

BIBLIOGRAPHY

Barash P, Cullen B, Stoelting R: Clinical Anesthesia, ed 2, Philadelphia, 1992, JB Lippincott.

Baue A: Glennis Thoracic and cardiovascular surgery, ed 5, Norwalk, Conn, 1991, Appleton & Lange.

Benumof J, Saidman L: Anesthesia and perioperative complications, St Louis, 1992, Mosby.

Dervan J, Goldberg S: Acute aortic regurgitation: pathophysiology and management, Cardiovasc Clin North Am 16(2):1281-1288, 1986.

Gerson M: Cardiac nuclear medicine, ed 2, New York, 1991, McGraw-Hill.

Goldberger E: Treatment of cardiac emergencies, ed 5, St Louis, 1990, Mosby.

Grossman W, Baem D: Cardiac catheterization, angiography, and intervention, ed 4, Philadelphia, 1991, Lea and Febiger.

Kaplan, J: Thoracic anesthesia, ed 2, New York, 1991, Churchill Livingstone.

Kapur P: Anesthesia and the beta-blocked patient, Semin Anesth 10(2):87-96, 1991.

Kayser S: Pharmacology and hematology: antithrombin III, heparin, and warfarin, Anesth Today 2(2):15-17, 1990.

Kirklin J, Baratt-Boyes B: Cardiac surgery, 1986, New York, John Wiley and Sons.

Miller R: Anesthesia, ed 3, New York, 1990, Churchill Livingstone.

Moreno-Cabral C, Mitchell R, Miller D: Manual of postoperative management in adult cardiac surgery, Baltimore, 1988, Williams & Wilkins.

Pelletier L, Carrier M: The immediate postoperative period. In Care of the patient with previous coronary bypass surgery, Philadelphia, 1991, FA Davis.

Rosow C, Eckhardt W: The pharmacology of cardiopulmonary bypass, Semin Anesth 10(2):122-128, 1991.

Smith P: Postoperative care in cardiac surgery. In Sabiston D, Spencer F: Surgery of the chest, ed 5, Philadelphia, 1990, WB Saunders.

Stinson E, Swerdlow C: Recurrent ventricular tachycardia, ventricular fibrillation: the ICD/PCD. In Austen W, Vlahake G, editors: Current therapy in cardiothoracic surgery, Philadelphia, 1990, BC Decker.

Topol E: Textbook of interventional cardiology, Philadelphia, 1990, WB Saunders.

Underhill SL, Woods SL, Sivarajan ES et al: Cardiac nursing, ed 2, Philadelphia, 1989, JB Lippincott.

Waller B: Pathology of coronary balloon angioplasty and related topics. In Topol E, editor: Textbook of interventional cardiology, Philadelphia, 1990, WB Saunders.

33

CARE OF THE VASCULAR SURGICAL PATIENT

Integrity and patency of the vascular system, including the arteries, veins, and lymphatic vessels, are essential to the life of human tissues. Before 1950, the patient with impaired vascular patency was treated only medically. Loss of limb or life from impaired blood flow was common, and surgery on the vascular system was only in the experimental stage. The advancement of vascular surgery from the experimental laboratory to accepted procedure in the clinical setting resulted from the successful development of diagnostic tools, such as arteriography, improvements in antibiotics and anticoagulants, and refinements in vascular surgical instruments and techniques.

In the past decade the field of vascular surgery has exploded. This explosion has resulted in the development of new methods of noninvasive diagnosis and the treatment of disease. Although arteriography continues to be the mainstay in invasive diagnosis, noninvasive procedures—including ultrasonography, computed tomographic scanning, magnetic resonance imaging, and subdigital arteriography—complement the picture. The nonsurgical treatment options include percutaneous transluminal angioplasty with and without laser and fibrinolytic therapy. Although these options are nonsurgical, these patients require close observation in the postanesthesia care unit (PACU). Therefore perianesthesia nurses must be aware of these new procedures so that adequate care can be delivered.

DEFINITIONS

Aneurysm: a localized, abnormal dilatation, distention, or sac in an artery.

Angiography (arteriography): the injection of radiopaque dye into the arteries followed by rapid-sequential radiographs of the vascular tree to determine abnormalities.

Angioscopy: a procedure that uses a specialized scope in the operating room to visualize the pathway within blood vessels and to assess graft patency after revascularization procedures.

Bypass: a rerouting of the vascular system by construction of another arterial route by use of a vein graft or a synthetic (Dacron or Teflon) artery, and reestablishment of functional integrity.

Embolectomy: the surgical removal of an embolus from a blood vessel.

Embolus: a bit of free-floating foreign matter (may be clotted blood, air, tumor, or other tissue cells; amniotic fluid; fat; or other foreign bodies) carried by the blood stream.

Endarterectomy: opening of the artery over an obstruction and removal of the obstruction, or excision of atheromatous material creating the blockage.

Fibrinolytic therapy: the injection of streptokinase or urokinase (plasminogen activators) through a catheter to dissolve a clot.

Ischemia: a lack of adequate blood supply to meet the tissue needs.

Ligation: tying or binding of a blood vessel; in vascular surgery, a technique used to prevent embolism (Fig. 33-1).

Percutaneous transluminal angioplasty (PTA): the use of a special catheter with a balloon at the distal tip that is passed percutaneously to the area of stenosis. The balloon is inflated and deflated to compress the area of stenosis and widen the vessel lumen.

Plication: the creation of folds in the wall of a vessel or other methods of reducing intraluminal size (see Fig. 33-1).

Subdigital arteriography: a procedure used in conjunction with arteriography to localize regions of peripheral arterial disease. The dye is injected through the catheter, and the computer subtracts all background

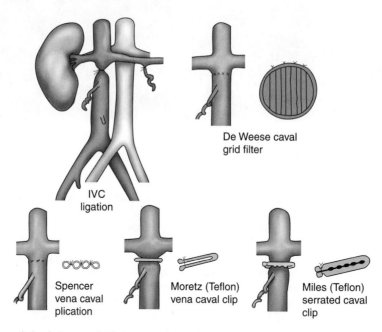

De Weese caval
grid filter

IVC
ligation

Spencer
vena caval
plication

Moretz (Teflon)
vena caval clip

Miles (Teflon)
serrated caval
clip

Fig. 33-1 Various surgical techniques available for preventing embolism from pelvic and lower extremity veins. *IVC,* Inferior vena cava. *(Redrawn from Fairbairn JF II, Juergens JL, Spittell JA, Jr: Allen-Barker-Hines peripheral vascular diseases, ed 4, Philadelphia, 1972, WB Saunders.)*

layers (i.e., bone), leaving only the image of dye-filled vessels.

Sympathectomy: the resection of selected portions of the sympathetic nervous system to denervate the vascular system, producing vasodilatation.

Thrombectomy: the surgical excision of a thrombus from within a blood vessel.

Thrombus: a stationary blood clot or atheromatous plaque that partially or totally occludes a blood vessel.

NONINVASIVE TREATMENT OF VASCULAR DISEASE

The three major noninvasive treatments for peripheral vascular disease include percutaneous transluminal angioplasty (PTA), PTA with laser (light amplification by the stimulated emission of radiation), and fibrinolytic therapy. These procedures are performed in the radiology department by the radiologist in conjunction with the surgeon. Although the aforementioned procedures are performed with local anesthesia, the patients require postprocedural nursing care in the PACU. The nursing care for this patient population is similar to that of patients undergoing other revascularization procedures. The catheter site has to be watched for bleeding and hematoma formation. Pulses, color, movement, sensation, and vital signs must be assessed frequently.

PTA has been performed on superficial femoral, iliac, popliteal, and tibial occlusions. Major complications that arise after PTA include bleeding, hematoma, and acute restenosis of the vessel. PTA is often used in conjunction with surgery and laser treatment.

Laser-assisted PTA is a well examined surgical procedure. The procedure is essentially the same as PTA, except that the laser is used first. It is coupled with angioplasty because it does not widen the vessel enough to significantly improve flow. A channel is created by the laser, and PTA follows to increase the diameter of the vessel. The major complication is vessel rupture. Because of the high incidence of vessel rupture, nurses must monitor the patient's cardiovascular status more closely, including hemoglobin and hematocrit levels and perfusion to the extremity. Research continues to improve both the equipment and the techniques in this area so that laser-assisted PTA can be applied to a broader patient population (see Chapter 44).

Another option to treating aneurysms is endovascular stent-grafting. Using this technique, the surgeon can repair the aneurysm by placing the graft inside the aneurysm through small incisions in the groin area. The grafts are packaged tightly into a small plastic tube and placed into the aorta to bypass the aneurysm with x-ray guidance. The outer tube, or sheath, is withdrawn; the graft is expanded; and the aneurysm is then fixed. In most cases, the patient will experience minimal morbidity and are usually able to go home the day after the surgical procedure was performed.

Fibrinolytic therapy is also used extensively. The specialized catheter is placed in the area of stenosis, and the infusion of urokinase or streptokinase is initiated. Urokinase is presently the drug of choice. This therapy is started in the radiology department; the patient may then be transferred to the PACU for close observation while the drug is being infused. Reperfusion is evident when the patient complains of a burning pain and the extremity is warm.

Arteriograms are performed at regular intervals to evaluate clot lysis. A successful outcome is complete lysis. Therapy is discontinued by the physician when (1) the clot is lysed; (2) symptomatology is increased; (3) bleeding that requires transfusion occurs; or (4) response is lacking. The major complication of therapy is bleeding. Nursing care revolves around monitoring for this complication. Because the agents used are plasminogen activators, prothrombin and partial thromboplastin times and hematocrit and hemoglobin levels must be monitored on admission and at least every 4 hours.

GENERAL CONSIDERATIONS

Vascular surgery is now commonly practiced in most institutions, and the perianesthesia nurse must be prepared to care for these patients postoperatively and to evaluate their vascular status. Vascular occlusive disease is most often treated with surgical revascularization procedures. Other forms of adjunct treatments—namely PTA, laser, and fibrinolytic therapies—are achieving increasing success. These noninvasive therapies are generally reserved for patients (1) who are poor surgical candidates because of their general health status; (2) whose surgical reconstructions are limited or prohibited; and (3) who sustain graft thrombosis after one or more revascularization procedures. These forms of therapy were briefly discussed in the previous section.

Many vascular impairments are amenable to surgery, especially when localized. Vascular surgery generally involves eliminating an obstruction by excision and removal of thrombi and emboli, the bypassing of atherosclerotic narrowing, and the resection of aneurysms. Occasionally, sympathectomy is performed to treat vasospastic disease, but its success is limited to patients whose vascular systems are still elastic enough to dilate. Veins may be ligated or plicated to prevent emboli from passing up the vena cava into the heart and lungs. Research in vascular disease continues, and new techniques and surgical devices are introduced for trial almost daily. The nurse should be familiar with all of the procedures being performed in the local setting and with any specific care involved postoperatively. Only the more common procedures will be discussed here.

Vascular problems may be acute and constitute a life-threatening or limb-threatening emergency; they may be chronic conditions for which surgery is performed only as a last resort after medical treatment has failed. In either instance, the perianesthesia nurse must be sensitive to the feelings of these patients and be prepared for the questions about limb viability that will invariably arise when the patient awakens.

Perianesthesia care of vascular surgical patients is determined by the surgical site, the extent of surgical revision, and the anesthesia used.

Method of Anesthesia

Anesthesia may be local, spinal, or general, depending on the surgical site and the patient's condition. Peripheral embolectomy may be accomplished with only local anesthesia and appropriate sedation, whereas an aortoiliac bypass graft requires prolonged general anesthesia. Anesthetic management of bypass graft patients is exceptionally important, because they are often elderly and in poor physical condition and present with many risk factors. Patients who undergo thoracic or abdominal aortic surgery are considerably more labile than patients who undergo peripheral vascular surgery, and they often are transferred directly from the operating suite to the intensive care unit for monitoring and special care. The thoracic aortic surgery patients will usually be transferred wherever the open-heart patients go, such as the ICU. However, in some cases, the open-heart surgical patients will go to the PACU. The goals of treatment in vascular surgical patients are to support the vascular system, to remove the cause of the problem, and to prevent further episodes of ischemia.

DIAGNOSTIC PROCEDURES

Arteriography is commonly performed before any vascular surgery to determine the exact location of the problem. It is usually accomplished within the radiology department. The patient may be returned to the PACU for a brief period of observation, depending on the policies of the hospital and the patient's postanesthesia recovery (PAR) score (see Chapter 3). Arteriography is generally accomplished with the use of only local anesthesia at the catheter insertion site.

Postarteriography care includes observation of the catheter site for bleeding. Usually, a pressure dressing is applied to the site for several hours. However, many patients will arrive to the PACU to have a sealed typed dressing that only requires a bandaid or clear dressing, with drainage being minimal. The injection site may become irritated or thrombosed, and occasionally the patient may have an allergic reaction to the radiopaque dye. Postarteriography care includes the following:

1. Observing the catheter site for bleeding and hematoma.
2. Palpating pulses distal to the catheter site (i.e., pedal pulses if the femoral artery is used).
3. Maintaining bed rest for 6 to 8 hours with the extremity kept straight.
4. Hydrating with intravenous fluids to clear the radiopaque dye.
5. Vision checks should be performed on the patient as visual problems have been reported in some patients undergoing carotid arteriograms.

The cardiovascular status of the patient should be carefully monitored if pulmonary arteriography is

performed because passage of the catheter may create myocardial irritability.

The patient is often apprehensive after arteriography and is anxious to know the results. The nurse should be familiar with the information given to the patient by the physician and be able to reinforce or reinterpret it for the patient if necessary.

PERIPHERAL VASCULAR SURGICAL PROCEDURES

Treatment for peripheral vascular disease may be performed directly on the involved vessels or sympathectomy may be done, depending on the nature of the problem and the age and general condition of the patient.

Peripheral procedures include embolectomy, thrombectomy, endarterectomy, and ligation and stripping of veins (see Fig. 33-1). Some specific procedures are the femoral-popliteal bypass graft (Fig. 33-2), peripheral artery embolectomy, carotid endarterectomy or bypass, and venous ligation and stripping of the lower extremities.

The method of anesthesia used may be local, as for embolectomy; spinal, as for surgery on the lower extremities; or general, as for more extensive procedures or when the patient cannot tolerate local or spinal anesthesia.

Perianesthesia Care

Positioning. On return to the PACU, the patient is placed in the supine position, with head of the bed maintained in a semi-Fowler's position and the head and neck turned to the side. Some controversy exists over the positioning of the patient after vein stripping. In this author's experience, surgeons have preferred to elevate the patient's legs slightly (20 to 30 degrees) to aid venous return. The surgeon's preference should be followed; if that preference is not specified, the nurse should ask for clarification.

Circulatory Status. Checking the circulation to the operated extremity is one of the most important nursing functions. Careful, explicit recording of observations is important for determining any changes. The circulatory status of the patient and the pulses present should be reported to the nurse by the surgeon. It is helpful to PACU personnel for the surgeon to mark on the skin those places where the pulses can be evaluated best.

All pulses on the affected extremity are evaluated frequently and compared with pulses on the

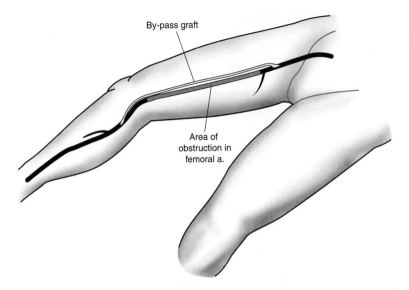

Fig. 33-2 Saphenous femoropopliteal bypass graft in place, going around the femoral artery obstruction. *(Redrawn from LeMaitre GD, Finnegan JA: The patient in surgery: a guide for nurses, ed 4, Philadelphia, 1980, WB Saunders.)*

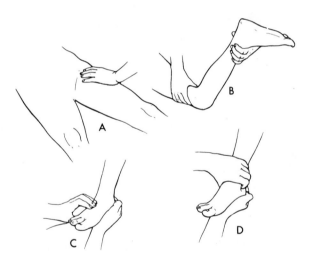

Fig. 33-3 Method of palpation for pulsations in the peripheral arteries. **A,** Femoral artery. **B,** Popliteal artery. **C,** Dorsalis pedis artery. **D,** Posterior tibial artery. *(From Fairbairn JF II, Juergens JL, Spittell JA, Jr: Allen-Barker-Hines peripheral vascular diseases, ed 4, Philadelphia, 1972, WB Saunders.)*

unaffected side (Fig. 33-3). The pulses should be checked not only for their presence but also for pulse volume and occlusion pressure. A reduction in pulse volume or occlusion pressure is more likely to be detected if the same nurse cares for the patient during the entire stay in the PACU.

If assignments need to be changed—for instance, if a shift change occurs—a direct report, with direct inspection, palpation, and evaluation of the pulses, should be made from nurse to nurse so that the relieving nurse has accurate baseline observations for future assessments.

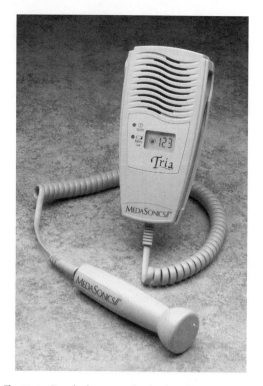

Fig. 33-4 Doppler instrument for the detection of blood flow. *(Courtesy of Cooper Surgical, Inc., Trumbull, Conn.)*

The PACU should have an ultrasonic Doppler device to assist with evaluating pulses (Fig. 33-4). The Doppler can indicate the presence of adequate blood flow even when pulses are not palpable. The affected part should remain warm, dry, and normal in color. Capillary refill should be checked by the examiner applying pressure on the skin surface and nail bed with his or her fingers, which should produce blanching. Normal pink color should return quickly when pressure is released (normal capillary refill is less than 3 seconds). Coolness, pallor, numbness, and tingling may be danger signs that vascular problems have developed. If pulses previously present become more difficult to palpate or are absent, the surgeon should be notified immediately.

Dressings.   All dressings should be checked for drainage. Dressings following bypass grafting and embolectomy are usually light, and they should remain dry and intact. If frank bleeding occurs, the surgeon should be notified, because this may indicate an interrupted arteriotomy or graft anastomosis site. A tourniquet or a blood pressure cuff should be kept at the bedside for immediate use if rupture on an arterial operative site should occur. If a cuff is used, it should be applied proximal to the incision site and inflated carefully and slowly until bleeding just stops. The pressure necessary to stop bleeding is normally just below the systemic systolic blood pressure.

After venous ligation and stripping, the legs are wrapped with Kerlix or similar elastic gauze dressings, and compression is applied with Ace wraps or antiembolism stockings from toes to groin. Some seepage of blood may occur but should not soak through the dressings. Excessive bleeding should be reported to the surgeon.

Pain Relief.   Pain following any of these procedures should be mild and easily controlled with moderate doses of the narcotic analgesics. Severe, unrelieved pain should be reported to the surgeon because it may indicate ischemia or graft occlusion. For a thorough discussion on pain relief please see Chapter 28.

Intake and Output.   The PACU course for these patients is usually smooth and uneventful. Fluids may be instituted orally as soon as the patient recovers the pharyngeal reflexes, and solids can then be given progressively as tolerated.

The patient may experience urinary retention, which is especially likely to occur after spinal anesthesia. Check for abdominal distention. Some surgeons allow male patients to stand for voiding. If measures to enhance the ability to void are not effective, a catheterization order must be obtained.

Sympathectomy

Some carefully selected patients with vasospastic disease are amenable to sympathectomy, which results in vasodilatation of the vessels in the extremity by removing the vasoconstrictive effects of the sympathetic nervous system.

Cervicodorsal Sympathectomy.   Cervicodorsal sympathectomy is performed to denervate the upper extremity and improve circulation. The most common approach used is the transaxillary-transpleural incision. Resection of the thoracic ganglia, T2-T6, and half of the stellate ganglia, C8-T1, is accomplished.

Anesthesia is general. On return to the PACU, the patient is placed in the supine position until sufficiently recovered from anesthesia to be able to tolerate the head of the bed being elevated 30 to 45 degrees. A chest tube is present because a thoracic incision has been made, and it should receive care as outlined in Chapter 25. Because the chest tube is inserted primarily to remove air to correct the surgically created pneumothorax, bleeding should be negligible. Accumulation of more than 200 ml of blood in the collection receptacle in 8 hours or less is excessive and should be reported to the surgeon.

Bilateral breath sounds should be evaluated. Circulation to the hand and arm must be assessed by evaluating pulses, temperature, and color. As soon as pharyngeal reflexes have returned, the patient may be started on oral fluids and the diet progressed as tolerated. The dressings should remain dry and intact. The patient's cardiovascular status should be assessed and any downward trends reported because these may indicate hemorrhage from the intercostal vessels, thoracic aorta, or subclavian artery. Damage to these vessels causes excessive bleeding, and hypovolemic shock can develop quickly.

Lumbar Sympathectomy. Lumbar sympathectomy is performed to denervate the lower extremity and improve circulation. A flank incision is used to approach the lumbar ganglia (L1-L4), and the ganglia are resected. This particular procedure is not commonly performed. Lumbar sympathectomy is accomplished under general anesthesia. The patient may be placed in the supine or side-lying position when returned to the PACU. The light flank dressing on the operative side should remain dry and intact. If bleeding occurs, the surgeon should be notified, because this may indicate damage to one of the lumbar veins. Drainage from the incision site must be carefully assessed. The presence of urine in the drainage suggests that damage to the ureter may have occurred during surgery.

Postoperative pain should be minimal and easily controlled with small dosages of narcotic analgesics. If the patient complains of severe flank pain not associated with the incision, the surgeon should be informed, because this may indicate inadvertent ligation of the ureter. Ligation of the ureter leads to dilatation of the renal pelvis with urine. If the patient is unable to void normally within 8 to 10 hours, catheterization will probably be required.

The patient may develop an ileus and should be given nothing by mouth for the first 24 hours postoperatively. Bowel sounds should be monitored for return. Fluid intake is provided intravenously. Occasionally, a nasogastric tube is required to decompress the stomach, and this should be cared for as outlined in Chapter 31. Circulation to the lower extremities should be assessed by evaluating the pulse, temperature, and color.

After sympathectomy, especially the lumbar type, the patient has an increased sensitivity to changes in body position; thus turning and sitting up should be accomplished slowly. This patient is also more sensitive to changes in room temperature and should be provided with warmed blankets or a Bair Hugger (forced warm air device) in the PACU to conserve body heat.

Carotid Endarterectomy

Special mention must be given to the postanesthesia nursing care after carotid endarterectomy.

Positioning. After surgery on the carotid arteries, the patient is placed in the supine position, with the head of the bed elevated 25 to 30 degrees to minimize venous oozing in the neck. Sudden changes in head position should be avoided during the immediate postoperative period. Raising the head suddenly or more than 30 degrees can precipitate hypotension, and lowering the head can precipitate hypertension as a result of a temporary inability of the great vessels to compensate for changes in head position.

Circulatory Status. After carotid endarterectomy or bypass, circulation to the head and neck is checked by assessing the patient's level of consciousness. If local anesthesia has been used, the patient's degree of orientation is a useful sign. If general anesthesia has been employed, consciousness is more difficult to evaluate; however, the pharyngeal reflexes, the lid (or blink) reflexes, and the patient's response to pain stimuli are helpful indicators of the level of consciousness. As the patient emerges from anesthesia, specific levels of response should be noted along with the time of response, so that any relapse will be detected. Check pupillary response and motion of the extremities to further assess neurologic status.

As with all surgical procedures, the dressing should be checked for excessive drainage, which should be reported to the physician. A Penrose

Table 33-1	Cranial Nerve Assessment for the Carotid Endarterectomy Patient	
Cranial Nerve	Function	Assessment
VII (facial)	Muscles of facial expression, saliva secretion	Smile, frown
IX (glossopharyngeal)	Swallowing, pharyngeal muscle	Pharyngeal reflexes, swallowing
X (vagus)	Pharyngeal and laryngeal muscles	Speech
XII (hypoglossopharyngeal)*	Muscles of tongue	Stick tongue out, move side to side

*This nerve traverses the internal carotid artery.

drain may be placed to facilitate drainage. Hematoma formation is a major complication. The nurse must assess neck size, comparing the operative side with the nonoperative side to determine if a hematoma is forming. Hematoma can compromise the airway, and the surgeon should be notified immediately. The patient may require reoperation for evacuation of the hematoma. Along with this, the position of the trachea should be checked to be sure it is midline and the hand grips should be evaluated to be sure they are equal bilaterally.

Neurologic Function.   All patients recovering from general anesthesia require close monitoring for the return of neurologic function. This aspect of care is vital with this group of patients because the carotid artery is the main blood supply for the brain. During surgery, plaque or microemboli from the surgical bed can become dislodged and travel to the brain. Assessing neurologic status includes level of consciousness, mentation, movement of extremities, and cranial nerve function to include bilateral and equal pupils (Table 33-1).

Meticulous blood pressure monitoring must be performed for these patients because of the risk of hypotension or hypertension during the immediate postoperative period. Postoperative carotid endarterectomy patients may exhibit a labile blood pressure because of manipulation of the carotid sinus. As a result of surgical trauma, the baroreceptor located in the carotid sinus may not function properly in the immediate postoperative period. Postoperative orders should include parameters indicating when to notify the physician.

Operations on the Large Vessels

Operations on the large vessels include embolectomy and thrombectomy; bypass procedures on the aorta, iliac arteries, and renal arteries; and ligation and plication of the vena cava (Figs. 33-5 to 33-7).

Surgery on the great vessels still is associated with rather high rates of morbidity and mortality. Because of the cardiovascular problem, patients are usually in a precarious physical state before surgery. These patients are often elderly, and, in addition to the specific problem for which surgery is being performed, they often have diffuse cardiovascular and respiratory diseases that affect all the vital organs. Vascular surgery on the large vessels—especially abdominal and thoracic aortic surgery—is often prolonged and is quite shocking to the system.

As with postoperative cardiac patients, these patients should be cared for in the immediate recovery period by at least two professional nurses if the patient is unstable. The decision on staffing these patients should be based on the patient's condition. All physiologic functions must be assessed accurately and continually. In some institutions, a special unit is set aside for the postoperative care of cardiac and vascular patients. If these patients are sent to the general PACU, adequate numbers of well-educated personnel must be available to manage their care. After recovery, these patients must be transferred to the surgical intensive care unit, where close monitoring and special care can be provided until they are fully stable and until the time has passed during which the most common complications occur.

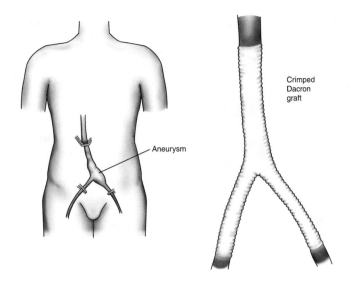

Fig. 33-5 Aneurysm of the distal aorta. Right, the crimped Dacron graft has been inserted. *(Redrawn from LeMaitre GD, Finnegan JA: The patient in surgery: a guide for nurses, ed 4, Philadelphia, 1980, WB Saunders.)*

Anesthesia for these procedures is general and may be prolonged. Surgery may take as long as 10 hours in some instances. The procedure may involve extensive blood loss, and the incisions used are commonly long and involve both thoracic and abdominal entrances. For a review of care of the patient and management of chest tubes after thoracic incisions, see Chapter 31.

Positioning and Initial Care. On return to the PACU, the patient is placed in the supine position with head and neck turned to the side. As soon as the patient can tolerate it, the head of the bed is elevated 30 to 45 degrees to promote respiratory function. After vena cava plication, the patient is kept supine, or the bed may be placed in the Trendelenburg position, as directed by the surgeon.

The surgeon and anesthesiologist should give the receiving nurse a detailed report on the anesthesia, the procedure accomplished, blood loss and replacement, other fluid replacement, the patient's overall condition, and any special instructions. At the same time, all necessary monitors and support systems should be hooked up, all drainage tubes and catheters cared for appropriately and baseline measurements of all physiologic functioning determined and documented.

Cardiopulmonary Status. Most commonly, owing to systemic shock from the procedure, the extent of anesthesia, and the general condition of the patient, respiratory support with a volume-controlled ventilator is provided postoperatively for at least 8 to 24 hours. A 24-hour period of assisted or controlled respiration gives the patient a rest and assists in stabilizing his or her condition more rapidly. The reader should review Chapter 27 for information on the care of the patient with an endotracheal airway and management of the respirator.

Because of the age of the average patient who undergoes this surgery, respiratory care is especially important. The patient should be suctioned frequently, following the guidelines in Chapter 27, and the patient's position should be changed at least every hour. Because thoracic and abdominal incisions are long and painful, adequate analgesia must be maintained to promote respiratory function as well as comfort. An order for pain medication (see Chapter 28) should give the perianesthesia nurse flexibility in medicating the patient appropriately for both of these purposes while controlled ventilation is still being used.

The patient's cardiac status should be monitored electronically. Any dysrhythmias not

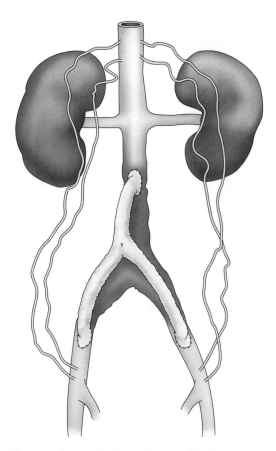

Fig. 33-6 An aortoiliac Dacron bypass graft in place.
*(Redrawn from LeMaitre GD, Finnegan JA: The patient
in surgery: a guide for nurses, ed 4, Philadelphia, 1980,
WB Saunders.)*

previously present must be investigated and an
explanation for their presence sought. The nurse
must, of course, be prepared to treat immediately
any lethal dysrhythmias that develop (see
Chapter 25). The cause of premature ventricular
contractions is often inadequate oxygenation.
Arterial samples for blood gas analysis are
commonly necessary to evaluate the patient's
cardiorespiratory status. It is therefore highly
advantageous to have an arterial line present
from which to draw specimens. The arterial line
is also helpful in monitoring the patient's systolic
blood pressure continuously. Systolic blood pressure should be recorded every 10 to 15 minutes
during the first 2 postoperative hours and every

30 minutes thereafter. Because these procedures
involve a moderate to extensive blood loss and
are shocking to the system, a systolic blood pressure of 100 mm Hg is generally acceptable if the
patient was not hypertensive preoperatively.

Control of hypertension is also essential when
surgery has been performed on the great vessels.
Extreme elevations in blood pressure can stress
the suture line, precipitating oozing and rupture
of the operative site. In some institutions, standard orders allow pharmacologic treatment of
systolic blood pressure higher than 150 mm Hg,
according to physician preference.

A pulse rate of 80 to 100 beats/min is generally acceptable. Moderate tachycardia is expected
as a result of the stress of surgery. Central venous
pressure or pulmonary artery monitoring may
also be instituted to assist in the evaluation of
the patient's cardiovascular function and fluid
balance.

Circulatory Status.   Circulation to the extremities must be checked every hour, and results must
be recorded along with the vital signs. All peripheral pulses should be present. The surgeon should
indicate the parameters within which he or she
would like the patient's vital signs to remain.
Trends in these measurements are more important indicators of the patient's status than is
any one number. Any indication of hypotension or impending shock should be reported to
the surgeon. Hemorrhage and shock are the
most common complications of vascular surgery
and may result from the primary surgery or from
associated injury to the aorta, the vena cava, or
the nearby vessels, including the iliac or renal
arteries and veins or the lumbar veins. Massive
bleeding is particularly likely if anticoagulant
therapy was instituted preoperatively.

Temperature.   The temperature should be
taken hourly for several hours postoperatively.
An electronic axillary or rectal temperature or
the core temperature from the pulmonary artery
catheter is most accurate as is the tympanic
temperature. Many PACUs use FirstTemp, a
product that provides a highly accurate measure
of core temperature. The presence of a nasogastric tube, an endotracheal tube, or a connected
respirator makes oral temperature readings
impossible, and the paraphernalia present make
rectal readings difficult. A temperature elevation
to 38.36°C or 38.86°C (101.6°F or 102.6°F) is

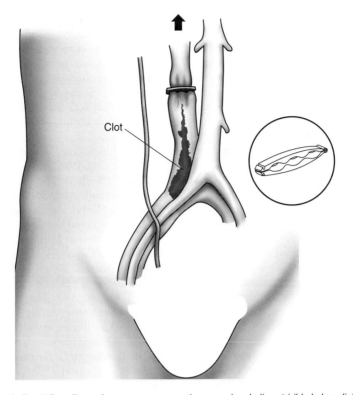

Fig. 33-7 A partially occluding Teflon clip on the vena cava preventing a caval embolism (visible below clip) from reaching lungs. *(Redrawn from LeMaitre GD, Finnegan JA: The patient in surgery: a guide for nurses, ed 4, Philadelphia, 1980, WB Saunders.)*

common after these extensive procedures and does not indicate infection. A temperature of 39.46°C (103.6°F), however, is significant and may indicate respiratory problems such as pulmonary atelectasis. In this instance, efforts at pulmonary toilet must be increased, and the surgeon may institute an antibiotic regimen if it has not already been ordered. Also, if the patient is hypothermic, the perianesthesia nurse should monitor the patient for possible infection and coagulation problems.

Intake and Output.   Adequate fluid intake is provided by intravenous infusions maintained throughout the postoperative period. The quantity and content of the fluids are determined by the surgeon, based on the patient's cardiovascular status and urine output. Blood replacement may be necessary. Hematocrit and hemoglobin determinations are usually performed 4 and 8 hours postoperatively. At least four units of

blood, typed and cross-matched for this patient, should be kept available in the blood bank until released by the surgeon.

A Foley catheter should be connected to straight gravitational drainage with a calibrated measuring device. Urine output is measured and recorded hourly. At least 0.5 ml/kg/hr (approximately 30 ml/hr) of urine output should be expected, and the surgeon should be notified if any downward trend occurs. Decreased or inadequate urine output may indicate hypotension caused by hypovolemia or impending shock with renal shutdown. The urine should be examined for the presence of blood or for cloudiness. Blood in the urine may indicate injury to a ureter or kidney, reaction to blood transfusion, or massive hemorrhage. Descending thoracic aneurysms may require cardiopulmonary bypass, which can cause hematuria secondary to red blood cell damage.

A nasogastric or long intestinal tube will be present and receives care as described in Chapter 37. It should be connected to low intermittent suction. The drainage and all stools should be given a guaiac test for occult blood, and its presence should be reported to the surgeon immediately. The presence of blood may indicate impending infarction of the colon, which must be treated immediately. Occasionally, a gastrostomy must be performed in this situation; it receives routine care.

All intake and output measurements must be conducted accurately and then recorded. The intake and output record assists in the evaluation of hypotensive states, pulmonary congestion, edema, and renal shutdown, all of which are common problems encountered after major vascular surgery.

Pain Relief. The incisions for major vascular surgery are long and painful, and significant dosages of narcotic analgesics are often required to keep the patient comfortable and promote respiratory effort. All vital signs must be monitored continuously after administration of medication, because the opioids commonly alter the patient's cardiorespiratory status (see Chapter 20). Transcutaneous electrical nerve stimulation (TENS) has been effective in controlling incision pain in these patients. Although not satisfactory as the sole pain relief modality, TENS, in conjunction with narcotic analgesia, may significantly reduce the dosage of narcotics necessary to control pain. This is advantageous because it allows the patient to breathe and ambulate more easily. Epidural or intrathecal pain management for these types of patients is discussed in Chapter 28.

Dressings. Abdominal incisions are not usually drained; thus all dressings should remain dry and intact. If dressings become soaked with serosanguineous drainage, the surgeon should be notified. The surgeon should change the dressing and inspect the incision.

Neurologic Status. The state of consciousness, facial function, movement, and strength of all extremities, as well as pupillary size and reaction and carotid pulses, must be evaluated frequently as parameters of cerebral function. Cerebrovascular accidents are not uncommon postoperatively because of the dislodgment of emboli during surgery.

BIBLIOGRAPHY

Alspach J: Core curriculum for critical care nursing, ed 5, Philadelphia, 1998, WB Saunders.

Atlee J: Complications in anesthesia, Philadelphia, 1999, WB Saunders.

Barash P, Cullen B, Stoelting R: Clinical anesthesia, ed 4, Philadelphia, 2000, Lippincott Williams & Wilkins.

Benumof J: Anesthesia and uncommon diseases, ed 4, Philadelphia, 1998, WB Saunders.

Benumof J, Saidman L: Anesthesia & perioperative complications, ed 2, St Louis, 1999, Mosby.

Bickley L, Hoekelman R: Bates' guide to physical examination and history taking, ed 7, Philadelphia, 1998, Lippincott Williams & Wilkins.

Bilodeau M, Capasso V: Peripheral arterial thrombolytic therapy, Crit Care Nurs Clin North Am 2(4):673-680, 1990.

Blank CA, Irwin GH: Peripheral vascular disorders, Nurs Clin North Am 25(4):777-793, 1990.

Bondy B: An overview of arterial disease, J Cardiovasc Nurs 1(2):1-11, 1987.

Borgini L, Almgren C: Peripheral vascular angioscopy, AORN J 52(3):543-550, 1990.

DeFazio-Quinn D: Ambulatory surgical nursing core curriculum, Philadelphia, 1999, WB Saunders.

Dixon MB, Nunnelee J: Arterial reconstruction for atherosclerotic occlusive disease, J Cardiovasc Nurs 1(12):36-49, 1987.

Durbin N: The application of Doppler techniques in critical care, Focus Crit Care 10(3):44-46, 1983.

Ernst C, Stanley J: Current therapy in vascular surgery, ed 4, Philadelphia, 2000, WB Saunders Company.

Estafanous F, Barash P, Reves J: Cardiac anesthesia, ed 2, Philadelphia, 2001, Lippincott Williams & Wilkins.

Fahey V: Vascular Nursing, Philadelphia, 1988, WB Saunders.

Fahey V, Riegel B: Advances in diagnostic testing for vascular disease, Cardiovasc Nurs 25(3):13-18, 1989.

Fode N: Carotid endarterectomy: nursing care and controversies, J Neurosci Nurs 22(1):25-31, 1990.

Ganong W: Review of medical physiology, ed 20, New York, 2001, McGraw-Hill Professional.

Guyton A, Hall J: Textbook of medical physiology, ed 10, Philadelphia, 2000, WB Saunders.

Hardman J, Limbird L: Goodman and Gilman's the pharmacological basis of therapeutics, ed 10, New York, 2001, McGraw-Hill Professional.

Katzung B, editor: Basic and clinical pharmacology, ed 8, Los Altos, Calif, 2000, Appleton & Lange.

Lake C, Hines R, Blitt C: Clinical monitoring: practical applications for anesthesia and critical care, St Louis, 2001, Mosby.

Longnecker D, Murphy F: Dripps/Eckenhoff/Vandam introduction to anesthesia, ed 9, Philadelphia, 1997, WB Saunders.

Longnecker D, Tinker J, Morgan G: Principles and practice of anesthesiology, ed 2, St Louis, 1998, Mosby.

Miller R, editor: Anesthesia, ed 5, New York, 2000, Churchill Livingstone.

Moore W: Vascular Surgery: A comprehensive review, ed 6, Philadelphia, 2001, WB Saunders.

Nagelhout J, Zaglaniczny K: Nurse anesthesia, ed 2, Philadelphia, 2001, WB Saunders.

Omoigui S: The anesthesia drugs handbook, ed 2, St Louis, 1995, Mosby.

Rutherford R, Gloviczki P, Cronenwett J, editors: Vascular surgery, ed 4, Orlando, 1999, Harcourt Brace & Company.

Sakalaris B: Laser therapy for cardiovascular disease, Heart Lung 16(5):465-471, 1987.

Seabrook G, Mewissen M, Schmitt D et al: Percutaneous intra-arterial thrombolysis in the treatment of thrombosis of lower extremity arterial reconstructions, J Vasc Surg 13:646-651, 1991.

Stoelting R: Pharmacology and physiology in anesthetic practice, ed 3, Philadelphia, 1999, Lippincott-Raven.

Stoelting R, Miller R: Basics of anesthesia, ed 4, New York, 2000, Churchill Livingstone.

Stone D: Perioperative Care: Anesthesia, medicine, and surgery, St Louis, 1998, Mosby.

Townsend C, Beauchamp R, Evers B et al: Sabiston textbook of surgery: the biological basis of modern surgical practice, ed 16, Philadelphia, 2001, WB Saunders.

Waugaman W, Foster S, Rigor B: Principles and practice of nurse anesthesia, ed 3, Norwalk, Conn, 1999, Appleton & Lange.

Whittemore A: Advances in vascular surgery, ed 10, St Louis, 2002, Mosby.

Orthopedic nursing in the postanesthesia care unit (PACU) is challenging and rigorous. In this highly technologic age, the care demanded by the orthopedic patient requires both vigilant general perianesthesia care and a sound knowledge of orthopedic surgical procedures. The perianesthesia nurse must possess astute nursing observation and inspection skills to ensure a low incidence of morbidity in this patient population. The psychosocial challenges are generally more evident within this group because, more commonly, the goal of the surgery is focused on restoring mobility and relieving pain and disability. The nurse must be sensitive to heightened anxieties and be empathetic to individual needs.

DEFINITIONS

Anesthesia: local or systemic loss of sensation caused by trauma or injury.

Arthrodesis: surgical fixation or fusion of a joint.

Arthroplasty: reconstruction of joints to restore motion and stability.

Arthroscopy: surgical examination of the interior of a joint by the insertion of an optic device (arthroscope) capable of providing an external view of an internal joint area.

Arthrotomy: surgical exploration of a joint.

Articulation: the connection of bones at the joint.

Cineplastic (kineplastic) amputation: an amputation that includes a skin flap built into a muscle; a portion of the prosthetic mechanism is activated by the muscle.

Disarticulation: amputation at a joint.

Diskectomy (discectomy): removal of herniated or extruded fragments of an intervertebral disk.

External fixators: equipment used to manage open fractures with soft-tissue damage (provides stabilization for the fracture while it permits treatment of soft-tissue damage).

Fasciotomy: surgical separation of the fascia (a fibrous membrane that covers, supports, or separates the muscles) to relieve muscle constriction or reduce fascia contracture.

Harrington rods: equipment used in spinal fixation for scoliosis and for some spinal fractures.

Hemiarthroplasty: replacement of the femoral head with a prosthesis.

Internal fixation: the stabilization of a reduced fracture by the use of metal screws, plates, nails, and pins.

Joint replacement: the substitution of joint surfaces with metal or plastic materials.

Laminectomy: removal of the lamina to expose the neural elements in the spinal canal or to relieve constriction.

Lordosis: abnormal anterior convexity of the lower part of the back.

Luque rods: spinal fixation that apply transverse force to treat scoliosis.

Meniscectomy: surgical removal of the damaged knee joint fibrocartilage.

Open reduction: the reduction and alignment of a fracture through surgical dissection and exposure of the fracture.

Osteoporosis: diminished amount of calcium in the bone.

Osteotomy: surgical cutting of the bone.

Paresthesia: numbness and a tingling sensation.

Scoliosis: lateral curvature of the spine.

Sequestrectomy: surgical removal of necrotic bone.

Spinal fusion: a fusion of the cervical, thoracic, or lumbar region of the spine with an iliac or other bone graft, primarily fusing the laminae and sometimes the joints, most often through the posterior approach.

Syme amputation: modified ankle disarticulation (below-the-ankle) amputation of the foot.

Volkmann contracture: the final state of unrelieved forearm compartment syndrome; contractures of tendons to wrist and hand.

GENERAL PERIANESTHESIA CARE

Specific nursing care related to the orthopedic patient that begins in the PACU includes positioning, neurovascular assessment, care of immobilization devices, wound care, range-of-motion exercises, and observation for complications.

Positioning

After the initial assessment of the orthopedic patient is made, attention is turned to positioning. Proper body alignment is important for all these patients and requires a sound knowledge of operative procedure and body mechanics. Each surgeon generally has specific directives for positioning, but general guidelines apply to all patients. The goal is to provide optimum comfort and safety for the operated limb. The upper extremities should be held close to the body; elevation should be achieved without undue pressure on the elbow or shoulder. The lower extremities are in a neutral position, with support provided for their entire length, and heels are off the bed.

Elevation of operative limbs is usually indicated to increase venous return, reduce swelling, and promote comfort. When elevating a hand or an arm, the hand must be higher than the heart; and no pressure should be placed on the elbow. This position can be achieved by the use of a stockinette device for suspension on an intravenous (IV) pole. Measure the stockinette from elbow to approximately 12 inches beyond the fingertips. Cut a piece double this length. Fold it in half, and rest the elbow in the fold. Using safety pins, close the sides around the limb to form a tube, while making sure the fingers are exposed (to assess neurovascular status). With the excess material, tie a knot and suspend the end from the IV pole. Be careful to properly support the elbow. If using a pillow for elevation, remember to allow the arm slight flexion for maximum comfort and provide additional support for the elbow and shoulder.

Lower extremity elevation is most effective if the toes are above the heart. If it is not in an immobilization device, the limb is kept in a position of extension. This position is achieved by elevating the foot of the bed rather than the use of pillows. If pillows are used, be sure to support the entire length of the limb and keep the heels off the bed.

Shoulder immobilization can be accomplished with a sling or shoulder immobilizer. An airplane splint may be applied for rotator cuff repairs. If a sling is used, the patient is instructed to keep his or her arm close to the chest with the wrist and elbow supported. The shoulder immobilizer requires special care to pad areas where skin contacts skin.

The patient with a hip pinning is positioned with proper body alignment, and the legs are in a proper neutral position. Care is given to avoid stress to the operative area with exaggerated flexion or rotation. A pillow is placed between the knees when turning to prevent adduction and rotation. For the patient with a total hip replacement, proper body alignment is achieved by placing an abduction pillow between the knees at all times. Most important with these patients is to avoid flexion and adduction of the newly placed joint. If the abduction pillow straps are not in use, it is necessary to support the lateral aspect of the leg to avoid external rotation. This can be accomplished by the use of rolled towels or sheets.

The perianesthesia nurse should also be familiar with various types of orthopedic equipment that may be used and that can affect positioning. Often, the patient with a total knee replacement and those with more extensive knee arthrotomy are placed in a continuous passive motion (CPM) machine. The purpose of CPM is to enhance the healing process by providing CPM to the joint, thus increasing circulation and movement. Traction may also be used with various patients to immobilize and align a specific area. The perianesthesia nurse is not usually involved in setting up the traction but should be aware of some basic principles for maintenance: (1) the traction must be continuous; (2) the patient is centered in bed in good alignment to maintain the line of pull in line with the long bone; (3) weights should hang freely, not resting on the floor or bed; and (4) the pulley ropes should be in alignment and free of knots. One type of traction is depicted in Figure 34-1.

Neurovascular Assessment

Critical to the care of the orthopedic patient is assessment of the neurovascular status of the operative limb. Any alteration in blood flow to the extremity or nerve compression requires

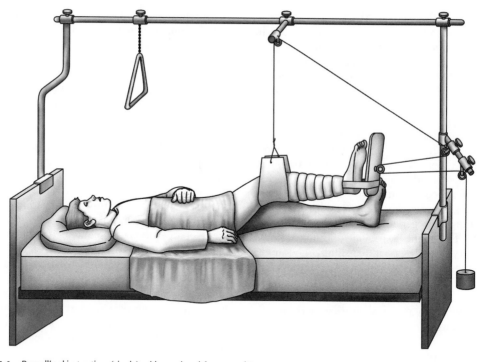

Fig. 34-1 Russell's skin traction (single) with overhead frame and trapeze.

immediate intervention. Assessment is recommended every 30 minutes because problems can occur as soon as 2 to 4 hours. Baseline neurovascular indicators should be noted in the admission nursing assessment. These can be used to establish whether or not there have been any deleterious effects from the surgery and to avoid the masking of potential complications. Both the affected and unaffected limbs are assessed.

The hallmarks of neurovascular changes due to constriction and circulatory embarrassment are pain, discoloration (skin that is pale or bluish), decreased mobility, coldness, diminished or absent pulses, altered capillary refilling, and swelling. Pain is common with orthopedic patients, and the approach to treatment must be individualized. Pain unrelieved by conventional methods, such as elevation and repositioning and the administration of narcotics, must be further assessed. Color indicates circulatory compromise. Cyanosis suggests venous obstruction; pallor suggests arterial obstruction. Mobility is assessed by determining the range of motion of the fingers or

toes and strongly indicates neural compromise. Fingers are flexed, extended, spread, and wiggled. Toes should be dorsiflexed, plantarflexed, and wiggled. Inability to move the fingers or toes, pain on extension of the hand or foot, or coldness of the extremity is indicative of ischemia. Sensation is described as normal, hypesthetic (dulled), paresthetic, or anesthetic. Alteration in sensation suggests nerve compression or circulatory compromise. Limb perfusion is further assessed by the presence of peripheral pulses and capillary refilling. Capillary refilling is assessed by compression of the nail bed, which causes it to blanch; when the compression is released, color briskly returns. Compromise delays the filling time. With the development of pulse oximetry, a more reliable method of perfusion assessment is available. With placement of the oximeter sensor on a finger or toe of the affected limb, the pulsation will be sensed and oxygen saturation displayed. This method is more reflective of perfusion than capillary refilling and is valuable when pulses cannot be assessed because of the presence of a cast or dressing.

Care of Immobilization Devices (Cast Care)

Immediate assessment of the orthopedic patient in the PACU should include the type of immobilization device applied. The soft knee immobilizer should be checked for proper placement and closure and the surgical dressing checked for drainage. For care involving traction, refer to the section on positioning earlier in this chapter.

The cast is a rigid immobilization device molded to the contours of the part to which it is applied. The cast has a dual purpose: to immobilize in a specific position and to provide uniform pressure on the encased soft tissue. The cast should be inspected for visibility of fingers and toes for neurovascular assessment. If the cast is bivalved, the edges should be inspected for roughness to avoid discomfort and potential skin breakdown. When the patient arrives in the PACU, the cast will probably still be wet, and special care must be taken to prevent indentations. A wet cast must be handled carefully with the palms of the hand to avoid pressure from fingertips. Support the cast on a pillow and avoid hard, flat surfaces. Improper handling and flat surfaces can cause indentations that may lead to the development of pressure sores. More frequently, a fiberglass cast is applied with quicker drying properties, but the same general principles still apply. Any drainage noted on the cast should be circled, and the time should be noted. This documentation can provide a guide for postoperative blood and fluid loss and can alert the nurse if the drainage appears to be excessive. Note that orthopedic wounds tend to ooze and bleed more than other surgical wounds.

Wound Care

All surgical dressings should be checked for drainage and closure. Orthopedic patients are highly susceptible to infection; therefore strict asepsis when changing dressings or handling drains is required. Drains may be placed in the wound to minimize blood accumulation and the possibility of infection. Care must be taken to attend these drains to maintain suction.

It is not uncommon for a patient with total joint replacement to have a large amount of blood loss in the immediate postoperative period. This loss can be as great as 250 to 300 ml in the first hour. The retrieval of this blood for reinfusion (autotransfusion), when coupled with pre-operative autologous blood donation, has substantially reduced the need for homologous transfusions. Autotransfusion is accomplished by the use of self-contained disposable systems that are designed for easy setup and safe use.

Range-of-Motion Exercises

Range-of-motion exercises can be initiated in the PACU as soon as the patient is alert and cooperative. Flexion, extension, and rotation of joints distal to the operative area assist in stimulating circulation and strengthening muscles. Prevention of venous stasis decreases the incidence of thromboembolism, and early movement of joints promotes healing and stabilization.

Observation for Complications

Postoperative complications for the orthopedic patient include deep vein thrombosis, pulmonary embolism, fat embolism syndrome, compartment syndrome, shock, and urinary retention.

Deep Vein Thrombosis. Thrombosis is the formation of a blood clot associated with three conditions outlined by Virchow in 1846: venous stasis, altered clotting mechanism, and altered vessel wall integrity. Immobilization and the insult of the surgical procedure place the orthopedic patient at high risk. Immobilization impairs the leg muscle action needed to move the blood sufficiently, and the surgical procedure injures vessel walls that activate and alter clotting mechanisms. An inflammation process begins within the vessel wall and leads to deep vein thrombosis. The patient usually complains of pain and tenderness. Signs include swelling and sometimes localized redness. Palpation of the calf reveals firmness or tension of the muscle. A positive Homans' sign may be exhibited.

Venous complications can usually be prevented by early initiation of exercise, but if they occur, exercise should cease; anticoagulant therapy is usually initiated. Anticoagulant therapy is routinely begun postoperatively on the higher risk patients, such as those with total joint replacements. Antiembolism stockings or pneumatic hose should be used on all patients who will not be ambulatory, who have hip or lower extremity injury, who are elderly, or who have a previous history of thrombophlebitis. These stockings provide compression that enhances venous flow rates. The pneumatic stockings (alternating–pressure-gradient stockings) provide automatically a consistent compression-decompression system. These stockings are growing in popularity and should be considered for the higher risk total hip replacement and spinal surgical patients.

Pulmonary Embolism. The most serious sequela of deep vein thrombosis is pulmonary embolism. If the patient has been inactive and movement has been restricted before surgery, the risk of clot formation is greatly enhanced. Embolization of this clot leads to pulmonary embolism. The severity of symptoms depends on the size and number of clots. Symptoms range from none if the clot is small to a myriad that may include—with increasing severity—anxiety, dyspnea, tachypnea, hemoptysis, substernal pain, stabbing "pleuritic" pain, tachycardia, cough, signs and symptoms of cerebral ischemia, fever, elevated sedimentation rate, shock, and sudden death. Immediate nursing care involves administration of oxygen and relief of pain.

Fat Embolism Syndrome. Fat embolism syndrome is a condition that leads to respiratory insufficiency and is related to multiple fractures, especially of the long bones. It is caused by fat droplets released into the circulation from the bone marrow and local tissue trauma. Similar to pulmonary embolism, these fat globules migrate to the lungs, where they cause occlusions. The fat globules break down into acids, thereby irritating vascular walls and causing extrusion of fluids into the alveoli. The lung involvement alters ventilation and leads to hypoxemia. Fat embolism syndrome may lead to adult respiratory distress syndrome. The symptoms related to lung involvement include tachypnea, tachycardia, anxiety, petechiae over the chest, PO_2 less than 60 mm Hg, fever, pallor, and confusion. Brain involvement is evidenced by agitation, confusion, delirium, and coma. Immediate nursing care of this sometimes-fatal complication includes administering oxygen, keeping the patient quiet, and preventing motion at the fracture site.

Compartment Syndrome. Compartment syndrome is a condition in which increased pressure within a muscle compartment causes circulatory compromise and leads to diminished function of the limb. Left undetected, the compression may cause permanent damage to the extremity. The compartment is described as a fascial sheath enclosing bone, muscle, nerves, blood vessels, and soft tissue. The two main causes of increased pressure to this space are (1) constriction from the outside, such as a cast or bandage that decreases the size of the compartment; or (2) increased pressure within the compartment, such as swelling. The hallmark symptoms of compartment syndrome include intense pain unrelieved by conventional methods, paresthesia, and sharp pain on passive stretching of the middle finger of the affected arm or the large toe of the affected leg. Progressive symptoms include decreased strength, decreased sensation (numbness and tingling), and decreased capillary refilling; peripheral pulses are not generally compromised. Immediate intervention includes elevation of the extremity, application of ice, and release of restrictive dressings. Fasciotomy may be required if conservative measures are unsuccessful.

Shock. Because of the highly vascular composition of bone and secondary injury to the soft tissue, hemorrhage is always a potential risk in the trauma and postoperative orthopedic patients. Vigilant observation of the operative area and blood pressure and pulse will alert the perianesthesia nurse to any impending danger. Immediate nursing measures include keeping the patient warm and flat in bed, monitoring vital signs, and replacing fluid volume. The surgeon is notified immediately, and more definitive treatment is initiated (see Chapter 51).

Urinary Retention. Urinary retention refers to the inability to void despite the urge or desire. This condition may occur in adult patients on whom hip or back surgery has been performed. The retention may be the result of spinal anesthesia or possibly inability to void in the supine position. These patients should be monitored for bladder distention and complaints of pain in the lower abdomen. The surgeon should be notified if distention occurs or if the patient is unable to void within 8 hours after the surgery is completed.

PERIANESTHESIA CARE AFTER HAND SURGERY

The hand surgical patient usually is admitted to the PACU with a large, bulky dressing in place on the hand and forearm. An elastic bandage to apply pressure may also be in place outside the dressing. The hand should be elevated above the level of the heart at all times to prevent edema and hemorrhage. The hand may be placed on pillows on the chest of the patient or suspended from the bed frame or IV pole by stockinette. The elbow should be supported with a pillow. Support under the shoulder and wrist aids in decreasing pressure to the elbow. If a drain is present, it should be checked to ensure that it is activated, or it may be connected to a vacuum blood tube. The drain is placed to minimize the bleeding into the wound and to reduce the possibility of infections. Drains should be checked every 1 or 2 hours to maintain a proper vacuum and the output recorded on the intake and output records. The tips of the fingers should be visible, and the neurovascular status should be assessed every 30 minutes for signs of change. It should be remembered that hand surgery is often done with the use of an axillary block and that sensation and movement may not fully return for several hours after surgery. Baseline neurovascular indicators should be noted in the admission nursing assessment. These can be used to establish whether any deleterious effects from the surgery have occurred.

PERIANESTHESIA CARE AFTER ARM AND FOREARM SURGERY

Postanesthesia care of the patient who is recovering from arm and forearm surgery centers on elevating the extremity, observing for excessive bleeding, and monitoring for neurovascular changes. The radial pulse should be taken every 30 minutes and compared with that of the unaffected limb. If pulses cannot be assessed because of a dressing or cast, the pulse oximeter sensor should be placed on a finger of the affected arm; the pulsation will reflect perfusion to the limb. Any decrease in intensity of the pulse or in bilateral strength of the hand, any excessive bleeding, and any changes in neurovascular status should be reported to the surgeon. Symptoms of excessive pain, weakness, or decreased sensation, especially on passive extension of the fingers, usually indicate compartment syndrome, which constitutes an orthopedic emergency. Patients should be encouraged to perform active range-of-motion exercises with their wrists and hands.

PERIANESTHESIA CARE AFTER SHOULDER SURGERY

Shoulder surgery may include arthroscopy, arthrotomy, or total shoulder joint replacement.

The patient is admitted to the PACU with a bulky pressure dressing in place along with a sling-style shoulder immobilizer. Make sure that the immobilizer does not interfere with chest expansion because this would inhibit adequate respiratory exchange. The surgical dressing should be inspected for bleeding because the shoulder is a vascular area in which hemorrhage is difficult to manage.

Inspection should include checking to see if any skin surface is in contact with another. If this is the case, a protective pad should be inserted between the two skin surfaces. The radial pulse should be monitored because flexion of the arm in the immobilizer can reduce blood flow to the hand. The immobilizer should be checked for areas that might be causing pressure to the shoulder and arm. Remember to support the elbow and wrist to prevent any undue pressure to the ulnar and radial nerves. Again, neurovascular observations are a critical part of the postanesthesia assessment of these patients. The patient should be encouraged to perform active range-of-motion exercises with that hand.

PERIANESTHESIA CARE AFTER HIP OR FEMORAL SURGERY

When the patient who has had hip or femoral surgery is admitted to the PACU, nursing assessment should include pulmonary and neurovascular function, body alignment, and the amount and type of bleeding from the surgical incision. Because of advancing age and long bone trauma, these patients represent the highest risk group for postorthopedic complications.

Preexisting medical conditions and the effects of anesthetic agents compromise respiratory function. Coughing and deep breathing, sustained maximal inspirations, and position changes, when possible, are of utmost importance. The incentive spirometer can be used to facilitate good lung expansion. Any change in the pulmonary dynamics should be reported to the anesthetist.

Because swelling at the operative site can reduce blood flow to the feet, neurologic signs along with pulses of the affected foot should be monitored and compared with those of the unaffected foot. The dorsalis pedis pulse can be palpated on the dorsum of the foot and lateral to the extensor tendon of the great toe. The posterior tibial pulse can be palpated just behind and slightly below the medial malleolus of the ankle. The extremity is elevated where indicated.

The body should be aligned as normally as possible. The legs and feet are maintained in a neutral position, elevated as indicated, and supported to avoid rotations of and pressure on the heels. Traction may be applied and has been discussed earlier in this chapter. Observe for peroneal nerve compression in any patient with lower limbs wrapped in elastic bandages or strapped as in an abductor pillow. Compression may occur where the peroneal nerve crosses the knee at the head of the fibula. Decreased sensation over the dorsum of the foot, tingling, extremity weakness, and an inability to bring the foot up are signs indicative of this injury, which is a common cause of foot-drop. The patient should be encouraged to perform active range-of-motion exercises of the ankle to enhance venous return.

The patient with total hip replacement has an abduction pillow placed between the knees at all times. This position must be maintained to avoid adduction and internal rotation of the newly placed joint. The patient should not be allowed to flex the hips at a greater than 30- to 40-degree angle or to adduct the leg of the affected side. The muscle groups are weakened, and dislocation of the joint is a potential risk. If turning is required, the patient may be turned to the unoperated side no more than 45 degrees with hip abduction maintained and total leg support provided. The head of the bed may be elevated no more than 45 degrees.

An autotransfusion system or Hemovac drain is usually inserted at the operative site to facilitate the removal of blood; the color and amount should be inspected frequently. If the color is bright red or the drainage is more than 300 ml in an 8-hour period, the surgeon should be notified. The patient with total hip replacement may experience a large blood loss, which becomes a problem if the loss is sustained or if it increases.

PERIANESTHESIA CARE AFTER KNEE SURGERY

Postanesthesia care of the patient who has had surgery of the knee involves observation for complications and proper knee positioning. The surgical procedure may involve repair of ligaments and tendons or removal of all or of a portion of the meniscal cartilage. Patients may undergo a total knee replacement when degenerative processes have caused the knee joint to become nonfunctional.

The knee joint is formed by the articulation of rounded condyles of the femur with shallow depressions in the tibia, also called condyles. At the periphery of the articulation between the femoral and tibial condyles are the wedge-shaped meniscal cartilages that function primarily in joint lubrication and in cushioning. Located within the joint capsules, the medial and lateral cruciate ligaments are primarily responsible for lateral stability, and the anterior and posterior cruciate ligaments within the intercondylar notch are primarily responsible for anteroposterior stability. Externally, the joint is strengthened by the tendons of the quadriceps muscle, which is stabilized by the patella.

After knee surgery, the patient arrives in the PACU with a bulky compression dressing in place. Ice over the surgical site may be ordered to provide comfort and minimize swelling. The leg should be elevated and positioned in full extension. This can be facilitated by elevation at the ankle so that maximum extension of the leg can be accomplished. Remember to avoid pressure to the heel. An effective means of providing compression and cold is the use of the CryoCuff (Fig. 34-2). The CryoCuff is a large vinyl bladder that fits over the knee. The cuff, anchored by Velcro straps to the leg, is then filled with ice water via a portable canister. When filled, safe cooling and compression are provided to the operative area.

Assessments of neurovascular status should be performed every 30 minutes. Any decrease in sensation over the dorsum of the foot should be noted because this can represent compression of the peroneal nerve where it crosses the fibula at the knee. The surgeon should be notified if any neurologic or circulatory change is found, because early detection and correction prevent permanent nerve deficit or ischemic muscular injury. If the patient received a spinal anesthetic, it will be necessary to wait for the motor function to return before neurologic assessment is initiated.

These patients should be encouraged to flex, extend, and rotate their ankles as soon as possi-

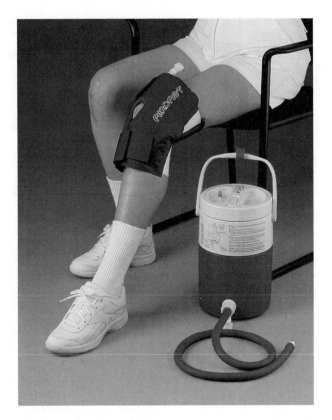

Fig. 34-2 CryoCuff system. *(Courtesy of Aircast, Summit, NJ.)*

ble to improve circulation. Knee-strengthening exercises may also be started in the PACU. Isometric exercises and quad sets aid in healing the muscle and providing stability to the joint. Isometrics involve a 6-second contraction of the entire leg followed by relaxation. The quad sets require contraction of the quadriceps muscle while pressing the knee to the bed for 5 to 10 seconds and then relaxation.

Arthroscopic examination of the knee is done to facilitate minor repairs and the diagnosis of more extensive damage to the knee; in general, fewer postoperative complications occur because this is a less invasive procedure. However, neurovascular assessment remains an important part of the postanesthesia care of these patients.

The patient with total knee replacement and those patients who have undergone extensive arthrotomy knee repairs are sometimes placed in a continuous passive motion (CPM) machine (Fig. 34-3). This device provides a safe method of elevation, comfort, and continuous range-of-motion to the operative knee. The CPM promotes healing by increasing circulation and movement of the knee joint. The machine should be inspected to ensure proper positioning of the limb. The flexion and extension settings of the machine should be determined by the physician and are generally 0 to 30 degrees at slow speed initially.

Extensive knee procedures generally have large amounts of drainage. An autotransfusion device or Hemovac drain is present to facilitate removal of drainage from the wound. The Hemovac drain is emptied and reactivated as necessary. Autotransfusion is discussed in Chapter 26. Drainage amounts of 250 to 300 ml in 1 to 2 hours are not uncommon.

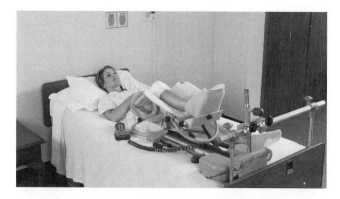

Fig. 34-3 An OptiFlex® Knee CPM with Bed Mount. *(Courtesy Chattanooga Group, Inc., Hixson, Tenn.)*

PERIANESTHESIA CARE AFTER FOOT SURGERY

The patient who has had a surgical procedure performed on the foot has either a cast or a bandage over the operative site. The amount and color of bleeding should be noted. Neurovascular signs should be monitored every 30 minutes. The extremity should be elevated above the level of the heart, with pillows supporting the entire length of the leg.

PERIANESTHESIA CARE AFTER SPINAL SURGERY

There are several types of spinal procedures. The important features of the postoperative assessment relate mostly to the surgical area of the spine. Patients who have had a cervical procedure should be monitored for neurologic signs of the upper extremities. Symptoms such as weakness and radiating pain should be reported to the surgeon. Patients in halo traction should be monitored for any deficiency in the sixth cranial (abducent) nerve. Any decrease in the lateral movement of the eye is indicative of injury to the abducent nerve.

If the surgical procedure involves C3, C4, or C5, respiratory movements should be monitored because the diaphragm muscle is innervated by the spinal outflow from these vertebrae. The patient with this nerve deficit exhibits lack of diaphragmatic excursion as well as shortness of breath and the use of intercostal and accessory muscles in breathing. If these symptoms appear, oxygen should be administered, and assistance in ventilation may be necessary.

Patients who have had midthoracic or lower spinal surgery may develop an ileus. This complication is signaled by abdominal distention, diminished or absent bowel sounds, and tympany on percussion of the abdomen. The usual treatment is to withhold oral food and fluids and to decompress the stomach with a nasogastric tube.

Patients who have had lumbar or sacral spinal surgery should be observed for loss of strength in the lower extremities and bladder distention. Bladder distention may be indicated by diaphoresis, hypertension, tachycardia, tachypnea, and a feeling of distress. If the patient has a catheter in place, it should be irrigated to remove any obstruction. If the patient has no urinary catheter and cannot urinate, the surgeon should be notified.

Patients with progressive curvature of the spine (scoliosis) may undergo a Harrington or Luque rod insertion for correction or stabilization of the spine. The procedure entails a spinal fusion followed by rod placement. The postanesthesia assessment entails those features included in the assessment of the thoracic and the lumbosacral spine surgical patient.

Patients who have surgery on the spine should also be observed for bleeding from the site of the operation. The patient should be turned from side to side to help reduce stasis of fluids in the lungs. The technique for turning the spinal patient is called logrolling. All parts of the patient's body should move in unison. To facilitate this, a pillow may be placed between the patient's knees and the knee opposite the side the patient will be turned to should be flexed. Using a draw sheet can also help to facilitate turning in one smooth motion. Pillows should be placed to support the length of the back and buttocks along with the pillow between the patient's knees. This method of turning the patient puts the least amount of pressure on the spine. With the advent of microdisk surgery, disturbance to the stability of the spine is minimal, and these patients are generally allowed activity as desired.

All spinal patients with restricted movement should have antiembolism or pneumatic stockings on, and ankle pumping and rotation should be encouraged to decrease the stasis of blood in the lower extremities. The patient should be encouraged to use the incentive spirometer every hour to reduce the stasis of fluids in the lungs. Neurovascular evaluation is performed every 30 minutes to assess any improvements or deficiencies. Pain is a relative experience for the spinal surgical patient. In many instances, the relief from nerve compression pain is so dramatic that the operative site pain is minimized. In other instances, the pain from spinal fusion is often difficult to manage. As discussed earlier in this chapter, the pain experience must be individualized and treated appropriately. The perianesthesia nurse's goal is to help the patient perceive the pain as something that can be controlled rather than a fearful, unrelenting burden.

PERIANESTHESIA CARE AFTER LIMB AMPUTATION

Patients who have had an amputation of the leg are admitted to the PACU with a dressing or a cast applied to the extremity. A cast is used to provide uniform pressure to the soft tissue, to control swelling, and to position the limb to avoid contracture. See cast care discussed earlier in this chapter in the section on immobilization devices. To prevent hip contracture, elevation of the lower extremity with a soft compression dressing should be achieved by elevating the foot of the bed rather than using a pillow. The patient with an amputation of the arm usually has a bulky compression dressing in place. The dressing should be assessed for drainage. The extremity should be elevated, and ice may be applied to reduce postoperative edema and discomfort.

BIBLIOGRAPHY

Allard JL, Dibble SL: Scoliosis surgery: a look at Luque rods, Am J Nurs 84(5):609-611, 1984.

Alspach J: Core curriculum for critical care nursing, ed 5, Philadelphia, 1998, WB Saunders.

Atlee J: Complications in anesthesia, Philadelphia, 1999, WB Saunders.

Barash P, Cullen B, Stoelting R: Clinical anesthesia, ed 4, Philadelphia, 2000, Lippincott Williams & Wilkins.

Benumof J: Anesthesia and uncommon diseases, ed 4, Philadelphia, 1998, WB Saunders.

Benumof J, Saidman L: Anesthesia & perioperative complications, ed 2, St Louis, 1999, Mosby.

Callahan J: Compartment syndrome, Orthop Nurs 4(4):11-14, 1985.

DeFazio-Quinn D: Ambulatory surgical nursing core curriculum, Philadelphia, 1999, WB Saunders.

Farrell J: Orthopedic pain: what does it mean? Am J Nurs 84(4):466-469, 1984.

Farrell J: Positioning postoperative orthopedic patients, Today's OR Nurse 6(10):12-16, 1984.

Herron D, Nance J: Emergency department nursing management of patients with orthopedic fractures resulting from motor vehicle accidents, Nurs Clin North Am 25(1):71-83, 1990.

Ganong W: Review of medical physiology, ed 20, New York, 2001, McGraw-Hill Professional.

Genge M: Orthopedic trauma: pelvic fractures, Orthop Nurs 5(1):11-18, 1986.

Gregory B, Van Valkenburgh J: The athlete's knee, J Post Anesth Nurs 5(6):414-417, 1990.

Guyton A, Hall J: Textbook of medical physiology, ed 10, Philadelphia, 2000, WB Saunders.

Hardman J, Limbird L: Goodman and Gilman's the pharmacological basis of therapeutics, ed 10, New York, 2001, McGraw-Hill Professional.

Johnson J: Respiratory complications of orthopedic injuries, Orthop Nurs 5(1):24-28, 1986.

Katzung B, editor: Basic and clinical pharmacology, ed 8, Los Altos, Calif, 2000, Appleton & Lange.

Lake C, Hines R, Blitt C: Clinical monitoring: practical applications for anesthesia and critical care, St Louis, 2001, Mosby.

Longnecker D, Murphy F: Dripps/Eckenhoff/Vandam introduction to anesthesia, ed 9, Philadelphia, 1997, WB Saunders.

Longnecker D, Tinker J, Morgan G: Principles and practice of anesthesiology, ed 2, St Louis, 1998, Mosby.

Maier P: Take the work out of range-of-motion exercises, RN 49(9):46-49, 1986.

Miller BK, Gregory M: Carpal tunnel syndrome, AORN J 38(3):525-537, 1983.

Miller R, editor: Anesthesia, ed 5, New York, 2000, Churchill Livingstone.

Mims B: Back surgery: helping your patient get through it, RN 48(5):26-32, 1985.

Nagelhout J, Zaglaniczny K: Nurse anesthesia, ed 2, Philadelphia, 2001, WB Saunders.

Rodts M: Orthopedic nursing and sports nursing, Nurs Clin North Am 26(1):1-240, 1991.

Shenkman B, Stechmiller J: Fat embolism syndrome: pathophysiology and current treatment, Focus Crit Care 11(6):26-35, 1984.

Stoelting R: Pharmacology and physiology in anesthetic practice, ed 3, Philadelphia, 1999, Lippincott-Raven.

Stoelting R, Miller R: Basics of anesthesia, ed 4, New York, 2000, Churchill Livingstone.

Stone D: Perioperative care: anesthesia, medicine, and surgery, St Louis, 1998, Mosby.

Tetzlaff J: Clinical orthopedic anesthesia, Boston, 1995, Butterworth-Heinemann.

Thompson MB: An overview of arthroscopy, Today's OR Nurse 4(11):9-13, 1983.

Townsend C, Beauchamp R, Evers B et al: Sabiston textbook of surgery: the biological basis of modern surgical practice, ed 16, Philadelphia, 2001, WB Saunders.

Turner P: Caring for emotional needs of orthopedic trauma patients, AORN J 36(4):566-570, 1982.

Urbanski PA: The orthopedic patient: identifying neurovascular injury, AORN J 40(5):707-711, 1984.

Waugaman W, Foster S, Rigor B: Principles and practice of nurse anesthesia, ed 3, Norwalk, Conn, 1999, Appleton & Lange.

Willert D, Barden R: Deep vein thrombosis, pulmonary embolism, and prophylaxis in the orthopedic patient, Orthop Nurs 4(4):27-32, 1985.

Wise L: A comparison of orthopedic casts: breaking the mold, MCN 11(3):174-176, 1986.

35

CARE OF THE NEUROSURGICAL PATIENT

Virginia C. Hawkins, MSN, RN, CCRN
John K. Hawkins, PhD, RN, CRNA, MHS

Many healthcare facilities have specialized neurologic care units that receive neurologic surgical patients directly from the operating room, but most facilities require that these patients first be recovered from anesthesia in the postanesthesia care unit (PACU) before they return to the routine care units. Neurosurgical patients, or those with underlying neurologic conditions, present a challenge to the perianesthesia nurse. In addition to being familiar with routine perianesthesia care, the nurse must have a basic understanding of the nervous system and pathologic conditions or injuries that may affect this system and must be able to translate this knowledge into the skills necessary to assess, provide care for, and evaluate the neurosurgical patient.

This chapter is divided into two sections: cranial surgery and spinal surgery. The division is made solely for this discussion, because some aspects of care related to each topic are common to both areas. In addition, disease or injury in any portion of the nervous system may also affect other organs and systems of the body. In caring for the neurosurgical patient, the nurse must consider each structure of the nervous system (see Chapter 8) as it relates to the individual as a whole.

DEFINITIONS

Baroreceptor: a sensory nerve cell aggregate present in the wall of a blood vessel that is stimulated by changes in blood pressure.

Compliance: the ability of the brain to yield when a pressure or force is applied.

Crepitus: a crackling sound produced by the rubbing together of fractured bone fragments or by the presence of subcutaneous emphysema.

Cranial surgery: Surgery classified by infratentorial and supratentorial location

Infratentorial: the area below the tentorium that includes the brain stem, cerebellum, and posterior fossa. This approach is used for lesions in the brain stem and cerebellum region.

Supratentorial: the area above the tentorium that includes the cerebrum. The supratentorial approach is used for frontal, temporal, parietal, and occipital lobe lesions.

Craniotomy: a surgical opening of the skull.

Craniectomy: removal of a portion of the skull without a replacement.

Cranioplasty: to repair the skull by replacing a part of the cranium with a synthetic material.

Decompensation: the inability of the heart to maintain adequate circulation because of an impairment in brain integrity.

Diabetes insipidus: a metabolic disorder caused by injury or disease of the posterior lobe of the pituitary gland (the hypophysis).

Focal deficit: any sign or symptom that indicates a specific or localized area of pathologic alteration.

Laminectomy: excision of the posterior arch of a vertebra to allow excision of a herniated nucleus pulposus.

Phrenic nucleus: a group of nerve cells located in the spinal cord between the levels of C3 and C5. Damage to this area abolishes or alters the function of the phrenic nerve.

Pyramidal signs: symptoms of dysfunction of the pyramidal tract, including spastic paralysis, Babinski's reflex, and increased deep tendon reflexes.

Rhizotomy: surgical interruption of the roots of the spinal nerves within the spinal canal.

Spinal shock: a state that occurs immediately after complete transection of the spinal cord. It may sometimes occur after only partial transections. All sensory, motor, and autonomic activities are lost below the level of the transection, and reflexes are absent. Paralysis is of a flaccid nature and includes the urinary bladder. Autonomic activity gradually resumes as spinal shock subsides. Once autonomic activity has returned, bladder and bowel training programs may be begun. Flaccid paralysis may develop into varying degrees of spastic paralysis, as evidenced by spasms of flexor or extensor muscle groups. The presence of autonomic activity also allows for episodes of autonomic hyperreflexia.

Subarachnoid block: the injection of a local anesthetic into the subarachnoid space around the spinal cord.

Subluxation: partial or incomplete dislocation.

Tonoclonic movements: tense muscular contractions alternating rapidly with muscular relaxation.

Valsalva maneuver: contraction of the thorax in forced expiration against the closed glottis; results in increases in intrathoracic and intraabdominal pressures.

CRANIAL SURGERY

Diagnostic Tools

Some of the techniques used to ascertain the presence and extent of cranial injury or disease include invasive and noninvasive techniques. A brief discussion of invasive as well as noninvasive diagnostic procedures is included here to familiarize the PACU nurse with the techniques and the special considerations necessary in the care of these patients.

Conventional Radiography. Skull films are not ordered as often as computed tomographic (CT) scans and magnetic resonance imaging (MRI) scans. They are most often ordered to diagnose the presence of a skull fracture and provide information about the size, shape, and integrity of the skull and facial bones and any unusual calcification, and presence of air (Fig. 35-1).

CT Scanning. CT scanning creates a cross-sectional picture that separates various densities in the brain by means of an external x-ray beam. A computer-based apparatus allows the assessment of brain-emitted radiation and stores this information in the computer. The computer performs thousands of simultaneous equations on the radiation input and output data stored on its

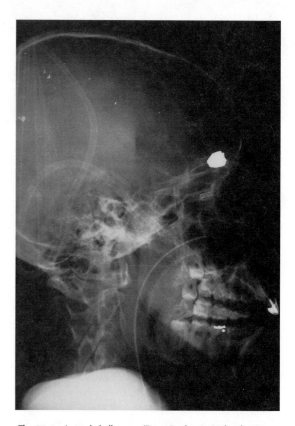

Fig. 35-1 Lateral skull x-ray. *(From Bucher L, Melander S: Critical nursing, Philadelphia, 1999, WB Saunders.)*

tapes and delivers an accurate, detailed picture of the brain and of any abnormalities (Fig. 35-2). The computer images correlate to tissue density. The dense structures, such as bone, will appear white in color. Air and cerebrospinal fluid (CSF) will appear as black area because they have much less density. The radiologist will look at the structures, changes in density, and any abnormalities in shape, size, or location of structures.

Contrast material may be used to enhance images. An iodinated radiopaque material will be injected intravenously. Scans are usually taken before and after the administration of the radiopaque material. CT scanning has the advantages of accuracy and rapidity; both are essential in emergency situations. The entire procedure may last 15 to 20 minutes and may be difficult to use in an agitated, confused, or restless patient.

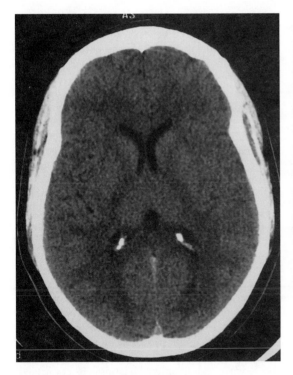

Fig. 35-2   CT scan. *(From Bucher L, Melander S: Critical nursing, Philadelphia, 1999, WB Saunders.)*

The CT scan is most helpful in diagnosing hematomas, subarachnoid hemorrhage, hydrocephalus, cerebral atrophy, and tumors.

Care before the CT scan should include an assessment of the patient's allergies—specifically allergies to shellfish, iodine, or contrast dye. A blood urea nitrogen and creatinine levels should be checked to assess kidney function. Some patients may experience a headache, feeling of warmth, salty taste in the mouth, nausea or vomiting when given contrast dye. After the procedure it is important for the patient to be well hydrated to help excrete the contrast dye.

Magnetic Resonance Imaging.   Also known as nuclear magnetic resonance imaging, MRI is a technique for obtaining cross-sectional pictures of the human body without exposure of the patient to ionizing radiation. MRI yields anatomic information comparable in many ways to the information supplied by a CT scan but is often able to more accurately discriminate between healthy and diseased tissues (Fig. 35-3). MRI is excellent in detecting soft tissue changes.

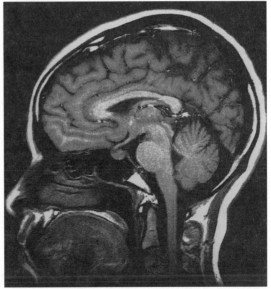

Fig. 35-3   Normal magnetic resonance imaging. *(From Bucher L, Melander S: Critical nursing, Philadelphia, 1999, WB Saunders.)*

It can detect necrotic tissue, small malignant tumors, and degenerative diseases.

The patient is placed within a cylindrical high-powered magnet. Body tissues are then subjected to a magnetic field, which causes some of the hydrogen ions to align themselves with the field. A burst of low-energy radio waves is then applied that knocks atomic protons within the tissues out of alignment. When the radio waves are discontinued, these protons release tiny amounts of energy that are "read" by a computer. Then the MRI generates an image based on this information, thus yielding a detailed picture of the structural content and contours of the internal organs.

Contraindications for MRI include claustrophobic, agitated, or obese patients and patients with metallic devices or fragments present in the body.

Positron Emission Tomography.   Positron emission tomographic (PET) scanning is used most often in major research facilities. The PET scan measures glucose uptake and metabolism, cerebral blood flow patterns, and oxygen uptake to ascertain the functioning of the tissues or organs. The patient is injected with a glucose analogue that is tagged with a radionuclide. As the radionuclide decays in the tissue, the protons emitted are recorded by detectors, and a computerized picture is generated. PET scans have been helpful in identifying schizophrenia, Alzheimer's disease, epilepsy, cardiovascular disease, head trauma, and other brain disorders.

Electroencephalography. An electroencephalogram (EEG) is the tracing and recording of the electrical activity at the surface of the brain. Aberrations in the rate and amplitude signal the presence of tumors, abscesses, scars, hematomas, or infection and may aid in the localization of such lesions.

Cerebral Angiography. Arteriography, or angiography, is the diagnostic tool for aneurysms, arteriovenous malformations, and other cerebrovascular abnormalities. A cannula is introduced into the femoral or axillary artery and threaded to the level of the common carotid artery. Radiopaque dye is then injected, and radiographs record its path through the cerebral vasculature (Fig. 35-4). During and after arteriography, the patient may experience an allergic reaction to the dye that may range from mild urticaria to anaphylaxis. Resuscitative equipment must be immediately available until the danger of allergic reaction has passed.

Irritation brought on by use of the dye may manifest itself in altered states of consciousness, hemiparesis, or speech difficulties that are usually transient. It is imperative that the site of injection be examined closely at frequent intervals for the presence of bleeding that may occur beneath the skin and defies casual detection. The effects of the local anesthetic agent often last for several hours and prevent the patient from detecting and reporting the pain caused by hemorrhage. Routine postprocedure care will include bedrest, observation of the puncture site for signs of bleeding, monitoring of vital signs and neurologic signs. Intravenous fluids are maintained until the danger of untoward reaction has passed and the patient no longer experiences the transient nausea that occasionally occurs.

Brain Scanning. A radioactive compound is injected intravenously and is taken up by brain tissue. The pattern of this uptake is detected by a scintillation scanner, and a visual record is made. Uptake may be altered at the site of a disorder and may reflect the presence of cerebral neoplasms, hematomas, abscesses, and AVMs.

Injuries and Pathologic Conditions of the Brain

Types of Injuries. When a head injury occurs, the most crucial concern is the extent of injury to the brain itself. Linear skull fractures in and of themselves are of little significance. The injury becomes more severe when the fracture involves depression of fragments into the brain, penetration of a foreign object, leakage of CSF, expanding hematomas, or signs and symptoms of herniation. The primary goal is to protect the brain and facilitate the patient returning to an optimal level of functioning.

Skull fractures are categorized as linear, depressed, or basilar. They are often described as simple, comminuted, and compound. The linear skull fracture is the most common. Most linear skull fractures are not depressed and do not require treatment. A depressed skull fracture is an inward depression of the skull and are classified as open or compound. Infection is a primary concern and surgery may be necessary to remove bony fragments, clean the wound, and elevate the depressed bone. Basilar skull fractures occur in the base of the skull and are difficult to diagnose with radiographs. Diagnosis is confirmed with clinical data. Patients will often present with "raccoon's eyes," periorbital ecchymosis, or "Battles sign," ecchymosis around the mastoid process, or CSF otorrhea.

Concussion is caused by a violent jar or shock to the skull, such as rapid acceleration-deceleration. The patient may be dazed, "see stars," or experience a period of impaired consciousness. When they regain consciousness, these patients may experience posttraumatic amnesia and remember nothing of the injury itself nor of the events immediately preceding the injury.

Contusion is a bruising of the brain or hemorrhage on its surface. The extent of severity depends on the site and degree of brain injury. Consciousness may or may not be lost, but coma indicates diffuse injury. Laceration is the tearing of the brain. Laceration and contusions of the brain are usually found in the frontal and parietal lobes.

Consequences of Injury. Traumatic head injury can cause hemorrhage beneath a skull fracture or from a shearing of the veins or cortical arteries and results in epidural, subdural, subarachnoid, or intraventricular hemorrhage (Fig. 35-5). The signs and symptoms of brain ischemia and increased ICP vary with the speed at which the

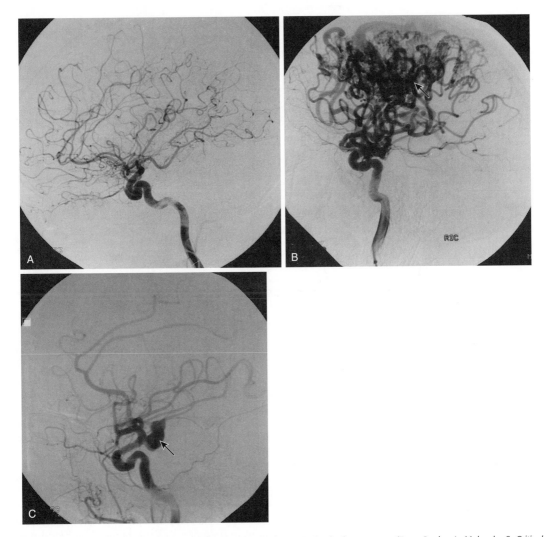

Fig. 35-4 Cerebral angiograms. **A,** Normal. **B,** Cerebral hemorrhage. **C,** Cerebral aneursym. *(From Bucher L, Melander S: Critical nursing, Philadelphia, 1999, WB Saunders.)*

functions of vital centers are altered. A small clot that accumulates rapidly may be fatal. On the other hand, the patient may survive a slowly developing, much larger hematoma through effective compensatory mechanisms.

An epidural hematoma, or extradural hematoma, accumulates in the epidural space (between the skull and the dura mater) and is arterial. Often the cause is the rupture or laceration of the middle meningeal artery, which runs between the dura and the skull in the temporal region. Epidural hematomas may also be seen in the frontal, occipital, and posterior fossa regions. Epidural hematomas require rapid emergency surgery. The patient usually loses consciousness, after which he or she experiences a lucid period then rapid deterioration. The hemorrhage may be massive, and treatment consists of evacuation of the clot through burr holes made in the skull.

Subdural hematoma may result from trauma and the shearing of the bridging veins. Venous blood usually accumulates beneath the dura and spreads over the surface of the brain. A subdural hematoma may be acute, subacute, or chronic,

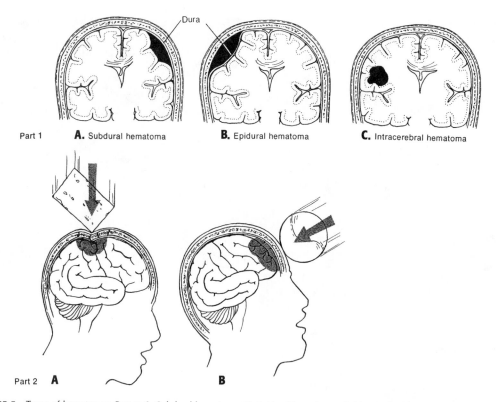

Fig. 35-5 Types of hematomas. Part 1: **A,** Subdural hematoma. **B,** Epidural hematoma. **C,** Intracerebral hematoma. Part 2: Mechanisms of head injury. **A,** Direct injury resulting in depressed skull fracture and compression injury. **B,** Blow to skull resulting in tearing of blood vessels. Shaded areas represent cerebral contusion. *(Part 1, In Clochesy J, Breu C, Cardin S et al: Critical care nursing, ed 2, Philadelphia, 1996, WB Saunders. Part 2, From Luckman J, Sorensen KC: Medical-surgical nursing: a psychophysiologic approach, ed 3, Philadelphia, 1987, WB Saunders.*

depending on the size of the vessel involved and the amount of blood present. Patients who present with acute subdural hematomas exhibit rapid deterioration in their condition and are critically ill.

Subacute subdural hematomas fail to show acute signs and symptoms at their onset. Brain swelling is not great, but the hematoma may become large enough to produce symptoms. Progressive hemiparesis, obtundation, and aphasia often appear 4 to 21 days after injury. The degree of ultimate recovery depends on the extent of damage produced at the time of injury.

Chronic subdural hematomas are seen most often in older adults. A history of head injury may be lacking because the causative injury is often minimal and long forgotten or deemed insignificant by the patient. The history is usually one of

progressive mental or personality changes with or without focal symptoms as blood slowly accumulates and compresses the brain. The blood itself becomes thicker and darker within 2 to 4 days and within a few weeks resembles motor oil in character and color. Papilledema may be present. Chronic subdural hematomas may mimic any disease that affects the brain or its coverings. Treatment consists of evacuation of the defibrinated blood through multiple burr holes or craniotomy incision.

Intracerebral hematomas are more commonly found in the elderly—often after a fall—but are also seen as a result of spontaneous rupture of a weakened blood vessel. Hemorrhaging may be scattered or isolated. Surgical evacuation of an isolated or well-defined clot may be attempted, but the mortality rate remains high.

Subarachnoid hemorrhage may occur as the result of traumatic brain injury. Bleeding into the subarachnoid space may result in a vasospasm. A vasospasm is the narrowing of the blood vessel lumen and places the patient at risk for a delayed ischemic event. The risk of developing vasospasms is greatest three to seven days after the bleed.

Intraventricular hemorrhage is bleeding into the ventricles caused by brain trauma such as penetrating wounds.

Supratentorial herniation is regarded as an emergency more severe than an epidural hematoma. The tentorium is an extension of the dura mater, which forms a transverse partition or shelf that divides the cerebral hemispheres from the cerebellum and brain stem. The superior portion of the brain stem passes upward through an aperture in the tentorium known as the tentorial hiatus. No space-occupying mass or lesion that expands within the cerebral hemispheres can escape upward or outward because of the confinement of the skull. Consequently, expansion within and compression of the hemispheres causes herniation of its contents (usually a portion of the temporal lobe known as the uncus) through the tentorial hiatus.

Uncal herniation is accompanied by compression of the lateral brain stem on the same side, thus shutting off its blood supply and suppressing certain basic functions. The third cranial nerve (oculomotor) is in close proximity to the herniated uncus, and the pupil on the injured side becomes fixed and dilated. The reticular-activating system located in the brain stem that is responsible for waking and alertness becomes affected, and the patient rapidly becomes less and less responsive. Displacement of the midbrain causes compression of the pyramidal tract, thus resulting in contralateral hemiparesis or hemiplegia and plantar extensor responses (Babinski's reflex). The respiratory center in the medulla may be affected, which will result in changes in the respiratory pattern or cessation of respiration altogether.

In addition to these changes, the cerebellum itself may be so compressed that the cerebellar tonsil herniates inferiorly through the foramen magnum. This usually results in immediate death, as the centers vital to life are compressed or sheared. The best treatment for supratentorial herniation is prevention through early detection and treatment of increased ICP and its causes.

If efforts to minimize edema and increased ICP fail, surgical intervention, if possible, is required as a life-saving measure.

Types of Pathologic Conditions. Cerebral aneurysms are round dilatations of the arterial wall that develop as a result of weakness of the wall due to defects in the media layer of the artery. Most cerebral aneurysms occur at bifurcations close to the circle of Willis, usually involving the anterior portion. Common bifurcations include those with the internal carotid, the middle cerebral, and the basilar arteries and in relation to the anterior and posterior communicating arteries. The exact cause or precipitating factor is not well defined but may be related to congenital abnormality, arteriosclerosis, embolus, or trauma. Aneurysms are usually asymptomatic and present no clinical problem to the patient unless rupture occurs, thus resulting in neurologic deficits. Ruptured cerebral aneurysm is the major cause of subarachnoid hemorrhage. Intracerebral hemorrhage may occur alone or with the subarachnoid bleed. Morbidity and mortality rates are high due to rebleeding of the aneurysm and cerebral vasospasm of adjacent arteries. Surgical intervention involves identification and clipping of the aneurysm through a craniotomy.

Arteriovenous malformation (AVM) is a vascular network appearing as a tangled mass of dilated vessels that create an abnormal communication between the arterial and venous systems. The communication may be singular or multiple and resembles an arteriovenous fistula in that no connecting capillary system between the arteries and the veins exists. AVMs most commonly occur in the supratentorial structures and usually involve the vessels of the middle cerebral arteries. AVMs are usually present at birth as the result of congenital abnormalities but may exhibit a delayed age of onset; symptoms most commonly occur between the ages of 10 and 20 years. Symptoms may include headache, seizures, altered level of consciousness (LOC), and intracranial hemorrhage with resultant increased ICP. The treatment of choice is complete surgical excision by dissection or obliteration by ligation of feeder vessels. Radiation is used to treat AVMs that are not surgically accessible.

Intracranial tumors are space-occupying lesions that destroy brain tissue and nerve structures by invasion, infiltration, and compression and produce increased ICP.

Intracranial tumors can be primary or metastatic. Primary tumors are classified as primary intracerebral (intraaxial) tumors, which originate from glia cells, or primary extracerebral (extraaxial) tumors, which originate from supporting structures of the nervous system. Metastatic tumors most commonly arise from breast malignancies in women and lung malignancies in men. Clinical manifestations can be both localized and generalized in nature. Local pathophysiologic changes—such as focal neurologic deficits, seizures, visual disturbances, cranial nerve dysfunction, and hormonal changes—result from the tumor itself destroying tissue at a particular site in the brain. Generalized pathophysiologic changes result from the effects of increased ICP. The treatment for cerebral tumors is surgical excision or surgical decompression if total excision is not possible. Surgery is often performed before, during, or after radiation treatment and chemotherapy.

Hydrocephalus in and of itself is not a disease entity but rather a clinical syndrome characterized by excess fluid within the cerebral ventricular system, the subarachnoid space, or both. Hydrocephalus occurs because of abnormalities in overproduction, circulation, or reabsorption of CSF. Hydrocephalus can be classified into two categories: noncommunicating (obstructive) or communicating (nonobstructive). Noncommunicating hydrocephalus is the result of an obstruction in the ventricular system or the subarachnoid space that prevents the flow of CSF to the location of the arachnoid villi, where reabsorption occurs. The obstruction may be caused by congenital abnormalities or space-occupying lesions. Communicating hydrocephalus occurs when the flow of CSF is normal but impaired absorption of the fluid at the arachnoid villi is impaired. Common causes of communicating hydrocephalus include inflammation of the meninges, subarachnoid hemorrhage, congenital malformation, and space-occupying lesions.

Intracranial Pressure Dynamics

ICP is pressure that is exerted against the skull by its contents: solid brain matter and intracellular water, CSF, and blood. These contents are essentially noncompressible, and a volume change in any compartment requires a reciprocal change to occur in one or both of the other compartments if the ICP is to remain constant (Monroe-Kellie hypothesis). Because of the communications between their intracranial and extracranial compartments, CSF and blood can be translocated extracranially in partial compensation for increased ICP. These compensation capabilities are limited because of the small amount of CSF that the spinal subarachnoid space can hold, and total displacement of cerebral blood results in cerebral ischemia. Normal ICP is 0 to 15 torr. Intracranial hypertension occurs when a sustained increased ICP at the level of the head occurs and exceeds 15 torr.

Volume may be added to any of the cerebral compartments and results in increased ICP when the compensatory capacity is exceeded. Brain volume can be increased by a tumor, a hematoma, or edema. Blood volume can be increased through dilatation of the vascular bed. CSF volume can be increased through obstruction in the ventricles, resistance to reabsorption, or, in rare instances, increased production of the CSF. Large brain tumors increase pressure by their mass, by blocking the rate of CSF reabsorption, or both. If the tumor is near the surface of the brain, it can cause inflamed meninges that may exude large quantities of fluid and protein into the CSF, thus increasing ICP. Hemorrhage or infection also causes increases in ICP. Large numbers of cells suddenly appear in the CSF and can almost totally block CSF absorption through the arachnoid villi. Regardless of the mechanism, when the volume added exceeds the volume that can be displaced, intracranial compliance is greatly reduced, and ICP begins to increase.

Figure 35-6 illustrates the relationship between intracranial volume and pressure. Phase I demonstrates the success of compensatory mechanisms in maintaining a constant ICP despite early increases in volume. In phase II, the limited capability of compensatory mechanisms has been exceeded, and ICP begins to rise. In phase III, even a slight increase in volume causes a dramatic rise in ICP, thus resulting in complete decompensation and death. The shape of the curve may be altered by the rate at which the volume increases. Slowly developing increases in volume broaden the curve, whereas rapid increases narrow it.

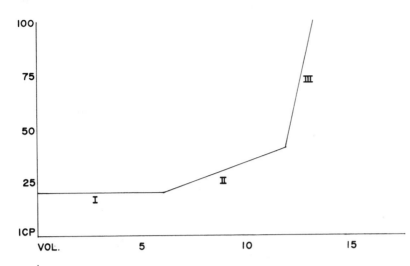

Fig. 35-6 Pressure-volume curve.

Perianesthesia care for the patients with the potential for increased ICP requires an understanding of cerebral blood flow (CBF) and the factors that affect it; these factors become defective during increased ICP and are manipulated to reduce ICP. CBF is directly proportional to cerebral perfusion pressure (CPP) and inversely proportional to cerebrovascular resistance. CPP is the difference between the mean arterial pressure (MAP) and the right atrial pressure. When ICP is greater than right atrial pressure, the CPP is determined by the difference between the MAP and ICP.

$$CPP = MAP - ICP$$

and

$$CBF = (MAP - ICP)\ CVR$$

CPP = cerebral perfusion pressure; MAP = mean arterial pressure; ICP = intracranial pressure; CBF = cerebral blood flow; and CVR = cerebrovascular resistance

Consequently, any increase in ICP or reduction in MAP reduces CPP and resultant CBF. Normal CBF is 45 to 60 ml/100 g/minute. The CBF below which cerebral ischemia occurs has been termed the critical CBF, which is at flow rate of 16 or 17 ml/100 g/min. Normal CPP is 80 to 100 torr. CBF begins to fail at a CPP of 30 to 40 torr. Irreversible hypoxia occurs at a CPP below 30 torr. When ICP equals MAP, CPP equals zero and CBF ceases.

Factors that influence CBF regulation are PaO_2 and $PaCO_2$ (metabolic regulation), arterial blood pressure and autoregulation, and venous blood pressure. Metabolic regulation works in two ways. The first is by regulation of blood flow based on the tissue needs for metabolic substrates—oxygen and glucose. As the activity of neuronal and glial cells in the brain increases, the demand for oxygen and glucose increases. The increased demand causes vasodilatation of arterioles, which increases CBF. Likewise, if the metabolic demand decreases, vasoconstriction occurs and CBF decreases.

The second—and most significant—way metabolic regulation affects CBF is by the presence of metabolic byproducts, specifically carbon dioxide. Carbon dioxide is the most potent vasodilator of cerebral blood vessels. Normal cerebral vessels respond to changes in carbon dioxide by dilating when carbon dioxide increases and constricting when carbon dioxide decreases. The relationship between CBF and carbon dioxide is linear, and changes in CBF are in direct proportion to changes in carbon dioxide. There is a decrease of 1 ml/100 g/min in CBF for every 1 torr decrease in carbon dioxide. When treating elevated ICP, carbon dioxide levels of 30 to 35 torr are used to lower CBF.

Autoregulation is the ability of the cerebral vasculature in normal brain tissue to alter its resistance so that CBF remains relatively constant over a wide range of CPP. This mechanism causes

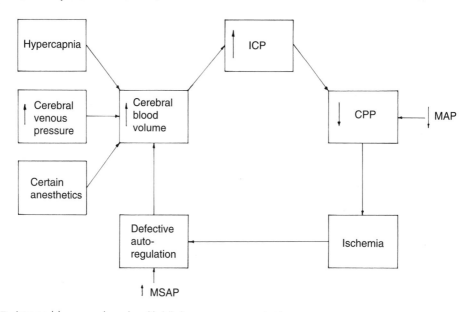

Fig. 35-7 Intracranial pressure dynamics with failed compensatory mechanisms.

vasoconstriction when perfusion pressure increases and vasodilatation when perfusion pressure decreases. The limits of autoregulation are at a CPP of approximately 60 torr at the lower end and 160 torr at the upper end. Beyond the limits of autoregulation, CBF becomes passively dependent on CPP. When CPP increases above the upper limit of autoregulation, it exceeds the ability of the vasculature to constrict; CBF becomes directly related to and possibly dependent on CPP.

The lower limit of CBF autoregulation is the blood pressure below which vasodilatation becomes inadequate and CBF decreases. When CPP decreases below 60 torr because of increases in ICP, autoregulation ceases to be beneficial or effective in regulating CBF. Defective autoregulation aggravates pressure increases and creates critical or irreversible levels of ICP by increasing the blood volume within the cranium in an effort to maintain CBF. Defective autoregulation generally occurs when ICP exceeds 30 to 35 torr. Eventually, autoregulation ceases altogether, and blood flow fluctuates passively with changes in arterial pressure, regardless of metabolic activity or regulation.

When ICP is increased, CPP and CBF are reduced, which renders the tissues ischemic.

Ischemic cerebral tissue releases acid metabolites that cause a relatively fixed reduction in cerebrovascular tone. Autoregulation ceases, and any increase in MAP causes further increase in cerebral blood volume and elicits a further increase in ICP. CPP is reduced, thus causing ischemic areas (such as those surrounding an expanding intracranial mass) to enlarge. As can be seen in Figure 35-7, a pathologic cycle ensues in which the outcome is that ICP and MAP eventually equilibrate, the CPP drops to zero, CBF stops, and death occurs.

Neurosurgical Procedures. With further developments in technology, neurosurgeons have more options in the treatment of their patients. Surgical procedures that use instrumentation, lasers, and radiation therapy have increased the surgeon's ability to treat neurologic disorders.

Stereotaxis. Stereotaxis is the precise location of deep brain lesions. A stereotactic frame is applied to the patient's head, and the target tissue is located with the stereotactic frames coordinates and CT scanning. Stereotaxis is also used for destruction of intracranial sensory pathways and is especially useful in the treatment of intractable chronic pain.

Stereotactic Radiosurgery. The most common approaches to stereotactic radiosurgery (SR) are gamma knife and medical linear accelerator units (LINAC). Stereotactic radiosurgery can destroy deep and surgically inaccessible areas. The goal of SR treatment is the delivery of high dose radiation to a specific target area without delivering the radiation to surrounding tissue. Regardless of the type of SR, a stereotactic frame is secured to the patient's head for accurate determination of target location. The placement of the stereotactic frame requires local anesthesia. Complications after SR may not appear for months to years later. Potential complications include permanent neurological deficit, rebleeding, and worsening clinical symptoms.

Laser Surgery. The benefit of laser surgery is that it enables the neurosurgeon to access areas that were surgically inaccessible with conventional surgery. Using laser surgery, the surgeon can dissect a structure without trauma to the surrounding tissue, shrink tumors, and coagulate blood vessels.

Anesthetic Agents and Intracranial Pressure. Anesthetic agents alter ICP by increasing or decreasing CBF and cerebral metabolic rate. In addition to their effects on ICP, some of these agents may also reduce systemic blood pressure and cause cerebral ischemia due to inadequate CPP.

Inhalation Anesthetics. The inhalation anesthetic agents generally decrease blood pressure and may increase ICP in the cranial surgical patient. They produce a clinically significant degree of cerebrovascular vasodilatation and metabolic depression and can modify autoregulation. In fact, high dosages of volatile anesthetic agents can cause a total loss of autoregulation. The resulting increase in CBF will ultimately lead to increased ICP. In patients with decreased intracranial compliance secondary to neurologic disease, anesthetic agents that increase CBF may produce marked changes in ICP.

In most modern facilities, halothane and enflurane are rarely used because of the availability of more recently developed volatile inhalation agents that offer the advantage of rapid uptake and elimination, thus providing a more rapid recovery. However, halothane and enflurane are still available and may be used in small facilities and/or more remote areas because they are relatively inexpensive in comparison to the newer inhalation agents. Therefore they will be discussed here.

Halothane (Fluothane) produces dose-related elevations in CBF. Low concentrations produce minimal changes in CBF and ICP, whereas higher concentrations can increase CBF nearly threefold. Introduction of halothane simultaneously with the initiation of mechanical hyperventilation sufficient to lower $PaCO_2$ to 25 torr does not reliably prevent drug-induced elevations in CBF and ICP. Conversely, establishment of hypocarbia before adding halothane prevents increases in ICP; however, this also may not be totally reliable. Presumably, prior hypocarbia attenuates or blocks the cerebral-vasodilating effects of halothane that lead to increased CBF.

Enflurane (Ethrane), like halothane, can cause abrupt increases in ICP. As with halothane, hypocarbia produced simultaneously with the administration of enflurane does not always protect against an increase in ICP. In addition to increased CBF, the increased ICP may reflect the ability of enflurane to increase both the rate of production and resistance to reabsorption of CSF. Enflurane also has the ability to produce central nervous system seizure activity that can occur in pathologic or nonpathologic conditions. The likelihood of enflurane-evoked seizure activity is increased when high concentrations are used or when hyperventilation of the lungs lowers $PaCO_2$ below 30 torr. These characteristics make enflurane unsuitable for patients who are undergoing neurosurgical procedures.

Isoflurane (Forane): at normocarbia, has been shown to increase ICP. Unlike halothane, the initiation of hyperventilation simultaneously with the introduction of isoflurane prevents the increase in ICP that occurs at normocarbia. Unlike enflurane, isoflurane does not alter production of CSF and actually decreases resistance to absorption. Isoflurane does not cause excitation of the central nervous system as enflurane does. Isoflurane produces reductions in cerebral metabolic rate that exceed those produced by an equivalent-dose concentration of halothane, and there is less impairment of autoregulation than with halothane. The greater decrease in cerebral metabolic rate may explain why CBF increases are minimal at low concentrations.

Although they have not been extensively studied, Desflurane and Sevoflurane, demonstrate essentially the same characteristics as isoflurane. During normocarbia, desflurane and sevoflurane cause cerebral vasodilation with resultant increases in CBF and ICP. The cerebrovascular response to CO_2 is maintained; therefore the increase in CBF can be attenuated with hyperventilation. The cerebral metabolic rate is reduced in a dose-dependent manner similar to that of isoflurane, and no neuronal excitation as is seen with enflurane seems to exist. Both agents cause cardiovascular depression and can be used with caution for controlled hypotension to reduce CBF. Desflurane, unlike sevoflurane, may result in an increase in MAP and heart rate when used for induction or at initially high concentrations. This affect may be attenuated by the use of narcotics and/or beta blockers. Both desflurane and sevoflurane have relatively low blood/gas partition coefficients that allow for rapid elimination of the agent, which makes them very desirable for use because of the more rapid recovery.

Nitrous oxide has become very controversial for use during intracranial surgical procedures. When used alone, nitrous oxide can cause an increase in CBF, ICP, and cerebral metabolic rate at normocarbia. These effects, however, are attenuated by the use of barbiturates, benzodiazepines, narcotics, and hyperventilation. To a small extent, nitrous oxide is a cerebral vasodilator and does not interfere with autoregulation of the CBF. For neurosurgical patients in whom increased ICP is not a problem, nitrous oxide may be an acceptable choice when combined with other agents to benefit from its rapid onset and elimination. However, it should be used cautiously in patients with increased ICP.

Intravenous Anesthetics. Intravenous anesthetic agents (with the exception of ketamine) are usually the anesthetics of choice in cranial surgery.

Barbiturates such as thiopental (Pentothal) are potent cerebral vasoconstrictors that can reduce CBF with subsequent reduction in elevated ICP. Cerebral vasoconstriction that is produced by barbiturates and the impact on CBF and ICP are dose-related. The reduction in CBF produced by barbiturates is even greater if hypocarbia is also present and is maintained at a constant level. Deep thiopental anesthesia during normo-

carbia results in about a 50% reduction in both cerebral metabolic rate and CBF.

Benzodiazepines, such as diazepam (Valium) and midazolam (Versed) produce sedation and amnesia by stimulating specific receptors in the brain. The benzodiazepines produce dose-related reductions in cerebral metabolic rate and CBF. When central benzodiazepine receptors are pharmacologically saturated, these drugs may decrease cerebral metabolic rate as much as 40%.

Narcotics, such as fentanyl, morphine, and meperidine, are typically classified as cerebral vasoconstrictors, with resultant reductions in CBF. This effect is readily abolished by vasodilatation that can accompany narcotic-induced ventilatory depression and the resultant increase in $PaCO_2$. In humans maintained at normocarbia, fentanyl does not alter CBF. During normocarbia, the combination of nitrous oxide and morphine does not significantly alter CBF or autoregulation. Fentanyl—and the combination of fentanyl and droperidol (Innovar)—causes a reduction in CBF and ICP in patients with normal CSF pathways. Alfentanil and sufentanil may in fact cause an increase in ICP in patients with compromised cerebral compliance.

Etomidate (Amidate) produces a maximal 45% decrease in cerebral metabolic rate and CBF; like the barbiturates, it can produce complete EEG suppression and appears to be comparable in lowering ICP. Unlike the barbiturates, etomidate has less effect on MAP and offers greater stability in hemodynamically compromised patients.

Propofol (Diprivan) reduces cerebral metabolic rate, CBF, and ICP and increases cerebrovascular resistance in a dose-dependent manner. The use of propofol in patients with elevated ICP may not be appropriate because of the substantial decrease in MAP and resultant decrease in CPP.

Ketamine (Ketalar, Ketaject) can rapidly increase ICP and often reduce CPP, despite mild increases in blood pressure. Ketamine is generally contraindicated for use in neurosurgical patients unless the fontanelles are open, CSF aspiration is instituted, or ventilatory control is maintained.

The use of controlled ventilation to produce $PaCO_2$ levels in the range of 25 to 30 torr and the administration of nitrous oxide and oxygen and possibly low concentrations of isoflurane, together with narcotics and muscle relaxants, is a generally accepted anesthetic technique for the neurosurgical patient.

Adjunctive Drugs Used to Reduce Intracranial Pressure

Diuretics. Mannitol and furosemide (Lasix) are diuretics often used to control increased ICP. Mannitol, an osmotic diuretic, is the agent of choice for ICP reduction. Mannitol is administered intravenously in doses of 0.25 to 1 g per kg in a 15% to 25% solution over 30 to 60 minutes, with the maximum effects occurring in 1 or 2 hours. Urine output can reach 1 or 2 L within 1 hour. Appropriate infusion of crystalloid and colloid solutions is often necessary to prevent adverse changes in plasma concentrations of electrolytes and intravascular fluid volume because of the rapidity of diuresis.

Potential complications of the use of mannitol include hyperosmolarity, electrolyte loss, changes in blood viscosity and coagulation, transient intravascular hypervolemia, and rebound or secondary elevation of ICP.

Furosemide is a loop diuretic. Furosemide is administered intravenously at a dose of 1 mg per kg to patients with normal ICP who are undergoing craniotomy and is more effective in reducing ICP than mannitol. Furosemide is the drug of choice in patients with congestive heart failure.

Furosemide, when combined with mannitol, has been shown to potentiate the ICP-reducing effects of mannitol at the cost of rapid loss of intravascular volume and electrolytes. The ICP effects of these drugs are lost after 1 or 2 hours.

Corticosteroids. The drugs most commonly used are dexamethasone and methylprednisolone. Steroids are effective in lowering increased ICP because of localized vasogenic cerebral edema associated with mass-type lesions, such as neoplasm, abscess, and intracerebral hematoma. It is controversial with head trauma and cerebral infarctions with edema. The mechanism for the beneficial effect of corticosteroids is not known but may involve stabilization of capillary membranes, reduction in CSF production, blood-brain barrier repair, prevention of lysosomal activity, enhanced cerebral electrolyte transport, improved brain metabolism, and promotion of water and electrolyte excretion.

Barbiturate Therapy. Initiation of barbiturate therapy is the last medication adjunct used in treating intracranial hypertension. The patient must have an intracranial pressure–monitoring device and usually started when ICP is above 30 mm Hg for 30 minutes and a CPP below 70 mm Hg. The most common barbiturate is Pentobarbital, which lowers the ICP by inhibiting free radical mediated lipid peroxidation, altering the vascular tone, and suppressing metabolism.

Intracranial Pressure Monitoring. The most precise indicator of the pressure state within the cranium is the CSF pressure. Monitoring of ICP is the standard of care for patients at risk for intracranial hypertension. Measurement of this pressure may be obtained from the lateral ventricles, subarachnoid space, epidural or subdural spaces, or the intraparenchymal. Values from these areas are meaningful indicators of ICP only if pressure is freely transmitted between these compartments. Because injury and disease of the brain often create obstruction in CSF flow, the most accurate values are those obtained from the ventricle.

Lumbar puncture values reflect only a relative index of the actual ICP. These values depend on the state of the spinal canal and all the factors that affect it. On the other hand, measurement of the ventricular fluid pressure gives a direct and absolute value of the ICP, regardless of the influence or condition of the spinal canal. Lumbar puncture has other limitations. Its use is limited to those patients without suspected intracranial mass or to those whose ICP is not elevated or is elevated only slightly. In patients with these conditions, herniation of the brain tissue with the removal of CSF is a risk. ICP monitoring does not present this risk and can be used in a variety of conditions.

ICP monitoring devices are categorized into two primary categories. The first category includes devices that use fluid or hydrostatic coupling to transmit to an external transducer. Ventricular catheters, subarachnoid bolts or screws, and subdural catheters fall into this group. The second group uses a transducer to directly monitor ICP. These intracranial devices use fiberoptics to transmit ICP pressures (Fig. 35-8).

The subarachnoid bolt or screw was developed in 1973 and requires only a twist-drill hole in the skull and a nick in the dura for insertion. As the name implies, the sensor lies in the subarachnoid space. The advantage of this type of monitoring device is less risk of infection and that it can be used in patients with small ventricles. However, in the presence of moderately severe cerebral

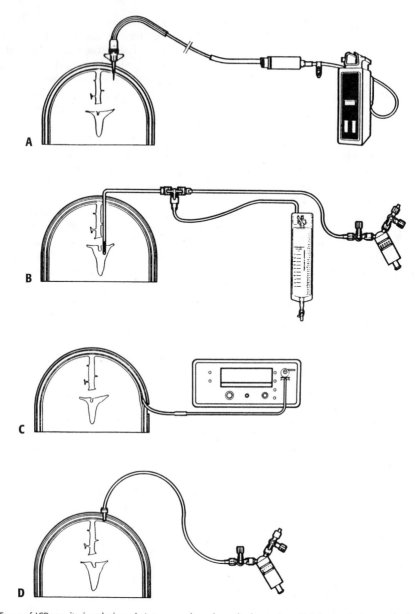

Fig. 35-8 Types of ICP monitoring devices. **A,** Intraparenchymal monitoring system. **B,** Intraventricular monitoring system. **C,** Epidural monitoring system. **D,** Subdural monitoring system. *(Sole ML, Lamborn ML, Hartshorn JC: Introduction to critical care nursing, ed 3, Philadelphia, 2001, WB Saunders. Courtesy Integra NeuroSciences, Camino, San Diego, Calif.)*

edema, a small piece of brain tissue may be driven into and occlude the proximal end of the screw, thus rendering it useless.

The intraventricular catheter (IVC) is introduced into a CSF-containing ventricle via a twist-drill burr hole and is connected to an external transducer that converts the hydrostatic pressure force into a graph and numeric readout. The advantages of the IVCs are that it provides a direct ICP reading and is easily kept patent.

Another advantage is that CSF can be drained through the catheter to treat ICP elevations. In this way it may serve as a temporary artificial extension of the CSF-shunting compensatory mechanism. Intracranial compliance can also be tested by injecting fluid into the cranium and reading the responding pressure. If an abrupt and steep rise in ICP occurs, it can be assumed that compliance no longer exists and that the volume-pressure curve is a steep one. When the patient's arterial pressure is being monitored simultaneously, exact CPP can be calculated at any time. The ventricular catheter also has the advantage of allowing instillation of contrast media or air to study the size and patency of the ventricle. The principal disadvantage of the IVC is the risk of infection and hemorrhage.

The fiberoptic catheter uses the fiberoptic transducer-tipped probe and can be placed in the ventricles as well as in subarachnoid, subdural, and intraparenchymal sites. The advantages are its easy placement and lack of relation to ventricular size. The major disadvantages are its expense, its inability to allow for CSF sampling or drainage, its possible need for probe replacement, and the fragility of the fiberoptic cable, which will break easily.

ICP monitoring is a valuable tool in assessing the efficacy of nursing interventions that are intended to decrease ICP and is essential in determining accurate assessments of the pressure state within the cranium and in treating elevations in ICP before the patient deteriorates.

Pressure Waves in Increased Intracranial Pressure.
Pressures waves are abnormal, spontaneous variations in ICP. Three patterns have been identified. The first and most significant type is the A wave, which is more commonly called a plateau wave. These waves are associated with increases in ICP between 50 and 100 torr that last for 5 to 20 minutes. They are seen only in advanced stages of increased ICP (the last phase of the volume-pressure curve) and superimpose themselves when the baseline ICP is elevated and exceeds 20 torr. Early increases in MSAP do not accompany plateau waves, and autoregulation is impaired. Thus plateau waves signal hypoxia of brain cells and a decrease in CPP. They may cause both transient and irreversible damage to the brain and may be premonitory signs of acute incidents. The cause of plateau waves is not

fully understood, but they probably result from a combination of transient blood volume alterations and CSF obstruction. Hypoventilation (by accumulating carbon dioxide and increasing intracranial blood volume) may be the cause, and the high ICP causes ischemia of the respiratory centers, thus resulting in irregular breathing.

The second type of pressure wave pattern is called the B wave. These waves are sharp, rhythmic oscillations with a sawtooth pattern occurring every 30 seconds to 2 minutes. These may indicate increases in ICP as much as 50 torr and are more commonly seen in patients with unstable increases.

The third type of pattern is the C wave. These waves are smaller rhythmic oscillations in ICP, which occur every 4 to 8 minutes, and they indicate increases in ICP as much as 20 torr. They are associated with respiratory influence on the blood pressure, but their significance is questionable.

Intracranial Pressure Assessment
Continuous ICP monitoring is the only accurate method of assessing ICP at any given time. This method has two advantages: (1) it provides an ongoing record of the ICP; and (2) it provides a means of assessing intracranial dynamics. The clinical signs of increased ICP are numerous. The early signs are often vague and overlooked, and research has demonstrated the unreliability of these signs in determining or recognizing increased ICP.

Early signs of increased ICP are increasing restlessness, confusion, and severe headache. Nausea, vomiting, paralysis, visual field deficits, conjugate deviation of the eyes, sensory loss, and nuchal rigidity are also early signs. Their presence may or may not confirm a diagnosis of increased ICP.

The late signs of increased ICP are decreasing responsiveness and LOC; pupillary changes; increased systolic blood pressure; bradycardia; widening pulse pressure; alteration in respiratory pattern; decorticate or decerebrate posturing; and absence of or decrease in cough, gag, corneal, and deep tendon reflexes. A positive Babinski's reflex is normal in infants younger than 18 months of age but indicates increased ICP in those older than 18 months.

Most of these signs are manifestations of brain shift, with resultant dysfunction of the reticular-activating system, brain stem, and medulla. Pressure would either have to elevate quite rapidly or be sustained at high levels to affect these structures so dramatically. Primary injury to these structures may elicit the same signs without appreciable increases in ICP. In this situation, they may well indicate the level of brain function and the gravity of the situation but not reflect the pressure dynamics that exist at that moment.

Just as these signs may be present without increase in ICP, ICP may be dangerously high with few, if any, signs. Classic brainstem signs (reflecting changes in cardiac, respiratory, or vasomotor function) usually occur late, after the onset of intracranial hypertension, if at all. The most important factor in determining the degree of secondary brain damage incurred by elevated ICP is the effect of altered CPP on the brain. Clinical research has shown that the level of CPP is the best indicator of outcome from severe head injuries. CPP lower than 40 torr has been associated with poor outcomes. CPP needs to be maintained no lower than 50 to 60 torr to provide a minimally adequate blood supply to the brain.

Most hospitals with the capacity for cranial surgery also have the capacity for continuous ICP monitoring. It is still very important to recognize signs and symptoms of intracranial hypertension without the assistance of an ICP monitor.

With this in mind, the traditional signs and symptoms of increased ICP are discussed here. These are not precise or infallible as indicators of increased ICP. At the very least, they indicate that something is not right and that constant vigilance and further investigation are necessary. Even the transient appearances of these pressure signs are important. They indicate development of a highly delicate and unstable intracranial situation, a sign that the patient may be experiencing plateau waves.

Postoperative Nursing Management

Four major areas of assessment are required in PACU care of the cranial surgical patient: vital signs, LOC, motor and sensory functioning, and pupillary signs. These should be routinely assessed at least every 15 minutes for the first 2 hours postoperatively. Then, if they are within normal limits or unchanged since surgery, they should be assessed every 30 minutes. If the patient's condition is unstable or deteriorating or if the surgeon specifies, assessments should

be made more frequently. If the patient's ICP is being monitored, correct calibration of the monitor must be ensured, ICP value recorded, and waveform described. The same approach is used for arterial pressure recording.

Reports should be taken from both the anesthesiologist and the surgeon. Of particular importance are surgical procedure, pathological findings, bone flap presence, allergies, preexisting medical problems, anesthetics, and any problems that occurred during surgery. Special positioning orders or restrictions, the presence of drains, and known CSF leaks must be noted. The Glasgow Coma Scale (GCS) (Table 35-1) is a widely used neurologic assessment tool because of its simplicity, consistency, and reliability between raters who use it. However, the GCS cannot assess subtle changes in the patient's neurologic status. When the GCS is used, the patient's responses are scored on a scale of 3 to 15. A score of 3 indicates coma, and a score of 15 indicates a fully alert, oriented person with all neurologic functions intact.

Vital Signs. Assessment of vital signs includes blood pressure, pulse, respirations, and ICP (if monitored). Changes in vital signs may indicate increasing ICP, shock, hemorrhage, electrolyte imbalance, or other disturbances. The perianesthesia nurse should keep in mind that the injured patient may have other pathophysiologic processes unrelated to his or her head injury. Temperature is always monitored, and an elevation usually represents an infectious process—most often in the respiratory or urinary tract. Infrequently, elevations are attributable to direct damage to the temperature-regulating center in the hypothalamus. Temperature elevation also increases the metabolic rate of the brain, which may further increase ICP.

Airway patency is ensured, and the rate, depth, and rhythm are noted. If the rhythm is irregular, try to determine its pattern. Changes in the respiratory pattern may indicate injury to the respiratory center of the brain and the severity of the neurologic injury (Table 35-2). If the patient is on a ventilator, check the machine for proper functioning and settings. It should be noted, however, that mechanical ventilation may mask changes in the respiratory pattern.

For many years the nursing literature has documented a relation between changes in blood pressure and pulse and increases in ICP. These

Table 35-1 **Glasgow Coma Scale**		
Category	Response	Score
Eye opening	Spontaneous	4
	To speech	3
	To pain	2
	None	1
Best verbal response	Oriented to person, place, and time	5
	Confused	4
	Inappropriate words	3
	Incomprehensible sounds	2
	No response	1
Best motor response	Obeys commands	6
	Localizes to pain	5
	Withdrawal from pain	4
	Abnormal flexion	3
	Abnormal extension	2
	Flaccid	1

changes are often referred to as Cushing's reflex and Cushing's triad. Cushing's reflex is described as an elevated systolic blood pressure, bradycardia, and widening pulse pressure. Further increases in ICP may lead to Cushing's triad, which is described as bradycardia, hypertension, and bradypnea. Cushing's reflex and triad are late clinical signs of increased ICP and may indicate brain stem herniation. Patients with head injury often have a higher than normal blood pressure and heart rate. This may be the result of pain, hypoxia, and agitation or the release of endogenous catecholamines.

Level of Consciousness. The most important indicator of brain function is the LOC, but it is not necessarily indicative of altered ICP. A decreased LOC in the PACU may be caused by the lingering effects of the anesthesia or by neuromuscular-blocking agents sometimes used with patients on positive pressure ventilation. A change in LOC may also be the result of hypoxia, hypoglycemia, vitamin deficiency, and fluid and electrolyte imbalances. Other underlying pathologic changes may cause alterations in LOC. To assess LOC, it is best to describe the patient's response instead of using vague terms such as stuporous, semiconscious, or unconscious. A standard assessment form such as the GCS (see Table 35-1) should be available for assessing the LOC. A change in LOC may also be indicative of deterioration or improvement in the patient's condition.

Motor and Sensory Functioning. Assessment of motor and sensory function is part of an ongoing neurologic assessment and is performed to note changes from the baseline assessment. It can also provide clues to extending hemorrhage or expanding edema. Focal changes, such as decreased hand strength unilaterally or an inability to move one side of the body, often accompany these events. Sensations may be decreased because of brain involvement, not just spinal cord injury (SCI). Observe whether the patient can move all four extremities. Check both hand grasps simultaneously. Are they weak or strong, equal or unequal? Foot strength can be tested by having the patient push or pull against the nurse's hands. (Be sure the patient uses only the foot and ankle, not the entire leg.) If the patient does not respond to simple commands, test to see whether a painful stimulus such as a pin prick or pinch will induce movement. (Test both sides to determine sensory impairment.) If the patient does not respond to pain, test for motor function by raising both arms or both legs and letting them fall together. A paralyzed limb will fall to the bed more quickly than an unaffected one. To further check leg motor ability, flex both of the patient's

Table 35-2 Respiratory Patterns

Pattern	Description	Location of Injury and Other Causes
Cheyne-Stokes respirations	Regular increase in the rate and depth of breathing that peaks and is followed by a decreasing rate and depth of breathing, which progresses to apnea; then the cycle repeats itself	Bilateral dysfunction of cerebral hemispheres Midbrain and upper pons
Central neurogenic hyperventilation	Deep, rapid, and regular pattern of breathing	Low midbrain and upper pons Increased ICP with head trauma
Apneusis breathing	A pause at full inspiration occurs; may see prolonged inspiratory pause alternating with a prolonged expiratory pause	Mid and low pons Hypoglycemia, anoxia, and meningitis
Cluster breathing	Periodic breathing with frequent apneic episodes	Low pons and high medulla
Ataxic breathing	Irregular breathing with shallow, deep respirations and irregular apneic episodes; usually slow in rate	Medulla

knees with the feet flat on the bed; release them at the same time. The normal leg will maintain its position momentarily and then resume the original position. The affected limb will abduct while falling and will maintain knee flexion.

Facial muscle movement should also be tested. If possible, ask patients to wrinkle their foreheads, shut their eyes tightly, smile, and show their teeth. Any asymmetry should be noted. If the patient is not responsive to verbal commands, noxious stimulation may elicit a grimace or other facial movement. The presence of a Babinski's reflex is pathologic and indicates pyramidal tract dysfunction in any person older than 18 months of age. Starting at the heel and using a moderately sharp object, such as the rounded tip of a bandage scissors or the tip of a retracted pen, stroke the lateral sole and proceed to the ball of the foot. Firm pressure is necessary to elicit an accurate response. The Babinski's reflex is present when the great toe dorsiflexes (bends toward the head) and the remaining toes "fan out." The Babinski's reflex is not present when the stimulus elicits a plantar or downward flexion of the great toe.

Motor response to a painful stimulus may be one of decerebrate or decorticate rigidity, or these postures may exist in the absence of any stimulation. Decerebrate posturing is characterized by rigidity and contraction of all the extensor muscles. The legs are stiffly extended with the feet plantar flexed. The arms are extended and hyperpronated. Decerebrate rigidity is usually the result of upper brain stem damage; this means that the cerebral hemispheres are functionally cut off. Decorticate posturing indicates that function has been cut off at a lower level and that the entire cortex is physiologically cut off. In this instance, the legs are extended and internally rotated, and the feet are plantar flexed. The arms are flexed at all joints, and the hands are often held beneath the chin.

Pupillary Activity. Pupillary reactions are controlled by the third cranial nerve. When assessing the pupils, the perianesthesia nurse should examine both simultaneously for shape, size, and equality. Normal pupils are round and, at a midpoint diameter, within the range of 1 to 9 mm. Instead of using terms like constricted or dilated, it is more precise to measure their diameters directly with a pocket millimeter ruler. Test the direct light reflex of each pupil with a small bright flashlight. Normally, the pupil will constrict briskly. If it reacts sluggishly or not at all, it is abnormal. To test the consensual light reflex, hold both eyelids open, shine the light in one eye, and observe the other pupil. The opposite pupil should constrict simultaneously with the lighted one, although perhaps not to the same degree.

Normal pupillary size and reactivity can be altered by some medical situations and by certain drugs. Previous surgery or direct injury to the eye may alter or abolish reactivity. Blindness abolishes reactivity to light because the sensory part of the reflex pathway is absent.

Unusual eye movements should be noted. Normal gaze in a person who is awake and alert is straight ahead, with no involuntary movements. This is generally true of unresponsive patients, although their eyes may rove slowly and in random fashion. (When detecting this movement, do not be misled into thinking that the patients are actually following you or your movements.) Their eyes should move together in the same direction (conjugate gaze). If the eyes are dysconjugate, they move in a jerky, oscillatory fashion (nystagmus) or the gaze deviates from the midline. These ocular movements are abnormal and should be detailed in the nursing notes.

Nursing Care

The PACU nurse has three primary responsibilities in the care of the neurosurgical patient: (1) to institute measures of care to sustain optimal physiologic function in the perianesthesia patient; (2) to recognize and prevent conditions that increase ICP beyond normal limits; and (3) to detect and communicate signs and symptoms of the patient's condition to the physician (Box 35-1).

SPINAL SURGERY

The goal of surgical intervention is to minimize complications related to spinal cord injuries (SCI), spinal cord tumors, or developmental abnormalities. Complete or incomplete SCI, bony fragments in the canal, unstable dislocation, and evidence of cord compression are some indications for immediate surgical intervention.

Diagnostic Tools

Several methods are used in diagnosing injury or disease involving the spine or spinal canal.

Conventional radiography and fluoroscopy identify fractures and fracture-dislocations. Narrowing of an intervertebral space is sometimes evident as a result of a herniated nucleus pulposus, or "slipped disk." Fluoroscopy is used to demonstrate instability of the injured part on manipulation. Splintered or displaced bone fragments and radiopaque foreign bodies (such as bullets or other metal fragments) are also seen on radiographs. Radiographs also demonstrate abnormalities such as scoliosis and osteoporotic and arthritic changes. Tumors may be evidenced by erosion, calcium deposits within the mass, increased interpediculate distance, enlargement of an intervertebral foramen, or collapse of a vertebra.

CT scanning is used to delineate mass lesions existing in the same plane as the spine and spinal cord. Large blood clots may also be localized with this method.

MRI is being used increasingly to accurately detect and assess space-occupying lesions of the spine, such as herniated nucleus pulposus and tumors.

Electromyography is employed in evaluating muscle function as a means of detecting the nature and location of motor unit lesions. Tumors and herniated nucleus pulposus compressing the cord or motor nerve roots affect the function of the muscle groups they innervate.

Myelography is one of the most valuable tools available in diagnosing compression of the spinal cord caused by tumor, fracture-dislocation, or herniated nucleus pulposus. A lumbar puncture is performed, at which time a Queckenstedt test may also be done.* The myelogram consists of the injection of a radiopaque dye into the CSF canal and the fluoroscopic observation of its flow in the suspected area (Fig. 35-9). Cord compression is evidenced by an interruption in the contour of the spinal cord. Disruption of the contours of the spinal nerve roots may also be found.

---

*In the Queckenstedt test, the veins of the neck are compressed on one or both sides. In a healthy person, the CSF pressure rises rapidly and then quickly returns to normal when the pressure is taken off the neck. In a patient whose spinal cord is obstructed, little or no increase in pressure is found. This test is diagnostically accurate for most cord compressions; however, false negative results may be obtained if the lesion is located high in the cervical spine area. The Queckenstedt test is not performed in patients with known or suspected increased ICP.

Box 35-1   Postoperative Nursing Management

Maintain Patent Airway

Encourage deep breathing and use of incentive spirometer

Avoid coughing to help prevent increased ICP

Administer oxygen

Provide ventilatory assistance if indicated

Monitor pulse oximetry

Monitor PO_2 and PCO_2

Provide oral and nasal airways as indicated

Position to prevent aspiration and obstruction

Suction as necessary

Monitor vital signs

Provide for baseline data

Investigate changes from baseline

Monitor for any signs of restlessness and evaluate for underlying cause

Maintain proper position of supertentorial craniotomy and head

Elevate head of bed 30 to 45 degrees to facilitate venous return, promote CSF circulation, and reduce cerebral edema

Maintain neutral head position and avoid neck flexion

Turn side to side and may position supine

Position on nonoperative side as indicated by specific surgical procedure and physician orders to

Prevent shifting and displacement of intracranial contents

Infratentorial craniotomy

Keep flat or slightly elevated

Position body in neutral position

May be turned side to side and do not position on back

Transphenoidal surgery

Elevate head of bed 30 to 45 degrees

Position body in neutral alignment

Maintain skin and mucous membrane

Provide mouth care frequently integrity

Turn every 2 hours and monitor bony prominences

Maintain body alignment with the use of positioning aids

For periorbital edema use cool compresses to eyes

Instill artificial tears, normal saline, or lubricate, to prevent corneal damage

Use an eye shield if necessary to prevent corneal abrasions

Prevent Infection

Observe dressing for signs of CSF drainage

Halo or ring sign (lighter colored rings on dressing or linen with blood in the center)

Check drainage for glucose (mucus does not contain glucose, CSF does)

Use sterile technique when changing dressings

Provide urinary catheter care if present with soap and water. Prevent undue stress on catheter

Monitor fluid and electrolyte balances

Maintain accurate I/O

Monitor serum osmolarity (290–320 mOsm/kg)

Maintain urine output greater than 30 cc/hr

Monitor urine specific gravity

Monitor skin turgor

Administer antiemetic to prevent vomiting and increased ICP

Maintain normothermia

Hyperthermia

Remove excessive layers of clothing or bed covers

Administer antipyretics

Sponge baths using tepid water

Hypothermia blanket

Prevent shivering (shivering increases ICP)

Administer chlorpromazine if indicated for shivering

Provide for pain relief and comfort

Administer analgesics as ordered (do not mask neurological signs, usually codeine or acetaminophen)

Do not cluster nursing activities together

Elevate head of bed to help prevent headache

Reduce environmental stimulation by keeping light low; reduce noise

Prevent thrombophlebitis

Apply thigh high elastic stockings and sequential compression boots

Inspect legs daily

Provide emotional and pyschosocial care

Explain all procedures and offer psychologic support and reassurance

Communicate with family and involve in plan of care

Speak quietly

Adapted from Shpritz DW: The neurosurgical patient. In Litwack K, editor: Core curriculum for perianesthesia nursing practice, Philadelphia, 1999, WB Saunders.

Injuries and Pathologic Conditions of the Spine

Injuries of the Spine. The spine protects the spinal cord and the terminal nerve roots. Injuries to the spine and spinal cord occur as a result of flexion, hyperextension, rotation with both flexion and extension, compression, and penetrating wounds (Fig. 35-10). Head injuries often accompany injuries to the spine and vice versa. The cervical spine is extremely mobile and therefore particularly susceptible to injuries that hyperflex or hyperextend the neck. Propulsion may occur anteroposteriorly or laterally. The spinal cord is relatively large in the cervical area and sustains damage fairly easily after injury. This area is unique in that the superior portion of C2 lacks a vertebral body. Instead, the neck has a dens, or projection, called the odontoid. Many injuries to the odontoid extend into C1, or atlas, which has no vertebral body at all.

The thoracic spine is fixed by the ribs, but the lumbar spine is not; thus there is an increased incidence of injury to the thoracic, lumbar, or sacral regions of the spine. Motor vehicle accidents are the leading cause of spinal cord injuries.

Consequences of injury to the spine are the result of the mechanical insult or biochemical and hemodynamic changes. Mechanical insult includes the direct injury and changes to the cord structure, motion stress on the cord, and continuous compression to the cord. This physical injury to the cord results in the primary or initial spinal cord dysfunction. Edema of the cord, which causes cellular changes and ischemia, may occur in the hours after the initial injury. This process is called secondary injury and may last up to 5 days.

The primary goal in the early treatment of spinal cord injuries is to prevent further compromise of spinal cord tissue from secondary injury. If the damage to tissue as the result of the direct injury cannot be altered, an attempt is made to protect the remaining tissue by alleviation of compression and movement of the spinal cord. Spinal cord immobilization, surgical intervention to alleviate cord compression, and pharmacological therapies to reduce edema are used as immediate therapies.

Complete Spinal Cord Lesion. The extent of injury to the spinal cord is described as complete or incomplete lesion. In a complete SCI there is no motor or sensory function more than

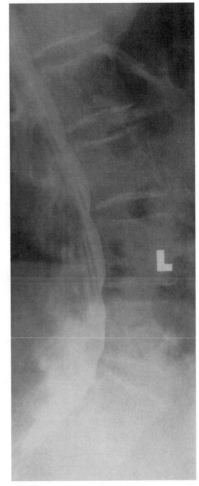

Fig. 35-9 Lumbar myelogram. *(From Bucher L, Melander S: Critical nursing, Philadelphia, 1999, WB Saunders.)*

three levels below the level of injury. When this type of injury lasts more than 24 hours, it indicates no recovery of distal function. Clinical findings during the acute phase after total cord transection include the following:

1. Immediate loss of all sensory, motor, autonomic, and reflex functions below the level of the injury from spinal shock. Spinal shock may persist for days or weeks, depending on the injury and the patient's general state of health. It usually lasts 4 to 8 weeks.
2. Urinary retention due to bladder sphincter paralysis.

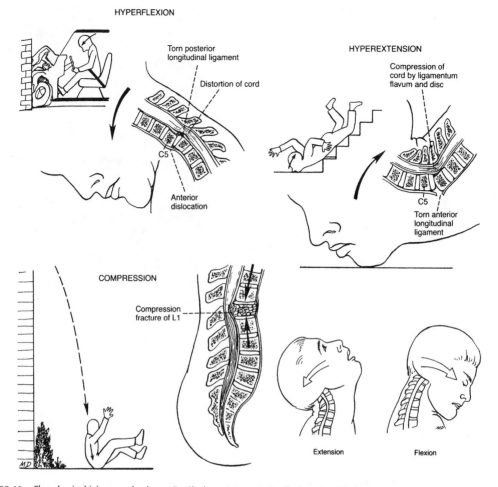

Fig. 35-10 Closed spinal injury mechanisms. *(In Clochesy J, Breu C, Cardin S et al: Critical care nursing, ed 2, Philadelphia, 1996, WB Saunders. From Luckman J, Sorensen KC: Medical-surgical nursing: a psychophysiologic approach, ed 3, Philadelphia, 1987, WB Saunders.)*

3. Paralytic ileus with progressive abdominal distention.
4. Respiratory insult or cessation. Injury to the lower cervical or upper thoracic spine results in cessation of intercostal function. In this event, respiration is under the sole stimulus of the phrenic nerve, and breathing is diaphragmatic. Injury to the cord at the levels of C3-C5 injures the phrenic nucleus, thus paralyzing the diaphragm and causing respiratory failure.
5. Loss of sweating below the level of the lesion.
6. Point tenderness over the injured part. Crepitus may or may not be present.

Initial therapeutic efforts are directed at preserving life. Mechanical stability, protection of nervous tissue, and freedom from pain are long-term therapeutic goals.

Incomplete Spinal Cord Lesion. Incomplete spinal cord lesion indicates residual motor or sensory function more than three segments below the level of injury. Indications of incomplete lesion are sensation, sense of position, or voluntary movement of the legs, sensation around the anus, voluntary rectal sphincter contraction, and/or voluntary toe flexion.

Various syndromes or types of incomplete lesions may result from the injury. Incomplete lesions include central cord syndrome, Brown-Sequard syndrome, anterior cord syndrome, and posterior cord syndrome.

Central cord syndrome (CCS) is the most common type of incomplete lesion. CCS occurs more commonly in older adults as a result of a hyperextension injury, such as a blow to the face or forehead. CCS from sports injuries are also seen in younger patients.

The center of the cord is contused and may hemorrhage, thus resulting in bilateral upper extremity weakness and a burning sensation. If CCS is caused by a contusion, lower extremity function will usual return first, bladder function next, upper extremities next, and finger movement last.

Brown-Sequard syndrome may occur after injuries that transect the cord such as knife or gunshot wounds, epidural hematoma, herniated cervical disc, spinal cord tumor, spinal AV malformation, and cervical spondylosis. Clinical signs are ipsilateral loss of motor, touch, pressure, and vibration below the lesion and contralateral loss of pain and temperature below the lesion. This type of lesion has the best functional recovery rate; many patients regain independent ambulation.

Anterior cord syndrome usually occurs as the result of compression of the anterior portion of the cord and loss of blood supply from the anterior spinal artery. Clinical signs are loss of motor function, pain, temperature, and sensation below the level of injury. Touch, position, and vibration sensation are still intact. Anterior cord syndrome is usually caused by flexion injuries in the cervical area.

Posterior cord syndrome is a rare disorder. Clinical signs are pain and paresthesias in the neck, upper arms, and torso. There may be mild paresis of the upper arms.

Surgical Intervention for Spinal Cord Injuries

Surgeons differ in their opinions about the optimal timing for surgical decompression and fusion. Early surgical intervention is indicated to decompress the spinal canal from bone or disk fragments, to provide stabilization, and to repair damage caused by penetrating objects.

Patients who require surgery may have exploration, insertion of Harrington rods or stabilization instruments, or decompression laminectomy procedures. Procedures may be performed through an anterior or posterior approach, depending on the cord lesion. Fusion is accomplished by the placement of a bone graft taken from tibial or iliac bone into the involved interspace or of a fixation device. External immobilization is often used postoperatively until osseous union is complete.

General contraindications to surgery are the existence of associated life-threatening injuries, depressed respiratory function caused by high cervical injuries, lack of skilled personnel and necessary equipment, and a patient with improved neurologic status.

Nursing Care and Considerations in the Patient with Spinal Cord Injury

In the United States alone, more than 10,000 people annually experience SCI. Of these people, 36% sustain injuries to their spinal cords in motor vehicle accidents. Permanent injuries of this nature are devastating to the patient and the patient's family. The nursing responsibilities are great during the acute, rehabilitative, and chronic phases. Patients with SCI may be sent to the PACU in any of these phases, and their care requires special consideration and knowledge of SCI pathophysiology.

The initial assessment of the patient with SCI in the PACU needs to focus on airway patency, adequate respiration, and maintenance of systemic and spinal cord perfusion. Vital signs should be assessed every 15 minutes until stable. Baseline neurologic assessment including motor and sensory evaluation should be completed with the initial and ongoing assessments (Fig. 35-11).

Immobilization is a primary intervention to help prevent the process of secondary injury. The standard of care for immobilization is to place the neck in a neutral position and in a rigid cervical collar. Stabilization of fractures may be accomplished by several devices that promote alignment.

Current pharmacologic treatments to help reduce spinal cord edema and secondary injury include the administration of Methylprednisolone. The current standardized treatment for patients with SCI treated within 8 hours is to receive a bolus and continuous IV infusion. Improvement in motor function has been directly associated to the administration of Methylprednisolone.

UNIVERSITY OF MARYLAND
MIEMSS—UMMS
SPINAL CORD INJURY FLOW SHEET

Muscle Strength

5   Normal
4   Active movement through range of motion
       against resistance
3   Active movement through range of motion
       against gravity
2   Active movement through range of motion
       with gravity eliminated
1   Palpable or visible contraction
0   Total paralysis
U   Unable to test strength of extremity

Rectal Tone, Proprioception, Diaphragm
P–Present   A–Absent   U–Untestable

Medication	Sensation
S—Sedation	N—Normal
PL—Paralytic	ABN—Abnormal
T—Tranquilizer	A—Absent
P—Pain	U—Untestable

MOTOR LEVEL   *Circled entry means to refer to nurses note*

Level of bony/ ligamentous injury														
Anatomical Classification														
Date														
Time														
Medications														
Diaphragm (R/L)	C_4													
Deltoid (raise arms) (R/L)	C_5													
Biceps (elbow flexion) (R/L)	$C_{5,6}$													
Wrist extensors (R/L)	C_6													
Triceps (elbow extension) (R/L)	C_7													
Flexer digitorum profundus (finger flexion) (R/L)	C_8													
Hand intrinsics (finger abduction) (R/L)	T_1													
Iliopsoas (hip flexion) (R/L)	L_2													
Quadriceps (knee extension) (R/L)	L_3													
Tibialis anterior (dorsiflex foot) (R/L)	L_4													
Extensor hallucis longus (great toe extension) (R/L)	L_5													
Gastrocnemius (ankle plantar flexion) (R/L)	S_1													
Function	Level													
Proprioception (finger) (R/L)														
Proprioception (toe) (R/L)														
Rectal Tone (P/A)														
Initials														
Initials/signature														

Medical Records No.

Fig. 35-11   Spinal cord assessment tool. *(From Cardona VD, Hurn PD, Mason PJB, Scanlon AM, Veise-Berry SW: Trauma Nursing, ed. 2, Philadelphia, 1994, WB Saunders.)*

SENSATION

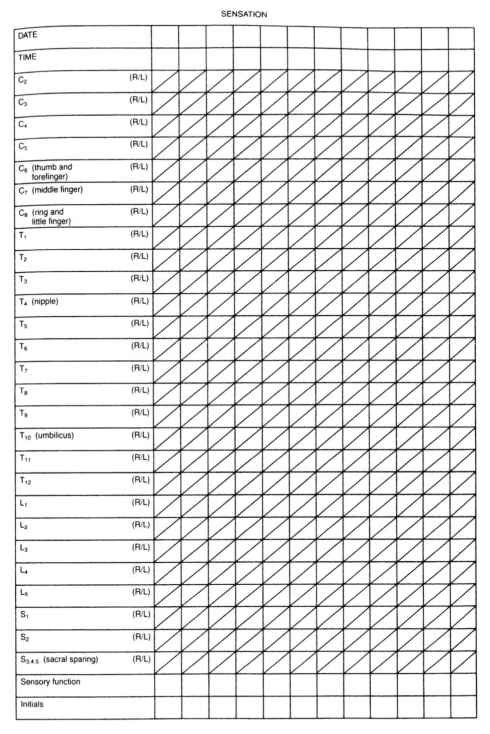

DATE													
TIME													
C₂	(R/L)												
C₃	(R/L)												
C₄	(R/L)												
C₅	(R/L)												
C₆ (thumb and forefinger)	(R/L)												
C₇ (middle finger)	(R/L)												
C₈ (ring and little finger)	(R/L)												
T₁	(R/L)												
T₂	(R/L)												
T₃	(R/L)												
T₄ (nipple)	(R/L)												
T₅	(R/L)												
T₆	(R/L)												
T₇	(R/L)												
T₈	(R/L)												
T₉	(R/L)												
T₁₀ (umbilicus)	(R/L)												
T₁₁	(R/L)												
T₁₂	(R/L)												
L₁	(R/L)												
L₂	(R/L)												
L₃	(R/L)												
L₄	(R/L)												
L₅	(R/L)												
S₁	(R/L)												
S₂	(R/L)												
S₃,₄,₅ (sacral sparing)	(R/L)												
Sensory function													
Initials													

Fig. 35-11 *Cont'd*

Complications Associated with SCI

Spinal Shock.   Spinal shock is a form of neurogenic shock characterized by a loss of motor, sensory, autonomic, and reflex activity below the level of the lesion and resulting in flaccid paralysis and paralytic ileus. The classic signs and symptoms of spinal shock include systemic hypotension, bradycardia, and hypothermia. Spinal shock is a condition that occurs immediately after injury and may last hours to months, depending on severity of the injury. Average recovery from spinal shock is 1 to 6 weeks.

Hypotension.   Hypotension is not uncommon because of vasodilation of the vessels below the level of the injury. The goal of treatment is to maintain systemic and renal perfusion. Bradycardia may accompany the hypotension. Dopamine is indicated for the treatment of hypotension and bradycardia. Other causes of hypotension, such as a GI hemorrhage, must be considered and ruled out. Hypotension is usually not caused by hemorrhagic shock; therefore the patient volume status should be monitored closely and not overloaded with intravenous fluids.

Bradycardia.   Bradycardia is associated with spinal shock and nursing interventions such as manipulation of an endotracheal tube, suctioning, turning, and insertion of a nasogastric tube may elicit a vasovagal response that leads to bradycardia. Nursing interventions should closely monitor for and provide prevention from a vasovagal response.

Thrombosis.   Conditions are optimal for the development of deep vein thrombosis and pulmonary embolus because of venous pooling and loss of movement below the level of injury. Calf measurements, use of antiembolism stockings, compression devices, low-dose heparin, and low molecular weight heparin are used to prevent these complications.

Autonomic Dysreflexia.   Autonomic dysreflexia usually occurs after the resolution of spinal shock and the return of reflex activity. It results from reflex stimulation of the sympathetic nerves below the level of injury. Causes of the reflex stimulation include bladder distension, fecal impaction, and noxious stimuli. Symptoms of autonomic dysreflexia are pounding headache, hypertension, profuse sweating and flushed skin above the level of injury, pallor and goose bumps

below the level of the injury, anxiety, and visual disturbances. Treatment is aimed at removing the noxious stimulus and preventing complications secondary to hypertension.

PACU care centers around the routine prevention of known precipitants of autonomic dysreflexia. For example, the bladder must not become distended, and skin breakdown must be prevented. If signs and symptoms appear, the stimulus must be sought and removed as rapidly as possible. If the symptoms cannot be alleviated, the nurse should notify the physician, elevate the head of the bed (if not contraindicated), and monitor the blood pressure every 5 minutes. Severe cases can require treatment by spinal anesthesia and the administration of ganglionic blocking agents. For chronic problems, subarachnoid blocks or rhizotomy may be necessary.

Pain Management.   Patients may experience pain in areas about the level of injury. The pain may be described as sharp, dull, or burning and often is associated with muscle spasms. Morphine for pain or Valium, Flexeril, or other antispasmodic agents may be ordered. Intramuscular medications should never be administered below the level of the lesion, because they will only cause local inflammation and tissue breakdown, and absorption will be negligible.

Concomitant Head Injury.   Every patient with acute injury to the spine must be observed for signs and symptoms that indicate head injury. Evaluation of cranial status should be done at the same intervals as the vital sign measurements. An abnormal neurological "check" should be reported to the physician immediately because it may indicate injury to the brain or increased ICP that results from the upward expansion of cord edema.

Respiratory Complications.   Respiratory insufficiency or failure is the most serious complication of SCI. Respiratory complications can be independent of the level of injury. C4 and higher injuries require mechanical ventilation because of the direct involvement of the phrenic nerves. Assessment of a patient's ventilation should include the following parameters: status, rate, depth, pattern, and oxygen saturation. Evaluation of pulmonary function should include tidal volume, inspiratory force, and vital capacity. Changes in pulmonary function are early indicators of deterioration in respiratory status and

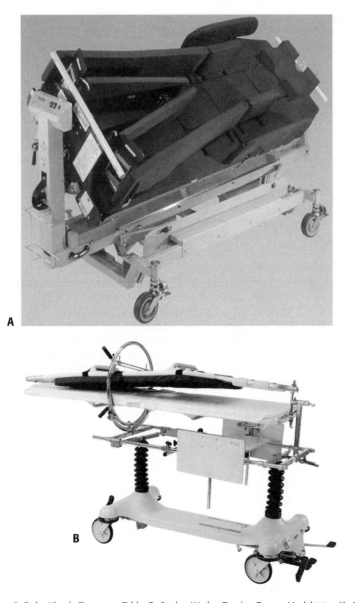

Fig. 35-12 **A,** Roto Rest® Delta Kinetic Treatment Table. **B,** Stryker Wedge Turning Frame, Model 965. *(A, Courtesy of KCI, San Antonio, Texas. B, Courtesy of Stryker Corporation, Kalamazoo, Mich. Used with permission of Stryker Corporation.)*

may necessitate ventilator support. Intubation of the patients may depend on their ability to clear secretions and to maintain adequate gas exchange. A program of chest physiotherapy and the use of pressure support ventilation and positive end expiratory pressure will assist with the prevention of atelectasis. Auscultation of lung sounds should also be performed routinely to assess the presence of abnormal lung sounds. Chest radiographic examinations and arterial blood gas determinations should be monitored routinely and ordered immediately if signs of deterioration occur. Potential respiratory complications that result from SCI include pneumonia, aspiration, pulmonary edema, and pulmonary embolism. Rotational beds before surgical stabilization will facilitate the mobilization of secretions and help prevent respiratory complications (Fig. 35-12). A team approach by nursing staff, physicians, respiratory therapists, and physical therapists is necessary in treating the SCI patient. Because of the rapid onset of pulmonary complications, the PACU nurse must be aggressive in caring for the patient with SCI.

Skin Breakdown. As with the cranial surgical patient, skin care for the patient with SCI is an important aspect of PACU nursing care. Skin breakdown is one of the most obvious, costly, and detrimental complications that a patient with SCI can experience. The patient must be turned and repositioned at least every 2 hours to prevent skin breakdown and damage to underlying body tissues. A specialty surface such as an air mattress or alternating pressure mattress may be necessary to prevent skin breakdown.

Bone Demineralization. Long-term immobility causes demineralization of bone tissue. Calcium is freed into the circulation and results in osteoporosis, or "silent fractures," and renal calculi.

Gastrointestinal Complications. Generalized atony and loss of motility render the stomach and intestine distended and highly susceptible to fecal impactions and obstructions. Distention is relieved by intermittent nasogastric suction. Programs of bowel training are initiated within twenty-four hours of admission.

There is a high incidence of stress ulcers among these patients, especially in quadriplegics. Here, parasympathetic vagal action is unopposed because of sympathetic block from the ascending and descending visceral nerve paths, and gastric acid secretion by the parietal cells of the stomach is increased. This stressful situation is further compounded by the administration of corticosteroids used to reduce cord edema that are singularly capable of inducing hyperacidity of gastric juices. Antacids or a histamine$_2$ antagonist, or both, are given prophylactically to prevent stress ulcers. If gastric juices are accessible through a nasogastric tube, gastric pH can be monitored as a guide to treatment. Serial hematocrit determinations establish a baseline and may be the first indication of a "silent" gastrointestinal hemorrhage.

Urologic Complications. After transection of the spinal cord, the bladder sphincter becomes paralyzed, and urinary stasis develops. Indwelling urinary catheterization is necessary to prevent bladder distention during the acute phase.

Long-term catheterization, osteoporosis, decreased muscle tone, fluid and electrolyte abnormalities, alterations in cardiovascular dynamics, anemia, and catabolism contribute to urologic complications. Stasis, calculi and fistula formation, and chronic urinary tract complications that lead to septicemia make urologic complications the leading cause of death in the paraplegic and quadriplegic populations.

Anesthetic Considerations. The most influential factors in the anesthetic management of the patient with SCI are the duration of the injury (acute or chronic), fluid and electrolyte status, airway management, and autonomic hyperreflexia.

The use of a depolarizing muscle relaxant (succinylcholine) for intubation purposes in the patient with SCI is conservatively contraindicated owing to the release of potassium. The succinylcholine-induced release of potassium is the result of proliferation of cholinergic receptors in muscle tissue below the level of transection. The resultant hyperkalemia, often as high as 14 mEq per L, can lead to ventricular fibrillation and cardiac arrest. The release of potassium caused by succinylcholine administration can be seen as early as 1 day after injury and as long as 9 months later. The degree of muscle involvement—not the dosage of succinylcholine—is the determining factor in the amount of potassium released.

Patients with SCI may experience some degree of hypotension because of a relative hypovolemia that results from sympathetic nervous system depression. The degree of the hypotension depends on the level of transection and the duration of the injury with regard to whether the patient is still experiencing spinal shock. The patient must be adequately resuscitated with fluids, and measures must be taken to monitor fluid status and to ensure adequate organ perfusion.

Airway management is a significant problem in patients with SCI whose injuries involve the cervical spine. Endotracheal intubation must be performed without manipulation of the cervical spine so as to avoid further irreversible damage. Intubation may be accomplished by awake, blind oral or nasal approach, fiberoptics, or retrograde intubation. When the airway obstruction is severe, tracheostomy or cricothyrotomy may be necessary. Patients may arrive in the PACU with the endotracheal tube in place and not be extu-

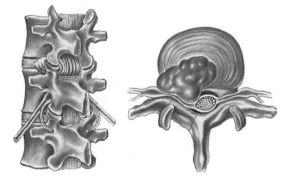

Fig. 35-13 Herniated nucleus pulposus and laminectomy. *(From Thompson JM, McFarland G, Kirsch J et al: Mosby's clinical nursing, ed 5, St Louis, 2002, Mosby.)*

bated until adequate management of the airway and ventilation are ensured.

Herniated Nucleus Pulposus

Herniated nucleus pulposus (Fig. 35-13) may occur in any of the intervertebral disks but is most commonly found in one of the last two lumbar interspaces. Pain and some degree of compromise in sensory or motor function along the distribution of the involved nerve are common preoperative findings. Before surgical intervention is undertaken, diagnostic confirmation is sought, and the suspected herniated nucleus pulposus is differentiated from tumor, subluxation of the facets, or rheumatoid spondylitis.

Surgery consists of partial hemilaminectomy and removal of the diseased disk. If fusion is necessary to prevent recurrence of pain or deformity, a bone graft is removed from the iliac crest or tibia and placed as a bridge over the defective space. Spinal fusion lengthens the operative procedure and requires a second operative wound site. Therefore a greater potential for postoperative complications exists, and the recuperative phase may be lengthened. The threat of shock is also greater because of increased blood loss and pain.

Movement restrictions in the PACU are determined by the surgeon and depend on the extent of the surgery and whether a fusion was done. If fusion was not done, the patient is often allowed to stand at the bedside, and ambulation is allowed as soon as the effects of the anesthetic have subsided. If the spine is fused, mobility restrictions are more severe. Usually, turning is allowed if done in the log-rolling fashion.

As in all spinal procedures, sensory function and motor strength of the extremities should be assessed along with the vital signs in the PACU. Evidence of CSF leaks must be sought on dressings and bed linens.

Intraspinal Neoplasms

Intraspinal neoplasms may occur at any level of the cord from the foramen magnum to the sacral canal. Most of the tumors are found in the thoracic region, because this is the longest subdivision of the spine. Cord compression and neurologic deficit produce symptoms similar to those produced by displaced fracture of the spine, but they usually develop and progress at a slower pace. Neurologic examination, myelography, and tomography determine the exact location of the lesion.

Intraspinal tumors may arise from the cord or its coverings, from fibrous tissue, or as a result of metastatic disease (Fig 35-14). For descriptive purposes they are placed in the following subdivisions:

- Intramedullary tumors: those arising solely from the substance of the cord.
- Extradural-extramedullary tumors: those arising outside the dura, either in the epidural space, vertebrae, or surrounding tissues.
- Intradural-extramedullary tumors: those arising within or under the dura but not invading the cord.
- Dumbbell tumors: those arising within the spinal canal and extending extraspinally along the nerve through the intervertebral foramen.

Early diagnosis and treatment are essential to prevent irreversible damage to the spinal cord. Eighty-five percent of intraspinal neoplasms are benign. The remainder are either primarily malignant or secondary to metastasis. The decision to intervene surgically is made after considering the patient's general condition and life expectancy. Also considered are other metastases and the type and location of the primary tumor.

Treatment consists of laminectomy, surgical exploration, and excision of the mass. Most benign tumors can be excised completely. Prognosis depends on the location of the tumor, the severity and duration of the preoperative neurologic deficit, and whether the tumor is completely

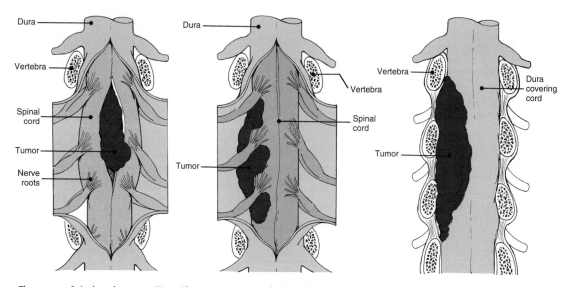

Fig. 35-14 Spinal cord tumors. *(From Thompson JM, McFarland G, Kirsch J et al: Mosby's clinical nursing, ed 5, St Louis, 2002, Mosby.)*

removable. Intramedullary tumors are associated with a more guarded prognosis, because they can rarely be excised without increasing the neurologic deficit.

Postoperative Care for SCI Surgical Interventions

Perianesthesia care of lumbar surgical patients should include keeping the head of the bed flat and log rolling the patient to help maintain proper body alignment, promote skin integrity, and minimize discomfort. The surgical site should be inspected for drainage and hematoma, and if spinal fusion was performed, the donor site should also be inspected. Assessment of the patient's comfort should be performed frequently because of muscle spasms that are often associated with lumbar surgery. The neurologic examination should include assessment of sensation in the lower extremities and should note the presence of tingling, numbness, or paralysis. The pedal pulses, color, temperature, and capillary refill of the lower extremities should also be assessed.

BIBLIOGRAPHY

Barash P, Cullen B, Stoelting R, editors: Clinical anesthesia, ed 2, Philadelphia, 1992, JB Lippincott.

Baumann C: Image guided surgery in the treatment of malignant brain tumors, J Neurosci Nurs 30(6):362-363, 1998.

Benumof J, Saidman L: Anesthesia and perioperative complications, St Louis, 1992, Mosby.

Buckley DA, Guanci MM: Spinal cord trauma, Nursing Clinics of North America 34(3):661-687, 1999.

Butcher L, Melander S: Critical care nursing, Philadelphia, 1999, WB Saunders.

Cottrell J, Smith D: Anesthesia and neurosurgery, ed 4, St Louis, 2001, Mosby.

Davis AE: Neurological patient assessment. In Kinney M, Packa D, Dunbar S, editors: AACN's clinical reference for critical care nursing, New York, 1998, McGraw-Hill.

Davis AE: Sensory and motor disorders. In Kinney M, Packa D, Dunbar S, editors: AACN's clinical reference for critical care nursing, New York, 1998, McGraw-Hill.

Davis AE, Brionbes TC: Intracranial disorders. In Kinney M, Packa D, Dunbar S, editors: AACN's clinical reference for critical care nursing, New York, 1998, McGraw-Hill.

Dodson B: Pharmacology of anesthetic agents and adjuncts used in neuroanesthesia, Anesthesia Today 6(2):15-19, 1995.

Duffy C, Matta B: Sevoflurane and anesthesia for neurosurgery: a review, J Neurosurg Anesthesiol 12(2):128-40, 2000.

Grande C, editor: Textbook of trauma anesthesia and critical care, St Louis, 1993, Mosby.

Hickey J: The clinical practice of neurological and neurosurgical nursing, ed 4, Philadelphia, 1997, Lippincott-Raven.

Hilton G, Frei J: High-dose methylprednisolone in the treatment of spinal cord injuries, Heart Lung 20(6):675-680.

Juarez VJ, Lyons M: Interrater reliability of the Glasgow coma scale, J Neurosci Nurs 27(5):283-286, 1995.

Kajs-Wyllie M: Antihypertensive treatment for the neurological patient: a nursing challenge, J Neurosci Nurs 31(3):141-151, 1999.

Katz J, Benumof J, Kadis L: Anesthesia and uncommon diseases, ed 3, Philadelphia, 1990, WB Saunders.

Kinney M, Packa D, Dunbar S: AACN's clinical reference for critical care nursing, ed 4, New York, 1998, McGraw-Hill.

Kirkness CJ, Mitchell PH, Burr RL et al: Intracranial pressure waveform analysis: clinical and research implications, J Neurosci Nurs 30(5):271-277, 2000.

Leith B: (1998). Pharmacological management of pain after intracranial surgery, J Neurosci Nurs, 30(1):220-224.

Lucke KT: Pulmonary management following SCI, J Neurosci Nurs 30(2):91-103, 1998.

Luchka S: Working with ICP monitors, RN 54(4):34-37, 1991.

McCance K, Huether S: Pathophysiology: the biologic basis for disease in adults and children, St Louis, 1990, Mosby.

Miller R: Anesthesia, ed 4, New York, 1994, Churchill Livingstone.

Minton MS, Hickey JV: A primer of neuroanatomy and neurophysiology, Nurs Clin North Am 34(3):555-572, 1999.

Neatherlin JS: Foundation for practice, Nurs Clin North Am 34(3):573-592, 1999.

Newfield P, Cottrell J: Handbook of neuroanesthesia, Philadelphia, 1999, Lippincott Williams and Wilkins.

Nikas DL: The neurologic system. In Alspach J, editor: AACN's core curriculum for critical care nursing, ed 5, Philadelphia, 1998, WB Saunders.

Pendergast V, Sullivan C: Acute spinal cord injury, Critical Care Nursing Clinics of North America, 12(4), 499-508, 2000.

Pope W: External ventriculostomy: a practical application for the acute care nurse, J Neurosci Nurs 30(3):185-190, 1998.

Schultz DL: The role of neuroscience nurse in lumbar fusion, J Neurosci Nurs 27(2):90-95, 1995.

Shpritz DW: The neurosurgical patient. In Litwack K, editor: ASPAN: core curriculum for perianesthesia nursing practice, ed 4, Philadelphia, 1999, WB Saunders.

Shpritz DW: Neurodiagnostic studies, Nurs Clin North Am 34(3):593-606, 1999.

Stoelting R: Pharmacology and physiology in anesthetic practice, ed 2, Philadelphia, 1991, JB Lippincott.

Sullivan J: Positioning of patients with severe traumatic brain injury: research-based practice, J Neurosci Nurs 32(4):204-209, 2000.

Tempelhoff R: The new inhalation anesthetics desflurane and sevoflurane are valuable additions to the practice of neuroanesthesia, J Neurosurg Anesthesiol 9(1):69-71, 1997.

Thompson JM, McFarland G, Kirsch J et al: Mosby's clinical nursing, ed 4, Philadelphia, 1997, Mosby.

Waugaman W, Foster S, Rigor B: Principles and practice of nurse anesthesia, ed 2, Norwalk, Conn, 1992, Appleton & Lange.

White CL, Pokrupa RP, Chan MH: An evaluation of the effectiveness of patient-controlled analgesia after spinal surgery, J Neurosci Nurs 30(1):225-232, 1998.

Wojner AW: Neurovascular Disease. In Kinney M, Packa D, Dunbar S, editors: AACN's clinical reference for critical care nursing, New York, 1998, McGraw-Hill.

Wood M, Wood A: Drugs and anesthesia: pharmacology for anesthesiologists, ed 2, Baltimore, 1990, Williams & Wilkins.

Young W: Effects of desflurane on the central nervous system, Anesthesia and Analgesia 75:S32-S37, 1992.

36

CARE OF THE THYROID AND PARATHYROID SURGICAL PATIENT

Kim Litwack, PhD, RN, FAAN, CPAN, CAPA, CFNP

Surgery of the thyroid gland was first performed around 500 AD, and the first successful removal of goiter occurred in 1000 AD. By the 1800s, numerous thyroidectomies had been performed; however, nearly half of the patients died secondary to tetany. This morbidity was secondary to the removal of the parathyroid glands, whose function was not well understood at the time. In the early 1900s, an understanding of the role of the parathyroid glands was gained, and the advocated procedure of subtotal thyroidectomy significantly reduced postoperative complications. In the late 1990s, the techniques of endoscopic thyroidectomy and minimally invasive radio-guided parathyroidectomy further reduced both perioperative and postoperative complications. For many patients, these techniques are performed on an outpatient basis. Note that the type of surgical procedure selected will depend on the patient's age, cell type of tumor, size of tumor, presence of encapsulated or extracapsular tumor, and any invasion of adjacent structures.

DEFINITIONS

Bilateral subtotal thyroidectomy: removal of majority of thyroid tissue of both lobes, leaving a small remnant of thyroid tissue at the back of the thyroid to protect the parathyroid glands and to prevent recurrent laryngeal nerve damage, a potential complication associated with total thyroidectomy.

Endoscopic thyroidectomy: minimally invasive surgical removal of small (<3 cm), single nodule thyroid lesions or cysts that show no evidence of malignancy on biopsy. Uses 3 to 4 small incisions, producing less pain, faster return to normal activity, less scarring, and magnification of the surgical site with the use of the endoscope. May be done on an outpatient basis.

Minimally invasive radio-guided parathyroidectomy (MIRP): pioneered in 1996, technique of minimal invasiveness to remove diseased parathyroid lobe with intraoperative nuclear mapping. Because 90% of patients have only one diseased lobe, this technique allows for preservation of the remaining healthy tissue and minimizes potential postoperative complications. May be performed on an outpatient basis.

Near total thyroidectomy: removal of all of the thyroid gland with the exception of a very small portion on the opposite side of the thyroid.

Parathyroidectomy: excision of one or more diseased parathyroid glands.

Thyroidectomy: total excision of the thyroid gland leaving the parathyroid glands. Total thyroidectomy is normally only performed in patients with medullary malignancy because total thyroidectomy renders the patient immediately unable to produce any thyroid hormone, thus requiring supplementation with thyroid hormone for the remainder of his or her life.

Thyroid lobectomy with isthmisectomy: removal of one lobe of the thyroid and the isthmus connecting the two lobes.

ANESTHESIA

Surgery on the thyroid and parathyroid glands is generally performed under general anesthesia. Therefore postoperative care indicated for a patient who receives general anesthesia is instituted. Minimally invasive radio-guided parathyroidectomy (MIRP) is performed under local anesthesia, thereby minimizing the recovery requirements.

PERIANESTHESIA NURSING CARE

Positioning

If the patient is minimally responsive on arrival to the PACU, the patient should be placed in a side-lying position to protect the airway. Once the patient is responsive—or if he or she is responsive on admission—the patient is placed in a semi-Fowler's position to promote venous return. The patient should be positioned with particular care and support to the head and neck, so that no undue tension is placed on the suture line. The patient should be taught to support the head and neck during position changes by placing their hands at the back of their neck.

Cardiopulmonary Assessment and Care

Immediate postoperative observations should include close attention to respiratory function, which may be compromised by hemorrhage, venous oozing, or laryngeal edema. A tracheostomy set should be readily available. Signs and symptoms of respiratory obstruction—such as stridor, air hunger, and/or falling oxygen saturations—should be reported immediately to the anesthesiologist and surgeon, and appropriate measures should be taken. Col-mist humidification is generally added to the oxygen provided to any patient who has received general anesthesia to ease the sore throat expected after endotracheal intubation and to promote general respiratory well-being.

Pain Management

Because many of these surgeries are being performed on an outpatient basis, pain should be minimal after thyroidectomy and parathyroidectomy. Small doses of a narcotic such as fentanyl or morphine may be required in the first 24 hours for patients who are being admitted. Severe pain is not a normal finding and should be reported immediately to the surgeon.

Dressings

Postoperative dressings are minimal, and drains are generally not required. Drainage should also be minimal and should not visibly soak through the dressing. The usual symptoms of hemorrhage should be assessed, and the nurse should watch for swelling of the neck and feel the back of the neck for drainage. Any excess bleeding should be reported immediately.

Intake and Output

As with any surgical patient, monitoring of intake and output is important in the evaluation of

cardiovascular stability. Because many of these surgeries will be performed on an outpatient basis, it will be particularly important to ensure that the patient is capable of tolerating oral fluids before discharge. Many facilities also require that the patient void before discharge.

Complications

With a greater understanding of thyroid and parathyroid function and improvement of surgical technique, postoperative complications after thyroidectomy and parathyroidectomy are rare. Complications may be caused by the surgery or changes in metabolism and may include obstruction of the airway, bleeding, damage to the recurrent laryngeal nerve, and hypoparathyroidism (tetany). Less frequently seen complications include thyroid storm and infection.

Laryngeal Nerve Injury. The recurrent laryngeal nerve may be injured from severing, clamping, compression, or stretching during surgery. Symptoms of bilateral recurrent laryngeal nerve injury may indicate life-threatening airway obstruction, which requires immediate intervention. Unilateral recurrent laryngeal nerve injury may present as voice changes and a weak cough. Aspiration is a potential risk. The injury is generally transient and may be treated with time and/or steroids.

Bleeding. As the surgical techniques have become more refined and less invasive, the risks of postoperative bleeding have been significantly reduced. However, bleeding may cause tracheal compression and subsequent airway obstruction. If a surgeon suspects that bleeding may be a problem, a drain is placed. Excessive bleeding, as discussed previously, should be reported to the surgeon.

Hypoparathyroidism (Tetany). Hypoparathyroidism is another complication that may occur after total thyroidectomy or total parathyroidectomy and that may be caused by intential removal of the parathyroid glands or inadvertent or unavoidable damage during thyroidectomy. This complication manifests itself as hypocalcemia and is usually transient. Signs of hypocalcemia will rarely manifest in the immediate postoperative period but may present 24 to 72 hours postoperatively. Symptoms include tingling of the fingers and toes, perioral tingling, muscle cramps (tetany), and spasm. If calcium levels are not restored, seizures and laryngeal stridor are imminent. Assessment of any patient who complains of tingling should include testing for the presence of Chvostek, s sign (the development of a lip twitch or facial spasm when the cheek is tapped over the facial nerve) and Trousseau's sign (the development of a carpal spasm when a blood pressure cuff is applied and circulation transiently occluded). Definitive treatment is the intravenous administration of calcium. Although both calcium chloride and calcium gluconate may be used, calcium gluconate is preferred for its greater bioavailability and less arrhythmogenic potential. If intravenous calcium is administered, it is given via slow push, with continuous electrocardiographic monitoring before, during, and after the infusion.

Thyroid Storm. Thyroid storm or crisis is a rare complication that may occur after surgical manipulation of a hyperactive thyroid during surgery. Under ideal conditions, an overactive thyroid has been controlled preoperatively with medications. The patient may develop fever and tachycardia intraoperatively. Postoperatively, additional symptoms of agitation, disorientation, and hypertension may present. Treatment includes the administration of beta antagonists as well as supplemental cooling and increased oxygenation.

Infection. Thyroid and parathyroid surgery is generally not considered "dirty" surgery, and rarely is the patient given postoperative antibiotics as a routine. Any symptoms of infection that appear postoperatively with surgical follow-up will be treated with appropriate antibiotic therapy and wound care.

BIBLIOGRAPHY

Coffey A, Petti G: Endocrinology. In Bailey B, Johnson J, Kohut R, Pillsbury H et al, editors: Head and neck surgery—Otolaryngology, Philadelphia, 1993, JB Lippincott.

Litwack-Saleh K: Practical points in the care of the patient post-thyroid surgery, J Post Anesth Nurs, 7:404-406, 1992.

McKennis A, Waddington C: Nursing interventions for potential complications after thyroidectomy. (Last accessed online at www.sohnnurse.com/thyroidectomy.html on April 8, 2002.)

Netterville J, Ossoff R: Evaluation and treatment of complications of thyroid and parathyroid surgery, Otolaryngologic Clinics and North America 23: 529-551, 1990.

Norman J: Minimally invasive radio-guided parathyroidectomy, Surgery 122:998-1004, 1997.

Shaha AR: Controversies in the management of thyroid nodule. Laryngoscope, 110:183-193, 2000.

Shaha AR: Thyroid cancer: extent of thyroidectomy, Cancer Control 7:240-245, 2000.

37

CARE OF THE GASTROINTESTINAL, ABDOMINAL, AND ANORECTAL SURGICAL PATIENT

Denise O'Brien, MSN(c), RN, CPAN, CAPA

Care of the patient after abdominal surgery or surgery on the gastrointestinal tract is an extremely broad subject. This chapter discusses the care involved after surgery on the gastrointestinal tract, including the esophagus and the anus, as well as the accessory organs—the liver, gallbladder, pancreas, and spleen (Fig. 37-1). Surgery on the female reproductive organs, which are also contained within the abdominal cavity, is reviewed in Chapter 39. The care common to all patients undergoing abdominal surgery is discussed, and only the most important variations related to specific procedures are included.

Surgical intervention within the abdominal cavity is generally directed toward restoring normal function and therefore involves repair of congenital abnormalities, reconstruction of deformities, removal of obstructions to restore patency of the gastrointestinal tract and the biliary tract, treatment of malignancies, and maintenance of the integrity of related organs, such as the liver, pancreas, and spleen.

DEFINITIONS

Antrectomy: removal of the lower part of the stomach.

Appendectomy: removal of the vermiform appendix.

Cecostomy: creation of an opening for insertion of a tube into the cecum to decompress the bowel by removing air and accumulations of digestive juices.

Cholecystectomy: removal of the gallbladder; the procedure may be performed with an open or a laparoscopic approach with electrosurgical cautery.

Cholecystostomy: establishment of an opening into the gallbladder to permit drainage of the organ and the removal of stones. This is performed infrequently

except to provide relief in an extremely debilitated and unstable patient.

Colostomy: opening of the colon onto the abdomen; may be permanent or temporary, single or double lumen. May be performed with either an open procedure or a laparoscopic approach.

Diverticulum: a "herniation" of mucosa/submucosa through a weakness in a muscular wall, most commonly in the sigmoid colon.

Endoscopic retrograde cholangiopancreatography (ERCP): a side-viewing fiberoptic endoscope is used to cannulate pancreatic and biliary ducts through the ampulla of Vater for cholangiography, pancreatography, stone removal, and invasive manipulation such as sphincterotomy.

Endoscopy: visualization of a body cavity with a lighted tube or scope.

Esophagogastroduodenoscopy (EGD): passage of a fiberoptic gastroscope, usually under topical anesthesia and intravenous sedation, to view the esophagus, stomach, and duodenum.

Esophagoscopy: direct visualization of the esophagus and cardia of the stomach by means of a lighted instrument (esophagoscope). Esophagoscopy may be used to obtain a tissue biopsy or secretions for study to aid in diagnosis.

Gastrectomy: removal of the stomach. Usually a subtotal gastrectomy is done, in which part of the stomach is removed, expressed as a percentage (usually 60% to 80% but can be much as 95%); also called gastric resection (Fig. 37-2A).

Gastroenterostomy: creation of an anastomosis between the posterior wall of the stomach and the small intestine (Fig. 37-2B).

Gastroscopy: direct inspection of the stomach with possible removal of a tissue specimen by means of a lighted instrument (gastroscope).

551

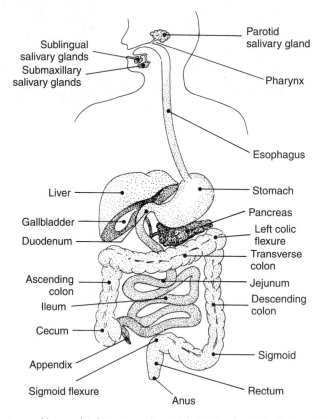

Fig. 37-1 The digestive system and its associated structures. *(From Sole ML, Lamborn ML, Hartshorn JC: Introduction to critical care nursing, ed 3, Philadelphia, 2001, WB Saunders.)*

Hemorrhoidectomy: surgical excision of dilated veins of the rectum.

Hernia: the displacement of any viscus (usually bowel) or tissue through a congenital or acquired opening or defect in the wall of its natural cavity. Usually this term is applied to protrusion of abdominal viscera; however, it is actually the defect itself through which abdominal contents have protruded.

Herniorrhaphy: correction of a hernia, also termed hernioplasty. Hernias and herniorrhaphies are classified according to their anatomic sites and the condition of the viscus that has protruded. Reducible hernias are those in which the bowel or contents of the hernial sac can be replaced into their normal cavity. An irreducible, or incarcerated, hernia is one in which the contents cannot be replaced. A strangulated hernia is one in which the blood supply to the protruding segment of bowel is obstructed. When a segment of bowel

becomes strangulated, it rapidly becomes necrotic. A strangulated hernia constitutes a surgical emergency.

Herniorrhaphy, diaphragmatic: replacement of abdominal contents that have entered the thorax through a defect in the diaphragm and repair of the diaphragmatic defect.

Herniorrhaphy, epigastric and hypogastric: repair and closure of the abdominal wall defect.

Herniorrhaphy, femoral: a defect in the region of the femoral ring, which is located just below Poupart's (inguinal) ligament and medial to the femoral vein. Femoral hernias are seldom found in children and occur most often in women.

Herniorrhaphy, incisional: reunion in layers of the abdominal wall that may also involve placement of prosthetic (synthetic) mesh (e.g., Marlex, Gore-Tex).

Herniorrhaphy, inguinal: repair of a defect in the inguinal region; may be direct (through Hesselbach's

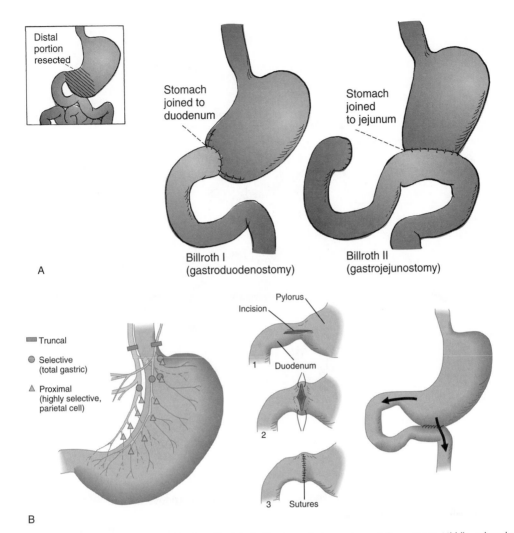

Fig. 37-2 **A,** Gastric surgical procedures: Billroth I, Billroth II. **B,** Gastric surgical procedures: Left, vagotomy. Middle, pyloroplasty. Right, gastroenterostomy. *(From Black JM, Hawks JH, Keene AM: Medical-surgical nursing: clinical management for positive outcomes, ed 6, Philadelphia, 2001, WB Saunders.)*

triangle) or an indirect (through the internal ring) inguinal hernia (Fig. 37-3).

Herniorrhaphy, umbilical: closure of the peritoneal opening and reconstruction of the abdominal wall beneath the umbilicus (umbilical ring); usually occurs in pediatric patients and is most common in African-American infants; often closes spontaneously in infants before 2 years of age.

Ileostomy: opening of the ileum to the surface of the abdomen. Used to treat inflammatory conditions of the bowel—such as ulcerative colitis and regional enteritis—

and to provide a permanent or temporary stoma after emergency surgery for obstruction or cancer.

Intussusception: telescoping of the bowel into itself.

Laparoscopy (peritoneoscopy): direct visualization of the peritoneal cavity by means of a lighted instrument (often connected to a color video monitor) inserted through the abdominal wall via a stab wound. An increasing number of abdominal procedures are performed assisted by laparoscopy (lap-assisted). Gastrointestinal or abdominal procedures currently performed via laparoscope include cholecystectomy, truncal

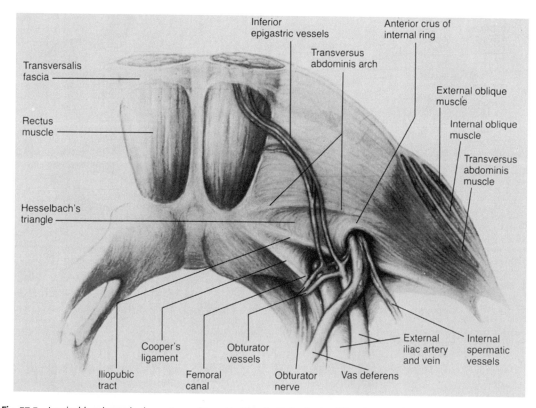

Labels in figure:
- Transversalis fascia
- Rectus muscle
- Hesselbach's triangle
- Inferior epigastric vessels
- Transversus abdominis arch
- Anterior crus of internal ring
- External oblique muscle
- Internal oblique muscle
- Transversus abdominis muscle
- Iliopubic tract
- Cooper's ligament
- Femoral canal
- Obturator vessels
- Obturator nerve
- Vas deferens
- External iliac artery and vein
- Internal spermatic vessels

Fig. 37-3 Inguinal hernia repair: the anatomy. *(From Madden JL: Abdominal wall hernias: an atlas of anatomy and repair, Philadelphia, 1989, WB Saunders.)*

vagotomy, gastrojejunostomy, Nissen fundoplication (Fig. 37-4), inguinal herniorrhaphy, appendectomy, jejunostomy, colostomy, and ileocolectomy.

Laparotomy (celiotomy): an opening made through the abdominal wall into the peritoneal cavity, usually for exploratory purposes. If an abnormality is found, the operation is usually named according to the procedure or procedures carried out.

Pancreaticoduodenectomy (Whipple procedure): removal of the head of the pancreas, the entire duodenum, a portion of the jejunum, the distal third of the stomach and the lower half of the common bile duct, with reestablishment of continuity of the biliary, pancreatic, and gastrointestinal systems. The procedure, which is used primarily for the treatment of malignancy of the pancreas and duodenum, is associated with a 2% to 5% risk of mortality. Sometimes a pylorus-sparing procedure is performed, thus leaving the entire stomach intact.

Percutaneous endoscopic gastrostomy (PEG): endoscopic procedure for the insertion of a gastrostomy tube, performed under local anesthesia and intravenous sedation.

Pyloromyotomy (Fredet-Ramstedt's operation): enlarging the lumen of the pylorus by longitudinally splitting the hypertrophied circular muscle without severing the mucosa; used as treatment for pyloric stenosis. Pyloric stenosis is most common in firstborn male infants.

Pyloroplasty: a longitudinal incision made in the pylorus and closed transversely to permit the muscle to relax and establish an enlarged outlet. Heineke-Mikulicz is the most common type of procedure (see Fig. 37-2B).

Splenectomy: removal of the spleen.

Transduodenal sphincterotomy: partial division of the sphincter of Oddi and exploration of the common duct to treat recurrent attacks of acute pancreatitis caused by formation of calculi in the pancreatic duct or blockage

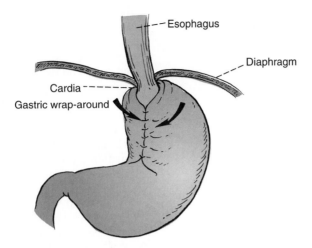

Fig. 37-4 Hiatal hernia repair with gastric wrap (Nissen fundoplication). *(From Black JM, Hawks JH, Keene AM: Medical-surgical nursing: clinical management for positive outcomes, ed 6, Philadelphia, 2001, WB Saunders.)*

of the sphincter of Oddi. May also be used to treat biliary stones.

Vagotomy: division (usually with frozen section) of branches of the vagus nerve that innervate the stomach to reduce secretions and movements (see Fig. 37-2B).

Volvulus: intestinal obstruction due to twisting of the bowel.

GENERAL CARE AFTER ABDOMINAL SURGERY

Abdominal or gastrointestinal surgery may be performed with local, regional, or general anesthesia. The choice of anesthesia varies with the type of procedure, the patient's cardiac and pulmonary status, and the surgeon's need for muscle relaxation. Usually, only the simpler procedures are performed under local or regional (spinal or epidural) anesthesia. Diagnostic procedures such as endoscopy, biopsy, and percutaneous gastrostomy often are performed under local anesthesia with appropriate sedation. Inguinal or femoral herniorrhaphies are often performed with local, spinal or epidural, or general anesthesia. Most other abdominal surgical and laparoscopic procedures are performed under general anesthesia.

A number of abdominopelvic incisions have been developed and are commonly used (Fig. 37-5). An ideal incision ensures ease of entrance, maximal exposure of the operative site, and minimal trauma. It should also provide good primary wound healing with maximal wound strength.

The reader should review Chapters 24 through 28 for general care after surgery.

Perianesthesia Care

As with any procedure, the surgeon and anesthesia care provider should give the perianesthesia nurse a full report on the anesthesia used and the procedure performed. With complicated abdominal procedures, especially those that involve extensive resection or rerouting of the gastrointestinal tract, or both, the surgeon may draw a diagram of the procedure performed, along with the incisions and drainage tubes that are present. This assists those who are caring for the patient in an assessment of the wounds, dressings, and expected drainage. The surgeon can draw this diagram on the nursing care plan, which should be initiated on the patient's admission to the PACU so that continuity of information is ensured.

Positioning.   After abdominal surgery, patients are often positioned on their sides until laryngeal reflexes have started to return. They are then placed in a semi-Fowler's position to ease the tension on suture lines and to promote respiratory effort. After some procedures on the esophagus, however, patients should be kept flat to avoid tension on the suture line. After hemor-

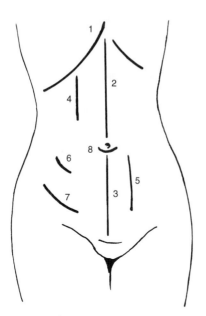

Fig. 37-5 Commonly used abdominal incisions: *1.* Kocher's incision: right side, gallbladder and biliary tract surgery; left side, splenectomy. *2.* Upper abdominal midline incision: rapid entry to control bleeding ulcer. *3.* Lower abdominal midline incision: female reproductive system. *4.* Upper paramedian incision: right side, biliary tract surgery, cholecystectomy; left side, splenectomy, gastrectomy, vagotomy, hiatal hernia repair. *5.* Lower paramedian incision: right side, appendectomy, small bowel resection; left side, sigmoid colon resection. *6.* McBurney's incision: appendectomy. *7.* Inguinal incision: inguinal herniorrhaphy. *8.* Infraumbilical: umbilical herniorrhaphy.

rhoidectomy, patients may assume any position of comfort, which will most likely be on their sides.
Dressings and Drains. All dressings should be checked. The nurse must know what kind of incision was used and whether any drains are in place. If drains are in place, considerably more drainage can be expected. Drains are discussed in more detail under the specific procedures. Drainage should be assessed for character, volume, and odor. The nurse should determine who can or should remove the dressing if needed. Some surgeons reinforce the abdominal incision and dressing with a binder. They believe that this gives the incision valuable support. Others, however, believe that binders restrict respiratory effort and that this disadvantage outweighs the limited advantage of incisional support.

Because drainage is often copious after gastrointestinal surgery, frequent reinforcement of dressings may be necessary. Ask the surgeon for anticipated or expected amounts of drainage for this patient and his or her procedure. If drainage becomes excessive (more than expected from the particular procedure), the surgeon should be notified and the incision directly inspected.

All tubes should be connected to the appropriate drainage devices, usually straight-gravity or suction drainage, as the surgeon specifies. Maintenance of the patency of these tubes is one of the most important nursing functions after gastrointestinal surgery. Irrigation of nasogastric tubes after esophageal or gastric surgery should be directed by the surgeon's orders.

Respiratory Function. The promotion of good respiratory function is a nursing priority for the patient who has had abdominal surgery. Painful abdominal incisions cause the patient to restrict chest expansion voluntarily. This is especially true with high abdominal incisions. The patient must be coached often in doing sustained maximal inspirations, coughing, and changing position to prevent respiratory complications. Assisting the patient by the splinting of the incision and judiciously using pain medications aid in deep breathing and coughing and prevent the development of atelectasis. Coughing and incentive spirometry in the PACU setting are valuable in promoting respiratory function.

Frequent assessment of breath sounds during the postoperative period can alert the nurse to impending respiratory problems. An accidental nick into the diaphragm during upper abdominal surgery is possible and can result in respiratory distress. Positive pressure ventilation during anesthesia can also lead to respiratory problems. Breath sounds must be monitored closely to assess for pneumothorax.

Fluid and Electrolyte Balance. Fluid and electrolyte shifts or losses can be substantial during gastrointestinal surgery. Losses continue postoperatively through gastrointestinal tubes or other drains. For this reason, accurate intake and output records are mandatory. This begins with the intake and output report from the anesthesia care provider, which should be the first PACU entry. All drainage from incisions should be included in the assessment of electrolyte balance. Frequent serum electrolyte determinations may be necessary if losses are great. Intravenous fluids are used for replacement for at least the first 24 hours postoperatively and until the nasogastric tube is removed. See Chapter 14 for discussion of the specific problems in electrolyte loss from the gastrointestinal tract.

Urinary retention may become a problem after abdominal surgery because of incisional pain, opioid analgesics, anesthetics, and physiologic splinting. Urine output should be checked frequently, and accurate records should be kept. The nurse should also check for bladder distention and document the findings. (The patient may not recognize the need to void, especially after spinal or epidural anesthesia.) The patient should void within 6 to 8 hours postoperatively. If the patient has not voided by the time of discharge from the PACU, notify the receiving unit to check specifically for urinary retention. If permissible, it may help the male patient to stand to void. If urinary retention causes pain, distends the abdomen, or becomes prolonged, urinary catheterization may become necessary. Patients who have had extensive surgery often return to the PACU with a urinary catheter in place. Accurate output records should be maintained.

Care of the Patient with Nasogastric or Intestinal Tubes

Anesthesia and manipulation of the viscera during surgery cause gastric and colonic peristalsis to diminish or disappear completely for up to 5 days after surgery. Nasogastrointestinal or nasogastric tubes are commonly used postoperatively to prevent the sequelae of this hypomotility. Edema at the operative site also can result in obstruction. Decompression of the stomach—with removal of accumulated fluid and air—not only prevents vomiting and eases tension on the abdominal suture line but also increases the area's vascularity and thus improves its nutrition and reduces the risk of gastric anastomotic leak.

If gastric decompression is needed, short tubes are generally used today; long intestinal tubes are no longer used. Short tubes used include the Levin, the Rehfuss, and the plastic Salem sump, which is a double-lumen nasogastric tube and is the most commonly used tube. The double lumen prevents excessive negative pressure from developing when the tube is connected to suction.

When the patient returns from the operating suite with a nasogastric tube in place, the nurse must ascertain why the tube was placed, where it was placed, and whether it should be connected to suction or to straight-gravity drainage. The physician often will order the tube to be connected to low-pressure, intermittent suction (20 to 80 mm Hg). Usually only low-pressure, intermittent suction is used because excessive negative pressure in either the stomach or the bowel pulls the mucosa into the lumen of the tube and can cause traumatic ulcers. For double-lumen nasogastric tubes, continuous suction at 40 to 60 mm Hg is usually ordered and necessary for the tube to function properly. Keeping the open lumen above the midline and fitted with an antireflux valve may help improve functioning of the double-lumen tube.

Tube Patency.   Patency of the tube must be ensured. The nurse should observe for drainage from the tube. All characteristics of the drainage must be noted: consistency, color, odor, quantity, and any deviations from the expected drainage. After gastrointestinal surgery, initial drainage is bright red in small volumes, but it should become dark after 24 hours. Bloody drainage should not be expected from a nasogastric tube placed only for decompression of the stomach after biliary tract, liver, or splenic surgery. If no drainage is present, if the patient's abdomen becomes distended or if the patient vomits around the nasogastric tube or complains of nausea, the tube may be clogged, or the suction apparatus may be malfunctioning; check both. To maintain the patency of the nasogastric tube, irrigation with 20 to 30 ml of normal saline may be done every hour—or more frequently if necessary. Plain water in 20-ml amounts may be used to irrigate the tube without creating electrolyte abnormalities. Larger amounts of plain water should not be used when irrigating for gastric bleeding because of the large volume and the risk of electrolyte alterations. Before any type of irrigation, check with the surgeon, especially after esophageal or gastric procedures. Frequent irrigations increase the loss of electrolytes from the gastrointestinal system. Some surgeons advocate the use of air to irrigate the nasogastric tube to maintain patency.

Irrigation.   The amount of irrigating solution instilled should be recorded as such, unless its equivalent is aspirated by syringe. All gastrointestinal drainage should be accurately measured and recorded. If irrigations do not increase drainage, the tubing should be checked for clogs by milking it toward the suction container to dislodge any obstruction. The suction apparatus is checked by disconnecting the nasogastric tube at the junction of the nasogastric tube and the drainage tube leading to the container. With the suction turned on, the end of the drainage tube is placed in a glass of water; if the water is sucked up, the suction device is functioning. If these measures fail, gastric mucosa may be occluding the lumen of the tube or the tube may be kinked. In this instance, the patient or the tube may need to be repositioned. If the patient has had gastric, pancreatic, or esophageal surgery, the tube should not be manipulated; the surgeon should be notified of the malfunctioning tube.

Patient Comfort. The presence of a nasogastric tube is a most uncomfortable experience for the patient. However, appropriate nursing care can relieve sore throat, dry mouth, hoarseness, earache, sore nose, and dry lips. Ensure that the tube is taped securely and properly (hypoallergenic tape is best) in a position to prevent pressure on the naris. The tube may be secured to the upper lip or nose in the position it naturally assumes. The tube should not be taped to the patient's nose and then to the forehead. This causes pressure on the underside of the nostril and can cause tissue necrosis. To lessen the pressure and pull on the patient's nose, either tape or pin the tube to the gown.

Apply petrolatum ointment to the tube where it enters the nose and around the nares. The outside portion of the tube is kept free of mucus or other drainage. This prevents encrustations from forming and reduces irritation of the nostril. Petrolatum ointment, cream, or lip balm is applied to the lips to keep them soft and prevent cracking. Good, frequent mouth care is essential for the comfort of the patient and to prevent parotitis. Moistened swabs, mouthwash, or even a toothbrush may be used to provide mouth care for the patient. Simply ensure that the patient understands not to swallow any of the material used. This, of course, would not be fatal but could be detrimental to fluid and electrolyte balance.

Gargles with warm tap water or warm saline—or with viscous lidocaine or applications of a local anesthetic spray—relieve the patient's sore throat. A physician's order should be provided for these measures. Some surgeons allow their patients to suck on isotonic ice chips or hard candy or to chew gum. Anesthetic throat lozenges, if allowed, are comforting to the patient. All patients with a gastrointestinal tube in place are given essentially nothing by mouth until the tube is removed. The only exception may be certain medications, given orally or through the tube, or ice chips, less than 200 ml every 8 hours.

DIAGNOSTIC STUDIES

Invasive diagnostic procedures are occasionally done at the patient's bedside on the nursing unit, but they are more commonly done in a special procedures room, often located within the surgical suite. They require local anesthesia and appropriate sedation or sometimes general anesthesia. Patients may be sent to the PACU for a brief observation period. Care after endoscopy includes all the general care afforded a perianesthesia patient. After esophagoscopy and gastroscopy, the nurse should be alert for the return of the gag reflex. When pharyngeal reflexes have returned, unless contraindicated by the diagnosis or in anticipation of further surgery, the patient may be started on liquids and may progress to a regular diet as tolerated. Rest is the most important treatment for this patient. There may be bleeding, swelling, or dysfunction of the involved area—indications of complications from the procedure.

Patients who have had laparoscopy have only small bandages or tape strip closures (Steri-Strips) over the stab wounds used for entry of the scope and its accessories. These bandages should remain clean and dry. These patients are probably apprehensive about what was discovered about their conditions during the diagnostic procedure; the surgeon should give accurate information after the procedure. The nurse should be familiar with what the patients have been told regarding findings of the diagnostic laparoscopy so that he or she can interpret or repeat the information for the patients, if necessary.

CARE AFTER SURGERY ON THE GASTROINTESTINAL TRACT

Esophagus

Surgery on the esophagus includes repair of hiatal hernia and various forms of tracheoesophageal fistulas, excision of esophageal diverticula, treatment of stenosis of the lower end of the esophagus, esophagomyotomy, esophagectomy, antireflux procedures, and cardiomyotomy.

Postoperative care depends on the kind of incision used to expose the operative site: abdominal, thoracic, or laparoscopic. Surgery on the esophagus frequently involves a thoracic incision. Care for the patient following a thoracic incision is discussed in Chapter 31. Procedures on the esophagus are performed under general anesthesia. A tracheostomy often is performed (see Chapter 29 for care of the patient after tracheostomy).

On arrival to the PACU, the patient should be placed in a semi-Fowler's position. This aids in the drainage of blood from the pleural space and prevents tension from impinging on the suture lines. The incision is generally long (from the tip of the scapula to the seventh or eighth rib area) and painful. Analgesics must be given in adequate doses to promote rest and adequate respiratory effort. An interpleural or epidural catheter often is in place for postoperative analgesia. Patient-controlled analgesia may be used. Transcutaneous electrical nerve stimulation (TENS) may also provide incisional pain relief.

A nasogastric tube will be in place and should be cared for as previously discussed. The nurse should not manipulate it. Chest tubes should be managed as discussed in Chapter 31. A large sterile dressing should be in place, and it should be checked frequently for drainage and reinforced as necessary. Excessive bloody drainage should be reported to the surgeon.

Stomach

Surgery on the stomach involves procedures to treat ulcers (antrectomy and vagotomy, gastric resection, gastrectomy), removal of portions of the stomach for malignancy, and rerouting of the gastrointestinal system at this point to treat pyloric obstruction. All postoperative care of the patient is generally the same, and anesthesia is general. The patient postoperatively should be placed in a semi-Fowler's position to relieve tension on the suture line and to promote drainage. The abdominal incisions are fairly high, long, and painful, and particular attention must be paid to pulmonary toilet. This type of patient must be encouraged more often than any other to expand the lungs and to cough and must generally have assistance to change position. Assistance in splinting the wound with the hands or with a firm pillow is most appreciated by the patient. These procedures generally produce considerable postoperative pain, and analgesics should be used generously but judiciously. Patient-controlled or epidural analgesia may be effective for upper abdominal incisional and visceral pain.

A nasogastric tube will be in place and should be cared for as previously discussed. Small volumes of bright, bloody drainage from the nasogastric tube can be expected for the first 2 to 3 hours, because it is not uncommon to have bleeding at the anastomotic site in these procedures. However, bright bleeding that does not decrease after this period or bleeding that becomes excessive (more than 75 ml/hr) should be reported immediately to the surgeon. Observe the nasogastric tube and its drainage closely because blood easily clots and clogs the tube; notify the surgeon immediately if the tube stops draining or appears obstructed with blood. Because blood loss may be highly significant in this patient, cardiovascular status must receive careful scrutiny. Vital signs are checked frequently, and a certain amount of hypotension and tachycardia is to be expected. If hypotension and tachycardia persist or maintain a downward trend, the surgeon should be notified.

Blood replacement may have to be instituted. Hemoglobin and hematocrit levels should be determined 4 to 6 hours postoperatively and the surgeon notified if they are significantly lower than previous determinations. Little or no drainage should be expected from the incision unless drains are in place. If drainage does appear, the dressing should be reinforced and the surgeon notified. The nurse in the PACU should not replace the initial dressing unless so directed by the surgeon. Drains with copious output may need a drainage device applied over them to protect the patient's skin and allow for accurate measurement of drainage.

Urinary retention is commonly a problem, and many surgeons prefer to insert a Foley catheter while the patient is in the operating room. Accurate measurements of output should be ascertained. If a urinary catheter is not in place, the patient should be checked frequently for bladder distention, which may indicate an over-full bladder and urinary retention. If the patient is unable to void, a catheterization order should be obtained.

Perforated Ulcer. Perforation of an ulcer is usually a surgical emergency, and neither the patient nor the family members will be adequately prepared—neither physically nor emotionally—for the surgery. This concerns the perianesthesia nurse because complications, especially hypovolemia and shock, may more readily occur in this patient.

Pyloric Stenosis. Specific care for infants following surgery for pyloric stenosis is detailed in pediatric texts. However, the perianesthesia nurse should be aware of their general care. Position is important. The infant should be kept either on the right side or on the abdomen until the danger of vomiting and aspiration has subsided, then should be placed in an upright position. Careful placement of the diaper is important to avoid contamination of the wound. It may also be helpful to apply a pediatric urine collector not only to prevent contamination of the wound with urine but also to determine accurate output. Feedings are usually begun for these infants 4 to 6 hours postoperatively, but the surgeon's instructions should be explicitly followed.

Small Bowel

Operations on the small bowel include exploratory laparotomy with lysis of adhesions and resection for obstruction or perforation. Care after these procedures is essentially the same as that already mentioned. No excessive drainage from incisions should be noted unless drains have been placed. Fluid and electrolyte balance must be monitored carefully. Remember that the loss of sodium and bicarbonate ions will be great—thus resulting in imbalance—and that fluid losses during surgery may be significant, but fluid overload must be avoided.

The patient with an ileostomy will enter the PACU with a bag in place over the stoma, and returns may be expected almost at once; these should be recorded. Particular attention must be paid to this stoma, the drainage, and the collection device; no leakage onto the skin should be allowed because this causes significant skin damage. Under the collection device, the peristomal skin is protected with a skin barrier that includes pectin-based and karaya-based wafers or paste.

Large Bowel

Surgery on the large bowel includes appendectomy, colostomy, various types of colonic resection for removal of tumors or correction of other problems, total proctocolectomy with ileoanal anastomosis (Fig. 37-6), and abdominoperineal resection (Fig. 37-7). Most of these surgical procedures are performed under general anesthesia. On return to the PACU, patients are kept flat and on one side until the reflexes have returned; they may then assume a position of comfort unless otherwise specified by the surgeon. Postoperative care is essentially the same as for small bowel surgery.

If the patient returns from surgery with a colostomy, some special care is required. It is unusual for the colostomy to start functioning immediately postoperatively; however, spillage must be prevented from contaminating the incision or excoriating the skin. A pouch or collection device may be in place over the colostomy. The skin around the stoma should be protected with an appropriate skin barrier if drainage is present. Check the color of the stoma—it should be bright red and moist—and document its appearance in the nursing record.

Fluid and electrolyte balance must be monitored carefully. Some blood-tinged urine may be expected after colectomy because retractors used in surgery may have caused contusions of the bladder; however, gross blood may indicate that the bladder was more severely injured. Dressings should remain dry, unless drains were placed in the wound. If drains were placed, some bloody drainage may be expected, and dressings should be reinforced as necessary. If dressings soak through, the drainage should be considered excessive and must be reported to the surgeon.

Incisions may be left open to heal with delayed primary closure or by secondary intent. Abdominal wounds for bowel surgery may be contaminated (e.g., traumatic penetrating injuries, colostomies) with an increased risk of infection. For a delay primary closure, the wound is left open, protected with moist gauze, and—when it is clean and red—closed with sutures that were placed during the original surgery and left slack. The cleanliness of the wound and the

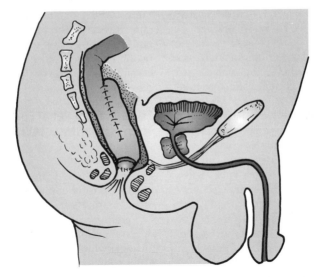

Fig. 37-6 Ileoanal anastomosis with J-pouch for treatment of ulcerative colitis. *(From Black JM, Hawks JH, Keene AM: Medical-surgical nursing: clinical management for positive outcomes, ed 6, Philadelphia, 2001, WB Saunders.)*

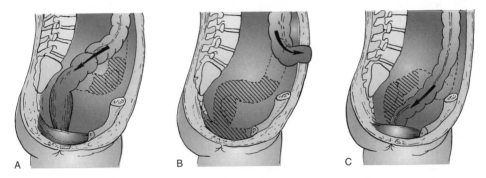

Fig. 37-7 Large bowel procedures for resection of malignancy: **A,** Anterior resection with primary anastomosis. **B,** Abdominoperineal (anteroposterior) resection with permanent colostomy. **C,** proctosigmoidectomy with "pull through." *(From Black JM, Hawks JH, Keene AM: Medical-surgical nursing: clinical management for positive outcomes, ed 6, Philadelphia, 2001, WB Saunders.)*

health of the granulation tissue in the wound generally determine the best time for closure.

Abdominoperineal Resection. Abdominoperineal resection for cancer of the rectum is a major procedure that results in permanent colostomy and two separate incisions. Vital signs are monitored carefully, and any adverse trend reported. Perineal drains will be in place and should be noted on the patient's chart and nursing care plan. The perineal dressings often become saturated with bloody drainage and must be reinforced. If drainage remains bright and obviously new bleeding is occurring and if frequent dressing changes are required, the surgeon should be notified. If sump catheters are used to drain the perineal wound, they may be attached to a grenade or bulb (Jackson-Pratt) device and an accurate measurement of drainage may be obtained.

The patient who has undergone abdominoperineal surgery will have a colostomy. Check the blood supply to the stoma frequently because impaired blood supply is an early and serious complication. Pain may be severe and should be relieved with adequate doses of opioid analgesics or use of an epidural catheter for analgesia to ensure comfort of the patient and promote respiratory sufficiency.

Appendectomy and Herniorrhaphy. Patients who have undergone surgery for appendectomy or herniorrhaphy usually return to the PACU almost fully awake and without serious postoperative complications. No nasogastric tube, Foley catheter, or drain will be in place, and recovery is generally uneventful. However, patients who have large ventral hernia repairs with mesh may have nasogastric tubes and drains in place. Patients may assume a position of comfort as soon as pharyngeal reflexes have returned, and they may start on a progressive diet as tolerated unless a nasogastric tube in is place. All the postoperative care outlined in Chapters 24 and 28 is applicable. When the laparoscopic approach is used, general anesthesia usually is given. Patients may complain of shoulder pain or bloating because of insufflation of air. They may also complain of sore throat from intubation and the neuromuscular blocking agents. Monitor fluid intake, and replace fluid losses appropriately. Dressings should remain dry and intact, and any postoperative incisional bleeding or drainage should be reported to the surgeon. The most important postoperative complication is bleeding. The nurse should also watch for urinary retention. If the patient has undergone inguinal hernia repair, the nurse should watch for development of scrotal edema or hematoma, which may indicate slow bleeding from the operative site.

Lower Rectum and Anus

Surgery on the lower rectum and anus includes excision of pilonidal cysts, rectal fissures, fistulas, rectal abscesses, tumors, and hemorrhoids. Perianesthesia nursing care is the same as for any patient who undergoes anesthesia, which may be local, regional, or general. Dressings should be checked frequently for excessive drainage and bleeding. The incisions may be closed but often are packed to facilitate drainage of infected material and aid in healing. Urinary retention may be a problem, because the proximity of the bladder and operative site may make urination difficult.

Pain can be exquisite, but patients are often embarrassed by the location of the operative site and may not ask for analgesia. The nurse should be alert to signs and symptoms of pain and discomfort and administer analgesia as necessary for relief.

SURGERY ON RELATED ORGANS WITHIN THE ABDOMINAL CAVITY

Liver

Surgery on the liver includes biopsy, small wedge biopsy, excision of tumors, major resection, repair of traumatic lacerations, and hepatic transplant.

Percutaneous liver biopsy is a common procedure, usually performed in the endoscopy suite, although the patient may be taken to the operating suite and may return to the PACU for a short period of observation. Postoperative care depends on the type of anesthesia used; it is usually local but may involve other types if the patient cannot or will not cooperate. The patient should remain positioned on the right side for at least 2 hours after the procedure. Vital signs should be determined frequently—every 10 to 15 minutes for the first hour and every 30 minutes for the second hour. Complications include hemorrhage due to penetration of a blood vessel and peritonitis due to accidental puncture of the bile duct. If the patient's vital signs begin a downward trend and if he or she reports severe abdominal pain or becomes febrile, the surgeon should be notified immediately.

Open surgery on the liver for the excision of tumors or the repair of lacerations is done under general anesthesia and involves a fairly long upper abdominal vertical or bilateral subcostal oblique (chevron) incision. All care previously discussed for patients after general anesthesia and upper abdominal incisions applies. Respiratory care is of paramount importance. The liver is an extremely vascular and friable organ. It is difficult to suture, and gross bleeding is common and often involves large blood losses, especially when surgery is necessitated by traumatic injury or large resection. Large drains of the Penrose or suction (grenade or bulb) type are placed in the region of the laceration or excision of the tumor and are brought through separate sites to the skin surface. For the first 8 hours, expect approximately 250 to 500 ml of sanguineous drainage from the drains.

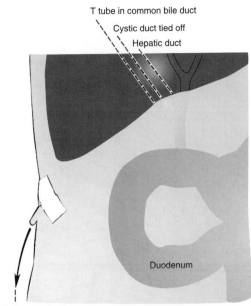

T tube in common bile duct

Cystic duct tied off

Hepatic duct

Duodenum

To drainage collection

Fig. 37-8 T-tube placement in common bile duct. *(From Black JM, Hawks JH, Keene AM: Medical-surgical nursing: clinical management for positive outcomes, ed 6, Philadelphia, 2001, WB Saunders.)*

Coagulation studies must be performed frequently and monitored closely because many patients develop coagulation abnormalities during and after liver surgery. Specific coagulation factors may be administered, according to the results of the coagulation tests. Hypoglycemia must be avoided. Patients are commonly started on peripheral intravenous dextrose 10% solutions, total parenteral nutrition, or feeding jejunostomy infusions.

Vital signs must be determined frequently and any downward trend reported to the surgeon at once. Blood replacement or hemostasis may be inadequate. Frequently, this patient will also have a T-tube in place in the common bile duct (Fig. 37-8). This tube should be attached to straight-gravity drainage, and accurate measurements of the output should be made. A nasogastric tube will be in place and should receive care as discussed previously. Pain is usually severe, and opioid analgesics or epidural analgesia are necessary to promote rest and respiratory effort.

Spleen

Surgery on the spleen involves general anesthesia and removal of the organ. The spleen is removed because of rupture from trauma; accidental trauma from associated surgery; diseases that cause damage, such as mononucleosis and malaria; a variety of hematologic malignancies; left-sided portal hypertension; and hypersplenism. A midline or left subcostal incision is used. Postoperative care for the patient after splenectomy is the same as that for the patient after repair of a lacerated liver. Dressings should remain dry and intact. A drain may be placed in the subdiaphragmatic space to prevent the collection of blood under the diaphragm and to detect unrecognized injury to the pancreas that may have occurred.

The perianesthesia nurse should know the circumstances that lead to the patient's splenectomy. If it was necessitated by trauma, the nurse must be particularly alert for signs that indicate development of unrecognized complications from the accident. Vital signs should be determined frequently and trends watched—especially those that indicate progressive bleeding. Neurologic signs should be checked, and the patient should be assessed carefully for any signs of injury to the extremities. Any arrhythmia should be reported because this may indicate cardiac injury.

Pancreas

Surgery on the pancreas is difficult and technically demanding. It involves general anesthesia, and care for these patients is the same as for other postoperative patients. If the operative procedure done is to remove malignant tumors, a mortality rate of 2% to 7% is not unreasonable because of extensive resection and poor general condition of the patient.

Postoperative care of the patient after a pancreaticoduodenectomy (Whipple or modified Whipple procedure) is a challenge. All postoperative care for the abdominal surgery patient applies. Particular attention must be paid to drains and catheters. Surgeons should augment their reports to the nurse by explaining exactly what procedure was performed, where drains or wound catheters were placed, and how to care for them. Surgeons should brief the nurse on expected drainage and what should be considered excessive. As with all abdominal surgical patients, intravenous lines and intravenous therapy will already have been initiated. Because of the generally poor nutritional status of these patients, hyperalimentation may be started almost immediately postoperatively.

All respiratory, cardiac, and renal functioning must be monitored carefully and the surgeon notified of any untoward signs. Assisted ventilation may be required for at least 24 hours following this procedure (this type of care is discussed in Chapter 25). If frequent arterial blood gas analysis is needed for this patient, an arterial line should be in place for this purpose. Blood gas analysis yields valuable information about the patient's respiratory acid-base status, which may be precarious. Urine output should be determined hourly, and at least 0.5 to 1 ml/kg/hr should be expected.

Frequent assays of blood glucose levels should be ordered on all patients after pancreatic surgery. Most of these patients need to receive intravenous insulin during the postoperative period. Insulin doses are titrated to maintain the blood glucose levels between 180 and 250 mg/dl. This aids in the prevention of hypoglycemia and hyperglycemia.

Large fluctuations in serum glucose levels or acid-base balance can precipitate electrolyte abnormalities in these patients. Potassium and calcium levels, in particular, should be monitored closely.

Biliary Tract

Surgery on the biliary tract includes exploration for removal of stones from the gallbladder and the ducts and removal of the gallbladder. It may also include repair of biliary tract injuries and resection for malignancy or benign strictures. Anesthesia is general, regional, or a combination of both. Currently, the standard is for laparoscopic cholecystectomy that may have been preceded by ERCP. Performed with a laparoscope, the patient has an umbilical incision and three or four abdominal stab wounds for instruments (Fig. 37-9). The open incision is either a right subcostal or a midline incision. On return to the PACU, the patient is placed in a semi-Fowler's position. All tubes must be cared for appropriately. A nasogastric tube will be placed intraoperatively and is often removed when the operative procedure ends. A T-tube will have been placed in the common bile duct if the common duct was opened during surgery. This tube is usually connected to straight-gravity drainage to a bile bag.

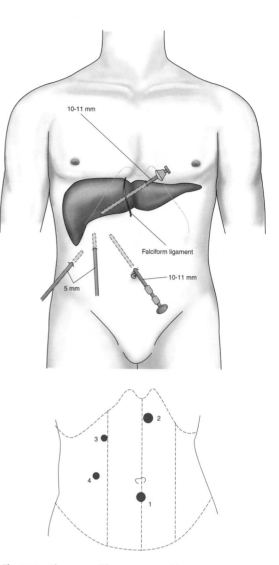

Fig. 37-9 Placement of laparoscope and instrument ports for laparoscopic cholecystectomy. *(Redrawn from Malt RA: The practice of surgery, Philadelphia, 1993, WB Saunders.)*

Careful attention must be paid to maintaining the patency of this tube and its attachment to the patient; the surgeon needs to be called immediately if the tube is dislodged.

Bile drainage should be carefully measured and accurately reported. Between 200 and 500 ml of bile drainage can be expected within a 24-hour period. Dressings should remain dry and intact, and dressings should be reinforced as necessary to keep the surrounding skin dry.

As with all upper abdominal incisions, pain is a problem, and analgesics (intermittent, continuous, or patient controlled), epidural analgesia, TENS, and relaxation exercises should be used to promote rest and respiratory effort. Any downward trend in vital signs, excessive bleeding from the incision, or bleeding noted in the bile drainage from the T-tube should be reported to the surgeon. Bleeding from the cystic artery is a serious complication and can lead to rapid deterioration in the patient's status.

After laparoscopic cholecystectomy, the patient may be one of the most stable of any seen in the PACU. Any patient with unexplained pain, oliguria, or hypotension should be immediately discussed with the surgeon. Complications of gas embolism, deep vein thrombophlebitis, subcutaneous emphysema, injuries to major vessels and intestine, and bile leakage all have been reported following laparoscopic procedures.

BIBLIOGRAPHY

Black JM, Hawks JH, Keene AM: Medical-surgical nursing: clinical management for positive outcomes, ed 6, Philadelphia, 2001, WB Saunders.

Etala E: Atlas of gastrointestinal surgery, Baltimore, 1997, Williams & Wilkins.

Given B, Simmons S: Gastroenterology in clinical nursing, ed 4, St Louis, 1984, Mosby.

O'Brien D: The gastrointestinal surgical patient. In Litwack K, editor: Core curriculum for perianesthesia nursing practice, ed 4, Philadelphia, 1999, WB Saunders.

O'Brien D, Walter V, Burden N: Special procedures in the ambulatory setting. In Burden N, Quinn D, O'Brien D et al, editors: Ambulatory surgical nursing, Philadelphia, 2000, WB Saunders.

Phippen ML, Wells MP: Patient care during operative and invasive procedures, Philadelphia, 2000, WB Saunders.

Schmieding NJ, Waldman RC: Gastric decompression in adult patients, Clinical Nursing Research 6(2):142-155, 1997.

Surratt S, Ryan AB, Hallenbeck P et al: Troubleshooting a sump tube, Am J Nurs 93(1):42-47, 1993.

Thompson JM, McFarland GK, Hirsch JE et al: Mosby's clinical nursing, ed 5, St Louis, 2002, Mosby.

Townsend CM, Beauchamp D, Evers BM et al, editors: Sabiston textbook of surgery: the biological basis of modern surgical practice, ed 16, Philadelphia, 2001, WB Saunders.

Genitourinary surgery involves procedures performed on the kidney, ureters, bladder, urethra, and male genitalia. Problems may be congenital or acquired. Adrenalectomy is included in this chapter for convenience and because of the proximity of the adrenal glands to the kidneys.

DEFINITIONS

Adrenalectomy: partial or total excision of one or both of the adrenal glands.

Bladder neck operation (Y-V plasty): a plastic repair of the bladder neck done to correct stricture.

Chordee: downward bowing of the penis due to congenital malformation or to hypospadias with fibrous bands.

Circumcision: excision of the foreskin (prepuce) of the glans penis.

Cystectomy: excision of the bladder and adjacent structures; may be partial, to excise a lesion, or total, to excise a malignant tumor. This operation usually involves the additional procedure of ureterostomy.

Cystolithotomy: opening of the bladder to remove stones.

Cystoscopy: direct visualization of the urethra, prostatic urethra, and bladder by means of a tubular lighted telescopic lens.

Cystotomy: an incision into the bladder.

Epididymectomy: excision of the epididymis from the testis. This procedure is rarely done but may occasionally be indicated to treat persistent infection.

Epispadias: urethral meatus situated in an abnormal position on the upper side of the penis. Surgical correction involves plastic repair.

Extracorporeal shock wave lithotripsy: use of shock waves through a liquid medium into the body to disintegrate stones.

Heminephrectomy: partial excision of the kidney.

Hydrocelectomy: excision of the tunica vaginalis of the testis to remove a hydrocele (a fluid-filled sac).

Hypospadias: a deformity of the penis and malformation of the urethral wall in which the urinary meatus is located on the underside of the penis, either short of its normal position at the tip of the glans or on the perineum or scrotum. This condition is often associated with chordee. Surgical correction involves plastic repair; penile straightening and urethral reconstruction (urethroplasty) are usually done in two or more stages.

Kidney transplant: removal of a donor kidney by means of a nephrectomy and ureterectomy, followed by transplantation of the donor kidney into the recipient's iliac fossa.

Nephrectomy: removal of a kidney; used to treat some congenital unilateral abnormalities that cause renal obstruction or hydronephrosis; sometimes necessitated by the presence of tumors and following severe injuries.

Nephrostomy: an opening into the kidney to maintain temporary or permanent drainage.

Nephrotomy: an incision into the kidney.

Nephroureterectomy: removal of a kidney and the entire ureter that drains it.

Orchiectomy: removal of the testis or testes. This procedure renders the patient sterile.

Orchiopexy: suspension of the testis within the scrotum. This procedure is used to treat an undescended or cryptorchid testis to bring it into the normal intrascrotal position.

Penile implant: a penile prosthesis implanted for treatment of organic sexual impotence.

Percutaneous nephrolithotomy: removal or disintegration of renal stones by passage of a nephroscope through a percutaneous nephrostomy tract.

Phimosis: tightness of the foreskin so that it cannot be drawn back from over the glans; also, the analogous condition in the clitoris.

Prostatectomy: enucleation of prostatic adenomas or hypertrophied masses.

Pyeloplasty: revision or reconstruction of the renal pelvis.

Pyelostomy: an incision into the renal pelvis to establish drainage or to permit irrigation of the renal pelvis.

Pyelotomy: incision into the renal pelvis.

Spermatocelectomy: the removal of a spermatocele, which usually appears as a cystic mass within the scrotum, attached to the upper pole of the epididymis. A spermatocele is usually caused by an obstruction of the tubular system that conveys the sperm.

Transurethral surgery: piecemeal resection of the prostate gland and of tumors of the bladder and bladder neck and fulguration of bleeding vessels and of tumors by means of a resectoscope passed into the bladder via the urethra.

Ureterectomy: complete removal of one or both of the ureters.

Ureterolithotomy: incision into the ureter and removal of stones.

Ureteroneocystostomy (ureterovesical anastomosis; vesicopsoas hitch procedure): division of the ureter from the urinary bladder and reimplantation of the ureter into the bladder at another site.

Ureteroplasty: reconstruction of the ureter.

Ureterostomy, cutaneous (anastomosis of transplant; Bricker operation; ureteroileostomy): diversion of the urinary stream by anastomosing the ureters into an isolated loop of ileum that is brought out through the abdominal wall as an ileostomy (Fig. 38-1).

Urethral dilatation and internal urethrotomy: gradual dilatation of the urethra and lysis of a urethral stricture.

Urethral meatotomy: incisional enlargement of the external urethral meatus to relieve stenosis or stricture.

Urethroplasty: reconstructive surgery of the urethra.

Varicocelectomy: ligation and partial excision of dilated veins in the scrotum.

Vasectomy: excision of a section of the vas deferens. This procedure is carried out electively for birth control or before prostatectomy to prevent the spread of infection from the urethra to the epididymis.

Vasoepididymostomy: anastomosis of the vas deferens to the epididymis.

Vasovasostomy: anastomosis of two separate segments of the vas deferens to reverse a vasectomy.

Vesicourethral suspension (Marshall-Marchetti operation): suspension of the bladder neck to the posterior surface of the pubis in women to treat stress incontinence.

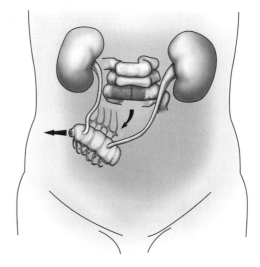

Fig. 38-1 Ileal conduit, showing ileal segment with anastomosed ureters. *(Redrawn from LeMaitre GD, Finnegan JA: The patient in surgery: a guide for nurses, ed 4, Philadelphia, 1980, WB Saunders.)*

NURSING CARE AFTER DIAGNOSTIC PROCEDURES

Several invasive diagnostic procedures are used for patients with genitourinary disease. If patients require general anesthesia, they are usually admitted to the postanesthesia care unit (PACU) for observation.

Renal Angiography

For a renal angiographic examination, a small catheter is threaded through the femoral artery into the aorta or renal artery; radiopaque dye is instilled; and radiographs are made. Local anesthesia is usually all that is needed; however, general anesthesia may be used for children or patients who cannot cooperate during the procedure. When the patient is admitted to the PACU, check the groin area for bleeding. A pressure type of dressing usually is present and may be replaced by a simple bandage after a few hours. Pedal pulses should be checked to ensure that no interruption of blood supply to the extremities has occurred. If possible, the leg should be kept straight. Fluids should be encouraged to facilitate excretion of the dye.

Renal Biopsy

Renal biopsy is usually performed at the bedside with only local anesthesia, although general anesthesia may be used for children. The patient should maintain bed rest in a flat, supine position for as long as 4 hours. A small pillow may be positioned under the head for comfort. Vital signs are monitored, and the site of biopsy is checked for bleeding. Coughing and other activities that increase abdominal venous pressure should be avoided. Fluids should be increased to 3000 ml daily, and the urine should be observed for occult blood.

Cystoscopy

Cystoscopy may be performed in a special-procedures room with only local anesthesia and appropriate sedation. Children and patients who cannot or will not cooperate during the procedure may need general anesthesia. This procedure may also be performed under spinal anesthesia. It may be performed simply for diagnostic purposes, or it may be used for treatment—such as resection of tumors, removal of stones and foreign bodies, and dilatation of the ureters.

On admission to the PACU, the patient is placed in a side-lying position if general anesthesia was used or flat on his or her back if spinal anesthesia was used. After the effects of anesthesia have been eliminated, the patient may assume a position of comfort. The patient may complain of back pain, a feeling of bladder fullness, and bladder spasms. These symptoms may become severe enough to require analgesia. Belladonna and opium suppositories or intravenous narcotics may be administered to relieve patient discomfort.

Fluid administration should be increased and started as soon as the effects of anesthesia are gone. Urine output should be monitored carefully. The patient can expect frequency of urination and a burning sensation because of trauma to the mucous membranes from the procedure, which may inadvertently cause voluntary retention. The urine may be pink-tinged for several voidings; this is to be expected. Bright blood or clots in the urine, however, should be reported to the surgeon. If the patient complains of severe abdominal pain, this should be reported because it may indicate accidental ureteral or bladder perforation or internal hemorrhage.

The patient should be observed for signs of sepsis. The spread of infection throughout the urinary tract or into the blood stream may occur following a cystoscopy. If symptoms of sepsis —such as chills, tachycardia, tachypnea, flushing, and temperature elevation—are noted, the surgeon should be notified.

GENERAL POSTOPERATIVE CARE

Assessment of the patient after genitourinary surgery involves particular attention to fluid and electrolyte balance. Intake and output records are especially important and must be accurately maintained. Postoperative care is directed primarily at maintenance of urinary tract function, which is second in importance only to cardiorespiratory function. Maintenance of patency of the urinary tract often depends on the use of catheters, which come in a variety of shapes and sizes (Fig. 38-2).

Urethral catheters are used to drain urine from the bladder to keep it decompressed and to measure urine output accurately. A retention catheter is used postoperatively and left in place until the patient is stable and the surgeon orders its removal. The catheter is attached to a sterile, closed gravitational-drainage collection system. The urine collection reservoir may be a large (usually 2000-ml) container or a small calibrated chamber that can be emptied into a large reservoir after timed urine output volumes have been determined and recorded (Fig. 38-3).

The catheter should be anchored securely to the patient's thigh with tape and the tubing brought over the leg. Loop the catheter over once before taping to prevent undue tension on the urinary meatus. Attach the connecting tubing to the bed linens so that no proximal loops of tubing lie below the distal tubing; this is a straight gravity drainage system. Check frequently for kinks; the tubing should never be under the patient because compression of the tubing obstructs the flow of urine. The urine receptacle should always be kept below the bladder level to prevent urine reflux up the tubing. Particular attention must be paid to this principle during the transfer of patients because attendants typically pick up the receptacle to transfer it to the new setting.

Mucus or blood, or both, can clog the tubing and prevent urine flow. Irrigations should be administered only according to the surgeon's orders. All irrigations are sterile procedures. A large sterile Toomey syringe and sterile irrigating

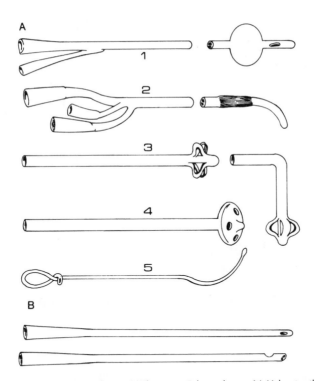

Fig. 38-2 A, Self-retaining catheters: *(1)* Foley catheter; *(2)* three-way Foley catheter; *(3)* Malecot catheter; and *(4)* Pezzer catheter. The self-retaining protuberance at the tip of the Malecot and Pezzer catheters must be elongated with a stylet *(5)*, which is passive through the lumen before insertion. After insertion, the stylet is removed, and the protuberance secures the catheter in place. **B,** Straight catheters. The straight catheter may have a single eye or many eyes; it may have a round tip or a whistle tip. These catheters are not self-retaining and must be secured with adhesive tape when being used as indwelling tubes. *(From Whitehead S: Nursing care of the adult urology patient, New York, 1970, Appleton-Century-Crofts.)*

solution (usually normal saline or normal saline with a selected antibiotic) are used. Care must be taken to keep all parts of the drainage system sterile. This may be accomplished by placing a small sterile plastic cover on the drainage tubing while the irrigation is performed. Irrigations should never be given under pressure, and when the bladder is irrigated, no more than 30 ml should be instilled at one time, unless ordered otherwise by the surgeon.

To obtain a urine specimen from the closed system, use a sterile syringe and needle. Some catheters have a small, specially constructed spot from which to draw specimens. On those that do not have such a spot, use the distal part of the catheter, close to the drainage tubing. Cleanse the area with alcohol or povidone-iodine

(Betadine), insert the needle, and withdraw a specimen.

Suprapubic Catheters

Suprapubic catheters are used to drain residual urine from the bladder. The catheter is introduced into the urinary bladder via a stab wound through the lower abdomen and into the anterior bladder wall. The catheter is sutured in place, and a dressing is applied. (Usually a type of dressing that allows direct observation of the puncture site is used.) The catheter is connected to a straight gravitational drainage system. Care of the suprapubic catheter is similar to that of the Foley catheter. The catheter should be securely taped with a loop made to prevent tension on the bladder wall or the abdomen. The skin around

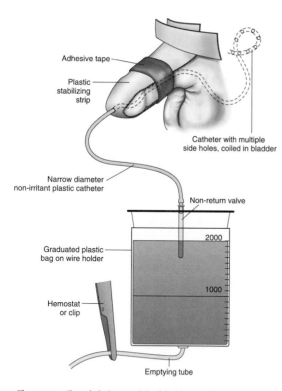

Adhesive tape

Plastic
stabilizing
strip

Catheter with multiple
side holes, coiled in bladder

Narrow diameter
non-irritant plastic catheter

Non-return valve

2000

Graduated plastic
bag on wire holder

1000

Hemostat
or clip

Emptying tube

Fig. 38-3 Closed drainage of the bladder. *(Redrawn from Douglas AP, Kerr DS: A short textbook of kidney disease, London, 1968, Pitman Medical.)*

the puncture site should be kept clean and dry. The catheter tubing should be checked periodically for kinks and to ensure that the stopcock valve is open to allow the urine to drain from the bladder.

Ureteral Catheters

Ureteral catheters are used to drain urine or to splint the ureters while they heal. They may be placed through the urethra or through abdominal or flank incisions. Care of these catheters is essentially the same as that for urethral catheters. Attention to patency must be especially scrupulous because the renal pelvis can hold only 5 ml without becoming overdistended and damaging the kidneys.

Sterile irrigations are undertaken only as ordered by the physician. Only 5 ml of fluid should be used for the irrigation via gravitational flow. Irrigations should never be given under

pressure, such as with a syringe and plunger. The nurse must be sure that situations that may cause dislodgment or displacement of these catheters are avoided because this could be disastrous to the outcome of the surgery. Special care must be taken during patient transfer to ensure that these catheters stay in place. One person should be assigned this responsibility during the transfer. If the catheters should become dislodged in spite of all the precautions taken, the surgeon must be notified immediately.

Intake

Optimal fluid intake is exceptionally important for this patient postoperatively; increased fluids are the general rule. If the patient can tolerate oral fluids, they should be given by this preferred route, and intake should be increased to total 3000 ml in a 24-hour period. Parenteral fluid therapy is indicated for a short time until the effects of anesthesia have passed, and it is continued only if the oral route of intake is inadequate.

Dressings

Care of dressings varies according to the procedure. Dressings applied after urinary tract surgery often become soaked with blood and urine. They should be reinforced as necessary, and the surrounding skin should be kept clean and dry to prevent unnecessary excoriation and breakdown. (If excessive staining is unexpected for a particular procedure and indicates a complication, it will be so indicated in the discussion of the specific procedure later in this chapter.) Excessive bleeding and hemorrhage are ever-present dangers of this surgery, because the kidneys and prostatic bed are extremely vascular. Vital signs must be monitored closely, and all avenues of output—especially the incisions and drainage tubes—should be evaluated frequently for bleeding.

Abdominal Distention

All patients should be assessed for abdominal distention after surgery that involves abdominal and flank incisions (see Chapter 37 for care of the patient after an abdominal incision because the same care applies after genitourinary surgery). These patients often arrive with nasogastric tubes, the care for which is discussed in Chapter 37. In addition, the patient should be assessed for distention caused by overfilling of the bladder because of an inability to void or a malfunction of the catheters.

Management of Discomfort and Pain

Discomfort after genitourinary surgery may be relieved with the administration of narcotics, including intravenous meperidine, belladonna, and opium suppositories. The physiology of the "need to void" should be explained to the patient preoperatively. The patient should be instructed not to attempt to void around the catheter because exerting pressure causes the bladder muscles to contract and results in painful bladder spasms. The avoidance of straining around the catheter and the intake of excessive fluids decrease bladder irritability and spasms. As the nerve endings become fatigued, the frequency and severity of the spasms diminish.

NURSING CARE AFTER SPECIFIC PROCEDURES

Renal and Ureteral Surgery

Procedures that involve the kidneys and ureters include excision of tumors and obstructions to urine flow (such as stones), reconstruction of urine outflow tracts, repair of lacerations, correction of deformities, excision of a kidney, and total organ transplant.

Anesthesia is almost always general for surgery on the kidneys and ureters. The kidneys are usually approached posteriorly through an incision that requires resection of the 11th or 12th rib. The surgical approach to the ureters is usually made through muscle-splitting flank incisions (Fig. 38-4). The perianesthesia course for these patients is usually smooth and involves general care for the perianesthesia patient and maintenance of urinary tract function. The patient should be placed in a position that avoids tension on suture lines or as indicated by the surgeon.

Exceptionally accurate intake and output records must be maintained. Low urine output should be reported to the surgeon.

Dressings should remain dry and intact unless drains are used, in which case dressings should be weighed when they are removed to determine output via this route. When determining output from the dressings, weigh the dressings before applying and again when removing, and subtract

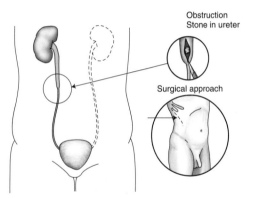

Fig. 38-4 Right hydroureter due to obstructing calculus. Inset shows incision in ureter for removal of stone. *(Redrawn from LeMaitre GD, Finnegan JA: The patient in surgery: a guide for nurses, ed 4, Philadelphia, 1980, WB Saunders.)*

the difference.* Patients with drains or stomas may require a small plastic bag over the area for collection of drainage that will consist primarily of urine. Drainage bags should be emptied frequently; if the bags are allowed to fill to capacity, the continual flow of urine will be interrupted.

Skin care for these patients is important. Urine should not be allowed to remain on the skin. Plain water should be used to cleanse the skin, and it should be carefully dried. No powders, lotions, or harsh skin preparations should be applied to the skin. If an ureteroileostomy has been performed, the stoma must be inspected frequently to ensure adequate vascularization. If it turns a bluish hue, the surgeon should be notified immediately.

A Foley catheter is generally in place and receives care as previously discussed. Fluid intake is increased both orally and parenterally to keep blood clots from forming in the ureters or bladder. Intestinal decompression may be necessary and is accomplished by nasogastric tube (see Chapter 37). This is essential when an ileal conduit procedure (ureterostomy) is performed to allow healing of the intestinal anastomosis. Any evidence of abdominal distention should be reported to the surgeon.

---

*One gram equals 1 ml of output.

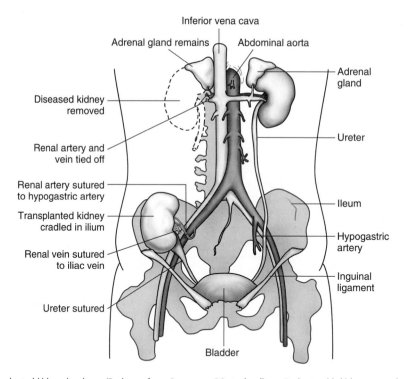

Fig. 38-5 Transplanted kidney in place. *(Redrawn from Bergersen BS et al, editors: Patients with kidney transplants, Curr Concepts Clin Nurs 1:1967.)*

Extracorporeal Shock Wave Lithotripsy. After extracorporeal shock wave lithotripsy the patient may be admitted to the PACU for a brief period of observation. Vital signs should be monitored as with any renal or ureteral surgery. Fluids should be increased and intake and output monitored carefully. Initially, the color of the urine may be cherry red to pink because of trauma from surgery; this may take several hours to clear. Petechiae, redness, and bruising may be seen on the skin at the site of lithotripsy. The patient may experience pain from the force of the shock waves. This pain is usually localized to the skin and may be relieved with ice packs. Renal colic pain may also be experienced as the fragments of pulverized stones pass through the lower urinary tract.

Kidney Transplantation. The kidney is the most commonly transplanted organ and the only one that can be preserved in a viable state for some time (Fig. 38-5). The kidney is relatively easy to remove and implant. Most people have two functioning kidneys and need only one to sustain life; therefore kidney transplantation is done only for patients who need the organ to replace a diseased or nonfunctioning solitary kidney. Transplantation can be accomplished two, three, or even more times in the same patient, with the use of hemodialysis when a functioning kidney is not in place.

Many kidney grafts come from cadaver donors. Some grafts, however, come from live donors, usually a blood relative of the recipient. The closer the recipient and donor in blood line, the better the chances for survival of the kidney graft. Postoperatively, the donor is usually the forgotten member. His or her care is essentially the same as that for the patient who has had a single kidney removed. All care considered previously for the urologic patient applies, as does care for the patient after abdominal incision. Because postoperative care is routine, this patient often feels a lack of self-esteem. Before surgery he or she was considered heroic and got a generous helping of attention and glory, whereas postoperatively, attention is directed primarily to the organ recipient. The donor patient feels this even in the PACU. For this reason, it is extremely important that the perianesthesia nurse be aware of the needs of the postoperative donor and demonstrate concern for his or her physical and psychologic well-being. The care of these patients should be assigned to separate teams, if possible. In addition to normal self-concern, the donor will be concerned about the recipient and should receive factual information.

General anesthesia is used for both the donor and the recipient in renal transplantation. If possible, these patients should be placed in a reverse or protective isolation room with all protective isolation measures instituted. Many PACUs do not have protective isolation capabilities; therefore these patients are returned directly from the operating suite to the surgical intensive care unit, where protective isolation can be instituted.

Protective isolation is necessary because these patients are placed on immunosuppressive therapy, which reduces the white blood cell count. The commonly used immunosuppressive agents—including azathioprine (Imuran), cyclophosphamide (Cytoxan), and cyclosporine (Sandimmune)—are nonspecific and suppress the entire immune system. Meticulous aseptic technique is therefore imperative when handling these patients to prevent the introduction of infection.

On admission to the PACU, the recipient should be kept in a flat position for 12 hours to allow the kidney to set. The head of the bed may be elevated 30 degrees to provide comfort and respiratory care. After 12 hours, the patient may turn to the side of the transplant. Turning to the opposite side may dislodge the graft.

All vital signs are monitored continuously. A Foley catheter will be in place, and all urine should be carefully monitored for volume and specific gravity. During the immediate postoperative period, the renal allograft is extremely sensitive to hypovolemia, and even a transient period of poor renal perfusion may result in oliguric renal failure. The kidney from a living donor may start to function almost immediately after transplantation, and diuresis will occur. The volume of urine output may be great enough to warrant measurement every 15 minutes. The cadaver kidney, on the other hand, reacts more

slowly, depending on the cold ischemic time spent during transportation.

Urine samples are generally collected hourly to ascertain electrolyte content, creatinine level, and osmolarity. Once daily, the total 24-hour urine collection (minus the small samples sent hourly) is sent to the laboratory for creatinine clearance test and culture. Urine output less than 1 ml per kg per hour should be reported to the surgeon because any decrease in urine output may be a sign of early rejection. Likewise, any gross hematuria should be reported immediately. A baseline postoperative weight should be ascertained as soon as feasible.

A nasogastric tube provides intestinal decompression and receives care as previously discussed.

A central venous pressure line is present to further assess the patient's cardiovascular status. Monitoring of these systems is imperative to ensure adequate renal perfusion.

Dressings over the incision site should evidence a minimal amount of drainage. The recipient may have a stenting catheter from the renal pelvis out through the urethra along with the Foley catheter for the first 36 to 48 hours to ensure ureteral patency.

Intravenous fluids provide most of the intake for these patients until the nasogastric tube can be removed. Intravenous replacement fluid composition is determined by the serum and urine electrolyte content, the hematocrit, and the clinical course of the patient. Volume is determined from necessary fluid requirements of the patient in normal status plus replacement on a volume-to-volume basis of drainage from the Foley catheter, nasogastric tube, ureterostomy, and cystostomy. For the first 72 hours after operation, the major source of output is from the ureterostomy. Meticulous handling of the closed urinary drainage system is mandatory to prevent the introduction of infection.

Vigorous pulmonary toilet should be instituted immediately to prevent atelectasis. The patient may be turned to the side of the kidney graft and back every 30 minutes to provide for change of position. The painful flank incision can be splinted either with the nurse's hands or with a firm pillow or a rolled blanket to assist the patient with coughing.

The threat of graft rejection is ever-present; therefore the healthcare professional must observe

Box 38-1	**Signs and Symptoms of Allograft Rejection**

Patient irritability
Anxiousness
Restlessness
Lethargy
Swollen, tender kidney
Decreased urine output
Fever; may be low grade
Increased blood pressure
Weight gain
Anorexia
Increased blood urea nitrogen and serum creatinine levels
Decreased creatinine clearance
Increased urine protein and lysozyme activity
Lymphocytes in the urine

closely for signs of rejection. Hyperacute allograft rejection can occur within minutes of the completion of the vascular anastomosis or in the first few postoperative hours. Signs and symptoms of hyperacute rejection are noted in Box 38-1. To prevent irreversible damage to the kidney, it is of the utmost importance to treat a threatened rejection as soon as it appears.

The patient may experience a strong fear of rejection while he or she is still in the PACU. Many patients view this surgery as the last chance to live a normal life after facing numerous physical, psychological, and socioeconomic stressors. The perianesthesia nurse may need to reassure the patient often that the kidney is functioning.

The postoperative kidney transplant patient is usually transferred to the surgical intensive care unit for several days after surgery for close observation and intensive care.

Bladder Surgery

The bladder is a smooth muscle storage tank that holds urine until a reflex—normally under voluntary control—releases the urine to pass through the urethra to be eliminated. Surgical procedures on the bladder include the removal of stones, foreign bodies, and tumors; the repair of strictures at the bladder neck and of injuries, such as lacerations; and the removal of the bladder itself.

Anesthesia for these procedures may be either spinal or general. On admission to the PACU, the patient is placed in a supine position. The head of the bed may be raised 30 degrees as soon as feasible. The removal of stones or foreign bodies and the resection of selected tumors may be accomplished via cystoscopy, which was discussed earlier. After the repair of lacerations or after cystotomy to remove stones, the patient will be admitted to the PACU with a Foley catheter in place, and a urinary diversion such as a suprapubic cystostomy will usually be in place. Urine from these drainage systems is pink-tinged but should not become grossly bloody. Dressings should remain dry and intact; fluids should be increased; and oral fluids should be started as soon as the effects of anesthesia have passed.

Lacerations or ruptures of the bladder are often the result of accidental trauma. They require emergency surgery, and the postoperative patient should be assessed carefully for any unrecognized associated injuries. Pain should be minimal for these patients and easily controlled with mild analgesics. If severe pain is present, it may represent a complication—such as internal hemorrhage and damage to a ureter—and should be reported to the surgeon.

Cystectomy requires the construction of an ileal conduit. Care for an ileal conduit was discussed in the section on ureteral surgery.

Prostatic Surgery

The prostate gland is a small, walnut-sized male reproductive organ. Its sole function is to manufacture a secretion that becomes part of the semen; it is a nonessential organ. Surgical procedures performed on the prostate gland include the excision of tumors and the resection or total removal of the gland.

The preferred anesthesia is spinal, although general anesthesia may be used. Several different approaches are common in surgery on the prostate. Most commonly, the transurethral approach is used, especially if only minor obstructive lesions or small portions of the gland are to be removed. A resectoscope is introduced through the urethra, and the surgeon excises the tissue with a moveable tungsten wire that operates on high-frequency current controlled with a foot pedal.

When the patient is admitted to the PACU after transurethral resection of the prostate (TURP), a three-way Foley catheter will be in place (see Fig. 38-2A). One lumen allows filling of the retention balloon; one lumen allows outflow of the urine and irrigation fluid from the bladder; and one lumen is attached to the irrigation fluid system. Irrigation fluid, which is usually normal saline at room temperature, is available in 3000-ml plastic bags, and it may be regulated like intravenous solutions. To avoid creating a hypothermic state by irrigating the bladder with this solution, the saline should be warmed before administration, and the patient's temperature should be monitored. The triple-lumen catheter is advantageous in that blood clots do not regularly form and block the system when the flow is continuous. The irrigation rate should be regulated so that drainage remains a light pink, watermelon color. If drainage becomes bright red, speed up the irrigation; if the returning fluid is clear, slow the irrigation down. Some institutions use a Y-connecting system with one arm of the Y connected to the irrigating fluid and the other to straight-gravitational drainage from the bladder. In either instance, because the prostatic bed is highly vascular, a fair amount of bleeding can be expected after TURP. This bleeding may also increase as the spinal anesthesia wears off and may require frequent irrigation to prevent clogging of the drainage tube.

If the catheter becomes clogged, it may be necessary to irrigate it with a piston syringe and the same normal saline irrigating solution. If patency of the catheter cannot be reestablished, the surgeon must be notified.

The patient's vital signs should be monitored closely. Observe for signs and symptoms of post-TURP syndrome (water intoxication) that may occur from venous absorption of the irrigation fluid through the venous sinuses. Serum sodium and potassium levels should be checked during the postoperative period because changes in fluid balance may affect these electrolytes. Signs and symptoms of water intoxication include a low serum sodium level, tachypnea, shortness of breath, nausea, vomiting, hypertension, bradycardia, increased pulse pressure, restlessness, apprehension, and mental disorientation. If this syndrome occurs, the perianesthesia nurse should administer oxygen to the patient, monitor blood loss

and electrocardiographic and fluid and electrolyte status, and administer intravenous fluid (hypertonic saline 3% or 5% in 100 ml per hour increments until the serum sodium level is satisfactory) and diuretics to mobilize the edema.

Oral fluids should be started and increased as tolerated as soon as possible. Diet may be progressed as tolerated.

Pain should be minimal and easily controlled with mild analgesics. Analgesics or tranquilizers may be administered to control the discomfort of bladder spasms and of the presence of the catheter, which makes the patient feel an urgency to void although the bladder is being emptied. Complaints of abdominal pain, abdominal rigidity, an increase in pulse rate, and other signs of shock should alert the nurse to the possibility that the bladder wall or the capsule of the prostate was accidentally perforated during surgery; these symptoms should be reported to the surgeon immediately.

Other approaches to prostatic surgery include the retrograde or suprapubic, perineal, and retropubic incisions. When the suprapubic approach is used, a midline vertical incision is made in the lowest part of the abdomen; the bladder is incised; and the tumors are removed. This is the procedure of choice when 60 g or more of tissue is to be removed. The patient is admitted to the PACU with a Foley catheter, which may or may not be attached to an irrigation system, in place. If it is not connected to an irrigation system, the catheter will have to be irrigated frequently by syringe to prevent clots from clogging the drainage system. The patient will also have a suprapubic catheter that should be connected to straight-gravitational drainage in place, and output should be measured carefully (Fig. 38-6). In addition, a small Penrose drain will have been inserted in the suprapubic space and brought out through a separate stab wound. A dressing of several layers of 4 × 4 sponges should cover the incision and the drain. A moderate amount of serosanguineous drainage can be expected owing to the presence of the drain. This dressing should be reinforced as necessary to keep the skin clean and dry. If excessive bright-red bleeding occurs, the surgeon must be notified.

The surgeon may apply traction to the Foley catheter by taping the catheter to the inner thigh. Because the traction puts tension against

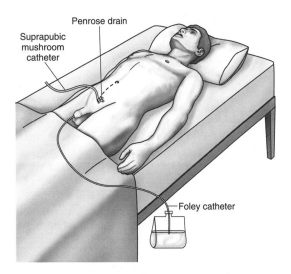

Suprapubic mushroom catheter

Penrose drain

Foley catheter

Fig. 38-6 Postoperative positions of drainage tubes after suprapubic prostatectomy. *(Redrawn from LeMaitre GD, Finnegan JA: The patient in surgery: a guide for nurses, ed 4, Philadelphia, 1980, WB Saunders.)*

the vesical outlet and promotes hemostasis, it may produce painful bladder spasms that may be relieved by the use of intravenous narcotics such as meperidine or belladonna and opium suppositories. After the traction is removed, a small increase in bleeding may be expected for a short time.

The perineal approach—used for removal of large amounts of tissue—is the approach of choice for prostatic cancer. A **V**-shaped incision is made above the rectum in this approach. The patient will be admitted to the PACU with a Foley catheter and a perineal drain in place. Because of the perineal drain, a moderate amount of serosanguineous drainage can be expected, and the dressing should be reinforced as necessary. No instrumentation—including thermometers—should be placed in the rectum during the immediate postoperative period.

When a retropubic approach is used, a small incision is made above the pubis, and a capsular incision is made into the upper surface of the prostate. A Foley catheter will be in place, and a small drain will have been inserted in the incision or brought out through a stab wound lateral to the incision.

As with all urologic patients, accurate intake and output records must be maintained after prostatic surgery. The perianesthesia nurse must be sure to indicate in the output data whether irrigation solution is included.

Most prostatic surgery is performed on adult men older than 50 years of age because prostatic hypertrophy most commonly occurs after 40 years of age. Therefore assessment of cardiorespiratory status should be performed frequently. Oxygen should be administered and weaned with pulse oximetry. All patients should be placed on a cardiac monitor to assess changes. Astute observation of vital signs is imperative to monitor cardiovascular function because postoperative bleeding may impair it. Observe carefully for decreasing blood pressure and increasing pulse rate, which may indicate impending shock.

One of the most common postoperative complications after the nerve-sparing radical prostatectomy is pulmonary embolism. For this reason, the surgeon may order low-dose heparin. Care in the PACU should include deep-breathing exercises and position changes along with passive or active movement of the extremities. Some type of antiembolism stocking should be used.

Scrotal Surgery

The scrotum is a sac separated into two pouches—externally by the median raphe and internally by the dartos tunic. Each pouch contains a testis, an epididymis, and a spermatic cord. The vas deferens—which is continuous with the epididymis at the lower end of the testis—as well as the arteries, veins, nerves, and lymphatic vessels that are held together by spermatic fascia form the spermatic cord. Operations on the scrotum include excision of masses and tumors, correction of deformities, and excision of diseased or abnormal structures that interfere with normal function.

Anesthesia for scrotal surgery may be local, general, or spinal. Spinal anesthesia is commonly used for adult patients, whereas general anesthesia is usually preferred for children younger than 12 years of age. Local anesthesia is often used for simple procedures such as vasectomy and epididymectomy.

The PACU course after surgery on the scrotal structures is usually uneventful. Care is dictated primarily by the agent of anesthesia and its method of administration.

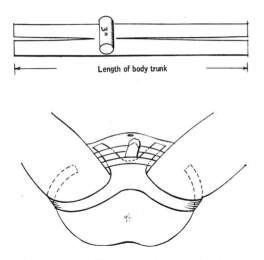

Fig. 38-7 Bellevue bridge for scrotal support. *(From Sutton AL: Bedside nursing techniques in medicine and surgery, ed 2, Philadelphia, 1969, WB Saunders.)*

The patient postoperatively may assume a position of comfort. Any dressings present should remain dry and intact. Oral food and fluids may be reinstituted as soon as the patient tolerates them. A Bellevue bridge commonly is applied to provide scrotal support and elevation (Fig. 38-7). This device is suspended from thigh to thigh with a tight sling across the expanse, upon which the scrotum is supported. A **T**-binder may also be used (Fig. 38-8).

The application of a light crushed-ice bag helps relieve scrotal edema, enhances hemostasis, and promotes comfort. Scrotal enlargement with apparent tension should be reported to the surgeon immediately. Progressive inguinal swelling may denote lymphatic obstruction after a varicocelectomy, and the surgeon must be notified. Pain should be minimal after these procedures and easily controlled by mild analgesics. Complaints of severe pain that is not controlled with mild analgesia should be reported to the surgeon.

As with any genital surgery, the patient's body image concerns and questions of fertility in particular may be of paramount importance. These concerns are not usually addressed in the PACU, but the nurse must be sensitive to them and prepared to assist the patient with factual information and reassurance, should they arise. Often, these patients feel an urgency to inspect the oper-

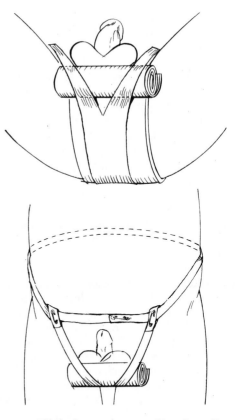

Fig. 38-8 T-binder for scrotal support. *(From Sutton AL: Bedside nursing techniques in medicine and surgery, ed 2, Philadelphia, 1969, WB Saunders.)*

ative site and should be assisted, if necessary, to do so.

The patient may be embarrassed by this type of surgery and reluctant to ask the nurse for assistance or to complain of pain, and he may hesitate to allow the nurse to inspect the incision area. A matter-of-fact attitude on the part of the nurse and efficient care promote a sense of well-being for the patient and may help alleviate these feelings. The nurse should keep in mind that preadolescent and adolescent boys are especially sensitive about the genital area. If at all possible, a male nurse should be assigned to these patients to alleviate their anxiety.

Penile and Urethral Surgery

Surgery on the penis and urethra involves removal of tumors or obstructions to urinary flow, plastic repair of deformities, and circumcision or excision of the foreskin. Partial or total amputation of the penis is rarely necessary for malignancy, which is essentially skin cancer. Laser technique is generally effective for the treatment of condyloma acuminata and squamous cell carcinoma of the penis.

Anesthesia for these procedures may be local, general, or spinal. The PACU course is usually smooth, and care is determined primarily by the anesthesia. Physical care of the patient who has had a plastic repair of hypospadias or epispadias is dictated by the surgeon. Care for the patient following cystoscopy was discussed at the beginning of this chapter; the same care applies for patients undergoing cystoscopy for the resection of tumors.

After circumcision—which may be performed for correction of phimosis or for elective reasons—the nurse should check for bleeding. Usually, only a small band of petrolatum-impregnated gauze is applied as a dressing around the glans and is changed as directed. Bleeding that soaks this dressing is excessive and should be reported.

Patients who have undergone surgery on the penis should avoid erection during the PACU phase and at least a week postoperatively. Patients with penile prostheses should be admitted to the PACU with the penis in a flaccid state, and the prosthesis should remain deflated. Inflation of the prosthesis should be avoided until after the first postoperative visit to the surgeon.

Pain may be significant but should not be severe. Scrotal and penile support with a Bellevue bridge and the application of a light ice pack provide some relief; however, analgesia with small doses of narcotics may be necessary. Food and fluids may be restarted as soon as the patient tolerates them. Urine output should be checked and recorded. Palpate for low abdominal distention, which may be caused by voluntary retention. This is not uncommon because of fear that micturition will create pain.

Adrenalectomy

Adrenalectomy involves the removal of one or both of the adrenal glands, which are situated on top of the kidneys. Adrenalectomy, an extensive and shock-producing procedure, may be performed for several reasons, including metastasized cancer from the reproductive organs, hyperfunc-

tion caused by hyperplasia of the organ, and adrenal tumors. Two adrenal tumors are of major consequence: pheochromocytoma, a usually benign tumor that causes hyperfunction resulting in severe symptoms, and neuroblastoma, a malignant tumor that is a leading cause of death in childhood.

General anesthesia is used for adrenalectomy and may include the use of cortisone titrated to maintain catecholamine levels and blood pressure. Cortisone is usually necessary only when bilateral adrenalectomy is performed or when the uninvolved adrenal gland has poor function. The administration of cortisone, which is continued in the PACU, is an extremely important nursing procedure. The anesthesiologist and surgeon should give specific instructions for titration of the solution. Failure to maintain postoperative levels of cortisone leads to hypovolemic and hyponatremic shock. Perianesthesia care of these patients is a nursing challenge; observations must be especially astute.

The surgical approach for adrenalectomy may be lateral, anterior, or posterior. On admission to the PACU, the patient is placed in the side-lying position until reactive from anesthesia, at which time he or she is placed in a semi-Fowler's position. The surgeon may prefer the patient be positioned on the operative side so that the perinephric space is obliterated to discourage bleeding. Assessment is aimed primarily at the cardiovascular status of the patient because hemorrhage and shock are the two most common and most disastrous complications. Profound shock may develop because of the reduction of circulating catecholamines that is precipitated by removal of the glands as well as to the effects of the drugs used for preoperative control of hypertension. The effects of these drugs usually last for a few hours after surgery. Because most of these drugs produce vasodilatation, they are usually a factor in postoperative hypotension. Therefore a fluid challenge usually is given in an attempt to treat hypotension. If fluid is not successful in increasing the blood pressure, then vasopressor drugs will be used. Epinephrine or norepinephrine in an intravenous solution may be titrated to maintain blood pressure, according to the surgeon's instructions.

Shock may also result from hemorrhage. The adrenal glands are extremely vascular. Intravenous fluids—including hypertonic saline solutions, blood, plasma, dextran, and glucose in water—may be used to maintain blood volume and prevent shock. Dressings over the bilateral incisions should remain relatively dry even though drains are placed. If these dressings become soaked, the surgeon should be notified, because this represents excessive bleeding. If the patient complains of abdominal pain, abdominal distention, nausea, or vomiting, development of an abdominal hematoma may be indicated; these signs should be reported to the surgeon.

Other parameters of the patient's status that may give clues to the development of shock should also be assessed. Dehydration (increased urine specific gravity) and restlessness may indicate developing shock. Central venous pressure should be checked. A Foley catheter will be in place, and urine output should be monitored hourly. The development of oliguria or output of less than 1 ml/kg/hr may indicate shock and subsequent renal shutdown. Serum and urine electrolyte levels—especially sodium—should be determined hourly.

All care outlined for the patient after high abdominal incisions in Chapter 37 is applicable to this patient. Good pulmonary toilet should be instituted immediately in the PACU. A nasogastric tube often is required until normal intestinal peristalsis returns. Incisional pain may require the use of narcotic analgesics. Because many narcotics have a hypotensive effect, they should be titrated judiciously, and blood pressure must be monitored continuously for at least 30 minutes after their administration.

The patient often is placed in protective isolation to avoid the introduction of infection. Meticulous sterile technique must be used when changing or reinforcing dressings. Because of their extreme lability, which lasts for approximately 48 hours, these patients should be transferred to the surgical intensive care unit for continuous monitoring.

BIBLIOGRAPHY

Alspach J: Core curriculum for critical care nursing, ed 5, Philadelphia, 1998, WB Saunders.

Atlee J: Complications in anesthesia, Philadelphia, 1999, WB Saunders.

Barash P, Cullen B, Stoelting R: Clinical anesthesia, ed 4, Philadelphia, 2000, Lippincott Williams & Wilkins.

Belker AM, Bennett AH: Applications of microsurgery in urology, Surg Clin North Am 65(5):1157-1178, 1988.

Benumof J: Anesthesia and uncommon diseases, ed 4, Philadelphia, 1998, WB Saunders.

Benumof J, Saidman L: Anesthesia & perioperative complications, ed 2, St Louis, 1999, Mosby.

Bickley L, Hoekelman R: Bates' guide to physical examination and history taking, ed 7, Philadelphia, 1998, Lippincott Williams & Wilkins.

Chambers JK: Fluid and electrolyte problems in renal and urologic disorders, Nurs Clin North Am, 22:815-825, 1987.

Cottrell J, Smith D: Anesthesia and neurosurgery, ed 4, St Louis, 2001, Mosby.

DeFazio-Quinn D: Ambulatory surgical nursing core curriculum, Philadelphia, 1999, WB Saunders, 1999.

Ganong W: Review of medical physiology, ed 20, New York, 2001, McGraw-Hill Professional.

Gharbieh PA: Renal transplant: surgical and psychologic hazards, Crit Care Nurse 8(6):58-71, 1988.

Glenn JF, editor: Urologic surgery, ed 4, Philadelphia, 1991, JB Lippincott.

Gruendemann BJ, Meeker MH: Alexander's care of the patient in surgery, ed 8, St Louis, 1987, Mosby.

Guyton A, Hall J: Textbook of medical physiology, ed 10, Philadelphia, 2000, WB Saunders.

Hardman J, Limbird L: Goodman and Gilman's the pharmacological basis of therapeutics, ed 10, New York, 2001, McGraw-Hill Professional.

Katzung B, editor: Basic and clinical pharmacology, ed 8, Los Altos, Calif, 2000, Appleton & Lange.

Keating MA, Cartwright PC, Duckett JW: Bladder mucosa in urethral reconstructions, J Urol 144(4):827-834, 1990.

Kelly MJ, Zimmern PE, Leach GE: Complications of bladder neck suspension procedures, Urol Clin North Am 18(2):339-347, 1991.

Lake C, Hines R, Blitt C: Clinical monitoring: practical applications for anesthesia and critical care, St Louis, 2001, Mosby.

Long BC, Phipps WJ, editors: Medical-surgical nursing: a nursing process approach, ed 2, St Louis, 1989, Mosby.

Longnecker D, Murphy F: Dripps/Eckenhoff/Vandam introduction to anesthesia, ed 9, Philadelphia, 1997, WB Saunders.

Longnecker D, Tinker J, Morgan G: Principles and practice of anesthesiology, ed 2, St Louis, 1998, Mosby.

Martin J: Positioning in anesthesia and surgery, ed 3, St Louis, 1997, Mosby.

Nagelhout J, Zaglaniczny K: Nurse anesthesia, ed 2, Philadelphia, 2001, WB Saunders.

Miller R, editor: Anesthesia, ed 5, New York, 2000, Churchill Livingstone.

Omoigui S: The anesthesia drugs handbook, ed 2, St Louis, 1995, Mosby.

Rauscher J, Parra RO: Vesico-psoas hitch procedure, AORN J 52(6):1177-1186, 1990.

Schaeffer AJ: Use of the CO_2 laser in urology, Urol Clin North Am 13(3):393-403, 1986.

Schick L: The patient with post-transurethral resection of the prostrate syndrome, J Post Anesth Nurs 6(2):136-142, 1991.

Stoelting R: Pharmacology and physiology in anesthetic practice, ed 3, Philadelphia, 1999, Lippincott-Raven.

Stoelting R, Miller R: Basics of anesthesia, ed 4, New York, 2000, Churchill Livingstone.

Stone D: Perioperative care: anesthesia, medicine, and surgery, St Louis, 1998, Mosby.

Townsend C, Beauchamp R, Evers B et al: Sabiston textbook of surgery: the biological basis of modern surgical practice, ed 16, Philadelphia, 2001, WB Saunders.

Walsh PC: Radical prostatectomy, preservation of sexual function, cancer control, Urol Clin North Am 14(4):663-673, 1987.

Waugaman W, Foster S, Rigor B: Principles and practice of nurse anesthesia, ed 3, Norwalk, Conn, 1999, Appleton & Lange.

39

CARE OF THE OBSTETRIC AND GYNECOLOGIC SURGICAL PATIENT

Wendy K. Winer, RN, BSN, CNOR

Surgery on organs of reproduction usually involves an adult patient. The perianesthesia nurse, however, may encounter pediatric or adolescent female patients who undergo gynecologic surgery for repair or correction of congenital, traumatic deformities or incapacitating pelvic pain (from causes such as endometriosis, ovarian cyst, or appendicitis). Surgery on the female genitalia may be conveniently divided into three major categories: (1) obstetric; (2) lower genital and vaginal; and (3) abdominal gynecologic. Abdominal surgery is then subdivided into either traditional surgery in the form of a laparotomy or into the category of operative laparoscopy. The area of operative laparoscopy in gynecologic surgery is expanding to such an enormous extent that most benign gynecologic surgery is moving in that direction. Most benign surgeries—except obstetrical surgeries—can be done in this way with many benefits for the patient. For this reason, the perianesthesia nurse must be aware of how the care of the patient differs with these procedures.

DEFINITIONS

Obstetrical surgery

Cerclage procedure: procedure for the treatment of incompetent cervix. The McDonald procedure involves the placement of a pursestring suture on the cervix at the level of the internal os; the Shirodkar procedure involves placement of a fascia lata (from the thigh) or a surgical band at the level of the internal os.

Cesarean hysterectomy: incision of the abdomen and the uterus, extraction of the infant and the placenta, and performance of a hysterectomy.

Cesarean section (C-section): delivery of an infant through an incision made in the abdominal and uterine walls.

C-section, classic: a midline incision between the umbilicus and the symphysis pubis and an anterior incision through the uterine wall.

C-section, low segment: an incision in the lower part of the uterus made after an abdominal incision.

Ectopic pregnancy: implantation of the fertilized ovum in any site other than the upper half of the uterus (Fig. 39-1).

Uterine aspiration (suction curettage): dilatation of the cervix and the vacuum removal of the uterine contents.

Lower genital surgery, vaginal surgery, abdominal surgery (laparotomy and laparoscopy)

Bartholin duct cyst: a cyst that results from chronic inflammation of one of the major vestibular glands at the vaginal introitus (Fig. 39-2).

Bartholinectomy: removal of a Bartholin duct cyst.

Cervical conization: removal of abnormal cervical tissue by scalpel, electrosurgical current, or laser.

Colporrhaphy: repair of the vaginal wall. May be anterior, as for cystocele repair, or posterior, as for rectocele repair or enterocele repair specifically for vaginal prolapse.

Culdoscopy: an operative diagnostic procedure in which an incision is made into the posterior vaginal cul-de-sac, through which a tubular instrument similar to a cystoscope is inserted for the purpose of visualizing the pelvic structures, including the uterus, fallopian tubes, broad ligaments, uterosacral ligaments, rectal wall, sigmoid colon, and, sometimes, the small intestine. A newer technique for this procedure is transvaginal hydrolaparoscopy, which uses normal saline and a camera attached to a small-diameter rigid endoscope.

Cystocele: prolapse of the bladder into the anterior vaginal wall.

Dilatation of the cervix and curettage of the uterus (D&C): introduction of instruments (dilators) through the vagina into the cervical canal and scraping of the

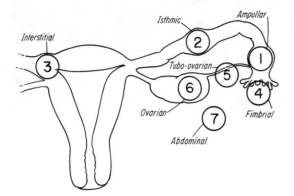

Fig. 39-1 Ectopic pregnancy. Diagram shows the various implantation sites, numbered in order of decreasing frequency of occurrence. *(From Townsend CM: Sabiston textbook of surgery: the biological basis of modern surgical practice, ed 16, Philadelphia, 2001, WB Saunders.)*

uterus with a curette to remove substances, including blood. This procedure is used for diagnostic purposes as well as for treating conditions such as incomplete abortion, abnormal uterine bleeding, and primary dysmenorrhea.

Enterocele: defect in the continuity of the endopelvic fascia most commonly seen after posthysterectomy when the anterior pubic fascia is not attached to the denoviellers fascia.

Hysterectomy: removal of the uterus; can be vaginal or abdominal (via laparotomy or laparoscopy).

Hysteroscopy: direct visualization of the canal of the uterine cervix and cavity of the uterus with an endoscope called a hysteroscope.

Procidentia: herniation of the uterus beyond the introitus.

Prolapse of the uterus: downward displacement of the uterus. Vaginal hysterectomy is often recommended for a prolapsed uterus when childbearing is no longer desired or when marked prolapse is present.

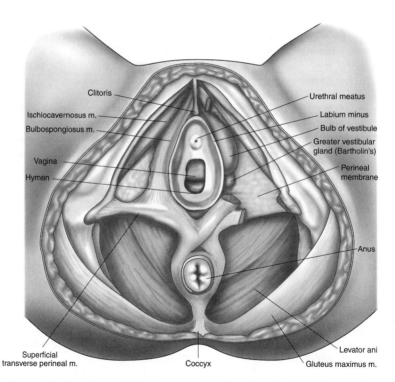

Fig. 39-2 Female perineum with skin and superficial fascia removed. *(Redrawn from Jacob SW, Francone CA, Lossow WJ: Structure and function in man, ed 5, Philadelphia, 1982, WB Saunders.)*

Rectocele: prolapse of the rectum into the posterior vaginal wall.

Trachelorrhaphy: removal of torn surfaces of the anterior and posterior cervical lips and reconstruction of the cervical canal.

Urethrocele: prolapse of the urethra into the anterior vaginal wall.

Vaginal plastic operation (anterior and posterior repair): reconstruction of the vaginal walls (colporrhaphy); the pelvic floor; and the muscles and fascia of the rectum, urethra, bladder, and perineum. Used to correct a cystocele or rectocele, restore the bladder to its normal position, and strengthen the vagina and the pelvic floor.

Abdominal gynecologic surgery (laparotomy and laparoscopy)

Abdominal myomectomy: removal of leiomyomas. Laparoscopy endoscopic visualization of the peritoneal cavity through a small incision in the anterior abdominal wall after the establishment of a pneumoperitoneum. A video camera is attached to the eye piece of the laparoscope so that the surgeon and team can visualize the procedure from a video monitor and have an enhanced, magnified view of the pelvis.

Oophorectomy: removal of an ovary.

Oophorocystectomy: removal of a cyst on the ovary.

Radical hysterectomy: removal of the uterus, the uterosacral and uterovesical ligaments, the upper third of the vagina, and all the peritoneum.

Salpingectomy: excision of the fallopian tube.

Salpingo-ophorectomy: removal of the fallopian tube and the associated ovary.

Salpingostomy (tubal plasty): removal of the obstructed portion of the fallopian tube and opening of the tube to establish patency. Tubal plasty or tubal reanastomosis can remove an obstructed portion of the tube and reconnect each normal end of the tube after the obstruction has been removed to establish patency. Note: tubal reanastomosis increases risk of ectopic pregnancy.

Total abdominal hysterectomy: removal of the uterus, including the corpus and the cervix—with or without the adnexa—through an abdominal incision.

Tubal ligation: interruption of fallopian tube continuity, which results in sterilization. The most common technique is the Pomeroy procedure, which is done through a laparoscope. A segment of the fallopian tube is ligated and excised. Reversal procedures are now being performed with microsurgery.

OBSTETRIC SURGERY

Obstetric surgery involves procedures on pregnant women to promote full-term pregnancy, to provide an alternative means of delivery when normal vaginal delivery is not feasible for reasons of fetal or maternal well-being, and to interrupt pregnancy.

Care after Specific Procedures.

Cesarean Section. Cesarean sections are performed both on emergency and elective bases. These patients have special physical and psychological needs. A selection of articles is included in the bibliography at the end of this chapter to assist the reader who provides care for families who experience cesarean birth.

Cesarean sections are indicated for dystocia (usually caused by cephalopelvic disproportion); antepartum bleeding; some toxemic conditions; certain medical complications, especially diabetes mellitus; and previous cesarean section. The low-segment cesarean section is usually the procedure of choice. Anesthesia may be general inhalation, spinal, or local infiltration of the operative field.

Postoperative care after cesarean section includes all care rendered to a patient who undergoes abdominal surgery as well as postpartum care.

On admission to the PACU, the patient should be placed in the side-lying position until she is reactive to prevent aspiration of stomach contents. As soon as her condition permits, she can assume any position of comfort. Oxygen should be delivered and monitored with the use of pulse oximetry.

Parenteral fluids are usually administered during the first 24 hours postoperatively, but oral fluids can usually be resumed as soon as bowel sounds are audible and the patient desires. Intravenous fluids often contain oxytocin to increase uterine muscle tone and stop excessive blood flow. Usually 10 to 20 units of oxytocin are added to 1000 ml of Ringer's lactate and are infused at 125 ml/hr. The main side effect of oxytocin is antidiuretic, and intake and output should be monitored accurately. A progressive diet is advised, pending the return of bowel sounds.

The patient will have an abdominal dressing as well as a perineal pad; both should be inspected for drainage. The abdominal dressing should remain dry and intact. A moderate amount of lochia rubra is normal, but saturation of two or more perineal pads with blood during the first hour is considered excessive. The area underneath the buttocks should be checked for pooling of blood.

The fundus should be checked frequently to ensure that it is firmly contracted. Checking the fundus is an uncomfortable procedure for the patient; therefore careful explanation should be provided before it is performed. The patient should be encouraged to relax her abdominal muscles as much as possible. Slow, deep breathing with an open mouth facilitates relaxation of those muscles. If the uterus is firmly contracted, it need not be massaged—and in fact should not be massaged—because this may cause uterine muscle fatigue and subsequent relaxation and bleeding. If the uterus is soft and "boggy," it should be gently but firmly massaged through the abdominal wall to stimulate contraction. The patient may be instructed to do this herself under supervision, which may allay anxiety and be more comfortable for her. Oxytocin often is administered intravenously and titrated to maintain the uterus in a state of contraction. If oxytocin is employed, the uterus should be checked for firmness but usually does not require frequent massage.

A full bladder is one cause of uterine atony. An indwelling urethral catheter commonly is left in place for the first 12 postoperative hours. A fundus palpated above the umbilicus or to the side of the abdomen (usually the right side) may indicate a nonfunctioning catheter. The catheter should be positioned for gravitational drainage and avoidance of kinks. The urine should be monitored for volume and color.

Many patients experience transient trembling or shivering after delivery. Several theories have been proposed with regard to this sense of chilling, although the actual cause remains unknown. This trembling is generally not associated with an elevation of temperature. Warmed blankets or warm-air therapy should be available as a comfort measure to the mother.

Many hospitals have separate PACUs for postpartum patients; thus the special considerations for the cesarean section patient pose no significant problems. The nurse who cares for the cesarean section patient within the general PACU must be judicious and often innovative to meet the needs of not only the mother but also the new family. The mother, the neonate, and the father should be together as soon as possible to allow for the bonding experience. This may be accomplished by using a quiet corner of the unit (if such a place exists), by drawing curtains around the family, or by expediting the discharge process to transfer the patient to the postpartum unit. The mother and father will be anxious to review the details of the birth together, and the perianesthesia nurse should be prepared to answer their questions. Consistent communication between the surgical nurse and the perianesthesia nursing staff makes answering these questions much easier.

Ectopic Pregnancy. Faulty implantation of the ovum may take place in the fallopian tube (in approximately 98% of all ectopic pregnancies), in the ovary, in any part of the abdominal cavity, or in the uterine cervix. The treatment of choice for this is laparoscopy (or laparotomy), with removal of the ectopic pregnancy. The ovary preferably is not resected or removed, but this may be necessary if the ovary is involved. If implantation occurs in the cervix, a hysterectomy is usually indicated to control hemorrhage. If abdominal implantation has occurred, the fetus is removed, and the placenta often is left within the cavity to be reabsorbed.

Laparoscopy (or laparotomy) is performed under general anesthesia. The perianesthesia nurse should be especially observant for signs of intraabdominal hemorrhage and shock, because these are not uncommon complications of ectopic pregnancy, especially one that has ruptured preoperatively. All patients with ectopic pregnancy should have complete typing and cross-matching for whole blood, which should be kept available in the laboratory for 24 hours. Rh-negative women should receive RhoGAM to prevent sensitization.

Cerclage Procedures. The McDonald or Shirodkar procedure is used to treat an incompetent cervix and is fairly successful in maintaining pregnancy. The suture is usually placed between the 14th and 18th week of gestation. These procedures may be accomplished under general, spinal, or regional anesthesia.

On admission to the PACU, the patient is placed in the side-lying position until she is reactive. Oxygen should be administered and weaned with pulse oximetry. Food and fluids may be resumed as soon as the patient is conscious and the laryngeal reflexes have returned. A perineal pad should be kept in place. Only a minimal amount of bloody spotting should be considered normal. Pain should be minimal and easily controlled with a simple analgesic such as acetaminophen. Any gross vaginal bleeding or abdominal cramping should be reported to the surgeon because this procedure may induce labor and expulsion of the uterine contents. The surgeon may order an external fetal monitor to assess the presence of uterine contractions and fetal heart tones. If labor begins, the suture must be removed immediately.

Uterine Aspiration. Uterine aspiration is used to terminate early pregnancy (i.e., first trimester) or to treat incomplete spontaneous abortion. It is a type of dilatation of the cervix and curettage of the uterus (D & C). A general anesthetic may be used, but the trend has been toward the use of a paracervical block and sedation only. Nursing care in the PACU is essentially the same as after D & C by conventional means. The woman who is Rh-negative should receive Rho-Gam to prevent sensitization. Complications from this procedure include incomplete evacuation and hemorrhage, which may be treated with oxytocin. Uterine perforation may occur and must be treated surgically.

GYNECOLOGIC SURGERY

Certain problems are inherent in gynecologic disease processes and the surgical procedures that deal with them. Because of prolonged or heavy menstrual periods, the patient often is more chronically anemic than even the peripheral blood indices indicate. Moreover, large amounts of blood may have accumulated within the pelvic organs at the time of the operation and may not be reflected in the external blood loss. Consequently, shock out of proportion to the estimated or measured blood loss may ensue. Although they are elective procedures, many gynecologic operations are associated with significant hemorrhage because of their location, the large vascular pedicles with their increased blood supply because of the menstrual cycles, and the large capillary bleeding that complicates hemostasis.

Because of the proximity of the female genitalia to the urinary tract, great care must be taken during surgery and in the observation period afterward to ensure the integrity of this system.

Therefore in addition to overall assessment and general care of these patients, the perianesthesia nurse should direct specific attention toward the patient's cardiovascular status, renal function, and fluid balance.

Laparoscopy

Operative laparoscopy commonly is performed as outpatient surgery to treat benign gynecologic problems. This may involve advanced operative laparoscopic procedures for more significant problems that involve the pelvic organs. A small incision (approximately 1 cm) is made at the subumbilical site for insertion of the primary trocar (typically 10 to 12 mm in diameter), which houses the laparoscope with attached video camera for visualization of the procedure (Fig. 39-3). After a pneumoperitoneum is established, the surgeon can visualize all the organs within the peritoneum. The video camera enables the

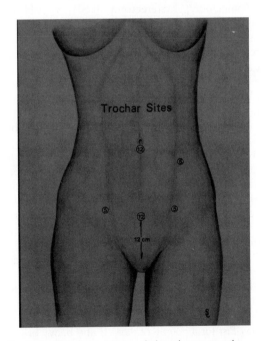

Fig. 39-3 Placement of trocars during advance operative laparoscopy. The trocar in the upper left quadrant is optional and only recommended in cases where the primary trocar is not sufficient because of severe adhesions. The laparoscope needs to be placed off to one side or the other for the purposes of taking down adhesions.

surgeon, first assistant, scrub tech, and entire team to view the procedure on the video monitor. The video camera provides excellent resolution and visualization of the pelvis. The surgeon is able to operate off the video monitor with instruments that are typically 5 mm in diameter (sometimes the instruments used are as small as 3 mm in diameter or as large as 12 mm in diameter, depending on the procedure. The surgeon can thoroughly examine the ovaries, fallopian tubes, and uterus after placing a second and third incision suprapubically in the right and left lower quadrant of the abdomen for additional instrumentation. Generally a fourth incision along the midsuprapubic area is used as well. During operative laparoscopy the surgeon may differentially diagnose pelvic inflammatory disease or perform relatively simple procedures, such as aspiration of an ovarian cyst, adhesiolysis, tissue biopsy, and tubal ligation. In addition, more advanced laparoscopic procedures may be done (i.e., extensive adhesiolysis; excision of endometriosis; myomectomy; hysterectomy [LSH, LAVH or total laparoscopic hysterectomy]; salpingectomy; salpingo-oophorectomy; removal of an ovarian remnant; ureterolysis; burch or colposuspension procedures; repair of pelvic floor relaxation, which may include cystocele, enterocele (high McCall's culdoplasty), posterior and/or paravaginal repairs; appendectomy; fimbriolysis and/or tubal reanastomosis) (Fig. 39-4). Closure of the skin wound involves only a few sutures to close the fascia at the subumbilical site and possibly sutures at the ancillary sites, depending on their size (incisional sites that house instrumentation 5 mm in diameter or less often may not need to be sutured and may only be closed using steristrips to approximate the edges of the skin incision). SteriStrips are used over all incision sites after a liquid adhesive is applied. A dressing of an eye pad is at the subumbilical site with clear adhesive type bandages over the other sites to allow the patients to shower. Some serous type drainage from these incision sites will occur and may last for a couple of days. If any heavy bright red bleeding occurs from any of these sites the physician should be notified immediately. Pain should be minimal to moderate initially in the PACU area and is generally successfully controlled with antiinflammatory agents or mild narcotics. Severe pain may indicate something more

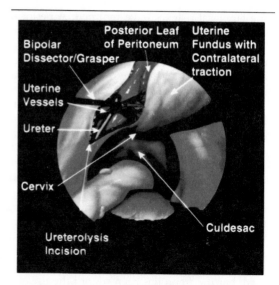

Fig. 39-4 Laparoscopic anatomy as seen through the laparoscope. This figure demonstrates the bipolar instrument used for uterine occlusion. (Courtesy Center for Women's Care and Reproductive Surgery, Atlanta.)

severe, and the surgeon should be notified immediately. A firm abdomen could indicate abdominal bleeding that would not be normal; severe pain, nausea, and/or vomiting could indicate a bowel perforation. If any of these conditions occur, the surgeon should be notified immediately. Postoperative care instructions, including an explanation of the possibility of referred chest or shoulder pain, should be discussed with the patient and a significant other. Instructions should always be written as well and given to the patient for review after discharge.

A follow-up phone call to the patient within 24 to 48 hours is recommended as well. Special care of the patient who undergoes outpatient surgery is outlined in Chapter 43.

Lower Genital and Vaginal Surgery

The conditions that require this type of surgery occur most often in parous and older women. They are caused primarily by exaggeration of the normal relaxation of the pelvic ligaments and support that occurs during childbirth and after menopause. A number of specific procedures, named after their developers, may be encountered and include the following:

- Baldy-Webster procedure: shortening the round ligaments and changing the direction of their pull by attaching them to the back of the uterus.
- Fothergill-Hunter procedure: complete repair of the vaginal wall—from above downward toward the vulva—to correct faulty supportive structures of the pelvic floor.
- Gilliam procedure: shortening the round ligaments by attaching them to the abdominal wall.
- LeFort operation (colpocleisis): closure of the vagina by approximation of the anterior and posterior vaginal walls with or without attendant vaginal hysterectomy.
- Radical vulvectomy: abdominal and perineal dissection of the superficial and deep inguinal nodes and portions of the saphenous veins, reconstruction of the vaginal walls and pelvic floor, and closure of the abdominal wounds.
- Vulvectomy: removal of the labia majora, labia minora, and possibly the clitoris and perianal area, with a Z-plasty closure. Used to treat leukoplakia vulva, carcinoma *in situ* of the vulva, and Paget's disease of the vulva.

Other vaginal surgical procedures include fistula repairs, those to correct urinary stress incontinence, excision of leiomyomata, and vaginal reconstruction to repair congenital or acquired defects. It is important to note that many of the pelvic floor repair procedures can be done laparoscopically if the surgeon knows laparoscopic suturing. If the surgeon can do this, it is done with permanent suture material for optimal results. In more severe cases in pelvic floor prolapse the surgeon may choose to use permanent mesh in addition to permanent suture.

General Perianesthesia Care

Anesthesia for lower genital and vaginal surgery may be local, general, or regional, depending on the amount of pelvic relaxation necessary to perform these procedures. On admission to the PACU, the patient should be placed in the side-lying position until the laryngopharyngeal reflexes have returned. She may then assume a position of comfort and be encouraged to move about frequently as part of antiembolism care. After making a general assessment of the patient's condition, check all dressings carefully. A vaginal packing often is in place with a perineal pad as the only dressing. Saturation of the vaginal packing may be expected after any vaginal surgery; however, saturation of the perineal pad when vaginal packing is in place should be considered excessive bleeding and should be reported. Vaginal and groin wounds often have drains, and care must be exercised to avoid dislodging them. If drains are in place, a moderate amount of drainage may be expected.

Food and fluids may be safely resumed after the minor procedures—such as D&C and bartholinectomy—once the pharyngeal reflexes have returned. After more extensive procedures, the patient is usually not given anything by mouth until peristalsis is reestablished; intake is supplied by intravenous fluids. Urine output should be monitored carefully for amount and for the presence of blood. If a Foley or suprapubic catheter is in place, care must be taken to ensure its patency and to avoid inadvertent dislodging.

Pain must be carefully evaluated and may be alleviated by appropriate analgesics. Abdominal cramping is common after gynecologic surgery. For these patients, relaxation exercises are often helpful if they have been learned preoperatively. Warm blankets over the abdomen may also aid in relaxation. Because the patient is often drowsy because of the anesthesia, she will need coaching, especially during the first hour. If cramping is not relieved by relaxation exercises, analgesics, or other comfort measures, the surgeon should be notified because this may indicate a perforated uterus or more severe problem. After removal of tumors or cysts from the vaginal area, ice may be applied to reduce edema and provide comfort.

ABDOMINAL GYNECOLOGIC SURGERY

Abdominal gynecologic surgery may be performed alone or in conjunction with vaginal surgery.

General Postoperative Care

Postoperative care after abdominal gynecologic surgery involves all the care and considerations rendered to the patient who undergoes any type of abdominal surgery. Anesthesia is most often general.

Overall assessment of the patient, with special emphasis on the cardiovascular status, should be undertaken as soon as the patient is admitted to the PACU.

The most common and dangerous complications of any obstetric or gynecologic surgery are excessive hemorrhage and shock. Therefore the perianesthesia nurse should direct assessment to a complete evaluation of the patient's circulatory status at frequent intervals. All dressings should be checked for drainage. Pain should be evaluated, and appropriate comfort measures and analgesics should be administered.

After hysterectomy and other major abdominal procedures, the patient is usually not given anything orally until peristalsis has returned and nausea has subsided. Intake is supplied by intravenous fluids. Occasionally, the patient is admitted to the PACU with a nasogastric tube in place to prevent abdominal distention. If abdominal distention develops, nasogastric and rectal tubes may be used to relieve it.

A Foley catheter is often in place, and its patency must be ensured. The perianesthesia nurse should accurately document the amount of urinary output as well as the presence of blood. A not uncommon complication of hysterectomy is accidental perforation or ligation of a ureter. Inadvertent injury to the bladder wall or the bowel may also occur.

To help prevent vascular disorders, especially in the lower extremities, the patient's position should be changed frequently; high-Fowler's position should be avoided; and active and passive range-of-motion exercises of the lower extremities should be instituted in the PACU as soon as possible.

It is important to note that if a hysterectomy is done laparoscopically and the uterus is removed vaginally (i.e., LAVH)—whether the vaginal cuff is repaired vaginally or laparoscopically—vaginal packing typically is not used. In addition, not only will patients encounter some vaginal bleeding after an LAVH but also after most laparoscopies because a uterine manipulator is used during the procedure. In addition, in hysteroscopy, patients will encounter postoperative vaginal bleeding as well. It is important to note, however, that in all of these cases the bleeding should not be heavier than that from a menstrual period; if heavier bleeding occurs, the surgeon should be notified immediately. In addition, patients postoperatively should be instructed to refrain from sexual intercourse and from vaginal insertion of foreign objects, including tampons; these instructions may vary among physicians. Patients may experience vaginal discharge in some form for several weeks after these procedures. After laparoscopic surgery the surgeon typically will see the patients in an office visit 2 weeks after the operation.

After laparoscopic surgery, patients should begin to feel significantly better within 48 to 72 hours. If they are still having a great deal of discomfort or if they begin to feel better and then a couple of days later start to feel much worse, the surgeon should be notified immediately. This could indicate a postoperative complication that could involve an injury to the bowel, bladder, or ureter. A bowel injury often does not present itself until the patient has gone home; this could be very serious, and the physician must identify and recognize it as soon as possible.

BIBLIOGRAPHY

Berger PH, Saul HM: Radical hysterectomy: treatment for advanced cervical carcinoma, AORN J 52(6):1212-1222, 1990.

Clark-Pearson DL, Dawood MY: Green's gynecology: essentials of clinical practice, ed 4, Boston, 1990, Little, Brown.

Combs CA, Murphy EL, Laros RK: Factors associated with hemorrhage in cesarean deliveries, Obstet Gynecol 77(1):77-82, 1991.

Dickason EJ, Schult MO, Silverman BL: Maternal-infant nursing care, St Louis, 1990, Mosby.

Edwards J: Lasers in gynecology, Nurs Clin North Am 25(3):673-683, 1990.

Frieden FJ, Ordorica SA, Hoskins IA et al: The Shirodkar operation: a reappraisal, Am J Obstet Gynecol 163(3):830-833, 1990.

Harris AP: The obstetric recovery room, Anesthesiol Clin North Am 8(2):311-323, 1990.

Iams JD, Zuspan FP, editors: Zuspan & Quilligan's manual of obstetrics and gynecology, St Louis, 1990, Mosby.

Janke JR: Prenatal cocaine use: effects on perinatal outcome, J Nurse Midwifery 35(2):74-77, 1990.

Jones, WB: Surgical approaches for advanced or recurrent cancer of the cervix, Cancer 60(8):2094-2103, 1987.

Lamb MA, Chu J: Invasive cancer of the vulva, AORN J 47(4):928-936, 1988.

Litwack K: Practical points in the care of obstetrical

surgical patients, J Post Anesth Nurs 5(3):182-185, 1990.

Long BC, Glazer G: The patient with reproductive problems. In Long BC, Phipps WJ, editors: Medical-surgical nursing, St Louis, 1990, Mosby.

Lyons TL, Winer WK: Posterior pelvic floor repair. In Cusmano PG, Deprest JA, editors: Advanced gynecologic laparoscopy: a practical guide, New York, 1996, Parthenon Publishing.

Lyons TL, Winer WK: Laparoscopic treatment of urinary stress incontinence. In Tulandi T: Atlas of laparoscopic and hysteroscopic techniques for gynecologists, ed 2, Philadelphia, 2000, WB Saunders.

Lyons TL, Lee T, Winer WK: Laparoscopic removal of a bladder leiomyoma, JAAGL 5(4):423-426, 1998.

Lyons TL, Winer WK: Clinical outcomes with laparoscopic approaches and open burch procedures for urinary stress incontinence, JAAGL, 2(2), 193-198, 1995.

Lyons TL, Winer WK: Transvaginal hydrolaparoscopy: a new technique for pelvic assessment, GyneTrends 2(2):4-5, 1998.

Lyons TL, Winer WK: Laparoscopic rectocele repair using polyglactin mesh, JAAGL 4(3):381-384, 1997.

Matthews NC, Greer G: Embolism during caesarean section, Anesthesia 45:964-965, 1990.

McLucas B: Intrauterine applications of the resectoscope, Surg Gynecol Obstet 172(6):425-431, 1991.

Peterfreund DO: Outpatient laparoscopy, J Post Anesth Nurs 3(3):185-188, 1988.

Rostad ME: The radical vulvectomy patient: preventing complications, DCCN 7(5):289-294, 1988.

Stanley ME, Seaton P, Trobaugh M: Post anesthesia care for the patient who has had a spontaneous abortion, J Post Anesth Nurs 3(5):317-320, 1988.

Winer WK: Role of the operating room nurse. In Sutton C, Diamond M, editors: Endoscopic surgery for gynecologists, ed 2, Philadelphia, 1998, WB Saunders.

Winer WK: Laparoscopic procedures: innovations and complications, Today's Surgical Nurse 21(1):15-19, 1999.

Winer WK: Endoscopy equipment: maintenance and management. In Soderstrom R, editor: In The masters' techniques in gynecologic surgery: operative laparoscopy, ed 2, Philadelphia, 1998, Lippincott-Raven.

Winer WK: Operating room personnel, In Sanfilippo JS and Levine RL, editors: Operative gynecologic endoscopy, ed 2, New York, 1996, Springer-Verlag Inc, Chapter 26, pp. 412-422.

Winer WK: Simple ways to save money when doing operative laparoscopy, NewsScope of AAGL, 3(3):4, 1998.

Breast cancer is a malignant tumor that has developed from cells of the breast. The disease occurs mostly in women but does occur rarely in men. With the newer forms of treatment of cancer of the breast—including better forms of diagnosis—surgical procedures on the breast have increased. However, with the advent of better radiation and chemotherapy, surgical procedures performed on the breast may not be as extensive as in years past. Nondisease breast procedures may be performed for cosmetic purposes. Breast surgery is most commonly performed on women; however, procedures are occasionally performed on males and children.

The incidence of breast cancer continues to increase. One in nine American women is expected to develop breast cancer during her lifetime, whereas 1 in 100 men is expected to develop breast cancer in his lifetime. Cancer of the breast continues to be one of the leading causes of cancer-related deaths in women.

As the patient's advocate, the perianesthesia nurse must be supportive, caring, and reassuring to the patient having breast surgery. Positive support is the start of the patient's rehabilitation process.

DEFINITIONS

Adenocarcinoma: a general type of cancer that starts in glandular tissues anywhere in the body. Nearly all breast cancers start in glandular tissue of the breast and therefore are adenocarcinomas. The two main types of breast adenocarcinomas are ductal carcinomas and lobular carcinomas.

Augmentation mammoplasty: surgery to enlarge or augment the size of the female breast with a breast implant. This is the most popular cosmetic procedure.

Breast biopsy: excision of breast tissue. The specimen is sent to pathology for frozen section. Also, a needle localization can be performed when a suspected lesion is identified on mammogram. The procedure involves placing a thin needle or guide into the breast under mammographic visualization. The lesion is then excised and taken to pathology for a frozen section to determine a diagnosis.

Breast reconstruction (mammoplasty): the breast is reconstructed after mastectomy.

Ductal carcinoma in situ (DCIS): Ductal carcinoma in situ (also known as intraductal carcinoma) is the most common type of noninvasive breast cancer. Cancer cells are inside the ducts but have not spread through the walls of the ducts into the fatty tissue of the breast. Nearly all women diagnosed at this early stage of breast cancer can be cured. The best way to find DCIS is with a mammogram. With more women getting mammograms each year, a diagnosis of DCIS is becoming more common. DCIS is sometimes subclassified based on its grade and type to help predict the risk of cancer returning after treatment and to help select the most appropriate treatment. Grade refers to how aggressive cancer cells appear under a microscope. Several types of DCIS exist, but the most important distinction among them is whether tumor cell necrosis (areas of dead or degenerating cancer cells) is present. The term comedocarcinoma is often used to describe a type of DCIS with necrosis.

Infiltrating (or invasive) ductal carcinoma (IDC): starting in a milk passage, or duct, of the breast, this cancer has broken through the wall of the duct and invades the fatty tissue of the breast. At this point, it has the potential to metastasize, or spread, to other parts of the body through the lymphatic system and bloodstream. Infiltrating ductal carcinoma accounts for about 80% of invasive breast cancers.

Infiltrating (or invasive) lobular carcinoma (ILC): ILC starts in the milk-producing glands. Similar to IDC, this cancer has the potential to spread (metastasize) elsewhere in the body. About 10% to 15% of invasive breast cancers are invasive lobular carcinomas. ILC may be more difficult to detect by mammogram than IDC.[1]

Inflammatory breast cancer: this rare type of invasive breast cancer accounts for about 1% of all breast cancers. Inflammatory breast cancer makes the skin of the breast look red and feel warm, as if it was infected and inflamed. The skin has a thick, pitted appearance that doctors often describe as resembling an orange peel. Sometimes the skin develops ridges and small bumps that look like hives. Doctors now know that these changes are not caused by inflammation or infection, but the name given to this type of cancer long ago still persists. Cancer cells that block lymph vessels or channels in the skin over the breast cause these symptoms.

In situ: this term is used for an early stage of cancer in which it is confined to the immediate area where it began. Specifically in breast cancer, in situ means that the cancer remains confined to ducts (ductal carcinoma in situ) or lobules (lobular carcinoma in situ). It has not invaded surrounding fatty tissues in the breast nor spread to other organs in the body.

Lobular carcinoma in situ (LCIS): although not a true cancer, LCIS (also called lobular neoplasia) is sometimes classified as a type of noninvasive breast cancer. It begins in the milk-producing glands but does not penetrate through the wall of the lobules. Most breast cancer specialists think that LCIS itself does not become an invasive cancer but that women with this condition have a higher risk of developing an invasive breast cancer in the same or the opposite breast. For this reason women with LCIS should have physical exams two or three times a year as well as an annual mammogram.

Lumpectomy: only the tumor and surrounding tissue of a "breast lump" are excised. The rest of the breast remains intact. The procedure includes dissection of the axillary lymph nodes. The lump is generally smaller than 4 cm in diameter.

Mastopexy (breast lift): reshaping (uplifting) the sagging breasts by surgically tightening the skin (Figs. 40-1 and 40-2).

Medullary carcinoma: this special type of infiltrating breast cancer has a relatively well defined, distinct boundary between tumor tissue and normal tissue. It also has some other special features, including the large size of the cancer cells and the presence of immune system cells at the edges of the tumor. Medullary carcinoma accounts for about 5% of breast cancers. The outlook, or prognosis, for this kind of breast cancer is better than for other types of invasive breast cancer.

Modified radical mastectomy: removal of the entire

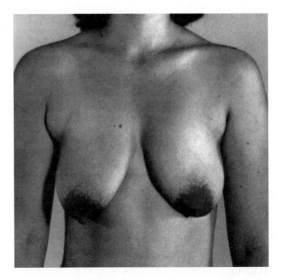

Fig. 40-1 Mastopexy (breast lift). Before surgery, this patient complained of sagging (ptosis) of the breasts.

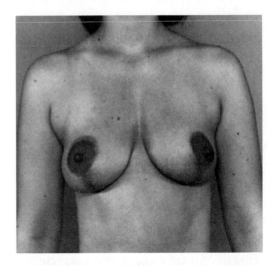

Fig. 40-2 Mastopexy, showing the same patient as in Fig. 40-1 several weeks postoperatively. The scars are beginning to fade.

breast and axillary lymph nodes; the pectoralis major muscle is left intact. In some instances, the pectoralis minor muscle is excised.

Mucinous carcinoma: this rare type of invasive breast cancer is formed by mucus-producing cancer cells. The prognosis for mucinous carcinoma is better than for the more common types of invasive breast cancer. Colloid carcinoma is another name for this type of breast cancer.

Paget's disease of the nipple: this type of breast cancer starts in the breast ducts and spreads to the skin of the nipple and then to the areola, the dark circle around the nipple. It is a rare type of breast cancer and occurs in only 1% of all cases. The skin of the nipple and areola often appears crusted, scaly, and red with areas of bleeding or oozing. The woman may notice burning or itching. Paget's disease may be associated with in situ carcinoma or with infiltrating breast carcinoma. If no lump can be felt in the breast tissue and the biopsy shows DCIS but no invasive cancer, the prognosis is excellent.

Phyllodes tumor: this very rare type of breast tumor forms from the stroma (connective tissue) of the breast, in contrast to carcinomas, which develop in the ducts or lobules. Phyllodes (also spelled hylloides) tumor are usually benign but rarely malignant (having the potential to metastasize). Benign phyllodes tumors are successfully treated by removing the mass and a narrow margin of normal breast tissue. A malignant phyllodes tumor is treated by removing it along with a wider margin of normal tissue or by mastectomy. These cancers do not respond to hormonal therapy and are not so likely to respond to chemotherapy or radiation therapy. In the past, both benign and malignant phyllodes tumors were called cystosarcoma phyllodes.

Radical mastectomy: removal of the entire breast, skin, nipple, areolar complex, and pectoralis major and minor muscles with axillary node dissection (Figs. 40-3 and 40-4).

Tubular carcinoma: accounting for about 2% of all breast cancers, tubular carcinomas are a special type of infiltrating breast carcinoma. They have a better prognosis than usual infiltrating ductal or lobular carcinomas.

PERIANESTHESIA CARE AFTER SPECIFIC PROCEDURES

Breast Biopsy

Lumps in the breast often are discovered during monthly self-examination or by routine mammograms. Lumps are aspirated or excised and sent for definitive diagnoses.

In approximately half of all female patients who undergo a biopsy, the diagnosis is fibrocystic disease. Fibrocystic disease describes a variety of benign and localized tumors or swelling within the breast tissues. Other nonfibrocystic conditions also may cause breast lumps. Inflammatory conditions—such as breast abscesses, fat necrosis, and lipomas of the skin (e.g., sebaceous cysts)—may cause breast lumps.

A breast biopsy can be a one-step (biopsy and mastectomy, if needed) or two-step procedure. Two-step procedures are now the most common practice. The two-step procedure allows the patient to be educated about the choices and the opportunity to make an informed decision regarding the type of surgery to be performed in the event of a positive biopsy finding.

The patient often is admitted as a same-day surgical patient. Because of the patient's natural apprehension, the patient may receive intravenous sedation along with local anesthesia (see the position statement on intravenous sedation in Chapter 3.)

The patient is usually awake on arrival in the PACU but drowsy because of the sedation. Routine admission procedures are accomplished. The head of the bed may be elevated 45 degrees.

The dressing is usually a 4×4 sponge held in place by the patient's bra. It should be inspected for excessive drainage, which occurs only rarely. The patient can resume fluid and food intake as soon as the cough and gag reflexes have fully returned and nausea has subsided. Pain should be minimal, if any, and easily controlled with minor analgesics.

If the patient has received midazolam (Versed), she may repeatedly ask the same questions. The perianesthesia nurse must patiently repeat the answers and also ensure that the person who will accompany the patient at discharge understands the home care instructions.

Surgical Choices for the Treatment of Cancer

Advances in early diagnosis and modifications in surgical techniques have increased the number of surgical choices in the treatment of breast cancer (see Fig. 40-3).

Lumpectomy. Lumpectomy is the surgical treatment of choice when the breast tumor is well defined and less than 5 cm in diameter. In clinical trials reported in 1988, the National Surgical Adjuvant Breast Cancer Project reported that lumpectomy followed by radiation therapy produced 8-year disease-free survival rates equal to those of modified radical mastectomy.

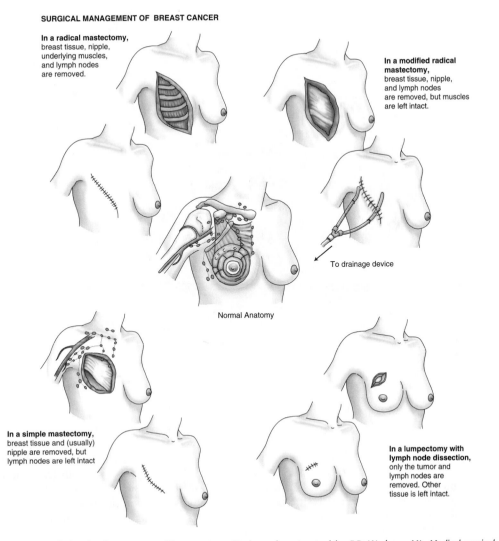

SURGICAL MANAGEMENT OF BREAST CANCER

In a radical mastectomy, breast tissue, nipple, underlying muscles, and lymph nodes are removed.

In a modified radical mastectomy, breast tissue, nipple, and lymph nodes are removed, but muscles are left intact.

To drainage device

Normal Anatomy

In a simple mastectomy, breast tissue and (usually) nipple are removed, but lymph nodes are left intact

In a lumpectomy with lymph node dissection, only the tumor and lymph nodes are removed. Other tissue is left intact.

Fig. 40-3 Surgical choices for the treatment of breast cancer. *(Redrawn from Ignatavicius DD, Workman ML: Medical-surgical nursing: critical thinking for collaborative care, ed 4, Philadelphia, 2002, WB Saunders.)*

Lumpectomy is usually performed under general anesthesia. The tumor is removed along with a margin of surrounding tissue. An axillary node dissection is performed through a separate incision. Axillary dissection involves taking a sample of 10 to 15 lymph nodes lateral and inferior to the pectoralis minor muscles.

When the patient is admitted to the PACU, all the initial assessment measures should be accomplished. The blood pressure cuff should be placed on the arm opposite the operative side.

The arm on the operative side should be elevated on a pillow because the removal of lymph nodes increases the risk of lymphedema. The operative-side arm should be assessed frequently for circulatory adequacy by monitoring color, temperature, capillary refill, and the presence and strength of the radial pulse. Venipunctures and injections should not be performed on the operative-side arm.

Dressings should be small, and bleeding or drainage should be minimal. A Hemovac or

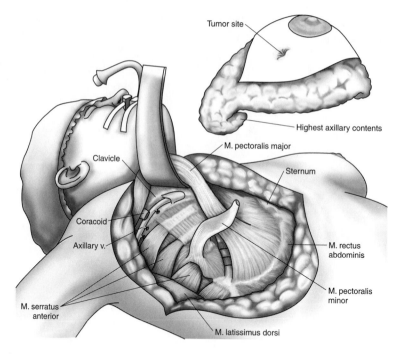

Fig. 40-4   Mastectomy.

Jackson-Pratt closed-drainage system may be connected to drains placed at the incision site.

Nursing personnel should be aware that although this procedure allows the patient to keep her breast, it does not eliminate her fear of the cancer diagnosis or concerns about whether the procedure was successful; thus the nurse must be provided factual reassurance.

Mastectomy

Modified Radical Mastectomy.   The modified radical mastectomy is the most commonly performed surgery to eliminate breast cancer. The entire breast and axillary nodes are removed. This procedure differs from the Halsted radical mastectomy in that the pectoralis major muscle is left intact.

Radical Mastectomy.   The radical mastectomy is seldom performed in the United States. Refined techniques for diagnosis and surgery, radiation therapy, and chemotherapy have made it unnecessary in most instances. Radical mastectomy may be performed in women (primarily

elderly women) who do not desire adjuvant therapy (radiation or chemotherapy).

Nursing care after either modified radical or radical mastectomy is essentially the same, except that, of course, the radical mastectomy involves more gross excision of tissue and demands more detailed observation of viability of remaining tissue.

Mastectomy is performed under general inhalation anesthesia. The patient will be admitted to the PACU with the head of her bed elevated 30 to 45 degrees. All admission assessments should be made, oxygen administered, and respiratory sufficiency determined by pulse oximetry.

Dressings are usually bulky and should be checked frequently for excessive serosanguineous drainage and for constriction. The most important postoperative complication is hematoma below the skin flaps. Attention to the drains and the maintenance of free drainage within the vacuum system prevent this occurrence. Drains are usually placed under the skin flaps to remove excess blood and serum that would ordinarily collect under the wound site, thus causing edema, infection, and sloughing of the skin graft. The drains may be connected to Hemovac or Jackson-Pratt devices. Generally, additional vacuum is needed the first 8 postoperative hours, and the Hemovac is connected to vacuum pressure of 20 to 30 mm Hg. These should be monitored for excessive bleeding, which must be reported to the surgeon. Dressings are necessarily snug but should not impair respiration or circulation to the upper extremity. The arm on the operative side should be supported and elevated on a pillow; it must be checked frequently for cyanosis or pallor, and the pulse must be palpated for intensity. If signs of respiratory distress or impaired circulation arise, the surgeon should be notified to rearrange the dressing. Unless an emergency arises, the perianesthesia nurse should not attempt to loosen the dressing, because skin grafts may inadvertently be disrupted.

When a radical mastectomy is performed, extensive excision and skin grafting are usually required (see Chapter 41). Donor sites (usually the thigh) should be checked for drainage and treated according to hospital policy.

The patient should be advised to avoid excessive motion in the immediate postoperative period. She should not strain the pectoral girdle by levering herself on the bed with her arms to change position. These patients usually need intravenous fluid augmentation for the first 24 postoperative hours. There is no reason to refrain from oral feeding after cough and gag reflexes have returned and if she is not experiencing nausea. Small sips of fluids may be offered and taken as desired and diet resumed as tolerated. Postoperative pain is moderate to severe and can usually be controlled with narcotics such as meperidine (Demerol) and morphine. Hypothermia may be a problem because of prolonged exposure in the operating room, and rewarming should be accomplished with additional warmed blankets or a BairHugger.

Postoperative instructions for patients who have axillary node dissections should include hand and arm care instructions. Consistent education and support are required. Emotional support may be sought through support groups such as the "Reach to Recovery" program (American Cancer Society on the Web at: www.cancer.org/ or phone: [800] ACS-2345).

Breast Reconstruction. One of the advances made in breast surgery during recent years is the availability of effective means of reconstructing the breast after removal for cancer. This can be done by a variety of methods in which the surgeon—in collaboration with a plastic surgeon—tailors the operation to the patient's deformity. Breast reconstruction may be accomplished in conjunction with mastectomy or at a later time.

For reconstructive augmentation mammoplasty, a pocket is made under the remaining tissues into which a soft silicone bag is made to simulate the natural contour (Figs. 40-5 and 40-6). The pocket can be made at the time of surgery or before the surgery by means of an inflatable tissue extender. The expander method requires the administration of several injections of gradually increasing volumes of saline over a period of weeks. The expander is then replaced surgically with a soft, silicone bag prosthesis.

Muscle-skin flap reconstruction (Figs. 40-7 and 40-8) involves moving nearby muscle and skin into the area of the mastectomy to replace the lost volume. Commonly used muscle and skin flaps include the latissimus dorsi and rectus abdominis muscles with attached skin. Nipple-areola reconstruction may be accomplished by using

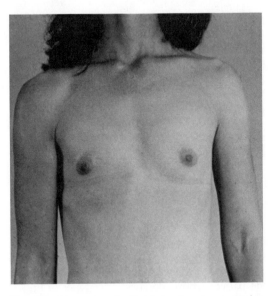

Fig. 40-5 Appearance of patient before breast augmentation.

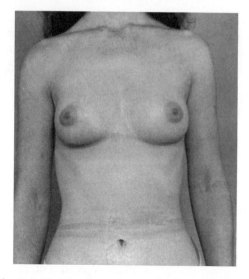

Fig. 40-6 Postoperative appearance of patient after breast augmentation with silicone bag prostheses.

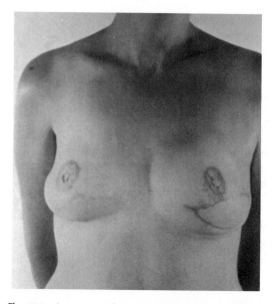

Fig. 40-8 Appearance of same patient as in Fig. 40-7 after muscle-skin flap (latissimus) and nipple reconstructions. The patient has gained considerable weight, and later she delivered a healthy baby. She is free of disease 6 years after the mastectomy.

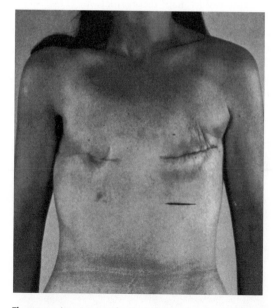

Fig. 40-7 Appearance of patient after healing from bilateral mastectomies for cancer.

small portions of the labia and grafting to the selected location.

Postoperative care is generally the same as for the patient who undergoes other types of breast surgery, with attention to graft and flap donor sites.

These operations have provided a measure of comfort to patients whose body image has been significantly disrupted by mastectomy. They report a return of their sense of femininity and confidence. Many women do not choose to undergo additional surgery after mastectomy, but knowing that the operation is available is reassuring.

Mastopexy (Breast Lift). Breast ptosis (sagging) is defined by the position of the nipple areolar complex related to the inframammary crease. The reshaping process differs from reduction mammoplasty in the amount of tissue removed. Generally less than 300 g of tissue removed is to be considered a mastopexy procedure.

Mastopexy is commonly being performed as a same-day procedure, and postoperative care following mastopexy is generally not demanding. General anesthesia is most commonly used, and only minor adjustments in breast tissue are made.

The patient is positioned postoperatively on her back and may assume a semi-Fowler's to high-Fowler's position for comfort as soon as she awakens. The motion of the arms is restricted to below shoulder level.

Postoperative dressings are minimal, and drains are rarely required, because the entire procedure, with the exception of nipple release, is at the level of the dermis. Drainage should be minimal, and if frank bleeding occurs, the surgeon should be notified. Pain is usually not a problem, and discomfort can be controlled with the mild analgesics. Food and fluids may be resumed as tolerated after nausea has disappeared.

Mammoplasty.   Perianesthesia nursing care for reduction and augmentation mammoplasties is essentially the same for both procedures.

Reduction mammoplasty is the surgical method of correcting mammary hypertrophy. Women who experience mammary hypertrophy often complain of shoulder strap discomfort; breast pain; back and neck pain; and an inability to participate in physical activities such as jogging, aerobics, and horseback riding.

A new method in reduction mammoplasty is the laser deepithelialization technique. When the carbon dioxide laser is used to remove the epidermis from the inferior pedicle, reduction mammoplasty can be performed with little blood loss. The inferior pedicle technique is a commonly used approach to reduction mammoplasty. When the inferior pedicle technique is used, the laser simplifies skin removal. The laser is preferred for pedicle deepithelialization in all patients especially in patients who have large ptotic breasts, because rigid stabilization is not necessary.

Anesthesia may be local—in combination with appropriate sedation—or general for breast augmentation. Breast reduction is usually performed under general anesthesia and may require more extensive manipulation of tissue. Regional anesthesia with intercostal block may be used for either procedure if the patient does not fear being conscious during the operation.

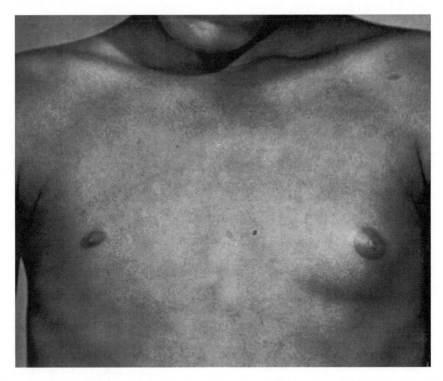

Fig. 40-9   Gynecomastia (idiopathic hypertrophy of the breast) in an 8-year-old boy. *(From Haagensen CD: Diseases of the breast, ed 3, Philadelphia, 1986, WB Saunders.)*

On admission to the PACU, the patient is positioned on her back, and as soon as her condition warrants, she is placed in a low-Fowler's position. Dressings may be of any variety, but most often, wide strips of Elastoplast, which readily conform to the patient's new skin contours, are used. A Velpeau bandage should be in place to restrain the patient from raising her arms, and she should be advised of this. Drains are rarely required, and drainage should be minimal. If drains are present, they should be connected to a vacuum source, such as the Hemovac. As after mastectomy, the patient should be advised to do nothing that puts strain on the pectoral girdle.

Pain after augmentation is generally minimal and can be relieved with mild analgesics. Light ice packs may be used to relieve discomfort and to minimize tissue swelling. Pain after reduction may be more significant and usually requires narcotic analgesia for the first 24 hours.

Surgery in Gynecomastia

Gynecomastia, or benign hypertrophy of one or both breasts in boys and men, is relatively common (Fig. 40-9). It may be bilateral or unilateral. The causes may be hormonal, systemic disease-oriented, drug-related, or idiopathic.

In extreme instances or when in cases in which gynecomastia causes problems in psychological adjustment, this excess tissue can be excised or removed with suction lipectomy. Suction lipectomy is useful when the gynecomastia is caused primarily by fat. Good cosmetic results are obtained. The surgical procedure is similar to that of breast reduction in women. A periareolar incision is made and tissue is removed. Suction drainage of the incision site is usually necessary and may be conveniently accomplished by use of a Hemovac.

Postoperative care is essentially the same as that for women who undergo breast surgery. If no drains are required, the patient can be discharged the day of surgery once reflexes have returned, nausea has subsided, and food and fluids can be taken.

BIBLIOGRAPHY

Alspach J: Core curriculum for critical care nursing, ed 5, Philadelphia, 1998, WB Saunders.

American Cancer Society: Cancer facts and figures: cancer reference information, Atlanta, 2002, American Cancer Society.

Atlee J: Complications in anesthesia, Philadelphia, 1999, WB Saunders.

Barash P, Cullen B, Stoelting R: Clinical anesthesia, ed 4, Philadelphia, 2000, Lippincott Williams & Wilkins.

Becker DW, Bunn JC: Laser deepithelialization: an adjunct to reduction mammoplasty, Plast Reconstr Surg 79(5):754-760, 1979.

Benumof J: Anesthesia and uncommon diseases, ed 4, Philadelphia, 1998, WB Saunders.

Benumof J, Saidman L: Anesthesia & perioperative complications, ed 2, St Louis, 1999, Mosby.

Bickley L, Hoekelman R: Bates' guide to physical examination and history taking, ed 7, Philadelphia, 1998, Lippincott Williams & Wilkins.

Cawley M, Kostic J, Cappello C: Information and psychological needs of women choosing conservative surgery, Cancer Nurs 13(2):90-94, 1990.

DeFazio-Quinn D: Ambulatory surgical nursing core curriculum, Philadelphia, 1999, WB Saunders.

Fisher B, Redmond C, Poisson R et al: Eight-year results of a randomized clinical trial comparing mastectomy and lumpectomy with or without radiation in the treatment of breast cancer, New Engl J Med 320:822-828, 1989.

Ganong W: Review of medical physiology, ed 20, New York, 2001, McGraw-Hill Professional.

Georgiade GS: Reconstructive and aesthetic breast surgery. In Sabiston DC Jr, editor: Textbook of surgery: the biological basis of modern surgical practice, ed 14, Philadelphia, 1991, WB Saunders.

Guyton A, Hall J: Textbook of medical physiology, ed 10, Philadelphia, 2000, WB Saunders.

Harris JR, Helman S, Henderson IC et al: Breast Diseases, ed 2, Philadelphia, 1991, JB Lippincott.

Iglehart JD: The breast. In Sabiston DC Jr, editor: Textbook of surgery: the biological basis of modern surgical practice, ed 14, Philadelphia, 1991, WB Saunders.

Katzung B, editor: Basic and clinical pharmacology, ed 8, Los Altos, Calif, 2000, Appleton & Lange.

Lake C, Hines R, Blitt C: Clinical monitoring: practical applications for anesthesia and critical care, St Louis, 2001, Mosby.

Longnecker D, Murphy F: Dripps/Eckenhoff/Vandam introduction to anesthesia, ed 9, Philadelphia, 1997, WB Saunders.

Longnecker D, Tinker J, Morgan G: Principles and practice of anesthesiology, ed 2, St Louis, 1998, Mosby.

Martin J: Positioning in anesthesia and surgery, ed 3, St Louis, 1997, Mosby.

Miller R, editor: Anesthesia, ed 5, New York, 2000, Churchill Livingstone.

Nagelhout J, Zaglaniczny K: Nurse anesthesia, ed 2, Philadelphia, 2001, WB Saunders.

Nielson BB, East D: Advances in breast cancer, Nurs Clin North Am 25(2):365-375, 1990.

Patrick M: Medical-surgical nursing, ed 2, Philadelphia, 1991, JB Lippincott.

Stein P, Zera RT: Breast cancer, AORN J 53(4):938-963, 1991.

Stoelting R: Pharmacology and physiology in anesthetic practice, ed 3, Philadelphia, 1999, Lippincott-Raven.

Stoelting R, Miller R: Basics of anesthesia, ed 4, New York, 2000, Churchill Livingstone.

Stone D: Perioperative care: anesthesia, medicine, and surgery, St Louis, 1998, Mosby.

Townsend C, Beauchamp R, Evers B, Mattox K: Sabiston textbook of surgery: the biological basis of modern surgical practice, ed 16, Philadelphia, 2001, WB Saunders.

Waugaman W, Foster S, Rigor B: Principles and practice of nurse anesthesia, ed 3, Norwalk, Conn, 1999, Appleton & Lange.

41

CARE OF THE PLASTIC SURGICAL PATIENT

The field of plastic surgery continues to grow and expand daily and presents numerous challenges to the surgeon who performs plastic and reconstructive surgery. This discipline has changed profoundly during the past 10 years, especially in the area of reconstructive surgery.

Plastic surgery derives its name from the Greek word *plastikos*, which means to mold or give shape. Plastic and reconstructive procedures correct acquired and congenital deformities. Corrective procedures deal with the body in its entirety and strive to restore normal appearance as well as function.

A deformity can be devastating not only to physical well-being but also to spiritual and psychological well-being. Each of us desires to be whole. The parents of a child with a congenital malformation often have a profound sense of guilt.

Few absolutes exist in plastic surgical techniques and in the associated preoperative or postoperative care. Therefore only the basic aspects of postoperative care for the plastic surgery patient are presented in this discussion. Some elements of care related to specific body parts are discussed in related chapters, and the reader should refer them.

The most basic techniques of plastic surgery relate to excision of skin lesions, to closure of skin wounds, and to placement of skin grafts and skin flaps. Minor plastic surgical procedures are often performed with local anesthesia. Postoperative nursing care is minimal and primarily involves observation of the surgical site for untoward symptoms. When the patient must undergo general anesthesia, postoperative care includes all the considerations discussed under general care of the postoperative patient, in addition to attention to the surgical site. Postoperative vital signs,

including accurate temperature measurement, are especially important in the care of the perianesthesia plastic surgical patient, because these signs provide baselines from which to judge the possible later complications of an immunologic reaction.

SKIN GRAFTS

Skin grafting is the most common method for covering open areas rapidly and permanently. A skin graft is a layer of epidermis with attached dermis of variable thickness that is completely isolated from its blood supply from the donor site. It is transferred to a recipient site elsewhere on the body without formal surgical revascularization.

The types of skin grafts are defined as follows:

1. A full-thickness graft includes all underlying dermis.
2. A split-thickness graft includes a portion of the underlying dermis. It may be thin, medium, or thick, depending on the amount of dermis that is included.
3. A composite graft comprises two or more tissue components and often skin and subcutaneous tissue, cartilage, or mucosa.
4. Autograft indicates that the donor and the recipient are the same person.
5. Isograft signifies that the donor and the recipient are genetically identical.
6. Allograft or homograft means that the donor and the recipient are of the same species.
7. Xenograft indicates that the donor and the recipient are of different species.

The most important factor in the success of a skin graft is adherence. The graft must have good contact with healthy tissue that has adequate vascularity. When the graft is properly placed on the recipient site, a fibrin layer forms that binds the graft to the recipient bed. A plasmalike fluid (extravasated from blood vessels in the area) collects at the graft site. This fluid contains sufficient nourishment for the graft to survive until new vascularization has been established.

For cosmetically pleasing results, the color, texture, thickness, and hair-bearing nature of the skin used for grafting must be chosen to match the recipient site. As a rule, the nearer the donor skin to the recipient area, the better the match.

It is important to check during the first 24 postoperative hours that serum or blood is present. Excess fluid may cause the graft to lift from its bed and must be removed. The donor site should be kept clean and will heal with a new layer of skin. Because of the variations in surgeons' preferences in the methods of dressing wounds, positioning of the patient, use of ice or antibiotic ointments, and handling of donor sites, the postanesthesia care unit (PACU) must have established policies related to the care of the plastic surgical patient as established by the individual plastic surgeon (see Chapter 42 for additional discussion of care for grafts and donor sites).

Generally, the grafted area should be elevated, if possible, and protected from both pressure and motion. The patient should be positioned to prevent pressure on—or other trauma to—either the graft or the donor site. The physician may order cold packs to reduce the metabolic requirements of the graft and enhance its survival. These can be made by partially filling a rubber glove with cracked ice and cool water or saline, which makes a light, moldable cold pack. Dressings over grafts should be observed closely for drainage, and any excess should be reported to the physician.

Full-thickness donor sites may be sutured closed and treated as a surgical wound if the donor site is small. If a large area is used for full-thickness grafting, it may be necessary to graft the donor site with split-thickness grafts (Fig. 41-1).

FLAPS

The term "flap" commonly refers to a skin flap; however, because of the advances in reconstructive surgery, flaps are not limited to skin tissue. Flaps are classified by their anatomic composition: skin with muscle fascia or bone, or both; skin alone; omentum; or a composite of these tissues.

Local Flaps

Flaps (Fig. 41-2) are the preferred treatment for covering wounds with vascularity inadequate to

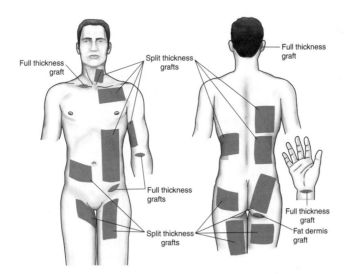

Fig. 41-1 Available donor sites of skin grafts. *(Redrawn from Converse JM: Reconstructive Plastic Surgery, Vol 1, ed 2, Philadelphia, 1977, WB Saunders.)*

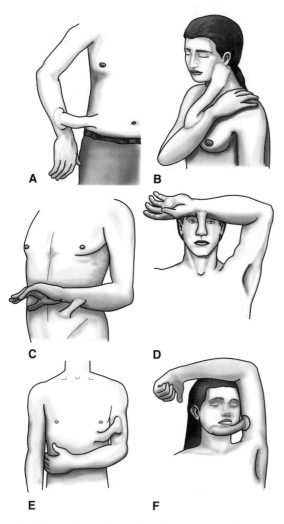

Fig. 41-2 Various methods of transfer of tubed pedicle flaps. **A** and **B**, Transfer via the wrist; **C** and **D**, the "salute" position of Kilner; **E** and **F**, transfer via the arm (Schuchardt). *(Redrawn from Converse JM: Reconstructive plastic surgery, Vol 1, ed 2, Philadelphia, 1977, WB Saunders.)*

support a skin graft; reconstructing full-thickness defects of specialized body parts such as ears, eyelids, nose and lips; and covering over gliding tendons. Reconstructions requiring tissue bulk, such as decubitus closure, are also done with flaps.

Microvascular Tissue Transfer

Microvascular tissue transfer is one of the most important advances in the field of reconstructive surgery. The surgeon who performs microvascular tissue transfer harvests tissue from one part of the body and transfers it to virtually any other part of the body to replace missing tissue or heal problem wounds.

Microvascular tissue transfer is possible only when the surgeon has access to a sophisticated operative microscope with high magnification. Whichever type of flap is used, the newly positioned flap is kept under constant observation by perianesthesia personnel. The most serious complication in the microvascular tissue transfer procedure is necrosis of the tissue. Tissue death occurs when either the artery or the vein supplying the flap develops a thrombus. Arterial thrombosis can result in complete flap failure within 4 hours of onset. Arterial occlusion is characterized by a pale, cool flap that does not bleed when stuck with a needle.

Venous thrombosis is more common, but it is not an immediate threat. It is identified by a congested, warm, mottled flap that continuously oozes dark blood. Objective assessment of the flap is possible through the use of fluorometry, laser Doppler, temperature monitoring, buried Doppler probe, and a photoplethysmograph (PPG) disk. The PPG disk monitors the blood flow. The perianesthesia nurse should notify the surgeon when the monitoring indicates occlusion is occurring.

Pain at the sites of skin grafting or flaps is usually minimal; donor sites ordinarily generate the more painful stimuli. Management includes mild analgesics and attention to comfort measures.

BONE GRAFTS

When bone grafts have been performed, the graft site must be immobilized and excessive movement of the patient avoided. The patient may experience considerable pain at the donor site and must be moved carefully. Pain can be managed with narcotic analgesics after an assessment of the patient's overall condition. If split-rib grafts are used, the patient should be placed in a low-Fowler's position; respiratory status should be checked frequently; and signs of possible pneumothorax, such as tachycardia and tachypnea, should be reported to the surgeon immediately. Graft sites may require elevation, and ice often is used for pain management and reduction of swelling.

COSMETIC SURGERY

Physical appearance affects self-image and can be extremely important psychologically. People seek cosmetic surgery to enhance their physical appearance, and this surgery has become commonplace. In the United States, this may be the result, in part, of the national preoccupation with youth and the desire to remain forever youthful in appearance.

Whatever the reasons, one must recognize that such surgery does take place and that, because it is a surgical procedure, it cannot be taken lightly. These patients have been screened by their surgeons and found to be acceptable in terms of risk, psychological testing, and "anatomic deformity." The patients place an enormous importance (and often expense) on their surgery and should not be judged or made the object of insensitive remarks about their vanity. Those associated with postoperative care of the cosmetic surgery patient should give the same professional care to that patient as to any other. If the nurse has significant biases against these procedures, reassignment should be considered.

Dermabrasion

Dermabrasion is the surgical planing of the skin, with removal of the epidermis and portions of the superficial dermis, to remove high spots or other irregularities in an uneven skin surface. Enough of the dermal and epidermal elements are preserved to allow reepithelialization, and the result is smooth healing and blending of the scarred areas with the surrounding skin surface.

Usually the dermabraded areas are treated by the open method, and postanesthesia care includes protection of those areas from abrasion caused by rubbing on pillows or bed clothing. Facial edema, especially of the eyelids, may be expected, and the patient must be reassured that this will subside rapidly. The dermabraded area should be observed closely for the development of moisture. If moisture develops, it should be dried with a heat lamp or a warm hair dryer. This procedure may produce an uncomfortable burning sensation for the patient and may be minimized by holding the lamp or dryer a considerable distance from the area to be dried. Analgesics should be administered as necessary to manage burning-type pain sensations.

Blepharoplasty

Blepharoplasty is a procedure to correct deformities of the upper or lower eyelid by excising redundant skin or protruding fat. The procedure is usually performed under local anesthesia with supplemental intravenous sedation. Iced compresses minimize swelling and bleeding. The patient may resume a regular diet postoperatively; however, hot liquids are contraindicated for 24 hours to prevent vasodilatation and bleeding. Activities such as bending and heavy lifting should be avoided. Pain is usually minimal and can be managed with mild analgesics. Aspirin should be avoided. Antibiotic ointment may be used for lubrication (see Chapter 30).

Rhytidoplasty (Face Lift)

The face-lift operation is usually done under local anesthesia with supplementary sedation. Although some "lift" is accomplished around the cheek areas, the most important and long-lasting change is in the loose skin of the neck. The facial-neck skin is freed from the underlying tissues and pulled upward and backward toward the postauricular scalp. Excess skin is trimmed off, and meticulous suturing is performed. The procedure takes from 2 to 5 hours, and the patient comes to the PACU with a large, fluffy bandage about the neck and cheeks. Surprisingly, such extensive surgery is not usually associated with significant pain. Pain, especially on one side, is unusual and may be the first sign of a complication. It may mean that the skin is being tightened by active bleeding—the most common serious complication of face lift. The surgeon should be notified at once, and he or she may decide to open the dressing to assess the situation. Bleeding is more common in patients with hypertension. Sedation, a quiet atmosphere, and continued elevation of the head of the bed are important measures in the prevention of complications.

Rhinoplasty

Rhinoplasty is performed to reshape or reconstruct the nose when its shape has been altered as a result of trauma or when the patient is unhappy with its form. Rhinoplasty may be performed under local anesthesia with supplemental narcotics and intravenous sedation or general anesthesia. On admission to the PACU, the patient's head is elevated 30 to 45 degrees. Humidified oxygen is administered. In addition to routine assessment, the nasal area is assessed for swelling and bleeding. Drip pads (2 × 2 s) may be lightly taped under the nostrils.

Otoplasty

Otoplasty is performed to reduce prominence of the ears. The patient has a head dressing for support. Generally, only minimal discomfort occurs and lasts postoperatively no longer than 12 hours. Pain that lasts longer suggests a hematoma or other complication and should be reported to the surgeon.

Liposuction

Suction lipectomy (liposuction) removes subcutaneous fat to improve facial or body contours. It may be used in conjunction with other techniques. Anesthesia may be local or general. Liposuction is commonly performed in the same-day surgical arena; however, if more than 2500 ml of fat is removed, an overnight stay and fluid replacement may be necessary.

Pain should be minimal. However, if large areas are treated, analgesia with meperidine may be required. Drugs that contain aspirin should be avoided so as not to increase bleeding time. If large areas are suctioned, the patient needs intravenous fluid replacement. The patient can usually start oral fluids and a progressive diet as soon as pharyngeal reflexes have returned.

Relatively few complications of this procedure have been reported; however, postoperative bleeding and infection are possible.

SURGICAL REPAIR OF INJURIES TO THE FACIAL BONES

Because of their protrusion and prominence, the facial bones often are broken in motor vehicle accidents, fights, and sporting events. Fractures vary in their location and complexity, and the repair may vary from closed reduction to the use of internal fixation with plates and screws, interosseous wiring, and bone grafting. Repair of injuries to the facial bones often requires general anesthesia. If the damage is extensive and airway obstruction or concomitant cranial or intrathoracic injury is present, a tracheostomy must be performed. All patients who have facial, jaw, or neck surgery should have a tracheostomy set kept

at the bedside in the PACU, in the event that an airway emergency should occur. If a tracheostomy is not performed, the endotracheal tube or nasotracheal tube should be left in place until the laryngopharyngeal reflexes have fully returned. Because the apparatus may be most uncomfortable, the nurse must explain the need for it to the patient and enlist his or her cooperation (see Chapters 17 and 27 for the essential procedures).

On admission to the PACU, the patient who has undergone repair of the facial bones is placed in a low-Fowler's position as soon as his or her condition warrants. This aids in minimizing the development of head and neck edema. Careful monitoring of the airway is mandatory.

If interdental wire fixation was performed, a pair of wire clippers should be affixed to the head of the bed (clearly visible to all personnel) in the event that rapid opening of the jaws is needed. Opening of the jaws may become necessary if an airway emergency develops (see Chapter 29 for care of the patient with interdental fixation).

Good oral hygiene is a priority for these patients and may be accomplished with lemon-glycerin swabs and a weak solution of hydrogen peroxide. Petrolatum ointment should be applied to the lips to prevent drying and cracking. Frequent suctioning of secretions may be necessary during the first postoperative hours. Once nausea has subsided and the gag reflex has fully returned, the patient may be allowed small sips of fluids.

SURGICAL REPAIR OF CLEFT LIP AND PALATE

Cleft lips and palates are common congenital defects that have many associated problems, including facial growth abnormalities, dental irregularities, speech difficulties, ear diseases, psychological disorders, and cosmetic problems. A cleft palate creates difficult nursing and swallowing for the infant.

Repair of the cleft lip (Figs. 41-3 and 41-4) is usually accomplished when the child is about 3 months old. He or she should weigh at least 10 lb and have a hemoglobin level of at least 10 g/dl. Repair is accomplished under general anesthesia. On admission to the PACU, the infant is placed in a semiprone position. The infant's arms should be restrained to avoid disruption of the newly repaired lip, and the infant should not be allowed to cry because crying puts excessive tension on

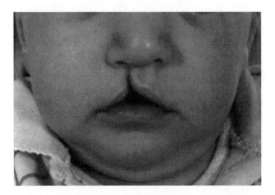

Fig. 41-3 Preoperative appearance of a unilateral cleft lip.

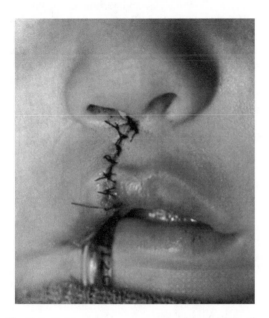

Fig. 41-4 Postoperative appearance of unilateral cleft lip. The incision is covered with an antibiotic ointment to prevent crusting.

the newly repaired lip. If possible, the mother or father should be allowed in the PACU to hold the child to help prevent crying. A rocking chair may prove invaluable in comforting the child, who may be sedated if necessary.

The most important nursing activity—in addition to preventing trauma to the lip—is airway management. A mist humidifier at the bedside (or near the rocking chair) should be used at least 12 hours postoperatively to aid in clearing of secretions and general respiratory well-being. Hemorrhage may occur as a complication but is rare; however, the loss of even a few milliliters of blood in an infant may be significant, and any bleeding requires definitive control. Once the child has fully awakened from anesthesia, small sips of clear fluids may be given.

Pain is usually minimal. Iced normal saline-soaked gauze may be applied to the suture areas to reduce swelling and promote comfort. Analgesia may be provided with the milder oral analgesics.

Repair of a cleft palate is usually completed when the child is 12 to 18 months of age, preferably before the beginning of speech. It is advantageous, again, to have a parent accompany the child in the PACU if possible. On admission to the PACU, the child is placed in the semiprone or "tonsil" position, and careful attention should be given to airway maintenance. As in cleft lip repair, the child's arms should be restrained and crying avoided. Because doing so tends to occlude the airway, the head should not be flexed.

Suctioning of secretions may be necessary but must be performed gently and only if the nurse's view is unobstructed. The catheter, plastic dental suction tip, or Yankauer suction tip should be passed over the dorsum of the tongue, and only minimal vacuum pressure should be used. A mist tent or cold-mist humidifier should be used for at least 12 hours postoperatively to aid in the elimination of tenacious secretions.

Hemorrhage may occur as a complication and requires control. Any bleeding should be recorded and reported to the surgeon. Pain may be managed with mild analgesics, such as acetaminophen elixir. Rarely, a stronger analgesic is needed.

MICROSURGERY

Microsurgery is performed with the aid of the dissecting microscope, which greatly improves visualization of the detail of small structures. Its greatest value in plastic surgery has been in the repair of small blood vessels and nerves. Postanesthesia care for the patient who has undergone microsurgery is the same as that for the principal procedure, with emphasis on notation of color changes in the skin at the operative site. White indicates that no blood is entering the area, usually because of arterial blockage. Pink is normal. Check for a blanch reflex; momentary pressure on the skin should produce white blanching, which should return to normal pink color within seconds after release of pressure. Blue indicates the presence of blood that is low in oxygen and suggests a problem. Dark blue to black with swelling indicates impending death of tissue caused by venous obstruction. Any color change from the normal pink should be reported to the surgeon immediately.

BIBLIOGRAPHY

Alspach J: Core curriculum for critical care nursing, ed 5, Philadelphia, 1998, WB Saunders.

Arnet GF, Basehore LM: Dentofacial reconstruction, Am J Nurs 84(12):1488-1490, 1984.

Atlee J: Complications in anesthesia, Philadelphia, 1999, WB Saunders.

Baj PA: Liposuction: "new wave" plastic surgery, Am J Nurs 84(7):892-893, 1984.

Barash P, Cullen B, Stoelting R: Clinical anesthesia, ed 4, Philadelphia, 2000, Lippincott Williams & Wilkins.

Benumof J, Saidman L: Anesthesia & perioperative complications, ed 2, St Louis, 1999, Mosby.

Butterworth J: Atlas of procedures in anesthesia and critical care, Philadelphia, 1992, WB Saunders.

Coté C, Todres I, Goudsouzian N, Ryan J: A practice of anesthesia for infants and children, ed 3, Philadelphia, 2001, WB Saunders.

DeFazio-Quinn D: Ambulatory surgical nursing core curriculum, Philadelphia, 1999, WB Saunders.

Fraulini KE: Nursing care of the plastic/reconstructive surgery patient, Curr Rev Recov Room Nurses 2(6):11-15, 1984.

Ganong W: Review of medical physiology, ed 20, New York, 2001, McGraw-Hill Professional.

Goodman R: Grafts and flaps in plastic surgery, AORN J 48(4):650-663, 1988.

Grossman JA: Body contouring, AORN J 48(4):713-714, 1988.

Guyton A, Hall J: Textbook of medical physiology, ed 10, Philadelphia, 2000, WB Saunders.

Jrukuwicz MJ, Drezek TJ, Mathes SG et al: Plastic surgery: principles and practices, ed 1, St Louis, 1990, Mosby.

Longnecker D, Murphy F: Dripps/Eckenhoff/Vandam introduction to anesthesia, ed 9, Philadelphia, 1997, WB Saunders.

Longnecker D, Tinker J, Morgan G: Principles and practice of anesthesiology, ed 2, St Louis, 1998, Mosby.

Motoyama E: Smith's anesthesia for infants and children, ed 6, St Louis, 1996, Mosby.

Mulliken JB: Principles and techniques of bilateral cleft lip repair, Plast Reconstr Surg 75:477-487, 1985.

Nagelhout J, Zaglaniczny K: Nurse anesthesia, ed 2, Philadelphia: W. B. Saunders, 2001.

Nagelhout J, Zaglaniczny K: Nurse anesthesia, ed 2, Philadelphia, 2001, WB Saunders.

Sauter SK: Cleft lips and palates, AORN J 50(4):813-823, 1989.

Stoelting R: Pharmacology and physiology in anesthetic practice, ed 3, Philadelphia, 1999, Lippincott-Raven.

Stoelting R, Miller R: Basics of anesthesia, ed 4, New York, 2000, Churchill Livingstone.

Stone D: Perioperative care: anesthesia, medicine, and surgery, St Louis, 1998, Mosby.

Swain D, Shell DH: Microvascular tissue transfer, AORN J 49(4):1032-1043, 1989.

Townsend C, Beauchamp R, Evers B, Mattox K: Sabiston textbook of surgery: the biological basis of modern surgical practice, ed 16, Philadelphia, 2001, WB Saunders.

Waugaman W, Foster S, Rigor B: Principles and practice of nurse anesthesia, ed 3, Norwalk, Conn, 1999, Appleton & Lange.

42

CARE OF THE THERMALLY INJURED PATIENT

Dennis M. Driscoll, PhD, RN, CCRN

A serious burn is one of the most devastating injuries that a human can sustain. It affects the skin and every organ system of the body, with the magnitude of the effect proportionate to the extent of burn. As the fifth most common cause of unintentional-injury death in the United States, thermal injury is a major health problem for which an estimated 1 million people seek medical attention annually. This represents a significant decline from estimates reported in the last decade. Approximately 45,000 are hospitalized, and an estimated 4500 die of the direct effects or complications associated with these injuries.[1] Nursing care for the thermally injured patient requires collaboration between members of a multidisciplinary healthcare team. Knowledge of the local and systemic manifestations of thermal injury is required to ensure a thorough assessment of the patient's condition and an evaluation of the patient's response.[1]

INTEGUMENTARY SYSTEM

To understand the physiologic reactions to a thermal injury, it is important to review the anatomy of the skin (Chapter 15). The skin is more than a simple hide that covers the body. It is a combination of tissues that form the largest organ of the body that provides a buffer between the internal and external environments. Skin is the body's first line of defense for protection against infection, prevention of loss of fluids, regulation of temperature, and provision of sensory input through the sense of touch.

The anatomic layers of the skin are the epidermis and the dermis. The epidermis is the outermost layer and comprises stratified squamous epithelial tissue that varies in depth from 0.07 to 0.12 mm, with the deepest areas being on the palms of the hands and the soles of the feet.[2] Histologically, the epidermis can be subdivided into five layers, the most important of which are the stratum corneum and the stratum germinativum. The stratum corneum, which is constantly shed, comprises densely packed dead cells, keratin, and surface lipids. The major function of this layer is to provide a barrier to prevent the loss of body fluids or the invasion of microbes or noxious agents from the environment. The stratum germinativum constantly undergoes subdivision to form new cells that replace those shed from surface layers. It is only in the germinativum layer that cells undergo mitosis that leads to new epithelium.

The dermis ranges in thickness from 1 to 2 mm and lies below the epidermis. This layer comprises collagen, connective tissues, smooth muscle, blood vessels, nerves, lymphatics, and glandular structures. Within the dermal layer, the sweat glands and hair follicles are lined with epithelial cells that generate epithelium to assist in the closure of partial-thickness wounds. The dermis provides nutrients and structure for the epidermis. Under the dermis lies the hypodermis, which contains fat, smooth muscle, and areolar tissue. This layer acts as a heat insulator and shock absorber.

THERMAL INJURY CLASSIFICATION

The classification of thermal injuries is based on the depth of the injury, which is directly related to the temperature and duration of exposure to the thermal energy.[3] The longer the tissue is in contact with a high temperature/heat source, the deeper the tissue destruction. Formerly, the depth of injury was identified as first-, second-, and third-degree. The preferred nomenclature for reporting depth of injury is superficial, partial-thickness, and full-thickness injury. Superficial injury involves the outermost layer of the epidermis and is usually caused by prolonged exposure to the sun. On presentation, the skin appears dry, erythematous, and usually without blisters; is painful; and has a rapid capillary refill. Systemic involvement is limited; complete healing occurs in 5 to 7 days. The magnitude of the physiologic response ranges from a minor alteration of the evaporative barrier to edema formation. The major debilitating symptom is pain. Patients with superficial injury usually do not require hospitalization.

Partial-thickness injury can be subdivided into superficial partial-thickness and deep-dermal partial-thickness injuries. These injuries are characterized by damage involving the epidermis and varying depths of the dermis. The superficial partial-thickness injury involves the epidermis with sparing of most dermal appendages. On presentation, the skin is pink or mottled red, may have formed blisters, or is wet with serous exudate. The rate of capillary refill decreases, and the wound is extremely painful. The margin of the wound is raised with respect to adjacent uninjured tissue because of the edema within the wound. This level of partial-thickness injury usually heals without skin grafting. Deep-dermal partial-thickness injury destroys the entire epidermis and most of the dermis, thus leaving only the epithelial lining of the hair follicles and sweat glands intact. On examination, the skin appears wet with serous exudate, is dark red or waxy white in color, and has a decreased sensitivity to touch. Because of the structures involved and the compromised perfusion that occurs in deep-dermal injury, mechanical trauma or infection may convert this injury to a full-thickness level.

Full-thickness injury involves the destruction of both layers of the skin to the level of hypodermis or subcutaneous tissue and may involve fat, fascia, muscle, and bone. All epithelial elements are destroyed. These wounds present as dry, charred, or pearly white and have a leathery texture. The wound is depressed relative to uninjured tissue or adjacent partial-thickness injury because of the lack of circulation, loss of elasticity, and coagulation necrosis. With the destruc-

tion of the dermal elements, these wounds are anesthetic and require autografting to close the wound.

EXTENT OF INJURY

Two methods are used to estimate the body surface area (extent) of thermal injury. The most commonly used method for rapid estimation for an adult victim is the Rule of Nines. This guideline reflects the fact that various body regions represent 9%—or multiples of 9%—of the total body surface area. The head and neck area represents 9%; the anterior and posterior trunk each represent 18%; each upper extremity represents 9%; each lower extremity represents 18%; and the perineum and genitalia represent 1% (Fig. 42-1). By determining the portion of each region involved, one can quickly estimate the percentage of injured body surface area. Because the percentage of the various regions differs with age, an age-adjusted tool is needed for infants and children. A more precise prediction can be accomplished with the Lund and Browder chart, which is an age-adjusted surface area chart (Fig. 42-2).

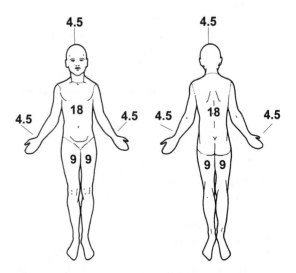

Fig. 42-1 Schematic outline of the Rule of Nines. Use of the rule provides a rapid method to determine the percentage of body surface burned, but it is of limited accuracy. *(From Townsend C, Beauchamp R, Evers B et al: Sabiston textbook of surgery: the biological basis of modern surgical practice, ed 16, Philadelphia, 2001, WB Saunders.)*

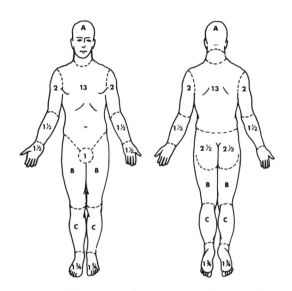

Relative Percentages of Areas Affected by Growth
(AGE IN YEARS)

	0	1	5	10	15	ADULT
A: 1/2 of head	9½	8½	6½	5½	4½	3½
B: 1/2 of thigh	2¾	3¼	4	4¼	4½	4¾
C: 1/2 of leg	2½	2½	2¾	3	3¼	3½

Total Per Cent Burned _____ 2° + _____ 3° = _____

Fig. 42-2 Classic Lund and Browder chart. The best method to determine the percentage of body surface burn is to mark the areas of injury on a chart and then compute the total percentage according to the patient's age. Every emergency department should have such a chart for plotting the burned area soon after the patient is admitted. *(From Sabiston DC Jr: Davis-Christopher textbook of surgery: the biological basis of modern surgical practice, ed 11, Philadelphia, 1977, WB Saunders.)*

TYPES OF THERMAL INJURY

Thermal injury may result from contact with heat, cold, chemicals, or electricity. Most thermal injuries are caused by flames, hot liquids, heated metals, or steam. Cold injuries may occur with immobility of body parts, even at temperatures above freezing when the humidity is high. Frostbite is characterized by the formation of intracellular fluid crystals. In patients with severe frostbite, regional ischemia with necrosis of the epidermis, the dermis, or the underlying structures occurs. Because the nursing management and wound care for frostbite are similar to the treatment for heat-related injuries, these patients may be treated in burn centers.

Chemical injury is caused by exposure to acids, alkali, or organic compounds. Acids and alkali often are used in industry for cleansing, curing, extracting, and preserving purposes. In the home, chemicals are commonly found in drain cleaners and cleaning solvents that may cause tissue damage. Most exposures to organic compounds are associated with use of fertilizers, pesticides, or petroleum products. The depth of chemical injury is the result of the concentration of the chemical and the duration of exposure. The proper use of protective clothing decreases the risk of dangerous exposure. The chemical neutralization of acids or alkali compounds is contraindicated because of the delay in treatment and risk of an exothermic reaction when acids and bases are combined.[4] Initial intervention should include removal of all dry chemical and then irrigation with copious amounts of water immediately to dilute and remove the agent. Patients who are exposed to chemical agents should be monitored for systemic toxicity, such as pulmonary insufficiency and hepatic or renal failure.[3]

Electric injuries are subdivided into low-voltage (less than 1000 V) and high-voltage (more than 1000 V) types. Electric injury is caused by the passage of electric current through the body and the conversion of electric current to heat.[5] Electrical current follows the path of least resistance, with the extent of injury related to the intensity of the current and the duration of contact time. Specific tissue resistance is irrelevant with high-voltage electric injury; the body acts as a volume conductor.[5] The contact points may be the only visible wounds, yet deep tissue damage is often sustained. The extent of injury is often difficult to assess immediately after injury and requires sequential assessment to appreciate the amount of tissue involved. Surgical exploration may be required if any indication of deep tissue damage exists, as assessed by palpation of the muscle compartments. Associated injuries such as fractures; cardiac dysrhythmias; soft tissue, vascular, and head injuries; cataracts; and neuropathies may occur secondary to electric current passage or associated falls.[6]

PATHOPHYSIOLOGY OF THERMAL INJURY

During the first 48 hours after thermal injury, systemic consequences are associated with a hypodynamic stage, followed by a hyperdynamic stage.[5,6] Organ system involvement, magnitude, and duration are proportional to the extent of the burn and reach a plateau when the injury is approximately 50% to 60% of the total body surface area.[5,6] Individuals with an injury to more than 25% of total body surface area will have immense fluid shifts from their intravascular space into the surrounding tissue because of changes in capillary permeability.[7] The initial changes in capillary integrity permit even large protein molecules to pass freely into the interstitium. For this reason, colloid-containing fluids are usually withheld until capillary integrity is restored around 24 hours after injury. Tissue edema occurs in both injured and uninjured tissue because of the changes in capillary permeability and hypoproteinemia and the volume and pressure effects of fluid resuscitation.

Redistribution of body water, electrolytes, and protein associated with the increased capillary permeability creates a decrease in the circulating blood volume. This intravascular depletion is accompanied by a sudden, abrupt decrease in cardiac output that does not correlate with the gradual reduction in blood volume.

Peripheral vascular resistance increases as a result of the neurohormonal stress response after injury. This increase in afterload contributes to the decreased cardiac output and curtails perfusion to major organ systems.

Cardiac output and organ perfusion improve with adequate fluid resuscitation. Within 36 hours after injury, cardiac function becomes supranormal. This hyperdynamic phase lasts until the burn wound is closed.[2,7]

Fluid management of the thermally injured patient requires attention to detail to prevent the potential morbidity associated with either underresuscitation or overresuscitation. Failure to deliver enough fluid may result in inadequate organ perfusion. Overresuscitation may lead to pulmonary or wound edema. Wound edema in a circumferentially injured extremity may decrease perfusion of uninjured tissue in the distal portion of that extremity.

During the early postinjury period, the individual may present symptoms of modest pulmonary hypertension. Even an individual without inhalation injury may have decreased lung compliance.[8] In the early stages of resuscitation, the minute ventilation may be decreased in a hypovolemic patient but commonly increases in proportion to the extent of burn as the resuscitative phase progresses.[5]

The kidneys experience a similar hypodynamic-hyperdynamic pattern. The consequences of diminished intravascular volume, plasma flow, and glomerular filtration rate result in decreased urine output. Acute renal failure, although rare, may result if fluid resuscitation is delayed. Approximately 24 hours after injury, vascular integrity is restored and fluid requirements decrease. This period is followed by the shift of interstitial fluid to the intravascular compartment; an ensuing diuresis occurs 48 to 72 hours after injury.[2]

The gastrointestinal tract exhibits decreased activity in patients with injuries that involve more than 25% of total body surface area.[3,9,10] A nasogastric tube should be inserted to decrease the risk of gastric dilatation, emesis, and aspiration. After adequate fluid resuscitation, normal functioning of the gastrointestinal system returns. Endoscopic studies have demonstrated that gastrointestinal ulcerations occur in 80% of critically ill patients with thermal injury without some form of prophylactic therapy. Because of the potential risk of acute stress ulcers, preventive modalities are employed for all thermally injured patients with total body surface area involvement of 35% or more.[7] Gastric pH is maintained between 3.5 and 4.5 with antacid or histamine blocker therapy.

Several hematologic changes follow a thermal injury. Although the number of red blood cells decreases after injury, the hematocrit level is usually elevated because hemoconcentration secondary to the fluid shifts occurs immediately after the injury. Some red blood cells are lysed because of direct thermal injury; however, hemolysis may continue for several days. Blood loss related to wound debridement, phlebotomy, or alterations in the coagulation system—such as thrombocytopenia, thrombocytosis, and disseminated intravascular coagulation—should be monitored closely.

The thermally injured patient is highly susceptible to infection because of alterations in host-defense mechanisms. The primary and secondary lines of defense against infection are limited with the loss of integument. Responsiveness of lymphocytes is depressed in thermally injured patients, and immunosuppressive substances can be isolated in the sera.[11] These changes occur immediately after injury and continue until the wound is closed. The immune response at the cellular level is unclear, and it can only be hypothesized whether changes are caused by the introduction of organisms or by a deficiency in components. What have been described are alterations in T-cell function, the humoral B-cell system, and nonspecific host defenses.[8,11] The immunologic responses result from complex interactions of multiple factors, including the thermal injury, nutritional deficits, stress, microbial products, and treatment.

Extensive thermal injury results in catabolism characterized by a significant elevation of the metabolic rate and loss of lean body mass.[10,12,13] Thermally injured patients manifest a negative nitrogen balance in response to the injury. The rate of catabolism may be further increased with infection. Aggressive nutritional support is needed to meet energy requirements, replace the protein losses, and promote wound healing.[9,10] Blood glucose levels increase in response to a stressful critical injury or illness. Wilmore reported that increased gluconeogenesis accounts for this hyperglycemia.[14] The gastrointestinal tract is the preferred route for feeding the thermally injured patient. If facial injury, altered levels of consciousness, or gastric ileus limit oral intake, initiation of tube feedings should be considered.[6] Total parenteral nutrition should be considered when enteral feeding is contraindicated.

WOUND MANAGEMENT

Twenty-five years ago, patients with extensive thermal injuries had a limited chance of survival. Those who survived the resuscitative phase often succumbed to overwhelming infection. Although wound treatment modalities are initiated at the time of admission, they become the focus of care during the acute phase. The goals of wound management are the prevention of infection, the preservation of tissue, timely wound closure, and the maintenance and restoration of function. Nursing care rendered in the postanesthesia care unit (PACU) is important in the attainment of these goals.

All the energies invested in the care of the thermally injured patient are directed at a single outcome: the transformation of a contaminated open wound to a clean closed wound. The open wound is associated with the hypermetabolic and physiologic stress responses that do not become corrected until the wound is closed.[5] Current wound management after resuscitation involves excision of the necrotic tissue and coverage of the wound.[15] Advantages of early excision include early mobilization, reduction of pain, early wound closure, reduced risk of infection, and reduced length of hospital stay. Disadvantages include exposure to surgical stress in the early postresuscitation period and the risk of excising viable tissue that might heal.[5,16,17]

The necrotic tissue, foreign material, and cellular debris are mechanically removed from the burn wound by either a tangential or full-thickness excision. Tangential excision is the sequential removal of thin layers of necrotic tissue until viable tissue with an adequate blood supply is reached. This débridement technique may be used for both superficial and deep-dermal partial-thickness injury.[5,16,17]

Full-thickness excision involves the removal of nonviable tissue to the level of viable tissue, usually down to subcutaneous fat or fascia, with scalpel or electrocautery techniques. Excision of an area of thermal injury that exceeds 20% of the total body surface at one time is not recommended because of surgical stress and the magnitude of blood loss. Each operative procedure is limited to 20% of the total body surface area or 2 hours of operative time. Time between procedures allows for recovery and reepithelialization of donor sites.[15,16]

After the excision is complete, hemostasis must be achieved. Topical thrombin may be sprayed onto the excised bed and are followed by the placement of warm, moist laparotomy pads. An alternative method is the application of gauze sponges soaked in 1:10,000 epinephrine solution to the wound bed.[17] Pressure is then applied by application of a circumferential gauze dressing. After approximately 10 minutes, the pressure dressing is gently removed. Specific sites of bleeding are identified and cauterized or ligated.

Many skin grafting techniques are available to the surgeon who manages the care of the thermally injured patient. For the purposes of this chapter, only the definitive closure of the wound is addressed. Once the necrotic tissue is removed, the exposed underlying tissues must be covered to provide protection and prevent infection. The definitive covering is autograft skin. A portion of the patient's epidermis with a partial layer of dermis is removed from a region of unburned tissue using a dermatome. This tissue is referred to as a split-thickness skin graft and can be applied as an intact sheet or with an expanded meshed sheet to the wound bed. A full-thickness skin graft is one in which a segment of full dermis and epidermis is transplanted to a recipient site.[12,13,17] The skin graft is secured in place by fibrin glue, staples, sutures, an immobilizing dressing and splints, or a combination of these methods.

Split-thickness grafts typically vary in thickness from 0.01 to 0.035 inches. Sheet grafts are preferred when the wound location has cosmetic or functional importance—such as on the face, neck, hands, and feet. In the postanesthesia period, nurses must assess the healing grafts for the presence of hematoma or seromas, which may prevent graft adherence.

Meshed autograft skin is indicated for patients with extensive thermal injury, because meshing allows for maximum coverage of wounds from limited donor sites. The mesh graft's interstices allow the escape of blood and plasma, thus decreasing the risk of interference with graft vascularization. The meshed autografts are usually expanded one and one half to four times their normal size. A layer of fine-mesh and coarse-mesh gauze soaked in an antimicrobial or saline solution is applied directly over the grafts and is secured with roller gauze. This dressing prevents the desiccation of the exposed wound bed until the interstices are closed by epithelial migration.

The donor site selection may be limited by the extent of the injury but cosmetic or functional outcomes should be considered, if possible. After the harvesting of the skin grafts, the newly created partial-thickness wound at the donor site must be protected against maceration and infection. Management of these wounds includes the application of various types of dressings or temporary coverings.[12,13,16,17] Fine-mesh gauze is often applied directly over the donor site. Blood is evacuated from beneath the gauze by using a straight edge such as scissors or scalpel handle, and the dressing is allowed to dry. Donor site care in the PACU requires the application of radiant heat to begin drying this dressing. Any insult—such as mechanical trauma, heat or cold injury, and infection—may convert this surgically created partial-thickness wound to a full-thickness injury.

Most operative procedures on thermally injured patients are performed with the patient under general anesthesia. Ketamine may be administered to the thermally injured patient for anesthesia or analgesia. The advantages of ketamine induction include the production of intense analgesia and maintenance of normal pharyngeal and laryngeal reflexes.

Regional anesthesia may be used for local débridement. If grafting is to be completed following the excision, regional anesthesia may not be adequate to allow harvest of donor sites from areas remote from the excision. For additional information on anesthetics, see Section III.

PERIANESTHESIA NURSING CARE

In healthcare facilities that have a specialty care unit for the treatment of thermally injured patients, perianesthesia care is typically provided in that unit. If a thermally injured patient must receive care in a PACU, selected factors in addition to standard perianesthesia care must be considered. Ambient room temperature should be maintained at 85°F to prevent hypothermia. Infection control policies—including isolation procedures, handwashing techniques, and a strict dress code—should be developed for the PACU that treats this unique patient population.

Perianesthesia nursing care for thermally injured patients includes recovery from anesthesia, proper positioning, immobilization to prevent autograft disruption, use of restraints as appropriate, prevention of hypothermia, inspection of dressings for signs of hemorrhage, and adequate pain management. Assessment and documentation are critical components of nursing management during the perianesthesia period. Assessment must be directed primarily toward the maintenance of a patent airway and adequate respiration and circulation. Standard procedures for the management of patients who are recovering from anesthesia should be used. The secondary assessment focuses on the donor and graft sites. Documentation should include a review of systems plus the location of graft and donor sites, the appearance of the dressings, patient position, and all medications administered.

Specific wound care depends on the operative procedure and the location of the operative site. The most common cause of graft loss is mechanical shear from movement of the grafted body part. Immobilizing the joint above and below the grafted region is necessary. Most split-thickness mesh grafts are dressed with a nonadherent material, covered by coarse-mesh gauze, and secured with roller gauze. Immobilization is accomplished by applying splints over the dressings. Although hemostasis is achieved intraoperatively, postoperative increases in blood pressure and movement may cause bleeding at the operative sites. If bleeding occurs, the surgeon should be notified.

Sheet skin grafts are generally not dressed to allow direct visualization. Sheet grafts must be assessed for the accumulation of blood or serum under the graft. Formation of hematomas or serous blebs between a graft and the wound bed requires evacuation to prevent graft loss. Fluid accumulations beneath the graft may be aspirated with a small syringe and needle. The surgeon may make a small incision near a bleb to allow the fluid to be expelled or use a cotton-tipped applicator to "roll" the fluid to the edges of the graft.[16]

In the immediate perianesthesia period, the donor sites should receive heat and aeration to promote drying. The nurse must ensure that donor sites remain clean, dry, and free from pressure. With proper care, multiple skin grafts can be harvested from the same location.[16]

Thermal injuries are one of the most painful forms of trauma that one can experience, and pain management provides a major challenge for the perianesthesia nurse. Astute nursing assessment and evaluation are required to differentiate restlessness caused by pain from other causes, such as hypoxia and bladder or gastric distention. Pain can be reduced by frequent intravenous administration of small doses of morphine sulfate (3 to 5 mg in adults).[2,18] Intramuscular injections should be avoided during the postoperative period because the normal fluid shifts may impair soft-tissue circulation, thus rendering analgesia ineffective. As circulatory integrity is restored, narcotics previously deposited in the muscles and subcutaneous tissue may be mobilized and possibly lead to an overdosage. Continuous infusion of intravenous narcotics may be an effective technique to produce a constant level of analgesia but requires careful monitoring for undesirable physiologic effects.[10,16]

SUMMARY

The nursing care of the thermally injured patient provides an exciting challenge for the perianesthesia nurse. With the advent of successful resuscitation formulas, new surgical techniques, improved nutritional delivery systems, and innovative wound management interventions, the survival rate of patients with major thermal injury has greatly improved. However, the nurse must continue to understand the rationale for intervention to provide optimal monitoring and evaluation of these patients in the perianesthesia period. Outcomes are enhanced when all members of the healthcare team provide collaborative care for the severely injured patient.

REFERENCES

1. Burn Foundation: Burn incidence and treatment in the U.S.: 2000 fact sheet (accessed online at www.ameriburn.org/pub/factsheet.htm).
2. Sheridan RL: Evaluating and managing burn wounds, Dermatology Nur 12:17, 2000.
3. National Burn Institute: Advanced burn life support course manual, Lincoln, Neb, 1990, National Burn Institute.
4. Bates N: Acid and alkali injury, Emerg Nur 7:21, 1999.
5. Pruitt BA Jr, Goodwin CW Jr: Thermal injuries. In Davis JH, Drucker WR, Foster RS et al, editors: Clinical surgery, St Louis, 1987, Mosby.
6. Pruitt BA Jr, Treat RG: The burn patient. In Dudrick SJ, Bave AE, Eiseman B et al, editors: Manual of preoperative and postoperative care, Philadelphia, 1983, WB Saunders.
7. Cummings J, Purdue GF, Hunt JL et al: Objective estimates of the incidence and consequences of multiple organ dysfunction and sepsis after burn trauma, J Trauma 50:510, 2001.
8. Arturson MG: The pathophysiology of severe thermal injury, J Burn Care Rehabil 6:129, 1985.
9. Carlson DE, Jordan BS: Implementing nutritional therapy in the thermally injured patient, Crit Care Nurs Clin North Am 3:221, 1991.
10. Romito RA: Early administration of enteral nutrients in critically ill patients, AACN Clin Issues 6:242, 1995.
11. Warden GD: Immunologic response to burn injury. In Boswick JA, editor: The Art and science of burn care, Rockville, Md, 1987, Aspen.
12. Gueugniaud PY, Carson H, Bertin-Mayht M et al: Current advances in the initial management of major thermal burns, Intensive Care Medicine 26:848, 2000.
13. Kao CC, Garner WL: Acute burns, Plastic Reconstructive Surgery 10:2482, 2000.
14. Wilmore DW: Metabolic changes after thermal injury. In Boswick JA, editor: The art and science of burn care, Rockville, Md, 1987, Aspen.
15. Kravitz, M: Thermal injuries. In Cardona VD, Hurn PD, Bastnagel Mason PJ et al, editors: Trauma nursing: from resuscitation through rehabilitation, Philadelphia, 1994, WB Saunders.
16. Duncan DJ, Driscoll DM: Burn wound management, Crit Care Nurs Clin North Am 3:199, 1991.
17. Heimbach DM: Early burn wound excision and grafting. In Boswick JA, editor: The art and science of burn care, Rockville, Md, 1987, Aspen.
18. Molter NC: Pain in the burn patient. In Punctillo KA, editor: Pain in the critically ill: assessment and management, Rockville, Md, 1991, Aspen.

BIBLIOGRAPHY

DeSantis D, Phillips P, Spath MA et al: Delayed appearance of a circulating myocardial depressant factor in burn patients, Ann Emerg Med 10:22-24, 1981.

How S, Chan HH, Ying SY, Cheng HS et al: Skin care in burn patients: a team approach, Burns 27:489, 2001.

Hunt JP, Calvert CT, Peck MD et al: Occupational-related burn injuries, J Burn Care Rehab 21:327, 2000.

Linneman PK, Terry BE, Burd RS: The efficacy and safety of fentanyl for the management of severe procedural pain in patients with burn injury, J Burn Care Rehab 6:519, 2000.

Meeker MH, Rothrock JL, Alexander EL: Alexander's care of the patient in surgery, St Louis, 1999, Mosby.

Still JM Jr, Law EJ: Primary excision of burn wounds, Clin Plas Surg 27:23, 2000.

Teodorczyk-Injeyon JA, Cembrzybske-Nowak M, Lolani S et al: Immune deficiency following thermal trauma is associated with apoptotic cell death, J Clin Immunology 15:318, 1995.

Wallace BH, Caldwell FT Jr, Cone JB: The interrelationships between wound management, thermal stress, energy metabolism, and temperature profiles of patients with burns, J Burn Care Rehab 15:499, 1994.

Weinberg K, Birdsell C, Vail D et al: Pain and anxiety with burn dressing changes: patient self report, J Burn Rehab 21:155, 2000.

Wolman R, Luterman A: The continuous infusion of morphine sulfate for analgesia in burn patients: extending the use of an established technique. In Proceedings of the American Burn Association, Seattle, 1988.

43

CARE OF THE AMBULATORY SURGICAL PATIENT

Nancy Burden, RN, MS, CPAN, CAPA

Ambulatory surgery continues as an area of growth, both in numbers of patients and in advancing knowledge and technology. Today more than half of all surgeries performed in the United States are done on an outpatient basis. Baby boomers are now hitting their late fifties, and we are beginning to see the effects of their assault on health care. Not only will this huge generation place demands on healthcare providers simply because of their numbers; they will also bring demands for the best and fastest care as typical of their generation. The great mobility of the population in the United States brings another challenge as families are scattered, thus reducing the stronger family support systems of years past.

A variety of factors drive the move toward outpatient surgery. Foremost, experience over the past thirty-plus years has shown the process to be successful and safe. Overall clinical outcomes have not suffered from shortened postoperative hospitalization in appropriate patients. In fact, avoiding a hospital stay can reduce the opportunity for nosocomial infection and medical errors.

Third-party payers—including insurance companies, health maintenance organizations, and the federal government—generally mandate that surgical procedures be performed in the lowest appropriate cost setting for payment eligibility. Thus the trend has been to push procedures from hospitals to outpatient settings to physician offices. Ambulatory surgery and hospital industry organizations continually work with federal agencies to lobby for appropriate placement of procedures. Federal payment decisions often result in managed care companies following suit; therefore this is a very important focus for administrators

in all levels of healthcare settings. A discrepancy still exists in government reimbursement for the same procedures done in a hospital outpatient department (HOPD) versus in a freestanding ambulatory surgery center (FASC), financially favoring the former.

In addition to the financial pressures of identifying and using the most cost-effective site for surgical procedures, other factors have contributed to the trend of same-day admission and early postoperative discharge. Technologic advances in instrumentation and equipment allow more complex procedures to be done with less invasiveness and physical trauma. Examples include lithotripsy and laparoscopic, endoscopic and arthroscopic approaches in a multitude of surgical specialties from sinus surgery to orthopedics, urology, gynecology, and more.

Innovative procedures have come on the market, although they are currently self-pay procedures because Medicare does not approve payment. They are outpatient procedures in the HOPD, FASC, or physician offices. Examples include orthotripsy—similar in concept to lithotripsy but for treatment of heel spurs—and cosmetic procedures such as new approaches to eliminate unsightly veins. Some of these procedures remain controversial in medical circles as to their merit.

The pharmacologic industry has developed shorter-acting anesthetic agents and adjunctive drugs that allow quicker return to alertness and self-care and have fewer unpleasant side effects. Also, consumers are more educated and sophisticated than in past generations, and current fast-paced lifestyles lend themselves to "in and out" care.

In response to the special needs of patients who require nursing care in a much shortened time span, ambulatory perianesthesia nursing addresses patient needs related to both anesthesia and surgery. Specific emphasis is placed on providing rapid yet comprehensive patient assessment along with complete, understandable patient and family education. Ambulatory surgical nurses encourage the patient's self-care and self-responsibility for preadmission and postdischarge compliance with the planned medical and nursing care, and then must assess the patient's ability, desire, and intentions to comply. In addition, these nurses emphasize the patient's early ambulation and return to normal life activities, patient teaching, and family involvement in the patient's care.

It is important to recognize and address the social, emotional, and educational needs of patients as well as the physical. Many people will ask all the questions they have, but in many cases unspoken questions linger for patients and their families. These may relate to the final outcome of the procedure relating to their health and well-being, financial burdens, doubts about the availability and quality of postoperative support at home, their vulnerability, and if and how quickly they will be able to resume full preoperative life activities. Nurses should provide open doors for these types of questions and discussions.

Home support is essential because the patient returns home so quickly after surgery. Involvement of the family or another responsible adult is integral to the overall plan of care. Postoperative complications such as nausea and vomiting might otherwise be considered minor or merely unpleasant for hospitalized patients who have nursing support. For ambulatory surgical patients, however, these problems become serious deterrents to discharge and can lead to costly, prolonged hospital stays, unplanned hospitalizations, or unpleasant home recuperations.

The basic tenet of nursing care in this setting is the promotion of wellness and self-care to the degree possible. Patients should be continually encouraged to think positively and to provide self-care as is appropriate and possible. Orem's general theory of nursing—the Self-Care Deficit Nursing Theory—can be used to describe nursing planning and intervention appropriate to the ambulatory surgical patient.[1] The nurse calculates the patient's self-care demand and shares with the patient what he or she must do to regain or promote health in relation to postoperative recovery. Nursing actions revolve around teaching the patient and family, gaining their acceptance of the prescribed actions, and then assessing the degree to which the nurse feels the patient can and will comply.

The concept of self-fulfilling prophecy is also an important tool that nurses can employ to help patients expect success and comfort. According to this concept, an outcome is more likely to happen just because the patient expects it. The outcome is "preprogrammed" by the patient's outlook; thus the nurse's programming of wellness and uneventful recovery can be an important tool to shape the patient's mindset.

Whether the patient has surgery in a hospital setting, a freestanding ambulatory surgical center, or in the physician's office, basic nursing needs remain the same. That care combines both critical assessment and monitoring during periods of high dependence, such as immediately after general anesthesia or sedation, with periods when the patient is encouraged and taught how to assume responsibility for self-care. This care often is provided through a two-phase recovery process: the initial postanesthesia care unit (PACU) and a less care-intensive second-phase unit from which the patient is eventually discharged.

The ambulatory surgical patient population has changed during the past thirty-plus years. More complex procedures are performed on sicker and older patients. Services such as 23-hour admission units and recovery care centers have provided a safety net of lengthier postoperative nursing care after more complex procedures, such as mastectomy, laparoscopically assisted vaginal hysterectomy, and open shoulder procedures. Some physicians are already discharging patients in a few hours or more after even these advanced procedures. Early discharge after more complex procedures becomes more common as we gain more history of patient outcomes, the frequency and extent of complications, and the level of patient acceptance based on experience and research.

Without several shifts of nurses to prepare and educate patients and families before ambulatory surgery or to tend to the patient's postoperative needs, it is important that ambulatory surgical nurses have certain characteristics. Foremost, clinical assessment skills must be accurate and rapid. Ambulatory surgical nurses should be self-motivated and able to communicate in professional terms with their peers and in lay terms with patients. The nurse's documentation skills and the forms used in the facility should allow for precise documentation of findings in minimal time. Probably most important from the patient's viewpoint, the nurse working in ambulatory surgery should present a positive, pleasant demeanor and show genuine concern for and interest in patients and their families.

ASSESSMENT AND PREPARATION OF THE PATIENT

Careful preoperative selection and preparation of patients for outpatient surgery help to reduce the risks of perioperative complications. Nonetheless many patients may be less than physically, emotionally, or socially ideal candidates yet return home soon after surgery or other procedures because of insurance requirements. In addition to systemic illnesses that limit their ability to care for themselves and possibly increase the risk of perioperative complications, many people have limited social or family support. Nurses are especially challenged to prepare these more complicated patients for an early transition to home.

The ultimate goals of complication-free recovery and early discharge are supported by what occurs preoperatively. Proper patient selection, preparation, and education all contribute significantly to eventual patient outcome. Nursing preparation must be comprehensive. Physical assessment, history taking, and evaluation of the patient's social, emotional, and cognitive status are all essential to that care. The challenge for the ambulatory surgical nurse, however, is completing all those evaluations in a condensed time frame.

Nursing care also must reach beyond the facility into the patient's home setting. This includes providing preoperative education that helps encourage preparation of a safe home setting for postoperative recuperation. Although nurses cannot be responsible for the actions of patients outside the facility, nurses do provide education, coaching, and suggestions for the patient's preoperative and postoperative care at home. The need to gain the patient's confidence and cooperation as well as to ensure the involvement of a responsible adult cannot be overstated.

Before the day of surgery, an on-site preadmission assessment is ideal for the nurse to establish a rapport with the patient, secure the patient's history, complete a physical assessment, help reduce patient anxiety, provide comprehensive preoperative instructions, identify potential risk factors, and take steps to reduce those risk factors on or before the day of surgery. However, because of the lifestyles of the patient population, the economic restrictions of healthcare providers, and the trend toward little or no diagnostic testing, a telephone contact before the day of the patient's procedure is much more common today. Although neither a physical assessment nor a facility tour can occur by telephone, all other components of the preadmission care can be provided.

High-risk patients can be identified and asked to come to the facility as appropriate for physical examination and anesthesia consultation. Identifying significant risk factors early allows time to correct any deficiencies or, if necessary, to cancel the surgery before the day it is scheduled to avoid day-of-surgery cancellations or unexpected postoperative admissions that are more costly to the institution, upsetting to the patient and physician, and generally time-consuming. For example, patients with a significant cardiac history warrant a careful cardiac assessment. Recent myocardial infarction of less than 6 weeks, unstable angina, decompensated congestive heart failure, and severe dysrhythmias or valvular disease are major predictors of perioperative risk[2] that should be considered before any surgery—but especially before elective surgery that could wait until a more stable cardiac status can be attained.

Specific instructions necessary before the day of the procedure include what arrangements the patient should make for transportation and adult support, the projected length of stay, and, in general, what to expect on the day of surgery. The patient also should be instructed in the proper clothing to wear for ease of dressing after surgery, how to prepare the home environment, what physical restrictions they may encounter postoperatively, and any equipment or supplies that he or she should purchase or secure before their arrival for surgery.

The Internet has become a common source of information for the population at large and specifically for preoperative patients. Nurses should be prepared to evaluate the value and accuracy of such information and advise the patient toward appropriate sites. An example of a valuable site for consumers who are considering surgery is that of the Agency for Healthcare Research and Quality at www.ahrq.gov. See Box 43-1 for content information. Other valuable Internet sites for patient information include the following:

- American Society of Anesthesiologists (www.asahq.org)
- American College of Surgeons (www.facs.org)
- Society for Ambulatory Anesthesia (www.sambahq.org)
- American Association of Nurse Anesthetists (www.aana.com)
- Association of Perioperative Registered Nurses (www.aorn.org)

- American Society of Perianesthesia Nurses (www.aspan.org).

The ASPAN site provides patient information on the following:

1. Preanesthetic interview/testing
2. What to expect on the day of surgery
3. Preoperative holding area
4. What to expect in the operating room
5. What to expect in the postanesthesia care unit
6. Admission to a facility
7. Outpatient surgery
8. What to expect if you are going home on the day of surgery
9. Pain management

Patients who take routine medications need instructions by the anesthesia provider about which medications should be taken on the morning of surgery, usually with a small sip of water. Medications most often continued until the

---

Box 43-1   Internet Sources of Patient Information

QUICK TIPS: WHEN PLANNING FOR SURGERY

The single most important way you can stay healthy is to be an active member of your own healthcare team. One way to get high-quality health care is to find and use information and take an active role in all of the decisions made about your care. This information will help you when planning for surgery.

No surgery is risk-free. It is important to learn about the possible benefits and risks involved in the surgical procedure you are about to have. Research has shown that patients who are informed about their procedures can better work with their doctors to make the right decisions.

Getting a second opinion is important. Your doctor, surgeon, health plan, or local medical society can help you find someone who can give you a second opinion. Before seeking a second opinion, make sure your health plan will cover this expense.

Before having surgery, ask your physician these questions:

- What operation are you recommending?
- Why do I need the operation?

- Are there alternatives to surgery?
- What are the benefits of having the operation?
- What are the risks of having the operation?
- What will happen if I don't have this operation?
- Where can I get a second opinion?
- What has been your experience in doing the operation? How many have you performed?
- Where will the operation be done?
- What kind of anesthesia will I need?
- How long will it take me to recover?
- How much will the operation cost?

Remember, quality matters, especially when it comes to your health. For more information on healthcare quality and materials to help you make healthcare decisions, please see *Quality of Health Care: "Q-Pack."*

Agency for Healthcare Research and Quality: Quick tips: when planning for surgery, AHRQ Publication No. 01–0040d, Rockville, Md, May 2002 (accessed online May 24, 2002 at www.ahrq.gov/consumer/quicktips/tipsurgery.htm).

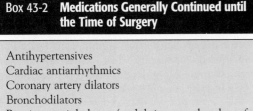

time of surgery are listed in Box 43-2. Precise instructions regarding insulin and diet on the day of surgery for patients with diabetes should be given. Although these instructions are the responsibility of the physician, they are often confirmed, reinforced, and explained by nursing personnel.

Patients should be encouraged to fill any prescriptions for postoperative medications before the day of surgery even if they believe they may not actually need analgesic medication after surgery. If patients have not yet received any prescriptions, they should know to bring money or insurance cards to obtain medications if it is likely that prescriptions will be given on the day of surgery.

Parents of small children are asked to have two adults accompany the child—one to drive and the other to attend to the child in transit to home. In some institutions, supporting adults are instructed that they must remain at the facility throughout the patient's stay. In others, only parents of minors or special needs adults are required to remain on site. Patients and families should be told about such expectations ahead of time.

The preparation of patients immediately before surgery is essentially the same as for all surgical patients. Physical assessment includes at least vital signs, breath sounds, peripheral pulses as indicated, baseline oxygen saturation levels, skin condition at the site of surgery or regional anesthetic injection, and other appropriate assessments. A valid, correct, and signed consent; verification of the fasting period, home support and driver; and careful preoperative identification of the operative site are essential.

Current pressure from government, industry, consumer and other groups to reduce medical errors and improve overall patient safety is

demonstrated by a Sentinel Event Alert regarding wrong site surgery published in December of 2001 by the Joint Commission on Accreditation of Healthcare Facilities. In their database of 150 reported cases of wrong site/person/procedure surgery collected from August 1998 through December 2001, the commission noted that 58% of errors had occurred in HOPDs and FASCs. Seventy-six percent involved surgery on the wrong body part or site; 13% involved surgery on the wrong patient; and 11% involved the wrong surgical procedure. Of the 126 cases, 41% relate to orthopedic/podiatric surgery.[3] Later clarification assigned a small percentage of those errors to FASC locations.

The Outcomes Monitoring Project of the Federated Ambulatory Surgery Association (FASA), which represents freestanding ASCs shows a low level of patient complications. For the second quarter of 2001, 68.2% of ASCs reported a complication rate of less than 3 per 1000 patient encounters, and 36.4% of ASCs reported a complication rate of 0 per 1000.[4]

Fasting Before Surgery

Fasting requirements as defined per facility by the department of anesthesia are decidedly more lenient that in the past. Traditional guidelines for "nothing after midnight" have been challenged and are now rarely used. Studies have found that prolonged fasting results in thirst, headache, irritability, hunger, and nonadherence and fails to reduce gastric volume and acidity as was formerly thought.[5] The American Society of Anesthesiologists advocates the following fasting guidelines for elective procedures that involve anesthesia and sedation[6]:

Clear liquids	2 hours for adults and children
Breast milk	4 hours preoperatively for both neonates and infants
Infant formula	6 or more hours
Light meal (e.g., toast and a clear liquid)	6 hours
Nonhuman milk	6 hours
Meal with fried or fatty foods or meat	8 or more hours

In the ambulatory surgical population, ensuring the required fasting period can be more challenging because the nurse has decidedly less opportunity to teach and less ability to control the patient who is not admitted to a hospital bed overnight. Adult patients and parents of pediatric patients must be thoroughly educated about the specifics of the fasting period. They should know that in addition to food and beverages, they should avoid water, gum, candy, coffee, and cough drops immediately before surgery. It may be helpful to explain in lay terms that although gum and hard candy are not swallowed, they stimulate the stomach to produce acids that may be harmful if aspirated. Although "scare tactics" are not appropriate, all patients must understand the seriousness of breaking the fasting period and of accurate reporting of nonadherence.

Parents should carefully monitor their children at home and in the automobile so that the child does not eat or drink without the parent's knowledge. Adolescents also may be at particular risk because of their tendency to resist authority and their misguided sense of immortality. On the day of surgery, the nurse must strive to elicit truthful and accurate verification of the patient's actual adherence.

Diagnostic Testing

Required preoperative diagnostic tests vary widely from one institution to another and are a matter both of clinical judgment by individual physicians and the policies set by the medical board that administers the ambulatory surgical program. Current trends are toward performing none or only essential diagnostic tests that are aimed at providing the basic information necessary for safe anesthesia and surgical interventions. The American Society of Anesthesiologists supports the concept that no routine or screening testing is necessary.[7] The use of generic screenings without clinical evidence of patient appropriateness has a significant financial impact on health care in the United States each year. Institutional policies prevail; however, patients should be informed before any diagnostics if a chance that their insurance will not cover specific testing (e.g., an Advanced Beneficiary Notice for Medicare recipients) exists.

Nurses responsible for preparing patients for surgery should carry out the policies of the facility for all diagnostic testing and ensure that results of any tests are included in the medical record. Abnormal results should be provided to the physician before the patient is medicated or transferred to surgery. Test results should be secured and the physician notified before the day of surgery whenever possible.

Preoperative Medications

Some providers prefer to avoid all premedications in the ambulatory surgical patient and may even encourage patients to walk to surgery to promote their sense of normalcy and self-control. Others believe that certain goals can be met pharmacologically to smooth the anesthetic course.

Preoperative medications may be given to decrease salivation; reduce anxiety; promote calmness before induction of general anesthesia; and, for children, reduce the fear and stress of separation from their parents. Antiemetic and gastrokinetic medications may be used to reduce the risk of vomiting and subsequent aspiration. Occasionally, opioids may be added to the regimen before painful procedures, although their penchant to promote nausea and vomiting often precludes their preoperative use.

When premedications are given, intravenous (IV) administration is certainly the trend. This route spares the patient from the pain of intramuscular injections and helps avoid prolonged sedative effects that can delay eventual postoperative discharge. Children particularly dread and fear "shots" and for many years may recall an injection more negatively than the surgical procedure itself. Also, many patients do not arrive at the surgical facility long enough before surgery to be given intramuscular medications and obtain the most effective results.

After the administration of any preoperative medications, patients should be monitored for allergic, atypical, or untoward drug reactions, such as respiratory or cardiac depression. Appropriate interventions to correct such situations should be initiated immediately with concurrent notification of the physician.

Emotional Support

Emotional support also helps reduce patient anxiety and potentially the associated complications—such as hypertension, tachycardia, vomiting, aspiration, and increased postoperative pain related to fear. The emotional component of nursing care while the patient is being prepared for surgery cannot be overstressed. All words spoken to the patient should be positive. Questions or statements should imply the positive aspects of recovery, particularly being able to go to a familiar and comfortable home soon after the surgery. The nurse also teaches the family directly and by example to speak in similar positive terms to encourage the patient's confident attitude. This approach supports a climate of wellness and positive outcome.

Preoperative Goals

The primary goals of preparing patients for ambulatory surgery are focused on identifying and reducing the potential risks related to surgery and anesthesia and promoting each patient's quick return to self-care. This includes a significant shift of responsibility to the patient and family by way of educating them and then encouraging and evaluating their actions. Although patient preparations may not necessarily be identical for inpatients and outpatients, they should meet the same quality standards of care. Nurses who admit and prepare patients for surgery must be thorough in their assessments; instructions must be prepared personally and with adequate equipment to intercede effectively in emergencies.

INTRAOPERATIVE PERIOD

Intraoperative care of the ambulatory surgical patient basically parallels that of all surgical patients. Specific nursing responsibilities include maintaining asepsis; properly preparing the operative site; providing for patient safety in identification, transfer and positioning; assisting the anesthesia team; maintaining confidentiality; protecting the patient's dignity; handling specimens; and documenting and reporting the intraoperative care and events.

Because of the trend to reduce or eliminate preoperative sedative medications and because a significant number of ambulatory surgical patients are given regional or local anesthesia, the perioperative nurse may care for more awake patients who are more aware of their surroundings than for those under general anesthesia. This increases the importance of monitoring and controlling the appropriateness of any discussions taking place near the patient.

Also the increased use of RN administered sedation/analgesia demands competency of the perioperative nurse in monitoring, arrhythmia detection, medication effects and side effects, and effective reversal agents. The nurse's knowledge base should also include related cardiac and respiratory anatomy and physiology, airway management, and resuscitative techniques. The availability of emergency supplies and support personnel must be ensured before the procedure begins. In particular, flumazenil and naloxone, specific reversal agents for benzodiazepines and opioids, respectively, should be immediately available to treat serious respiratory or cardiac depression related to the sedative drugs.

Anesthesia Considerations

Anesthesia for the ambulatory surgical patient incorporates the traditional goals of adequate analgesia, muscle relaxation, amnesia, and—in the event of general anesthesia—loss of consciousness to accomplish the intended procedure. Because the ambulatory surgical patient is discharged soon after the procedure, the anesthesia plan should promote reduced postoperative hangover and complications. Both general and regional anesthesia approaches are used and are sometimes combined. Regional and local techniques are favored by many clinicians because the patient does not lose consciousness, can usually be discharged sooner after the procedure, and often has the advantage of prolonged pain relief in the operative site or extremity.

The ongoing development of new and shorter-acting general anesthetic agents has significantly reduced complications such as postoperative nausea and vomiting and has encouraged rapid return to alertness, thus making general anesthesia as likely to be used as other techniques.

PERIANESTHESIA PERIOD

Recovery of ambulatory surgical patients often occurs in several stages. After general or major regional anesthesia or after intraoperative complications in any patient, a two-phase recovery is typical. Phase I begins when the patient arrives in a fully equipped and staffed PACU. Once the patient regains consciousness, lucidity, and physiologic stability and meets PACU discharge criteria, transfer to a less-intensive care unit is appropriate. Phase II of recovery is usually completed in a department equipped with lounge chairs and more homelike surroundings where families reunite and where the patient's self-care is encouraged. After local or regional anesthesia, which has a limited effect on physiologic stability, the patient is often transferred from the OR directly to the Phase II level of care.

Perianesthesia Care

After receiving a report from the OR and anesthesia personnel, the nurse applies all the usual parameters of PACU care to the ambulatory surgical patient. Airway and respiratory management are paramount. The patient is closely observed for untoward cardiac, respiratory, or other effects from anesthetic agents. The operative site and any related areas are monitored for bleeding, and any existing parenteral fluids are maintained. Further nursing duties include oxygen delivery, monitoring of vital signs and oxygen saturation, and periodic stir-up of the patient to move and deep breathe. Observation for any complications of surgery or anesthesia is coupled with rapid and appropriate nursing interventions should problems be identified.

These parameters are essential to the care of all PACU patients, but certain specific needs of ambulatory surgical patients must be met as well. Nursing care should be planned in a manner that not only identifies, reports, and treats complications in their early stages but that also reduces the risk of unpleasant complications that would delay the patient's discharge to home. For instance, the speed of progressive head elevation should be paced to the individual patient's responses. Faintness, lightheadedness, hypotension, pallor, nausea, or vomiting implies the need to lower the patient's head and begin the process again. Adequate parenteral hydration before having the patient sit upright may reduce the patient's risk of developing gastrointestinal symptoms related to hypovolemia or hypotension. Oral fluids are given slowly—with adequate time between drinks—to assess the patient's tolerance.

Pain should be managed aggressively and immediately not only because it is humane and kind to do so but also because preventing pain is easier than controlling it when it has become severe. Again, intramuscular injections may be unpleasant and, for some patients, can interfere with the goal of imminent discharge. Patients who have more complex procedures may benefit from the long action of an intramuscular injection, but for most patients, the IV route is the first choice because of its immediate effects and the shortened observation time for related complications such as respiratory depression. Provision of adequate analgesia with oral medications and general comfort measures is usually attained before the patient is transferred to the Phase II perianesthesia area.

The goal of adequate patient comfort is supported when the patient knows, before surgery, that the nurse is concerned about and eager to provide adequate pain relief. Patients should be encouraged to discuss their usual tolerance for pain and should not be judged in that regard based on the attitudes and prior experiences of the staff. They should also know that although total absence of postoperative discomfort may not be a realistic goal, acute pain should be reported and will be treated. Patient comfort—supported by positive thinking, general comfort measures, and oral analgesics—is one of the criteria by which eventual discharge readiness is measured, and this goal must be addressed even in the early stages of recovery.

In pediatric patients, some potential postoperative problems include bleeding, croup, nausea and vomiting, and fever of unknown origin—any of which can result in unplanned hospitalization. Children need gentle care and strong emotional support. The presence of one or both parents in the PACU can be quite reassuring both to the child and the parents.

Emergence delirium is more common in children than in adults. The child who is agitated and thrashing should be gently restrained to prevent self-injury. Parents who observe this behavior need explanation and support. In both children and adults, it is essential to accurately differentiate the restlessness associated with emergence delirium from other physiologic complications—such as hypoxia, bladder distention, and pain—that must be treated appropriately.

Progressive or Phase II Care

Patients who do not require the intensity of PACU care are transferred to the Phase II unit of the ambulatory surgical facility. This area is generally furnished with lounge chairs, and the decor is more homelike than in the PACU so as to encourage a sense of wellness and normalcy. The Phase II area includes a nourishment center, patient bathrooms and changing areas, and ready access to an outside door for patient discharge. As in all acute healthcare settings, emergency equipment and support personnel must be readily available.

The goals of nursing care in this setting address the patient's physical, emotional, social, educational, and spiritual needs. These are summarized in Box 43-3. The comprehensive goals also include meeting the needs of the family or other responsible adult. Close nursing observation for potential complications is ongoing during the patient's stay. Expediting a safe discharge and complication-free recuperation is the ultimate objective of all nursing and medical interventions.

Specific areas of concern in the Phase II unit include observation of cardiorespiratory status and other vital signs to ensure stability in relation to the patient's preoperative normal levels. Other goals are to ensure adequate nutrition and fluid status, provide effective pain management, avoid unpleasant gastrointestinal symptoms, observe the operative site and associated symptoms, and encourage ambulation. Observation of the patient sitting up and then walking without orthostatic hypotension, faintness, or dizziness

provides some element of confidence that he or she will be able to maneuver in a similar manner at home. Patients should be able to demonstrate proper use and care of ambulatory aids such as walkers, crutches, and casts. Existing parenteral fluids or IV access ports should be maintained until the patient is able to ambulate without faintness and discharge readiness is ensured.

The tradition of requiring a certain level of oral intake before discharge has come under scrutiny. Certainly the patient's level of hydration must be considered, but forcing oral intake on someone who has no desire or interest can be self-defeating and result in poor tolerance. The patient's appetite and desire to eat or drink are often considered the best indicators of readiness. In deciding whether to delay discharge until the patient can tolerate oral fluids, the physician considers the patient's overall condition—including gastrointestinal status, the amount of IV fluid replacement given, and the patient's likeliness to report and to handle any inability to tolerate food or fluids at home. Extensive nausea or vomiting should be effectively treated before the patient is discharged.

It is most often in the Phase II unit that patients reunite with family members or the responsible adults who will accompany and care for them at home. Early reunion should be

---

Box 43-3 **Goals of Nursing Care in Phase II Recovery Unit**

1. To provide close assessment of and attention to the patient's physical, emotional, and educational needs in the postoperative period
2. To provide an environment and personnel who are prepared for emergency interventions at all times
3. To provide family-oriented care that stresses the concept of wellness and acknowledges the integral relationship of the patient and family or other supporting adult
4. To encourage the patient toward as much self-sufficiency as possible, given the type of surgery and anesthesia performed
5. To respect the patient's right to confidentiality, privacy, and respectful, compassionate nursing care

6. To maintain accurate records of patient-related care and environmental preparedness
7. To interact with physicians and other healthcare providers in a professional manner that results in high-quality patient care
8. To provide patients and families with a resource for questions, comments, and nursing information during their stay and in the immediate period after discharge
9. To offer an environment that encourages the professional growth of nursing personnel

Adapted from Smith S: Progressive postanesthesia care: phase II recovery. In Burden N, DeFazio D, O'Brien D et al, editors: Ambulatory surgical nursing, ed 2, Philadelphia, 2000, WB Saunders.

encouraged, and nurses in this setting must purposefully involve such support people. The responsible adult may need to learn how to care for the patient's physical needs, such as changing a dressing, observing extremity circulation, or emptying drains. Encouraging a return demonstration of manual skills or having the caretaker repeat information is a good way to reinforce learning and to evaluate the person's ability to provide support. The nurse also helps the responsible adult understand that the patient should perform self-care to the extent of his or her ability and that encouraging such behavior is in the best interest of the patient for both a speedy recuperation and a positive mental outlook.

Discharging patients to home after anesthesia and invasive procedures is a serious responsibility. Planning for that discharge should begin well before the actual time of discharge, hopefully at the time the patient is scheduled for surgery. Still, it is the discharging nurse who ensures that all those plans come together. Ensuring patient safety at home and in transit may require the nurse to discuss problems with the physician and to enlist the assistance of home health agencies or transportation sources. Whatever is necessary, the nurse is ethically obliged to intervene for the patient's safety before his or her discharge.

The physician is ultimately responsible for the decision to discharge a patient; however, the nurse's application of written discharge criteria that have been previously approved by the physician staff does meet the standards of the Joint Commission on Accreditation of Healthcare Organizations.

Specific written criteria that patients must attain before discharge are included in the policies of the institution. In most facilities, it is now within the scope of the nurse's job description to apply those criteria that have been ratified by the medical oversight board when discharging patients, although any special concern about the patient's actual condition or ability to safely recuperate at home should prompt the nurse to solicit direct physician involvement in the discharge process.[8] Various areas of concern typically included in discharge criteria include vital signs; level of consciousness; comfort (pain, nausea, use of oral analgesics); activity level; surgical site; instructions; the support of a responsible adult and driver; and, to a lesser

degree, nourishment, hydration and ability to urinate.

Any patient who does not meet the facility's predetermined discharge criteria requires a specific physician's order for discharge. The nurse's notes should reflect why or how the patient did not meet existing criteria and what was done about it. For example, the criteria may require that all patients void before discharge, but a certain patient is eager to leave, cannot void after several hours of recovery, and has been discharged by the physician without meeting the criterion. The nurse should document the involvement of the physician, notification of the responsible adult about the problem area, an assessment of the patient's abdomen, the specific guidelines and instructions given to the patient about what symptoms might indicate a full bladder, the importance of avoiding over distention of the bladder, how long to wait at home without voiding before seeking care, telephone numbers given to the patient for obtaining medical assistance, and any other instructions given.

The eventual closure of documentation also should include a nursing notation regarding the patient's status related to unmet discharge criteria on the following day or later that day as ascertained by telephone contact. This last portion of comprehensive care and documentation is possible only if the person making the postdischarge telephone call is aware of such an issue. Therefore it is essential that a mechanism be in place for communication of information from one nurse to the next or that discharging nurses are personally responsible for the eventual postdischarge follow-up of patients in their care.

Before discharge, written and verbal instructions for home care should be provided. Anxiety, discomfort, and the amnesic effects of many medications given to patients can result in poor or absent recall of information from the day of surgery; therefore whenever possible, instructions should be given both to the patient and to the adult responsible for the patient after discharge.

Most facilities have developed preprinted discharge instruction sheets with carbonless copies that remain on the chart after being signed by the patient, the accompanying adult, or both, as proof that the instructions were given. In addition to the usual instructions about eating, hygiene, wound care, ambulation, return physician visit, and telephone numbers for assistance, the patient should receive a description of what symptoms may be usual and what should be reported to the physician. For instance, knowing that a slight sore throat or generalized sore muscles may follow general anesthesia helps the patient avoid worry. When those same discharge instructions have been followed by suggestions for alleviating possible minor symptoms, the patient has an even greater chance of recuperating comfortably.

The individual patient's specific needs must be addressed as well. The nurse should ensure that the physician's discharge instructions have included areas such as the following:

When should the diabetic patient resume taking insulin—and how much?
When should oral medications be resumed?
When can the patient drive, watch television, have a glass of wine?

Although it may not be verbalized by the patient or partner, many patients also want to know whether sexual intercourse should be avoided and for how long and why. Providing comprehensive discharge instructions means individualizing information for each patient.

Postdischarge Follow-Up

Mechanisms should exist for assessing and documenting patient outcomes as well as patient and family satisfaction with the care provided by the ambulatory surgical unit. Telephone calls and written surveys that can be returned by mail are two means of providing that follow-up. Written surveys most often address satisfaction issues, but evaluating the patient's recuperation from anesthesia and surgery requires a more aggressive and timely approach.

In many communities it has become a standard of care that patients are telephoned on the day after surgery to ascertain their clinical condition, safety, and comfort level. Such a contact often serves as a valuable resource for patients who may have symptoms that should be evaluated by their physicians or questions about which they are embarrassed or reluctant to telephone and ask their physicians. Not only is the patient's safety and medical condition supported, the nursing staff also can identify the effectiveness of current modes of care. Other reasons for a postdischarge call include promotion of the facility's caring attitude, identifying and reducing medicolegal issues, marketing, meeting accrediting and regulatory standards, and providing the nurse with closure and a sense of job satisfaction.

In some instances, a second call may be made at a date several weeks after the patient's discharge for the goal of assessing a particular concern related to a quality improvement or risk management study. Documentation of patient contacts via telephone should become a permanent part of the medical record. This level of follow-up after the patient's discharge closes the loop of the evaluation phase of the nursing process in the ambulatory surgery setting.

REFERENCES

1. Orem D: Nursing: concepts of practice, ed 5, St Louis, 1995, Mosby.
2. Marley RA, Kremer MJ, Alves SL: Perioperative evaluation and preparation of the patient. In Nagelhout JJ, Zaglaniczny KL, editors: Nurse anesthesia, ed 2, Philadelphia, 2001, WB Saunders.
3. Joint Commission on Accreditation of Healthcare Facilities: Sentinel Event Alert, Issue 24, Chicago, 2001, JCAHO (accessed online May 25, 2002 at www.jcaho.org/sentinel/sentevnt_frm. html).
4. Federated Ambulatory Surgery Association: FASA responds to JCAHO alert on wrong site surgery, Alexandria, Va, December 7, 2001, FASA (accessed online May 25, 2002 at www.fasa.org/ pr120701.htm).
5. Green CR, Pandit SK, Schorck MA: Preoperative fasting time: are the traditional guidelines changing? Anesth Analg 83:123-128, 1996.
6. American Society of Anesthesiologists: Practice guidelines for preoperative fasting and the use of pharmacologic agents to reduce the risk of pulmonary aspiration: application to healthy patients undergoing elective procedure, Park Ridge, Ill, American Society of Anesthesiologists (accessed online May 25, 2002 at www.asahq.org /practice/npo/npoguide.html).

7. American Society of Anesthesiologists: Statement on routine preoperative laboratory and diagnostic screening. Approved by House of Delegates October 14, 1987. (Last amended October 13, 1993, Park Ridge, Ill.)

8. Joint Commission on Accreditation of Healthcare Organizations: 2002-2003 Standards for Ambulatory Care, Chicago, 2002, JCAHO, PE 1.8.4.1: 47, 176.

CARE OF THE LASER/LAPAROSCOPIC SURGICAL PATIENT

Vallire Hooper, MSN, RN, CPAN

The evolution of laser and laparoscopic procedures over the last decade has greatly changed the face and pace of perianesthesia nursing care. More and more procedures are done on an outpatient basis. Patients who undergo procedures that 10 years ago required lengthy hospitalizations are now discharged within 24 to 48 hours. Much of this increase in ambulatory surgery and rapid hospital discharge has been driven by reimbursement and insurance issues. Anesthetic innovations such as BIS monitoring, improved inhalational agents and muscle relaxants, and advances in pain management and regional anesthetic/analgesic techniques have also had a positive impact. Technologic advances in surgical techniques, however, have had the greatest impact because these advances allow more complex procedures with less trauma to the patient. Laser and laparoscopic techniques form the foundation for many of these surgeries.

This chapter will provide an overview of laser and laparoscopic technologies and how use of this technology affects perianesthesia patient care. Details of the care of patients undergoing specific procedures may be found in the appropriate systems chapters throughout the book.

LASER SURGERY

The term "laser" is actually an acronym for *light amplification by stimulated emission of radiation.* It describes a process by which energy is converted into a light form or light energy. The theory on which laser technology is based was developed by Albert Einstein in 1917. Schawlow and Townes further explored this theory and developed the LASER principle in 1958; the first true laser device was built by Dr. Theodore H.

Maiman in 1960. Laser devices, although initially controversial, revolutionized surgical procedures; technology and use continue to expand.[1] The benefits of laser assisted surgery are many (Box 44-1).

Laser Light

Ordinary light travels in waves that have four distinct properties: wavelength, amplitude, velocity, and frequency. Laser light differs from ordinary light in three ways that makes it both unique and effective in the surgical setting.[2-4]

1. Ordinary light is polychromatic, which means that it comprises a multiple array of colors or wavelengths. Laser light, on the other hand, is monochromatic and thus is all one color or wavelength. This pure color of the laser beam can determine how it will react with certain tissues.
2. Laser light is also collimated. The light waves travel parallel to each other as they travel and do not diverge or spread. Ordinary light spreads out in space as it travels (Fig. 44-1). Collimation reduces the loss of power and allows for better focus and precision.
3. Laser light is coherent. All of the waves travel in the same phase and direction and all of the peaks and troughs of the waves are synchronized. Ordinary light, on the other hand, is incoherent as its waves travel out in random directions (Fig. 44-2). This coherence gives the laser beam its power.

Tissue Interaction

Four different interactions can occur when laser energy comes into contact with human tissue

627

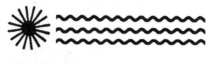

Box 44-1 The Benefits of Laser Surgery[2]

- Seals small blood vessels, thus reducing intraoperative and postoperative blood loss
- Decreases postoperative edema and the chance of the spread of malignant cells by sealing lymphatics
- Seals nerve endings, thus reducing postoperative pain in certain procedures
- Sterilizes tissue as a result of the heat generated by the laser
- Decreases scarring through the reduction of postoperative stenosis
- Laser beam precision minimizes tissue damage
- Decreased operative and anesthesia time
- Increased use of local anesthetic techniques as opposed to general anesthesia
- More procedures can be done on an ambulatory basis
- Quicker recovery and return to activities of daily living

Fig. 44-2 Coherent versus incoherent light. *(From Ball K: Lasers: the perioperative challenge, ed 2, St Louis, 1995, Mosby.)*

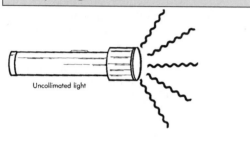

Uncollimated light

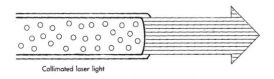

Collimated laser light

Fig. 44-1 Collimated versus uncollimated light. *(From Ball K: Lasers: the perioperative challenge, ed 2, St Louis, 1995, Mosby.)*

(Fig. 44-3). The extent this interaction is dependent on the wavelength of the laser, power settings, spot size, contact time of the laser beam with the tissue, and the characteristics of the tissue. These interactions can have both positive and negative effects.[1-4]

1. Reflection. Reflection occurs when the direction of the laser beam is changed after it comes in contact with an area. This direction change can be intentional or accidental and thus can have both positive and negative effects. Mirrors can be used to intentionally reflect the laser beam to direct the beam to a hard-to-reach area. This must be done carefully, however, to prevent an inadvertent strike and possible damage to a nontargeted area. Reflection can also occur if the laser beam hits an obstacle (such as a surgical instrument) and then is inadvertently reflected to another area, thus causing a tissue burn.

2. Scattering. The laser beam can also scatter as it comes into contact with certain tissues. This scattering causes the beam to disperse over a

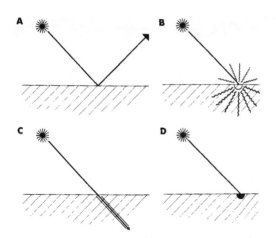

Fig. 44-3 Laser tissue interaction: **A,** Reflection. **B,** Scattering. **C,** Transmission. **D,** Absorption. *(From Ball KA: Surgical modalities. In Meeker MH, Rothrock JC, editors: Alexander's care of the surgical patient, St Louis, 1999, Mosby.)*

Table 44-1	**Tissue Changes with Temperature Increases**	
Temperature	Visual Change	Biologic Change
37°C-60°C	No visual change	Warming, welding
60°C-65°C	Blanching	Coagulation
65°C-90°C	White/gray	Protein denaturization
90°C-100°C	Puckering	Drying
100°C	Smoke plume	Vaporization, carbonization

From Ball KA: Endoscopic surgery, St Louis, 1997, Mosby.

large area and weakens its strength. Backscattering can also occur as the beam scatters backward up the endoscope, thus causing damage to the operator's eye and/or the optics or distal end of the scope.

3. Transmission. Transmission occurs when the laser beam passes or is transmitted through fluids or tissue with little or no thermal effect. Transmission depends on the active medium of the laser and the tissue that it comes in contact with. For example, an argon laser beam can be transmitted through the clear structures and solutions of the eye to coagulate a bleeding vessel on the retina. This occurs because the argon energy is not absorbed by clear structures and solutions; therefore no thermal effect is noted on these tissues.

4. Absorption. Thermal effects and tissue response occur only when tissue absorbs the energy of the laser that contacts it. The amount of absorption and penetration depends on the beam's wavelength and power, the characteristics of the contact tissue (color, consistency, and water content), the duration of the beam exposure, and the beam spot size. As the tissue absorbs the laser energy, a thermal response occurs, and the contact cells are heated. The degree of tissue change or thermal damage depends on the temperature to which the cells are heated. This temperature change is purposely regulated to effect the desired tissue response (Table 44-1).

Types of Lasers
Lasers are classified by the four active mediums (gas, solid, liquid, and semiconductor crystals) used to generate the laser energy. In a gas medium, electrical energy is pumped through a gas (such as argon) to produce the laser energy. A solid medium uses a special rod doped with an element that is activated by exposure to flash lamps to create the laser energy. Liquid mediums are organic dyes that produce a wide range of wavelengths when activated by another laser beam. Semiconductor crystals are used in the medical field as well as in consumer products and fiberoptic communication systems. Experimental mediums that are currently being explored include metal vapor and free electrons. The actual laser name is derived from the medium substance that is used to generate the laser energy.[3,5] A summary of the various lasers currently in use can be found in Table 44-2.

Preoperative Care
Preoperative care, as with any procedure, focuses on the adequate preoperative assessment and preparation of the patient. Although procedure specific issues are addressed in other chapters,

Table 44-2 Summary of Laser Types and Uses[1,2,6-22,41]

Name	Active Medium	Special Characteristics	Uses
Ruby Laser	Solid	First successful medical laser Has been replaced by newer technology	Tattoo and hair removal
Nd:YAG	Solid	Transmitted through clear fluids and structures and more highly absorbed by darker tissue Can be focused to a precise diameter for precise procedures in tight areas such as the middle ear Also provides good penetration depth, although the energy is not highly focused and the laser light tends to scatter, thus causing thermal damage to approximately 5 mm Can be delivered in a contact and noncontact mode	Primary function is coagulation Special pulsed mode also used in ophthalmology Used for skin rejuvenation and removal of pigmented lesions and tattoos in dermatology Interstitial laser prostatectomy Various applications also used in gastroenterology, pulmonary, oral surgery, and gynecology
Erbium:YAG	Solid	Highly absorbed by water Shallow depth of penetration	Used for oral surgery, ophthalmic surgery, dermatology Used with endoscopes
Holium:YAG	Solid	Produces a vapor bubble to transmit the beam to the tissue in fluid environments Shallow depth of penetration Ablates tissue very precisely Can be conducted through a flexible fiber	Transmyocardial revascularization Oral surgery Many other applications in the surgical arena
Frequency-doubled (KTP) YAG	Solid	Depth of penetration dependent on wavelength	Used with flexible or rigid endoscopes Used for general surgery, urology, gastroenterology, neurosurgery, otorhinolaryngology, dermatology, cosmetic surgery
CO_2	Gas	Most versatile laser Can be operated in continuous or pulsed modes Different tissue and thermal effects can be created by varying the length and frequency of each pulse Highly absorbed by water Requires an articulating arm system for delivery	Performs coagulation, cutting, and vaporization functions Transmyocardial revascularization Popular for use in cutaneous laser resurfacing Also used in the following surgical specialties: general, gynecology, ENT, neurosurgery, plastic surgery, dermatology, oral surgery

Table 44-2 Summary of Laser Types and Uses[1,2,6–22,41]—cont'd

Name	Active Medium	Special Characteristics	Uses
Argon	Gas	Transmitted through clear structures and solutions Moderate depth of penetration Highly selective to pigmented tissue such as hemoglobin, melanin, and other similar tissues Because of the high selectivity of the beam to pigmented tissues, adjacent tissue injury is significantly reduced	Used with rigid endoscopes Very well suited for ophthalmic surgery Used in dermatology for the ablation of vascular and pigmented lesions Also used in gastroenterology, gynecology, and otology
Krypton	Gas	Used in ophthalmology as an alternative to the argon laser	Very effective for selective photocoagulation procedures Used primarily in ophthalmology Also used for the removal of pigmented lesions
Dye	Liquid	Patient is injected with dye 24 to 48 hours before procedure Abnormal tissues retain the dye, and the laser selectively destroys that tissue Variable wavelengths and depth of penetration varies according to the dye used	Used primarily in ophthalmology and dermatology Limited applications such as photodynamic therapy and for vascular lesions Used with flexible or rigid endoscopes
Excimer	Excited dimer (argon-fluoride)	Complex delivery system Gases are extremely toxic and require appropriate laser housings and exhausts Very large and require more floor space	Excellent cutting capabilities with no significant damage to the adjacent tissue Has been used very successfully to sculpt corneas for refractive purposes and to ablate plaque in arteries Also used for phototherapeutic keratectomy procedures Other uses in orthopedics and dermatology also being explored
Diode	Semiconductor crystals	Extremely compact, efficient, and reliable	Often used in consumer products such as video disc players and computers Now being used for surgical lasers primarily in ophthalmic and urologic applications such as interstitial laser prostatectomy

Continued

Table 44-2 Summary of Laser Types and Uses[1,2,6–22,41]—*cont'd*

Name	Active Medium	Special Characteristics	Uses
			Other applications—including pain management, oral surgery, and treatment of leg vein telangiectasia—are being explored
Free-electron	Relativistic electron beam		Investigations of use in photodynamic therapy of tumors, neurosurgery, treatment of psoriasis, and possible treatment of hyperbilirubinemia are being explored

certain issues unique to laser surgery must be addressed in this discussion. One of those issues is appropriate patient selection. Procedure specific requirements and contraindications must be evaluated.

For example, transmyocardial laser revascularization (TMLR) is generally limited to patients with advanced cardiovascular disease and who are hemodynamically stable and not candidates for traditional bypass surgery. Several thallium-201 scans must be conducted preoperatively to differentiate healthy and ischemic tissues and determine the number of channels needed.[14,20,23] Dermatologic procedures may require extensive skin prepping at home, preoperative administration of prophylactic antibiotics and/or antivirals, multiple treatments, and extensive postoperative skin care regimens that may last postoperatively up to a month or more.[10,12,16,22] Preoperative care must include education concerning these issues and must determine whether the patient will be able to comply with the treatment regimen.

The patient must also be prepared for what to expect both during and after surgery. Many of these procedures are conducted without any anesthesia or with moderate sedation. The patient must be prepared for the sights, smells, and other sensations that he or she will experience. Eye protection must be worn by all people in the operating room, including the patient. Odors may include the smell of flesh burning or vaporizing.

The patient may also experience burning and/or stinging types of painful sensations with certain procedures.

Intraoperative Issues

Intraoperative issues concerning laser procedures primarily concern safety. Lasers are considered a class III medical device and, as such, are subject to U.S. Food and Drug Administration (FDA) jurisdiction. Many other regulatory, industry, and professional bodies also address the safe use of lasers. Regulations addressed include the registration of laser devices, training requirements, laser safety officer responsibilities, and safety rules.[4,5]

A laser safety program should be in place in any facility in which laser procedures are conducted. This includes freestanding ambulatory facilities and physician's offices. A laser safety committee complete with a laser safety officer should be established and responsible for guiding and overseeing all laser use in the facility. Issues that should be addressed include staff education, physician credentialing, and the monitoring of quality and safety issues. All staff involved in laser use must receive appropriate education before using or being involved in laser procedures. Topics included in these special training classes include laser biophysics, laser equipment, laser-tissue interaction, safety procedures, and clinical applications. Knowledge and skills should be verified through a competency based credentialing program and the skills reassessed and updated on a regular basis.[1,4,5]

The three most important areas of safe laser use include eye protection, smoke evacuation, and fire safety. The eyes are very susceptible to damage from laser radiation. The damage may occur acutely or may go unnoticed and develop gradually over time. The type of damage will also vary with the type of laser. Anyone who enters an operating room where a laser is in use (including the patient) is at risk for eye damage and therefore should wear protective eyewear specific to the laser in use. Filtering devices should also be placed on operative microscopes and endoscopes. The patient's eyes should also be protected with either the appropriate eyewear or moist gauze pads.[1,2,4]

Another major safety concern with the use of laser technology is the control of the smoke that the laser produces. This smoke is called the laser or surgical plume and can contain particles of vaporized tissues, toxins, and steam that are extremely small and capable of coating the alveoli over time, thus leading to respiratory conditions and complications. Even short exposure may be related to headaches, nausea, myalgia, rhinitis, and conjunctivitis. Patients may also experience these symptoms. As such, a smoke evacuation system with high-efficiency particulate air filters should be used whenever a smoke plume is generated. This system should be maintained as close to the laser-tissue impact site as possible. All persons in the room should also wear high-filtration masks because routine surgical masks do not provide adequate filtration.[1,2,4,24]

Whenever a laser is in use, risk of fire is increased. A fire can be triggered anytime a reflected laser beam or a direct beam comes in contact with any dry, combustible item. The oxygen, anesthetic gases, and vapors from alcohol-based prep solutions also contribute to the possible danger. All members of the laser team must be trained in fire safety and be able to respond quickly should a fire occur. All combustibles near the laser tissue impact site should be kept wet to prevent ignition. Use of flammable draping materials and skin prep solutions should be avoided. Sterile water or saline should be immediately available to douse any small fires, should they occur. Airway fires are of particular

concern because polyvinyl chloride (PVC) endotracheal tubes (ETT) are highly flammable, particularly when combined with the high oxygen flows running through them during anesthesia. Specific laser-retardant ETT, special ETT protective wraps, or foil-wrapped red rubber ETT should be used during oral, tracheal, or esophageal laser procedures that require general anesthesia, and the cuffs should be inflated with sterile saline to provide a heat sink and retard a fire.[1,2,4]

Postoperative Care

A laser procedure does not in and of itself require any technique-specific postoperative care. Patient management should include routine PACU and Phase II care that is geared to the type of anesthesia administered and the given procedure. Specific surgical procedure issues are addressed in the systems appropriate chapters throughout this book.

LAPAROSCOPIC SURGERY

Laparoscopic surgery is a form of endoscopic surgery that uses a fiberoptic laparoscope inserted into the peritoneum to surgically assess and/or treat a wide and continually expanding range of conditions.[25] To understand the history of laparoscopy, one must first examine the origins of endoscopy, which began in ancient times and was driven by the innate human curiosity to peer inside body cavities. Speculums were first developed and used to examine various areas of the body such as the rectum and vagina as early as 400 BC. An Arabian physician first used a mirror to reflect light and examine the cervix in 1012 AD. The first crude endoscope was developed in 1585 and used the sun as a light source to examine the nasal cavity.[1,5,26]

The 1800s saw the addition of more reliable—but crude—light sources to these endoscopic examinations. An Italian physician, Phillip Bozinni, developed a device that used a candle for illumination to examine the urethra of a living patient. Later devices used alcohol lamps and a wick. Edison's development of the incandescent light bulb in 1880, however, truly spurred the evolution of modern endoscopy and laparoscopy as we know it today.[5,26]

True laparoscopy was first accomplished by George Kelling in 1901, when he viewed the abdominal viscera of a living dog using a cysto-scope. Kelling is also credited with performing the first pneumoperitoneum with this procedure. Equipment and techniques continued to evolve and the first laparoscopic tubal ligation was performed in 1941. By 1973, more than 500,000 gynecologic laparoscopic procedures had been performed. Laparoscopic cholecystectomy procedures all but replaced open procedures within 3 years of its introduction in 1987. The technology continues to expand today into multiple therapeutic and diagnostic procedures across most surgical specialties, and many experts believe that as much as 80% of all abdominal surgeries will be performed laparoscopically in the next few decades.[5,26-28] An overview of these procedures can be found in Table 44-3.

Table 44-3	Therapeutic and Diagnostic Indications for Laparoscopy	
Therapeutic	**Diagnostic**
Cholecystectomy	Chronic liver disease
Deroofing of hepatic cyst	Fever of unknown origin
Hernia repair	Neoplasms
Appendectomy	Staging of lymphoma
Colectomy	Gastrointestinal hemorrhage
Jejunostomy	Benign peritoneum
Nephrectomy	Acute abdominal pain
Peptic ulcer disease	Chronic abdominal pain
Antireflux surgery	Acute abdominal process
Hysterectomy	Second-look laparoscopy
Tubal ligation	Abdominal trauma
Retrieval of ova	Pancreatic disease
Pelvic lymphadenectomy	
Vascular surgery	
Cardiomyotomy	
Presacral neurectomy	
Peritoneal dialysis	
Cryptorchidism	
Variocele	

From Sharma K, Kabinoff G, Ducheine Y et al: Laparoscopic surgery and its potential for medical complications, Heart and Lung: The Journal of Acute and Critical Care 26:52-67, 1997.

Preoperative Issues

Preoperative care should be focused on the adequate assessment and preparation of the patient. Routine diagnostics and assessments that are conducted for all general anesthesia and/or surgical patients should be completed. Special attention should be paid to establishing the appropriateness of a laparoscopic procedure for this patient as laparoscopy, and the creation of a pneumoperitoneum brings its own inherent risks and problems. A recommended preoperative checklist should include the following[26]:

- History and physical examination
- Evaluation of medical problems
- Thorough evaluation of the cardiac and respiratory systems
- Normalization of fluids and electrolytes
- Antibiotics
- Deep vein thrombosis prophylaxis
- Genitourinary system evaluation
- Appropriate laboratory and radiologic studies
- Informed consent

Numerous relative and absolute contraindications to laparoscopic procedures (Table 44-4) are well established, and the patient should be closely evaluated with regards to these issues. Previous abdominal surgery should be thoroughly evaluated as possible scarring and/or adhesions may impact the performance of the laparoscope. A comprehensive evaluation of the cardiovascular and pulmonary systems is mandated before any laparoscopic procedure because a pneumoperitoneum may greatly stress these systems. Large abdominal wall hernias, diaphragmatic defects, and previous scars may affect trocar placement. Pregnancy was once considered an absolute contraindication to laparoscopic surgery; however, these procedures have now been shown to be safe and effective well into the second trimester.[26,29]

Intraoperative Issues

The primary difference between laparoscopic surgeries and their open counterparts are patient positioning and the creation of a pneumoperitoneum, both of which can create patient management challenges during the operative and recovery phases.

Pneumoperitoneum. The creation of a pneumoperitoneum involves the insufflation of the

Table 44-4	**Contraindications to Laparoscopic Surgery**[10,21,36]
Relative	**Absolute**
Prior abdominal or pelvic surgery	Hypovolemic shock
Previous peritonitis or pelvic fibrosis	Large pelvic or abdominal mass
Obesity	Severe cardiac decompensation
Diaphragmatic hernia	Hemodynamic instability
Umbilical abnormality	Massive bleeding
Abdominal/iliac aneurysm	Inability to tolerate laparotomy
Severe pulmonary disease	Inexperienced surgeon
Bowel obstruction	Unfit for general anesthesia
Intolerance to positioning	
Abdominal wall hernia	
Uncorrected coagulopathies	
Portal hypertension	
Late pregnancy	
Severe acute cholecystis	
Ductal calculi	
Sepsis	
Thickened gallbladder, >4 mm	
Jaundice	
Acute pancreatitis	

abdomen with a gas. The most commonly used gas for insufflation is CO_2 because of its relatively low risk of venous gas embolism and noncombustibilty. Other gases that have been evaluated in clinical and experimental settings include nitrous oxide, helium, and argon as described in Table 44-5.[28,30]

A pneumoperitoneum is used during laparoscopic surgery to allow the surgical team to visualize the abdomen and perform the indicated procedure. Unfortunately, however, the creation and maintenance of this pneumoperitoneum can have varying effects on the patient and is associated with many of the complications generally associated with laparoscopic surgery. The patient's position during surgery can exacerbate these adverse affects.[28]

The pneumoperitoneum is created when gas is insufflated into the abdominal cavity by puncturing the abdominal wall with a Veress needle and then using a mechanical insufflator with a pressure-limiting function to inflate the peritoneum. Normal insufflation pressures are 15 to 18 cm H_2O. Insufficient pressure produces an inadequate pneumoperitoneum and impairs surgical visualization. Excessive pressure creates even greater cardiovascular and respiratory compromise than that commonly associated with the procedure.[31]

Cardiovascular Changes. A wide variety of hemodynamic effects have been reported with the insufflation of a CO_2 pneumoperitoneum. The increased abdominal pressure compresses veins within the abdominal cavity and results in an initial increase in preload; however, true preload is ultimately decreased because of impaired venous return. Afterload is also increased as a result of the increased abdominal pressure and the resultant neurohumoral reflexes. The most common net effects from these changes include increases in heart rate, systemic vascular resistance (SVR), and central venous pressure (CVP). Cardiac output (CO) drops, and mean arterial pressure (MAP) may increase, decrease, or remain unchanged, depending on the relative changes in CO and SVR. Hemodynamic monitoring may be used to monitor for pressure changes and myocardial compromise in extremely high-risk patients. Pneumoperitoneum can cause dysrhythmias to include sinus tachycardia, bigeminy, and premature ventricular contractions. Once pneumoperitoneum has been established there will be a resultant increase in the abdominal pressure causing vagal stimulation that can lead to severe bradycardia and possible asystole.[26,28,31]

Respiratory Changes. The creation of a CO_2 pneumoperitoneum will also have several adverse effects on the respiratory system. Oxygenation may be impaired because of reductions in lung volume and the associated atelectasis that results from an elevated diaphragm. Ventilation may also be impaired and result in CO_2 retention and hypercarbia. Other untoward effects include

Table 44-5	**Advantages and Disadvantages of Insufflation Gases**	
Gas	Advantages	Disadvantages
Carbon dioxide	Low risk of gas embolism Noncombustible	Hypercarbia Acidosis Pain
Nitrous oxide	Low risk of gas embolism Decreased pain	Supports combustion
Helium	Stable acid-base status Does not support combustion	Subcutaneous emphysema Unknown risk of venous gas embolism
Argon	Stable acid-base status Does not support combustion	Possible cardiac depression

From Corwin CL: Pneumoperitoneum, Society of American Gastrointestinal Endoscopic Surgeons, Primary Care Physician's Resource Center, 2001 (accessed online November 1, 2001, at www.sages.org/primarycare/chapter5.html).

Table 44-6	**Cardiopulmonary Effects of a Pneumoperitoneum**[10,36]	
	Elevated	Reduced
Respiratory	Respiratory rate $PaCO_2$, mixed venous CO_2 tension, alveolar CO_2 tension Arterial-venous CO_2 difference Peak airway pressure Plateau airway pressure Intrathoracic pressure Airway resistance Atelectasis	PH Forced expiratory volume Forced vital capacity Functional residual capacity Total lung capacity Compliance
Cardiovascular	Heart rate with initial insufflation Systemic blood pressure MAP CVP Pulmonary artery pressure SVR Myocardial oxygen demand	Stroke volume CO Venous return unchanged or reduced Bradycardia with maintenance of pneumoperitoneum

reduced pulmonary compliance, increased airway resistance, and reduced vital capacity. All of these effects will be exacerbated by the commonly used Trendelenburg position. These respiratory changes are also further exacerbated by the following: surgery that lasts more than four hours, a history of COPD, age, obesity, and an ASA physical status of III or greater.[26,28,31] A summary of these effects can be found in Table 44-6.

Other System Effects. In addition to the extensive cardiopulmonary changes affected by the creation of a pneumoperitoneum, various other body systems may be impacted as well. The patient should be closely monitored for the development of hypothermia and preventative measures taken to prevent this complication.[32] Hypercarbia may lead to increased cerebral blood flow with a net result of increased intracranial blood pressure, possible cerebral edema, and potential brain stem herniation. Renal failure may result from the impaired renal blood flow caused by the increased abdominal pressure (IAP) and/or hypercarbia. IAP also compromises venous return and puts the patient at risk for development of deep vein thrombosis (DVT). Stress hormones are also elevated because of peritoneal distention, increased anesthetic time, pain, decreased venous return, and acidosis. This release of epinephrine, norepinephrine, and plasma cortisol may all contribute to numerous adverse effects.[26,38] Concerns about the effect of a pneumoperitoneum on the implantation and spread of tumor cells also arise. The role of laparoscopic surgery for the treatment of cancer remains controversial; however, animal studies have shown no increase in the spread of tumor cells as a result of the laparoscopic versus open surgical approach.[33,34]

Gasless Laparoscopy. Several systems are currently being evaluated for use in gasless laparoscopy. These systems work with various slings and retractors to lift the abdominal wall away from the intraabdominal contents to create a surgical space in which to perform the procedure. The primary advantage of this technique, of course, is the elimination of the need for a pneumoperitoneum. Disadvantages center around the inability to establish adequate surgical field exposure. Patient indications for gasless laparoscopy essentially parallel those for similar open and pneumoperitoneum cases. The gasless approach is better suited to lower abdominal cases, however, because greater abdominal distension can be accomplished in this area, particularly with women.[26]

Patient Positioning. Exaggerated surgical positions are often necessary with laparoscopic surgery to effect adequate organ exposure. The two most commonly used positions are the Trendelenburg, or head-down, position for bowel surgery and the reverse Trendelenburg, or head-up tilt, for upper abdominal procedures. Both positions result in changes in cardiac filling pressures and lung volumes that affect ventilation, oxygenation, and lower extremity venous stasis. These changes are exacerbated with the addition of a pneumoperitoneum (Table 44-7).[26]

Postoperative Issues

Care of the patient immediately after any laparoscopic procedure should include basic PACU care and monitoring specific to the procedure and type of anesthesia administered. Postoperative pain management is typically easier after laparoscopic procedures than after open procedures and can often be accomplished with a small amount of opioids in combination with nonsteroidals and local anesthetics. Visceral discomfort is often more difficult to treat and more unpredictable.

Table 44-7 **Physiologic Effects of Patient Position during Laparoscopic Surgery**		
System	Trendelenburg	Reverse Trendelenburg
Cardiovascular	Increased central filling pressures Increased MAP No change in CO	Decreased central filling pressures Decreased MAP Decreased CO
Pulmonary	No change in oxygenation No change in ventilation	No change in oxygenation No change in ventilation
Venous Stasis	No change in lower extremity venous blood flow	No change in lower extremity venous blood flow

From Eubanks WS, Swanstrom LL, Soper NJ, editors: Mastery of endoscopic and laparoscopic surgery, Philadelphia, 2000, Lippincott Williams & Wilkins.

This pain is triggered by the retained gas in the peritoneal cavity and the resulting irritation of peritoneal surfaces. It commonly presents as shoulder pain and may persist for several days after surgery. The patient should be prepared for this discomfort as a part of his or her preoperative education. The pain can generally be managed with oral analgesics.[26,27,31]

Postoperative nausea and vomiting can pose a significant problem with any intraabdominal surgery. Routine drainage of the stomach at the end of the case before removal of the NG tube will help to reduce the incidence, although it will not completely eliminate it. Prophylactic treatment with an antiemetic is not indicated for all laparoscopic cases, although it may be appropriate when multiple risk factors for postoperative nausea and vomiting are present.[31]

In addition to basic PACU care, careful attention should be paid to monitoring the patient for any complications associated with laparoscopic intervention. Laparoscopic procedures are remarkably safe when correctly performed; their major complication rate is less than 1%, and the overall mortality rate is 4 to 8 deaths per 1000 procedures.[26] Complications can occur, however, and can be divided into two categories: those associated with the procedure and those associated with the pneumoperitoneum.

Pneumoperitoneum Complications. The complications associated with the creation of the surgical pneumoperitoneum are directly related to the physiological changes associated with this procedure. Most complications occur during the initiation and maintenance of the pneumoperitoneum; however, it may be the perianesthesia nurse that picks up on the complication and/or will be responsible for the continued care and management of the patient. Table 44-8 provides a summary of pneumoperitoneum complications and their causes. Care should be based on the complication presented.

Laparoscopy Complications. Complications associated with laparoscopic technique are usually trocar-related injuries and involve the bowel, vasculature, or bladder.[26,28,35,36] Early recognition and treatment in the operating room, of course, results in the best outcome; however, up to two-thirds of injuries may go unrecognized at the time of surgery,[37] thus making vigilant

Table 44-8	**Pneumoperitoneum Complications**	
System	Complication	Possible Mechanism
Cardiovascular	Tension pneumothorax	Diaphragm injury
		Dissection near esophageal hiatus
		Barotrauma
	Myocardial infarction	Inadequate perfusion to meet increased demand
	Metabolic acidosis	Inadequate tissue perfusion due to reduced CO
		Hypercarbia
	Visceral organ ischemia	Impaired visceral blood flow
	Venous stasis/	Impaired lower extremity venous return
	thromboembolism	Endothelial damage from increased IAP
Pulmonary	Hypoxia	Atelectasis and reduced lung volume
	Hypercarbia	CO_2 retention
	Respiratory acidosis	Hypercarbia
	Aspiration	Increased risk of regurgitation of gastric contents due to increased IAP
Other	CO_2 gas embolus	Entry of CO_2 bubbles through injured blood vessels

Adapted from Eubanks WS, Swanstrom LL, Soper NJ, editors: Mastery of endoscopic and laparoscopic surgery, Philadelphia, 2000, Lippincott Williams & Wilkins.

PACU assessment and care as well as thorough discharge teaching essential to positive patient outcome.

Bowel Injuries. Bowel injuries are most troubling because they tend to go unrecognized at the time of surgery. The most common bowel injury involves perforation of the small intestine. Injury to the colon, duodenum, and stomach also occur. Perforations that go unrecognized in the operating room may present as peritonitis sometime after discharge. Delayed onset of sepsis is also quite common with these injuries. The mortality rate associated with unrecognized bowel injuries can be as high as 5%.[26] These injuries may also go unrecognized in the PACU because the patient may be asymptomatic at the time. Discharge teaching that emphasizes reporting of unrelieved pain, nausea and vomiting, and unresolved fever is particularly important in the recognition and resolution of this complication.

Vascular Injuries. Vascular injuries are most commonly associated with pelvic procedures and tend to occur in the vicinity of the distal aorta and its branches, the inferior vena cava, or iliac veins. Abdominal wall hemorrhage may also occur from inadvertent trocar insertion. Major vascular injury during laparoscopic procedures is rare. Most injuries are generally rapidly recognized and repaired in the operating room with direct suture ligation, although a patch or synthetic graft may be required for more extensive damage.[26,28] Injuries that go unrecognized in the operating room again pose the greatest challenge to the perianesthesia nurse. Unresolved tachycardia and hypotension must be closely evaluated as possible signs and symptoms of hemorrhage. Unresolved or extremely severe postoperative pain and/or abdominal distension are also possible signs and symptoms. Recognition of surgical hemorrhage and immediate surgical evaluation is critical to a positive patient outcome.

Bladder Injuries. The risk of bladder injury can be decreased by the routine insertion of a Foley catheter and decompression of the bladder with all laparoscopic procedures. Even with the routine insertion of a catheter, however, occasional bladder perforation will occur. The risk of perforation is greatest in those patients with previous abdominal or bladder surgery; risks are also elevated in those patients with congenital anomalies. The most common signs and symptoms are the appearance of air in the Foley bag or unexplained urinary tract bleeding during the procedure. Diagnosis can be confirmed with a retrograde cystogram, and surgical repair can be pursued.[26]

Other Complications. Other complications of interest include postoperative infection and laparoscopic electrosurgery complications. Antibiotic prophylaxis is a well established standard for all laparoscopic procedures, and studies have shown that postoperative infections after laparoscopic surgery in both clean and infected cases are lower than in open cases.[38] Electrosurgery has replaced laser energy as the preferred power supply during laparoscopic surgery because it is less expensive and provides for better tissue coagulation. This technique, however, has been associated with secondary thermal injuries that may go unrecognized because they occur outside of the surgeon's view through the laparoscope. As with bowel perforations, these injuries often present days to weeks postoperatively as peritonitis or sepsis, which again highlights the importance of thorough discharge instructions regarding the signs, symptoms, and management of postoperative infections.[39,40]

REFERENCES

1. Ball KA: Endoscopic surgery, St Louis, 1997, Mosby.
2. Ball KA: Surgical modalities. In Meeker MH, Rothrock JC, editors: Alexander's care of the surgical patient, St Louis, 1999, Mosby.
3. Ball K: Lasers: the perioperative challenge, ed 2, St Louis, 1995, Mosby.
4. Miller G: Minimally invasive surgery, laser, and other technologies. In Burden N, Quinn DMD, O'Brien D et al, editors: Ambulatory surgical nursing, ed 2, Philadelphia, 2000, WB Saunders.
5. Miller G: Laparoscopic and minimally invasive surgery. In Quinn DMD, editor: Ambulatory surgical nursing core curriculum, Philadelphia, 1999, WB Saunders.
6. Alora MBT, Dover JS, Arndt KA: Lasers for vascular lesions, Dermatology Nursing 11:97-102, 105-107, 1999.
7. Bates B: Repeated ruby laser tx zaps most hair, Skin and Allergy News 30(6):5, 1999.

8. Campos VB, Anderson RR, Dierickx CC: Use of an 800 mm high-power diode laser for the treatment of leg vein telangiectasia, Boston, 2001, Wellman Laboratories of Photomedicine, Harvard Medical School.

9. Fairchild SS: Patient care management: intraoperative phase. In Fairchild SS, editor: Perioperative nursing: principles and practice, ed 2, Philadelphia, 1996, Lippincott.

10. Formica K, Alster TS: Complications of cutaneous laser resurfacing: a nursing guide, Dermatology Nursing 10:353-356, 1998.

11. Formica K, Alster TS: Cutaneous laser resurfacing: a nursing guide, Dermatology Nursing 9:19-22, 1997.

12. Gill KS, Sitbon JRR, Trocme S: Phototherapeutic keratectomy: ophthalmic surgery update, AORN J 66:242-252, 1997.

13. Goldman MP, Marchell N, Fitzpatrick RE: Laser skin resurfacing of the face with a combined CO_2/Er:YAG laser, Dermatol Surg 26(2):102-104, 2000.

14. Hayden AM: Transmyocardial revascularization: evolutions/revolutions, RN 61(5):44-48, 1998.

15. Kaufman H: Caution: lasers in use (Microsoft PowerPoint presentation), 1997 (online at www.umc.sunysb.edu/oralbio/lasers/index.htm).

16. LeRoy L: Laser resurfacing: the nurse's role, Dermatology Nursing 9:173-175, 1997.

17. Mannino G, Papale A, DeBella F et al: Use of erbium: YAG laser in the treatment of palpebral xanthelasmas, Ophthalmic Surgery and Lasers 32(2):129-133, 2001 (online at www.slackinc.com/eye/os/stor3031/Mannino.htm).

18. Neckel C: Lasers in oral surgery [Online], 2001. http://www.oralia.com/wwwgb/neckel.html.

19. Perlmutter AP, Muschter R: Insterstitial laser prostatectomy: symposium on benign prostatic hyperplasia, Part IV, Mayo Clinic Proceeding 73:903-907, 1998.

20. Piatek YM, Atzori M: PTMR, Am J Nurs 99:64-66, 1999.

21. Ramian G: The world wide web virtual library: free electron laser research and applications (accessed online in 2001 at http://sbfel3.ucsb.edu/www/vl_fel.html).

22. Romero P, Alster TS: Skin rejuvenation with cool touch 1320 nm Nd:YAG laser: the nurse's role, Dermatology Nursing 13:122-127, 2001.

23. Norman E: A new treatment of myocardial ischemia, Am J Nurs 98:16FF, 1998.

24. Giordano BP: Don't be a victim of surgical smoke, AORN J 63:520-522, 1996.

25. Venes D, editor: Taber's cyclopedic medical dictionary, ed 19, Philadelphia, 2001, FA Davis.

26. Eubanks WS, Swanstrom LL, Soper NJ, editors: Mastery of endoscopic and laparoscopic surgery, Philadelphia, 2000, Lippincott Williams & Wilkins.

27. Sharma K, Kabinoff G, Ducheine Y et al: Laparoscopic surgery and its potential for medical complications, Heart and Lung: The Journal of Acute and Critical Care 26:52-67, 1997.

28. Steuer K: Pneumoperitoneum: physiology and nursing interventions, AORN J 68:410-436, 1998.

29. Hooper VD: Laparoscopic hernia repair (EDA 201-0419), Carrolton, Texas, 2000, Health & Sciences Television Network.

30. Corwin CL: Pneumoperitoneum, Society of American Gastrointestinal Endoscopic Surgeons, Primary Care Physician's Resource Center, 2001 (accessed online November 1, 2001 at www.sages.org/primarycare/chapter5.html).

31. Bogdonoff DL, Schirmer B: Laparoscopic surgery. In Stone DJ, Bogdonoff DL, Leisure GS et al, editors: Perioperative care: anesthesia, medicine, and surgery, St Louis, 1998, Mosby.

32. ASPAN: Clinical guideline for the prevention of unplanned perioperative hypothermia, JOPAN 16:305-314, 2001.

33. Gutt CN, Riemer V, Kim ZG et al: Impact of laparoscopic colonic resection on tumour growth and spread in an experimental model, Br J Surg 86:1180-1184, 1999.

34. Tsivian A, Shtabsky A, Issakov J et al: The effect of pneumoperitoneum on dissemination and scar implantation of intra-abdominal tumor cells, J Urol 164:2096-2098, 2000.

35. Fahlenkamp D, Rassweiler J, Fornara P et al: Complications of laparoscopic procedures in urology: experience with 2407 procedures at four German centers, J Urol 162:765-770, 1999.

36. Rantanen TK, Salo JA, Sipponen JT: Fatal and life-threatening complications in antireflux surgery: analysis of 5502 operations, Br J Surg 86:1573-1577, 1999.

37. Ferriman A: Laparoscopic surgery: two thirds of injuries initially missed, BMJ 321:784, 2000.

38. Targarona EM, Balague C, Knook MM et al: Laparoscopic surgery and surgical infection, Br J Surg 87:536-544, 2000.

39. Munro MG: Complications of laparoscopic electrosurgery. In Ponsky JL, editor: Complication of endoscopic and laparoscopic surgery: prevention and management, 1997, Lippincott-Raven.

40. Tucker RD, Voyles CR: Laparoscopic electrosurgical complications and their prevention, AORN J 62:49-78, 1995.

41. Marcus J, Goldbert DJ: Lasers in dermatology: a nursing perspective. Dermatology Nursing 8:181-195, 204, 1996.

CHRONIC OBSTRUCTIVE PULMONARY DISEASE

Chronic obstructive pulmonary disease (COPD) describes bronchial obstructive respiratory diseases. It is characterized by dyspnea with or without cough and sputum. The two major clinical manifestations of COPD are airway obstruction and airway destruction. The magnitude of the various disease entities that the term COPD includes is great. Therefore it is difficult to elaborate individually on the diseases because each deserves separate attention. Rather, this chapter briefly describes the overall characteristics of COPD and general care required in the postanesthesia care unit (PACU). Variations between COPD patients exist. It is important for the perianesthesia nurse to consult with the physician about the specific nursing care to be administered to the patient with COPD. For discussion of specific COPD diseases, see the bibliography at the end of the chapter.

Description of COPD

Three major diseases are part of COPD: asthma, emphysema, and chronic bronchitis. All are characterized by airway obstruction. These diseases may have medically reversible components—such as bronchospasm—or they may have irreversible components, such as alveolar septal destruction. Some of the reversible components of asthma—such as retained secretions, bronchospasms, and infections—can be corrected by the interaction of the physician, nurse, physical therapist, and respiratory therapist. The treatment of asthma may include oxygen therapy, bronchodilators, chest physiotherapy, and proper hydration.

Chronic bronchitis is associated with chronic cigarette smoking. The nurse can contribute greatly to the patient's future health by strongly influencing him or her to refrain from smoking. Other therapy for the reversible components may include the use of bronchodilators, chest physiotherapy, and oxygen.

The patient with emphysema usually has airway destruction that is irreversible. As the alveolar septa are destroyed, insufficient alveolar ventilation ensues and eventually leads to hypercarbia. As the disease progresses, carbon dioxide cannot be expelled from the lungs and is retained there. The patient usually increases minute ventilation to try to compensate for the hypercarbia. Respiratory acidosis develops slowly as the various acid-base buffer systems try to neutralize the accumulated acid. In this compensated state, the patient usually has a near-normal pH, high plasma bicarbonate, low chloride concentrations, and a high total carbon dioxide level. The $PaCO_2$ usually is low because some inspired oxygen is unable to cross into the blood from the lungs because of the decreased respiratory diffusion membrane surface area in the lungs. Pulmonary hypertension usually appears as the disease progresses. Cor pulmonale may develop, and because of the pulmonary venous engorgement, the right heart may begin to fail. The patient with emphysema who has irreversible destruction may be treated with chest physiotherapy, bronchodilators, and steroids.

Surgical Considerations

The incidence of pulmonary complications in patients who have undergone abdominal or thoracic surgery is high. Changes occur in the pulmonary status of the patient who undergoes anesthesia and surgery. In the postoperative phase, these changes are characterized by gradual or abrupt alveolar collapse. The patient with

COPD, when subjected to surgery, then represents an even higher risk for postoperative complications. It is important that these patients be given meticulous preoperative care so that they are in the best possible health when they enter surgery. This preoperative medical treatment usually includes hydration, nutrition, chest physiotherapy, bronchodilators, and prophylactic antibiotics if an infection is present. Serial pulmonary function tests and arterial blood gas determinations are used to monitor the progression of the preoperative treatment.

When the patient's pulmonary function reaches a peak preoperatively (i.e., when the pulmonary function tests and arterial blood gas test results no longer show continued improvement), surgery is considered because the patient has reached his or her optimal pulmonary status.

Care of the COPD Patient

Perianesthesia care centers on prevention of complications. The modified stir-up regimen should include frequent cascade coughing, sustained maximal inspirations (SMIs), and repositioning of the patient (see Chapters 10 and 26). An appropriately implemented modified stir-up regimen is of great importance, especially in patients who are recovering from upper abdominal or thoracic operations. Surgery at these sites can cause decreased ventilatory effort and a complete absence of sighs by the patient. Given that the patient already has compromised respiratory function, the possibility of retained secretions and atelectasis is magnified. Hence these patients represent a significant challenge to the perianesthesia nurse.

When the patient is completely reactive, the use of the incentive spirometer may be helpful in reducing the incidence of atelectasis. Consequently, the perianesthesia nurse who is responsible for supportive measures should assist and encourage the patient in using the SMI with or without the incentive spirometer. Based on subjective research findings, it is believed that if the perianesthesia nurse explains the rationale of the SMI maneuver and properly instructs the patient in the use of the technique preoperatively, the patient is more likely to correctly use the SMI maneuver postoperatively with or without coaching. The performance of the SMI maneuver— with or without mechanical devices—should be monitored by the nurse to ensure proper production of a sustained inspiration with a 3-second inspiratory hold. The perianesthesia nurse should also encourage and monitor the patient's performance of the cascade cough to facilitate early secretion clearance.

Patients with COPD have some component of reactive airways disease. Consequently, their airways become compliant and can become compressed during a forced expiratory maneuver. This dynamic compression of the airways is a function of the equal pressure point theory as discussed in Chapter 10. To reduce the amount of dynamic compression of the airway during exhalation, the patient should be encouraged to use pursed-lip breathing. Breathing through pursed lips during exhalation can be the same as adding 5 to 10 cm H_2O of positive end-expiratory pressure. Increasing the pressure inside the airway during exhalation reduces the amount of dynamic compression of the airways and decreases the amount of air trapping that commonly occurs in patients with COPD.

The cardiac status should be monitored meticulously because of the frequent involvement of the heart in the pathologic disorders of these patients. Kidney function should also be monitored because it may be altered, especially in patients who exhibit fluid retention and edema of the extremities.

The patient with severe COPD who has marked hypercarbia can present difficulties in the PACU. Patients who have severe emphysema usually fit into this category. Their ventilatory effort is stimulated by the hypoxic drive, in which lack of oxygen stimulates ventilation. Hypoxia indirectly stimulates the respiratory center by means of chemoreceptors in the carotid bodies located at the bifurcation of the carotid artery. When the patient receives 100% oxygen to breathe in the PACU, oxygen tensions rise in the inspired gas; the carotid and aortic chemoreceptors will cease to function; and the patient will quickly become apneic. The patient's respiratory status should be assessed carefully and the physician consulted before 100% oxygen is administered. Mist therapy postoperatively aids in liquefying the secretions and helps in the all-important maintenance of a patent tracheobronchial tree. If excessive bronchial drainage is not removed, it will provide a convenient avenue for bacteria and it might also obstruct the airways, thus leading to insufficient alveolar ventilation and hypoxia.

The patient with COPD should be under constant surveillance for signs of cardiopulmonary decompensation, including shallow, rapid, gasping respirations; severe dyspnea; substernal retraction; and disorientation. Blood pressure may be elevated or low, but the patient usually has tachycardia, fever, and muscle rigidity. Cyanosis may or may not be present.

Respiratory depressant drugs, such as narcotics, should be given in low dosages, or if the COPD is severe, they should be avoided completely. Repositioning of the patient and splinting of the incision site—in addition to reducing the anxiety usually seen in these patients—reduces the need for narcotic drugs. Some form of regional analgesia may be extremely beneficial for these patients.

MYASTHENIA GRAVIS

The patient with myasthenia gravis (MG) deserves special consideration in the PACU because of the respiratory dysfunction and possible pharmacological ramifications of the disease. MG is a chronic disease characterized by progressive muscle weakness and easy fatigability. Most patients with MG have developed antibodies to muscle acetylcholine receptors. The antibody does not bind exactly on the site that binds the acetylcholine, but it does bind close to it. The acetylcholine receptors are steadily destroyed, with a resulting reduction in the binding of acetylcholine at the postsynaptic myoneural junction. The myasthenic patient will sometimes have a lesion in the myocardium that is a spotty, focal necrosis accompanied by an inflammatory reaction. An alteration in the S-T segment and T wave is sometimes seen in these patients.

The incidence of MG has been estimated to be between 1 in 15,000 and 1 in 40,000. It occurs twice as often in females than in males and at earlier ages. The main symptom is weakness in one or more of the muscle groups; ptosis of the eyelid is the most common sign of the disease.

Ptosis is usually accompanied by diplopia, blurred vision, or nystagmus. Ocular signs and symptoms often are worsened by bright light. The patient may also have "myasthenic facies," which is caused by weakness of the facial muscles. This can progress to dysphagia and difficulties in speech.

Respiration is often affected in the myasthenic patient. Dyspnea can be either inspiratory—if the diaphragm is involved—or expiratory, if the intercostal and abdominal muscles are affected. The patient may also have emotional disturbances caused by anxiety and depression.

Diagnosis of MG is made on the clinical symptoms and the characteristic electromyogram. The clinical symptoms can be assessed by the neostigmine test or by the edrophonium test, both of which involve anticholinesterases that increase the strength of the myasthenic muscle. Muscle relaxants—such as d-tubocurarine chloride (curare) or gallamine triethiodide (Flaxedil)—given in very small dosages exaggerate MG symptoms and can be used in the patient's workup.

Treatment for this disease consists of various pharmacologic interventions designed to enhance neuromuscular transmission and slow the progression of the disease. Anticholinesterase drugs, which slow down the enzymatic destruction of acetylcholine at the neuromuscular junction, are commonly used. Oral pyridostigmine and the shorter-acting neostigmine are the anticholinesterases of choice. Myasthenic patients seem to favor pyridostigmine over neostigmine because of its length of action and its less unpleasant side effects. Steroids and other immunosuppressive agents may be used in some patients to reduce antibody production responsible for the disease.

Thymectomy seems to be an appropriate therapeutic mode because the thymus gland appears to be intimately involved in the disease process. About 67% of the myasthenic patients who do not have thymoma experience improvement after thymectomy. On the other hand, about 25% of the myasthenic patients with thymoma show improvement in the disease process after thymectomy.

Because thymectomy has been used as a therapeutic intervention in the treatment of MG, the perianesthesia nurse will probably render nursing care to many patients with MG. Because of the location of the incision, the myasthenic patient does not usually receive any intraoperative skeletal muscle relaxants. These myasthenic patients can experience an exacerbation of symptoms in the PACU. Hence critical monitoring of the patient's ventilatory status should be the primary focus of the perianesthesia nursing care. Myasthenic patients who are recovering from any type of surgical procedure and who have been administered any form of anesthesia (general, inhalation, or regional) can develop exacerbated symptoms and myasthenic crisis in the PACU. Consequently, respiratory support should always be available for these patients.

Care of the Myasthenic Patient
The patient with MG can present various difficulties because of an impaired respiratory system, possible poor nutrition, susceptibility to infection, altered psychiatric status, and possible altered response to drugs used during anesthesia. The patient should be placed in a quiet area, where no direct light will shine in his or her eyes. The patient's respiratory effort and exchange should be monitored continuously. Oxygen should be administered with humidification, and secretions should be removed by frequent suctioning and postural drainage. Oxygen saturation levels for these patients should be maintained above 96%. Any change in respiratory status should be reported to the physician immediately. Because cardiac mechanisms may be responsible for some sudden deaths in this patient population, cardiac monitoring should be instituted for every myasthenic patient in the PACU. It is also important to monitor the fluids administered to myasthenic patients. Hypovolemia and hypervolemia must be avoided because of their deleterious effects on the already compromised heart and lungs.

The patient should be kept as pain-free as possible to facilitate good respiratory exchange. Morphine and other narcotics are often potentiated by anticholinesterases. Therefore the initial narcotic dose should be reduced to half the normal dose and then increased if required. If the patient is receiving continuous mechanical ventilation, the normal amount of medication can be given without compromising the patient's respiratory status.

The emotional status of the myasthenic patient is of considerable importance. As few clinicians as possible should be responsible for the myasthenic patient throughout the emergent phase because the patient is likely to be distrustful of anyone he or she does not know. Communication is important, and the patient should be informed about any nursing procedure to be performed. If the myasthenic patient has a tracheostomy, paper and pencil should be used to facilitate communication between nurse and patient.

DIABETES MELLITUS
Diabetes mellitus is a chronic metabolic disease associated with insulin deficiency or insensitivity, hyperglycemia, and glycosuria. It occurs in about 2% to 3% of the general population. One important aspect of this disease is an associated degeneration of the small blood vessels (microangiopathy) that is most marked in the retina, kidneys, and nervous system.

The focus of the physiologic activity of insulin is to "open the door" of the cell to let glucose enter. In the diabetic state, the patient has an elevated blood glucose level because of a defect in the cellular response to insulin, and the "door" remains closed. Sources of the excess glucose are dietary carbohydrate, liver glycogen, and glucose formed by the fatty acids metabolized to acetone, or beta-hydroxybutyric acid. These three products are known as ketone bodies. The patient's degree of insulin deficiency is reflected by hyperglycemia, glycosuria, and ketoacidosis.

Anesthesia and Diabetes
The goal of perianesthetic management of the patient with diabetes is maintenance of the serum glucose level less than 200 mg/dl and to prevent hypoglycemia and severe fluid loss. Clinicians' stances regarding specific methods to accomplish these goals differ. One method is to withhold the usual dose of long-acting or intermediate-acting insulin. Two liters of 5% dextrose, with 10 to 15 units of crystalline regular insulin added to each liter, is given to the patient during surgery. In another method, the patient is administered 5% dextrose in Ringer's lactate at 125 ml/hr. Regular insulin, in 5-unit increments, is administered as needed to keep the patient's blood glucose level at or above 200 mg/dl. A more widely used method consists of giving half the daily dose of insulin on the morning of surgery or one third of the daily dose if the surgery is scheduled later in the day. The patient is given 500 to 1000 ml of

5% dextrose and water before surgery and at least 1000 ml of 5% dextrose and water during surgery. This method avoids hypoglycemia during surgery but increases the need for careful nursing attention in the PACU.

These methods are used in the patient who is undergoing elective surgery. Emergency surgery for the uncontrolled diabetic patient is an entirely different situation. Before the patient undergoes anesthesia and surgery, treatment of the diabetes should be instituted, if possible. Blood glucose and blood urea nitrogen levels often are determined to indicate the proper amount of regular insulin to be administered intraoperatively on a sliding scale. Intravenous solutions are given to treat dehydration.

Care of the Patient with Diabetes

The patient should be monitored for fluid and electrolyte balance and degree of glycosuria. Most authors agree that mild glycosuria is more desirable than glucose-free urine. Hypoglycemia should be avoided. Patients who have had a stressful problem relieved (e.g, the removal of an intraabdominal abscess) may have reduced postoperative insulin requirements. This reduction may be as much as 50% in the first 24 hours. However, because of the stress of surgery, postoperative insulin requirements are usually increased.

Urine glucose levels can be monitored by the Clinitest method. This method does not monitor the blood glucose level directly but provides a rough indicator of insulin requirements. Consequently, because the urinary glucose concentration is considered a late indicator of blood glucose levels, it should not be used in patients with significant insulin-dependent diabetes. Blood glucose levels can be monitored closely in the PACU by using a Dextrostix (glucose oxidase) with blood from a finger stick. Blood glucose laboratory determinations should be done at least twice daily for 2 to 3 postoperative days. A sliding scale that is usually used for the Clinitest method is shown in Table 45-1. If the Dextrostix method is being used to monitor the glucose level, the objective during the PACU period is to prevent hypoglycemia and to accept mild hyperglycemia, with the aim of maintaining the blood glucose concentration between 150 and 200 mg/dl.

Table 45-1	Sliding Scale for Insulin Determinations
Urine Glucose (Trace %)	Regular Insulin Dose (Units)
0.25	5
0.50	8
1	10
2	15

Respiratory acidosis should be prevented by aiding the patient to cough and breathe deeply to promote adequate pulmonary ventilation and carbon dioxide elimination. Metabolic acidosis must be prevented by the administration of fluid and electrolytes. Therefore strict monitoring of intake and output measurements should be instituted on every diabetic patient admitted to the PACU.

The patient with diabetes is very likely to receive an insulin preparation in the PACU. The types of insulin and their times of onset, peak effects, and duration of action are summarized in Table 45-2.

Observation of the diabetic patient for possible diabetic coma (as a result of hyperglycemia) or insulin reaction ensures his or her proper emergence from anesthesia. The symptoms of each complication are summarized in Table 45-3. It is sometimes difficult to detect hyperglycemia or hypoglycemia by symptoms when a patient is recovering from an anesthetic. Therefore frequent tests of blood and urine glucose are most helpful in determining the patient's state. It is also important to keep in mind that any patient who arrives in the PACU, especially in the older age groups, may have undiagnosed diabetes.

RHEUMATOID ARTHRITIS

Rheumatoid arthritis is a relatively common disease that affects the connective tissue of the body. The clinical course varies, but it tends to be progressive and leads to characteristic deformities. Many patients become incapacitated over time. The disease affects more women than men, and its incidence in temperate climates is about 3%. The cause is not completely understood, but

Table 45-2 Time of Action of Various Insulin Preparations

Types of Insulin	Time of Onset (Minutes)	Peak Effects (Minutes)	Duration of Action (Hours)
Insulin injection, USP (regular)	0.30	2-4	6
Crystalline zinc insulin	1	2-4	8
Globin zinc insulin	2-4	8	18-24
Isophane insulin injection (NPH)	0.5-1	2-12	24
Protamine zinc injection (PZI)	1	2-3	24
Lente insulin (insulin zinc suspension)	2-4	8-20	20-28

Table 45-3 Characteristics of Diabetic Complications

Category	Diabetic Coma	Insulin Reaction
Onset	Slow	Sudden
Skin	Flushed, dry, hot	Pale, moist
Behavior	Drowsy	Excited
Breath	Acetone (sweet)	Normal
Respirations	Kussmaul's (air hunger)	Normal-rapid, shallow
Pulse	Rapid, weak	Normal-slow, full bounding
Blood pressure	Low	Normal
Vomiting	Present	Absent
Hunger	Absent	Present
Thirst	Present	Absent
Urine glucose level	Large amount	Absent

it is thought to be an autoimmune phenomenon. The outstanding clinical feature of this disease is proliferative inflammation. The patient often appears chronically ill, undernourished, and anemic.

These patients often undergo surgery to correct restrictive deformities caused by the disease process (Table 45-4). On arrival in the PACU, they require comprehensive nursing management. Some of the hazards to be aware of in patients with rheumatoid arthritis are listed in Table 45-5.

Care of the Patient with Rheumatoid Arthritis

Airway. Extubation is often deferred in these patients until they are unquestionably able to maintain their own airways. This is of prime importance because these patients are often extremely difficult to intubate and are prone to airway obstruction.

Lungs. The patient with rheumatoid arthritis usually has pulmonary dysfunction such as diffuse interstitial fibrosis, granulomatous lesions, or large silicotic nodules. These pulmonary dysfunctions lead to what is termed stiff lungs, and these patients are prone to atelectasis, hypoxemia, and hypercarbia in the PACU (see Chapter 10). Postoperative blood gas analysis and good pulmonary support are therefore important. Respiratory depressant narcotics should be given with caution, if at all. Deaths in rheumatoid arthritic patients have resulted from drug-induced respiratory failure during this period.

Heart. Disease of the pericardium, myocardium, endocardium, and coronary vessels is usually associated with rheumatoid arthritis.

Table 45-4 Corrective Surgery for Rheumatoid Arthritis	
Operative Site	Common Operative Procedure
Neck	Atlantoaxial arthrodesis
Shoulder	Synovectomy and partial excision of acromion
Elbow	Synovectomy and radial head excision; resection arthroplasty
Wrist	Synovectomy and excision of distal ulna
Hand	Metacarpal phalangeal arthroplasty and flexor and extensor tenosynovectomy
Hip	Cup or total replacement, arthroplasty
Knee	Synovectomy (often bilateral), arthroplasty
Foot	Resection arthroplasty (often bilateral)

From Jenkins LC, McGraw RW: Anaesthetic management of the patient with rheumatoid arthritis, Can Anaesth Soc J 16:408, 1969.

Table 45-5 Perianesthesia Hazards in Patients with Rheumatoid Arthritis	
Area of Concern	Complication
Respiratory system	
Airway	Hypoplastic mandible restriction, cervical spine motion, atlantoaxial subluxation, laryngeal tissue damage
Ventilation	Rheumatoid nodules in lung, chronic diffuse interstitial fibrosis, costovertebral joint disorder that inhibits ventilation, thoracic vertebrae flexion deformity that inhibits ventilation, tuberculous lung
Cardiovascular system	Pericardial, myocardial, coronary artery disorders, aortic valve regurgitation, arrhythmias
Hemopoietic, hepatic, and renal systems	Anemia, leukopenia, bleeding tendency (decreased platelets), renal amyloidosis
Miscellaneous	Skin fragility; postoperative chest complications, such as atelectasis, hypercarbia, and hypoxia; multiple joint disease

Modified from Jenkins LC, McGraw RW: Anaesthetic management of the patient with rheumatoid arthritis, Can Anaesth Soc J 16:408, 1969.

Therefore cardiovascular status should be monitored continuously in the PACU. Hypotension should be avoided because it may lead to left ventricular decompensation and acute heart failure.

Blood. The arthritic patient usually exhibits anemia, most commonly of the hypochromic microcytic variety. In most instances, this type of anemia can be treated with blood transfusion.

Postoperative hematocrit and hemoglobin levels should be determined when the patient arrives in the PACU. Blood loss should be extensively monitored, including observation of the stools for blood. The contents recovered from the nasogastric tube (if present) should be checked for blood because these patients may have a bleeding peptic ulcer secondary to long-term aspirin and steroid therapy.

Fluid Balance. Renal function is usually impaired in the patient with chronic rheumatoid arthritis. Therefore drugs that are primarily excreted by the kidneys should be avoided, and urinary output should be monitored at regular, perhaps hourly, intervals.

OBESITY

Obesity, the most common nutritional disorder in the world today, presents many difficulties to the perianesthesia nurse. Many definitions of obesity can be found in the literature. The American Life Insurance Company states that a person is obese if he or she exceeds the expected or ideal weight, corrected by age and sex, by more than 10%. Morbid obesity is a term that denotes a weight twice as much as that predicted for age, sex, body build, and height. Morbidly obese patients can be divided into two groups. Obesity with normal levels of arterial carbon dioxide tension is called simple obesity and includes 90% to 95% of morbidly obese patients. The other group, which represents 5% to 10% of obese patients, has the obesity-hypoventilation (pickwickian) syndrome. This is characterized by extreme obesity; episodic somnolence; and by hypoventilation (increased $PaCO_2$ level) with twitching, plethora, edema, periodic respiration, secondary polycythemia, right ventricular hypertrophy, and right ventricular failure.

The most useful anthropometric index for determining obesity is the body mass index (BMI). This measurement employs the person's weight (in kilograms) divided by height squared (in meters):

$$BMI = weight\ (kg)/height\ (m)^2$$

The patient with a BMI of 27 (25% to 30% overweight) usually presents minimal risks in the perioperative period. A BMI higher than 30 is associated with an increased perioperative mortality.

Physiologic Considerations in Obesity

Respiratory System. Preoperative evaluation of obese patients reveals that 85% of them have exertional dyspnea and some degree of orthopnea. Periodic breathing, especially when sleeping, may also be present.

Obese patients tend to develop some degree of thoracic kyphosis and lumbar lordosis because of a protuberant abdomen. In addition, the layers of fat on the chest and abdomen reduce the bellows action of the thoracic cage. The overall lung-thorax compliance is reduced, thus leading to increased elastic resistance of the system. Usually the diaphragm is elevated, and the total work of breathing is increased as a result of the deposition of abdominal fat. Because of these factors, the oxygen cost of breathing is three or more times that of normal, even at rest.

The primary respiratory defect of obese patients is a marked reduction in the expiratory reserve volume. The reason for the decrease in expiratory reserve volume and other lung volumes is that the obese patient is unable to expand his or her chest in a normal fashion. Therefore diaphragmatic movement must account for the changes in lung volume to a much greater extent than thoracic expansion does. As previously discussed, the diaphragmatic movement is moderately limited by the anatomic changes of obesity, which account for the decreased lung volumes.

In the obese patient, the functional residual capacity may be below the closing capacity in the sitting and supine positions. Therefore the dependent lung zones may be effectively closed throughout the respiratory cycle (see Chapter 10). Consequently, inspired gas is distributed mainly to the upper or nondependent lung zones. The resulting mismatch of ventilation to perfusion produces systemic arterial hypoxemia (Fig. 45-1).

The hypoventilation and ventilation-perfusion abnormalities that contribute to systemic arterial hypoxemia also contribute to retained carbon dioxide, thus leading to hypercarbia, which can be observed in the pickwickian syndrome.

Cardiovascular System. It has been estimated that 30 pounds of fat contain 25 miles of blood vessels and that the increased body mass in obesity leads to an increased oxygen consumption and carbon dioxide production. It is not surprising that the cardiac output and the total blood volume are increased in the obese state. This increase in cardiac output is a result of an increase in stroke volume rather than an increase in heart rate; the latter usually remains normal.

The transverse cardiac diameter has been shown to be greater than normal in approxi-

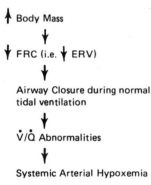

Fig. 45-1 The relationship of body mass to systemic arterial hypoxemia. *FRC,* Functional residual capacity; *ERV,* expiratory reserve volume; *V/Q,* ventilation/perfusion. *(From Drain C, Vaughan R: Anesthetic considerations of morbid obesity, AANA J 47:556–565, 1979.)*

mately two-thirds of obese patients. A linear relationship seems to exist between cardiac diameter and body weight.

It has been suggested that obesity predisposes to electrocardiographic changes. The Q-T interval is often prolonged and the QRS voltage is reduced (because of the increased distance between the heart and the electrodes). Finally, likelihood of ventricular arrhythmias is increased in the obese patient.

A positive correlation exists between an increase in body weight and increased arterial pressure. A weight gain of 28 pounds can increase the systolic and diastolic blood pressure by 10 and 7 mm Hg, respectively. The increase in blood pressure is probably caused by the increased cardiac output.

Chronic heart failure, although uncommon, can occur in persons with long-standing morbid obesity with or without hypertension. It is usually characterized by high output and biventricular dysfunction, with the left ventricle predominating. Clinically, heart failure may be difficult to diagnose because pedal edema may be chronically present.

Cerebral blood flow in obese persons does not differ significantly from that in persons of normal weight. Oxygen uptake of the brain remains normal in the obese person. However, the fraction of the total body oxygen represented in the cerebral metabolism is less than normal because

the total body oxygen requirement is increased. Although the kidneys of obese subjects weigh more than those of nonobese counterparts, renal blood flow is the same or slightly lower than that found in patients of normal weight.

Pregnancy. Problems associated with obesity in pregnancy occur relatively commonly. Studies indicate that patients who weigh at least 250 pounds have a 35% chance of operative obstetrics. In fact, some form of obstetric complication may be observed in 63% of obese patients. Seven times more toxemia, five times more pyelonephritis, and ten times more diabetes mellitus occurs in obese patients than in similar groups of nonobese pregnant patients.

Other Disorders. Diabetes mellitus has been associated with obesity. It is the third most prevalent preoperative pathologic condition found in obese patients. Adult patients with diabetes are often obese, and an improved glucose tolerance test follows weight reduction. Other associated problems that may be clinically present include abnormal liver function tests, fatty infiltration of the liver, gallstones, hiatal hernia, and varicose veins.

Care of the Obese Patient
Respiratory. Significant problems arise in the PACU phase of the perioperative care of the obese patient. In fact, the problems associated with obesity are becoming more apparent to all perianesthesia nurses since the advent of the jejunoileal bypass and gastric stapling procedures for the treatment of morbid obesity. A direct correlation exists between the incidence of postoperative pulmonary complications and the degree of obesity. The mortality rate after upper abdominal operations in obese patients is 2.5 times that of their nonobese counterparts.

Positioning can be a valuable therapeutic tool to improve arterial oxygenation. It has been demonstrated that position significantly affects PaO$_2$ levels for 48 hours postoperatively. The obese patient should be cared for in a semi-Fowler's position unless cardiovascular instability exists. Routine use of the supine position should be avoided because the functional residual capacity can decrease below the closing capacity and thus reduce the number of ventilated alveoli, which will ultimately lead to hypoxemia. Moreover, early ambulation in the PACU is of great value in enhancing lung volumes of the obese patient.

In the postoperative period, the position of the operative incision is a factor, because it has been demonstrated that obese patients with a vertical incision have a more marked postoperative hypoxemia than obese patients who receive a transverse incision. Therefore supplemental inspired oxygen may be postoperatively necessary for 3 to 4 days in patients with a vertical incision. Serial arterial blood gas determinations can serve as a guide to supplemental oxygen administration. Moreover, after the patient's arterial line is in place, arterial blood gas determinations should be done to provide a baseline guide for proper ventilation. If the patient arrives in the PACU with the endotracheal tube in place, the patient should be started on a ventilator. The nurse should then auscultate for bilateral breath sounds to ensure proper placement of the endotracheal tube. Because of the many technical difficulties associated with tracheal intubation of the obese patient, the perianesthesia nurse should constantly monitor the patient for proper placement of the tube. If it becomes displaced, the patient should be ventilated with a bag-valve-mask system, and the anesthesia personnel should be summoned immediately.

Cardiovascular pathophysiology may reduce cardiac reserve, especially in the older obese patient. A reduction in arterial oxygen tension caused by incision site or postoperative position causes an increase in cardiac output to facilitate tissue oxygen delivery. This could lead to cardiac decompensation in an already compromised cardiovascular system. Arterial hypoxemia should be avoided because many obese patients cannot compensate for the increased cardiac output demand and the concomitant pulmonary vasoconstriction caused by the reduced arterial oxygen tension.

Early postoperative ambulation is important not only in enhancing lung volumes but also in helping reduce the incidence of venous thrombosis. Indeed, relatively immobile obese persons are particularly susceptible to the development of pulmonary emboli.

Cardiovascular. The obese patient has a higher incidence of hypertension, coronary artery disease, myocardial infarction, and cardiomegaly. Therefore careful electrocardiographic monitor-

ing should be employed. If an arterial line was not used intraoperatively, a blood pressure cuff that covers one-third to half the length of the upper arm should be employed. A baseline blood pressure measurement when the patient arrives in the PACU will prove valuable in comparison to the intraoperative measurements to assess the accuracy of the blood pressure reading.

Fluid Dynamics. Because fatty tissue is 6% to 10% water—in comparison to lean tissue, which comprises 70% to 80% percent—alteration in fluid requirements is likely to occur in the obese patient. In the normal person, the percentage of body water is 65; in the obese person, the body water is about 40% of total weight. Calculations of fluid requirements must be adjusted to compensate for this reduction in total body water.

Psychologic Aspects. Psychologic support of the obese patient should not be overlooked when perianesthesia care is administered. Many of these patients have become obese because of repeated episodes of emotional stress. Body image, along with the ability to interact with others, may be a problem for obese patients; they may appear to be demanding and aloof from others. It is important for the perianesthesia personnel to establish a positive rapport with the obese patient preoperatively. Along with this, it is important that the perianesthesia staff not express any negative feelings about the patient or about morbid obesity in general. Hence the added psychologic support will serve to minimize fear and anxiety and ultimately improve the outcome of the obese patient.

CIGARETTE SMOKING

Cigarette smoking affects the manner in which a patient recovers from an anesthetic. The perianesthesia nurse should be aware of the diverse reactions that smoking can have on the patient who is emerging from an inhalation anesthetic.

Although studies on the relationship between smoking and its effects on anesthesia are meager, they indicate an increase in the risk factor in the patient who smokes.

Respiratory Effects of Smoking

A growing body of convincing scientific literature suggests that almost all pulmonary disease is related in some way to the inhalation of infectious or irritant particulate material. Cigarette smoke in its gaseous phase contains nitrogen, oxygen, carbon dioxide, carbon monoxide, hydrogen, argon, methane, hydrogen cyanide, ammonia, nitrogen dioxide, and acetone. In the particulate phase, cigarette smoke contains nicotine, tar, acids, alcohol, phenols, and hydrocarbons. Smokers who inhale nicotine from a cigarette into the lungs actually receive 25% to 30% of the nicotine contained in the cigarette. Thirty percent is destroyed by combustion, and 40% is lost in the side stream. Therefore if a person inhales the smoke from a cigarette that contains 2.5 mg of nicotine, 1 mg of nicotine will actually be absorbed by the lungs. It is also known that filters make little difference in this absorption. Contrary to some opinions, smoking cigars and pipes also presents risk for pulmonary disease. Carbon monoxide combines with the hemoglobin molecule at the same point as oxygen does. It has an affinity for this receptor point that is 210 times greater than that of oxygen. Therefore the oxygen-carrying capacity of hemoglobin is reduced, and the end result is that less oxygen is given up to the tissues by the hemoglobin. When carbon monoxide combines with hemoglobin, a compound called carboxyhemoglobin is formed. The amount of carboxyhemoglobin in the blood is especially important in the patient who has a diseased myocardium because myocardial oxygenation is limited by the flow of the blood through the coronary arteries. During stress, such as in surgery and anesthesia, the amount of carboxyhemoglobin saturation could lead to severe myocardial hypoxia in heavy-smoking patients with coronary artery disease because the diseased coronary arteries cannot increase the flow significantly. The only means of preventing hypoxia is to increase the extraction of oxygen from the hemoglobin. Small amounts of carboxyhemoglobin may hinder the uncoupling of the oxygen, thus resulting in yet more oxygen retention at any given tension. This effect clearly would be greater when the oxygen tension is further reduced by local ischemia and any additional vasoconstriction associated with smoking.

Smoking is an important causative factor in chronic pulmonary disease, especially the obstructive type. The pulmonary function alterations characteristic of smokers usually include a reduction in vital capacity, an increase in residual volume to total lung capacity, an uneven distribution of inspired gas, a decrease in dynamic compliance, and an increase in nonelastic resistance.

Chronic bronchitis is the disease most often associated with smoking and is seen often by the perianesthesia nurse. Hypertrophy of bronchial mucous glands with production of excessive mucus is the hallmark of this disease. A vicious cycle develops as this failure to remove the mucus leads to retention of pathogenic organisms and irritants. The resulting distorted alveolar septa and the increased pressure on the alveoli from chronic bronchitis can lead to emphysema.

Cigarette smoke can cause a progression from hyperplasia to metaplasia to neoplasia in the lungs. Sometimes associated with bronchial carcinoma is the Eaton-Lambert syndrome, often called the myasthenic syndrome because its symptoms resemble those of MG. This syndrome in some way affects neuromuscular transmission, and patients experience the classic symptoms of muscle weakness. These patients are especially sensitive to the skeletal neuromuscular blocking agents used in clinical anesthesia. If the anesthetist is unaware of this syndrome and administers the normal dosage of skeletal muscle relaxants, the patient will probably be unable to ventilate spontaneously on emergence from anesthesia even when pharmacologic reversal of the muscle relaxant is attempted. In this situation, postoperative mechanical ventilation is necessary.

Cardiovascular Effects of Smoking

The correlation between vascular disease and smoking is strong. Smoking may influence thrombosis, and because thrombi and platelets contribute to the development of arteriosclerosis, smoking can contribute to arteriosclerosis and its complications.

Inhalation of nicotine produces a release of catecholamines, activates the carotid and aortic chemoreceptor bodies, and directly stimulates the muscles of the vessel walls. As a result, the immediate effects of smoking even a small number of cigarettes can be fairly marked—producing increases in heart rate, peripheral resistance, cardiac workload, and blood pressure. Each of these actions causes a greater myocardial oxygen demand. Furthermore, because the smoker's hemoglobin can provide less oxygen to the myocardium, it is unsurprising that smoking can cause cardiac arrhythmias, either through myocardial anoxia or epinephrine release.

Care of the Patient Who Smokes

Many investigations have demonstrated that patients who smoke have a significant increase in pulmonary complications in comparison to nonsmokers. Patients who smoke more than two packs of cigarettes a day are especially prone to perianesthetic complications. Many of these complications develop when cigarette smokers have a preexisting chronic respiratory disease, usually bronchitis. The major postoperative complications associated with smoking are infection, atelectasis, pleural effusion, pulmonary infarction, and bronchitis.

Complications associated with chronic cigarette smoking revolve around the inability of the patient to clear secretions. The goal of nursing care in the PACU centers on clearing the tracheobronchial tree. This necessitates frequent suctioning, cascade coughing, and the SMI maneuver. If rales and rhonchi are heard on auscultation, percussion and postural drainage should be initiated.

Because cardiovascular disease is associated with a long history of cigarette smoking, the patient should have continuous electrocardiographic monitoring. Arrhythmias, such as premature ventricular contractions, should be sought because they may be the first signs of decreased myocardial oxygenation in the cigarette smoker.

SICKLE CELL ANEMIA

Sickle cell anemia is an inherited type of hemolytic anemia. It is a chronic disease marked by exacerbations. The clinical manifestations are based entirely on sickling of the red blood cells and its consequences.

More than 100 abnormal hemoglobins have been described in humans. When it is exposed to low oxygen tensions, this particular form of hemoglobin causes the red blood cell to distort its shape (sickle) and to cause infarction and other complications. Normal hemoglobin is labeled hemoglobin A, whereas this sickling hemoglobin is labeled hemoglobin S.

Hemoglobin S is thought to have arisen in Arabia in Neolithic times and from there to have spread eastward and westward; it is found today in parts of India, east and west Africa, and the West Indies as well as among African-Americans.

The common sickle cell disorders are sickle cell trait (SA), homozygous sickle cell disease (SS), sickle cell-hemoglobin C disease, and sickle cell-thalassemia. A combination of thalassemia and sickle cell anemia occurs in sickle cell-beta thalassemia.

Sickle cell trait is found in about 8% to 12% of the African-American population, who are heterozygous for sickling, and represents a combination of sickle hemoglobin (SA) and normal hemoglobin (AA). The red blood cells of such persons contain from 20% to 40% hemoglobin S but are not misshapen under normal living conditions. The person may experience sickling if he or she is exposed to any conditions that cause hypoxia, such as depressed respiratory function from anesthetics in the PACU.

The most common form of sickle cell disease is the homozygous sickle cell disease. It occurs in about 1 in 400 to 500 African-Americans. These persons have inherited sickling genes from both parents, and they usually have 80% to 100% hemoglobin S. Sickling is present all the time, and minor reductions in oxygen tension can cause a sickle cell crisis. The onset of symptoms occurs around the age of 2, and rarely do these persons live past the age of 40.

Sickle cell-hemoglobin C disease is caused by the presence of the gene for sickle hemoglobin and the gene for hemoglobin C. The course of the disease is usually milder than that of the homozygous sickle cell disease, although the person will experience discomfort and occasional sickle cell crises.

Sickle cell-thalassemia—which occurs in persons who have traits for sickle cell-thalassemia and beta-thalassemia—has a less severe course and symptoms in comparison with the other forms of these diseases. The sickle cell crises are not seen as commonly in this disease.

Pathogenesis of Sickle Cell Anemia

To understand the pathogenesis of this disease, it is helpful to know what happens to the red blood cell when sickling occurs. If oxygen tension is lowered, long crystals called tactoids are formed within the red blood cells because of rearrangement of the amino acid chains or polymers. The cell membrane becomes distorted by the twisting of the polymers. The result is the sickle cell shape for which the disease is named. The process can be reversed if the oxygen tension is increased.

The actual pathologic action of sickling occurs in the microcirculation. Because of increased viscosity and the distortion of the red blood cells with the formation of tactoids—which prevents the cells from molding to the size and structure of the capillaries—the sickled cells are wedged in the capillary bed, thus occluding normal flow. As the cells aggregate, a thrombus is formed. Symptoms depend on whether the thrombus becomes an embolus and, if so, on where it becomes lodged; infarctive episodes will be caused in that tissue. Areas of infarctive crisis are the spleen, myocardium, kidney, liver, mesentery, bone marrow, and brain.

Oxygen tension causes sickling, but several other precipitating factors are also involved, such as acidosis, hypotension, regional vasodilatation, dehydration, hemoconcentration, stasis of blood, hypothermia, sepsis, decreased cardiac output, and respiratory impairment.

Sickle Cell Anemia and Anesthesia

It is generally believed that anesthesia is not hazardous to patients with sickle cell trait. Nevertheless, it must be kept in mind that sufficiently adverse hypoxic conditions can precipitate a sickling crisis. Definite hazards arise with anesthesia in patients with sickle cell and sickle cell–hemoglobin C disease. Because of its ability to cause the intravascular sickling syndrome, general anesthesia has been the subject of much research. The most important factor in this syndrome is hypoxemia, which generally occurs during the emergent period rather than intraoperatively. Local anesthesia or nerve block is the technique of choice. Epidural and spinal techniques should be avoided because of the possibility of hypotension with these two methods.

Care of the Patient with Sickle Cell Disease

Prevention of sickle cell crisis is the main objective in the PACU phase. If diagnostic procedures are not available or if emergency surgery prevents testing for the sickling trait, all African-Americans patients should be treated as possible carriers of the trait because the incidence of this disease is relatively high among African-Americans.

In the patient with sickle cell disease, the postoperative period is critically important because incisional pain, analgesics, pulmonary infections, and low arterial oxygen partial pressures all are predisposing factors to the formation of sickle cells. Hence in the PACU, supplemental humidified oxygen—along with appropriate monitoring of intravascular volume and core temperature—is of utmost importance for ensuring the positive outcomes of the patient.

Temperature regulation is important for the patient with sickle cell disease. Although cold reduces tactoid formation, it also reduces body metabolism, which may lead to crisis. Hyperthermia causes excess sweating, however, and may lead to dehydration, which can also cause sickling. Temperature monitoring and the use of hypothermia and hyperthermia blankets can allow maintenance of body temperature in the optimal range of 36°C to 37°C.

Cardiac monitoring is important because the occurrence of arrhythmias—such as extrasystole and prolonged P-R interval—in sickling patients is high. Vasodilators or vasoconstrictors should be avoided, if possible, because the dilators may cause hypotension and the vasoconstrictors may cause circulatory stasis.

Respiratory rate and volume should be monitored closely so that hypoxia can be avoided. Oxygen saturation or arterial blood gas monitoring can aid in assessing respiratory status, and postoperative pain should be managed with drugs that do not depress respiratory function.

Kidney function should be monitored because the renal tubules will become blocked by the hemolyzed red blood cells if crisis occurs, and infarcts may occur in some areas of the kidney. Insertion of a urinary catheter to monitor urinary output at regular intervals will prove useful.

SICKLE CELL CRISIS

The types of crisis seen in sickle cell anemia are vasoocclusive, aplastic, sequestration, and hemolytic. The vasoocclusive crisis is the most common type and is characterized by tissue ischemia, infarction, and necrosis. The bones, tendons, synovia, spleen, liver, and intestine are common sites of occlusion. Infections, dehydration, high altitudes, extreme physical exertion, and emotional upsets can trigger this type of crisis.

The aplastic crisis is most grave and constitutes a medical emergency. It is characterized by a sudden drastic decrease in red blood cell production. The patient will initially appear weak and have signs of cardiac decompensation.

The spleen is involved in sequestration crisis. A large amount of blood becomes trapped in the spleen, thus causing hypovolemia and shock; this constitutes a medical emergency. Clinically, the patient's blood pressure decreases and the pulse rate increases. Palpation and percussion reveal an enlarged mass in the right upper quadrant of the abdomen.

Bacterial infections, poisons, and medications—such as phenothiazines and sulfonamides, aspirin in large quantities, and quinine—can produce hemolysis of the red blood cell. The patient also has an enzyme deficiency (glucose-6-phosphodehydrogenase) in this type of sickle cell anemia.

If crisis occurs, the following modes of treatment are recommended: keep the patient warm; treat infections; and maintain oxygenation, hydration, and alkalinization. Heparin may be administered to reduce the risks of embolus formation, and magnesium sulfate may also be indicated for its vasodilator and anticoagulant properties.

NAUSEA AND VOMITING

One of the most perplexing problems for the perianesthesia nurse is the syndrome of postoperative nausea and vomiting (PONV). Most often, patients who experience nausea and vomiting have a history of chronic gastrointestinal irritability. Although the incidence of nausea and vomiting has decreased through the years, the problem remains perennial in every PACU. The surgeon hopes that nausea and vomiting will be minimal because disturbances in electrolyte balance and wound healing are associated with such upsets. The perianesthesia nurse also appreciates a decreased incidence of these upsets because when patients are vomiting, airway management can become most difficult.

Mechanism of Action

The vomiting (emetic) center is located in the medulla near the dorsal nucleus of the vagus

nerve (Fig. 45-2). It can be excited by reflex impulses that arise in the pharynx, stomach, or other portions of the gastrointestinal tract. Foreign materials—such as blood and mucus or irritant gases in the stomach or other portions of the gastrointestinal tract—can produce this syndrome. The vomiting center can be excited by impulses received from cerebral centers. This is because the vomiting center is located very close to the fourth cerebral ventricle (see Chapter 8) and it receives impulses from the chemoreceptor trigger zone (CTZ), cerebral cortex, labyrinthovestibular center, and the neurovegetative system of the hypothalamus. Of these physiologic centers, the CTZ has the greatest impact on the vomiting center. In fact, the CTZ, when stimulated by the appropriate stimuli,

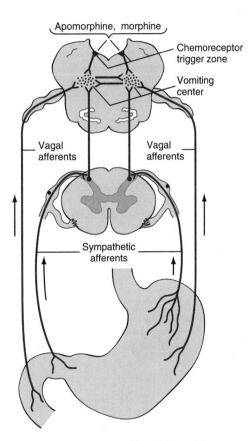

Fig. 45-2 The afferent connections of the vomiting center. *(From Guyton AC, Hall JE: Textbook of medical physiology, ed 10, Philadelphia, 2000, WB Saunders.)*

can initiate vomiting independent of the vomiting center. The CTZ is rich in the receptors serotonin, dopamine, histamine, and opioids and is not protected by the blood-brain barrier. This lack of protection allows the CTZ to be directly stimulated by chemical stimuli from the systemic circulation or the cerebral spinal fluid (CSF).

Drugs such as anesthetic agents and narcotics sensitize the vestibular apparatus, the organ of balance. This explains why two of the principal causative factors of nausea and vomiting are rough handling of the patient during transportation and regular changes of position in the immediate recovery period.

The vomiting center as well as the CTZ can be excited by chemical materials carried to it in the blood. Drugs such as apomorphine, morphine, and meperidine (Demerol) arrive this way and directly excite the vomiting center. This is designated as central vomiting. The vomiting center can be excited by interference with its blood supply. Severe cerebral anoxia and increased intracranial pressure are such examples. Finally, the vomiting center can be excited by dehydration and electrolyte imbalance.

Incidence of PONV

Studies indicate that the incidence of nausea and vomiting is higher in women than in men. A lower incidence occurs in those patients who were premedicated with morphine than in those who receive meperidine. Of great interest is that patients who receive their anesthetic by mask have a higher incidence of nausea and vomiting than do patients who receive their anesthetic by endotracheal tube. This is because some of the anesthetic gases are inadvertently "pumped" into the stomach and cause gastric distension. Many clinicians report that when nitrous oxide is used intraoperatively, the incidence of PONV rises significantly. Hence from a clinical point of view, patients who receive intraoperative nitrous oxide should be monitored extensively for PONV in the PACU. Other possible causes of nausea and vomiting of statistical significance are hypotension during surgery, intraabdominal surgery, increased duration of surgery, obesity, and a history of motion sickness.

Many authors agree that postoperative nausea is related to pain. Opiates of sufficient dosage tend to reduce pain and abate nausea, and they seldom provoke nausea. If the dosage of the analgesic is inadequate, the nausea may persist, and further supplemental doses of analgesic may be required. Other techniques for relief of pain that should be instituted concomitant with the administration of opiate are repositioning the postoperative patient, encouraging the patient to cough and breathe deeply, and administering oxygen.

Patients who received a nitrous-narcotic anesthetic and whose state was reversed postoperatively with an excessive dose of naloxone (Narcan) usually exhibit nausea and vomiting in the emergent phase. Naloxone does not possess any emetic properties. Therefore the analgesic state should be reestablished to eliminate the vomiting reaction caused by pain when the opiate receptors are occupied by naloxone rather than opiates.

Care

In most cases, vomiting is preceded by nausea. Nausea is a feeling of impending vomiting. Several signs accompany the feelings of nausea. The patient will usually have excessive salivation, dilated pupils, tachypnea, swallowing, pallor, sweating, and tachycardia. If the patient's nausea worsens, retching will usually occur, and the tachycardia may change to bradycardia. If patients complain of nausea, they should be encouraged to perform the SMI and the cascade cough, and oxygen should be administered if hypoxemia is suspected. A cold washcloth placed on the patient's forehead, and words of encouragement sometimes extinguish the nausea. It is mandatory for the nurse to remain with the patient because the patient can go into the vomiting stage at a moment's notice, and the danger of aspiration of vomitus and obstructed airway is always present.

Phamacologic Interventions. If the above does not relieve the nausea and vomiting, a pharmacologic intervention will be needed (Table 45-6). As previously discussed, the following receptors are in the CTZ: serotonin (5-HT$_3$), dopamine (D$_2$), histamine, and muscarinic. Drugs that block serotonin (5-HT$_3$) are ondansetron (Zofran) and dolasetron (Anzement), and the drugs that block the dopamine (D$_2$) receptor are droperidol (Inapsine) or metoclopramide (Reglan). For the histamine receptors, pro-

Table 45-6   Drugs Used to Control Nausea

Drug	Category/Action	Route of Administration	Dosage	Side Effects
Dolasetron (Anzement)	Serotonin (5-HT$_3$) Antagonist Antiemetic	PO IV	50-100 mg 12.5 mg	Minor changes in ECG intervals, headache, dizziness, diarrhea
Ondansetron (Zofran)	Serotonin (5-HT$_3$) Antagonist Antiemetic	PO IV	8-16 mg 2-8 mg	Minor changes in ECG intervals, headache, dizziness, diarrhea
Granisetron (Kytril)	Serotonin (5-HT$_3$) Antagonist Antiemetic	PO IV	1-2 mg 1-3 mg	Minor changes in ECG intervals, headache, dizziness, diarrhea
Tropisetron (Navoban)	Serotonin (5-HT$_3$) Antagonist Antiemetic	IV	2-5 mg	Minor changes in ECG intervals, headache, dizziness, diarrhea
Droperidol (Inapsine)	Dopamine (D$_2$) receptor Antagonist Butyrophenone	IV	0.625 mg	Prolonged emergence, hypotension, extrapyramidal reactions
Metoclopramide (Reglan)	Dopamine (D$_2$) receptor Antagonist Gastrokinetic	IV	10-20 mg	Prolonged emergence, hypotension, extrapyramidal reactions
Promethazine (Phenergan)	Antihistamine	PO IM IV	25 mg 12.5-25 mg 12.5-25 mg	Drowsiness Dry mouth Blurred vision
Diphenhydramine (Benadryl)	Antihistamine	IM or IV	10-50 mg	Drowsiness Dry mouth Blurred vision
Atropine	Anticholinergic	IV	0.4 mg	Drowsiness Dry mouth Blurred vision Tachycardia
Glycopyrrolate (Robinul)	Anticholinergic	PO IM IV	1-2 mg 0.1-0.2 mg 0.2 mg	Drowsiness Dry mouth Blurred vision
Scopolamine patches	Anticholinergic	Transdermal patch	1.5 mg	Drowsiness Dry mouth Blurred vision Confusion

Continued

		Route of		
Table 45-6 **Drugs Used to Control Nausea**—*cont'd*				
Drug	Category/Action	Route of Administration	Dosage	Side Effects
Dexamethasone (Decadron)	Steroid/enhance effects of 5-HT₃ antagonists	IV	8 mg	Hypocalcemia Hypokalemia with potassium depleting diuretics
Prochlorperazine (Compazine)	Antiemetic Phenothiazine	PO IM IV Rectal	5-10 mg (tabs) 25-50 mg 25-50 mg 50-100 mg	Drowsiness, dizziness, hypotension, extrapyramidal reactions
Hydroxyzine (Atarax or Vistaril)	Antiemetic Antihistamine	IV	10-25 mg	Potentiation of narcotics and barbiturates, and other central nervous system depressants; drowsiness, dry mouth

IM, Intramuscular; *IV*, intravenous; *PO*, oral.

methazine (Phenergan) or diphenhydramine (Benadryl) can be given. For the muscarinic receptors, atropine, glycopyrrolate (Robinul), or scopolamine patches may be given. It should be stated that because of the antiinflammatory properties of steroids, the drug dexamethasone (Decadron) is often administered in combination with a serotonin (5-HT₃) blocking drug and dopamine blocking (D₂) agent. It is difficult to state exactly what drug protocol is effective for PONV because the drugs that are used vary widely between clinicians. Hence all drugs are in Table 45-6.

Airway Management. Perianesthesia care of the patient who is vomiting focuses on airway management. The patient should be placed in a head-down position so that the vomitus will drain away from the lungs. Oral suctioning should be instituted if the patient is not completely able to control his or her airway. Oxygen should be administered when any question of compromise of the respiratory status arises. Rapid assessment of the patient's respiratory status should be made during and after the vomiting episode. This is done by bilateral auscultation of

the chest for adventitious sounds. Any possible aspiration of vomitus should be reported immediately to the physician. If the airway becomes obstructed, place the patient in a head-down position, turn his or her head to one side, and try to remove foreign material by suctioning or with the finger. While performing this maneuver, the nurse should send another person for an anesthesia care provider. A third person should remain to assist the nurse.

BIBLIOGRAPHY

Alspach J: Core curriculum for critical care nursing, ed 5, Philadelphia, 1998, WB Saunders.

Anderson R, Krogh K: Pain as a major cause of postoperative nausea, Can Anaesth Soc J 23(4):366, 1976.

Aronson R, Weiss S, Ben R et al: Association between cigarette smoking and acute respiratory tract infections in young adults, JAMA 248:181-183, 1982.

Atlee J: Complications in anesthesia, Philadelphia, 1999, WB Saunders.

Austin R: Cigarette smoking and chronic bronchitis, Br Med J 2(6046):1261, 1976.

Ayres S: Cigarette smoking and lung diseases: an update. In Basics of respiratory disease, New York, American Lung Association, 1975.

Barash P, Cullen B, Stoelting R: Clinical anesthesia, ed 4, Philadelphia, 2000, Lippincott Williams & Wilkins.

Bayes J: Asymptomatic smokers: ASA I or II? Anesthesiology 56:76, 1982.

Benumof J: Anesthesia and uncommon diseases, ed 4, Philadelphia, 1998, WB Saunders.

Benumof J, Saidman L: Anesthesia & perioperative complications, ed 2, St Louis, 1999, Mosby.

Berman L: Cigarettes, coronary occlusions, and myocardial infarctions, JAMA 246:871-872, 1981.

Bickley L, Hoekelman R: Bates' guide to physical examination and history taking, ed 7, Philadelphia, 1998, Lippincott Williams & Wilkins.

Biddle C, Biddle W: A survey of perianesthetic complications in the asymptomatic smoker, AANA J 51(5):481-484, 1983.

Biddle C, Hernandez S: Perioperative control of diabetes mellitus-revised, AANA J 51(2):138-141, 1983.

Bowdle T, Horita A, Kharasch E: The pharmacologic basis of anesthesiology, New York, 1994, Churchill Livingstone.

Braunwald E: Harrison's principles of internal medicine, ed 12, New York, 1991, McGraw-Hill.

Breslow M, Miller C, Rogers M: Perioperative management, St Louis, 1990, Mosby.

Brown B, editor: Anesthesia and the obese patient, Philadelphia, 1981, FA Davis.

Burrows B, Knudson R, Quan S et al: Respiratory disorders: a pathophysiologic approach, ed 2, Chicago, 1983, Year Book Medical Publishers.

Cameron L, Kirsch J: Myasthenia gravis pharmacologic management, Crit Care Rep 1:157-163, 1989.

DeFazio-Quinn D: Ambulatory surgical nursing core curriculum, Philadelphia, 1999, WB Saunders.

Drain C: Physiology of the respiratory system related to anesthesia, CRNA: The Clinical Forum for Nurse Anesthetists 7(4):163-180, 1996.

Drain C: Pathophysiology of the respiratory system related to anesthesia, CRNA: The Clinical Forum for Nurse Anesthetists 7(4):181-192, 1996.

Drain C, Robinson S: The pharmacology of respiratory disorders related to anesthesia, CRNA: The Clinical Forum for Nurse Anesthetists 7(4):193-199, 1996.

Drain C: Anesthesia care of the patient with reactive airways disease, CRNA: The Clinical Forum for Nurse Anesthetists 7(4):207-212, 1996.

Erikssen J, Hellen A, Stormorken H: Chronic effect of smoking on platelet count and platelet adhesiveness in presumably healthy middle-aged men, Thromb Haemost 38(3):606-611, 1977.

Ferrara-Love R, Sekeres L, Bircher N: Nonpharmacologic treatment of postoperative nausea, J PeriAnesth Nurs 11(6):378-383, 1996.

Fink D, Raymon R: Rheumatoid arthritis of the cricoarytenoid joints: an airway hazard, Anesth Analg 54(6):742, 1975.

Friedman F: Mortality in cigarette smokers and quitters: effects of baseline differences, N Engl J Med 30:1407-1410, 1981.

Frost E: Preanesthetic assessment of the patient with respiratory disease, Anesthesiol Clin North Am 8:657-676, 1990.

Ganong W: Review of medical physiology, ed 20, New York, 2001, McGraw-Hill Professional.

Gibson J: Anesthesia for the sickle cell diseases and other hemoglobinopathies, Semin Anesth 6(1):27-35, 1987.

Guyton A, Hall J: Textbook of medical physiology, ed 10, Philadelphia, 2000, WB Saunders.

Hardman J, Limbird L: Goodman and Gilman's the pharmacological basis of therapeutics, ed 10, New York, 2001, McGraw-Hill.

Lake C, Hines R, Blitt C: Clinical monitoring: practical applications for anesthesia and critical care, St Louis, 2001, Mosby.

Longnecker D, Murphy F: Dripps/Eckenhoff/Vandam introduction to anesthesia, ed 9, Philadelphia, 1997, WB Saunders.

Longnecker D, Tinker J, Morgan G: Principles and practice of anesthesiology, ed 2, St Louis, 1998, Mosby.

Lynch J: Preoperative and intraoperative insulin needs in diabetic patients, AANA J 52(3):275-279, 1984.

Maduska A: Sickling dynamics of red blood cells and other physiologic studies during anesthesia, Anesth Analg 54(3):361-364, 1975.

McIntosh L: Essentials of nurse anesthesia, New York, 1997, McGraw-Hill.

Miller R, editor: Anesthesia, ed 5, New York, 2000, Churchill Livingstone.

Nagelhout J, Zaglaniczny K: Nurse anesthesia, ed 2, Philadelphia, 2001, WB Saunders.

Schenker M, Samet J, Spiezer E: Effect of cigarette tar content and smoking habits on respiratory symptoms in women, Am Rev Respir Dis 125:684-690, 1982.

Spindler J, Mehlisch D, Brown C: Intramuscular ketorolac and morphine in the treatment of moderate to severe pain after major surgery, Pharmacotherapy 10:51S-58S, 1990.

Stoelting R: Pharmacology and physiology in anesthetic practice, ed 3, Philadelphia, 1999, Lippincott-Raven.

Stoelting R, Miller R: Basics of anesthesia, ed 4, New York, 2000, Churchill Livingstone.

Stone D: Perioperative care: anesthesia, medicine, and surgery, St Louis, 1998, Mosby.

Townsend C, Beauchamp R, Evers B et al: Sabiston textbook of surgery: the biological basis of modern surgical practice, ed 16, Philadelphia, 2001, WB Saunders.

Traver G, Tremper Mitchell J, Glodquist-Priestley G: Respiratory care: a clinical approach, Gaithersburg, Md, 1991, Aspen Publishers.

Vaughan R, Engelhardt RC, Wise L: Postoperative hypoxemia in obese patients, Ann Surg 180(6):877, 1974.

Walker J: Efficacy of single-dose intravenous dolasetron versus ondansetron in the prevention of postoperative nausea and vomiting, Clin Ther 23(6):932-938, 2001.

Waugaman W, Foster S, Rigor B: Principles and practice of nurse anesthesia, ed 3, Norwalk, Conn, 1999, Appleton & Lange.

Waxman SJ, Waxman SG: Correlative neuroanatomy, ed 24, Norwalk, Conn, 1999, Lange Medical Publishers.

White P: What's new in intravenous anesthesia: 1990 International Anesthesia Research Society Review Course Lectures, Cleveland, 1990, IARS.

Weinberg G: Basic science review of anesthesiology, New York, 1997, McGraw-Hill.

Wightman J: A prospective survey of the incidence of postoperative pulmonary complications, Br J Surg 55:81-91, 1968.

46

CARE OF THE PEDIATRIC PATIENT

Donna L. Johnson, RN, CRNA, MSNA

Pediatric anesthesia is a popular subspecialty in the practice of anesthesiology. For clarification, the "newly born" or "newborn" is defined as younger than 72 hours old; the neonate is an infant during the first 28 days of life; the infant includes the neonatal period and extends through 12 months of age; and a child is younger than 13 years of age. Because their immaturity presents various definite physiologic differences, infants and children cannot be regarded as simply small adults. Some of the main differences lie in the respiratory and cardiovascular systems and in the regulation of body temperature.

Anesthetic management of the pediatric patient has been revised in several areas as comprehension of pediatric physiology and pathophysiology has improved. Along with this increased depth of knowledge, pediatric anesthesiology and perianesthesia care are increasingly more challenging and rewarding. The information within this chapter will provide information regarding perianesthesia care for children of all ages that hopefully can make it both rewarding and enjoyable.

ANATOMIC AND PHYSIOLOGIC CONSIDERATIONS

Respiratory System

Newborns are usually obligate nose breathers and are prone to airway obstruction. This is because the newborn has small nares, a large tongue, a small mandible, a short neck, and a large amount of upper airway lymphoid tissue.[1-3] Consequently, when ventilating a newborn by use of a face mask, the nurse should be careful not to apply too much pressure over the soft tissue of the neck

because pressure of this kind can easily obstruct the airway. Also, the epiglottis is at the level of the first cervical (C1) vertebra in the neonatal period.[3] By 6 months of age the epiglottis usually has moved down to the level of C3, thus making oral breathing more feasible.[3]

The vocal cords of the newborn are situated at approximately the level of C4, as opposed to the location at C6 in the adult.[3] The shape of a child's larynx is that of an inverted cone, whereas in the adult it is more cylindrical.[3] The opening of the vocal cords in the adult normally is the narrowest portion of the trachea, but in the newborn the narrowest portion of the trachea is the cricoid cartilage.[3] The clinical implications of this anatomic feature are that if edema around the cricoid cartilage occurs—because of infection or mechanical irritation from an endotracheal tube (ETT)—significant narrowing of the airway may occur. Also, because the cricoid ring is the narrowest part of the larynx, this limits the size of the ETT to be used. An uncuffed ETT is used until the age of 8 to 10.[3] The endotracheal tube should allow a slight leakage (20-25 cm of water pressure) around itself when positive pressure is applied by use of an anesthesia bag.

The epiglottis of the newborn is U-shaped, hard, short, and narrow, whereas it is flatter in the adult. Generally, a straight laryngoscope blade would be used for intubation in the PACU. Finally, the tracheal length is relatively short, particularly in the infant less than 6 months of age, which makes proper placement and taping critical to avoid bronchial intubation or accidental extubation. Once the endotracheal tube position is secured, the nurse should reconfirm the presence of bilateral breath sounds.

Newborns are diaphragmatic breathers. This is because the ribs are situated horizontally in a cylindrical thorax, which limits thorax expansion. Consequently, the ventilatory effort results almost entirely of the movement of the diaphragm. Because newborns are diaphragmatic breathers, they are susceptible to ventilatory problems, such as hypoventilation when excursion of the diaphragm is impeded. Hence, gastric distention caused by faulty bag and mask ventilation, improper positioning, or bowel obstruction can produce inadequate ventilation. In addition, the sternum and anterior rib cage are compliant, and the intercostal and accessory muscles of respiration are poorly developed. In the premature infant, the sternum may be retracted deeply with each inspiration leading to impaired ventilation. The respiratory rate of infants and young children is faster for multiple reasons. The perianesthesia care provider should be knowledgeable of the normal values of respiratory rate for infants and children (Table 46-1).

As in the adult, the newborn's primary drive to ventilation is carbon dioxide. However, the secondary drive in the newborn is different from that of the adult. The newborn younger than 1 week of age responds to a reduction in the partial pressure of oxygen by transient hyperventilation followed by hypoventilation.[3,4] Therefore hypoxia does not stimulate but rather depresses ventilation in the newborn.[3] This secondary drive response is aggravated by hypothermia, a condition that can occur in the postanesthesia care unit (PACU). The respiratory rate is higher and the tidal volume lower in infants and children. When ventilation equipment, such as a mask, is used, dead space is increased.

The respiratory control center in both fullterm and premature infants may easily fatigue; therefore ventilatory reaction to high carbon dioxide tensions or to low percentage of oxygen is not as rapid in the newborn.[3,4] As a result, the newborn may not be able to compensate for rapid changes in arterial blood gas levels. By three weeks of age, hypoxemia induces sustained hyperventilation, as in older children and adults.[3,4] Along with this, newborns and infants may breathe irregularly because of their lack of a mature respiratory center, and periodic breathing is often seen in this age group.[3]

Endotracheal intubation is more widely used in pediatric anesthesia today (Table 46-2). The advantages of endotracheal intubation include decreased dead space, avoidance of laryngospasm and gastric distention, and prevention of aspiration. However, the incidence of postintubation edema from trauma and infection may be increased.

Cardiovascular System

A multitude of factors influence changes in myocardial function in association with age. Normally the respiratory rate and heart rate decreases with increasing age. Systolic and diastolic blood pressure increase with age and body size. The cardiovascular age-related changes for newborns, infants, and children is summarized in Table 46-1. The newborn heart function is at

Table 46-1	Cardiovascular Age-Related Changes in Children					
Age	Respiratory Rate (per Minute)	Heart Rate Awake (BPM)	Heart Rate Asleep	Heart Rate Exercise/ Fever	Systolic Blood Pressure	Diastolic Blood Pressure
Newborn	45-60	100-180 (140)	80-160	<220	65	40
12 months	40	80-160 (120)	70-120	<200	95	65
3 years	30	80-120 (100)	60-90	<200	100	70
6 years	25	70-115 (100)	60-90	<200	90	60
12 years	20	65-90 (80)	50-90	<200	110	60

Adapted from Motoyama E, Davis P: Smith's anesthesia for infants and children, ed 6, St Louis, 1996, Mosby, pp. 87-89.

Table 46-2 Pediatric Airway Equipment

Age	Weight (kg)	Internal Diameter (mm)	Length Oral (cm)	Length Nasal (cm)	Suction Catheter (French)	LMA Size (#)	LMA Cuff Volume (Ml)	Oral Airway Size*
Premature	0.7-1.0	2.5 uncuffed	7-8	9	5	—	—	000-00
Premature	1.0-2.5	3.0 uncuffed	8-9	9-10	5	—	—	000 (30 mm)
Newborn	2.5-3.0	3.5 uncuffed	9-10	11-12	6	1	2-5	00 (40 mm)
3 months	3.5-5.0	3.5 uncuffed	10-11	12	6	1	2-5	0 (50 mm)
3-9 months	5.0-8.0	3.5-4.0 uncuffed	11-12	13-14	6	1.5	7	0 (50 mm)
9-18 months	8.0-11.0	4.0-4.5 uncuffed	12-13	14-15	8	1.5	7	1 (60 mm)
1.5-3 years	11.0-15.0	4.5-5.0 uncuffed	12-14	16-17	8	2	10	1 (60 mm)
4-5 years	15.0-18.0	5.0-5.5 uncuffed	14-16	18-19	10	2	10	2 (70 mm)
6-7 years	19.0-23.0	5.5-6.0 uncuffed	16-18	19-20	10	2.5	14	2 (70 mm)
8-10 years	24.0-30.0	6.0-6.5 cuffed	17-19	21-23	10	2.5	14	2 (70 mm)
10-11 years	30.0-35.0	6.0-6.5 cuffed	18-20	22-24	12	3.0	15-20	3 (80 mm)
12-13 years	35.0-40.0	6.5-7.0 cuffed	19-21	23-25	12	3.0	15-20	3 (80 mm)
14-16 years	45.0-55.0	7.0-7.5 cuffed	20-22	24-25	12	3.0	15-20	3 (80 mm)

Adapted from Motoyama E, Davis P: Smith's anesthesia for infants and children, ed 6, St Louis, 1996, Mosby, p. 296.
LMA, Laryngeal mask airway.
*Oral airway size as a guide. A quick method of determining oral airway size is by placing the airway along the side of the face. The oral airway length should extend from the lips to the angle of the mandible.

near peak ventricular function and therefore has little cardiac reserve. Heart rate plays a major role in determining cardiac function.[3] The newborn is relatively unable to compensate for suboptimal conditions such as hypoxemia, acidosis, or myocardial depression.[3] With the advent of more sophisticated blood pressure monitoring devices, measurements in infants can be taken with greater accuracy. The pediatric patient ordinarily demonstrates the usual signs of impending shock or airway obstruction, yet if the problem is not rectified quickly, physiologic status will deteriorate rapidly. Hence the perianesthesia nurse should closely observe children for subtle changes in status; if abnormalities arise, prompt intervention is essential.

Fetal hemoglobin is high in the newborn. The hemoglobin level and number of blood cells are high at birth. Also, remember that fetal hemoglobin in the newborn has a high oxygen affinity but a low ability to unload oxygen to the tissues. Values then decrease progressively until age 3 months. A physiologic anemia occurs at approximately 3 months of age from reduction in the fetal hemoglobin present at birth and primarily from a decrease in erthyropoiesis production.[1,3] Also, plasma volume increases which has a dilutional effect on Hb level.[2] The rates then rise slowly to the normal adult values. Oxygen delivery to the tissues may not necessarily be compromised because the oxyhemoglobin dissociation curve shifts to the right and because concentrations of 2,3-diphosphoglycerate increase.[1,3] These changes will help to ensure oxygen delivery to the tissues.

Composition and Regulation of Body Fluids

The kidney of the newborn matures rapidly. In the neonate renal function is characterized with obligate salt loss, slow clearance of fluid overload, and an inability to conserve fluid.[5] Consequently, newborns are intolerant of both dehydration and fluid overload. The newborn can conserve sodium to some degree despite a low glomerular filtration rate and limited tubular function;[6] however, premature infants are prone to hyponatremia as well as water overloading. Dehydration in the neonate of any gestational age has harmful effects on renal function.[3,6] Moreover, decreased renal function can delay the excretion of drugs primarily eliminated by renal clearance. At 20

weeks after birth, maturation of glomerular filtration and tubular function is nearly complete.[4]

The blood volume of the newborn younger than 1 month of age is approximately 80 to 90 ml/kg. However, the blood volume of the premature newborn will be as high as 100 ml/kg.[1] The estimated blood volume of an infant from 3 months until 3 years of age is 75 to 80 ml/kg. In children older than 6 years of age, the estimated blood volume approximates that of an adult (65 ml/kg in the adult female, 70 ml/kg in the adult male).

Water distribution in the various body compartments is markedly different among the premature newborn, the fullterm newborn, the child, and the adult. Water distribution is significant because body water composition will impact the volume of drug distribution. Premature infants have the highest percentage of fluid in their extracellular fluid compartment. A progressive decrease in total body water and distribution to the extracellular fluid compartment will decrease during the first year of life. Complete maturation of renal function occurs when the child reaches 2 to 3 years of age (Table 46-3).[4]

Thermal Regulation. Newborns and infants are sensitive to heat loss because they have a relatively large body surface area, a relatively small amount of subcutaneous fat, poor vasomotor control, and a decreased ability to produce heat.[5] The primary mechanism of heat production in a

Table 46-3	Formula for Hourly Maintenance Fluid Requirements in Infants and Children
Body Weight (kg)	**Hourly Fluid Requirements**
0-10 kg	4 ml/kg/hr for each kg body weight
10-20 kg	40 ml + 2 ml/kg/hr for each kg > 10 kg
>20 kg	60 ml + 1 ml/kg/hr for each kg > 20 kg

Adapted from Motoyama E, Davis P: Smith's anesthesia for infants and children, ed 6, St Louis, 1996, Mosby, p. 319. Based on 1 ml of fluid per 1 kcal of caloric expenditure.

neonate is nonshivering thermogenesis mediated by brown fat.[5] Shivering is of little significance to thermal regulation. When ambient temperature falls (<33°C), epinephrine is released by the sympathetic nervous system to activate thermogenesis. The preterm newborn will require a higher ambient temperature (35°C) to minimize oxygen consumption.[7] Ordinarily, to maintain a body temperature within normal limits, they metabolize brown fat, cry, and move about vigorously. Thus newborns and infants respond to a cold environment by increasing their metabolism, which ultimately leads to an increase in oxygen consumption and to the production of organic acids.

PREMATURITY

A premature newborn is defined as birth before 37 weeks' gestation. The often labile condition of premature neonates demands meticulous and vigilant perianesthesia care. Careful attention must be given to airway maintenance, medication dosage, fluid management, and temperature regulation. The premature infants as well as infants younger than 6 months of age are prone to airway obstruction and apneic episodes. The majority of infants who develop postanesthesia apnea are under 46 weeks' postconceptual age (PCA). However, apnea has been reported in infants up to 60 weeks' PCA.[4] In addition to apneic spells pulmonary complications include hyaline membrane disease and bronchopulmonary dysplagia. Also, the premature neonate is immunocompromised and at greater risk for postoperative infection. In the sick premature neonate the likelihood of blood transfusions, artificial ventilation, and the need for parenteral nutrition is greater.[4] The risk of apnea in the PACU may be decreased by intravenous administration of caffeine (10 mg/kg).[2] In neonates the half-life of caffeine is between 37 to 231 hours.[2] By 4 months of age, the half-life of caffeine drops dramatically to approximately 6 hours and is similar to that of an adult. Also, several authors cite the initial discovery of xanthine derivatives, such as theophylline or aminophylline, as a respiratory stimulant to decrease the frequency of apneic episodes in the newborn.[2,8]

Retinopathy of Prematurity

Retrolental fibroplasia is a fibrovascularization and scarring of the retina. Although this disease is associated with hyperoxia, a multitude of other risk factors may be involved, and the role of oxygen is controversial.[2,3] The risk of this retinal disorder is to newborns—especially premature infants who are born before 36 weeks' gestation and weigh less than 1000 to 1500 g.[2] Vascularization of the retina is complete at approximately 44 weeks' gestation.[3] The extreme prematurity may be the single most important factor in the development of retinopathy of prematurity (ROP). The normal PaO_2 in neonates is between 60 to 80 mm Hg. It has been recommended that oxygenation is continuously monitored with pulse oximetry and that hyperoxia should be avoided. A saturation of 90% to 95% would result in a PaO_2 in the range of 60 to 80 mm Hg.[9] In addition, it is important that the pulse oximeter probe be placed on the right upper extremity or ear lobe, in case of a patent ductus arteriosus. It may be helpful to place two pulse oximeter probes on the premature infant.[9] Moreover, when an arterial catheter is indicated it also should be placed in the right upper extremity.

In susceptible patients who are exposed to a hyperoxic environment, blood gas tension should be measured and an oxygen analyzer used to confirm the oxygen concentration. It is not known at what level of oxygenation, nor the exact length of exposure time, which may lead to the development of ROP.[2] One must consider that attempts to prevent arterial hyperoxia and visual impairment must be tempered with the realization that unrecognized arterial hypoxemia can result in irreversible brain damage.

Infant Respiratory Distress Syndrome

Infant respiratory distress syndrome (IRDS)—once called hyaline membrane disease—is a severe disorder of the lungs of the newborn. The incidence of IRDS increases in premature infants. The basis of the pathogenesis of IRDS is insufficient surfactant levels.[10] Surfactant is beneficial for following the two functions: (1) reducing surface tension so that less pressure is required to hold the alveoli open; and (2) maintaining alveolar stability by adjusting surface tension to changes in alveolar size. Insufficient surfactant levels increase surface tension at the alveolar air-liquid interface—resulting in alveolar collapse, an inordinate increase in the work of breathing, and impaired gas exchange. This impaired gas exchange results in hypoxemia and hypercarbia. Along with this, the pulmonary vascular resistance is increased and results in hypoperfusion of pulmonary and systemic circulation. This hypoperfusion, along with hypoxemia, causes tissue hypoxia and metabolic acidosis. An increase in survival with a decrease in serious complications is associated with administration of surfactant into the lungs at birth.[2] As lung compliance improves, a progressive decrease in tidal volume and ventilation pressure will help to prevent further lung injury.

Treatment for neonates with severe IRDS includes oxygen therapy, maintenance of intravenous fluids and nutritional support, temperature regulation, arterial blood gas monitoring, and lab sampling.[10] Extremely preterm infants and those with severe disease often require intubation during delivery room resuscitation or shortly after birth.[10] Also, intermittent positive pressure mechanical ventilation with positive end-expiratory pressure may be necessary to ventilate the exceptionally stiff lungs of these neonates. Chronic air trapping in preterm infants can occur and excessive inflation pressures must be avoided.[3]

PEDIATRIC ANESTHESIA TECHNIQUES

Administration of anesthetic inhalational agents to the pediatric patient has progressed from the technique of open-drop ether, to the nonrebreathing technique, and finally to the pediatric circle system. The Bain system is the coaxial modification of the Mapleson D breathing circuit and was primarily used for the neonate and infant until the development of the pediatric circle system. The Bain system does not have valves and therefore offers the advantages of being light in weight with decreased resistance to breathing. Also, spontaneous ventilation is more easily permitted. A high fresh gas flow rate—2 to 3 times the child's minute ventilation—is required with the Bain system, which is not as economical particularly for older children. In the PACU one might expect the body temperature to be slightly lower in part because of the use of high fresh gas flow rates with decreased ability to conserve heat loss. Advantages of the pediatric circle system include conservation of potent inhalation agents and body heat, ability to retain humidity, and easy collection and scavenging of waste gases.

The pediatric circle system has a smaller diameter than the adult tubing and has a low compression volume,[1] which allows for accurate delivery of desired tidal volume. The pediatric circle system can safely be used for the neonate and infant who weighs less than 10 kg if ventilation is controlled.[8]

The laryngeal mask airway (LMA) has been widely used for anesthesia in infants and children. The LMA is not a substitute for the endotracheal tube, but it can maintain upper airway patency, especially in spontaneously breathing patients. Also, it can serve as an emergency airway when the patient cannot be adequately ventilated with a bag and mask system or if intubation is unsuccessful. Successful endotracheal intubation can occur through the LMA with a fiberoptic bronchoscope. The appropriate LMA size—based on the patient's kg weight, and guidelines for cuff volume inflation—are included in Table 46-2.

Children 1 year of age and older will benefit from anxiolytic premedication to decrease preoperative anxiety and modify behavioral changes following discharge.[11] Many anesthesia practitioners will use oral midazolam premedication in pediatric patients 1 year of age and older, in whom a greater likelihood of uncontrollable separation anxiety exists. Also, midazolam can be given intramuscular, intravenous, rectal, or intranasal as an alternative route of administration for pediatric premedicant.[12] However, the oral route is generally preferred unless preoperative intravenous access is available. Flumazenil is a competitive antagonist at the benzodiazepine receptor and is used as a reversal agent for midazolam.[9,13] Flumazenil may be administered intravenously at a dose of 10 µg/kg over 15 seconds. If necessary, the dose of flumazenil can be repeated up to four times, at 1 to 3 minute intervals. However, the total dose should not exceed 50 µg/kg.[9]

An anticholinergic drug, such as glycopyrrolate or atropine, may be given to protect against bradycardia that can occur after succinylcholine administration or in association with induction of anesthesia. The most popular inhalation anesthetic agents used for pediatric anesthesia are halothane, sevoflurane, isoflurane, and desflurane. Halothane and sevoflurane are the most common induction inhalation agents. Once the child reaches the maintenance phase of general anesthesia, the anesthetist may switch to either isoflurane or desflurane. All inhalation anesthetic agents offer a relatively rapid emergence. Halothane was the most popular pediatric inhalation agent because of its relative freedom from airway irritation and smooth emergence. Sevoflurane offers a similar smooth induction with also a very rapid emergence with minimal potential risk and has somewhat replaced halothane in certain circumstances. Although sevoflurane and desflurane offer the advantage of rapid emergence, both may be associated with increased incidence of agitation or delirium upon emergence and into the PACU, especially in young children. It is imperative to have an analgesic base, when indicated, in place before this rapid emergence and transfer to the PACU.

Ketamine, a dissociative anesthetic, is sometimes used in pediatrics as an induction agent or for short procedures that do not require muscle relaxation. Emergence time depends on route of administration and whether the drug was repeated during the operation. The most serious disadvantage to ketamine is a high incidence of emergence delirium, hallucinations, and possible psychosis. Also, nystagmus may occur. After the use of ketamine, the postanesthesia recovery area should be quiet and conducive to a slow peaceful emergence and recovery.[14] A premedicant with a tranquilizing drug, such as midazolam, can significantly reduce these side effects.[14] Ketamine has the advantage of providing analgesia as well and caution should be used when additional narcotics are given in the PACU. For uncooperative children or in patients with Down syndrome or mental retardation, an intramuscular injection of midazolam combined with ketamine may be helpful.[8]

Fentanyl can be given as a premedicant in the form of a lollipop called an Oralet (5-15 µg/kg).[8] Once the child becomes sedate the Oralet will naturally fall away from the child's mouth. The fentanyl Oralet had fallen out of favor because of the potential for children to associate it with candy. It is important to note that fentanyl levels will continue to rise intraoperatively and will contribute to postoperative analgesia.

The introduction of the intravenous agent propofol has dramatically assisted the anesthesia provider to provide anesthesia with minimal recovery time. Propofol can be used in remote locations and provides deep sedation for painful or frightening procedures.[9,14] This drug has advanced anesthesia care for children in remote locations such as magnetic resonance imaging or for hematology and oncology patients.[15] Propofol provides rapid onset of action and quick emergence from anesthesia with minimal residual effects.[16] Earlier discharge and decreased recovery time is particularly notable when propofol is the only anesthetic agent used.[17] Maintenance of anesthesia can be accomplished through repeated dosing or continuous infusion.[15] Also, propofol has an antiemetic effect, and postoperative nausea is rare.

POSTOPERATIVE CARE OF THE PEDIATRIC PATIENT

When children require hospitalization and surgery an associated potential for organ system dysfunction of respiratory, circulatory, or neurologic function may be present.[4] The greatest vital organ dysfunction predominantly involves the respiratory system. The greatest focus of postoperative care initially should be directed towards the respiratory function with the administration of supplemental oxygen delivery, and maintenance of a patent airway. Ultimately, nutritional support will be the primary focus to meet the metabolic needs of the pediatric patient to promote healing and recovery from the stress of surgery and anesthesia. When the pediatric patient arrives in the PACU, the initial assessment should include identification of a patent airway, and vital signs, including temperature, should be obtained and recorded. A humidified air-oxygen mixture (high flow) should be administered along with securing a safe environment before report from the anesthetist is given. In a restless child or in one with a history of seizure disorder, side rail pads may be used. The patient will be placed in the lateral position in the operating room before transfer to PACU (Fig. 46-1). However, after an intraoral surgical procedure, the patient may be placed in the ¾ prone position—more commonly known as the tonsillar position—to facilitate adequate drainage of secretions and blood.

During the report, dressings should be checked for drainage and the intravenous infusion line should be checked for patency and for assurance

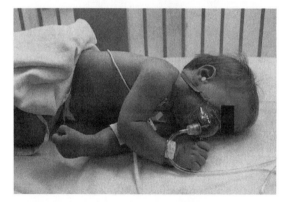

Fig. 46-1 An infant is transported to the PACU in the lateral position. *(From Motoyama E, Davis P: Smith's anesthesia for infants and children, ed 6, St Louis, 1996, Mosby.)*

that the line is adequately secured. Also, children's teeth should be checked routinely on admission to the PACU, especially if loose teeth are present, and again before discharge. It is important to note that in the event of loss, all teeth should be saved and given to the parents, if possible.

Over the years, anesthesia techniques have improved and when combined with rapid-acting anesthetic agents, the pediatric patient will usually arrive in the PACU awake, responsive, and with good abdominal muscle tone. These patients are usually quickly responsive to verbal and tactile stimulation. However, about 10% to 15% of pediatric patients who are recovering from general anesthesia exhibit hyperactive behavior. They require constant nursing care to prevent injury to themselves because they are extremely restless and quite vocal. This agitation or excitement may be related to hypoxemia, the pharmacologic side effects of certain drugs, pain, or awakening in strange surroundings. Therefore if a pediatric patient demonstrates hyperactive behavior, the perianesthesia nurse should assess the patient in the aforementioned areas before providing interventions.

Psychosocial Considerations

It is important that the nurse address issues of parental and child anxiety. By addressing the needs of the parents you will also help to lessen the stress on the child.[18] The parents should be allowed to be with the child as soon as is practical and preferably before the child awakens.[18] Remember that all surgical procedures and hospitalization are extremely stressful for a family. When the pediatric patient emerges from anesthesia, the perianesthesia nurse should meet certain emotional needs of all children to facilitate positive outcomes of the perioperative experience. It is important to provide explanations to the child in terms he or she can understand. Also, always be completely honest with the child. The developmental age of the child will determine which areas are of greatest concern (Table 46-4). For example, infants can become distressed when physical needs are not met. Taking into consideration the type of surgery and the degree of emergence from anesthesia, the primary care giver should hold or rock the patient—if it is age-appropriate—or do both. This will usually relax the patient, and infants especially enjoy being swaddled in a warm blanket, cuddling, rocking, having their heads or backs rubbed, and hearing the voice of the nurse. In the infant younger than 6 months of age, the nurse is "mom."[3] Because the infant mimics facial expressions, the nurse should smile and use facial expressions of happiness when caring for all children. Another consideration is that the PACU is a strange environment for the child. Often, dolls, teddy bears, and other familiar objects from home are taken to surgery and will arrive with the patient in the PACU. These special toys should remain with the child, especially during emergence, to help cope with the environmental change.

In the older infant and preschool child, stranger anxiety remains the greatest fear. This is a particularly vulnerable stage in childhood development. Children at ages 2 to 3 years are at the stage of autonomy versus self-doubt. They may exhibit independence that alternates with sudden dependence and the need for periodic cuddling and reassurance. Their greatest fears include separation from parents, pain, physical harm, strange environments, and the unknown.[3] Often the only mechanism of self-expression is through crying. Negativism may be the child's means of demonstrating control; thus "no" may actually mean "yes." Children of this age are prone to temper tantrums, ritualistic behavior, and breathholding spells. The perianesthesia nurse should be sure to differentiate apnea from

Table 46-4	**Classic Stages of Development Theories for Children**		
Theory Based on Age	Freud Psychosexual	Erikson Psychosocial	Piaget Cognitive
Infancy (0-1 year)	Oral	Basic trust	Sensorimotor (stages 1-5)
Toddlerhood (2-3 years)	Anal	Autonomy versus shame and doubt	Sensorimotor (stages V, VI)
Preschool (3-6 years)	Oedipal	Initiative versus guilt	Preoperational
School Age (6-12 years)	Latency	Industry versus inferiority	Concrete operations
Adolescence (12-20 years)	Adolescence	Identity versus identity diffusion	Formal operations

Adapted from Behrman R, Kliegman R, Jenson H: Nelson's textbook of pediatrics, ed 16, Philadelphia, 2000, WB Saunders, p. 26.

breathholding spells when assessing the respiratory status of the patient. Three-year-old children are certainly special children: lovable but stormy. They are too young to use their own reason and become impatient at times. It is therefore important for the perianesthesia nurse to avoid criticism and provide acceptable behavior alternatives to the patient.

Between the ages of 3 and 6 years, the child begins to become independent. However, in the PACU, dependency can occur because of pain, course of disease, or immobilization. Guilt can occur when the child desires to remain dependent.[4] Consequently, the perianesthesia nurse should provide as much opportunity for independence as possible. The nurse can foster independence by allowing the child to select alternatives in care.

The ages of 6 to 12 years coincide with school entrance. These children are striving for approval when tasks are completed and usually do not tolerate failure because it promotes their sense of inferiority and inadequacy. The hospital environment is new to them, and the child may be unprepared to handle the situation and thus demonstrate difficulty with impulse control. Because children lose control when they are immobilized or ill, the nurse should allow as much individualization and self-care as possible. The nurse should also encourage self-expression and compliment the child on accomplishments during recovery from anesthesia. Also, remember

that a child of this age has a vivid imagination and could easily distort reality.[4]

The adolescent years of ages 12 to 20 are a transitory time characterized by vacillations between dependence and independence, idealism and realism, confidence and uncertainty. The adolescent may experience anxiety over issues related to privacy, loss of control, autonomy, and competence. Privacy is of utmost importance to these patients; therefore the adolescent's body should be covered as much as possible to prevent exposure and resulting embarrassment.

Remember that the individual perioperative experience of each child will greatly impact the success of future medical encounters. Addressing the developmental needs of the child and support of parental involvement can go a long way to meet the needs of the child and lead to a positive experience for the whole family. A preoperative program for elective surgical procedures including a tour of the postanesthesia care unit can help to reduce preoperative anxiety and minimize postoperative negative behaviors.

Monitoring

Initially, monitoring in the PACU includes respiratory rate, blood pressure, pulse oximetry, ECG, fluid balance, and temperature control.[9] When the vital signs are obtained, the PACU values should be first compared with the preoperative and intraoperative recordings of vital signs. After the initial blood pressure is ascertained, particularly for outpatients, pulse oxime-try monitoring may be all that is needed. The pulse oximeter is superior to clinical judgment in providing the earliest warning of a desaturation event.[19] The frequency in measurement of other physiologic parameters depends on the status of the patient and the surgical procedure.[2]

The rate and depth of ventilation should be monitored in the PACU. Respiratory depression occurs with greater frequency if muscle relaxants are used during anesthesia. Because of the rapid ventilatory changes that can occur in the PACU, an oxygen saturation monitor should be used on all pediatric patients. A variable rate of fraction of inspired oxygen content with supplemental oxygen secondary to delivery techniques and depth of ventilation can occur.

The most likely causes of respiratory failure in children with surgical disease include extra-thoracic airway swelling and injury, thoracic dystrophy consistent with congenital disease or intraabdominal swelling, respiratory control abnormality such as occurs with congenital anomalies or drug induced, and loss of functional residual capacity that results in atelectasis.[4] The most common etiology involves the extratho-racic airway with swelling of the pharynx, larynx, or trachea. Infants and small children usually have a low incidence of postoperative atelectasis because crying from pain or awakening in an unfamiliar environment stimulates ventilation. Older children tend to remain in one position and not to move about. They must be encouraged to cough and to perform the sustained maximal inspiration (SMI) maneuver to prevent atelecta-sis. If the pediatric patient is unable to perform the SMI maneuver, deep breathing should be encouraged.[14]

Changes in the heart rate of the pediatric patient are one of the first clues of impending physiologic dysfunction. The PACU provider should initially consider hypoxia as the most likely cause of bradycardia. In the PACU, the heart rate of infants and children is influenced by physical activity and by the administration of atropine, glycopyrrolate, and anesthetic agents. Glycopyrrolate (Robinul), an anticholinergic atropine-like drug, may elevate the heart rate mildly, and not to the same degree as atropine. Also, crying, struggling, or pain can increase the heart rate.

In the event of respiratory dysfunction the designated PACU attending anesthesia provider should be immediately notified. An ongoing airway assessment should be performed, and emergency airway management may be necessary. An oral airway must be of proper size in order to relieve airway obstruction (Fig. 46-2). In addi-tion, correct positioning will assist the provider to ventilate and intubate when necessary. However, correct positioning will vary depending on the age of the child. For instance, children six years of age and older will benefit from a folded towel or small pillow placed under the occiput in combination with extension of the head (Fig. 46-3). This position has often been referred to as the "sniffing" position. In infants and younger children, in most instances, the size of the head is large relative to the trunk and hyperflexion of the neck occurs when lying flat on a bed. Further elevation of the occiput with a folded towel most likely will hinder airway management. Mild flexion of the neck, with slight extension of the head, may be accom-plished with placement of a shoulder roll. Optimal positioning of the head should assist in maintenance of a patent airway or help to ensure successful bag-mask ventilation when indicated. Excessive elevation of the occiput or exaggerated extension of the head should be avoided.

It is always advisable to keep reversal agents such as flumazenil (0.1 mg/kg, IV) and naloxone (1-10 µg/kg, titrated IV) readily available in the event of hypoventilation unresponsive to stimu-lation and for ventilatory assistance.[2,8] In addi-tion, the anesthesia care team providers should be notified in order to offer additional assistance and follow-up care. Pressure cycled ventilators are used in the neonatal intensive care unit to prevent barotrauma.[1] With a pressure cycled ventilator the risk of pressure trauma to the lungs is reduced by allowing the peak airway pressure to be varied to support optimum ventilation. However, a peak airway pressure limit must be maintained to decrease the risk of trauma to the lungs. Therefore in the event of needing postoperative mechanical ventilation of an infant, the settings would most likely be an intermittent mandatory ventilation rate of 20 to 40 breaths per minute, with a peak positive inspi-ratory airway pressure set at approximately 20 to 24 cm H_2O.[1]

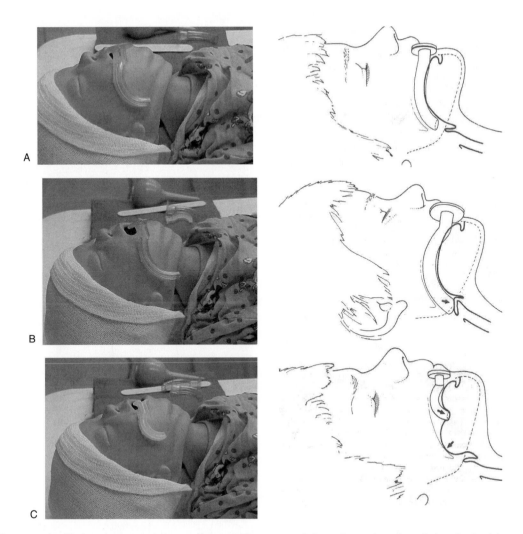

Fig. 46-2 Identification of correct oral airway selection. **A,** The correct oral airway size can be estimated when the tip of the airway ends just cephalad to the angle of the mandible. **B,** If the oral airway is too large the tip of the oral airway may obstruct the glottic opening by pushing down on the epiglottis. **C,** If the oral airway is too small, the tip of the airway may lead to obstruction by pushing down on the base of the tongue. *(Courtesy Department of Nurse Anesthesia, Virginia Commonwealth University. Also adapted from Cote' CJ, Ryan JF, Todres ID, Goudsouzian NG: A practice of anesthesia for infants and children, WB Saunders, 2001, p. 90.)*

A patent intravenous line (IV) should be maintained in the postoperative care unit. In ambulatory surgery with short-stay recovery rooms, additional IV fluids may not be necessary if the intraoperative total fluid volume is sufficient to cover the initial postoperative recovery. However, a patent IV line should be maintained throughout recovery. In the event of postoperative vomiting, additional fluids may be necessary.

Initially, the care provider should administer an isotonic maintenance hourly fluid rate based on the kilogram weight of the patient. If the pediatric patient is moderately to severely ill, monitors for central venous pressure, ECG status, urine output, specific gravity, and an arterial line may be used.

The most likely indications for a central venous catheter would include: the need to

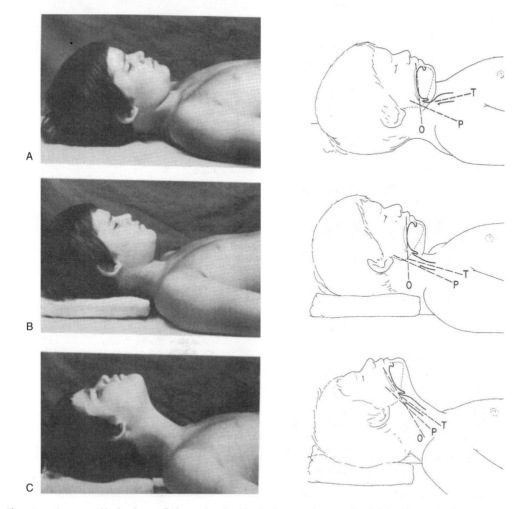

Fig. 46-3 Correct positioning for ventilation and tracheal intubation. **A,** When a patient is lying flat on a bed or stretcher, the oral *(O)*, pharyngeal *(P)*, and tracheal *(T)* axes pass through three divergent planes. **B,** When a folded sheet or towel is placed under the occiput of the head, the pharyngeal *(P)*, and tracheal axes align. **C,** With added extension of the atlanto-occipital joint, all three planes align to correct positioning for ventilation and tracheal intubation. *(Courtesy Department of Nurse Anesthesia, Virginia Commonwealth University. Also adapted from Cote' CJ, Ryan JF, Todres ID, Goudsouzian NG: A practice of anesthesia for infants and children, WB Saunders, 2001, p. 91.)*

monitor central venous pressure, cardiac surgery, inotropic drug administration, neurosurgery (with the potential risk of air embolism), major orthopedic procedures (such as spinal fusion), and abdominal surgical procedures when massive fluid shifting or blood loss is expected.[9] The central venous pressure line may be inserted via the internal jugular, external jugular, subclavian, femoral, basilic, or axillary veins.[9] It provides information on blood volume and serves as an avenue for fluid replacement. Remember, all

rapid infusions of blood products or fluids should be warmed before administration. A fluid or blood warming device should have a visible thermometer and an audible warning indicating excessive heating greater than 42°C.[1] The arterial line, which is inserted through the umbilical (neonate) or radial artery, can measure blood pressure and heart rate and provide for instantaneous blood gas or lab sampling. The ECG provides information on cardiac rate and rhythm. In the event of circulatory abnormalities, blood pressure and pulse should be ascertained and recorded frequently. Any deviation in the cardiac or pulmonary physiologic parameters should be reported immediately to the attending physician.

Newborns and infants expend a great amount of energy maintaining alveolar ventilation, cardiac output, muscular activity, and an appropriate temperature. Because of these high-energy metabolic processes, glycogen and fat stores may be mobilized and depleted rapidly.[3,4] Consequently, cold, stress, pain, and increased muscle activity compound the need for adequate caloric intake in the PACU. In high-risk situations, plasma glucose concentrations should be monitored.[13] Also, the patient's clinical condition dictates the final fluid and electrolyte requirements incurred as a result of trauma or complications from surgery. A glucose-containing infusion can be used for postoperative maintenance fluid replacement for children in high-risk circumstances.[4,6,13] However, rapid infusion of glucose-containing solutions should be avoided.[13] During the administration of fluids, the perianesthesia nurse should ensure that the indwelling catheter is patent and not infiltrated and should use a constant infusion pump to facilitate the proper administration of the correct volume and rate of fluids. To prevent inadvertent overhydration, not more than one third of the day's maintenance intravenous fluid volume should be measured into the intravenous bag at any time.

Important considerations for fluid management of the pediatric patient include monitoring for hypervolemia or hypovolemia. It is important to ensure proper administration of fluids. When attending to issues related to hydration additional areas of assessment and monitoring can be helpful and include the following: (1) urine output, specific gravity, and osmolality; (2) temperature; (3) electrocardiographic (ECG) status, pulse, and blood pressure; (4) hydration of the mucosa; (5) assessment of the fontanelles, in the newborn, for bulging or depression; and (6) blood loss. It is essential to make an accurate assessment of blood loss intraoperatively and postoperatively, because a small miscalculation of a few milliliters can have a serious impact on the total blood volume of an infant.

Permissible blood loss should be defined individually for each patient and is based on the patient's current medical condition, surgical procedure, and cardiovascular and respiratory function.[1] In healthy children with normal cardiovascular function, a lower hematocrit should be tolerated by increasing cardiac output when ventilation is not compromised. A higher inspired oxygen concentration should be provided. In the neonate or child with significant cardiac or pulmonary disease, initiation of blood loss replacement would occur earlier because of the patient's inability to compensate with increased potential morbidity. Initially, ongoing blood loss is replaced with isotonic crystalloid at a ratio of 1:3; for every 1 ml of blood lost, 3 ml of isotonic fluid, such as lactated Ringer's, is given. When losses are high, the usual blood replacement is such that for each 1 ml lost, 1 ml of packed red blood cells are administered (1:1) to the patient. Alternatively, if a colloid solution is used it would be replaced at the same ratio (1:1) as that for blood products—1 ml of 5% albumin per 1 ml of blood lost—until the patient's hematocrit reached a predetermined critical level that requires packed red blood cells.[3,4,9]

Dressings should be watched for excessive bleeding. Such bleeding should be reported at once to the attending physician, because infants and small children will have a narrower time span in which to compensate for loss. The leading cause of circulatory abnormalities in the postoperative pediatric patient is hemorrhage. Second most common is plasma redistribution. Rarely is the cause cardiogenic in nature. Urine output and specific gravity may yield additional information on kidney function and volume expansion.

Thermal Regulation in the PACU

Hypothermia can delay emergence from anesthesia and prolong the stay in the postoperative care unit. Hypothermia can have a detrimental affect on termination of neuromuscular blockade, metabolic balance, coagulation, and ventilatory control.[13] If an infant or small child arrives in the PACU with inadvertent hypothermia, the nurse should assess the patient for (1) vital signs (core temperature, pulse, and respiratory rate); (2) pulse oximetry waveform and saturation; and (3) the degree of emergence from anesthesia. If the patient is experiencing a delayed emergence from anesthesia, the nurse should protect the patient from aspiration of gastric contents and from hypoventilation by positioning (see Fig. 46-1) and stimulation. Dysrhythmias and cardiovascular depression are associated with profound hypothermia. Also, hypothermia may lead to a detrimental affect on coagulation, ventilatory control, and metabolism.[13] A profoundly hypothermic child should remain intubated and sedate. Continuous ECG monitoring will be necessary until the core temperature reaches at least 35°C.[1] Finally, to avoid excess oxygen demand and acidosis associated with hypothermia, newborns and infants should be maintained in a neutral thermal environment in the PACU by the use of incubators, warm blankets, infrared heating lamps, warm-air heating blankets, or elevated room temperature when possible. Care should be taken to minimize environmental exposure during physical assessment, and the head should remain covered.

A word of warning is needed here. If a water mattress is to be used to rewarm the patient, the temperature setting should be no higher than 37°C, and a layer of sheets between the mattress and the skin will aid as a barrier to prevent burns. Also, when a warm-air heating device is used, following the manufacturer's guidelines for proper use is imperative. Only the manufacturer's recommended blanket should be attached to the warm-air tube. Never place the warm-air heating tube between two blankets or directly blowing onto the infant or child for this has resulted in burns. Also, overly vigorous warming can cause a burn injury in infants.[2] Whatever rewarming method is used, the temperature of the device should be monitored frequently to prevent overwarming or injury. Records should be kept of core body temperature (rectal, esophageal, or tympanic), room temperature, and device temperature.

Postoperative Pain Management and Regional Anesthesia

The primary goals of recovery from anesthesia include the ability of the child to maintain their airway and return to baseline mental status. As one would anticipate, if the perioperative plan includes hospital admission more flexibility is afforded in pharmacologic intervention when access to medical personnel is available. Issues related to intravenous hydration and pain management are critical when discharge is planned from the PACU.

The issues related to pain management for children have received increased attention in recent years.[20] Choices for pain management include parenteral narcotics, regional anesthesia, and even patient-controlled analgesia (PCA), depending on the age and maturity of the child. Alternative medications such as nonsteroidal antiinflammatory drugs (NSAIDs), and oral or rectal acetaminophen in combination with parenteral narcotics may be helpful to control pain in the postoperative period as well. In fact, ketorolac in combination with morphine patient-controlled analgesia (PCA) in children has been shown to provide superior analgesia.[21] The overall opioid dose and incidence of opioid side effects decreased.[21] Ketorolac is the only NSAID approved by the Food and Drug Administration for parenteral use (0.5 mg/kg, IV/IM, q6h).[9,21] The recommended dosing of ibuprofen is 8 to 10 mg/kg, orally, every 6 hours. Acetaminophen is a nonopioid analgesic and antipyretic that can be given by the oral (10-15 mg/kg q4 hr) or rectal (20 mg/kg q4h) route.[2]

Opioids are administered for moderate to severe pain. Routes of administration for opioids include oral, rectal, oral transmucosal (under the tongue), intramuscular, intravenous, transdermal, epidural, subarachnoid, and subcutaneous.[13] The most common postoperative parenteral narcotics used in the pediatric population would include meperidine (0.5-1 mg/kg, IV/IM, q2-3h) and morphine (0.05-0.1 mg/kg, IV/IM, q2-4h).[9] However, meperidine use is limited because its metabolite normeperidine can cause dysphoria, agitation, and seizures.[13] Meperidine in low doses can be used for the treatment of rigors and shivering in the PACU. As mentioned previously, ketamine will lower postoperative opioid requirements. Also, extreme caution should be noted with use of the more potent opioids fentanyl or sufentanil in the PACU for fear of severe respiratory depression. Also, fentanyl and its analogs can produce chest wall rigidity when administered as a bolus, which will make mask ventilation extremely difficult.

Patient-controlled analgesia has been successfully used for children as young as six years of age but it requires the understanding and cooperation of the patient.[2,8,9,22] The inherent safety of PCA is based on the idea that if the child becomes too sleepy, he or she will not be able to push the button. It is imperative that family members and nurses do not push the button for the child.

Usually the PCA will have a loading dose that is administered with the medical staff in attendance. By pushing a button, the child is able to deliver a precise opioid dose preprogrammed into the infusion pump. A minimum interval between dosing (a lock-out mechanism) and a maximum dose delivered over a set period of time are also preprogrammed to prevent overdose. A basal metabolic rate may be preprogrammed into the infusion pump to prevent severe breakthrough pain. In some cases a basal infusion rate is not suggested for fear of additive sedation and to prevent respiratory depression. The overall total drug consumption with PCA use is less.[9,22,23] The potential complications associated with PCA include overdose from incorrect programming of parameters and very rarely mechanical malfunction of the device.[8] The perianesthesia care provider should assess the child for side effects associated with opioids (nausea, vomiting, itching, and ileus). An order should be written to discontinue all previous pain medications. In addition, all pain medication orders should be written by the Anesthesia Pain Service.[9] Children should be instructed on the use of a pain score method, such as the Visual Analogue Scale, and a record for assessment of pain should be included on the vital sign sheet (Table 46-5). Pediatric PCA with morphine has been shown to provide better analgesia with lower pain scores in comparison to meperidine.[24] Morphine will most likely be the opioid of choice for postoperative PCA use in children.[24] All nurses should be trained in PCA use.[9]

Regional anesthesia in children can dramatically improve pain management and lower general anesthesia requirements. The most common regional blocks in children include a penile block for circumcision, ilioinguinal block for hernia repair, spinal anesthesia (most often in the very ill neonate), and caudal epidural. Caudal block has been used for a variety of surgical procedures—including circumcision, inguinal herniorrhaphy, hypospadias repair, clubfoot repair, anal surgery, and other procedures below the umbilicus and of the lower extremities.[8] A caudal catheter can be threaded to the thoracic epidural space and can provide a thoracic level block for pain relief in small children (particularly useful for control of pain after open heart surgery).

SELECTED POSTOPERATIVE CONCERNS IN PEDIATRICS

The most common reasons for postdischarge readmission to the hospital are protracted vomiting and surgery-related complications. Recovery room nursing care of children must provide constant assessment of airway patency, ventilation, and circulatory stability.[13] In addition, common postoperative concerns in children include the potential for a postanesthetic excitement phase, and pain management.[13] Because the pediatric patient does not have the physiologic reserves of the adult patient, when complications occur, serious untoward sequelae will take place. Hence, the perianesthesia nurse must monitor for and react to any complication in a timely fashion.

Laryngospasm

Laryngospasm is caused by sensory stimulation of the superior laryngeal nerve.[8] A forceful involuntary spasm of the laryngeal musculature occurs. In the PACU laryngospasm can occur as the child awakens and is usually caused by blood or pharyngeal secretions draining toward the vocal cords.[25] For this reason, children are placed in the ¾ prone position to promote drainage of oral secretions away from the vocal cords. Posterior oral pharyngeal suctioning can cause additional trauma and should be avoided after the child has been extubated.

Initial treatment of laryngospasm includes positive pressure ventilation with an Ambu bag and mask (Fig. 46-4). The two-person bag-mask ventilation technique may provide superior ventilation in the event of significant airway obstruction or poor lung compliance. Intravenous Lidocaine (1-1.5 mg/kg) also can be helpful.[8] If hypoxia develops and the laryngospasm is not relieved from positive pressure ventilation by mask, then succinylcholine (0.25-1 mg/kg) should be given to allow control of ventilation with paralysis of the laryngeal muscles. The perianesthesia care providers should be ready to reintubate if necessary. When laryngospasm develops, large intrathoracic pressures are generated. A negative pressure pulmonary edema can result even in healthy children, and close attention should be given to further respiratory compromise after the laryngospasm has resolved.[8,26] Positive pressure ventilation will be used to treat pulmonary edema after a laryngospasm.

Table 46-5   Age-Specific Pain Measurement Tools for Children

Name	Features	Age Range	Advantages	Limitations
Visual Analog Scale (VAS)	Horizontal 10 cm ruler; subject marks between "no pain" and "worst pain imaginable"	≥8 years	Good psychometric properties; gold standard	Cannot be used in younger children or those with cognitive limitations
Faces scales (e.g., Wong, Baker, Oucher, Bieri, McGrath)	Subjects compare their pain to line drawings of faces or photos of children	≥4 years	Useful for younger ages than VAS	Choice of anchors affects responses (neutral versus smiling)
Color analog scales	Horizontal or vertical ruler, on which increasing intensity of red signifies more pain	≥4 years	Useful for younger ages Converges to VAS at older ages	Cannot be used in toddlers or those with cognitive limitations
Behavioral or combined behavioral-physiologic scales (e.g., CHEOPS, OPS, FACS, NIPS)	Scoring of observed behaviors (e.g., facial expression, limb movement) ± heart rate and blood pressure	Some work for any age; others are age-specific	Can be used even for infants and nonverbal children	Overrates fear in toddlers and preschool children Underrates persistent pain Some inconvenient measures requiring videotaping & complex processing
Autonomic measures (e.g., heart rate, blood pressure, heart rate spectral analyses)	Scores changes in heart rate, blood pressure, or measures of heart rate variability (e.g., "vagal tone")	All ages	All ages Useful for mechanically ventilated patients	Nonspecific; changes can occur unrelated to pain
Hormonal-metabolic measures	Plasma or salivary sampling of hormones (e.g., cortisol, epinephrine)	All ages	Can be used at all ages	Nonspecific; changes can occur unrelated to pain Inconvenient, cannot provide real-time information

Adapted from Behrman R, Kliegman R, Jenson H: Nelson's textbook of pediatrics, ed 16, Philadelphia, 2000, WB Saunders, p. 307.

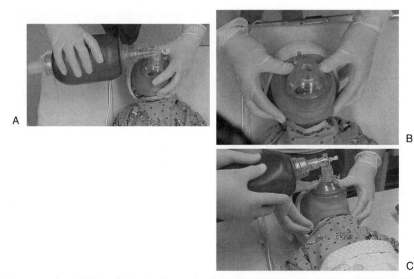

Fig. 46-4 **A,** One-person bag-mask ventilation. **B,** The two-handed technique for mask ventilation may be useful to improve mask fit and therefore ventilation when one-person bag-mask ventilation is difficult or inadequate. A modified jaw-thrust/chin-lift maneuver is demonstrated. The tips of the index and ring fingers are applied to the ascending ramus of the mandible behind the pinnae of the ear. The thumbs apply downward pressure to the facemask to ensure a tight seal. The mouth should open helping to maintain airway patency. The soft structures of the airway should be avoided. **C,** One person uses both hands to open the airway and maintain a tight mask-to-face seal while the assistant compresses the ventilation bag. *(Courtesy Department of Nurse Anesthesia, Virginia Commonwealth University.)*

Airway Obstruction

In the PACU, every pediatric patient, particularly children who have been intubated during anesthesia, should be monitored for signs of airway obstruction. Postintubation croup is caused by glottic or tracheal edema. When laryngeal swelling occurs, the diameter of the airway of the infant or small child can become significantly reduced; in fact, 1 mm of edema in the infant's trachea at the cricoid level decreases the diameter of the airway by 75%. The symptoms of laryngeal obstruction—in order of appearance—are croupy cough, hoarseness, inspiratory stridor, and aphonia. These symptoms are accompanied by increasing restlessness, tachypnea, use of accessory muscles of respiration, retraction of the suprasternal notch and intercostal spaces, and drawing in of the upper abdomen.[2] If these symptoms appear, the perianesthesia nurse should act immediately to relieve the obstruction, administer supplemental oxygen, and send someone to notify the PACU anesthesia provider. The progression of these symptoms can be rapid.

Treatment of postintubation croup involves use of a high-humidity atmosphere that is oxygen-enriched. Nebulized racemic epinephrine (0.5 ml of a 2.25% solution in 2.5 ml of normal saline) has been useful in the treatment of postintubation croup. Also, corticosteroids such as dexamethasone (Decadron, 0.2 mg/kg, IV) have been useful to decrease the laryngeal inflammation associated with other causes of croup.[7] However, corticosteroid use for postintubation croup remains controversial.[8] If laryngeal edema is allowed to progress, the patient may require reintubation, although this occurs very rarely.

Nausea and Vomiting

Nausea and vomiting is a leading cause of delayed discharge from the PACU. Children who are undergoing tonsillectomy, strabismus, or orchiopexy surgery are at greater risk.[27] If there is a greater likelihood of postoperative nausea or vomiting, it is best to administer prophylactic antiemetics whenever possible.[14] In the majority of cases, vomiting can successfully be treated with the use of phenothiazines (rectal promethazine, 0.5 mg/kg), metoclopramide (0.15 mg/kg, IV), or the newer serotonin-3 antagonist, ondansetron (0.05-0.15 mg/kg, IV, maximum dose 4 mg). Phenothiazines and metoclopramide can cause dystonic reactions which may be treated with diphenhydramine (0.5-1 mg/kg, IV).[13] Ondansetron has been shown to be the most effective drug once postoperative nausea and vomiting is present.[14] In the absence of an IV, ondansetron can be given under the tongue for quick absorption without the need for swallowing.[2] Ondansetron is less likely to be given as a preemptive antiemetic because of its higher cost. Propofol used alone for heavy sedation has antiemetic properties, and when it is combined with other drugs for maintaining anesthesia, it will decrease nausea and vomiting.[27]

Malignant Hyperthermia

Although malignant hyperthermia (MH) will be discussed in detail in Chapter 50, a brief description of the condition is given here. The incidence of MH is approximately 1:3000 to 1:15,000 in children, in comparison to 1:40,000 to 1:100,000 in adults.[2,3,9,28] Halogenated inhalation anesthetic agents, such as halothane, and the depolarizing muscle relaxant succinylcholine trigger this genetically determined condition. The pathophysiology of the condition centers on the enhanced release and diminished reuptake of calcium in the skeletal muscle. This causes sustained skeletal muscle contraction and, ultimately, profound hyperthermia. The muscle cells convert to anaerobic metabolism and lactic acidosis ensues. Ultimately, muscle cell breakdown occurs. The drug dantrolene effectively treats MH by inhibiting further release of calcium in the skeletal muscle. In most instances, MH occurs in the operating room; however, a patient may first experience the disorder in the PACU, or the successfully treated MH patient may have an exacerbation of MH symptoms later in the recovery process.

The earliest clinical feature of MH will be a rising end-tidal carbon dioxide level ($ETCO_2$); however, this will not be readily apparent in the PACU unless the patient is intubated and $ETCO_2$ is being monitored. Therefore in most cases of MH in the PACU, the first clinical sign is tachycardia with or without other dysrhyth-

mias; tachypnea and a profound increase in tidal volume are then observed in the spontaneously breathing PACU patient. Generalized muscle rigidity may or may not occur. Hyperthermia is often a late sign. Additional signs include arrhythmias, hypertension, sweating, and mottled skin. It may be difficult to diagnose MH in the PACU because of variable presentation. For example, fever is often an inconsistent and late sign.

Blood chemistry studies reveal an elevated potassium level and an initially elevated calcium level before it falls. Arterial blood gas levels demonstrate a severe fall in bicarbonate and pH and an elevated $PaCO_2$. The PaO_2 may be normal, depending on the FIO_2. Serum myoglobin, creatine kinase, lactic dehydrogenase, and aldolase levels usually rise.

To facilitate a reversal of this condition, the perianesthesia nurse must understand the pathophysiology of MH and should know exactly where the MH emergency cart is located. If a patient appears to be developing MH, the nurse should send for help immediately. He or she should start to assist ventilation of the patient with high-flow 100% oxygen and check to be sure the intravenous line is patent. Once the appropriate personnel arrive, have more than one person mix the dantrolene (20 mg/60 ml of sterile water). A note of warning is needed to ensure that the sterile water does not contain preservatives because much sterile water will be used. The usual starting dose of dantrolene is 2.5 mg/kg, IV. This can be repeated up to 10 mg/kg over 45 minutes or until the patient's condition stabilizes and temperature is reduced.

Once the protocol is initiated, the need for endotracheal intubation and active cooling with frequent temperature monitoring begins. Recognition and treatment of arrhythmias along with correction of the associated acidosis and electrolyte imbalance (hyperkalemia) should be anticipated. Most likely an arterial line, nasogastric tube, and three-way Foley catheter will be placed. The most successful outcome occurs when the syndrome is identified and treated early.[8,28] The child will be transferred to a pediatric intensive care unit to closely monitor and continue therapy for at least 24 hours.

SPECIAL CONSIDERATIONS

Otolaryngologic Surgery

The most common surgical procedures performed in pediatrics involve the ear, nose, and throat (ENT). The leading cause of obstructive sleep apnea (OSA) and hypoventilation in children is adenotonsillar hypertrophy.[13] Other anatomic factors that lead to OSA include micrognathia, retrognathia, or macroglossia. Also, morbid obesity in children or a congenitally small airway will narrow the nasopharynx. Chronic OSA can disrupt sleep and breathing patterns, thus leading to impaired daytime performance as well as more serious complications such as polycythemia, growth failure, heart failure, pulmonary hypertension, and arrhythmias.[13]

Pediatric patients who have tonsillectomies and other operations on the pharynx, larynx, and esophagus require intensive PACU care because the airway can become obstructed postoperatively as a result of surgical manipulation and bleeding. When the patient is admitted to the PACU, the laryngeal and pharyngeal reflexes should be present. The patient should be placed in the tonsillar position, $\frac{3}{4}$ prone with the arm and leg flexed and the head turned to the side. This position improves drainage of secretions and blood from the mouth, preventing possible aspiration or laryngospasm. The patient should be kept in this position until the gag reflex has returned completely.

Nausea with vomiting can lead to bleeding and airway compromise in the recovery room. During report the nurse should note whether an antiemetic was given perioperatively. The combination of propofol and ondansetron is extremely effective in reducing the incidence of vomiting in children after tonsillectomy. Before emergence and extubation in the operating room, it is common practice for the surgeon to suction gastric content and the oral pharynx and to assess for hemostasis. After the child has been extubated it is best to avoid deep oral pharyngeal suctioning to prevent trauma and bleeding.

Trauma Victim

Special consideration should be considered with airway management for the child with head or cervical spine injury. When assisted airway support is needed to relieve airway obstruction in the PACU, the jaw-thrust maneuver is indicated to open the airway (see Figs. 46-3 to 46-5).[2,29] An anesthesia provider should be notified at once to offer assistance and airway management. If a second care provider is available, assistance should be placed with emphasis on immobilization of the cervical spine by maintaining a neutral alignment. The head tilt-chin lift is contraindicated in the presence of cervical spine

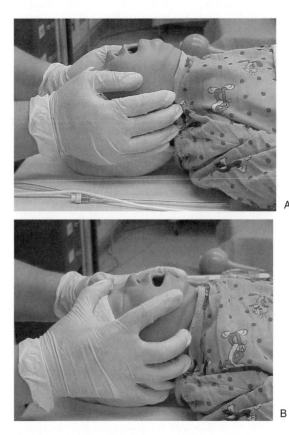

Fig. 46-5 A, Jaw thrust maneuver. It is important to elevate the jaw by placing the tips of the index and ring fingers along the ramus of the mandible (on the bony prominences of the face) while avoiding the soft structures overlying the larynx and glottic opening, which potentially can lead to airway obstruction. **B,** Spine immobilization with airway opening in an infant with potential head and neck trauma. A combined jaw thrust and spinal stabilization maneuver. *(Courtesy Department of Nurse Anesthesia, Virginia Commonwealth University.)*

injury.[29] Once the airway is controlled, a semi-rigid cervical collar, spine board, linen rolls, and tape can be used to immobilize the child. To support oxygenation and ventilation, inline traction and spine immobilization will be necessary for intubation and during transport.

DISCHARGE FROM THE PACU

With the advancement in pharmacologic drugs and inhalational agents for general anesthesia, rapid recovery with decreased side effects has led to earlier discharge from the PACU for children. Certain criteria must be met for safe transition from the PACU to a short-stay recovery unit or hospital ward; however, the goals of recovery will vary depending on the discharge location planned for the patient.[9] When evaluating a child for possible discharge from the PACU, the perianesthesia nurse should observe for each of the following: 1) an alert and easily arousable child; 2) protective airway reflexes; 3) strong muscle strength; 4) the oxygen saturation should be maintained above 95% on room air, or at the baseline preoperative level; 5) normothermia; 6) pain under control; 7) absence of vomiting; 8) no sign of active bleeding; and 9) stable vital signs. Children will continue to recover in an ambulatory or short-stay recovery unit after outpatient procedures.

Steward developed a simplified scale to determine when pediatric patients can be discharged from the PACU (Table 46-6).[2,30] This scale scores airway, consciousness, and movement, from 0 to 2. The maximum number of points is 6. Discharge depends on the overall functional status of the child. However, after procedures involving the airway, such as tonsillectomies, the child may stay in the hospital for a longer period of time for observation.

Factors that will delay postoperative recovery in children include residual anesthetic or neuromuscular blockade, hypothermia, hypoxemia, acid-base imbalance, hypocarbia, hypercarbia, hypovolemia, and elevated intracranial pressure.[2] It is never advisable to force fluids by mouth to facilitate discharge and indeed one should wait until the child vocalizes a desire. Early administration of liquids may cause vomiting. Also, it is not necessary to delay discharge until the child has voided. The anesthesia provider should be notified to assess the child, write the

Table 46-6 Steward's Postanesthesia Recovery Score	
Criterion	Score
CONSCIOUSNESS	
Awake	2
Responding to stimuli	1
Not responding	0
AIRWAY	
Coughing on command or crying	2
Maintaining good airway	1
Airway requires maintenance	0
MOVEMENT	
Moving limbs purposefully	2
Nonpurposeful movements	1
Not moving	0

From Steward D: A simplified scoring system for the post-operative recovery room, Can Anaesth Soc J 22(1):111-113, 1975.

discharge notes including any findings or recommendations for postoperative care and sign for discharge from the PACU. It is imperative that the parents or guardian be instructed concerning discharge care. A phone number should be included with written information on what to do in case of an emergency or for further clarification of postdischarge questions or concerns.

REFERENCES

1. Aker J: Pediatric anesthesia. In Nagelhout J, Zaglaniczny K, editors: Nurse anesthesia, ed 2, WB Saunders, 2001, p. 1132.
2. Gregory G: Pediatric anesthesia, ed 4, New York, 2002, Churchill Livingstone.
3. Motoyama E, Davis P: Smith's anesthesia for infants and children, ed 6, St Louis, 1996, Mosby.
4. Miller R: Anesthesia, ed 4, New York, 1994, Churchill Livingstone.
5. Stoelting R, Dierdorf S: Anesthesia and coexisting disease, ed 3, New York, 1993, Churchill Livingstone.
6. Dabbagh S, Ellis D, Gruskin A: Regulation of

fluids and electrolytes in infants and children. In Motoyama EK, Davis PJ, editors: Smith's anesthesia for infants and children, ed 6, St Louis, 1996, Mosby.

7. Longnecker D, Murphy F: Dripps/Eckenhoff/Vandam introduction to anesthesia, ed 9, Philadelphia, 1997, WB Saunders.

8. Morgan G, Mikhail M, Murray M: Clinical anesthesiology, ed 3, New York, 2002, Lange Medical Books.

9. Badgwell JM: Clinical pediatric anesthesia, Philadelphia, 1997, Lippincott-Raven Publishers.

10. Berman S: Pediatric decision making, ed 3, St Louis, 1996, Mosby.

11. Eckhenhoff J: Relationship of anesthesia to postoperative personality changes in children, American J of Dis Childhood 86:587-591, 1953.

12. Walbergh E: Plasma concentrations of midazolam in children following intranasal administration, Anesthesiology 74(2):233-236, 1991.

13. Behrman R, Kliegman R, Jenson H: Nelson's textbook of pediatrics, ed 16, Philadelphia, 2000, WB Saunders.

14. Steward D: Manual of pediatric anesthesia, ed 5, New York, 2001, Churchill Livingstone.

15. Martin L, Pasternak L, Pudimat M: Total intravenous anesthesia with propofol in pediatric patients outside the operating room, Anesth Analg 74:609-612, 1992.

16. Westrin P: The induction dose of propofol in infants 1-6 months and children 10-16 years of age, Anesthesiology 74(3):455-459, 1991.

17. Hannallah R: Propofol: effective dose and induction characteristics in unpremedicated children, Anesthesiology 74(2):217-219, 1991.

18. Bevin J, Johnston C, Tousignant G et al: Preoperative parental anxiety predicts behavioral and emotional responses to induction of anaesthesia in children, Can J Anaesth 37:177-182, 1990.

19. Cote C: A single-blind study of combined pulse oximetry and capnography in children, Anesthesiology 74(6):980-988, 1991.

20. Mubroy J: Safety and efficacy of alfentanil and halothane in paediatric surgical patients, Can J Anaesth 38(4):445-449, 1991.

21. Sutters K, Shaw B, Gerardi J et al: Comparison of morphine patient-controlled analgesia with and without ketorolac for postoperative analgesia in pediatric orthopedic surgery, Am J Orthop 28(6):351-358, 1999.

22. Vesely C: Pediatric-patient-controlled analgesia: enhancing the self-care construct, Pediatr Nurs Review 21(2):124-128, 1995.

23. Gillespie J, Morton N: Patient controlled analgesia for children: a review, Paediatr Anaesth 2:51-59, 1992.

24. Vetter T: Pediatric patient-controlled analgesia with morphine versus meperidine, J Pain Symptom Manage 7(4):204-208, 1992.

25. Roy W, Lerman J: Laryngospasm in paediatric anaesthesia, Can J Anaesth 35:93-98, 1988.

26. Lee K, Downes J: Pulmonary edema secondary to laryngospasm in children, Anesthesiology 59:347-349, 1983.

27. Barash P, Cullen B, Stoelting R: Handbook of clinical anesthesia, ed 3, Philadelphia, 1997, JB Lippincott.

28. Hopkins P: Malignant hyperthermia: advances in clinical management and diagnosis, Br J Anaesth 85:118, 2000.

29. Guidelines 2000 for Cardiopulmonary Resuscitation and Emergency Cardiovascular Care. International Consensus on Science, Dallas, American Heart Association. Parts 9-11.

30. Steward D: A simplified scoring system for the post-operative recovery room, Can Anaesth Soc J 22:111-113, 1975.

47

I t is difficult to define chronologically when old age begins because some persons age much more quickly than their chronologic age indicates. Legally, however, old age is defined as 65 years or older. The geriatric population (older than 65 years) constitutes approximately 11% of the population, and projections suggest that they will constitute 13% by 2000 and 17% by 2030. Because of the refinements in surgical and perianesthesia care, a greater percentage of geriatric patients will undergo anesthesia and surgery in the future. This category of patients presents a challenge to the perianesthesia nurse because 80% of the patients older than 65 years of age have one or more chronic diseases when they present for anesthesia and surgery.

Care of the geriatric patient is particularly important in the postanesthesia care unit (PACU) because of the physiologic changes that usually occur during the later years. These include congestive heart failure, insufficient oxygenation of the blood, improper elimination of carbon dioxide, fluid and electrolyte imbalance, drug toxicity, nerve palsies, and psychologic changes. To ensure that the geriatric patient will have a positive surgical outcome, the perianesthesia nurse must have the knowledge of the physiologic alterations caused by aging and the effects of anesthesia on the aged patient.

AGE-RELATED PROBLEMS

Cardiovascular System

When first admitted to the PACU, the geriatric patient often presents many physiologic and psychologic problems. With advancing age, the cardiovascular system often undergoes some changes. The aged heart has less reserve and less ability to adjust to stress. Coronary sclerosis is common and some atrophy of the myocardial fibers usually occurs. The recovery from excitability in the aged heart muscle is delayed, and it is more susceptible to dysrhythmias. Cardiac output in the aged is lower than it is in the young, and is less able to increase it during periods of stress.

The systolic blood pressure is usually higher in the geriatric patient because of degenerative arterial disease, which decreases elasticity of the large arteries. This disease makes it difficult for the cardiovascular system to react to stress. Hypotension should be avoided because of the danger of thrombosis and the reduced amount of oxygen that can be transported to the vital organs. Hypertension, on the other hand, must be equally avoided. The most immediate problem of hypertension in the aged is damage from a cerebral vascular hemorrhage. Other areas of concern are hypovolemia, increased susceptibility to hemorrhage, and anemia.

When geriatric patients arrive in the PACU, they may experience some degree of cardiovascular depression because of the anesthetic agents administered intraoperatively. With an age-related decrease in cardiac index, these patients require less inhalation anesthesia and, consequently, usually wake up faster in the PACU. However, because of this, these patients are particularly susceptible to hypotension and bradycardia during emergence from anesthesia. Because glycopyrrolate does not cross the blood-brain barrier, the bradycardia should be treated with that drug. With this approach, the confusion that can be produced by atropine is avoided. Also, because the circulation times are decreased in the aged, intravenous agents usually take a longer time to produce their effects. Consequently, drugs such as succinylcholine have a longer onset and duration of action.

Respiratory System

The aging process frequently affects the respiratory system. The thoracic bone structure usually becomes calcified, a condition that decreases the elastic recoil properties of the chest wall, which causes a premature balance in the elastic forces of the lungs and the chest wall. Thus the functional residual capacity, vital capacity, and total lung capacity are decreased (see Chapter 10). As a person ages, the ratio of residual volume to total lung capacity progressively rises, making ventilation less and less adequate. Senile emphysema causes the intrapulmonary mixing of gases to become less effective, thus leading to hypoxemia and hypercarbia. The upper respiratory tract is also affected by advancing age, thus leading to increased secretions and airway resistance.

In the PACU, the geriatric patient's ventilation should be constantly assessed. The modified stir-up regimen of reposition, cascade cough, and sustained maximal inspiration (SMI) is mandatory for the geriatric patient (see Chapter 26) to reduce the incidence of postoperative pulmonary complications. Along with this, secretions should be removed by assisting the patient to cough and, if required, by suctioning. Positioning to facilitate good ventilatory excursion may be difficult in the geriatric patient because of bone deformity, arthritis, or both. Usually, head-up positions promote proper ventilation.

Neuromuscular System

The weight of the brain decreases with advancing age. Along with this, the loss of neurons caused by the aging process is particularly marked in the cerebral cortex. These atrophic changes interfere with the basic neuronal process and are responsible for the increased susceptibility of the elderly to central nervous system side effects of drugs that are seen clinically in the PACU.

In relation to anesthesia, aging is associated with a progressive decrease in the minimum alveolar concentration for general inhalation anesthetic agents (see Chapter 18). Hence in the PACU, patients of advanced age may experience a prolonged emergence after the administration of an inhalation anesthetic. There seems to be a loss of neurotransmitters and synaptic function, along with a decrease in the number of axons supplying peripheral muscles and muscles innervated

by each axon. Consequently, over time, denervation and atrophy of the skeletal muscles become apparent, which leads to a reduction in conduction velocity in peripheral nerves. This is the reason that the dose requirement for regional anesthetics progressively declines with advancing age.

Renal System

As in other organ systems, renal function and mass progressively decreases with advancing age, which includes a decrease in the glomerular filtration rate and renal blood flow. Thus with reduced cardiac and renal function, the geriatric patient is especially susceptible to fluid overload. Along with this, the mechanisms involved in maintaining the constancy and volume in the extracellular fluid are progressively blunted with advancing age. This reduction in functional adaptive renal mechanisms is responsible in part for the problems in fluid and electrolyte balance seen in geriatric patients. An electrolyte of particular importance in the context of advancing age is sodium. The geriatric patient has a progressively blunted response to sodium deficiency—that is, patients in this age group lose the ability to conserve sodium in response to acute reduction in sodium intake. Because of the salt-losing tendency, the geriatric patient may experience symptoms such as confusion, loss of thirst, and disorientation in the PACU. This is particularly true when a transurethral resection of the prostate is performed or, for that matter, when any surgical procedure in which urinary irrigation is used. The geriatric patient who has experienced this type of surgical procedure should be monitored in the PACU for a deficiency in this electrolyte.

The first symptom of sodium deficiency is probably disorientation. Because some patients in the geriatric population may be somewhat disoriented, it is important that the perianesthesia nurse differentiate among the possible types of disorientation. Blood for electrolyte determination should be drawn and analyzed immediately before any sedation is administered to the patient. If the level of sodium is below normal, intravenous sodium will resolve the clinical picture of disorientation rather rapidly.

Another electrolyte of concern for the geriatric patient is potassium. Advancing age is associated with a progressive decrease in plasma renin concentration. Along with this, an equal reduction in the concentration of aldosterone—which acts on the distal tubule to increase sodium reabsorption and to enhance the excretion of potassium, thereby protecting against hyperkalemia—occurs. With advancing age, the protective mechanism that prevents hyperkalemia during periods of potassium challenge is lost. Given that the glomerular filtration rate is reduced in the geriatric patient, hyperkalemia may result when potassium is administered. Therefore along with monitoring the electrocardiogram for the peaking of T waves, electrolytes should be monitored particularly when a geriatric patient has received potassium salts intravenously in the perioperative period.

Because of the reduction in physiologic function of the renal system associated with advancing age, kidney function should be monitored in the PACU, including fluid and electrolyte balance. Fluid intake and output measurements should be monitored meticulously to ensure an adequate urinary output of 0.5 to 1 ml/kg/hr, because these patients are subject to oliguria and—in some instances—anuria. Also, drugs dependent on renal excretion for their elimination (such as gallamine) are affected by the decrease in kidney function, thus leading to a prolonged plasma concentration and ultimately to prolonged effect of the drug.

Hepatobiliary System

Advancing age is associated with a progressive reduction in hepatobiliary function. Hepatic blood flow is progressively reduced, and an age-related decrease in the functioning of the hepatic microsomal enzymes has been demonstrated. This ultimately leads to an age-related reduction in the biotransformation actions of the liver, and drugs that depend to a major extent on hepatic metabolism usually have a prolonged effect in the elderly population. Because considerable danger of hepatic injury from drugs, hypoxia, and blood transfusions in the routine perianesthesia care of the geriatric patient exist, careful attention should be given to appropriate airway care to enhance oxygenation and to ensure that the appropriate dosage of depressant drugs is given.

Drug Interactions

The physiologic response to a drug occurs in a twofold manner. The first process deals with the drug concentration at the site of action and is termed pharmacokinetics. The second process deals with the ability of the drug to react with a specific receptor and to translate that effect on the receptor into a physiologic response, which is called pharmacodynamics. Advancing age is associated with progressive alterations in both the pharmacokinetics and the pharmacodynamics of drug therapy. Furthermore, the geriatric patient may experience pharmacologic problems because of the multiple types of drugs being taken and the adverse drug interactions that may occur. Table 47-1 may be used to determine the possible adverse effects or drug interactions that may take place in the geriatric patient during the perioperative period.

Psychologic Aspects

The psychologic aspects of perianesthesia care of the geriatric patient center on maintaining the patient's self-esteem. Feelings of uselessness and lack of self-worth promote tension and anxiety, which in turn can affect the patient's physiologic status. Geriatric patients are usually set in their ways, and it is important for them to be able to contribute to their own care. Because their hearing and vision may be impaired, these patients tend to isolate themselves and may not be able to understand oral communication well. Therefore, when conversing with a geriatric patient with possible or documented hearing loss, the nurse should speak slowly and distinctly and in a loud voice.

Alzheimer's Disease

Senile dementia of the Alzheimer type (SDAT)—or Alzheimer's disease—is presently receiving a great deal of attention by medical researchers. This disease consists of a multiplicity of neuronal pathway degenerative processes that result in impairment of cognition and behavioral changes such as depression, aggression, paranoia, anxiety, agitation, and insomnia. No treatment or identification of risk factors exists for this disease.

General anesthesia is usually administered to the patient with SDAT. This is because SDAT

Table 47-1 Adverse Effects or Drug Interactions Associated with the Geriatric Patient

Drug	Adverse Effect or Drug Interaction
Antibiotics	Prolongation of muscle relaxants
Antidysrhythmics	Prolongation of muscle relaxants
Benzodiazepines	
Diazepam	Decreased metabolism
Chlordiazepoxide	Increased CNS effects
Flurazepam	Prolonged drowsiness
Digoxin	Decreased renal excretion with increased CNS disorientation, anorexia, nausea, and cardiotoxicity; blood levels two to three times higher in the elderly with any given dose
Diuretics	Hypokalemia Hypovolemia
Halothane	Decreased anesthetic requirement
Lithium	Clearance decreased by 65% and effective dose by 30% in comparison with patients at age 25 Increased side effects of tremor, diarrhea, and edema
Meperidine	Markedly elevated plasma levels and decreased red blood cell and plasma binding of drug Increased incidence of nausea, respiratory distress, and hypotension
Methyldopa	Enhanced hypotensive effects
Pancuronium	Decreased clearance from plasma
Propranolol	Plasma level approximately three to four times higher in the elderly because of decreased metabolism Bradycardia, congestive heart failure, bronchospasm, mental confusion, and attenuation of autonomic nervous system activity
Tricyclic antidepressants	Increased anticholinergic effects—confusion, agitation, and disorientation Cardiac conduction disturbances Increased anesthetic requirements
Warfarin	Enhanced sensitivity

Adapted from Krechel S, editor: Anesthesia and the geriatric patient, New York, 1984, Grune & Stratton and Miller R, editor: Anesthesia, ed 5, New York, 2000, Churchill Livingstone.
CNS, Central nervous system.

patients lack the cognitive function and cooperative skills necessary for the successful performance of regional anesthesia. These patients are sensitive to the effects of all medications—including the anesthetic agents—and therefore require reduced dosages. Because of this, delayed emergence from anesthesia is not uncommon.

SDAT patients usually require a longer time in the PACU. The perianesthesia nurse should take every step to keep the patient normothermic because hypothermia prolongs emergence. Along with this, maintaining adequate hydration optimizes the emergence process and helps reduce the incidence of confusion. Finally, drugs in the anticholinergic category should be avoided in the SDAT patient. This is because drugs such as scopolamine and atropine exacerbate the behavioral symptoms of SDAT.

PERIANESTHESIA CARE

The geriatric patient can be challenging to care for in the PACU. Patients must be monitored for postoperative pulmonary complications and require positive nursing interventions. Oxygen should be administered by high-flow mask. For the geriatric patient with chronic obstructive pulmonary disease, a Venturi-type mask at a specific low percentage should be administered (see Chapter 26). Oxygen saturation should be monitored closely to detect hypoxemia. If the geriatric patient becomes delirious, hypoxemia should be suspected. If the oxygen saturation is normal and the patient received an anticholinergic drug such as atropine, 1 or 2 mg of physostigmine should be administered to reverse the anticholinergic toxicity. The modified stir-up regimen must be instituted on the patient on arrival in the PACU. More specifically, the cascade cough should be encouraged and tracheal suctioning must be used if the cascade cough is ineffective. Aggressive use of the SMI also helps reduce the chance of the geriatric patient developing atelectasis. Finally, if possible, early ambulation should be encouraged in these patients because it prevents clot formation in the lower extremities and enhances lung function.

Hypothermia is a common outcome of the intraoperative surgical procedure. This is because the geriatric patient has a lower metabolic rate and a reduced peripheral circulatory status.

The aged population has an increased sensitivity to the depressant effects of anesthetic drugs. Prolonged emergence from general anesthesia can be expected. Consequently, airway management and rapid institution of the modified stir-up regimen are required. Along with this, the geriatric patient should receive a reduced dosage of postoperative analgesics because the usual dosage can have a profound respiratory depressant effect. It is best to titrate to effect with the intended outcome being a reduction in pain and restlessness with minimal reduction in respiratory status.

A reduced renal function along with an increased output of antidiuretic hormone during and after surgery places the geriatric patient at increased risk of postoperative overhydration. Therefore, urinary output along with the amount of fluid administered to the patient should be monitored closely.

Finally, in an effort to facilitate psychologic security, personal items such as dentures, glasses, and hearing aids should be returned to the patient as soon as possible.

BIBLIOGRAPHY

Alspach J: Core curriculum for critical care nursing, ed 5, Philadelphia, 1998, WB Saunders.

Atlee J: Complications in anesthesia, Philadelphia, 1999, WB Saunders.

Barash P, Cullen B, Stoelting R: Clinical anesthesia, ed 4, Philadelphia, 2000, Lippincott Williams & Wilkins.

Benumof J: Anesthesia and uncommon diseases, ed 4, Philadelphia, 1998, WB Saunders.

Benumof J, Saidman L: Anesthesia & perioperative complications, ed 2, St Louis, 1999, Mosby.

Bickley L, Hoekelman R: Bates' guide to physical examination and history taking, ed 7, Philadelphia, 1998, Lippincott Williams & Wilkins.

Code W, Roth S: Anesthesia in the geriatric patient, Gerontology 2(2):11-13, 1987.

Cusack B: Drug metabolism in the elderly, J Clin Pharmacol 28(6):571-576, 1988.

Del Portzer M: Geriatric cardiovascular problems, AANA J 44(6):609, 1976.

DeFazio-Quinn D: Ambulatory surgical nursing core curriculum, Philadelphia, 1999, WB Saunders.

Ganong W: Review of medical physiology, ed 20, New York, 2001, McGraw-Hill Professional.

Guyton A, Hall J: Textbook of medical physiology, ed 10, Philadelphia, 2000, WB Saunders.

Hardman J, Limbird L: Goodman and Gilman's the pharmacological basis of therapeutics, ed 10, New York, 2001, McGraw-Hill Professional.

Hazzard W, Andres R, Bierman E et al, editors: Principles of geriatric medicine and gerontology, ed 4, New York, 1998, McGraw-Hill.

Jansen V: The TURP syndrome, Can J Anaesth 38(1):90-97, 1991.

Katzung B, editor: Basic and clinical pharmacology, ed 8, Los Altos, Calif, 2000, Appleton & Lange.

Krechel S, editor: Anesthesia and the geriatric patient, New York, 1984, Grune & Stratton.

Lake C, Hines R, Blitt C: Clinical monitoring: practical applications for anesthesia and critical care, St Louis, 2001, Mosby.

Lee E: Disposition of drugs in the elderly, Ann Acad Med 16(1):128-132, 1987.

Longnecker D, Murphy F: Dripps/Eckenhoff/Vandam introduction to anesthesia, ed 9, Philadelphia, 1997, WB Saunders.

Longnecker D, Tinker J, Morgan G: Principles and practice of anesthesiology, ed 2, St Louis, 1998, Mosby.

McLeskey C, editor: Geriatric anesthesiology, Philadelphia, 1996, Williams and Wilkins.

Miller R, editor: Anesthesia, ed 5, New York, 2000, Churchill Livingstone.

Muravchick S: Geroanesthesia: principles for management of the elderly patient, St Louis, 1997, Mosby.

Murray J, Nadel J: Textbook of respiratory medicine, ed 3, Philadelphia, 2001, WB Saunders.

Nagelhout J, Zaglaniczny K: Nurse anesthesia, ed 2, Philadelphia, 2001, WB Saunders.

Stoelting R: Pharmacology and physiology in anesthetic practice, ed 3, Philadelphia, 1999, Lippincott-Raven.

Stoelting R, Miller R: Basics of anesthesia, ed 4, New York, 2000, Churchill Livingstone.

Stone D: Perioperative care: anesthesia, medicine, and surgery, St Louis, 1998, Mosby.

Townsend C, Beauchamp R, Evers B, Mattox K: Sabiston textbook of surgery: the biological basis of modern surgical practice, ed 16, Philadelphia, 2001, WB Saunders.

Traver G, Tremper Mitchell J, Glodquist-Priestley G: Respiratory care: a clinical approach, Gaithersburg, 1991, Aspen Publishers.

Waugaman W: Preoperative and postoperative considerations for patients with Alzheimer's disease, Geriatr Nurs 9:227-230, 1988.

Waugaman W, Foster S, Rigor B: Principles and practice of nurse anesthesia, ed 3, Norwalk, Conn, 1999, Appleton & Lange.

The incidence of surgery performed on pregnant women for reasons unrelated to the pregnancy itself has been reported to be as high as 40,000 to 50,000 cases per year. The most common conditions that require surgical intervention are acute appendicitis, ovarian cysts, and breast tumors. However, more complicated procedures have been reported and include craniotomy, open-heart surgery, and aneurysm repair that have been performed successfully in pregnant patients.

When caring for the pregnant patient postoperatively, one must remember that two patients require nursing care and assessment: the mother and the fetus. Perianesthesia nursing care should be directed toward providing emotional support for the mother as well as avoiding uterine stimulation that could produce preterm labor. Also of prime importance are preventing respiratory depression in the mother and maintaining normal uterine placental blood flow to ensure adequate fetal supply of oxygen and nutrients.

PHYSIOLOGIC CHANGES OF PREGNANCY

Almost every system in the body is affected in some way during pregnancy, either by hormonal changes or because of the increasing size of the uterus. The changes that affect perianesthesia nursing care are outlined in Box 48-1 and discussed in the following sections.

Cardiovascular Changes

Hemodynamic Alterations. The cardiovascular system undergoes significant change as pregnancy advances. Cardiac output and heart rate increase progressively during pregnancy until, at 30 to 34 weeks' gestation, the cardiac output is 30% to 50% higher than normal and the heart

rate is about 15% above the nonpregnant normal level, with electrocardiographic changes and heart sounds possibly developing (Box 48-2). The systolic blood pressure decreases to about 20 mm Hg below the nonpregnant level at about 20 weeks' gestation and then increases to about 10 mm Hg below the nonpregnant level at term. The diastolic blood pressure is reduced to about 15 mm Hg below the nonpregnant level at 20 weeks' gestation and then slowly returns to the nonpregnant level at term.

Perhaps the most significant effect on the cardiovascular system for the nurse to consider in routine postanesthesia management is obstruction of the inferior vena cava and the pelvic veins by the enlarging uterus (Figs. 48-1 and 48-2). This condition, known as aortocaval compression or Scott's syndrome, can develop by the second trimester and cause supine hypotension. It becomes mandatory to avoid the supine position postoperatively because it can significantly aggravate the obstruction. The side-lying position is the one of choice in the postanesthesia care unit (PACU) (Fig. 48-3).

Collateral circulation for venous return develops through the intervertebral venous plexus and the azygos vein. This condition reduces the volume of the epidural and subarachnoid spaces. Therefore the amount of drug required during regional anesthesia should be decreased. Keeping this in mind, the perianesthesia nurse should assess the patient on admission for a high block and monitor dermatone levels frequently thereafter (see Chapter 23).

In the nonpregnant patient, the sympathetic nervous system plays a role in promoting venous return to the heart from the lower extremities. This sympathetic stimulation of vasomotor tone is enhanced during pregnancy in an effort to

Box 48-1	**Physiologic Changes in Pregnancy**

CARDIOVASCULAR SYSTEM

Flow and pressure changes

Cardiac output increases from 20% at the end of the first trimester to 40% at term

Heart rate >15% of nonpregnant level

Stroke volume increases

Ejection fraction increases

Pulmonary capillary wedge pressure has no significant change

Central venous pressure has no significant change

Systolic blood pressure decreases to about 10 mm Hg below nonpregnant level at term

Diastolic blood pressure decreases by 10 to 15 mm Hg in early gestation through 30 weeks and then returns to pregestation levels at term

Blood volume and constituents

Total blood volume increases to about 45% above nonpregnant levels

Total plasma volume increases to about 55% above nonpregnant levels

Red blood cell mass increases to about 30% above nonpregnant levels

Hematocrit levels decrease to about 36 mg/dl during gestation

Hemoglobin levels decrease to about 11.6 g/dl

Plasma cholinesterase levels decrease as much as 80% of nonpregnant levels

Coagulation

Prothrombin time and partial thromboplastin time decreases 20%; platelet count decreases 15%; bleeding time decreases 10%

RESPIRATORY SYSTEM

Anatomic changes

Capillary engorgement of the nasal and oropharyngeal mucosa and larynx

Increased circumference of the thoracic cage

Elevated diaphragm

Respiratory system flow, volume, and ventilation changes

No change in FEV_1

No change in flow-volume loop

Total pulmonary resistance decreases

Tidal volume increases from 20% to 45% above nonpregnant levels

Functional residual capacity decreases by 20% to 60% below the nonpregnant level

Alveolar ventilation increases by 30% to 45% above nonpregnant level

Minute ventilation increases by 45% above nonpregnant level

Changes in blood gases

$PaCO_2$ decreases to about 30 mm Hg

PaO_2 increases to about 103 to 105 mm Hg

Arterial pH from 10 weeks' gestation until delivery is about 7.44

Metabolic rate and acid-base status

Metabolic rate is depressed during first 12 to 16 weeks

Metabolic rate is 15% above nonpregnant level at term

Oxygen consumption is 35% above nonpregnant level at term

Oxygen consumption is 40% above nonpregnant level during first stage of labor

Oxygen consumption is 75% above nonpregnant level during second stage of labor

Respiratory alkalosis with some metabolic compensation is present

GASTROINTESTINAL SYSTEM

Gastric emptying delays after 34 weeks' gestation

Gastric volume increases

Gastric pH decreases

Pyrosis (heartburn) is present in >50% of pregnant women

Intragastric pressure increases

Hepatic blood flow and function not altered

RENAL SYSTEM

Glomerular filtration rate increases

Urine output increases

FEV_1, Forced expiratory volume in 1 second

Box 48-2   Possible Alterations in Cardiovascular Parameters

Heart sounds are louder with the development of a
    split S_2
Short systolic murmur
More forceful apical impulse
Inverted T waves in leads III, V_1, and V_2
Left axis deviation in months 2-6
Flattened T waves
Depressed ST segments

If findings develop during pregnancy, they usually disappear
after delivery.

counteract the negative effects of uterine compression of the vena cava. Clinically, this protective mechanism is abolished by spinal or epidural
anesthesia because it acts as a pharmacologic
sympathectomy. Without an appropriate preload
of fluids, the pregnant patient may experience a
30% to 50% decrease in blood pressure during the
anesthesia. Therefore it is extremely important
that the pregnant patient receive an appropriate
preload of fluids before epidural or spinal anesthesia. Hemodynamic stability can be secured
by the infusion of 15 ml/kg of colloid solution or
30 ml/kg of crystalloid solution. If the patient is
to receive an inhalation anesthetic agent such as
enflurane, similar fluid preloading is given
because the inhalation anesthetic agents produce
peripheral vasodilatation.

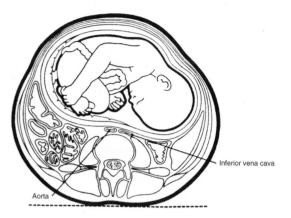

Fig. 48-2   The pregnant uterus compressing the aorta and
the inferior vena cava (aortocaval compression). The patient is
in the supine position. *(From Ostheimer SW: Regional
anesthesia techniques in obstetrics, New York, 1980, Breon
Laboratories.)*

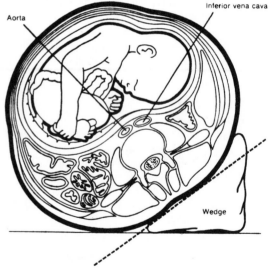

Fig. 48-3   Uterine displacement with a wedge under the hip
to relieve aortocaval compression. *(From Ostheimer SW:
Regional anesthesia techniques in obstetrics, New York, 1980,
Breon Laboratories.)*

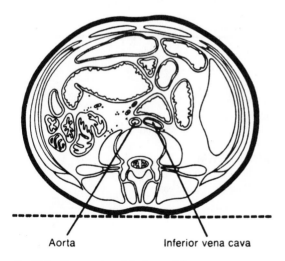

Fig. 48-1   Cross section of the lower abdomen
(nonpregnant). *(From Ostheimer SW: Regional anesthesia
techniques in obstetrics, New York, 1980, Breon Laboratories.)*

This increased fluid requirement has significant implications for the perianesthesia care of the pregnant patient. Consequently, the patient's cardiac and hydration status must be monitored closely throughout the emergence phase of regional anesthesia (see Chapter 23).

Hematologic Alterations. Blood volume increases along with the number of platelets, fibrinogen levels, and the level of activity of several clotting factors. However, a smaller rise in the number of circulating red blood cells occurs. This difference results in lower hematocrit and hemoglobin levels (see Box 48-1), although red blood cell mass actually increases. This condition is known as physiologic anemia of pregnancy.

The plasma concentration of the enzyme cholinesterase is decreased during pregnancy, and because plasma cholinesterase is involved in the mechanisms of clotting, the perianesthesia nurse should monitor the pregnant patient for thromboembolism. Plasma cholinesterase is also involved in the destruction of the depolarizing muscle relaxant succinylcholine. The recovery time from succinylcholine is unaltered and in fact may even be somewhat faster in pregnant women. This is explained by the fact that the volume distribution of succinylcholine increases during pregnancy because of an elevation in the plasma volume. In the immediate postpartum period, the plasma cholinesterase concentration and the plasma volume distribution are further reduced. Consequently, between postpartum days 1 and 2, prolonged paralysis and apnea after the administration of succinylcholine can occur, and the dosage of succinylcholine during this period should be reduced by about 50%.

Respiratory Changes
Upper Airway Anatomy. During pregnancy, there is capillary engorgement of the upper respiratory tract to include the nasal and oropharyngeal mucosa and larynx, and pregnant women may complain of nasal stuffiness. Along with this, nose breathing is difficult, and nosebleeds can occur.

Lung Mechanics and Ventilation. The diaphragm elevates, and the rib cage flares; therefore at term 85% of respiratory effort is intercostal and 15% diaphragmatic. (Normally, approximately 70% is intercostal, and 30% is diaphragmatic.) Because of the mechanical changes in the lungs and chest wall, the lung volumes and capacities do change during pregnancy. Overall, the inspiratory lung volumes and capacities moderately increase, and the expiratory lung volumes and capacities decrease. The inspiratory reserve volume and the inspiratory capacity increase by 5% to 15%. The functional residual capacity (FRC) decreases by approximately 20% to 60%. Also, the residual volume and expiratory reserve volume, which make up the FRC, are also decreased.

The tidal volume also increases about 20% to 45%, and the respiratory rate does not change, thus leading to a 30% to 45% increase in the alveolar ventilation and the minute ventilation. Therefore during pregnancy, the arterial oxygen level ranges from 95 to 105 mm Hg and the arterial carbon dioxide level is approximately 30 mm Hg with an arterial pH of 7.44. Consequently, the pregnant patient has some respiratory alkalosis for which the renal excretion of bicarbonate compensates. Hence, the normal bicarbonate level during pregnancy is about 19 mEq/L, and the base excess is reduced by 2 mEq/L.

In regard to flow rate changes, the forced expiratory volume in 1 second and the flow-volume loop remain unchanged. Along with this, the closing capacity (see Chapter 10) does not change during gestation. Consequently, it can be said that the small and large airways conductance and resistance do not change during pregnancy.

Gastrointestinal Changes
Motility and Secretions. Gastric emptying slows during pregnancy because the stomach is displaced as the uterus enlarges. Along with this, the gastric volume increases during hours 1 to 8 in the postpartum period. Therefore the perianesthesia nurse must be cognizant of the potential for vomiting and aspiration, particularly in patients who have had general anesthesia. Muscle relaxants may have been used and may result in the patient's normal protective mechanisms being obtunded. Once again, the side-lying position becomes of significant importance.

Hepatic System. Liver function test results are abnormal, but no evidence suggests alteration in liver function. Hepatic blood flow remains constant. Therefore those anesthetic agents that are metabolized in the liver should have the same duration of effect.

Renal Changes

Early in pregnancy, the kidneys receive an increased blood flow; therefore glomerular filtration and urine formation rates increase. This is necessary to handle the increased amount of waste products produced. Monitoring of output should reflect this expected increase in volume. Intervention may be required for hypovolemia even though the urine output is within ranges acceptable in a nonpregnant patient.

INTRAOPERATIVE ANESTHESIA CARE OF THE OBSTETRIC PATIENT

Because the effects of anesthesia have such a profound effect on the emergence of the pregnant patient, a complete review of the techniques and procedures of general and regional anesthesia are presented.

Positioning

Because the supine position causes a reduction in uterine blood flow in the pregnant patient, the semi-Fowler's position is used when possible. To prevent aortocaval compression, the patient is placed in the lateral decubitus position, and the right hip is elevated with a pillow or the uterus is displaced to the left with devices on the operating table.

Gastrointestinal Considerations

The pregnant patient has a reduced gastric emptying time and a reduced gastric pH. However, research has demonstrated that gastric volume and acidity in the pregnant patient do not differ significantly from those in the nonpregnant patient. However, many anesthesia clinicians believe strongly that the pregnant patient—especially the patient with pyrosis—is at risk of developing aspiration pneumonitis. Consequently, preoperative pharmacologic interventions are usually taken. Drugs that may be administered include a nonparticulate antacid such as sodium citrate (Bicitra) to increase the gastric pH, cimetidine (Tagamet), or ranitidine (Zantac), which are histamine-2 receptor blockers that reduce gastric acid secretion, and metoclopramide (Reglan), which speeds up gastric emptying time and elevates lower esophageal tone.

General Anesthesia

Induction.   Because of the strong full-stomach considerations, the pregnant patient is intubated with a rapid-sequence endotracheal intubation technique (see Chapter 27) that includes intravenous (IV) thiopental, etomidate, or ketamine followed by succinylcholine. A defasciculation dose of a nondepolarizing muscle relaxant may be given before the administration of the succinylcholine to avoid the increase in intragastric pressure. Some clinicians do not administer a defasciculating dose of a nondepolarizing muscle relaxant because it can delay the onset, reduce the intensity, and shorten the duration of action of succinylcholine. Cricoid pressure (Sellick maneuver) is used once the barbiturate is administered and is released after confirmation of appropriate placement of the endotracheal tube.

The endotracheal tube should be a small tube, usually 7 mm in diameter or smaller, because of increased mucosal engorgement in the nasal and oropharyngeal areas. Along with this, nasotracheal intubation is not used because of the high risk of tissue trauma.

Maintenance.   Nitrous oxide in 50% concentration with oxygen is usually administered. Inhalation agents such as halothane, isoflurane, and enflurane can be used. Analgesic concentrations of 0.5 minimum alveolar concentration (see Chapter 18) or less to avoid significant uterine relaxation can be used safely for these inhalation drugs. However, these inhalation agents, particularly halothane, may be used in high concentrations for a short period to produce uterine relaxation for intrauterine manipulation of the fetus or removal of a retained placenta. The clinical implication in the PACU for the patient who received a high concentration of an inhalation agent—even for a short period (<2 minutes)—is to monitor for postpartum hemorrhage and maternal hypotension. Also, the uterine response to oxytocic drugs is reduced when high concentrations of these inhalation agents are used.

In regard to skeletal muscle relaxation, succinylcholine infusion or short-acting nondepolarizing muscle relaxants such as atracurium and vecuronium can be used safely because they lack autonomic side effects and have a low degree of placental transfer. In the immediate postpartum period, the neuromuscular-blocking effects of vecuronium are prolonged.

Emergence.   At the end of the surgical procedure, the residual effects of the nondepolarizing muscle relaxants are reversed and the inhalation anesthetic agents are discontinued. When the patient is awake, responsive, and able to ventilate without assistance, she is extubated.

Regional Anesthesia

Regional anesthesia, primarily spinal and epidural, is used extensively for anesthesia in the pregnant patient because it produces analgesia without causing neonatal depression. This technique also reduces the risk of maternal hypoventilation and the need for narcotics and sedatives. Regional anesthesia does not require airway management, preserves airway reflexes, and allows the mother to remain awake during birth. It is contraindicated in patients with severe coagulation problems, severe hypovolemia, sepsis, and infection at the needle insertion site; in situations in which immediate delivery is crucial, such as in fetal distress; and when the patient refuses the procedure.

The level of sensory blockade for either spinal or epidural anesthesia for cesarean section is from T4 to S4. The commonly used local anesthetic drugs for spinal anesthesia are lidocaine, bupivacaine, and tetracaine (see Chapter 22). For epidural anesthesia, the commonly used local anesthetic agents are 2-chloroprocaine (Nesacaine), lidocaine with epinephrine, and bupivacaine.

In comparison to the spinal approach, the epidural approach is the preferred technique because drugs can be administered throughout the surgical procedure via a continuous epidural catheter. The anesthesia clinician then has the ability to control the onset, distribution, and duration of anesthesia. Along with this, the incidence of postdural puncture is much lower in comparison to the spinal technique.

PERIANESTHESIA CARE OF THE MOTHER AND THE FETUS

Studies have not shown one anesthetic technique to be better than another in the gravid patient. As with nonpregnant patients, the choice of technique is determined by the following:

1. Surgery to be performed
2. American Society of Anesthesiologists classification of the patient

3. Anesthetist's preference
4. Patient's preference
5. Underlying disease entities

The care of the pregnant patient postoperatively should be the same as for any patient who undergoes that procedure or for one who recovers from that particular anesthetic. However, additions to the routine nursing care must be instituted for all pregnant patients.

Positioning

To alleviate compression of the vena cava, the uterus should be displaced to the left, either by positioning the patient on her left side or by tilting the pelvis with a folded sheet or bath towel under the woman's right iliac crest. Slight elevation of the legs and the use of thigh-high elastic stockings should be standard.

Psychologic and Emotional Support

The mother's concern for her unborn child is paramount. Constant reassurance is mandatory. If possible, allow the mother to listen to the fetal heartbeat frequently during the recovery phase. Explain all procedures and why they are being done before they are carried out. If your PACU allows visitors, involvement of the father should also be considered.

Fetal Monitoring

The fetal heart rate must be monitored every 15 minutes if the fetus has reached viability (Table 48-1). If available, an indirect fetal monitoring system should be used for constant assessment of fetal stability (Fig. 48-4).

The second type of monitoring required is to observe the patient closely for signs of premature

Table 48-1 **Fetal Heart Rates**	
Description	Rate (beats/min)
Normal fetal heart rate	120-160
Moderate tachycardia	160-180
Marked tachycardia	>180
Moderate bradycardia	100-120
Marked bradycardia	<100

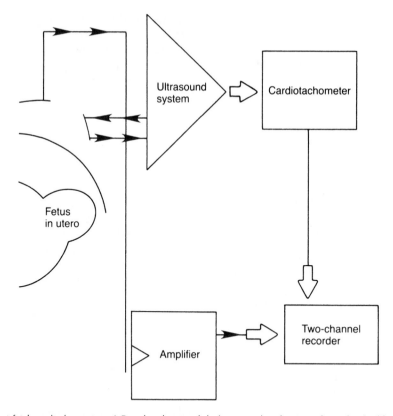

Fig. 48-4 Indirect fetal monitoring system. A Doppler ultrasound device transmits a beam to determine fetal heart rate. When the beam strikes a moving object within the fetus, such as a mitral valve leaflet, the frequency of the transmitted beam is shifted up or down, depending on which way the leaflet is moving. This valve movement is counted and displayed as a heart rate on the recorder.

labor. These include spontaneous rupture of membranes, increased fetal heart rate, presenting of vaginal mucus plug, uterine palpitations, uterine contractions, and restlessness of the mother.

Initially, the patient may not feel the contractions or be aware of membrane rupture; therefore palpation of the abdomen and assessment of vaginal discharge must be performed by the nurse. If premature labor begins, transfer of the patient to the labor and delivery area as soon as possible is recommended. A drug may have to be given to stop labor. These drugs should be administered by personnel familiar with proper protocols for administration and their side effects.

Pain Management
The Post-Cesarean Section Patient.

The post-cesarean section patient presents unique challenges in regard to pain management. More specifically, more women desire to care for their newborns within the first 24 hours. Heavy sedation with opioids and IV or epidural catheters inhibit the mother's ability to care for the infant. Also, the infant can be affected through the transfer of the drug in breast milk.

Patient-controlled analgesia (PCA) is becoming quite popular in pain management of the post-cesarean section patient (see Chapters 20, 25, and 28). It is well documented that the PCA interrupts the pain cycle, gives the patient a feeling of control, hastens the time to ambulation, and reduces the length of stay in the hospital. Morphine is the preferred drug to be administered by PCA. The usual dose is 1 to 1.5 mg, a lockout of 10 minutes, and an hourly limit of 10 to 12 mg.

Epidural administration of opioids is another option that can be used for the control of pain in the PACU. Morphine is the preferred drug because of its demonstrated safety and prolonged duration of action after a single dose of 5 mg. The primary side effects of epidural morphine are pruritus and nausea. Some clinicians have advocated using the narcotic antagonist naloxone (5 to 10 μg/kg/hr) to treat these side effects. However, problems arise with some reversal of the analgesia. Most clinicians treat the nausea with 0.5 mg of IV droperidol (Inapsine) and the pruritus with 12.5 mg of IV diphenhydramine (Benadryl).

Fentanyl is an alternative to morphine for epidural analgesia. The difficulty with fentanyl is that its duration of action is less than 5 hours and must be administered by continuous infusion or intermittent boluses. The epidural fentanyl technique provides excellent analgesia; however, most women desire to be ambulatory as soon as possible and do not like to be encumbered with the catheter, tape, and pump.

When administered epidurally with opioids, 2-chloroprocaine inhibits the analgesic effects of the opioids. This inhibitory action of 2-chloroprocaine is probably caused by the ethylenediaminetetraacetic acid (EDTA) that is used in the solution of the drug. EDTA is an antioxidant that has analgesic antagonism properties because it is a strong chelator of calcium. Therefore clinically epidural opioids should be avoided for at least 6 to 8 hours after 2-chloroprocaine has been administered.

A variety of receptor specific drugs to include opioids, alpha$_2$-adrenergic agonists, and local anesthetics are being evaluated for use via the intraspinal approach. With the refining of the spinal technique to include the use of small needles and ultrafine catheters, this technique is gaining in popularity for post–cesarean section pain relief. Morphine, 0.3 mg administered intrathecally, has a longer duration of action than 4 mg of morphine administered via the epidural route. Some anesthesia clinicians are now adding morphine to bupivacaine intraoperatively, with

the outcome being excellent analgesia that lasts well into the postanesthesia period.

The Pregnant Patient. Because of the growth in consumer awareness, the administration of medication during pregnancy has become a controversial issue that must be addressed on an individual basis. For pain management in the PACU, when the pregnant patient is in a hypersuggestive state, distraction techniques such as guided imagery and breathing exercises have had favorable results in place of drugs.

If a mild analgesic is required, the drug of choice is acetaminophen (Tylenol) and, for moderate pain management, propoxyphene (Darvon). Both drugs have been evaluated through prospective studies and have been shown to pose minimal risks to the fetus if used appropriately for short-term pain management. Narcotic analgesia may be warranted for severe pain but must be used judiciously, keeping in mind the respiratory depressive effects.

Ketorolac (Toradol), a prostaglandin synthetase inhibitor, is becoming quite popular in postoperative pain therapy. However, because prostaglandins have a profound effect on the neonatal cardiovascular and renal systems, research must be conducted to determine if ketorolac has a negative effect on those systems before its use can be instituted in the postanesthesia period.

The gravid patient in the PACU is a rare occurrence that requires the nurse to have a great deal of knowledge and the ability to provide continual support during this stressful situation. The nurse must be able to provide a quiet, calm, reassuring atmosphere for the patient. The objective of the care delivered is an optimum environment for both the mother and the fetus.

BIBLIOGRAPHY

Abboud T: Nonobstetric surgery during pregnancy, Semin Anesth 11(1):51-54, 1992.

Alspach J: Core curriculum for critical care nursing, ed 5, Philadelphia, 1998, WB Saunders.

Atlee J: Complications in anesthesia, Philadelphia, 1999, WB Saunders.

Barash P, Cullen B, Stoelting R: Clinical anesthesia, ed 4, Philadelphia, 2000, Lippincott Williams & Wilkins.

Benumof J: Anesthesia and uncommon diseases, ed 4, Philadelphia, 1998, WB Saunders.

Benumof J, Saidman L: Anesthesia & perioperative complications, ed 2, St Louis, 1999, Mosby.

Bickley L, Hoekelman R: Bates' guide to physical examination and history taking, ed 7, Philadelphia, 1998, Lippincott Williams & Wilkins.

Bowdle T, Horita A, Kharasch E: The pharmacologic basis of anesthesiology, New York, 1994, Churchill Livingstone.

Conklin K: Maternal physiological adaptations during gestation, labor, and the puerperium, Semin Anesth 10(4):221-234, 1991.

Coté C, Todres I, Goudsouzian N et al: A practice of anesthesia for infants and children, ed 3, Philadelphia, 2001, WB Saunders.

DeFazio-Quinn D: Ambulatory surgical nursing core curriculum, Philadelphia, 1999, WB Saunders.

Eisenach J: Pain management in the parturient: theoretical and practical aspects, Semin Anesth 11(1):55-65, 1992.

Estafanous F: Opioids in anesthesia: II, Boston, 1991, Butterworth-Heinemann.

Estafanous F, Barash P, Reves J: Cardiac anesthesia, ed 2, Philadelphia, 2001, Lippincott Williams & Wilkins.

Ganong W: Review of medical physiology, ed 20, New York, 2001, McGraw-Hill Professional.

Guyton A, Hall J: Textbook of medical physiology, ed 10, Philadelphia, 2000, WB Saunders.

Hardman J, Limbird L: Goodman and Gilman's the pharmacological basis of therapeutics, ed 10, New York, 2001, McGraw-Hill Professional.

Johnson M, Ostheimer G: Airway management in obstetric patients, Semin Anesth 11(1):1-12, 1992.

Katzung B, editor: Basic and clinical pharmacology, ed 8, Los Altos, Calif, 2000, Appleton & Lange.

Kelly M: Maternal position and blood pressure during pregnancy and delivery, Am J Nurs 82:809-812, 1982.

Lake C, Hines R, Blitt C: Clinical monitoring: practical applications for anesthesia and critical care, St Louis, 2001, Mosby.

Longnecker D, Murphy F: Dripps/Eckenhoff/Vandam introduction to anesthesia, ed 9, Philadelphia, 1997, WB Saunders.

Longnecker D, Tinker J, Morgan G: Principles and practice of anesthesiology, ed 2, St Louis, 1998, Mosby.

Martin J: Positioning in anesthesia and surgery, ed 3, St Louis, 1997, Mosby.

Miller R, editor: Anesthesia, ed 5, New York, 2000, Churchill Livingstone.

Moran D, Dewan D: Anesthesia for cesarean delivery, Semin Anesth 10(4):286-294, 1991.

Motoyama E: Smith's anesthesia for infants and children, ed 6, St Louis, 1996, Mosby.

Murray J, Nadel J: Textbook of respiratory medicine, ed 3, Philadelphia, 2001, WB Saunders.

Nagelhout J, Zaglaniczny K: Nurse anesthesia, ed 2, Philadelphia, 2001, WB Saunders.

Norris M, editor: Obstetric anesthesia, Philadelphia, 1993, Lippincott.

Shnider S, Levinson G: Anesthesia for obstetrics, ed 3, Baltimore, 1993, Williams & Wilkins.

Stoelting R: Pharmacology and physiology in anesthetic practice, ed 3, Philadelphia, 1999, Lippincott-Raven.

Stoelting R, Miller R: Basics of anesthesia, ed 4, New York, 2000, Churchill Livingstone.

Stone D: Perioperative care: anesthesia, medicine, and surgery, St Louis, 1998, Mosby.

Traver G, Tremper Mitchell J et al: Respiratory care: a clinical approach, Gaithersburg, Md, 1991, Aspen Publishers Inc.

Waugaman W, Foster S, Rigor B: Principles and practice of nurse anesthesia, ed 3, Norwalk, Conn, 1999, Appleton & Lange.

Ziadlourad F, Conklin K: Anesthesia for obstetric emergencies, Semin Anesth 8(3):222-231, 1989.

CARE OF THE SUBSTANCE ABUSER

The great increase in the number of persons who use narcotics, amphetamines, cocaine, hallucinogens, barbiturates, and date rape drugs has created new problems in perianesthesia nursing care.

Drug abuse is the nonmedical use of a drug and consists of the self-administration of any drug in a manner that deviates from the approved medical or social practices within a given culture. Physical dependence is an altered physiologic state caused by repeated administration of a drug that necessitates the continued administration of the drug to prevent the appearance of the withdrawal or abstinence syndrome characteristic for that drug. Psychologic dependence is habituation-compulsive drug use. In this type of abuse, a drug is used to alter mood and feeling, and eventually, dependent people come to believe that the effects of the drug are necessary to maintain an optimal state of well-being. Another term that should be defined in discussions of substance abuse is tolerance. Drug tolerance is a state in which, after repeated administration of a drug, a given dose produces a decreased effect or, on the other hand, in which increasingly larger doses are needed to obtain the same effect as that of the original dose.

The pharmacologic agents that are most commonly abused can be grouped as follows: (1) opioid analgesics; (2) general central nervous system (CNS) depressants, such as alcohol and the barbiturates; (3) CNS sympathomimetics, such as amphetamines and cocaine; (4) cannabinoids, such as marijuana; and (5) psychedelics—of which lysergic acid diethylamide (LSD) and phencyclidine are the prototypic drugs (Table 49-1)—inhalants, club drugs, and date-rape drugs.

OPIOID ANALGESICS

Opioid analgesics (narcotics) cause strong psychologic dependence. Physical dependence is manifested by the withdrawal syndrome of autonomic storm and CNS irritability. Also, a strong tolerance for these drugs and a cross-tolerance with other drugs of the same classification of opioid analgesics develop. Studies indicate that in people who are chronically addicted to opioid analgesics such as morphine, the minimum alveolar concentration of halothane (Fluothane) is increased, which indicates that a cross-tolerance with general inhalation anesthetics may exist.

Heroin, an opioid analgesic that is derived from morphine, is degraded in the body to morphine about 30 minutes after injection. The most common problem associated with the use of heroin and other opioid analgesics is pulmonary edema; other dysfunctions include superficial bacterial infections, adrenal insufficiency, bacterial endocarditis, liver disease, urinary abnormalities (proteinuria and glycosuria), and false-positive serology. In addition, about 30% of the opiate abusers have positive results on the Venereal Disease Research Laboratory test for syphilis, but only about 25% of these are true-positive when checked by the *Treponema* immobilization test.

Perianesthesia nursing care of an opiate abuser, such as the heroin addict, centers around monitoring the patient for complications. Probably foremost is monitoring for the withdrawal (abstinence) syndrome. The abstinence syndrome after opiate abuse occurs in two phases. The acute phase occurs during the first few days. The protracted phase, which is not readily treat-

Table 49-1	**Categories of Substance Abuse: Effects and Signs of Abuse and Withdrawal**		
Category	Possible Effects	Signs of Abuse	Signs of Withdrawal
OPIOID ANALGESICS			
Opium Morphine Codeine Heroin Meperidine (Demerol) Sublimaze (Fentanyl) Methadone (Dolophine)	Euphoria, "rush" with IV injection, feeling of detachment, drowsiness, miosis, nausea, respiratory depression Tolerance, physical and psychologic dependence	Injection scars or needle marks, usually on inner surfaces of arms Thrombophlebitis at injection sites, cellulitis Pinpoint pupils Uncoordinated movements Confusion, disorientation Heavy smoking	Watery eyes, runny nose, scratching, yawning, anorexia, irritability, tremors, panic, chills and sweating, muscle pains and cramps, nausea, vomiting, diarrhea
GENERAL CNS DEPRESSANTS			
Alcohol	Loss of inhibitions Impaired judgment Carefree mood Impaired motor coordination, concentration, memory Ataxia, incoherence Stupor, coma Tolerance and physical dependence	Reported intake: Heavy drinker* Alcohol-addicted† GI disturbances Malnutrition Heavy smoking Trauma Psychologic problems Social maladjustment	8 hours after abstinence: Tremors, GI disturbances, anxiety, jittery feeling, and headache 24-72 hours or longer of withdrawal: Increased tremors, hyperactivity, irritability, nervousness, insomnia, delusions, hallucinations, seizures, delirium tremens (DTs), high fever, profuse sweating, tachycardia, hyperventilation, nausea and vomiting
Barbiturates Amytal Butisol Nembutal Seconal Tuinal Phenobarbital	Euphoria, reduced anxiety, dry intoxication (drunken behavior without odor of alcohol) Tolerance, physical and psychologic dependence	Drowsiness, lack of interest, fatigue, irritability Changes in personality and behavior Possession of pills of varying colors and shapes	Range from anxiety, weakness, confusion, anorexia, and mild tremors to delirium disorientation, hallucinations, and convulsions

Table 49-1	**Categories of Substance Abuse: Effects and Signs of Abuse and Withdrawal**–*cont'd*		
Category	Possible Effects	Signs of Abuse	Signs of Withdrawal
Benzodiazepines 　Valium 　Librium 　Serax 　Ativan 　Versed	Same as barbiturates	Same as barbiturates	Same as barbiturates
CNS SYMPATHOMIMETICS			
Amphetamines	Increased alertness, euphoria, anorexia, insomnia, elevated blood pressure, tachycardia, anxiety Tolerance, psychologic dependence	Possession of pills of varying color Injection scars, needle marks Compulsion to talk, extreme activity, chain smoking Frequent nose rubbing or scratching, licking of dry lips, bad breath Changed eating and sleeping habits Projected sense of prowess or capability Possible aggressive or antisocial behavior	"Crashing" (response produced when stimulant effect ends); hunger, extreme lethargy, profound depression, and sleep disturbance
Cocaine	Same as amphetamines Possible tolerance, no physical dependence, high psychologic dependence	Same as amphetamines Inflamed nasal mucosa	Same as amphetamines "Crashing" may be profound
CANNABINOIDS			
Marijuana (hashish)	Sense of relaxation and well-being Distorted orientation to time and space Altered sensory perception Occasional excitement and spontaneous (often uncontrolled) laughter Increased appetite Tolerance and psychologic dependence, degree of physical dependence unknown	Possession of off-white or brown cigarette papers and coarse brownish-green tobacco Conjunctival congestion, dilated pupils Wearing of dark glasses because of light sensitivity	Reported abstinence symptoms: hyperexcitability, insomnia, decreased appetite

Continued

Table 49-1	**Categories of Substance Abuse: Effects and Signs of Abuse and Withdrawal**—*cont'd*		
Category	Possible Effects	Signs of Abuse	Signs of Withdrawal
PSYCHEDELICS			
Lysergic acid diethylamide (LSD) Phencyclidine (PCP)	Illusions Distorted perceptions of time, distance, body image, mood, affect Depersonalization and ego dissociation Psychotic behavior Tolerance, degree of psychologic dependence unknown	Possession of perforated small squares of blotter paper with colored designs, ampules of clear liquid, or capsules of white or colored powder, or tablets Unusual body odor Marked mood changes Dreamlike or trancelike state	None reported

From Knor E: Substance abuse. In Decision making in obstetrical nursing, Toronto, 1987, BC Decker.
CNS, Central nervous system; *IV*, intravenous; *GI*, gastrointestinal.
*Heavy drinker: a person who consumes five or more drinks on some occasions and at least 45 drinks a month.
†Alcohol-addicted: a person who consumes approximately 20 drinks of beer, wine, or liquor a day and has developed physiologic tolerance.

able, can persist for as long as 2 to 6 months. The acute opiate abstinence phase is not dangerous to life because it usually is not associated with convulsions and delirium. Instead, the symptoms are anxiety, nervousness, jittery behavior, anorexia, rhinorrhea, hypotension, muscle twitching, insomnia, sweating, pupillary dilation, gooseflesh, and nausea and vomiting. Symptoms during the protracted phase include those of the acute phase, along with convulsions and delirium. Treatment for the acute opiate abstinence phase is accomplished with any narcotic analgesic; reports indicate that clonidine has proved to be most effective in attenuating the symptoms. Treatment for the protracted phase centers around protection of the patient and abatement of the symptoms demonstrated by the patient. If a patient is a suspected opiate abuser, narcotic antagonists such as naloxone (Narcan) should not be administered because the withdrawal syndrome can be precipitated. No attempt should be made at withdrawal of the active abuser during the PACU period. Liberal use of morphine or methadone in the PACU appears to be satisfactory. The former abuser should not receive nar-

cotics; analgesics such as pentazocine (Talwin) and butorphanol (Stadol) should be used in their place.

GENERAL CNS DEPRESSANTS

The barbiturate addict may present only as nervous and anxious before surgery. However, the patient should be monitored postoperatively for anxiety, tremors, and hallucinations. These symptoms usually develop on the second or third postoperative day and can be treated with a barbiturate until acute illness has passed. These patients also appear to have an increased tolerance to anesthesia and therefore have an increased chance of anesthetic toxicity.

The use and abuse of the benzodiazepine compounds have increased significantly during the last decade. The benzodiazepine drug is usually taken in combination with marijuana or alcohol to obtain a "high." Chronic intoxication has been reported with the use of these compounds. The most abused benzodiazepine is diazepam (Valium); however, midazolam (Versed) will soon rank at the same level as diazepam. These drugs are becoming popular because of their rapid onset of action coupled with their pleasure-giving effects. The pharmacologic effects of the benzodiazepines are similar to those of the barbiturates. This classification of drugs is somewhat addictive and includes withdrawal syndromes.

To treat mild to moderate overdosages of benzodiazepines, the drug physostigmine in an adult dosage of 1 to 2 mg given intravenously can be used. A new antagonist with a longer action and fewer side effects has been introduced into clinical practice. This drug, flumazenil (Romazicon), is a true benzodiazepine receptor antagonist. The usual adult dosage is 0.1 to 0.2 mg given intravenously. As with naloxone for narcotic-addicted patients, flumazenil must be used with caution with benzodiazepine-dependent patients. More specifically, reversal of benzodiazepine-dependent patients is associated with precipitating the withdrawal syndrome, including seizures.

Alcoholism has long been widespread, yet it is difficult to define. An alcoholic, for purposes of this discussion, is a person who is excessively dependent on alcohol and who has developed a noticeable degree of mental, physical, psychologic, or pathologic disorders. Alcohol was the first anesthetic; it can produce anesthesia, respiratory depression, and hypotension.

Alcohol affects many of the body's major systems. It is well known that in the later stages of alcoholism, cirrhosis of the liver is quite common. This is of importance to the perianesthesia nurse because the liver detoxifies many drugs administered during the perioperative period (see Chapter 14). Hepatic cirrhosis may produce significant alterations in pulmonary and cardiovascular functions. Hyperventilation and arterial oxygen desaturation are common findings caused by an increase in shunting of blood away from areas in the lung where diffusion of oxygen takes place. Concomitant with this is an increase in blood volume that may lead to cardiac hypertrophy and eventually to congestive heart failure. Fluid balance is affected by the presence of alcohol because alcohol exhibits antidiuretic effects by inhibiting the release of antidiuretic hormone. Alcoholic cirrhosis (Laennec's cirrhosis) is also associated with portal vein hypertension, renal failure, hypoglycemia, duodenal ulcer, esophageal varices, and hepatic encephalopathy.

The alcoholic—in comparison to the nonalcoholic—usually requires a larger amount of sodium thiopental for induction and a higher concentration of anesthetic agents during surgery. It is difficult to predict the time or the character of emergence from anesthesia in the alcoholic patient. This patient may be anxious and may have a stormy emergence and postoperative phase.

During the PACU phase, the alcoholic patient should be monitored for withdrawal symptoms. The minor alcohol withdrawal syndrome is characterized by symptoms such as tremulousness, insomnia, and irritability. Because of autonomic nervous system imbalance, signs such as tachycardia, hypertension, and cardiac dysrhythmias are often observed. The minor alcohol withdrawal syndrome can occur within 6 to 8 hours after abstinence by the alcoholic patient. The signs and symptoms of this syndrome usually disappear within 48 hours without treatment.

In about 5% of the alcoholic population, the severe alcohol withdrawal syndrome, or delirium tremens, will occur with abrupt cessation of alcohol ingestion. The mortality rate from this syndrome is about 15%, and it is considered a medical emergency. The time of onset of delirium tremens is about 48 to 72 hours after the abrupt discontinuation of alcohol ingestion.

The patient is difficult to manage if withdrawal symptoms are allowed to develop. The severe withdrawal syndrome should be suspected if symptoms—such as restlessness, disorientation, tremulousness, and hallucinations—occur. In addition, because of activation of the sympathetic nervous system, symptoms such as diaphoresis, hyperpyrexia, tachycardia, and hypertension are seen. When any of these symptoms is observed, hypoxia should first be ruled out because the symptoms of withdrawal can be confused with those of hypoxia. The treatment used to control the withdrawal symptoms is sedation with diazepam, along with intravenous fluids and electrolytes, vitamin replacement (i.e, thiamine), and glucose. If deemed necessary by the attending physician, propranolol may be given to suppress the clinical manifestations of the increased sympathetic nervous system activity. Along with this, should cardiac dysrhythmias occur, lidocaine may be administered intravenously.

CNS SYMPATHOMIMETICS

Cocaine has a two-pronged effect—vasoconstriction and mood alteration—because it inhibits the reuptake of catecholamines. The mood-altering effect is similar to the psychologic effect produced by amphetamines. Cocaine is steadily becoming one of the most popular drugs among substance abusers. Patients who are known abusers of cocaine should be closely monitored in the PACU for hypertension and cardiac arrhythmias. Also, these patients are quite prone to nosebleeds. Hence care should be taken in administering nursing care near or directly to the nose and nasal cavity.

CNS stimulants, which include amphetamines, tend to be long-acting vasopressors. The patient will have dilated pupils, tachycardia, palpitations, cardiac arrhythmias, and changes in temperature regulation and will appear to be extremely anxious. If the stimulant is wearing off, the patient will be lethargic and very depressed. Continuous electrocardiographic monitoring for cardiac arrhythmias is necessary and is coupled with frequent blood pressure and pulse measurements. The mental sensorium should also be monitored throughout the patient's stay in the PACU.

CANNABINOIDS

The hemp plants, of which cannabis is the generic name, contain about 30 active substances that are called cannabinoids. Of these, tetrahydrocannabinol (THC) is the most active. Marijuana is the generic term applied to the hemp plants. The marijuana cigarette contains rolled-up or crushed, dried leaves from the hemp plant. Each marijuana cigarette contains about 0.005 g of THC. The cannabinoids are three times more potent when inhaled than when ingested orally. Psychologic changes occur minutes after inhalation of marijuana, and the effects peak in an hour, with a duration as long as 3 hours.

The peripheral effects of THC on the autonomic nervous system include vagal blockade and beta-adrenergic stimulation. Hence the abuser of marijuana experiences tachycardia, peripheral vascular dilatation, bronchodilatation, conjunctival congestion, and a dry mouth. The actual effects of THC on the CNS are not known.

Because of the rapid effects of the drug—along with the short duration of action and the absence of physiologic dysfunction or changes—abusers of marijuana do not seem to present any added problems in the PACU. However, because of the chronic irritation produced by the inhalation of smoke from the marijuana cigarette, chronic abusers should be monitored for chronic bronchitis.

PSYCHEDELICS

Phencyclidine is the hallucinogen most commonly used today. This drug is a popular veterinary anesthetic agent (Sernylan) and is related pharmacologically to the drug ketamine. It can be ingested, taken parenterally, or inhaled. The sensory effects have a rapid onset and last approximately 1 to 2 hours, and the CNS effects can last for 1 or more days. The CNS activation usually produces sympathetic nervous system activation.

It is unlikely that the perianesthesia nurse will have much contact with a patient under the influence of this drug. However, if a patient who abuses this drug should require perianesthesia care, the nurse must monitor this patient for sympathetic activation, and symptoms such as dilated pupils, increased pulse, and elevated blood pressure should be reported immediately to the attending physician.

LSD is a hallucinogen that reached its peak of use in the late 1960s and is now becoming a popular drug in the 1990s. This drug is ingested orally, and its major effects occur in a dose-related manner. Moderate dosage of the drug causes euphoria, marked sensory distortion (including heightened awareness of sensory stimuli), and occasional visual hallucinations. Large doses of LSD usually lead to frightening hallucinations and a distorted body image—commonly known as a "bad trip." This drug also produces some hypertension, dilated pupils, and increased temperature, by virtue of its stimulation of the central hypothalamic area of the brain. The onset of the psychologic effects of LSD is after about 40 minutes, and the duration is about 2 hours. Some of the milder effects of LSD have been reported to last as long as 8 hours after ingestion.

The primary focus of perianesthesia nursing care for the patient who is in the hallucinogenic state is to prevent self-injury and sedation. The "bad trip" effects can be managed with chlorpromazine (Thorazine) or diazepam. Other considerations in regard to the patient who has ingested LSD are that the analgesic effects of narcotics are potentiated by LSD and that the plasma cholinesterases are somewhat inhibited by LSD. Hence, narcotic dosage may need to be reduced in these patients, and if succinylcholine is to be administered to the patient, the possibility of prolonged apnea exists.

INHALANTS

Inhalants are extremely abused drugs and consist of breathable chemical vapors that produce mind-altering effects. Inhalants are likely to be abused by young people because they are easily accessible and inexpensive. Inhalants are classified into three categories: solvents, gases, or nitrates.

The solvents consist of paint thinners or solvents, electronic contact cleaners, and felt-tip-marker fluid. The gases consist of such household products and commercial products as butane lighters and propane tanks, whipping cream aerosols, spray paints, hair or deodorant sprays, and fabric protector sprays. Gases used for anesthetic medical purposes—such as ether, chloroform, halothane and nitrous oxide (see Chapter 18)—are now being abused. The nitrates, such as cyclohexyl nitrite and butyl nitrite, which are available to the public, and amyl nitrite, which is only available by prescription, are now being used as abused substances.

The abused inhalants produce effects that are similar to the anesthetics described in the signs and stages section of Chapter 18. Basically, these inhalants cause an intoxicating effect when they are inhaled through the nose or mouth into the lungs. When inhaled in high concentrations, these inhalants can induce heart failure and even death. Some of the irreversible effects of these inhalants can include hearing loss, peripheral neuropathies or limb spasms, central nervous system damage, and/or bone marrow damage. Some of the serious yet potentially reversible effects include hemoglobin oxygen depletion and liver and/or kidney damage.

The implications to the perianesthesia care of a patient that is using inhalants can be great. Given the fact that these substances can cause reversible and irreversible effects, each patient should be evaluated individually for use of these drugs. Health care professionals who care for these patients should remember that these inhalants are mainly used by children—with the highest usage between the 6th and 12th grades—and that it continues to be a significant problem among our country's youth. For perianesthesia nursing, the deliberate misuse of these volatile substances poses a significant risk or considerable morbidity and mortality in the adolescent population in the PACU.

CLUB DRUGS

Club drugs are most popular in the teenage and young adult population who are part of the nightclub, bar, rave, or trance scenes. Raves and trance parties are usually nightlong events that include adolescents who may not use the specific drugs; however, those who do are attracted to the use of these rather low-cost agents that appear to produce increased stamina and intoxicating highs. Research now demonstrates that these drugs can change critical parts of the brain. Along with this, because of their effects on the E-C coupling mechanisms of muscles (see Chapter 21), these agents are not implicated in malignant hyperthermia (see Chapter 50).

MDMA is a psychoactive drug that has both stimulant (amphetamine-like) and hallucinogenic (LSD-like) properties. This drug has many street names such as "Ecstasy," "Adam," "XTC," "hug," "beans," and "love drug." MDMA has many routes of administration, including oral, rectal, intravenous, or inhalation.

The problems associated with MDMA are similar to those found with the use of amphetamines and cocaine, which were discussed previously. The psychologic difficulties may include such phenomena as confusion, depression, sleep problems, severe anxiety, and paranoia. The physical difficulties include such things as muscle tension, involuntary teeth clenching, nausea, blurred vision, faintness, and chills or sweating. Physiologic concerns are that this category of drugs can cause hypertension and tachycardia, and long-term use may result in damage to the brain in the parts that focus on thought, memory, and pleasure.

Research on the impact of MDMA on the patient recovering from anesthesia is desperately needed. The reader is encouraged to review the effects of cocaine and their impact on recovery of the patient taking this class of drugs.

DATE-RAPE DRUGS

Gamma hydroxybutyrate (GHB) is a euphoric, sedative, and anabolic. It is a widely used drug that was obtained over the counter in health food stores until 1992. It has street names of "liquid Ecstasy," "soap," "easy lay," and "Georgia home boy." Coma and seizures can occur after the abuse of GHB. Combined with alcohol, GHB can cause nausea and dyspnea. GHB has been associated with poisonings, overdoses, date rapes, and deaths. This drug has a short duration of action and is not easily detectable on routine hospital toxicology screening tests. Research needs to be conducted on this drug to determine its long-term effects.

Flunitrazepam (Rohypnol) is a benzodiazepine that when mixed with alcohol incapacitates victims and prevents them from resisting sexual assault. This drug, like midazolam, produces anterograde amnesia. This drug is not approved for use in the United States and its importation is illegal. The street names for this drug include "rophies," "roofies," "roach," and "rope," and its illegal use continues to be a problem in the border states, particularly Texas.

Ketamine is an intravenous anesthetic drug (see Chapter 19) that is used illegally in the club and rave scenes and has been used as a date rape drug. It can be injected or snorted and is known on the street as "Special K" or "vitamin K." This drug produces a dreamlike state and hallucinations. In high street doses, ketamine will cause delirium, amnesia, impaired motor function, high blood pressure, depression, and apnea. The veterinary form of this drug appears to be the most abused, and its frequency of use is steadily increasing.

BIBLIOGRAPHY

Alspach J: Core curriculum for critical care nursing, ed 5, Philadelphia, 1998, WB Saunders.

Atlee J: Complications in anesthesia, Philadelphia, 1999, WB Saunders.

Barash P, Cullen B, Stoelting R: Clinical anesthesia, ed 4, Philadelphia, 2000, Lippincott Williams & Wilkins.

Benumof J, Saidman L: Anesthesia & perioperative complications, ed 2, St Louis, 1999, Mosby.

Brouette T, Anton R: Clinical review of inhalants, Am J Addict 10(1):79-94, 2001.

DeFazio-Quinn D: Ambulatory surgical nursing core curriculum, Philadelphia, 1999, WB Saunders.

Frost E, Seidel M: Preanesthetic assessment of the drug abuse patient, Anesthesiol Clin North Am 8(4):829-842, 1990.

Ganong W: Review of medical physiology, ed 20, New York, 2001, McGraw-Hill Professional.

Guyton A, Hall J: Textbook of medical physiology, ed 10, Philadelphia, 2000, WB Saunders.

Hardman J, Limbird L: Goodman and Gilman's the pharmacological basis of therapeutics, ed 10, New York, 2001, McGraw-Hill Professional.

Huckabee M: Perioperative care of the active substance abuser, J Post Anesth Nurs 3(4):254-259, 1988.

Katzung B, editor: Basic and clinical pharmacology, ed 8, Los Altos, Calif, 2000, Appleton & Lange.

Knor E: Substance abuse. In Knor E: Decision making in obstetrical nursing, Toronto, 1987, BC Decker.

Kurtzman T, Otsuka K: Inhalant abuse by adolescents, J Adolesc Health 28(3):170-180, 2001.

Longnecker D, Murphy F: Dripps/Eckenhoff/Vandam introduction to anesthesia, ed 9, Philadelphia, 1997, WB Saunders.

Longnecker D, Tinker J, Morgan G: Principles and practice of anesthesiology, ed 2, St Louis, 1998, Mosby.

Miller R, editor: Anesthesia, ed 5, New York, 2000, Churchill Livingstone.

Morgan M: Ecstasy (MDMA): a review of its possible persistent psychologic effects, Psychopharmacology (Berl) 152(3):230-248, 2000.

Nagelhout J, Zaglaniczny K: Nurse anesthesia, ed 2, Philadelphia, 2001, WB Saunders.

Pharm J, Puzantian T: Ecstasy: dangers and controversies, Pharmacotherapy 21(12):1561-1565, 2001.

Rogers E: Post anesthesia care of the cocaine abuser, J Post Anesth Nurs 6(2):102-107, 1991.

Stoelting R: Pharmacology and physiology in anesthetic practice, ed 3, Philadelphia, 1999, Lippincott-Raven.

Stoelting R, Miller R: Basics of anesthesia, ed 4, New York, 2000, Churchill Livingstone.

Stone D: Perioperative care: anesthesia, medicine, and surgery, St Louis, 1998, Mosby.

Teter C, Guthrie S: A comprehensive review of MDMA and GHB: two common club drugs, Pharmacotherapy 21(12):1486-1513, 2001.

Waugaman W, Foster S, Rigor B: Principles and practice of nurse anesthesia, ed 3, Norwalk, Conn, 1999, Appleton & Lange.

Weiss S: Anesthesia for the alcoholic and addict, AANA J 47(3):309-312, 1979.

Patients admitted to the postanesthesia care unit (PACU) usually experience some form of thermal imbalance. Thermal imbalance is defined as body core temperature that is outside the normothermic rage of 36°C to 38°C. Patients most likely experience hypothermia because of the combination of anesthetic drugs and a cold intraoperative environment. This chapter reviews the current concepts of hypothermia and hyperthermia and their impact on the care of the PACU patient.

OVERVIEW OF THERMOREGULATION

The body maintains its temperature between the narrow range of 36°C and 38°C. This is done by a balance of heat production and heat loss that is controlled by thermoregulatory mechanisms in the central nervous system (CNS). These mechanisms receive input from various thermoreceptors located in the skin, nose, oral cavity, thoracic viscera, and spinal cord. These thermoreceptors send sensory information in hierarchical order: spinal cord, reticular formation, and the primary control in the preoptic hypothalamic region of the brain.

The central temperature controls maintain body temperature by two primary responses: physiologic and behavioral. The physiologic thermoregulatory response consists of sweating, shivering, and alterations in the peripheral vasomotor tone. These responses fine-control the regulatory process of body temperature; consequently, heat loss is reduced by vasoconstriction and increased by vasodilatation and sweating. They also work by reducing heat production, lowering the metabolic rate, and increasing muscle tone and shivering to enhance heat production. The behavioral thermoregulation is run by subjective feelings of discomfort or comfort. For example, if in a hot environment, a person seeks air conditioning, and in a cold environment the person seeks heat. It is a stronger response mechanism but does not exhibit fine control such as in the physiologic thermoregulatory response system.

Body heat is produced by metabolism, and it has a circadian cycle, with the core temperature being lower in the morning than in the afternoon. Body heat is removed by four methods of heat transfer: radiation, conduction, convection, and evaporation (see Chapter 10), of which radiation is the major method of heat transfer.

POSTOPERATIVE HYPOTHERMIA

Hypothermia is defined as a core body temperature lower than 36°C. About 60% of the patients who arrive in the PACU experience some degree of hypothermia, and of those hypothermic patients, 18% to 23% actively shiver in the PACU. However, the relationship between hypothermia and shivering is not clear. Patients older than 60 years of age usually have lower admission and discharge temperatures in the PACU than younger patients do. However, elderly patients appear to have a delayed ability to compensate for the hypothermia. Patients who have general anesthesia experience a more rapid increase in postanesthesia temperature and a shorter duration of hypothermia in the PACU than the patients who receive intraoperative spinal or epidural anesthetics.

Body temperature is assessed by one of three methods. The thermistor responds to increased heat by emitting a lower voltage. The thermocouple, which has two dissimilar metals, responds to increased heat by sending out an increased voltage. The last sensor is called the direct-reading liquid crystal colorimetric sensor. This sensor is placed on the skin, usually the forehead, and the temperature is read directly from the sensor. The colorimetric sensor is not a good estimate of core temperature because of many uncontrollable factors such as vasoconstriction and environmental temperature.

Body temperature varies by the site being monitored (see Chapter 25). For example, the rectal temperature is usually 0.5°C to 0.7°C higher than the axillary or oral temperature. Axillary monitoring sites are used in many countries but less often in the United States, and the tympanic probe is associated with perforation of the tympanic membrane. However, well-designed tympanic membrane probes are the route of choice to monitor the core temperature. It should be noted that the oral route for measuring the temperature will usually render lower temperatures than the other routes; it probably is not the route of choice for monitoring core temperature. However, for continuous monitoring of the body temperature, the axillary devices are the preferred route of choice and have proven to be quite adequate because this method is an excellent predictor of trends in body temperature. For children, the rectal site is the route of choice.

Hypothermia is the most common problem for patients recovering from anesthesia in the PACU. Moderate hypothermia in the PACU is generally well tolerated. However, in the medically compromised patient or if the hypothermia is unrecognized, major problems can ensue.

Postanesthesia shivering (PAS) is caused by intraoperative exposure to a cold environment and the CNS depressant and peripheral vasodilatation effects of anesthesia. Muscles of the trunk and extremities can be involved; however, the PAS may be more obvious in the jaw and the shoulders. PAS can increase the metabolic rate 400% to 500%. This will cause the minute volume and cardiac output to increase, and if cardiopulmonary compensation does not occur, anaerobic cellular metabolism can result. Consequently, patients with ischemic disease of the myocardium, kidneys, or brain can be at risk during PAS. In fact, PAS has been associated with death in the PACU from myocardial infarction.

On arrival in the PACU, the patient should be assessed for hypothermia. This is particularly true if the intraoperative procedure lasted longer than 1 hour. Oxygen should be administered by mask, and pulse oximetry monitoring should be instituted to detect possible hypoxemia. After the oral or axillary temperature is obtained, the rewarming therapy should be instituted. The goal is to return the patient to a temperature of 36°C. Various rewarming techniques are available for use in the PACU. Warmed cotton blankets do not increase core body temperature or decrease the duration of hypothermia. Water-circulating warming mattresses have been found to be about as effective as warmed cotton blankets in the treatment of hypothermia. Moreover, complications such as burns and pressure necrosis have been reported with the water-circulating warming mattress. Infrared heat lamps are effective for the patient who is experiencing PAS. However, the most successful intervention for hypothermia is the use of convective warming (warm air therapy). This therapy is most effective because about 70% of the body surface area is exposed to the warm air that is circulating in a blanket.

MALIGNANT HYPERTHERMIA

In the past, reports in the medical literature discussed young, healthy persons who, after exercise in hot weather, developed "heat stroke" that was followed by death. Clinical reports of this syndrome continued to appear—especially of patients in the operating room developing an accelerated temperature during induction of anesthesia. By the 1950s, more information had become available. Because of research, the morbidity and mortality from this syndrome have now been reduced. Its cause is a genetically determined condition called malignant hyperthermia (MH). MH is precipitated by certain general inhalation anesthetics, depolarizing skeletal muscle relaxants, amide local anesthetics, and stress. The incidence of MH ranges from 1 in 14,000 to 15,000 in children and 1 in 50,000 in adults. The onset of MH usually occurs during induction of anesthesia. Once the acute episode is treated in the operating room, the patient may be admitted to the PACU. Reports of MH recurring in the PACU have been made. Because successful management of MH depends on early assessment and prompt intervention, the perianesthesia nurse must be knowledgeable in the pathophysiology and treatment of this syndrome.

Identification of MH-Susceptible Patients

Genetics. Humans probably inherit susceptibility to MH with more than one gene or more
than one group of possible mutational forms of a
gene. The pattern of inheritance may range from
recessive to dominant, with graded variations in
between. The ease of initiation of an episode of
MH seems to depend on the degree of genetic susceptibility and on environmental factors; this
explains why some patients who are known to be
susceptible show no signs of MH when exposed
to confirmed MH-triggering agents. It is also possible that an MH-susceptible (MHS) patient
could be given an anesthetic in the presence of
trigger agents; this patient might not experience
an acute MH reaction intraoperatively, but it
could develop instead in the PACU.

Evaluation of Susceptibility. Before anesthesia is administered, identifying patients who may
be susceptible to MH is of major therapeutic
importance. On history and physical examination, MHS patients usually demonstrate some
subclinical muscle weakness or abnormality, such
as deficient fine motor control. Many MHS
patients complain of muscle cramps that occur
spontaneously, during an infectious illness, or
during or after exercise. When these cramps are
present, they may be so severe that they are
almost incapacitating. The patient may also
describe heat prostration during physical exertion
that is associated with environmental heat stress.
In addition, there may be a positive patient
history or a positive genealogy going back two
generations (i.e., the patient or immediate rela-
tives may show MH symptoms during an anesthetic experience). Physical examination of the
MHS person may reveal myopathies such as
wasting of the distal ends of the vastus muscles
and hypertrophy of the proximal femoral muscles
of the thigh. Other myopathies that are associated with MH susceptibility are cryptorchidism,
pectus carinatum, kyphosis, lordosis, ptosis, and
hypoplastic mandible. Electromyographic
changes are seen in fewer than half of MHS
patients. Electrocardiograms of MHS patients
may reveal ventricular or atrial hypertrophy (or
both), bundle branch block, myocardial
ischemia, and ventricular dysrhythmias. Measurements of blood creatine phosphokinase
(CPK) are usually about 70% reliable in estimating susceptibility to MH.

The most definitive test for detecting MH
susceptibility is the biopsy of skeletal muscle.
Samples are obtained from the quadriceps muscle
and are subjected to isometric contracture
testing. The skeletal muscle of the MHS patient
has an increased isometric tension when exposed
to caffeine or halothane.

Patients at high risk for development of an
acute MH crisis have been classified as follows:
(1) patients who have an MH-positive muscle
biopsy or who have survived an acute MH crisis;
(2) patients who have a first-degree relative
known to be MHS or to have had a positive
muscle biopsy; (3) patients whose family
members have a clinically demonstrated muscle
abnormality; and (4) patients who are members
of a family whose plasma CPK measurements
have been found to be elevated in one or more
samples (taken on at least three occasions).

Normal Skeletal Muscle Physiology

Although a complete discussion of skeletal
muscle contraction can be found in Chapter 21,
a brief synopsis is presented here. The events
leading to the contraction of a skeletal muscle
begin with an electrical impulse that is transmitted down the axon to the motor nerve terminal,
where vesicles that contain acetylcholine are
located. On stimulation, the contents of the vesicles are released. This quantum of acetylcholine
crosses the myoneural junction and interacts
with its receptor on the postsynaptic membrane.
This receptor activation causes a transient
increase in the permeability for sodium and
potassium ions, which ultimately creates an electrical action potential (nerve impulse) that is
propagated along the muscle membrane. This
action potential electrically excites the sarcolemma and releases into the myoplasm calcium
ions that are stored in the sarcoplasmic reticulum. These calcium ions then attach to troponin
C, an inhibitory muscle protein that, when stimulated by the calcium, permits the actin and
myosin protein filaments to interact and cause
muscle contraction. The calcium ions in the
myoplasm are then taken up by a reuptake mechanism into the sarcoplasmic reticulum. The
process by which the electrically excited sarcolemma is coupled to the calcium released
from the sarcoplasmic reticulum is known as
excitation-contraction (E-C) coupling.

Pathophysiology of Malignant Hyperthermia

When a susceptible patient is exposed to a trigger agent—such as halothane—that causes MH to occur, the clinical features are produced by an excess of calcium ions in the myoplasm. Although the exact pathophysiology of MH is not known, it appears that in MH the reuptake of calcium from the myoplasm by the sarcoplasmic reticulum is decreased; it has also been suggested that the E-C coupling mechanism is defective. With an elevated calcium ion concentration in the myoplasm, the skeletal muscle contraction will be intense and prolonged, finally leading to a hypermetabolic state of acid and heat production. More specifically, heat is produced by the accelerated and continued synthesis and use of adenosine triphosphate (ATP) during glycolysis. The metabolic by-product of glycolysis, lactic acid, is transported to the liver, where part of it is oxidized to provide the ATP necessary to help make glucose. This glucose, along with glycogen, is released from the liver and transported back to the metabolically active muscle, where the entire cycle repeats. This revolving process liberates much heat and produces a significant amount of metabolic acid. Respiratory and metabolic acidosis develop because of this hypermetabolic state, and symptoms such as tachycardia, tachypnea, ventricular dysrhythmias, and unstable blood pressure appear. Because of intense vasoconstriction, the skin is mottled and cyanotic (Box 50-1). Elevated body temperature can actually be a late sign of MH; for this reason, the nurse should not prolong the assessment of the patient on the assumption that the patient's temperature must be significantly elevated before intervention is attempted. Once the patient's temperature begins to rise, it may increase at a rate of 0.5°C every 15 minutes and may approach levels as high as 46°C.

Muscle rigidity occurs in about 75% of the patients who experience MH. This is especially true in MHS patients after the administration of succinylcholine. In fact, the spasm of the masseter muscles following the injection of succinylcholine may be so severe that the nurse cannot open the patient's mouth to insert an airway. The onset of skeletal muscle rigidity after the administration of succinylcholine could be a sign of the impending development of MH.

Box 50-1 Signs and Symptoms of Malignant Hyperthermia

SIGNS (OBJECTIVE FINDINGS)
Central venous desaturation
Central venous hypercapnia
Metabolic acidosis
Respiratory acidosis
Hyperkalemia
Myoglobinemia
Elevated creatine phosphokinase

SYMPTOMS (SUBJECTIVE FINDINGS)
Tachycardia
Tachypnea
Ventricular dysrhythmias
Cyanosis
Skin mottling
Fever-hot, flushed skin
Rigidity
Profuse sweating
Unstable blood pressure

Primary signs and symptoms are italicized.

Triggering of Malignant Hyperthermia. Various environmental stimuli and pharmacologic agents can stimulate an acute episode of MH (Box 50-2). Fatigue, emotional upset, or very hot and humid weather can trigger a waking febrile episode. Patients usually respond to dantrolene, surface cooling, and other symptomatic treatment. The anesthetic agents that trigger MH seem to affect the sarcoplasmic reticulum or the E-C coupling mechanism, or both. Because of their wide use, halothane and succinylcholine are the most common trigger agents. Amide local anesthetics, such as lidocaine, are also trigger agents; it has been demonstrated that lidocaine causes the release of calcium ions into the myoplasm *in vitro*. In MHS patients or in patients who have had an episode of acute MH in the operating room, all possible trigger agents should be stringently avoided. As another precaution, because emotional upsets trigger MH, the perianesthesia nurse should provide a stress-free environment for the MHS patient.

Box 50-2 Environmental Stimuli and Pharmacologic Agents that may Trigger Malignant Hyperthermia

PSYCHOLOGIC/PHYSIOLOGIC STIMULI

Extensive skeletal muscle injury
Emotional crisis
Very hot and humid weather
Strenuous and prolonged exercise
Anoxia or hypoxia
Infection

PHARMACOLOGIC AGENTS

Halothane
Enflurane
Isoflurane (?)
Succinylcholine
d-Tubocurarine
Gallamine (?)
Amide local anesthetics-lidocaine, mepivacaine,
    bupivacaine, etidocaine
Caffeine
Carbon tetrachloride
Ethanol
Quinidine
Calcium salts

Pharmacologic Agents Associated with Malignant Hyperthermia

Dantrolene Sodium (Dantrium). Dantrolene is a muscle relaxant that is chemically and pharmacologically unrelated to other muscle relaxants. It is the only known pharmacologic agent that is effective in the treatment of MH. The site of action of this drug is distal to the end plate within the muscle fiber. The main pharmacologic action of dantrolene reduces the release of calcium by the sarcoplasmic reticulum without affecting reuptake. Consequently, the concentration of calcium in the myoplasm is reduced, thus inhibiting the E-C coupling mechanism and causing muscle contraction to cease. When administered orally, dantrolene has a half-life of 8 hours; when administered intravenously, the half-life is 5 hours. When it is used in the treatment of acute MH, the intravenous dosage is 1 to 2 mg/kg, which can be repeated every 5 to 10 minutes with a maximum dose of 10 mg/kg. If the

acute episode of MH occurs in the operating room and the patient is treated successfully, dantrolene therapy will be continued into the recovery (PACU) period to prevent recurrence of MH. After the acute period in the PACU has passed, the patient will be given oral dantrolene in four divided doses. Because dantrolene is poorly soluble, it is supplied in vials in the form of a lyophilized powder. To reconstitute a vial of lyophilized powder, 60 ml of sterile water for injection, USP, is added to the vial, and it is shaken until the solution is clear; many compatibility problems arise when dantrolene is mixed with solutions other than sterile water for injection, USP. Also, the sterile water for injection, USP, used to reconstitute the dantrolene should not contain any bacteriostatic agents because it is not unusual to use more than 2000 ml of diluent during the treatment of acute MH in an adult weighing 70 kg.

Procainamide (Procamide, Procapan, Pronestyl). Procainamide once was the main drug in the treatment of MH. The use of procainamide is controversial, particularly because the recommended initial dose is two to five times its cardiotoxic dose. Some authors suggest that if this drug is used in the treatment of MH, isoproterenol should be administered to maintain cardiac function. The recommended dose of procainamide is 0.5 to 1 mg/kg/min, up to a maximum dose of 15 to 30 mg/kg. The dosage should be lowered when the heart rate or dysrhythmias are reduced. At a lower dose range, procainamide may be useful in the treatment of the dysrhythmias during the acute episode of MH.

Perioperative Management of the MH-Susceptible Patient

Preoperatively, the MHS patient may be given oral dantrolene in four divided doses of 4 to 7 mg/kg daily for 1 to 3 days before the administration of the anesthetic. The patient is usually well premedicated; however, anticholinergics, such as atropine, should be avoided because they interfere with the normal heat loss mechanisms and, in the case of atropine, can cause tachycardia that may cause confusion in the diagnosis of acute MH. Also, phenothiazines should be avoided in the perioperative period because they may cause a release of calcium from the sarcoplasmic reticulum. Intraoperative anesthesia requires the use of agents that will not trigger an episode of MH (Box 50-3). Although regional anesthesia avoids the use of the general inhalation anesthetic agents and skeletal muscle relaxants, elevated temperatures in MHS patients have been reported with its use. If local anesthetic agents are to be used, amides such as lidocaine and mepivacaine should be avoided.

Intraoperative monitoring of the MHS patient includes the electrocardiographic, temperature, arterial blood gas (including acid-base), and precordial stethoscope determinations. These monitoring parameters should be continued into the PACU period (Box 50-4). Because some MHS patients have had MH triggered in the postoperative period, they should be followed for a minimum of 24 hours postoperatively and should not be subjected to anxiety or stress. These patients should be reassured that physicians and nurses have reliable instruments to monitor for MH and that prompt and effective treatment will be provided if it develops.

Treatment of Acute Malignant Hyperthermia in the PACU

The cornerstone of the successful treatment of MH is early detection (see Box 50-1). Box 50-5 lists the suggested equipment and drugs that should be kept in the PACU to be used in the treatment of acute MH. Chapter 1 also provides information on equipment and drugs that should be available for the treatment of acute MH. If the assessment indicates that the patient is developing acute MH, the following steps should be taken:

1. Discontinue the use of any trigger agent (see Box 50-3), and send for help.
2. Rapidly ventilate the patient with large tidal volumes by using a bag-valve-mask system and oxygen (total oxygen flow should exceed 15 L/min). Oral endotracheal intubation should be performed if the patient's airway is compromised.
3. Insert arterial and central venous lines, and send venous and arterial blood samples to the laboratory for immediate results on electrolyte and arterial blood gas analysis.
4. Start reconstituting the dantrolene as soon as possible.
5. Administer the intravenous dantrolene-1 to 2 mg/kg over 1 to 2 minutes, up to 10 mg/kg or until the patient's temperature starts to decrease.
6. Cool the patient. Cover all exposed surfaces with towels soaked in water. Cover the wet towels with ice. Use cooling blankets and fans if possible. Use cold gastric lavage and hydrate with iced intravenous fluids. To avoid hypothermia, discontinue all the cooling interventions when body temperature decreases to 38°C.
7. Administer sodium bicarbonate intravenously at a dosage of 1 to 2 mEq/kg. When

---

Box 50-3	**Drugs that are Considered Safe to Administer to a Malignant Hyperthermia-Susceptible Patient**

Nitrous oxide
Diazepam
Droperidol
Pancuronium
Thiopental
Ketamine
Fentanyl
Morphine
Ester local anesthetics-procaine, tetracaine, 2-chloroprocaine

---

Box 50-4	**Suggested Components of Monitoring of the Patient with Acute Malignant Hyperthermia**

Continuous ECG (consider 12-lead ECG and EEG after acute phase)
Core and axillary temperature
Urine output
Arterial pressure line
Pulse and blood pressure
Central venous pressure*
Swan-Ganz catheters*

ECG, Electrocardiogram; EEG, electroencephalogram.
*Should be considered; however, do not delay treatment if the insertion of these monitors is physically or technically difficult.

results of the arterial blood gas analysis are available, correct the base deficit using sodium bicarbonate according to the following formula:

$$base\ deficit = 0.3 \times weight\ (kg)$$
$$\times base\ excess\ (mEq/L)$$

If the $PaCO_2$ is elevated, increase the tidal ventilation of the patient. Do not administer sodium bicarbonate to correct respiratory acidosis because the $PaCO_2$ will only increase, which may lead to ventricular fibrillation.

8. Constantly monitor the patient's core temperature, blood pressure, pulse, cardiac rhythm, and pupil size and reactivity, and watch for cyanosis (see Box 50-4).

9. The hyperkalemia can be treated with intravenous insulin and glucose (0.25 to 0.5 U/kg of insulin to 0.25 to 0.5 g/kg of glucose).

10. If possible, catheterize the bladder and monitor urinary output and appearance. To secure a high urinary output, furosemide (1 mg/kg) or mannitol (1 g/kg) may be given.

11. Do *not* treat dysrhythmias with lidocaine because it is a trigger agent. Do not give intravenous calcium because it may also cause dysrhythmias.

12. Hypotension can be treated by the infusion of cold crystalloid solution.

13. Continue to send arterial and venous blood samples to the laboratory for prompt determination of arterial blood gases and electrolytes.

14. Look for such hopeful prognostic signs as a lessening coma, hyperactive tendon reflexes, and a stabilization of the temperature. Once the temperature returns to normal, continue constant observation of the patient.

Complications Following Acute Malignant Hyperthermia

Renal failure can occur because of myoglobinuria or hypotension. Consumption coagulopathies, such as disseminated intravascular coagulation, have been reported along with acute heart failure and pulmonary edema. Because the brain is the organ most sensitive to hyperthermia (permanent brain damage at $\geq 41°C$), brain deterioration can occur in patients who are not promptly diagnosed and treated for MH.

Box 50-5 Suggested Equipment and Drugs to be Used in the Treatment of Acute Malignant Hyperthermia

Equipment Needed
Intravenous lines with assorted cannula gauges
Central venous pressure sets (2)
Sterile venous and arterial strain gauge
Swan-Ganz catheter
Laboratory test tubes for blood chemistry analysis
Crystalloid solution (10 1000-ml bottles)—labeled _for hyperthermia only_ and stored in the PACU refrigerator
Bucket of cracked ice—labeled _for hyperthermia only_ and stored in freezer of the PACU refrigerator
Cooling blanket
Fan

Drugs Needed
Sodium bicarbonate (12 ampules of 8.4% strength)
Mannitol (4 ampules—12.4 g/50 ml)
Furosemide (4 vials)
Calcium gluconate (2 ampules—100 mg/10 ml)
Potassium chloride (2 ampules)
Glucose (2 bottles of 50% strength)
Iced intravenous saline (10 1000-ml bottles in refrigerator)
Procainamide (2000 mg)
Short-acting beta blocker such as Esmolol
Regular insulin (1 ampule of 100 units)
Dantrolene (Dantrium) intravenous—36 vials of lyophilized powder with at least 2200 ml of sterile water for injection, USP (without a bacteriostatic agent), to reconstitute the dantrolene

Note: All the equipment and drugs listed in the box should be stored in a box or cart in the PACU. The box or cart should be labeled **"hyperthermia."**

BIBLIOGRAPHY

Alspach J: Core curriculum for critical care nursing, ed 5, Philadelphia, 1998, WB Saunders.

Atlee J: Complications in anesthesia, Philadelphia, 1999, WB Saunders.

Augustine S: Hypothermia therapy in the post anesthesia care unit: a review, J Post Anesth Nurs 5(4):254-263, 1990.

Barash P, Cullen B, Stoelting R: Clinical anesthesia, ed 4, Philadelphia, 2000, Lippincott Williams & Wilkins.

Barker S: Trauma and malignant hyperthermia, Audio-Digest Anesthesiology, 43(1):1-3, 2001.

Burns S, Bostek C: Avoiding unintentional hypothermia: anesthesia implications, Nurse Anesth 1(3):128-133, 1990.

Benumof J: Anesthesia and uncommon diseases, ed 4, Philadelphia, 1998, WB Saunders.

Benumof J, Saidman L: Anesthesia & perioperative complications, ed 2, St Louis, 1999, Mosby.

Cory M, Fossum S et al: Constant temperature monitoring: a study of temperature patterns in the Postanesthesia Care Unit, J PeriAnesth Nurs 13(5):292-300, 1998.

Coté C, Todres I, Goudsouzian N, Ryan J: A practice of anesthesia for infants and children, ed 3, Philadelphia, WB Saunders.

DeFazio-Quinn D: Ambulatory surgical nursing core curriculum, Philadelphia, 1999, WB Saunders.

Ganong W: Review of medical physiology, ed 20, New York, 2001, McGraw-Hill Professional.

Guyton A, Hall J: Textbook of medical physiology, ed 10, Philadelphia, 2000, WB Saunders.

Hardman J, Limbird L: Goodman and Gilman's the pharmacological basis of therapeutics, ed 10, New York, 2001, McGraw-Hill Professional.

Hardy E, Cirillo B, Gutzeit N: Rewarming patients in the PACU: can we make a difference? J Post Anesth Nurs 3(5):313-316, 1988.

Krenzischeck D, Frank S, Kelly S: Forced-air warming versus routine thermal care and core temperature measurement sites, J Post Anesth Nurs 10(2):69-78, 1995.

Lake C, Hines R, Blitt C: Clinical monitoring: practical applications for anesthesia and critical care, St Louis, 2001, Mosby.

Lipton J, Giesecke A: Body temperature and shivering in the perioperative patient, Semin Anesth 7(1):3-10, 1988.

Litwack K: Practical points in the management of hypothermia, J Post Anesth Nurs 3(5):339-341, 1988.

Longnecker D, Murphy F: Dripps/Eckenhoff/Vandam introduction to anesthesia, ed 9, Philadelphia, 1997, WB Saunders.

Longnecker D, Tinker J, Morgan G: Principles and practice of anesthesiology, ed 2, St Louis, 1998, Mosby.

McIntosh L: Essentials of nurse anesthesia, New York, 1997, McGraw-Hill.

Miller R, editor: Anesthesia, ed 5, New York, 2000, Churchill Livingstone.

Morrison R: Hypothermia in the elderly, Int Anesthesiol Clin 26(2):124-133, 1988.

Motoyama E: Smith's anesthesia for infants and children, ed 6, St Louis, 1996, Mosby.

Nagelhout J, Zaglaniczny K: Nurse anesthesia, ed 2, Philadelphia, 2001, WB Saunders.

Stoelting R: Pharmacology and physiology in anesthetic practice, ed 3, Philadelphia, 1999, Lippincott Raven.

Stoelting R, Miller R: Basics of anesthesia, ed 4, New York, 2000, Churchill Livingstone.

Stone D: Perioperative care: anesthesia, medicine, and surgery, St Louis, 1998, Mosby.

Vaughan M, Vaughan R, Cork R: Postoperative hypothermia in adults: relationship of age, anesthesia, and shivering to rewarming, Anesth Analg 60(10):746-751, 1981.

Waugaman W, Foster S, Rigor B: Principles and practice of nurse anesthesia, ed 3, Norwalk, Conn, 1999, Appleton & Lange.

51

CARE OF THE SHOCK TRAUMA PATIENT

Judy Stevenson, RN, BSN, CCRN

In the United States, trauma continues to affect the lives of more than 70 million people each year and results in over 147,000 deaths, more than 400 per day.[1] Swiftly and without warning, traumatic injuries span all ages, cultures, and races and reach epidemic proportions. Furthermore, trauma accounts for more deaths in the United States during the first four decades of life than any other disease and is the fourth leading cause of death among the entire population of the United States.[2] Mortality from trauma is the tip of the iceberg; many patients survive trauma and thus require intervention from surgery.

Although 50% of all deaths attributed to trauma occur within minutes to hours after the injury, 30% die within 2 days from neurologic injury; the remaining 20% of deaths occur as a result of complications.[1] All complications that can occur in the anesthetized patient can occur in the postoperative trauma patient.[3] Overwhelming infection and sepsis result from these traumatic injuries, and trauma patients are at risk for multiple complications, including but not limited to respiratory, circulatory, and renal failure. Numerous pathologic conditions may contribute to this high incidence of late mortality due to sepsis.

PREHOSPITAL PHASE

During the past 20 years, the ultimate goal of emergency medical services has been to improve the field stabilization, resuscitation, and subsequent transportation of the multitrauma patient to the appropriate-level trauma center.[4] The concept of the "golden hour," which was introduced by R. Adams Cowley, MD, emphasizes the importance of the time in which resuscitation of severely injured patients must begin so as to survive.[2] It is the window of opportunity in which

to institute life and limb measures and can be as varying as minutes for some patients to hours for others.[1] During the prehospital phase, vital information regarding the trauma patient's condition at the scene and mechanism of injury reveal important clues to how the patient will present later. For example, if the patient experienced a prolonged extrication period at the scene, his or her airway may have been compromised; he or she may have had active or uncontrolled bleeding or have been exposed to environmental elements, thus decreasing core temperature.

Other conditions at the scene that may influence the trauma patient's outcome include such considerations as (1) whether restraint devices were used; (2) if airbags were deployed during impact; (3) whether the passenger was ejected from the car; (4) what position the patient was found in; (5) whether the car rolled over; (6) whether the windshield was broken; (7) the speed at which the vehicle was traveling; (8) where on the car was the impact; (9) whether the patient wore a motorcycle helmet; (10) whether there were other fatalities at the scene; and (11) what, if anything, bystanders did to assist the victim. All these observations by the first providers help piece each part of the trauma puzzle together to ensure a comprehensive approach to the management of the trauma patient.

Mechanisms of Injury

To accurately assess the trauma patient in the postanesthesia care unit (PACU), the nurse needs a basic understanding of the different mechanisms of injury. Mechanisms of injury are related to the type of injuring force and subsequent tissue response. A thorough understanding of these aspects of injury helps in determining the extent and nature of the potential injuries. The major factors that influence injury are the velocity of the objects and the force in terms of physical motion to moving or stationary bodies.[5] (Force is the mass of an object times acceleration.) Mechanism of injury can help identify common injury combinations, predict eventual outcomes, and explain the type of injury.[2] Although a certain pattern of injury may be predictable for specific injuries, all trauma patients can have other injuries. A thorough assessment to identify all injuries is needed.[6]

Various forms of traumatic injuries are blunt (high velocity); penetrating, such as those that cut or pierce; falls from great heights; firearms; and chemical, electrical, radiant, and thermal burns. Motor vehicle crashes create impressive forces that can fracture extremities, crush organs, and lead to massive blood loss and soft-tissue damage. At the time of a crash, three impacts occur: (1) vehicle to object; (2) body to vehicle; and (3) organs within body. Finally, forces are depicted in relation to acceleration, deceleration, shearing, and compression.[7]

Blunt Trauma. Blunt trauma may best be described as a wounding force that does not communicate to the outside of the body. High-velocity motor vehicle crashes and falls from great heights cause blunt-trauma injuries that are associated with direct impact, deceleration, continuous pressure, and shearing and rotary forces.[2] These blunt-trauma injuries are usually more serious and life-threatening than other types of trauma because the extent of the injuries is less obvious and diagnosis is more difficult. Because blunt injuries can leave little outward evidence of the extent of internal damage, the nurse must be extremely thorough in making observations and ongoing assessments.

When the body decelerates, the organs continue to move forward at the original speed. As the body's organs move in the forward direction, they are torn from their attachments by rotary and shearing forces.[2] Furthermore, blunt forces disrupt blood vessels and nerves. This mechanism of injury to the microcirculation causes widespread epithelial and endothelial damage, thus stimulating cells to release their constituents and further activating the complement, the arachidonic acid, and the coagulation cascades. Finally, blunt trauma may mask more serious complications related to the pathophysiology of the injury.

Penetrating Trauma. Penetrating wounds such as stab wounds and firearms are produced by a foreign body. The mechanism of injury causes the penetration and crushing of underlying tissues. Tissue damage inflicted by bullets depend on the bullet's size, velocity, range, mass, and trajectory. Knives often cause stab wounds, but other impaling objects can cause damage. Tissue injury depends on length of the object, force applied, and the angle of entry. These penetrating wounds cause disruption of tissues and cellular function, thus resulting in the introduction of debris and foreign bodies into the wound.[5] Finally, the insult to the body may occur as local ischemia, or it may extend to a fulminant hemorrhage from these penetrating injuries.

Contusion of Tissues

When blunt trauma is significant enough to produce capillary injury and destruction, contusion of tissues occurs. Consequently, the extravasation of blood causes discoloration, pain, and swelling.[8] If a large vessel ruptures, a hematoma may produce a distinct, palpable lesion. With a massive contusion or hematoma, an increase in myofascial pressures often results in sequelae known as compartment syndrome.[3] A compartment is a section of muscle enclosed in a confined, supportive membrane called fascia, and compartment syndrome is a condition in which increased pressure inside an osteofascial compartment impedes circulation impairing capillary blood flow and cellular ischemia, resulting in an alteration in neurovascular function. It occurs more frequently in the lower leg or forearm but can occur in any fascial compartment. Damaged vessels in the ischemic muscle dilate in response to histamine and other vasoactive chemical substances, such as the arachidonic cascade and oxygen free radicals. This dilatation, with resultant leakage of fluid into the tissues causing loss of capillary integrity, impedes the microvascular perfusion and results in increased edema and tissue pressure.[8] These pathologic changes cause a repetitive cycle within the confined tissues, increasing swelling and leading to increased compartment pressures. Fascial compartment syndrome can be measured if indicated. Normal pressure is over 10 but a reading over 35 suggests possible anoxia.[9] A fasciotomy may be indicated to prevent muscle or neurovascular damage.

SCORING SYSTEMS

Numerous scoring mechanisms have been designed to assist in determining severity of injuries and likelihood of outcomes. However, their accuracy can be limited despite the score.

STABILIZATION PHASE

The initial assessment, resuscitation, and stabilization processes that are initiated in the emergency department and trauma center (Fig. 51-1) extend into the operating room (OR), the PACU

(Fig. 51-2), and the critical care unit. Because the most common cause of shock (Table 51-1) in the trauma patient is hypovolemia from acute blood loss, the ultimate goal in fluid resuscitation is prompt restoration of blood volume through replacement of fluids so that tissue perfusion and delivery of oxygen to the tissues are maintained.[10] Although hypovolemia is the most common form of shock in the trauma patient, cardiogenic shock, obstructive shock (tension pneumothorax, cardiac tamponade), neurogenic shock (spinal cord injury), and septic shock (usually late due to infection) can occur. Rapid-volume infusors, such as the Bard 37 and the level 1 fluid warmer,

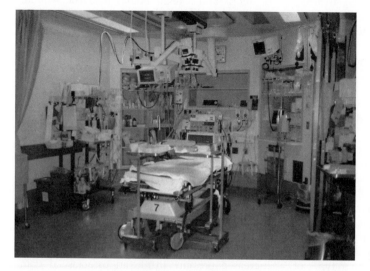

Fig. 51-1   Trauma Resuscitation Unit in the Admitting Area at the R. Adams Cowley Shock Trauma Center at the Maryland Institute of Emergency Medical Services Systems, Baltimore, Maryland.

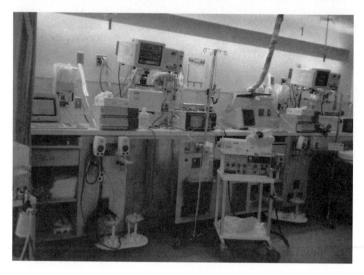

Fig. 51-2   Patient unit in the postanesthesia care unit at the Maryland Institute of Emergency Medical Services Systems, Baltimore, Maryland.

Table 51-1	**Types of Shock**			
Types	Definition	Causes	Signs	Treatment
Hypovolemic	Decrease in intravascular volume	Internal or external hemorrhage, third spacing of fluids, plasma volume loss	Increased HR Decreased BP Decreased CVP Decreased PCWP Increased Respirations Visible signs of bleeding or fluid loss Pallor Diaphoresis Anxiety Decreased urine output	Fluids and/or blood administration
Cardiogenic	Circulatory failure from impairment of contractility	Blunt chest trauma Cardiac contusion Injury to heart muscle Myocardial infarction	Decreased BP Cardiac ischemia Anxiety Confusion Tachypnea Decreased pulse pressure Cool and clammy skin Elevated CVP Elevated PCWP	Support cardiac rhythm Increase cardiac output Inotropics Vasoactive drugs Decrease afterload
Distributive	Neurogenic: Vasodilatation due to decreased neurogenic tone to vessels Anaphylactic: Histamine release into bloodstream following allergic reaction, increased in capillary permeability and vasodilatation	Bacteria Allergens Spinal cord injury Spinal anesthesia	Warm skin Flushed color Increased HR Decreased HR (if neurologic in origin) Increased temp Decreased BP Increased cardiac output Laryngeal edema with bronchospasm (anaphylaxis)	Treat cause Fluids Antibiotics Vasopressors Steroids Epinephrine Antihistamines

Continued

Table 51-1	**Types of Shock**–*cont'd*			
Types	Definition	Causes	Signs	Treatment
	Septic: Massive infection resulting in vasodilation and inadequate tissue perfusion			
Obstructive	Decreased cardiac output from compression to the aorta or great vessels preventing atria from filling and decrease in stroke volume	Cardiac tamponade Tension pneumothorax	Decreased BP Increased HR JVD Tracheal shift Muffled heart sounds Diminished or absent lung sounds Tachypnea	Treat cause, needle decompression and chest tube Pericardial centesis and surgical intervention

deliver warmed intravenous fluids at a rate of 500 to 700 ml/min.[9] The fluids should be warmed to prevent hypothermia. Crystalloids, colloids, or blood products may be used effectively to reverse hypovolemia, which can decrease the effectiveness of shock resuscitation.[10]

Crystalloids are electrolyte solutions that diffuse through the capillary endothelium and can be distributed evenly throughout the extracellular compartment. Examples of crystalloid solutions are lactated Ringer's injection, Plasma-Lyte, and normal saline solution. Although controversy exists between crystalloid versus colloid fluid resuscitation in multiple trauma, the American College of Surgeons' Committee on Trauma recommends that isotonic crystalloid solutions of lactated Ringer's or normal saline be used for that purpose. Furthermore, crystalloids are much cheaper than colloids. Administration of crystalloids should be 3 to 4 times the blood loss.[3,11]

Colloid solutions contain protein or starch molecules or aggregates of molecules that remain uniformly distributed in fluid and fail to form a true solution.[12] When colloid solutions are administered, the molecules remain in the intravascular space, thereby increasing the osmotic pressure gradient within the vascular compartment. Volume for volume, the half-life of colloids is much longer than that of crystalloids. Colloid solutions commonly used are plasma protein fraction, dextran, normal human serum albumin, and hetastarch.

New studies of several human trials have used hypertonic solutions to resuscitate patients in shock. Hypertonic saline or isotonic saline, 250 ml of 7.5% sodium chloride, increased blood pressure more effectively. In addition, patients with low Glasgow coma scale scores from head injuries have improved survival rates in the hospital.[1]

Although crystalloid and colloid solutions serve as primary resuscitation fluids for volume depletion, blood transfusions are necessary to restore the capacity of the blood to carry adequate amounts of oxygen. Furthermore, blood component therapy is considered after the trauma patient's response to the initial resuscitative fluids has been evaluated.[11] In an emergency, universal donor blood (type O negative for women in childbearing years), packed red blood cells can be administered for patients with exsanguinating hemorrhage. Other blood products—such as platelets and fresh frozen plasma—may need to be given to the trauma patient because of a consumption coagulopathy. Type-specific blood often times is available within 10 minutes and would be preferred over universal donor blood. Fully cross-matched blood is preferred in situations that can warrant awaiting type and cross-match, which often will take up to 1 hour.[11] Finally, the therapeutic goal of all blood component therapy is to restore the circulating blood volume, to give back other needed blood with red blood cells, and to correct coagulation deficiencies.[12]

In summary, fluid resuscitation of the trauma patient may be administered early and rapidly to ensure that adequate circulating volume as well as vital oxygen and nutrients are delivered to the tissues. Delay of resuscitation of patients in hemorrhagic patients until the start of surgery has recently been advocated. Early fluid administration has been criticized because it delays transport of the patient. Restoration of blood volume before hemostasis can have the adverse complication of exacerbation of blood loss due to increase in blood pressure.[16]

Diagnostic Studies and Protocols

Diagnostic tests and laboratory studies play a vital role in establishing the patient's baseline as well as current status. The results of these tests predicate the treatment protocols that will be initiated.

Comprehensive diagnostic studies are required to establish an accurate diagnosis and to plan effective treatment of the patient with multiple injuries. The initial routine studies may be arterial blood gas determinations, urinalysis, complete blood count, electrolyte levels, prothrombin and partial thromboplastin times, and type and cross-match. Other diagnostic studies that may be ordered for suspected injuries include but are not limited to lateral cervical spine, upright anteroposterior chest, and anteroposterior pelvic radiographs, computed tomographic (CT) scan, 12-lead electrocardiogram, ultrasound, and toxicology laboratory studies. Diagnostic peritoneal lavage is done only on the

severely injured hypotensive patient especially if the abdominal examination is suggestive of injury or is unreliable.[6] Pregnancy tests should be performed on all women of childbearing age, but do not delay treatment of life-threatening injuries.

Collaborative Approach

Collaborative practice is essential in the care of the trauma patient. During the initial prehospital phase, vital communication with the trauma team is initiated at the trauma center. Subsequently, when the patient is first admitted, a comprehensive approach to patient care is initiated. Together, the perianesthesia nurse, anesthesiologist, respiratory therapist, surgeon, and radiology technician form a collaborative environment so that care becomes focused and directed. This collaborative practice continues through the intraoperative as well as the postanesthesia periods.

The anesthesia provider or OR nurse communicates a comprehensive systems report to the perianesthesia nurse and verbally reviews any definitive findings of the CT scan, including whether there is generalized edema or a lesion. Vital nursing information is communicated to the appropriate OR and perianesthesia nurses caring for the trauma patient.

PERIANESTHESIA PHASE

Anesthesia Report

The anesthesiologist's report provides valuable information concerning the trauma patient's presenting status to the perianesthesia nurse. This report includes significant facts pertaining to the mechanism of injury, prehospital phase, admitting and stabilization period, operative report, intubation, anesthetic agents, estimated blood loss, fluid resuscitation, cardiopulmonary status, and treatment abnormalities.

When reviewing the anesthesia report, the nurse should note any difficulty intubating the patient. The nurse should be suspicious if the secretions are pink-tinged or bloody, which may otherwise indicate an infectious process, pulmonary edema, trauma, or uncontrolled hemorrhage.

A detailed operative report reveals the surgical insult to the patient. It also presents a comprehensive review of all anesthetic agents that reflects a rapid sequence of induction, balanced analgesia, and heavy use of narcotics, including the time these agents were given as well as the amount and type of muscle relaxants and reversal agents used.

The anesthesia report should reveal any untoward events that occurred during surgery, such as hypothermic or hypotensive events and significant dysrhythmias, including ischemic changes.

Another important aspect of the anesthesia report is the estimated blood loss and fluid replacement, which are carefully monitored through the hemodynamic status of the trauma patient. With the use of arterial lines and Swan-Ganz catheters, the anesthesiologist can closely monitor the patient's hemodynamic status. In severe chest injuries, Thora-Drain or other chest drainage units as well as autotransfusions or Cell Saver blood recovery systems may be used to conserve the vital, life-sustaining resource-blood. Because the goal of treatment is to keep the patient in a hyperdynamic state, the intraoperative trending should reveal that the patient is volume-supported. This is because the body responds hypermetabolically to trauma, and achieving that state ensures the delivery of oxygen and other nutrients to essential tissues in the body. End-organ perfusion is monitored and measured by the urinary output. Foley catheters are essential in managing fluids in the trauma patient.

Nursing Assessment

Nursing assessment of the shock trauma patient in the PACU begins with evaluating the patency of the airway. This may begin by proper positioning of the patient's head, always maintaining the cervical spine protection if injury is suspected. Do not remove cervical collars unless specifically directed by the trauma or neurosurgeon after confirming the absence of spinal cord injury. Also, the patient may need to have the airway cleared by suctioning and removal of secretions. Finally, the use of airway adjuncts—such as oropharyngeal and nasopharyngeal airways—may be needed.

Next, the nurse evaluates the patient's breathing. Recalling the mechanism of injury, such as blunt or penetrating trauma to the chest, the nurse should be highly suspicious of pulmonary contusions, fractured ribs, or shearing forces. By observation, the nurse assesses spontaneous

respirations, respiratory excursion, chest wall integrity, symmetry, depth, respiratory rate, use of accessory muscles, and the work of breathing. By palpation the nurse should evaluate for the presence of subcutaneous emphysema or tracheal deviation. By auscultation, the nurse assesses the lungs for bilateral breath sounds and evaluates for adventitious breath sounds. In addition, pulse oximetry and end-tidal CO_2 monitoring augment the complete respiratory assessment of the trauma patient.

After thoroughly evaluating the airway and breathing, the nurse begins the circulatory assessment. With the use of palpation, the nurse evaluates the circulation, checking the quality, location, and rate of the pulses, comparing the right to the left and the upper extremities to the lower extremities. If the nurse can palpate a radial pulse, the arterial pressure is at least 80 mm Hg. If no radial pulse is palpable, the nurse then palpates the femoral pulse (a situation that indicates a pressure of 70 mm Hg). If only a carotid pulse is palpable, the arterial pressure is approximately 60 mm Hg. The patient's blood pressure and pulse (rate and rhythm) should be monitored via the cardiac monitor. Any changes in patients appearance should be investigated and prompt the nurse to reassess. Be aware that pulseless electrical activity (PEA) may show as electrical impulses on the cardiac monitor without the presence of a palpable pulse. PEA can be seen in the trauma patient related to pneumothorax, cardiac tamponade, hypovolemia, or hypothermia.

Simultaneously, during the palpation of pulses, the nurse assesses the patient's skin temperature, color, and capillary refill. Capillary refill is a good indicator of tissue perfusion, especially in children.

Another aspect of assessment is circulatory access. The nurse should inspect the peripheral, central, and arterial lines to ensure the patency of the lines and healthy intravenous sites. Each line should be identified and labeled to distinguish the type of parenteral fluid and medication administration in use.

The operative site and all dressings and drains should be assessed and described. Furthermore, all drains should be labeled, drainage of fluid measured, and color and consistency described. Precise documentation of all fluid output is essential for accurate fluid replacement.

After completing the initial primary survey, the perianesthesia nurse begins the secondary comprehensive survey with a high degree of suspicion concerning the trauma patient's mechanism of injury for specific perianesthesia problems. The initial surgery often is directed at repairing the major life-threatening injuries. During the comprehensive secondary survey, head-to-toe assessment is performed as the trauma patient is emerging from anesthesia. The perianesthesia nurse may discover other injuries, such as pulmonary, cardiac, or renal contusions and compartment syndrome of different extremities. Additional injuries can manifest themselves at a later time after allowing swelling or bruising an opportunity to appear.

The head-to-toe assessment begins with a neurologic assessment, including the patient's level of consciousness; the appropriateness of verbal response; pupillary reactivity, size, and shape; equality of pupillary response to light and accommodation; movement; sensation; and pain response in the extremities. Each aspect is carefully evaluated and documented. Next, the head and face are inspected for abrasions, lacerations, puncture wounds, ecchymosis, and edema. These structures are palpated for subcutaneous emphysema or tenderness. The eyes are assessed for gross vision by asking the patient to identify the number of fingers the nurse is holding up. Furthermore, the eyes are evaluated for ecchymosis, "raccoon's eyes," and possible conjunctival hemorrhage. Extraocular movements are also evaluated by asking the patient to follow the nurse's finger in six directions. The nurse determines whether the patient is wearing contacts. The presence of maxillofacial injuries can be of great concern because of the potential to compromise the patient's airway.

The ears are inspected for Battle's sign (ecchymosis behind the ears). The nose is examined for drainage of blood or clear fluid. Clear fluid draining from the nose or ears should be checked for the presence of cerebrospinal fluid (CSF). Never pack a draining nose or ears. If CSF is suspected or in the presence of Battle's sign, a nasogastric tube should never be inserted through the patient's nose. An oral gastric tube would be the placement of choice.

The neck should be evaluated for edema, ecchymosis, tracheal deviation, pulsating or distended neck veins, and subcutaneous emphysema. As the perianesthesia nurse continues the assessment of the chest, the anterior as well as the lateral thorax and axilla are inspected for lacerations, abrasions, contusions, puncture wounds, ecchymosis, and edema. The nurse carefully palpates the chest for tenderness and subcutaneous emphysema. The chest wall is observed for symmetry, depth, and equality of expansion and excursion. Again, breathing is observed for rate, degree of effort, use of accessory muscles, or paradoxic chest wall movements. Breath and heart sounds are auscultated, noting adventitious lung sounds (such as wheezing, rales, and friction rubs) or murmurs, bruits, and muffled heart sounds. The perianesthesia nurse carefully notes the patient's facial expressions or body reactions that may suggest possible cardiac contusions or rib fractures.

The next areas to be inspected are the abdomen, pelvis, and genitalia. Again, all abrasions, contusions, edema, and ecchymosis are noted. The abdomen is auscultated for bowel sounds before palpating for tenderness and rigidity. The nasogastric tube, jejunostomy, or tube drainage is examined for color, consistency, and amount of fluid. In suspected internal hemorrhage, abdominal girth measurements should be assessed. The pelvis is palpated for stability and tenderness, especially over the crests and the pubis. Priapism,[5] which is persistent abnormal erection, may be noted. In addition, preexisting genital herpes may also be present. The urinary catheter is inspected for color and amount of drainage. Hematuria may indicate kidney or bladder trauma. Furthermore, urinary output must be vigilantly monitored to ensure a minimum of 30 ml/hr in adults so that the patient does not develop acute renal failure due to rhabdomyolysis, which can occur following traumatic injuries. The vagina and rectum are checked carefully for neurologic function and bloody drainage.

All extremities are examined for circulatory, sensory, and motor functions with range of motion. Because the trauma patient is rushed to the OR to correct life-threatening injuries, minor soft-tissue injuries often may be missed. Later, however, in the PACU, these soft-tissue and musculoskeletal injuries may develop into compartment syndrome. Again, each extremity must be thoroughly examined for abrasions, contusions, puncture wounds, ecchymosis, and edema. If there is neurovascular compromise, an arteriogram or venogram may be performed as a conclusive diagnostic study.

The patient is then log-rolled onto his or her side, maintaining cervical spine integrity, to assess the back, flanks, and buttocks for abrasions, contusions, and tenderness. Rectal tone is noted if spinal cord injury is suspected. Posterior chest assessment is completed as a last step in the head-to-toe assessment. Finally, a detailed, succinct description of the primary and secondary assessment is documented.

Preoperative medications given in the emergency department are noted. Included in medications before arriving in the OR may be tetanus prophylaxis, depending on the condition of the wound and the patient's past vaccination history.

Pain

Assessment and management of pain are important parts of the scope of care provided to the trauma patient in the PACU. The trauma patient experiences severe musculoskeletal injuries or even ruptured organs, thus causing severe pain. Pain may include more than the surgical site. The perianesthesia nurse needs to recognize that because pain is subjective, verbal, nonverbal, and hemodynamic, changes that indicate the patient may be exhibiting signs of pain should be noted. Pain can manifest itself with increased heart rate, increased blood pressure, pallor, tachypnea, guarding or splinting, and nausea and vomiting. Pain scales should be used to augment the nursing assessment of pain.

Optimal management of acute pain may employ the following techniques: (1) patient-controlled analgesia with intravenous or epidural infusions; (2) intravenous intermittent doses for pain or sedation; and (3) major plexus blocks. Guidance for medications should be based on choosing drugs that minimize cardiovascular depression and intracranial hypertension. A higher incidence of substance abuse—both alcohol and recreational or addictive mind-altering drugs—in the trauma patient population, may require higher doses of narcotics or analgesics.[4] PACU patients can emerge from anesthesia in a confused or combative state because of pain and disorientation. Other relaxation techniques—such as music therapy and guided imagery—may be initiated and used as adjuncts when the trauma patient returns for subsequent surgical procedures or wound débridement. Finally, continual pain assessment is vital to the patient's optimal care.

Nausea

Nausea can be of concern for the trauma patient. Seldom are trauma patients NPO before their traumatic event and therefore enter anesthesia with a potentially full stomach. Vomiting can lead to aspiration and another host of issues. Extubation of trauma patients should be delayed until the patient resumes his or her gag reflex to avoid aspiration. Many times nasogastric tubes are present but if the patient has consumed food before the event, particles may be too large to be evacuated. Nausea needs to be treated postoperatively and will be seen in higher incidence in the traumatized patient.

Psychologic Assessment

Often, the psychologic and emotional condition of the trauma patient is not considered a priority because the initial events are life-threatening. However, when the patient regains consciousness in the PACU, this aspect of the patient's care may prove to be the most challenging.

As the patient emerges from anesthesia, the perianesthesia nurse orients him or her to place and time. Because the patient may not even remember or recall the event that caused the accident, the nurse orients the patient to the hospital. Fear of death, mutilation, or change in body image may increase the patient's anxiety. The trauma patient may regain consciousness only to find that his or her extremities are immobilized or even amputated. Because a high incidence of injuries is related to alcohol or substance abuse, the patient may have no memory of events before, during, or after the injury. The patient may experience alterations in visual and auditory functions. If the patient was alert at the scene and remembers that loved ones were severely injured or killed, the patient may become upset or hysterical, often reliving the tragic event. Consequently, the patient not only experiences loss of body integrity and control but also the loss of loved ones.

The perianesthesia nurse needs to be supportive but also focused on maintaining the patient's integrity and coping skills. The nurse needs to speak to the patient calmly, slowly, and clearly, using simple language that is easily understood. Often the same information has to be repeated as the patient emerges from anesthesia. The practitioner should be honest with the patient. Psychologic aspects of trauma care should include the following three concepts, according to the Emergency Nurses Association: (1) need for information; (2) need for compassionate care; and (3) the need for hope.[6]

Infectious Risk

Because trauma patients represent the unknown population, infectious or communicable diseases—such as HIV, hepatitis, venereal diseases, or viruses such as chickenpox—may be transmitted by these patients. The nurse needs to use universal precautions (see Chapter 15) to decrease the risk of exposure to pathogens. Gloves, protective eyewear, masks, impervious gowns, and frequent hand-washing are important in reducing the risk of exposure to blood and body fluids.

Nursing Diagnosis

Nursing diagnoses are identified, such as ineffective airway clearance, ineffective gas exchange, alteration in cardiac output, alteration in tissue perfusion, high risk for fluid volume deficit, high risk for hypothermia, high risk for injury, altered comfort, altered thought processes, communication, high risk for anxiety, ineffective coping, disturbance in self-concept, and posttraumatic stress disorder. After nursing diagnoses are formulated, a plan of care is developed and implemented, and patient outcomes are evaluated.

The focus of the nursing care of the trauma patient is on vigilant, continuous reassessment. Consequently, treatment priorities are established on the basis of presenting signs and symptoms as well as abnormal laboratory values and diagnostic studies. The perianesthesia nurse must be cognizant of the complex pathophysiologic responses to the traumatic injury and should always anticipate that the trauma patient might exhibit subtle or overt signs of shock. Furthermore, if shock progresses, the perianesthesia nurse should be aware of other complications, such as adult respiratory distress syndrome, acute renal failure, and multisystem organ failure. Nursing care of the trauma patient provides a special challenge because of the unique physiologic responses.

SHOCK AS A COMPLICATION IN THE MULTITRAUMA PATIENT

The most common complication associated with traumatic injuries is shock. Although different types of shock exist, all exhibit a profound problem with inadequate delivery of oxygen and nutrients to the cells and result in inadequate tissue perfusion.[13,14] A measure of the body's overall metabolism is expressed as oxygen consumption (VO_2).[15] When VO_2 is inadequate, cellular hypoxia evolves. The magnitude of oxygen debt correlates with the lactic acid levels; indeed, this measure quantifies the severity and prognosis in different shock states.[13] Consequently, this complex syndrome of disequilibrium between oxygen supply and demand causes a functional impairment in cells, tissues, organs, and, eventually, body systems.[14] Important tissues such as the heart, brain, liver, kidneys, and lungs require large amounts of oxygen to support their specialized functions. Furthermore, these functions can be maintained only by energy derived from aerobic metabolism, and they cease when oxygen is in short supply.

Unfortunately, ischemia rapidly initiates a complex series of events that affect every organelle and subcellular system in the body. As cells become anoxic, adenosine triphosphate stores are depleted, and virtually all energy-dependent functions cease. Protein synthesis is depleted. Changes in ion transport and glycolysis result in the loss of intracellular potassium and the production of lactic acid. This may result in lethal complications for the ischemic heart. Finally, irreversible anoxic cellular injury kills vital tissues.

Clinical manifestations of shock include signs and symptoms of decreased end-organ perfusion: cool, clammy skin; cyanosis; restlessness; altered level of consciousness; altered skin temperature; tachycardia; dysrhythmias; tachypnea; pulmonary edema; decreased urinary output; increased platelet, leukocyte, and erythrocyte counts; sludging of blood; and metabolic acidosis.[13]

Types of Shock

The four major types of shock are the following: (1) hypovolemic; (2) cardiogenic; (3) distributive; and (4) obstructive. The first and most common type of shock, hypovolemic, results from an acute hemorrhagic loss in circulating blood volume that decreases vascular filling pressure.[14] The second type of shock is cardiogenic, which results from an inadequate contractility of the cardiac muscle. It is rare in the trauma patient but may be secondary to blunt cardiac injury or myocardial infarction (MI). The third type of shock is distributive, which causes an abnormality in the vascular system and produces a maldistribution of blood volume.[14] Distributive shock includes neurogenic, anaphylactic, and septic types. The most common among trauma patients is neurogenic shock from spinal cord injuries. The fourth type of shock is obstructive. Obstruction or compression of great vessels or the heart itself is the cause. Both tension pneumothorax and cardiac tamponade can cause obstructive shock.[6]

Hypovolemic Shock.   Hypovolemic shock may be defined as a decrease in intravascular volume, resulting in the fluid volume ineffectively filling the intravascular compartment.[14] Consequently, hypovolemic shock may evolve from many causes, such as internal and external hemorrhage, plasma volume loss, third spacing of fluids, and decreased venous return.[15]

Classifications of Hemorrhage.   As hemorrhage progresses, the cardiovascular system produces characteristic clinical manifestations that are classified according to approximate blood loss.[2] The following hemorrhagic classifications are described in the conceptual framework of the Committee on Trauma of the American College of Surgeons' Advanced Trauma Life Support Course.[11]

Class I hemorrhage, or the early phase, may be defined as a loss of as much as 750 ml of blood, or approximately 1% to 15% of the body's total blood volume. Minimal physiologic changes occur in heart rate, blood pressure, capillary refill, respiratory rate, and urinary output. However, the patient may experience mild anxiety in response to the sympathetic nervous system.

Class II hemorrhage, or the moderate phase, may be described as a loss of 750 to 1500 ml of blood, or approximately 15% to 30% of blood volume. In this phase, multiple, incremental physiologic changes occur. The patient may experience increased anxiety and restlessness as a result of cerebral stimulation by the sympathetic nervous system and subsequent catecholamine release. The heart rate may be higher than 100 beats per minute. Although minimal changes in blood pressure occur, peripheral vasoconstriction does develop, and a rise in diastolic blood pressure results, decreasing pulse pressure. Capillary refill is delayed slightly, and the skin is cool and pale. Finally, urinary output may be slightly depressed.

Class III hemorrhage, or the progressive phase, may be described as a loss of 1500 to 2000 ml of

blood, or a 30% to 40% loss of blood volume. These patients exhibit signs of cerebral hypoperfusion, hypoxia, and acidosis that create a progressive reduction in the level of consciousness. The patient may be confused, agitated, and anxious, and the heart rate may be higher than 120 beats per minute. The patient may experience systolic as well as diastolic hypotension. Capillary refill time may be delayed more than 2 seconds. Deep, rapid respirations result from the ensuing metabolic acidosis. As renal perfusion decreases, urinary output may be 5 to 15 ml per hr.

Class IV hemorrhage is described as a blood loss of more than 2000 ml of blood, or approximately 40% of the body's blood volume. This significant blood loss profoundly impacts the trauma patient. The patient's level of consciousness may be lethargic, stuporous, or unresponsive. The heart rate may be 140 beats per minute or higher, and the peripheral pulses may be weak and difficult to palpate. The capillary refill time may be more than 10 seconds. The patient may experience severe hypotension, and the blood pressure may be difficult to obtain. The skin may be cold, clammy, diaphoretic, and even cyanotic. The respiratory rate is shallow, irregular, and higher than 35 breaths per minute. Finally, there is no renal end-organ perfusion, thus resulting in anuria.[11]

According to the American College of Surgeons and Advanced Trauma Life Support Course, the treatment of patients experiencing blood loss hemorrhage is infusion of crystalloids and possibly blood. A rough guideline for the total volume of replacement fluid is 3 cc of crystalloid for each 1 cc of blood loss. This is referred to as the 3:1 rule. When the blood loss results in a class III hemorrhage, blood should be considered, whereas the patient in a class IV hemorrhage will require blood administration and without aggressive measures will die within minutes. The goal is to assess the patient's response to fluid resuscitation and evidence of adequate end-organ perfusion and oxygenation (e.g., urinary output, level of consciousness, and tissue perfusion). The same signs and symptoms alerting the presence of shock must be reassessed to determine the patient's response.[11] The first hour after injury is termed the "golden hour," in which treatment of shock successfully is associated with lower mortality.[16]

Treatment.   The primary goal of treating patients with hypovolemic shock is fluid replacement. By filling the vascular "tank," the heart is able to generate adequate cardiac output and produce enough hydrostatic pressure to allow perfusion of the tissues.

Cardiogenic Shock. Cardiogenic shock induced by inadequate cardiac output usually occurs in the trauma patient secondary to blunt injury to the heart muscle (e.g., contusions, and ruptured heart or injury to heart valves or septa) or occasionally MI.[6] MIs, however, may either precipitate or precede the traumatic event. Consequently, the patient with a history of heart disease or age-related cardiac reserve limitations or who requires myocardial depressants, such as anesthesia, has a high propensity for cardiogenic shock.[17] Finally, this trauma patient population is also at greater risk for developing cardiac failure because of the rapid fluid resuscitation.

Cardiogenic shock is circulatory failure caused by a consequence of impairment of cardiac contractility, not by a loss of intravascular fluid volume. This impaired pumping ability of the heart may result from destruction of contractility of the ventricles, as in MI. Another cause of pump failure occurs from the disruption of normal conduction sequence, as in heart blocks or dysrhythmias. Myocardial depression that results from the release of vasoactive substances like myocardial depressant factor during septic shock causes dysfunction and decreased myocardial contractility.

Another method of classifying causes of cardiogenic shock is to identify the shock as either coronary or noncoronary. Rice described coronary cardiogenic shock as an obstructive coronary artery disease process that interrupts blood flow and oxygen delivery to heart muscle cells, thus resulting in ischemia and death.[14] The infarcted area of heart muscle is necrotic and dead, thus providing no function. Because the area of infarction and the surrounding area of ischemic heart muscle do not contract normally, the heart's ability to pump blood is compromised.

Patients with acute MIs are at greatest risk of developing cardiogenic shock, especially when a significant portion (more than 40%) of the left ventricle is involved. This loss of contractility reveals a low cardiac output, elevated left-ventricular filling pressure, peripheral vasoconstriction, and arterial hypotension. Another problem involves the volume of blood accumulating in the left ventricle after systolic ejection,

increasing the left-ventricular filling pressure. This back-pressure mechanism causes the following sequence of events: (1) an increased left-atrial pressure; (2) an increased pulmonary venous pressure; and (3) an increased pulmonary capillary pressure that results in pulmonary interstitial edema and intra-alveolar edema.[14] A small percentage of MIs, however, do involve the damaged right ventricle, which does not propel sufficient blood forward through the lungs into the left heart.[14] Again, cardiac output decreases, and systemic circulation is insufficient to maintain the body's needs.

As discussed previously, noncoronary cardiogenic shock may develop in the absence of coronary artery disease and heart muscle damage, such as cardiomyopathies, valvular heart abnormalities, cardiac tamponade, and dysrhythmias.[14]

Cardiogenic shock may be defined as shock secondary to acute myocardial dysfunction, including the following clinical and diagnostic criteria: systolic blood pressure less than 80 mm Hg, or less than 30 mm Hg of baseline in the hypertensive patient; cardiac index less than 2.1 L per min per m^2; urinary output less than 20 ml per hr; diminished cerebral perfusion evidenced by confusion or obtundation; and cold, clammy, cyanotic skin characteristic of a low cardiac output state.[12] However, classic signs and symptoms of cardiogenic shock, such as pulmonary congestion, edema, neck vein distention, and hepatic congestion, may not be seen in the trauma patient with coexisting acute hypovolemia.

Other clinical indicators may be obtained through hemodynamic monitoring. Cardiac, stroke, and left-ventricular stroke work indexes are decreased because of pump failure. Pulmonary artery and pulmonary capillary wedge pressures are increased, thus indicating an increased left-ventricular end-diastolic pressure. Systemic vascular resistance is increased, reflecting vasoconstriction. Systemic venous oxygen saturation is decreased because of decreased cardiac output and increased oxygen extraction from the capillary bed. Arterial blood gas determinations reveal respiratory and metabolic acidosis that is associated with hypoxemia. Consequently, cardiogenic shock is the most lethal and results in mortality rates ranging from 80% to 100%.

Treatment. The importance of early recognition and treatment of cardiogenic shock cannot be overemphasized. Prompt improvement of myocardial oxygen supply and tissue perfusion, thus decreasing myocardial oxygen demand, is vital not only to minimizing heart damage but also to increasing the trauma patient's chance of survival. The goals of treatment for cardiogenic shock are to establish an airway, maintain ventilation and oxygenation, provide proper positioning, relieve pain, correct acidosis, monitor urinary output, and deliver pharmacologic support to improve or correct cardiac rhythm. Furthermore, increasing cardiac output may be achieved by judiciously increasing intravascular volume to improve preload. The heart rate and myocardial contractility may be increased with the inotropic and vasoactive drugs such as epinephrine, dopamine, and dobutamine. Another goal of therapy is to decrease afterload, which may be accomplished by lowering peripheral vascular resistance. Other important pharmacologic agents that may be employed in cardiogenic shock are vasopressors, vasodilators, adrenergic blocking agents, corticosteroids, digitalis, and thrombolytic agents.

When pharmacologic support fails to improve the oxygen supply and demand balance, alternative methods such as the intraaortic balloon pump and the right-ventricular and left-ventricular assist devices help increase myocardial oxygen supply, decrease myocardial VO_2, relieve pulmonary congestion, and improve organ perfusion.[18]

Distributive Shock. Distributive, or vasogenic, shock is an abnormal placement or a maldistribution of the vascular volume.[14] Indeed, the heart's ability to pump blood, as well as the body's blood volume, is normal. Therefore, this category of shock describes a unique pathologic condition existing within the vascular circulatory network that causes an alteration in blood vessels. The three types of distributive shock are neurogenic, anaphylactic, and septic.

Neurogenic Shock. Neurogenic shock is described as a tremendous increase in the vascular capacity such that even the normal amount of blood becomes incapable of adequately filling the circulatory system.[19] When the body experiences an increase in vascular capacity, the mean systemic pressure decreases, causing a decreased venous return to the heart. Because the sympathetic nervous system causes vasoconstriction to maintain vascular tone, the loss of sympathetic

innervation results in domination of the parasympathetic nerves, causing vascular dilatation, or "venous pooling." This massive vasodilatation of veins occurs as a result of the loss of sympathetic vasomotor tone. Neurogenic shock, however, often is transitory and does not commonly occur.

Although neurogenic shock may be caused by deep general or spinal anesthesia, loss of sympathetic vasomotor tone in the trauma patient may occur directly from a brain concussion or contusion of the basal regions of the brain or secondary to spinal cord injury above the level of T6.

Because massive, unopposed vasodilatation induces arterioles to dilate, decreasing peripheral vascular resistance, venules and veins also dilate, thus causing blood to pool in the venous vasculature and decreasing venous return to the right heart.[14] Consequently, the following series of events occurs: (1) decreased ventricular filling pressure; (2) decreased stroke volume; (3) decreased cardiac output; (4) decreased blood pressure; (5) decreased peripheral vascular resistance; and (6) decreased tissue perfusion.

The clinical presentation in neurogenic shock is quite different from that in hypovolemic shock, even though the blood pressure is low. The patient is frequently bradycardic, and the skin is warm, dry, and even flushed. Hemodynamic monitoring reveals a decrease in cardiac output, secondary to a decrease in resistance in arteriolar vasculature, and also a decrease in venous tone.

Treatment. The treatment of neurogenic shock may require extensive volume expansion as well as the use of vasopressors, such as ephedrine. In the case of spinal anesthesia, the perianesthesia nurse should place the patient in a supine position and, if possible, decrease the HOB and elevate the legs. Finally, the goal of treatment in neurogenic shock is to balance volume expansion with the titration of vasopressor administration.[21]

Anaphylactic Shock. Anaphylactic shock results from a severe antigen-antibody reaction. Although this type of shock is not commonly seen in the trauma patient, the condition may occur as an iatrogenic complication during resuscitation.[13] Other causes of anaphylactic shock are reactions to antibiotics, contrast media, and blood transfusions.

The pathophysiologic response of anaphylaxis relates to the inflammatory process and the activation of the complement and arachidonic cascades. The sequence of events involved in the development of anaphylactic shock may be divided into three phases, as follows[20]:

1. The sensitization phase, in which immunoglobulin E antibody is produced in response to an antigen and binds to mast cells and basophils.
2. The activation phase, in which reexposure to the specific antigen triggers mast cells to release their vasoactive contents.
3. The effector phase, in which the complex response of anaphylaxis occurs as a result of the histamine and vasoactive mediators released by the mast cells and basophils.

These vasoactive mediators act on blood vessels and cause massive vasodilatation and increased capillary permeability, which allows fluid to leak from the intravascular space to the interstitial space.[22]

Clinical symptoms of anaphylactic shock include conjunctivitis, angioedema, hypotension, laryngeal edema, urticaria, bronchoconstriction, dysrhythmias, and cardiac arrest. One or all of these symptoms may occur. Therefore immediate and effective life-saving treatment must be initiated.

Treatment. The initial treatment of the patient in anaphylactic shock is identification and removal of the specific antigen that has caused the allergic reaction. Furthermore, if the patient is receiving an infusion of blood or blood products, the perianesthesia nurse should immediately discontinue the transfusion and initiate an intravenous infusion with normal saline. Administration of oxygen by facemask should be started. The initial pharmacologic agent of choice is epinephrine, a bronchodilator that helps restore vascular tone as well as increase arterial blood pressure.

Aminophylline may be administered to reduce bronchial constriction and wheezing and to minimize respiratory distress.[23] Diphenhydramine (Benadryl), an antihistamine, is another drug of choice. Corticosteroids may be used to decrease the inflammatory response. Finally, gastric acid blockers such as ranitidine (Zantac) are given.

Septic Shock. Septic shock, the most common type of distributive shock, results from an acute systemic response to invading bloodborne microorganisms. The sepsis may be caused by gram positive bacteria; however, the most common cause is gram negative bacteria. Other pathogens that may cause septic shock are viruses, fungi, parasites, or *rickettsiae*. The trauma patient is predisposed to the following determinants that affect the outcome of septic shock: infection as a result of contaminated wounds, poor nutritional status, preexisting disease state, and altered integrity of the body's defense mechanisms.[15] Furthermore, sepsis-associated tissue damage is a major complication and remains the principal cause of death in the trauma patient surviving the first 3 days after the injury.[6]

Septic shock may be defined as a clinical syndrome that, on a continuum, begins with sepsis and ends with multisystem organ dysfunction or failure. Septic shock is primarily a complex cellular disease that results in a loss of autoregulation and tissue dysfunction that occurs early and persists despite increased cardiac output. Interactions between bacterial toxins and the body's cellular, humoral, and immunologic systems are considered to activate the kinins and complement, arachidonic, and coagulation cascades, which generate other endogenous mediators that only intensify regional malperfusion.[24]

The profound hemodynamic instability of septic shock is revealed in the body's biphasic response. The first phase, or the hyperdynamic response, is characterized by a high cardiac output and a low systemic vascular resistance, whereas the second phase, the hypodynamic response, reflects the classic shock picture with a low cardiac output and an extremely high systemic vascular resistance.[24] These phases may also be referred to as early shock—or a warm, hyperdynamic phase—and late shock, or a cold, hypodynamic phase. During early shock, the patient's skin is pink, warm, and dry because of the increased cardiac output and peripheral vasodilatation. With progressing shock, fluid leaks from the vascular compartment, and the patient develops relative hypovolemia, decreasing cardiac output, and increasing peripheral vasoconstriction.[14] The clinical manifestations of late shock are cold, clammy skin; decreased cardiac output; severe hypotension; and extreme vasoconstriction.[14]

In septic shock, the degree of myocardial depression is directly related to the severity of sepsis. Decreased force of contractions may be due to the release of vasoactive chemical mediators, such as myocardial depressant factor, endotoxins, tumor necrosis factor, complement, leukotrienes, and endorphins.[14] Furthermore, decreased ventricular preload resulting from increased capillary permeability augments the myocardial depression.

Rice describes alterations in peripheral circulation as massive vasodilatation, occurring secondary to mediator activation of the bradykinins, histamines, endorphins, complement split products, platelet-activating factor, and prostaglandins.[24] Another aspect of altered circulation is observed in the maldistribution of blood volume that occurs when some tissues receive more blood flow than is needed and other tissues are deprived of needed oxygen and nutrients. Finally, increased capillary permeability causes reduced circulating blood volume, increased blood viscosity, hypoalbuminemia, and interstitial edema.[14]

One of the first target organs to be affected in septic shock is the lung.[24] Endotoxin stimulates the production of complement split products, producing bronchoconstriction, and the release of other vasoactive mediators that cause neutrophil and platelet aggregation to the lungs increases capillary permeability. Consequently, fluid collects in the interstitium, thus increasing diffusion distance, decreasing compliance, and thereby causing hypoxemia. Pulmonary vasoconstriction may be caused by thromboxane A2, which augments capillary permeability and leads to acute respiratory distress syndrome or acute lung injury (ALI).

Septic shock also causes a profound alteration in metabolism. This metabolic dysfunction is attributed to the following: (1) increasing oxygen debt and rising blood lactate levels; (2) sustained proteolysis; (3) altered gluconeogenesis with concurrent insulin resistance; and (4) liberation of free fatty acids.[24]

Treatment. The treatment of septic shock consists of identifying and eliminating the focus of infection. With culturing of the blood, urine, sputum, wound drainage, and invasive lines, the organism can be identified, and the proper definitive antimicrobial therapy can be initiated. Hemodynamic monitoring ensures an accurate means to assess the patient's circulatory status as well as the patient's response to therapeutic interventions. Initially, the perianesthesia nurse may elect to use supplemental oxygen and

encourage the patient to breathe deeply. However, as the shock state progresses, the patient's respiratory status becomes compromised. Aggressive ventilator support must be established to maintain adequate oxygenation and tissue perfusion. Proper selection of parenteral fluid administration is important not only in correcting the cause of shock but also in supporting tissue perfusion.[24]

Pharmacologic support, including the use of positive inotropes (primarily dopamine, dobutrex and norepinephrine), and vasodilators (primarily nipride and nitroglycerin), may be indicated to augment contractility, preload, and afterload.[23]

Obstructive Shock. Obstructive shock is caused by an obstructive source such as acute pulmonary embolism, dissecting aortic aneurysm, vena cava obstruction, cardiac tamponade, or tension pneumothorax. The result of all these pathologic mechanisms is decreased cardiac output from compression to the atria, which prevents the atrium from filling and thus leads to decreased stroke volume. Cardiac tamponade may compress the atria during diastole so that the atria cannot fill completely and thus decrease in stroke volume results. Displacement of the inferior vena cava can obstruct return of venous blood to the heart, building up pressure as in a tension pneumothorax. Clinical manifestations will be in alignment with causative mechanisms.

Treatment. Interventions should be aimed toward correcting the cause. Tension pneumothorax may need a needle decompression and chest tube. Cardiac tamponade may need pericardialcentesis and surgical intervention. Without prompt and appropriate treatment, obstructive shock is fatal.

SUMMARY

The perianesthesia nurse must be cognizant of the complex pathophysiologic responses in the trauma patient. The focus of nursing care is on vigilant, continuous assessment. The perianesthesia nurse must anticipate and identify the patient at risk of developing shock. Furthermore, prevention of shock must be the primary goal in caring for the trauma patient. Consequently, the challenge of caring for the critically ill trauma patient demands that the perianesthesia nurse be familiar with current research concerning the pathophysiology and clinical manifestations of the condition as well as with new therapeutic regimens.[24]

REFERENCES

1. Feliciano D, Moore E, Mattox K: Trauma, Stamford, Conn, 1996, Appleton & Lange.
2. Stene JK, Grande CM: Trauma anesthesia, Baltimore, 1991, Williams & Wilkins.
3. Barker SJ: Anesthesia for trauma, AudioDigest Anesthesia, 40(6), 1998.
4. Weigelt JA, McCormack AF: Mechanism of injury. In Cardona VD, Hurn PD, Mason PJB et al, editors: Trauma nursing: from resuscitation through rehabilitation, Philadelphia, 1988, WB Saunders.
5. Childs SA: Musculoskeletal injury in the trauma patient: the role of free oxygen radicals, published master's thesis, Baltimore, 1990, University of Maryland.
6. Trauma Nursing Core Course, ed 5, Des Plaines, Ill, 2000, Emergency Nurses Association.
7. Barash PG, Cullen BF, Stoelting RK: Handbook of clinical anesthesia, Philadelphia, 1991, JB Lippincott.
8. Childs SA: Nailgun injury, Orthop Nurs 10:60-66, 1991.
9. American College of Surgeons Committee on Trauma, Guidelines for the operation of a burn unit. In Resources for the optimal care of the injured patient, Chicago, 1999.
10. Miller RD, editor: Anesthesia, ed 5, Philadelphia, 2000, Churchill Livingstone.
11. Advanced Trauma Life Support for Doctors, American College of Surgeons Committee on Trauma, Chicago, 1997.
12. Sommers MS: Fluid resuscitation following multiple trauma, Crit Care Nurse 10:74-81, 1990.
13. Houston MC: Pathophysiology of shock, Crit Care Nurs Clin North Am 2:143-149, 1990.
14. Rice V: Shock, a clinical syndrome: an update, I: an overview of shock, Crit Care Nurse 11:20-27, 1991.
15. Summers G: The clinical and hemodynamic presentation of the shock patient, Crit Care Nurse 11:161-166, 1991.
16. Capan LM, Miller SM, Turndorf H: Trauma: anesthesia and intensive care, Philadelphia, 1991, JB Lippincott.
17. DeAngelis R: The cardiovascular system. In Alspach JG, editor: Core curriculum for critical care nursing, ed 4, Philadelphia, 1991, WB Saunders.
18. Rice V: Shock, a clinical syndrome: an update, IV: nursing care of the shock patient, Crit Care Nurse 11:40-51, 1991.
19. Guyton AC: Textbook of medical physiology, ed 7, Philadelphia, 1986, WB Saunders.
20. Atlee J: Complications in anesthesia, Philadelphia, 1999, WB Saunders.
21. Littleton MT: Complications of multiple trauma, Crit Care Clin North Am 1:75-84, 1989.
22. Littleton MT: Pathophysiology and assessment of sepsis and septic shock, Crit Care Nurs Q 11:30-47, 1988.
23. Rice V: Shock, a clinical syndrome: an update, III: therapeutic management, Crit Care Nurse 11:34-39, 1991.
24. Committee on Trauma of the American College of Surgeons: Advanced Trauma Life Support Course, Chicago, 1997, American College of Surgeons.

BIBLIOGRAPHY

Barker SJ: Trauma and malignant hyperthermia, AudioDigest Anesthesia 43(1), 2001.

Benjamini E, Leskowitz S: Immunology: a short course, ed 2, New York, Wiley-Liss, 1991.

Chulay M, Guzzetta C, Dossey B: AACN handbook of critical care nursing, Stamford, Conn, 1996, Appleton & Lange.

Litwack K: Core curriculum for perianesthesia nursing practice, ed 4, Philadelphia, 1999, WB Saunders.

Moore PF, Mullins AJ: Treatment of acidosis in the critically ill and injured, Semin Anesth 13(3):205-212, 1994.

Peitzman AB: Shock. In Simmons RL, Steed DL, editors: Basic science review for surgeons, Philadelphia, 1990, WB Saunders.

Peruzzi WT, Shapiro BA: Perioperative mechanical ventilation for trauma patients, Semin Anesth 13(3):226-246, 1994.

Rigoni JA: Trauma anesthesia presentation, Department of Nurse Anesthesia, Virginia Commonwealth University, Richmond, VA, 1992.

Swearingen PL, Keen JH, editors: Manual of critical care nursing, ed 4, St Louis, 2001, Mosby.

Urden KD, Stacy KM: Priorities in critical care nursing, ed 3, St Louis, 2000, Mosby.

52

BIOTERRORISM AND ITS IMPACT ON THE PACU

Gordon Green, MD, MPH

In the past hundred years, we have witnessed major developments in the protection of the health of human beings. Many infectious disease threats have yielded to innovations in sanitation, water treatment plants, remarkable antibiotic discoveries, vaccines, and considerable understanding of the factors that affect our health. Smallpox has been eradicated from natural occurrence, and tuberculosis has been dramatically reduced. In this country, polio is quite rare. Deaths from childhood dysentery are few, and death in childbirth is uncommon. But some old problems remain, and new ones emerge. Until recent years, no one had heard of AIDS, hantavirus, Legionnaires disease, or toxic shock syndrome. The latest threat is bioterrorism. The recent anthrax cases and the epidemic of fear that accompanied them created a substantial problem for many health professionals. Much time and effort have been spent in counseling and in reassuring our patients about this disease. The very infrastructure of the national public health system has been called into question.

BIOLOGIC WARFARE

Biologic warfare has a long and ignoble history. In the 14th century, bodies of individuals who had died of plague were catapulted over the walls of cities in an effort to infect the defenders and thus attenuate the defenses. In the 18th century, blankets that had been used to wrap smallpox victims were subsequently distributed to Native Americans, in an effort to reduce their numbers through the spread of disease.

In the 1940s, the United States established a biologic warfare program. In 1969 the offensive aspects of the program were disestablished as worldwide sentiment against biologic warfare increased. Behind the Iron Curtain, however, this

was not so. In 1979, an incident involving the spread of anthrax from a production facility at Sverdlovsk revealed to the world the efforts by the Soviet Union to prepare offensive bioweapons. More recent defections from that political regime have led to further revelations about the extent of preparations for biologic warfare.

Numerous agents have been proposed over time. The intentional use of microorganisms, or toxins derived from living organisms, to produce death or disease in humans, animals, and plants have led to consideration of the agents in Box 52-1, which represents only a partial list.

It is clear that bioterrorist acts are, in many cases, quite unlike the usual "mass casualty" disasters that we have faced and with which we have considerable experience. In the case of an act like the destruction of the Murrah federal office building in Oklahoma in 1995 or an airplane crash like that in Lockerbie, Scotland, in 1988, all of the survivors are immediate and potential customers for the trauma service in hospital emergency rooms. But in the case of a bioterrorist release of an infectious disease agent or toxin, the effects may not be apparent for several days and may be widely distributed throughout the community. Victims of such an attack might turn up in widely dispersed emergency rooms and physician offices in ones, or twos, or threes and may not be immediately recognized as a mass casualty event. Each physician office must serve as an alert sentinel. In cases of bioterrorism, personnel from neither the fire department nor the police department are first responders. Practicing physicians and health professionals are the first responders.

In the event of a bioterrorist attack, such as anthrax attacks on the East coast in October 2001, the impact on communities and hospitals

Box 52-1	**Agents That Produce Death or Disease in Humans, Animals, and Plants**

Anthrax
Botulism
Plague
Smallpox
Tularemia
Brucellosis
Fungal mycotoxins
Various encephalitides
Marburg virus
Ebola
Typhus
Q Fever

would largely depend on how effectively the local health department responded to the crisis. Expert local health officers at the head of strong health departments in Florida, New York, and Washington, DC rapidly recognized the anthrax problem and used local, state, and federal resources to manage the problem effectively, thus limiting the adverse impact.

Planning for Care

We must develop plans for early detection and streamlining responses to bioterrorism, avoiding duplication of effort, and defining responsibilities and jurisdictional authority; develop a plan to administer mass vaccination and chemoprophylaxis, should they be required, with inclusion of both public and private resources; and develop, in conjunction with appropriate city, county, and state agencies and the Centers for Disease Control and Prevention, updated plans for quarantine, hospitalization, and evacuation procedures.

Planning for bioterrorism response should include the possibility that victims could number in the tens of thousands. Hospital capacity, generally numbering in the hundreds, would be quickly overrun; therefore we must consider emergency use of stadiums, convention centers, school gymnasiums, hotels, nursing homes, and the like for care or quarantine.

Reporting.   A major issue is reporting of cases, an important step in identifying a potential bioterrorist threat.

Disease reporting by physicians, emergency rooms, and laboratories is a key element in any bioterrorist threat detection system. Disease surveillance depends on accumulation of accurate, timely reports of disease incidence; however, our system of disease reporting is widely held to be inefficient, incomplete, and irrelevant. When data are aggregated from several—or many—reporting sites, the true dimensions of a bioterrorist attack may be recognized. The timely collection of information, analysis, and pattern recognition can only be accomplished by a designated public health agency.

City and county governments must work through local health departments to ensure that efficient reporting mechanisms are in place and that a two-way flow of information exists to help provide incentives for collaboration by primary care providers. This may include mechanisms for the health department to update area health professionals routinely with relevant information about immunization, local patterns of antibiotic resistance, seasonal changes in disease incidence monitored by the department, and information of immediate clinical relevance such as rapid notification of a newly recognized outbreak of illness in the area. At best, these would be *active* reporting and surveillance systems, with providers communicating with local health authorities on a real-time basis.

Nonetheless, the effectiveness of any surveillance system depends upon an available, competent local health agency to collect and analyze data, and (most importantly) to initiate appropriate and timely action to intervene.

Response.   In the event of biowarfare introduction of a dramatic disease, the key is strong leadership by the health officer in a well-resourced local health department, strong personal reporting relationships with the local health professionals of the community, and cost-effective local surveillance systems.

Tremendous resources are being pumped into bioterrorist response systems. The FBI, the Department of Defense, Centers for Disease Control and Prevention, the Federal Emergency Management Agency, and states and municipalities are all receiving funds to develop their responses. Computerized communications systems, large quantities of antibiotic dose-packs, vaccines, decontamination systems, hazardous materials suits, biosafety laboratories all can be made available on short notice. These vast resources are only called into play if an alert health professional detects an unusual situation and notifies the local health department. That local health department must have the epidemiologic and laboratory support to confirm or deny the possibility of a threat. Only then can this array of resources be called into play.

Strong local health departments and outfront local health officers generally are not in place over the country. This problem has been widely recognized. The need to upgrade our local health departments becomes obvious when bioterrorism is considered, but an upgrade would have salutary effects upon all of the public health challenges that confront us, now, and in the future.

Anthrax

In the postanesthesia care unit (PACU), patients may appear with any of a wide variety of syndromes. Many, but not all of them, are related to the respiratory tract. For example, anthrax has three identifiable symptom clusters. *Bacillus anthracis*, a spore forming bacterium, can lead to inhalational anthrax, which may appear much like a case of influenza, atypical pneumonia, or even pneumonic plague. In its classical form, it may appear in two phases. The first phase follows an incubation period of up to six days, and is characterized by a nonspecific syndrome of fever, muscle pain, a nonproductive cough (a diagnostic clue), malaise, and abdominal or chest pain. It then progresses to a second phase over two or three days, with progressive fever, diaphoresis, severe dyspnea, and possibly cyanosis. A further diagnostic clue is the finding of mediastinal widening, as revealed on chest radiographs or tomography. The patient may experience stridor and subcutaneous edema of the upper thorax or neck. This syndrome may progress to obtundation and coma, with hypothermia, circulatory failure, and death within 2 to 3 days. Prompt treatment with antibiotics may result in survival.

For therapy of inhalational anthrax in an adult patient, the current recommendation is for ciprofloxacin, 400 mg intravenously every twelve hours; if the bacterial strain is susceptible, continuing therapy with penicillin G, 40 million U intravenously every four hours, or doxycycline, 100 mg intravenously every 12 hours, should be used.

Because of the deposition of spores into skin breaks or abrasions, the cutaneous form of anthrax is much less difficult to treat, although it may not be easily recognized. It may be confused with various skin infections, insect bites, and nonspecific viral rashes. It is generally painless, although it may present with itching. With proper antibiotic therapy, death is uncommon.

Finally, gastrointestinal anthrax may occur if spores find their way into the GI tract. It may lead to ulcers in the upper tract (oropharynx) or in the terminal ileum or cecum. Presenting symptoms may include fever, sore throat, difficulty swallowing, nausea, vomiting, bloody diarrhea, or total body sepsis. Mortality may be higher than 50%. The gastrointestinal disease can easily be confused with nonspecific gastroenteritis and other bacterial or viral syndromes.

Laboratory diagnosis of anthrax will depend upon a high index of suspicion, so that the clinical microbiologist may be prepared for identification of *Bacillus anthracis*.

Pneumonic Plague

Another disease that may be encountered in the PACU is pneumonic plague. One should suspect plague in the patient who has rapid onset of pneumonia, high fever, headache, and chills, combined with a history of exposure to possibly infected animals or fleas. The pneumonic form of the disease can spread by the dispersion of *Yersinia pestis* to the bloodstream from infected lymph nodes of the bubonic form of the disease or through inhalation of the bacilli (so-called primary plague pneumonia). Diagnosis is facilitated by the finding of bipolar or gram negative coccobacilli on a smear from a lymph node, from aspirate from trachea or lung, or in the blood. The diagnosis may be confirmed with the more specific fluorescent-antibody test.

Pneumonic plague may be transmitted from person to person by droplets from the respiratory tract, spread on a face-to-face basis. Veterinarians are at special risk of pneumonic plague by treating abscesses caused by *Yersinia pestis* in cats.

It is important to treat cases of pneumonic plague rapidly. Recommended antibiotics include tetracycline, streptomycin, gentamicin, doxycycline, and chloramphenicol. Individuals who have had close contact with infected persons should be treated with appropriate antibiotics for one week.

Botulism

The disease of botulism is caused not by the bacterium itself but by bacterial toxin produced by *Clostridium botulinum*, a spore-forming organism. The toxin is generally elaborated under anaerobic conditions and results in a syndrome characterized by the triad of descending flaccid paralysis with bulbar palsies, clear sensorium, and no fever. Initial symptoms may be the sudden onset of visual difficulties, the result of paralysis of cranial nerves. Paralysis may then progress downward and result in difficulty swallowing and dry mouth and manifestations of further paralysis of motor and autonomic nerves. The lack of fever and clear mentation are characteristic and frightening aspects of the disease. Most of the fatalities occur from respiratory failure, and those who survive may have respiratory symptoms for many years thereafter.

The diagnosis is confirmed by the demonstration of the botulinum toxin in the serum, gastric juices, or food. Because the standard test is a bioassay that requires several days to complete, the clinical findings and a high index of suspicion are the best assets for diagnosis. Electromyogram may be useful in ruling out other paralytic conditions.

Most cases of botulism result from eating the preformed toxin in foods that have been canned or fermented at home or prepared unsafely. Uncommonly, toxins may be produced in wounds or in the gastrointestinal tract. Finally, the toxins theoretically may be distributed by a terrorist through aerosolization.

The management of cases of botulism consists largely of supportive care, augmented by immunization with botulism antitoxin (available from the Centers for Disease Control and Prevention). This antitoxin may reduce the severity of symptoms if administered sufficiently early in the course of the disease. Patients may require weeks or even months of respiratory care. Ventilatory support is the key to survival.

Smallpox

The nurse in the PACU is unlikely to encounter smallpox because this contagious systemic viral illness with its characteristic skin rash would likely be treated as an international emergency, with mandatory treatment at home, under isolation conditions. Patients would be treated with vaccines and with antiviral medication, but the case fatality rate may be as high as 50%. Contacts of cases should be vaccinated as soon as possible after exposure. Because smallpox no longer is a naturally occurring disease, the appearance of a case of smallpox would be no secret.

SUMMARY

Other bacterial and viral agents may be encountered as a result of bioterrorist events, and the critical care unit should have a plan which is both responsive and flexible. In considering the large numbers of individuals who may require care, the establishment of temporary care units in various community locations may be required, with logistic support from a wide variety of sources. The use of mechanical ventilators may be augmented through manually assisted ventilation if large numbers of victims are identified. Perianesthesia nurses should develop plans that include other health professionals and perhaps even nonprofessionals who can be given immediate on-the-job training in operation of life-saving techniques. Nonhealthcare workers can supply logistic support, patient data recording, and appropriate security and crowd management.

The old adage applies in this case, as in so many others: "If we fail to plan, then we must plan to fail."

BIBLIOGRAPHY

Arnon SS, Schechter R, Inglesby TV et al: Botulinum toxin as a biological weapon: medical and public health management, JAMA 285(8):1059-1070, 2001.

Chin J, editor: Control of communicable diseases manual, ed 17, Washington DC, 2000, APHA.

Henderson DA, Inglesby TV, Bartlett JG et al: Small-pox as a biological weapon: medical and public health management, JAMA 281(22):2127-2137, 1999.

Inglesby TV, Dennis DT, Henderson DA et al: Plague as a biological weapon: medical and public health management, JAMA 283(17):2281-2290, 2000.

Inglesby TV, Henderson DA, Barlett JG et al: Anthrax as a biological weapon: medical and public health management, JAMA 281(18):1735-1745, 1999.

Schwartz MN: Recognition and management of anthrax: an update, N Eng J Med 345(22):1621-1626, 2001.

Shafazand S, Doyle R, Ruoss S et al: Inhalational anthrax, Chest 116:1369-1376, 1999.

WEB RESOURCES

www.bt.cdc.gov
www.hhs.org

53

CARDIOPULMONARY RESUSCITATION IN THE PACU

William Hartland, Jr., PhD, CRNA

A nurse working in the postanesthesia care unit (PACU) must be ever vigilant to the possibility of being confronted with a patient who may require cardiopulmonary resuscitation. In February 2000, the International Guidelines 2000 Conference on Cardiopulmonary Resuscitation (CPR) and Emergency Cardiovascular Care was held to create valid, widely accepted international resuscitation guidelines. Those who attended this conference included representatives from the American Heart Association (AHA), the European Resuscitation Council, and various other resuscitation experts, councils, and organizations throughout the world.[1]

This chapter will look at cardiopulmonary resuscitation as it applies to the PACU. Although this chapter highlights the responsibilities of the healthcare provider during a cardiopulmonary emergency, it is not designed to replace formal training in either basic life support (BLS) or advanced cardiopulmonary life support (ACLS).

ETHICAL ISSUES RELATED TO CARDIOPULMONARY RESUSCITATION

Many patients are becoming increasingly concerned about the inappropriate use of life-sustaining procedures that can have a dramatic effect on the length and quality of life. Consequently, increasing numbers of patients are placing limitations on medical treatments that may impact their lives in the future. This is being accomplished through the use of living wills, advanced directives, Do Not Attempt Resuscitation orders (DNAR) and the no-CPR Program. Living wills allow a person to express preferences concerning their end-of-life medical care. Some states have adopted DNAP and no-CPR programs with focus on the use or extent of resuscitation efforts. Advanced directives are usually prepared by the physician attending critically/terminally ill patients who are unable to make decisions for themselves. These directives are based on the patient's living will, if one exists. The patient's right to limit medical interventions is firmly established in modern medical practice.[2,3] The operating room, however, is one area where restrictions on cardiopulmonary resuscitation have caused considerable ethical conflicts between patients and healthcare providers.

Approximately 75% of all cardiac arrests in the operating room are related to specific anesthesia or surgical causes such as an accidental overdose of an anesthetic agent. Resuscitation in such instances has been found to be highly successful. In such instances, many healthcare providers view honoring DNARs as failure to treat a reversible process and thus similar to committing murder.[3,4] One could argue that the same ethical dilemma exists in the PACU because this unit is so closely aligned with surgery. It is beyond the scope of this chapter to delve into all the ethical dilemmas concerning DNARs that may arise in the PACU and other topics related to advanced directives. It is very important that the PACU nurse be familiar with his/her institution's policies and guidelines concerning these issues.

CARDIOPULMONARY RESUSCITATION

Urgency of Cardiopulmonary Resuscitation

During a cardiopulmonary arrest, time is a major factor that influences patient outcomes. When a patient arrests, the probability of survival decreases rapidly with each minute of cardiopulmonary compromise. The survival rate from cardiac arrest caused by ventricular tachycardia decreases approximately 7% to 10% for each minute the patient is deprived of defibrillation. At 12 minutes, this survival rate decreases to 2% to 5%. It therefore is crucial that the PACU nurse responds quickly and efficiently during all cardiopulmonary emergencies.[5,6]

Indications for Resuscitation

Numerous precipitating events are associated with cardiopulmonary arrest. These events include respiratory compromise, circulatory/cardiac compromise, metabolic imbalances, medication/anesthetic overdoses or toxicity, and anaphylaxis. All these events can occur in the PACU.

Respiratory compromise appears to be the primary cause of morbidity in the PACU. Respiratory compromise can result from residual anesthesia, upper airway obstruction, laryngeal edema, laryngospasm, bronchospasm, noncardiogenic pulmonary edema, and aspiration.

One of the most common causes of upper airway obstruction in the postanesthetic patient results from mechanical obstruction from the tongue. This occurs when the tongue falls back into a position that mechanically obstructs the pharynx, thus blocking the passage of air to and from the lungs. The underlying cause of this obstruction may be the result of residual anesthetics, narcotics, or muscle relaxants administered during surgery. The tongue may also be edematous from surgical manipulation, anatomical deformities, or an allergic reaction. Clinical signs of this type of obstruction include snoring, flaring of the nostrils, use of accessory muscles for ventilation, retraction of the intercostal spaces and suprasternal notch, asynchronous movements of the chest and abdomen, tachycardia from hypoxia, and decreased oxygen saturation.[7] Arterial carbon dioxide pressure ($PaCO_2$) increases 6 mm Hg during the first minute of total obstruction with an additional 3 to 4 mm Hg increase each passing minute.[8] If the obstruction is not corrected, the patient's condition will continue to deteriorate and lead to cardiopulmonary arrest. This is especially tragic when the obstruction could have been corrected by simply stimulating the patient to take deep breaths or by repositioning the airway via a chin lift or jaw thrust. More advanced measures may include the use of a nasal or oral airway, remembering that the nasal airway is usually less stimulating and thus tolerated better in the patient emerging from general anesthesia. If the obstruction remains unrelieved, advanced airway management procedures such as the Laryngeal Mask Airway (LMA) or use of an endotracheal tube (ETT) may be indicated. Obviously, prevention of cardiopulmonary arrest is more desirable than treatment. When a cardiopulmonary arrest does occur, emergency procedures must be administered rapidly and decisively before irreversible damage occurs.

Emergency Equipment

The PACU nurse, faced with a cardiopulmonary event, will have an advantage over a layman or healthcare provider faced with a similar event outside the hospital. This advantage is rooted in the fact that the PACU nurse has immediate access to numerous resources to aid in the diagnosis and treatment of an actual or pending adverse cardiopulmonary event. These resources include the immediate availability of various monitoring modalities, emergency medications, essential emergency equipment, and access to the patient's medical history which can give valuable insight into possible underlying causes and pathology leading up to the adverse event. Another advantage is the availability of other healthcare providers for assistance and consultation.

The routine use of various monitoring modalities in the PACU is invaluable to nurses for the diagnosis of many developing patient complications that could precipitate a cardiopulmonary arrest. The use of pulse oximetry, for example, can be extremely helpful in the diagnosis of problems concerning patient oxygenation, as in the case of a progressing airway obstruction. The routine use of an ECC monitor allows the PACU nurse to identify life-threatening arrhythmias such as pulseless ventricular tachycardia (VT), ventricular fibrillation (VF), or asystole. Both these monitoring modalities provide the PACU nurse a more definitive means of diagnosis and opportunity for early intervention.

All advanced cardiac life support equipment should be immediately available to the PACU nurse. This equipment is usually found on a designated code cart or tray that is located in a designated area of the PACU. The cart should contain such emergency items as a defibrillator/monitor, emergency pharmacologic agents, equipment for circulatory and airway/respiratory management, and specialty trays for various emergency procedures. Usually the individual unit or healthcare institution establishes the general setup and contents of the cart. It is essential that each PACU nurse be familiar with not only the location of the cart but also with its contents and their proper use. The immediate availability of necessary emergency equipment and pharmacologic agents is essential for any possibility of patient survival.

Steps in Cardiopulmonary Resuscitation

Usually some event occurs that leads the PACU nurse to suspect a possible cardiopulmonary arrest. This event could be in the form of a witnessed or unwitnessed collapse of a patient. In the PACU this event may involve the development of a life-threatening arrhythmia such as VT, VF, or asystole. At the first sign of potential trouble, the nurse should immediately assess the responsiveness of the patient.[9] It is not the desire of any nurse to prematurely initiate a code and start CPR only to find out that the patient had fallen asleep and that one of his/her ECG leads was loose or disconnected. If the patient is unresponsive, the PACU nurse should immediately activate the unit's emergency response system. This can easily be done in the PACU by enlisting a coworker's help. Activation of this system will bring help in the form of necessary emergency equipment and essential personnel to the patient's bedside. Assistance from other healthcare team members serves many purposes, including the ability to perform many essential tasks simultaneously, availability of various knowledge backgrounds and experience levels for consultation, and overall support. Nursing personnel should be thoroughly familiar with their units' specific protocols for initiating a code and obtaining needed assistance.

Once unresponsiveness has been confirmed and the emergency system activated, the PACU nurse should immediately proceed with the AHA's Primary and Secondary ABCD Surveys. The primary survey is associated with the AHA's

BLS, whereas the secondary survey involves more ACLS procedures. Each of these surveys consists of 4 steps identified as the A-B-C-Ds of cardiopulmonary resuscitation. The A-B-C-Ds of the primary survey consists of Airway, Breathing, Circulation and Defibrillation. The A-B-C-Ds of the secondary survey stand for Airway, Breathing, Circulation and Differential Diagnosis.[1,2]

Primary A-B-C-D Survey

A: Primary Airway. The first step in the primary survey is airway assessment. In this step, the patient's airway is manually opened and breathing is assessed. A large majority of postoperative airway obstructions result from the mechanical obstruction of a patient's tongue and epiglottis obstructing the pharynx.[7] When a patient is unresponsive, possibly from residual anesthesia, decreased muscle tone may result in obstruction of the pharynx by the tongue and epiglottis. Because the tongue is attached to the lower jaw, the tongue can be lifted away from the back of the throat by moving the lower jaw forward, thus relieving the obstruction. To rule out the possibility of an airway obstruction, the nurse should mechanically open the patient's airway. This can be accomplished in a number of ways, depending on the patient's condition. Unless medically contraindicated, as in the case of a suspected neck injury, the PACU nurse can open the patient's airway by performing the headtilt maneuver. This maneuver is accomplished by simply tilting the patient's head backward and hyperextending the neck (Fig. 53-1). As stated previously, this maneuver should not be performed if the patient is suspected of having a cervical injury. Other techniques that can be used to open the patient's airway are the chin lift and jaw thrust. The chin lift involves placing two fingers under the bony portion of the lower jaw, near the chin, and pushing the patient's chin upward with moderate pressure (Fig. 53-2). The head tilt and chin lift maneuver are often done collectively (Fig. 53-3). With the jaw thrust, the rescuer positions himself or herself at the head of the patient. The rescuer places one hand on each side of the patient's head. The rescuer grasps the angles of the patient's lower jaw and lifts with both hands. The jaw thrust can be done together with the head tilt, or it can be done alone without the head tilt. The jaw thrust without head tilt is

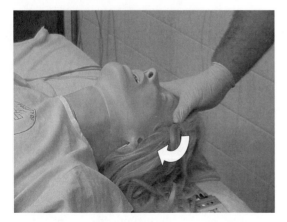

Fig. 53-1   Head Tilt: The patient's head is tilted backwards and the neck is hyperextended. This maneuver is contraindicated in the presence of possible cervical injury. *(Courtesy Department of Nurse Anesthesia, Virginia Commonwealth University, Richmond, Va.)*

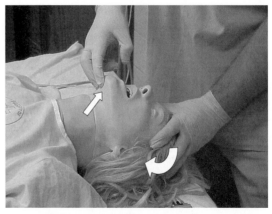

Fig. 53-3   The head tilt and chin lift maneuver are often done collectively. *(Courtesy Department of Nurse Anesthesia, Virginia Commonwealth University, Richmond, Va.)*

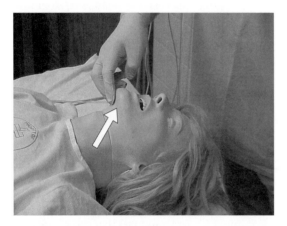

Fig. 53-2   Chin Lift: The rescuer places two fingers under the bony portion of the lower jaw, near the chin, and pushes the patient's chin upward with moderate pressure. *(Courtesy Department of Nurse Anesthesia, Virginia Commonwealth University, Richmond, Va.)*

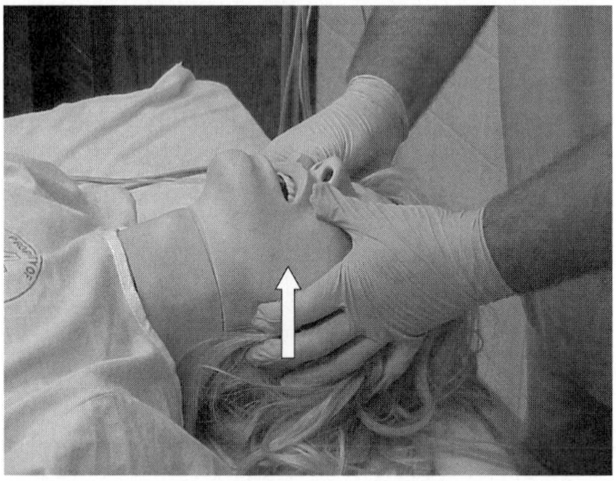

Fig. 53-4   Jaw Thrust: The rescuer grasps the angles of the patient's lower jaw and lifts with both hands. The jaw thrust can be done with the head tilt *(as pictured)*, or it can be done alone without the head tilt. The jaw thrust without head tilt is the technique of choice for a patient with a suspected neck injury because it causes the least movement of the cervical spine. *(Courtesy Department of Nurse Anesthesia, Virginia Commonwealth University, Richmond, Va.)*

the technique of choice for a patient with a suspected neck injury since it causes the least movement of the cervical spine[1] (Fig. 53-4). Many times, in the case of an obstruction, these maneuvers are all that is required for spontaneous respirations to occur. As soon as the airway is opened, breathing should be assessed. This can be accomplished by simply observing chest rise while listening for ventilatory sounds at the patient's nose and mouth.

B: Primary Breathing.   If no ventilations are detected, the PACU nurse should progress to the second step of the survey—Breathing. In this step, the patient should be immediately given two slow breaths. These two initial breaths can be performed with the use of a bag-mask device, such as an Ambu-Bag, which should be connected to a minimum supplemental oxygen source of 10 L/min as soon as possible.

If continuous ventilation is indicated, the patient should be ventilated at a rate of 10 to 12 times per minute (1 breath every 4 to 5 seconds). Infants and children 1 to 8 years of age should be ventilated approximately 20 times per minute at a volume large enough to raise their chests on inspiration. The AHA recommends that the adult patient be given tidal volumes of 10 ml/kg over 2 seconds during ventilation with bag-mask ventilation without the availability of supplemental oxygen. This tidal volume should result in a noticeable rise in the patient's chest. If supplemental oxygen is available and connected to the bag-mask device or given via nasal cannula, the rescuer should deliver lower tidal volumes (6-7 ml/kg) to reduce the risk of gastric distention with its potential complications. This reduction in tidal volume should only be performed if adequate chest rise and patient oxygen saturation can be maintained.[1,2]

If for some reason a bag-valve-mask system is not available, the PACU nurse should have access to a mouth-to-patient barrier device so ventilation can be started until appropriate airway support devices can be secured. While using these barrier devices, the rescuer must be sure to maintain a patent airway and an airtight seal to adequately ventilate the patient. When ventilating an infant, the rescuer must remember that the infant's neck is very pliable. As a result, the rescuer may actually cause an airway obstruction if the infant's head is forcefully flexed.

During the initial ventilation of the patient, an assistant should assess the adequacy of the ventilation by auscultation of the chest. If an assistant is not present, the nurse should check to see whether the chest rises and falls and whether air escapes during expiration. If properly trained personnel are available and the patient cannot be ventilated by these methods, advanced airway techniques such as endotracheal intubation should be performed immediately.

In today's climate of potential infectious disease, the AHA discourages the practice of mouth-to-mouth ventilation. An exception would be if the patient is a relative or someone the rescuer is certain has a negative prearrest infection state.[2] With the increased availability of barrier and bag-valve devices in the PACU, it is highly unlikely that the PACU nurse will ever be faced with a decision concerning mouth-to-mouth ventilation while on duty. Many hospitals have airway rescue breathing devices available in each patient room. Many healthcare workers routinely carry a small barrier device on their person in the event of such an emergency.

C: Primary Circulation. After the initial two slow breaths have been given, the rescuer should move to the third step of the survey—Circulation. During this step the patient's circulatory status should be evaluated. This is accomplished by assessing the patient's pulse. For an adult and child, this is accomplished by feeling the carotid artery for no more than 10 seconds. With an infant, it is best to check the brachial artery. If no pulse is detected, chest compressions should be started immediately.[9]

External cardiac compression should be performed with the patient in a horizontal position on a firm surface, and the lower extremities elevated to promote venous return. The rescuer should be positioned at the patient's side. To begin compressions, the rescuer should place the heel of one of his/her hands over the lower half of the patient's sternum, about 1.5 to 2 inches (approximately 2 finger widths) above the tip of the xiphoid process (Fig. 53-5). The rescuer's free hand should be placed on top of the hand already positioned on the patient's chest. The rescuer should keep his/her arms straight and shoulders directly over the adult patient's sternum while depressing down on the lower sternum a minimum of 1.5 to 2 inches (Fig. 53-6). The chest compression rate for adult patients should be approximately 100 compressions per minute. Evidence appears to support the premise that this rapid compression rate effectively benefits the patient in terms of blood flow and blood pressure.[1]

In children, the sternum is compressed with the heel of one hand only. In infants, the sternum is compressed with the tips of two fingers for one rescuer or the thumbs of the encircling hands of the rescuer when two healthcare providers are present (Figs. 53-7 and 53-8). In infants and

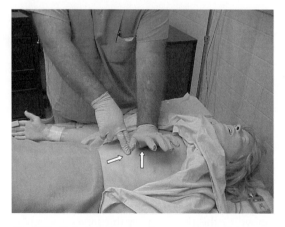

Fig. 53-5 To begin external cardiac compressions, the rescuer should place the heel of one of his or her hands over the lower half of the patient's sternum, about 1.5 to 2 inches (approximately 2 finger widths) above the tip of the xiphoid process. *(Courtesy Department of Nurse Anesthesia, Virginia Commonwealth University, Richmond, Va.)*

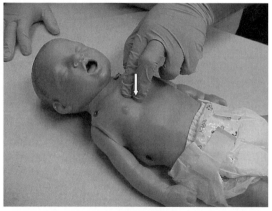

Fig. 53-7 In infants, the sternum is compressed with the tips of two fingers when only one rescuer is present. This frees the rescuer's other hand to open the airway for ventilations. *(Courtesy Department of Nurse Anesthesia, Virginia Commonwealth University, Richmond, Va.)*

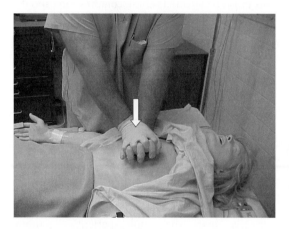

Fig. 53-6 The rescuer's free hand should be placed on top of the hand already positioned on the patient's chest. The rescuer should keep his/her arms straight and shoulders directly over the adult patient's sternum while pressing down on the lower sternum a minimum of 1.5 to 2 inches. *(Courtesy Department of Nurse Anesthesia, Virginia Commonwealth University, Richmond, Va.)*

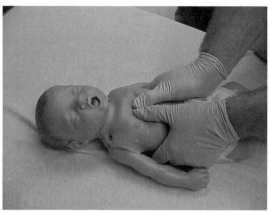

Fig. 53-8 If two rescuers are present, one rescuer can perform compressions with the thumbs of his or her encircling hands while the other rescuer performs ventilations. *(Courtesy Department of Nurse Anesthesia, Virginia Commonwealth University, Richmond, Va.)*

children a rate of 100 compressions per minute is recommended.[9]

If external cardiac compression is done correctly, systolic blood pressure will reach 60 to 80 mm Hg and diastolic pressure will be zero.

Mean blood pressure in the carotid artery seldom exceeds 40 mm Hg. Cardiac output from chest compression is approximately one fourth to one third normal. As a result, compressions must be regular, smooth, and uninterrupted.[1]

External cardiac compression must be combined with ventilation of the lungs. Evidence suggests that adult cardiopulmonary arrest patients are more likely to survive if a higher number of chest compressions are delivered even if the patient receives fewer ventilations. Because coronary perfusion pressure gradually rises with consecutive compressions it is recommended that a ratio of 15 compressions to two ventilations be administered whether there are one or two rescuers present. Once the patient's airway is secured and protected, as the case with oral tracheal intubation, compression rate should be continuous and uninterrupted with ventilations administered between compressions at a ratio of 1 ventilation every 5 compressions.[1] To assess the effectiveness of chest compressions, the nurse ventilating the patient should periodically check the patient's pulse during the compressions. Compression should be stopped for 10 seconds during the first minute of CPR and every few minutes afterwards to assess for spontaneous breathing or circulation. If adequate spontaneous circulation returns without spontaneous breathing, compressions should be terminated, but ventilations should continue at a rate of one breath every 5 seconds. If the patient is attempting to breathe but his or her spontaneous ventilations are inadequate, the nurse can assist the patient with the bag-mask device.[9] This is accomplished by ventilating the patient when he or she

attempts to inhale. Depending on the adequacy of the patient's own ventilations, the rescuer can assist with every ventilation, every other ventilation, or as needed. Once the patient's spontaneous ventilations are adequate, positive pressure ventilation can be discontinued, but supplemental oxygen should be continued via a mask or nasal cannula. A summary that compares resuscitation interventions across age groups is presented in Table 53-1.

D: Primary Defibrillation. Once ventilation and compressions have been initiated, the rescuer's attention should move toward Defibrillation—the most important determinant for survival in adult VF/VT. If he or she is not already being monitored, the patient should be connected to an ECG monitor or defibrillator with monitoring capabilities. Rhythm assessment is imperative for the detection of VF or VT. The PACU nurse must remember that for each minute of persistent VF, the patient's chance of survival decreases. Once VF/VT have been identified, the defibrillation sequence should start immediately.[1]

Two basic defibrillators are available to the healthcare provider. These are the conventional monitor/defibrillator and the automated external defibrillator (AED). Although AEDs are gaining popularity in some hospital settings, the

Table 53-1	**A Comparison of Ventilation and Chest Compressions for the Newborn, Infant, Child, and Adult Patient**			
	Newborn	Infant	Child	Adult
Ventilations (approximate)	30-60/min	20/min	20/min	12/min
Compressions (approximate)	90/min with 30 ventilations/min	100/min (at least)	100/min	100/min
Compression depth (approximate)	1/3 the depth of the chest	1/3 to 1/2 the depth of the chest (1/2 to 1 in)	1 to 1 1/2 in (1/3 to 1/2 the depth of the chest)	1 1/2 to 2 in
Compression/ ventilation ratio (1 or 2 rescuers)	3:1	5:1	5:1	15:2 (unless 2 rescuers with a protected patient airway, then 5:1)

conventional defibrillator is still used in most PACUs and other hospital specialty areas. PACU nurses must have a working knowledge of all defibrillator(s) available in their respective units.

When the nurse uses the conventional (manual) defibrillator, basic protocol should be followed. Upon arrival to the patient's bedside, the defibrillator should be immediately turned on. An energy level of 200J for the traditional monophasic defibrillators should be selected. When determining energy levels for the newer biphasic defibrillators, the nurse should follow the manufacturer's recommendations and the institution's protocol. The lead selection switch should be switched to "paddles." If monitor leads are used, lead I, II, or III should be selected. Paddles should have gel or paste made specifically for defibrillation applied to them before they are positioned on the patient's chest. This gel or paste will maximize current flow by reducing transthoracic impedence between the paddles and the patient's chest. If the defibrillator uses adhesive conductor pads instead of paddles, they should be positioned on the patient's chest at this time. One paddle or pad should be positioned just to the right of the patient's upper sternal border, below the clavicle. The second paddle or pad should be placed on the left side of the patient's chest slightly to the left of their nipple with the center of the electrode in the mid-axillary line (Fig. 53-9). Often the defibrillator's manufacturer will mark their paddles or pads to designate their position on the patient. Once positioned, the monitor display should be visually checked for rhythm assessment. If VF or VT is present, the operator should announce to the team members that the defibrillator is being charged and everyone should stand clear. The charge button on the defibrillator or apex paddle should be pressed. As soon as the defibrillator is charged, the operator should firmly and forcefully announce to all present that the patient is about to be shocked. To protect fellow rescuers, it is imperative that no one is in direct or indirect contact with the patient during defibrillation. This means that no one is touching the patient or any item or apparatus coming in contact with the patient including the stretcher or bed. If an individual is in direct or indirect contact with the patient during defibrillation, it is possible the electrical shock may pass through the individual as well as the

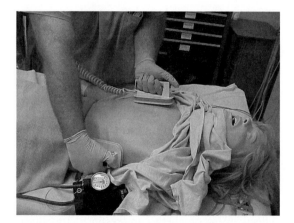

Fig. 53-9 During defibrillation, the operator should apply approximately 25 lbs of pressure on the paddles while simultaneously pressing both paddle discharge buttons with the rescuer's thumbs. *(Courtesy Department of Nurse Anesthesia, Virginia Commonwealth University, Richmond, Va.)*

patient. To alleviate this danger, the AHA suggests the following chant be used. First the defibrillator operator states loudly and clearly, "I am going to shock on three. One, I'm clear." At this time the operator checks to be sure he or she is clear of any contact with the patient. Next the operator states, "Two, you're clear" while making a visual check to ensure that no one else is touching the patient or any item that is in contact with the patient. Finally the operator states, "Three, everybody's clear." At this point the operator checks everyone—including himself or herself—one last time before administering the shock to the patient. If pads are used instead of paddles, pressing the defibrillator discharge button discharges the defibrillator. Using paddles, the operator should apply approximately 25 pounds of pressure on the paddles while simultaneously pressing both paddle discharge buttons.[1]

After the charge has been delivered to the patient, the patient's rhythm on the monitor is again evaluated. If any question concerning the displayed rhythm arises, the patient's pulse should be checked. If VF/VT persists, the defibrillator is immediately charged and the discharge sequence and warnings repeated. During the second shock, with a monophasic defibrillator, the energy level should be increased to 200-300 J. If the second shock is also unsuccessful, a third shock should be administered at an increased energy level of 360 J. Clinically equivalent levels should be used for biphasic defibrillators. Delay between any of the three-stacked shocks should be avoided. Stacked shocks—given close together with escalating current—have been shown to be more successful than shocks interrupted by drug therapy or CPR.[1]

If after the third shock VF/VT persists, CPR is to be continued for 1 minute and is followed by another stack of three shocks. As long as VF/VT persist, attempts to defibrillate must continue. The PACU nurse must remember that as long as the patient's myocardium has the energy to produce VF/VT, it should have the energy to produce a perfusing rhythm.[2]

As soon as the primary survey has been completed, the secondary survey must be addressed. The secondary survey builds on the primary survey, with more advanced assessments and treatments. In the presence of more than one rescuer, which is usually the case in the PACU, it is often possible to start the secondary survey before the primary survey is complete.

Secondary A-B-C-D Survey

A: Secondary Airway. If not previously intubated, the patient should be intubated as soon as possible. Endotracheal intubation should be performed by someone trained and experienced with this technique. In the PACU, this responsibility usually rests with the anesthesiologist or certified nurse anesthetist.

B: Secondary Breathing. Once the patient is intubated, confirmation of proper endotracheal tube placement should be assessed. This can be done by auscultation of the lungs to determine whether breath sounds are present and bilaterally equal in both lungs. Auscultation over the epigastric region is an additional means to assess accidental esophageal intubation. If a capnogram is available, the presence of end-tidal carbon dioxide should be confirmed along with oxygen saturation by way of an oxygen saturation monitor. Once proper tube placement has been confirmed, the tube should be secured in place to prevent dislodgment. This can be accomplished with tape or specially designed endotracheal tube holders.

C: Secondary Circulation. If not already present, intravenous access should be secured with a large-bore needle, and the patient should be connected to an ECG monitor. Cardiac rhythm analysis should be performed with appropriate pharmacological interventions. Vital signs such as blood pressure, pulse rate, and temperature should also be monitored and assessed.

In the case of VT/VF, we have seen from the primary survey that a stack of three shocks is delivered. If these three initial stacked shocks from the primary survey are unsuccessful in alleviating the VT/VF, the secondary survey suggests the patient be given epinephrine 1 mg IV or vasopressin 40 U IV as CPR continues for up to one minute. If after the epinephrine or vasopressin is administered during one minute of CPR it is assessed that the VT/VF persists, the patient should again be defibrillated. This second defibrillation routine should again follow the previous three shock series with the exception that all three shocks are delivered at 360 J. This cycle of stacked shocks, CPR/drugs, stacked shocks, and CPR/drugs should continue until the patient recovers or a physician declares him or her deceased.[1]

If the first dose of epinephrine has no effect it should be repeated every 3 to 5 minutes. If the single dose of vasopressin is administered with no resulting response after 10 to 20 minutes, the rescuer may give 1 mg IV push of epinephrine that can be repeated every 3 to 5 minutes. Additional pharmacologic interventions that might be considered include the administration of such drugs as amiodarone, lidocaine, magnesium, procainamide, and buffers.[2]

D: Differential Diagnosis. The differential diagnosis consists of determining the underlying cause(s) of the arrest. The primary purpose of the differential diagnosis is to identify reversible causes that have a specific therapy. For the PACU nurse this may involve looking at the patient's preoperative history and physical condition, preoperative and postoperative lab values, postoperative diagnosis, surgical procedure performed, and the patient's condition upon arrival into the PACU. It should also involve the patient's intraoperative course, including unexpected surgical events such as excessive blood loss, fluid replacement, pharmacological management, and any other intraoperative surgical/anesthetic events.

Any of these factors may add some insight into the underlying question of why the patient arrested. Potentially reversible causes of an arrest may include hypovolemia, hypoxia, acidosis, hypokalemia, hyperkalemia, hypothermia, drug overdoses, cardiac tamponade, pneumothorax, and coronary/pulmonary thrombosis. The PACU nurse should remember that successful resuscitation outcomes usually depend on the discovery and treatment of these or other reversible underlying causes.

Asystole

Thus far this discussion of the AHA's primary and secondary surveys has focused on pulseless ventricular tachycardia and ventricular fibrillation. The following examines another common arrhythmia—asystole. It is not an uncommon occurrence for the PACU nurse to check his or her patient, only to notice that the patient's rhythm on the EKG monitor is flat or straight-line. The nurse should remember that asystole is a specific diagnosis but that a flat line is not.[2] Many nonphysiological reasons could explain why the monitor may be flat or straight-line. One of the most common causes is one of the monitor leads becoming disconnected or unplugged. Monitor failure or an insufficient gain setting may also cause a straight-line wave. Although it lacks significant confirmation in human studies, a theory called "VF-has-a-vector" states that VF may present as a flat line in any lead recording at 90 degrees to the VF waves that are moving through the myocardium with a specific vector. This theory can be ruled out by selecting different leads on the ECG monitor.[1] Changing lead selection may also assist the nurse in identifying a disconnected lead.

A straight-line ECG rhythm may also indicate that the patient is in cardiopulmonary arrest. The PACU nurse should approach this situation the same way as he or she would approach other potential cardiopulmonary emergencies—by using the AHA's primary and secondary ABCD surveys. The first step to be taken is to assess patient consciousness. If the patient is awake and talking, without any distress, it is very unlikely he or she is in true asystole. By assessing consciousness, the nurse may find the patient was merely sleeping and has inadvertently disconnected one of his or her monitor leads. If, however, the nurse

confirms that the patient is unconscious and unresponsive, help should be called by activating the unit's emergency response system. The nurse should then immediately move into the primary A, B, C, D survey. It should be noted that at the beginning of the primary survey, asystole has not been established as a definite diagnosis. It is possible the patient is actually in VT or VF in addition to having a disconnected monitor lead. This disconnect should be discovered during the defibrillation stage of the survey. It is during this stage that the patient will be connected to a monitor/defibrillator to assess the necessity of defibrillation. If during the primary survey it is confirmed that instead of asystole, the patient is in VT/VF, defibrillation should be performed immediately. If the patient is confirmed to be true asystole, defibrillation may not be recommended, depending on the institution's policies.

Should the nurse shock a patient who is in confirmed asystole? This continues to be a controversial topic. Some practitioners argue that shocks for confirmed asystole cannot hurt and may help. At this time, however, no valid adult human research data support this rationale. During asystole, shocks may be harmful by producing a "stunned heart" and profound parasympathetic discharge. In this situation it would appear that such shocks would actually be counterproductive to promoting spontaneous cardiac activity. As a result, the AHA considers the practice of empiric shocking of asystole to have no evidence of support and to be potentially harmful to the patient.[1] The PACU nurse should consult their unit's or institution's policy concerning this practice.

Steps that should be followed with confirmed asystole include continuous CPR with epinephrine 1 mg IV push every 3-5 minutes and atropine 1 mg IV can be given every 3-5 minutes up to a maximum total dose of 0.04 mg/kg. Early transcutaneous pacing should also be considered.[2] During this process, the rescuers must always remember to continuously search for and treat identified reversible causes of the arrest as outlined in the secondary surveys differential diagnosis.

PHARMACOLOGIC THERAPY

The following is a short summary based on the AHA's recommendations concerning various drugs that are commonly used during cardiovascular resuscitation.[1,2] As the PACU nurse is aware, a thorough understanding of each drug—including its indications, contraindications, interactions, dosage, and adverse reactions—should be obtained before its use. It is also important that the nurse have the same understanding for all additional drugs found in the PACU's code cart.

Vasopressin

Vasopressin is a naturally occurring antidiuretic hormone. In high doses, higher than those needed for antidiuretic effects, vasopressin acts as a nonadrenergic peripheral smooth muscle vasoconstrictor. Vasopressin has been found useful as an alternative to epinephrine for the treatment of adult shock-refractory VF and to encourage the return of spontaneous circulation in the event of asystole or pulseless electrical activity. Use of vasopressin is based on research that shows high serum ADH levels in patients who have survived CPR. For patients in VT or VF, the recommended one time adult dose of vasopressin is 40 units IV. This can be given alone or in addition to epinephrine.

Epinephrine

The adrenergic effect of epinephrine increases myocardial and cerebral blood flow and may improve return of spontaneous circulation during CPR. The recommended dose of epinephrine hydrochloride is 1.0 mg (10 ml of a 10:000 solution) IV every 3 to 5 minutes during resuscitation. Epinephrine may also be administered via the endotracheal tube if IV access has not been secured. Although the optimal dose for tracheal delivery is unknown, a dose 2 to 2.5 times the IV dose may be needed. Only a physician trained in this technique should perform intracardiac injection of this drug. With the increased risk of coronary artery laceration, cardiac tamponade, and pneumothorax, intracardiac injection of epinephrine should only be used during open cardiac massage or when other routes of administration are unavailable.

Amiodarone

Amiodarone is useful in the treatment of atrial and ventricular arrhythmias—especially in the patient presenting with severely impaired heart function. For cardiopulmonary arrest, amiodarone is usually administered in a dose of 300 mg IV. A repeat dose of 150 IV may be considered in 3 to 5 minutes, with a maximum cumulative dose of 2.2 g IV per 24 hours. The primary adverse effects of amiodarone are hypotension and bradycardia. These adverse effects can usually be prevented by slowing the drug's rate of infusion. If these adverse effects develop, the patient's cardiovascular status can be stabilized with fluids, pressors, chronotropic agents, or temporary pacing.

Lidocaine

Lidocaine is useful as an antiarrhythmic agent for the treatment of ventricular ectomy, VT, and VF. During a cardiac arrest, it is administered as a bolus of 1.0 to 1.5 mg/kg IV, not to exceed 3 mg/kg. The administration of a prophylactic continuous infusion after circulation has been restored is controversial. If it is used, the infusion can be administered up to a maximum rate of 4 mg/min. Side effects include slurred speech, muscle twitching, altered consciousness, respiratory compromise, seizures, and tachycardia.

Magnesium

Magnesium is only used during a cardiac arrest when the arrhythmias are suspected to be caused from magnesium deficiency or in the presence of torsades de pointes. The usual dose in these states is 1 to 2 g IV. Rapid infusion of magnesium can cause clinically significant hypotension and possible asystole.

Procainamide

Procainamide hydrochloride is used to suppress both atrial and ventricular arrhythmias. It is used when VF or pulseless VT recurs after periods of non-VF rhythms. The intravenous dosage of procainamide is 20 mg/min. The bolus administration of procainamide should be stopped when the dysrhythmia is suppressed, when the QRS complex is widened by 50%, when hypotension occurs, or when the maximum total dose of the procainamide reaches 17 mg/kg. In urgent situations, 50 mg/min may be administered up to the maximum total dose. Procainamide should be avoided in the presence of a prolonged QT interval and torsades de pointes. Severe hypotension can result from rapid injection.

Atropine Sulfate

Atropine sulfate as an anticholinergic agent is very useful in treating symptomatic sinus bradycardia. It may also be useful with AV block at the nodal level and ventricular asystole. Atropine sulfate should not be used when Mobiz type II block is suspected. It should always be used with caution in a patient who presents with an acute myocardial infarction because acceleration of heart rate may increase ischemia. The recommended dose of atropine sulfate in the presence of bradycardia is 0.5 to 1.0 mg IV every 3 to 5 minutes up to a total dose of 0.04 mg/kg. For asystole and slow pulseless electrical activity, a dose of 1.0 mg is administered IV. This dose may be repeated in 3 to 5 minutes if asystole persists up to a maximum dose of 0.03-0.04 mg/kg.

Sodium Bicarbonate

Hyperventilation corrects respiratory acidosis by removing carbon dioxide. Acidemia during cardiac arrest and resuscitation primarily results from low blood flow. To maintain acid base balance, it is important that adequate alveolar ventilation and tissue perfusion is maintained during cardiac arrest. Clinical/laboratory data has not conclusively demonstrated that acidosis interferes with defibrillation, restoration of spontaneous circulation, or short-term survival. Few data indicate that the use of buffers improves outcome. Data does, however, indicate that bicarbonate can compromise coronary perfusion pressure and induce hypernatremia. Additionally, it can exacerbate central venous acidosis and cause adverse effects from extracellular alkalosis.

Sodium bicarbonate can be beneficial in patients with hyperkalemia, tricyclic/phenobarbitone overdose, or preexisting metabolic acidosis. Bicarbonate may also have some benefit during long resuscitative efforts or when confirmed interventions such as defibrillation, cardiac compressions, and intubation have been ineffective. If used, bicarbonate should be administered with an initial dose of 1 mEq/kg. Administration of bicarbonate should be guided by blood gas analysis or laboratory measurement.

SUMMARY

Whenever faced with a possible cardiopulmonary emergency, the PACU nurse should immediately institute the AHA's Primary and Secondary ABCD's of cardiopulmonary resuscitation. First consciousness must be assessed. If the patient is unconscious, help must be called, and the primary survey of Airway, Breathing, Circulation, and Defibrillation efficiently followed. Immediately after the primary survey the secondary survey of advanced Airway, Breathing, Circulation, and Differential Diagnosis should be performed.

A cardiopulmonary emergency is not an event that any healthcare provider looks forward to handling. It is, however, an event that is more common in highly specialized acute nursing units such as the PACU. As such, every nurse working in the PACU must always be prepared for such life-threatening emergencies.

REFERENCES

1. The American Heart Association in collaboration with the International Liaison Committee on Resuscitation: Guidelines 2000 for cardiopulmonary resuscitation and emergency cardiovascular care, international consensus on science, Circulation supplement I, 102:8, 2000.
2. Cummins RO, editor: ACLS Provider Manual, Dallas, 2001, American Heart Association.
3. Barash P, Cullen B, Stoelting R: Clinical anesthesia, ed 3, Philadelphia, 1997, JB Lippincott.
4. Walker R: DNR in the OR: resuscitation as an operating room risk, JAMA 266:2407, 1991.
5. Cummins R, Ornato J, Thies W et al: Improving survival from sudden cardiac arrest: the 'chain of survival' concept, Circulation 83:1833-1847, 1991.
6. Cummins R: From concept to standard-of-care? Review of the clinical experience with automated external defibrillators, Annual of Emergency Medicine 4:721-727, 1993.
7. Odom J: Airway emergencies in the post anesthesia care unit, Post Anesthesia Care Nursing 28:483-491, 1993.
8. Nagelhout J, Zaglaniczny K, editors: Nurse anesthesia, ed 2, Philadelphia, 2000, WB Saunders.
9. Aufderheide TP, Stapleton ED, editors: Instructor's manual: basic life support, Dallas, 2000, American Heart Association.

INDEX

A

A fibers, of afferent nerve, 340
A wave, 126, 531
Abdominal distention
  adrenalectomy and, 579
  genitourinary surgery and, 570-571
  gynecologic surgery and, 588
  laparoscopic perforation and, 639
  trauma injury and, 721
Abdominal myomectomy, definition of, 583
Abdominal pressure, increased, during
  laparoscopy, 637
Abdominal surgery
  COPD and, 643
  diagnostic studies, 558
  of female reproductive organs, terms used
    in, 581-583
  general care after, 555-558
  nausea, vomiting and, 656
Abdominoperineal resection, 560, 561-562
Abducent (abducens) nerve (VI), *101*,
    102
  cervical spine surgery and, 514
ABO blood groups, 209, 211
Abrasions, from trauma wounds, 720, 721
Absorption, laser beam, 629
Abstinence syndrome, 697; *see also*
  Withdrawal syndrome
Acceleration forces, trauma and, 715
Accessory nerve (XI), medulla oblongata
    and, 102
Accolate, respiratory care and, 266t
Acetaminophen (Tylenol)
  after ophthalmic surgery, 460
  after pediatric surgery, 674
  for analgesia in pregnant patient, 695
  for oral analgesia, 431
Acetazolamide, 197
Acetonuria, definition of, 189
Acetylcholine, 135-136
  biochemistry, 136
  magnesium and, 207
  neuromuscular transmission and, 317,
    318, 708
Acetylcholinesterase, 137-138, 318
  muscle relaxant reversal and, 325

Acetylcysteine (Mucomyst), respiratory care
    and, 266t
Achalasia, 221-222
Achlorhydria, definition of, 221
Acid-base balance
  kidneys role in, 194-195
  monitoring after pancreatic surgery, 564
Acid-base buffers, 174
  phosphate, 206
Acid-base relationships, 174-176
  metabolic imbalances in, 176, 176b
  respiratory imbalances in, 175-176
Acidemia, definition of, 150
Acidosis; *see also* Metabolic acidosis;
    Respiratory acidosis
  cardiopulmonary arrest and, 744
  definition of, 150
  malignant hyperthermia and, 678
  in newborns, 664
  progressive phase hemorrhage and, 724
  sodium bicarbonate and, 746
Acoustic nerves (VII), 102
  type and functions of, 103t
Acoustic reflexes, 101
Acquired immunity, 239
  cellular/cell-mediated, 239, 241-242
  definition of, 238
  humoral, 239-241
Acromegaly, 215
Actin, neuromuscular transmission and, 319
Action potential
  cardiac muscle transmission of, 129-130
  muscle transmission of, 708
  pain information from, 339
Activated coagulation time (ACT), after
    cardiac surgery, 490
Activated partial thromboplastin time
    (APTT), 207, 208
  cardiac surgery and, 490
Activation, definition of, 317
Activation phase, of anaphylactic shock,
    726
Active acquired immunity, definition of,
    238
Acuity of inpatients, perianesthesia nursing
    and, 11

Acute isovolemic hemodilution, autologous
    blood transfusions and, 210
Acute tubular necrosis, 198
Adalat, 141
  for hypertension, 145, 146t
"Adam," abuse of, 703-704
Adam's apple, 152
Addisonian crisis, 218-219
Additive effect, definition of, 248
Adenocarcinoma, definition of, 590
Adenohypophysis, 214
  hormones of, 214-215
Adenoidectomy; *see* Tonsillectomy and
    adenoidectomy
Adenosine (Adenocard), 252t
3', 5'-Adenosine monophosphate (cyclic
    AMP), 140-141, *142*; *see also* Cyclic
    adenosine monophosphate
Adenosine triphosphate (ATP), 213
  action of, *142*
  beta receptors and, 140
  in donated blood, 209
  malignant hyperthermia and, 709
  phosphate and, 206
  shock and, 723
  sodium-potassium ion exchange and,
    204
Adenotonsillar hypertrophy in children,
    679
Adenylate cyclase
  action of, *142*
  beta receptors and, 140
  as messenger hormone, 213
Adolescents
  fasting before ambulatory surgery and,
    620
  postoperative psychosocial support for,
    669
  succinylcholine contraindications for,
    327-328
Adrenal glands, 217
Adrenal medulla, 136
Adrenalectomy
  care after, 578-579
  definition of, 566
Adrenalin; *see* Epinephrine

Page numbers in *italics* refer to illustrations; page numbers followed by b indicate boxes; t, tables.

Adrenergic, definition of, 125
Adrenergic agents, 144t, 266t
   alpha₂ agonists for post C-section pain
      relief, 695
   for malignant hyperthermia treatment,
      712b
   respiratory care and, 266t
Adrenergic blocking agents, for cardiogenic
   shock, 725
Adrenergic nerves, 136b
   drugs that interfere with transmission by,
      142t
   norepinephrine and, 136
Adrenergic neurotransmitters, biochemistry
   of, 136-137, 137b
Adrenergic receptors, 139-141, 141t
   hepatocytes and, 226
Adrenocorticotropin (ACTH), 215
   glucocorticoids and, 217
   panhypopituitarism and, 218
   pituitary gland and, 214
Advanced cardiac life support (ACLS), 15,
   735
   eye surgery and, 452
   secondary ABCD survey and, 737
Advanced directives, cardiopulmonary
   resuscitation and, 735
Adventitious sounds, definition of, 150
AeroBid, respiratory care and, 266t
Aerosolized administration of drugs,
   systemic absorption of, 251
Afferent, definition of, 93
Afferent fibers, of reticular formation, 104
Afferent nerve impulses, spinal cord and,
   117-118, 121
African Americans, sickle cell anemia and,
   653, 654
Afterload, definition of, 125
Agency for Health Care Policy and
   Research, on pain management, 426
Agency for Healthcare Research and
   Quality, website, 618
Agglutination
   antibody, 241
   of RBCs in hemolytic reactions to
      transfusions, 398
Aggression, limbic system and, 99
Aging; see also Geriatric patients
   cardiac surgery complications and, 487
   eye surgery and, 452
   meperidine for pain management in, 423
   nursing population and, 24-25
   pain management for, 429
   perianesthesia nursing and, 11
   postoperative pulmonary complications
      and, 184
Agonists, definition of, 248
Airborne-transmission precautions, 40b
Airway(s)
   artificial, 362
   assessment and management, 409-421
      (see also Endotracheal intubation;
      Tracheal intubation)
   after ambulatory surgery, 622
   after shock trauma, 719
   for cardiopulmonary resuscitation,
      737-738, 743
   malignant hyperthermia and, 711

Airway(s) (Continued)
   nausea and, 659
   oral, 409-411
   pediatric, 667
      equipment for, 663t
      with head or cervical spine injury,
         679, 679-680
      postoperative, 670, 671, 672
      in premature infants, 665
   with rheumatoid arthritis, 647
   spinal cord injuries and, 544
   suggested PACU equipment for, 412b
   vomiting and, 655, 659
   closure, lung volumes and, 160-161
   destruction, 642
Airway obstruction; see also Laryngospasm
   in children, 664, 677
   COPD and, 642
   functional residual capacity and, 159
   inspiration versus exhalation and, 362
   in newborns, 661
   postoperative, 361, 362-363
   respiratory compromise and, 736
Akathisia, 98
Albumin
   for acute volume expansion, 211
   colloid osmotic pressure and, 204
   liver and, 226-227
   plasma oncotic pressure and, 208-209
   transfusion of, 399
Albuminuria, definition of, 189
Albuterol (Proventil, Ventolin), 252t
   respiratory care and, 266t
Alcohol
   abuse of, 697, 701
      effects and signs of, 698t
      benzodiazepines and, 700
      gamma hydroxybutyrate and, 704
Alcuronium chloride (Alloferin), 325
Aldactone, 196
Aldomet, sympathetic nerve stimulation
   and, 141
Aldosterone, 217; see also Renin-
   angiotensin-aldosterone mechanism
   during cardiopulmonary bypass, 484
   geriatric patients and, 684
   water balance and, 203
Aldosterone antagonists, 195, 196
Alerting process, limbic system and, 100
Alfentanil (Alfenta), 252t, 308
   intracranial pressure and, 528
Alkalemia, definition of, 150
Alkalosis; see also Metabolic alkalosis
   definition of, 150
   loop diuretics and, 196
   sodium bicarbonate and, 746
Allen test, 128-129, 373
   definition of, 491
Allergies; see also Hypersensitivity reactions
   CT scans and, 519
   immunosuppression for, 246
   local anesthetic esters and, 341
   shock from, 717t
   transfusion reactions and, 211, 398
   d-tubocurarine chloride and, 321
Alloferin, 325
Allograft rejection, as delayed
   hypersensitivity reaction, 243

Alpha-adrenergic receptors, 140
Alphadolone acetate, for steroid anesthesia,
   302
Alphaxalone, for steroid anesthesia, 302
Althesin, 302
Alveolar ducts, 157
   pulmonary hysteresis and, 160-161,
      161
Alveolar hypoxia, pulmonary vascular
   resistance and, 167
Alveolar partial pressure, inhalation
   anesthetics and, 278
Alveolar recoil pressure, 162
Alveolar sac, 157
Alveolar ventilation, 278
Alveolar-arterial CO₂ difference, 367
Alveoli, 157
Alzheimer's disease
   aging and, 684-685
   PET scans and diagnosis of, 520
Ambu-Bag, 739
Ambulation; see also Mobilization,
   postoperative
   after geriatric surgery, 686
Ambulatory surgery, 615-626; see also
   Laparoscopy; Laser surgery
   assessment and preparation for, 617-621
   diagnostic testing, 620
   emotional support, 620-621
   factors in, 615
   fasting before, 619-620
   intraoperative care, 621
   patient information on Internet for, 618,
      618b
   patient medications and, 618-619, 619b
   perianesthesia nursing care, 616-617
      recovery periods, 621-622
      specific tasks in, 622
   postdischarge follow-up, 625
   preoperative goals, 621
   preoperative medications, 620
   progressive or phase II care, 622-625
      discharge planning, 624
      goals of, 623b
      oral intake issues, 623
      reunions with family, 623-624
   risk factors, 617
   Sentinel Event Alert and, 619
Ambulatory surgical centers (ASCs), 16
   hospital outpatient departments versus
      freestanding, 615
American Association of Critical Care
   Nurses (CCRN), certification by, 15t
American Association of Nurse
   Anesthetists
   closed-claims study on medical
      malpractice, 66
   latex allergies web site, 244
American Cancer Society, 595
American Heart Association
   on blood pressure monitoring, 371
   cardiopulmonary resuscitation guidelines,
      737
   Guidelines for 2000 for Cardiopulmonary
      Resuscitation and Emergency
      Cardiovascular Care for Advanced
      Cardiac Life Support (ACLS),
      418

American Nursing Association (ANA)
certification by, 15t
Social Policy Statement of 1997, 13b
American Society of Anesthesiologists (ASA)
closed-claims study on medical malpractice by, 66
on diagnostic testing, 620
Ethics Committee guidelines on DNR orders during surgery, 84
on fasting before elective procedures, 619
herbal products caution by, 273
latex allergy task force, 244
on practice parameters and medical malpractice, 72
American Society of PeriAnesthesia Nurses (ASPAN)
certification by, 15t
clinical guidelines by, 60
PACU staffing recommendations, 3-4
patient information website, 618
patient reporting recommendations, 355
Position Paper on Pain Management, 430-431b
Scope of Perianesthesia Nursing Practice, 13-14b
Scope of Practice, 12
Standards for PeriAnesthesia Nursing Practice 2002, 39-40
on ECG monitoring, 374
on PACU staffing, 17
on PACU standard equipment, 7
Standards of Postanesthesia Nursing Practice 1991, on pulse oximetry, 363
Amidate; *see* Etomidate
Amides, local anesthetic, 341, 342t
Amiloride, 196
Amino acids, glucagon and, 218
Aminocaproic acid (Amicar), 252t
Aminoglycosides, anesthetic agents interactions with, 271
Aminophylline, 252t
for anaphylactic shock, 726
for apnea in premature infants, 665
as bronchodilator, 141
d-tubocurarine interaction with, 269t
Amiodarone, for cardiopulmonary resuscitation, 743, 745
Amnesia
anesthesia and, 276
date-rape drugs and, 704
diazepam and, 295
Amphetamines, abuse of, 697, 702
effects and signs of, 699t
Amputation
cineplastic (kineplastic), definition of, 506
perianesthesia care after, 515
Syme, definition of, 506
Amrinone (Inocor), 252t
for hypotension, 144
Amygdala, 96, 96
Amygdaloid body, 99
Amyl nitrite, abuse of, 703
Amytal, abuse of, effects and signs of, 698t

Analgesia; *see also* Patient-controlled analgesia
after anesthesia with enflurane, 285
after geriatric surgery, 686
after penile surgery, 578
after vascular surgery, 501
as anesthesia Stage I, 276
anesthetics *versus*, 427
for pediatric anesthesia emergence, 667
Analgesics
comparison of, 310t
oral, after ambulatory surgery, 429, 431
sickle cell anemia and, 654
sound level in PACU and, 60
Anaphylaxis, 717t, 723, 725, 726-727
definition of, 248
hypersensitivity reaction, 242
local anesthetics and, 344
latex allergic reaction and, 245
from morphine for pain management, 423
slow-reacting substance of, 242
systemic, as immediate hypersensitivity reaction, 243
Anastomosis
ileoanal
with J-pouch for ulcerative colitis, 561
proctocolectomy, total, with, 560
of transplant, definition of, 567
ureterovesical, definition of, 567
Androgens, 217
Anectine; *see* Succinylcholine
Anemia; *see also* Sickle cell anemia
hemolytic, as cytotoxic hypersensitivity reaction, 243
physiologic, of pregnancy, 691
rheumatoid arthritis and, 648
Anesthesia; *see also* Anesthetic agents
for ambulatory surgery, 621
analgesia *versus*, 427
axial nerve block, 352
barbiturate addiction and, 700
brachial plexus nerve block, 352
for cardiac surgery, 485
definition of, 506
diabetes mellitus and, 645-646
epidural, 351-352
pregnancy, blood pressure and, 690
for eye surgery, 456-458
inhalation, 276-291
administration of, 281-283
emergence from, 280
kidney disease and, 197
pharmacokinetics of, 278-280
potency of, 280-281
signs and reflex reactions of stages of, 276-278, 277f
slow lung units and, 163-164
intravenous
nonopioid, 292-303
mechanism of action, 292
opioid, 304-316
concepts of, 304-305
regional, 352-353
local, 339-345
allergic reactions to, 344
emergence from, 340b
for eye surgery, 456

Anesthesia (*Continued*)
and opioids for pain management, 425
overdosage of, 344-345, 344b
physiology of nerves and nerve conduction in, 339-341
nausea, vomiting and, 656
neurogenic shock and, 726
for pediatric patients, 666-667
for pregnant patients, 692-693
regional, 346-353
for ambulatory surgery, 621
for burn injuries, 612-613
definition of, 339
epidural, 351-352
intravenous, 352-353
malignant hyperthermia and, 711
for pediatric patients, 674, 675
for pregnant patients, 688, 693
spinal, 346-352
respiratory compromise and, 736
sickle cell anemia and, 654
spinal, 117
administration techniques, 346-348
combined spinal-epidural, 351
complications, 349-351
lidocaine for, 343
mechanism of action, 348-349
neurogenic shock and, 726
PACU care after, 351-352
for pediatric patients, 675
pregnancy, blood pressure and, 690
shock from, 717t
sickle cell anemia and, 654
spinal cord injuries and, 544
for thyroid and parathyroid surgery, 548
topical, 339
definition of, 456
for eye surgery, 456-457
for thoracic surgery, 467
for vascular surgery, 495-496, 501
Anesthesia machines, 281, 281-283
circuit in, 282
Anesthesia Patient Safety Foundation, 46
Anesthesia provider, patient reports by, 356b
Anesthesia-assisted rapid opiate detoxification (AAROD), 315-316
Anesthetic agents
alcoholism and, 701
ambulatory surgery and, 615
antibiotics interactions with, 271
blood and tissue uptake of, 279-280
blood-brain barrier and, 112, 280
brachial or pudendal plexuses and, 121-122
dermatomes and spinal or regional, 121, 348-349, 349
heart effects of, 131-132
inhalant, 283-289 (*see also* specific agent, e.g. Halothane)
assessing effects in PACU of, 289-290
intracranial pressure and, 527-528
malignant hyperthermia and, 707
muscle relaxant interactions with, 270t
opioids cross-tolerance with, 697

Anesthetic agents (Continued)
intravenous
nonopioid
barbiturates, 292-293
benzodiazepine antagonists, 298-299
benzodiazepines, 295-298
butyrophenones, 299-301
for children, 667
dissociative agents, 301-302
intracranial pressure and, 528-529
nonbarbiturates, 293-295
propanidid, 302
tranquilizers, 295-301
opioid
descriptions of specific, 305-312
detoxification in PACU from, 315-316
intracranial pressure and, 528-529
intrathecal and epidural
administration of, 312-313
local
for analgesia, 422-423
intermediate-duration, 341, 343
long-duration, 343-344
short-duration, 341
sickle cell anemia and, 654
properties of, 279t
shorter-acting, 61
Aneurysms
aortic, obstructive shock and, 728
cerebral, 521, 523
definition of, 493
of distal aorta, 501
noninvasive repair, 494-495
thoracic, after vascular surgery, 503
ventricular repair, 484
definition of, 483
Angina pectoris, definition of, 125
Angioedema, anaphylactic shock and, 726
Angiography
cerebral, for cranial surgery diagnosis,
520, 521
definition of, 493
renal, for renal surgery diagnosis, 567
Angioneurotic edema, local anesthetics
and, 344
Angioscopy, definition of, 493
Angiotensin; see Renin-angiotensin-
aldosterone mechanism
Angiotensin I, caveoli and, 167
Anions
definition of, 201
fluid distribution and, 204
Ankyloglossia ("tongue tied"), definition of,
433
Annuloplasty, definition of, 473
Anoxia, malignant hyperthermia and, 710b
Antacids
esophageal resting pressure and, 221
for vomiting/regurgitation, 223
Antagonists
definition of, 248
for pain management side effects, 424
Anterior clinoid process, 105
Anterior commissure, 96, 99
Anterior cord syndrome, 539
Anterior gray horns, 121

Anterior median fissure, 120
Anterior segment, ocular
definition of, 453
pain management after surgery on, 460
Anterior thalamic nuclei, 99, 99
Anthrax, as biological warfare agent, 730-
731, 731b, 732
Antiasthmatic agents, 266t
for pain management side effects, 424
respiratory care and, 266t
Antibiotics
anaphylactic shock and, 726
drug-drug interactions in PACU and,
268t, 271
geriatric patients and, 685t
muscle relaxants and, 330, 330b
neuromuscular blocking properties of,
330, 330b
for plague, 733
postoperative bleeding and, 135
for transfusion reactions from bacterial
contamination, 398
Antibodies
definition of, 238
humoral immunity and, 239, 240-241
Anticholinergic agents, 266t
Alzheimer's disease and, 685
for hypotension, 144
malignant hyperthermia and, 710
respiratory care and, 266t
d-tubocurarine chloride reversal with, 321
vecuronium reversal with, 323
for vomiting/regurgitation, 223
Anticholinergic antiparkinsonian drugs, 98
Anticholinesterase drugs
muscle contraction and, 317
for muscle relaxant reversal, 325
for myasthenia gravis, 644
d-tubocurarine chloride reversal with,
321
vecuronium reversal with, 323
Anticoagulant therapy
epidural block contraindication for, 351
prothrombin time and, 134-135
Antidepressants, tricyclic
geriatric patients and, 685t
for pain management, 424
physostigmine salicylate and, 138
Antidiuretic hormone (ADH), 192t, 215;
see also Vasopressin
alcohol abuse and, 701
anesthesia and release of, 197
blood volume, electrolytes and, 193
during cardiopulmonary bypass, 484
syndrome of inappropriate secretion of
(SIADH), 219
water balance and, 203
Anti-dumping statute, 79
Antidysrhythmics, geriatric patients and,
685t
Antiembolism stockings, spinal surgery and,
515
Antiemetics
ear surgery and, 435
for pain management side effects, 424
Antigen-antibody reactions, anaphylactic
shock and, 726

Antigens
B lymphocytes and, 239-240
definition of, 238
phagocytosis and, 239
T lymphocytes and, 242
Antihypertensive agents, 141
during ambulatory surgery, 619b
drug-drug interactions with, 267t, 272
Antiinfective agents, respiratory care and,
266t
Antiinflammatories, for analgesia, 422-423
Antilirium; see Physostigmine
Antimuscarinic drugs, for muscle relaxant
reversal, 325-326
Antiparkinsonian agents, 98
droperidol and, 299-300
physostigmine salicylate and, 138
Antispasmodic agents, for spinal cord
injuries, 540, 543
Antitoxin, botulism, 733
Antrectomy, 559
definition of, 551
Antrostomy, radical, definition of, 433
Anuria, Class IV hemorrhage and, 724
Anus, 225
care after surgery of, 562
Anxiety; see also Psychosocial assessment,
postoperative
club drugs abuse and, 703
eye surgery and, 457
hypertension and, 145
limbic system and, 99
postoperative, 362, 388-390
preoperative interview indications of,
427
signs and symptoms of, 389b
state versus trait, 428-429
Anxiolytics
for pain management, 424
for premedication with pediatric
anesthesia, 666
Anzement, 657t, 658
Aorta
arterial blood pressure and, 128
bypass procedures on, 500
coarctation of, definition of, 476
Aortic bodies, breathing regulation and,
179-180
Aortic regurgitation, definition of, 473
Aortic stenosis
definition of, 473-474
types of, 474
Aortic valve disease, definition of, 474
Aortic valves, 129
Aortocaval compression, 688, 690
uterine displacement to relieve, 690
Aortocoronary bypass grafts, 479
definition of, 474
Aplastic crisis, in sickle cell anemia, 655
Apnea
definition of, 150
epidural morphine and, 351
muscle relaxants and, 334
nasal intubation and, 181
obstructive sleep, in children, 679
pediatric breathholding spells versus,
668-669

Apnea (*Continued*)
  postanesthesia, in infants, 665
  propofol and, 294-295
Apnea monitors, 313
  patient-controlled epidural analgesia and,
    314
Apneustic breathing, 183, 534t
  definition of, 150
Apneustic center, 183
Apomorphine, vomiting center excitation
    and, 656
Appendectomy
  care after, 560, 562
  definition of, 551
Appendix, 225
Appetite, hypothalamus and, 101
Apresoline; *see* Hydralazine
Aprotinin, after cardiac surgery, 490
Aqueduct of Sylvius, 109; *see also* Cerebral
    aqueduct
Arachidonic acid cascade, pain
    management and, 423
Arachidonic cascade, blunt trauma and, 715
Arachnoid, 108, *109, 110,* 110-111, 346
Arachnoid granulations, *107,* 108
Arachnoid mater, *102, 106*
Arachnoid membrane, 117
Arachnoid trabecula, *109*
Arachnoid villus/villa, *106,* 108, *109, 110*
  blood-brain and blood-CSF barrier and,
    112
Aramine; *see* Metaraminol
Arato v. Avedon, 80-82
Arch, of vertebrae, 115
Arcuate (arciform) arteries, renal, 190, *191*
Arduran, 262t, 320t, 323
Arfonad, 264t
  for hypertension, 146t, 147-148
Argon
  for laser surgery, 631t
  for pneumoperitoneum in laparoscopy,
    635, 636t
Aristolochia, anesthesia interaction with,
    274t
Arms
  motor control of, 96
  perianesthesia care after surgery on, 511
  positioning after surgery on, 507
Arousal process, limbic system and, 100
Arrhythmias; *see also* Asystole; Cardiac
    dysrhythmias
  amiodarone for, 745
  amphetamines abuse and, 702
  cardiac surgery complications and, 487,
    489
  cocaine abuse and, 702
  CPR after, 737
  definition of, 125
  droperidol and, 300
  magnesium for, 745
  malignant hyperthermia and, 678
  procainamide for, 745
  sickle cell anemia and, 654
  smoking and, 653
  superventricular, *376,* 376-377, *377*
  ventricular, *377,* 377-378, *378*
    obesity and, 650

Artane; *see* Trihexyphenidyl
Arterial blood gas; *see also* Gas exchange
  cardiogenic shock and, 725
  malignant hyperthermia and, 678, 711-
    712
  in newborns, 662
  obesity and monitoring of, 651
  pediatric surgery and, 672
  sickle cell anemia and, 654
  spinal cord injuries and, 543
  vascular surgery and, 502
  Whipple procedure and, 564
Arterial blood pressure, 128-129
  cerebral blood flow and, 525
  mean, postoperative monitoring of, 384
  obesity and, 650
  partial, inhalation anesthetics and, 278
  pediatric surgery and, 672
Arterial catheter transducer systems
  hypertension detection and, 145
  hypotension detection and, 143
Arterial oxygen saturation, 363
  pregnancy and, 691
Arteries, 135
  laparoscopic perforation of, 639
Arteriograms, fibrinolytic therapy and,
    495
Arteriography
  care after, 496
  definition of, 493
Arterioles, 135
Arteriosclerosis
  definition of, 125
  smoking and, 652
Arteriovenous malformations (AVMs),
    523
Arthritis, rheumatoid, 646-649
Arthrodesis, definition of, 506
Arthroplasty, definition of, 506
Arthroscopy
  ambulatory surgery and, 615
  definition of, 506
  of knee, 513-514
  of shoulder, 511
Arthrotomy
  continuous passive motion machines
    and, 514
  definition of, 506
  of shoulder, 511
Articular process, of vertebrae, 115
Arytenoid cartilages, 152-153, *153*
ASA Difficult Airway Algorithm, 418
Aseptic technique, 233-234, 236
  ear surgery and, 434-435
  immunologic defense and, 239
  immunosuppression and, 246
  kidney transplantation and, 573
Aspiration
  of gastrointestinal contents after tracheal
    intubation, 418
  intermaxillary facial fixation and, 450
  LMA device and, 420
  pneumoperitoneum and, 638t
  postoperative, 361
  respiratory compromise and, 736
Aspiration pneumonitis, 223, 224
  in pregnant patient, 692

Aspirin
  sickle cell anemia and, 655
  surgical bleeding and, 207
Association areas, 99
Association fibers, 95
  in cerebral cortex, 96
Association of Operating Room Nurses,
    certification by, 15t
Association tracts, in spinal cord, 121
Asthma, 642
  allergic, as immediate hypersensitivity
    reaction, 243
  ketamine as anesthetic agent with, 301
  pathogenesis of, 182
  preexisting, postoperative complications
    and, 183
  sulfite allergy and dezocine
    contraindication with, 311
  d-tubocurarine chloride and, 321
Asystole, 744
  CPR after, 737
  during laparoscopy, 635
Atarax, 658t
Ataxic breathing, 534t
Atelectasis
  definition of, 150, 465
  functional residual capacity and, 159
  postoperative, 185, 361, 400
    in infants and children, 670
  pulmonary vascular resistance and, 167
  rheumatoid arthritis and, 647
  smoking and, 653
Atenolol (Tenormin), 252t
Ativan; *see* Lorazepam
Atlas, *105,* 116, *116*
Atracurium (Tracrium), 252t, 320t, 324
  for anesthesia maintenance in pregnant
    patients, 692
Atria, heart, 126
Atrial contraction, premature, 374, 376,
    376
Atrial gallop, myocardial infarction and,
    132
Atrial muscle, 129
Atrial pressure curve, 126
Atrial septal defect (ASD), *475*
  definition of, 474-475
Atrial standstill, postoperative monitoring
    for, 376
Atrial syncytia, 129
Atrioventricular (AV) valves, 126, 129
Atropine, 252t
  Alzheimer's disease and, 685
  for asystole, 744
  blood-brain barrier effects of, 138
  for bradycardia in high spinal block, 350
  for cardiopulmonary resuscitation, 746
  droperidol and, 299
  esophageal resting pressure and, 221
  geriatric patients and, 686
  heart rate after pediatric surgery and, 670
  for hypotension, 144
  kidney disease and, 197
  malignant hyperthermia and, 710
  muscarine responses and, 137, 142t
  for muscle relaxant reversal, 325, 326
  myocardial infarction and, 133

Atropine (Continued)
  nasal intubation and, 181
  for nausea, 657t, 658
  postoperative excitement from, 395
Atropine sulfate, succinylcholine for
    children/adolescents and, 328
Atrovent, 257t
  respiratory care and, 266t
Auditory area, in cerebral cortex, 97, 99
Augmentation mammoplasty, 597-598
  definition of, 590
  reconstructive, 595-596, 595-596
Auscultation, of chest
  in CPR ventilation
    primary, 739
    secondary, 743
  postoperative, 362-363
    nausea and vomiting assessment and,
      659
  in trauma patient, 719
Auscultatory gap, blood pressure
    monitoring and, 371
Autograft skin, meshed, 612
Autoimmune diseases
  drug-induced immunosuppression for,
    246
  T lymphocytes and, 242
Autologous, definition of, 201
Autologous blood transfusions, 209-210,
    395
Automated external defibrillator (AED),
    741-742
Automatic blood pressure monitoring, 372-
    373
Automatic skeletal movements, cerebral
    control of, 97
Automaticity, definition of, 125
Autonomic dysreflexia, spinal cord injuries
    and, 540
Autonomic functions
  diencephalon and, 100
  limbic system and, 99
  for pain measurement in children, 676t
  prefrontal area and, 98
Autonomic nervous system, 123
  spinal nerves and, 121
Autoregulation
  cerebral blood flow and, 525, 526
  definition of, 93
  inhalant anesthetic agents and, 527
  microcirculation and, 135
Autotransfusion system(s)
  after hip or femoral surgery, 512
  after knee surgery, 514
  for severe chest injuries, 719
AV (atrioventricular) bundle, 129
AV (atrioventricular) node, 129, 130
Axial nerve block, 352
Axid; see Nizatidine
Axis, 105, 116, 116
Axons
  pyramidal cell, 97
  spinal nerve, 121
Ayre T-piece, for inhalation anesthesia
    administration, 282, 283
Azathioprine (Imuran), for
    immunosuppression, 246, 573

Azotemia, 198
  definition of, 189
AZT, 41

B

B fibers, of afferent nerve, 340
B lymphocytes
  definition of, 238
  humoral immunity and, 239-240
B wave, 531
Babinski's reflex, 523, 534
Baby Boomers, 21, 22-24t
Bacillus anthracis, 732
Back, trauma nurse's assessment of, 721
Bag-valve–mask
  for apnea from nasal intubation, 181
  cardiac compression for CPR and, 741
  complications with newborns, 662
  for CPR, 739
  for infant and child ventilation, 671, 677
  nausea, vomiting and, 656
  obesity and, 651
  for positive-pressure breathing, 409, 410
    in children, 675
  requirements for, 410b
Bain anesthesia circuit, for inhalation
    anesthesia administration, 282, 283,
    284, 666
Balance, cerebellum and, 102
Balanced technique, of anesthetic agent
    administration
  morphine in, 306
  narcotics in, 305
  nitrous oxide in, 288, 307
Baldy-Webster procedure, 587
Balloon valvotomy/valvuloplasty, definition
    of, 475
Barbital; see also Phenobarbital
  kidney disease and, 197
Barbiturates, 292-293
  abuse of, 697, 700-701
    effects and signs of, 698t
  droperidol contraindication with, 301
  drug biotransformation and, 271
  intracranial pressure and, 528, 529
  for pain management, 424
  short-acting, Stage II anesthesia and,
    276
  sufentanil with, 308
Baroreceptors
  arterial blood pressure and, 128
  definition of, 517
  ventilation and, 182
Bartholin duct cyst, definition of, 581
Bartholinectomy, definition of, 581
Basal cell cancer, 231
Basal ganglia, 94, 95-96, 96, 100
  premotor area neurons and, 97
  pyramidal cell axons and, 97
Basement membrane, blood-brain barrier
    and, 112
Basic cardiac life support (BCLS), 15
Basic life support (BLS), 735
  primary ABCD survey and, 737
Basilar skull fractures, 520
Bathmotropic, definition of, 125
Bathmotropism, 129

Battles sign, basilar skull fractures and,
    520
Battle's sign, after trauma injury, 720
"Beans," abuse of, 703-704
Beclomethasone (Vanceril), respiratory care
    and, 266t
Behavioral responses
  diencephalon and endocrine control of,
    100
  limbic system and, 99
Behavioral scales, for pain measurement in
    children, 676t
Behavioral-physiologic scales, for pain
    measurement in children, 676t
Belladonna alkaloids
  after cystoscopy, 568
  kidney disease and, 197
  physostigmine salicylate and, 138
Bellevue bridge, for scrotal support, 577,
    577, 578
Benadryl; see Diphenhydramine
Beneficence, medical ethics and, 77, 78
Benzodiazepine antagonists, 298-299
  for ambulatory surgery, 621
Benzodiazepine receptors
  limbic system and, 99
  nonopioid drug interaction with, 292
Benzodiazepines, 295-298
  abuse of, 700-701
    effects and signs of, 699t
  flumazenil and, 298-299
  intracranial pressure and, 528
  for pain management, 424
  postoperative excitement from, 395
  sufentanil with, 308
Benzthiazide, 196
Benztropine (Cogentin)
  for acute dystonic reactions, 98
  droperidol and, 299-300
  for drug-induced parkinsonism, 98
Benzylisoquinolines, 304
Beractant (Survanta), respiratory care and,
    266t
Best interests test, informed consent/refusal
    and, 82
Beta-adrenergic receptors, 140
Betapace, 264t
Bicarbonate
  in carbon dioxide transport, 172, 173-174
  central chemoreceptors in breathing
    regulation and, 179
  kidney regulation of, 194-195
  pregnancy and, 691
Bicitra, 263t, 264t
  for aspiration pneumonitis in pregnant
    patients, 692
  for vomiting/regurgitation, 223
Bier block, 352-353
Bigeminy
  definition of, 125
  during laparoscopy, 635
Bilateral subtotal thyroidectomy, definition
    of, 548
Biliary, definition of, 221
Biliary lithotripsy, cholecystectomy versus,
    227-228
Biliary tract, care after surgery of, 564-565

Bilirubin, metabolism of, 226
Billroth I (gastroduodenostomy), 553
Billroth II (gastrojejunostomy), 553
Bioethical mandates, patient, family, and
　　ICU needs and, 87-88
Biofeedback, for pain management, 426
Biologic rhythms, limbic system and, 100
Bioterrorism, 730-733
　anthrax, 732
　botulism, 733
　planning for care, 731-732
　pneumonic plague, 732-733
　smallpox, 733
Bitolterol (Tornalate), respiratory care and,
　　266t
Black cohosh, anesthesia interaction with,
　　274t
Bladder injuries, after laparoscopy, 639
Bladder neck operation (Y-V plasty), 574
　definition of, 566
Bladder surgery
　care after, 574
　laparoscopic perforation after, 639
Blankets, warmed cotton, postanesthetic
　　warming and, 707
Bleeding; see also Hemorrhage
　after abdominal surgery, 559
　after ambulatory surgery, 622
　after appendectomy or herniorrhaphy,
　　562
　after cerclage procedure, 585
　after cystoscopy, 568
　after hysteroscopy, 588
　after laparoscopic cholecystectomy, 565
　after laparoscopy, 586
　after mastopexy, 597
　after pediatric surgery, 673
　after penile surgery, 578
　after radical mastectomy, 595
　after T&A, tonsil tray for, 440, 440b
　after thoracic surgery, 471
　after thyroid surgery, 549
　gynecologic surgery and, 585
　noninvasive vascular procedures and, 495
　with prostate surgery, 575, 576
　tracheostomy and, 445
　transfusion reactions and, 211
Bleeding time (BT), 134, 207
Blepharoplasty, definition of, 453
Blind nasotracheal intubation, 416
Blood
　perioperative replacement of, 207-208
　universal donor, 718
Blood component therapy, 209-210
　after multiple trauma, 718
　types, 210-211
Blood fluid balance, 201-203
Blood gas transport, 165, 169-170; see also
　　Arterial blood gas
Blood plasma, 203
Blood platelets, 134-135
Blood pressure
　after carotid endarterectomy, 500
　after cranial surgery, 532, 533
　after pediatric surgery, 669
　after vascular surgery, 502
　amphetamines abuse and, 702

Blood pressure (Continued)
　cardiac compression for CPR and, 740
　cardiac output and, 128
　Class IV hemorrhage and, 724
　fluid resuscitation after multiple trauma
　　and, 718
　hypertension detection and, 144-145
　hypotension detection and, 143
　hypothalamus and, 101
　in infants and young children, 662, 662t
　invasive measurement, 373
　limbic system and, 99
　malignant hyperthermia and, 709, 709b,
　　711b, 712
　microcirculation and, 135
　monitoring, 371-373, 372
　naloxone dosage and, 312
　neurogenic shock and, 726
　noninvasive automatic monitoring, 372-
　　373
　noninvasive manual monitoring, 371-372
　obesity and, 651
　phencyclidine abuse and, 702
　physostigmine salicylate and, 139
　pregnancy, anesthesia and, 690
　in trauma patient, 720
Blood urea nitrogen (BUN), 199
　diabetes mellitus and, 646
Blood vessels, 135
Blood volume; see also Hypervolemia;
　　Hypovolemia
　alcohol abuse and, 701
　distributive shock and, 723
　in infants and children, 664, 673
　kidney regulation of, 192-193
　maldistribution of, septic shock and, 727
　obesity and, 649
　pregnancy and, 689b, 691
　trauma and loss of, 716, 719
Bloodborne diseases, transmission
　　prevention of, 41
Blood-brain barrier, 111-112
　chemoreceptor trigger zone and, 656
Blood-CSF barrier, 111-112
Blood-gas partition coefficient, 279, 279t,
　　289-290
　for enflurane, 285
Blunt trauma, 715
　cardiogenic shock and, 724
　shock from, 717t
Blunted response, to carbon dioxide
　　response test, 181, 185
Body mass index, 649
　obesity, hypoxemia and, 650
Body of fornix, 99
Body Substance Isolation, 40
Body temperature; see also Hyperthermia;
　　Hypothermia; Temperature; Thermal
　　imbalance
　amphetamines abuse and, 702
　assessment, 706-707
　cardiac surgery and, 486-487, 491
　during cardiopulmonary bypass, 484-485
　club drugs abuse and, 703
　cranial surgery and, 532-533
　diencephalon and regulation of, 100
　hypertension and, 145

Body temperature (Continued)
　hypothalamus and, 101
　in infants and children, 664-665
　　blood products or fluids infusion and,
　　　672
　　pediatric circle system and, 666
　　postoperative, 667, 669, 673
　inhalation agents and, 290
　LSD and, 702
　malignant hyperthermia and, 709, 711b
　muscle relaxants and, 331
　oxygen transport and, 171
　PACU patient influences on, 386b
　pediatric surgery and, 669
　postoperative monitoring of, 385-386
　pulse oximetry interpretation and, 364
　regulation of, 232, 232, 706
　shock and, 723
　sickle cell anemia and, 654
　sympathectomy and, 499
　thermal burns and, 236
　transfusion reactions and, 211
　vascular surgery and, 502-503
Bohr effect, 172
Bone demineralization, spinal cord injuries
　　and, 544
Bone marrow
　damage, inhalant abuse and, 703
　depression, thiazide diuretics and, 196
Botulinus toxin, neurohumoral transmission
　　and, 142t
Botulism, as biological warfare agent, 731b,
　　733
Bowel perforation, after laparoscopy, 586,
　　588, 639
Bowman's capsule, 190, 191
Brachial plexus, 121
　nerve block, 352
　postsurgical injuries, 358
Bradycardia
　definition of, 125
　fentanyl and, 307
　during laparoscopy, 635
　muscle relaxants and, 336
　nasal intubation and, 181
　neurogenic shock and, 726
　PACU ventilation and, 181
　pediatric surgery and, 670
　propofol and, 294
　rectal examination and, 225
　sinus, postoperative monitoring for, 375,
　　375
　spinal cord injuries and, 540
　symptomatic sinus, atropine for, 746
Bradykinesia, drug-induced parkinsonism
　　and, 98
Bradykinin
　caveoli and, 167
　septic shock and, 727
Bradypnea, definition of, 150
Brain, 93-115; see also Cranial surgery
　arterial blood supply to, 112, 113, 114
　basal view, 95
　cerebral blood flow regulation, 112-113
　concussion, neurogenic shock and, 726
　coronal section, 109
　cranial nerves and their functions, 103t

Brain (Continued)
 CSF circulation through, 107
 forebrain, 94-101
 hindbrain, 102, 104
 inhalation anesthesia and, 280
 injury consequences, 520-523
 injury types, 520
 intercranial pressure and, 113-115
 lateral view, 94
 malignant hyperthermia and, 712
 meninges covering section of, 106
 midbrain, 94
 partial pressure, inhalation anesthetics
  and, 278
 parts of, 93-94
 pathologic condition types, 523-524
 protection of, 104-112
 venous drainage of, 108
Brain scan, for cranial surgery diagnosis, 520
Brain stem, 99, 101
 breathing regulation and, 182-183
 cerebellum and, 102
 foramen magnum and, 106
 functional description of, 104
 limbic system and, 100
 pyramidal cell axons and, 97
Breast biopsy
 care after, 592
 definition of, 590
Breast cancer, inflammatory, definition of,
  591
Breast lift, 591
 definition of, 591
Breast reconstruction, 595-596, 595-596
 definition of, 590
 muscle-skin flap, 595-596, 596
Breast surgery, 590-599
 lumpectomy, 592-594, 593
 mammoplasty, 597-598
 mastectomy, 593, 594, 594-595
 mastopexy, 591, 596-597
 perianesthetic care after, 592-598
 reconstruction, 595-596
Breathing; see also Respiration; Sustained
  maximum inspiration
 apneustic, 183
  definition of, 150
 for cardiopulmonary resuscitation
  primary survey, 738-739
  secondary survey, 743
 cranial surgery and, 534t
 deep
  after pediatric surgery, 670
  respiratory compromise and, 736
 depth of anesthesia and patterns of, 278
 eye surgery and, 459
 by newborns, 661, 662
 obesity and, 649
 positive-pressure, 409
 regulation of, 179-183
  carbon dioxide response in, 181
  central chemoreceptors in, 180-181
  controllers in, 182-183
  lung receptors in, 182
  peripheral chemoreceptors in, 179-180
  sensors in, 179-182
  upper airways receptors in, 181-182

Breathing (Continued)
 in stir-up regimen, 393-394
 trauma injuries and, 719, 720-721
Brethine; see Terbutaline
Bretylium (Bretylol), 252t
 d-tubocurarine interaction with, 267t
Brevibloc; see Esmolol
Brevital, 259t, 293
Bricker operation, definition of, 567
Broca's area, 97, 98
Bronchi, 156-157
 distribution in lungs, 156
Bronchial arteries, 157
Bronchial bifurcation angles, 155, 155-156,
  155t
Bronchial circulation, nutrition and, 167
Bronchiectasis, definition of, 150
Bronchiolar lumen, 156
Bronchioles, 156, 157
Bronchitis, chronic, 642
 marijuana abuse and, 702
 preexisting, postoperative complications
  and, 183
 smoking and, 652, 653
Bronchoconstriction
 anaphylactic shock and, 726
 septic shock and, 727
Bronchodilatation
 cyclic AMP and, 140
 marijuana abuse and, 702
Bronchodilators, during ambulatory surgery,
  619b
Bronchopulmonary dysplasia, prematurity
  and, 665
Bronchoscope, flexible fiber-optic, 466
Bronchoscopy
 bleeding after, 471
 definition of, 465
 positioning after, 467
 topical anesthesia for, 467
Bronchospasm, 157
 definition of, 150
 local anesthetics and, 344
 postoperative, 363
 respiratory compromise and, 736
Bronkosol, respiratory care and, 266t
Brown-Sequard syndrome, 539
Brucellosis, as biological warfare agent,
  731b
Bubonic plague, 732
Budesonide (Rhinocort), respiratory care
  and, 266t
Buffers; see also Acid-base buffers
 for cardiopulmonary resuscitation, 743
Bulb catheters, after abdominoperineal
  resection, 561
Bumetanide, 196
Bumetanide (Bumex), 252t
Bumex, 196
Bundle of His, 130
Bupivacaine (Marcaine, Sensorcaine), 252t,
  341, 342t, 343
 for cesarean section, 693
 for eye surgery, 456
 malignant hyperthermia and, 710b
 and morphine, for post C-section pain
  relief, 695

Buprenorphine (Buprenex), 311
Burn injuries, 607-614
 aseptic technique for, 233-234, 236
 carboxyhemoglobin and, 365
 classification of, 607-608
 extent of, 608
 pathophysiology of, 610-611
 perianesthesia nursing care, 613
 succinylcholine contraindications in, 328
 types, 609-610
 wound management, 611-613
Burnout; see Stress
Bursa-dependent cells, 239
 definition of, 238
Butane lighter gases, abuse of, 703
Butisol, abuse of, effects and signs of, 698t
Butorphanol (Stadol), 253t, 309, 310t
 opiate abuse and, 700
Buttocks, trauma nurse's assessment of, 721
Butyl nitrite, abuse of, 703
Butyrophenones, 299-301
 extrapyramidal reactions and, 98
Bypass, 500
 definition of, 493

C

C fibers, of afferent nerve, 340
C wave, 126, 531
Caffeine
 for apnea in premature infants, 665
 bronchodilatation and, 141
 malignant hyperthermia and, 710b
Calan, for hypertension, 146t
Calcitonin, 216
Calcium, 206
 after thyroid surgery, 550
 dantrolene and, 710
 magnesium and, 207
 malignant hyperthermia and, 709, 712
 muscle relaxants and, 268t, 330
 neuromuscular transmission and, 318,
  319, 708
 regulatory mechanisms of, 216-217
Calcium channel blockers, 141, 143
 for cardiac surgery complications, 488
 muscle relaxants and, 331
Calcium chloride
 digitalis interaction with, 269t
 for malignant hyperthermia cart, 8b
Calcium gluconate, for malignant
  hyperthermia treatment, 712b
Calcium salts, malignant hyperthermia and,
  710b
Caldwell-Luc operation, definition of,
  433
Calices, renal, 189, 191
Cancer
 drug-induced immunosuppression for,
  246
 laparoscopy and, 637
 of penis, 578
 smoking and, 652
Cannabinoids, abuse of, 697, 702
 effects and signs of, 699t
Capillaries, 135
 in alveoli, 157
 blood-brain barrier and, 112

Capillary hydrostatic pressure (P_{cap}), 168
Capillary leak syndrome, after cardiac
  surgery, 490
Capillary refilling
  Class IV hemorrhage and, 724
  moderate phase hemorrhage and, 723
  orthopedic surgery and, 508
  progressive phase hemorrhage and, 724
  in trauma patient, 720
Capnographs, 366
  for CPR assessment, 743
  end-tidal *versus* arterial carbon dioxide,
    367
Capnography, 362, 366-371
  clinical issues in, 368-371
  interpreting changes in, 367-368, 368,
    369, 370
  normal capnogram, 367, 367
  technology overview, 366-367
Capnometers, 366
Captopril (Capoten), 253t
Carbaminohemoglobin, carbon dioxide
  transport and, 172-173
Carbocaine; *see* Mepivacaine
Carbohydrate metabolism, hypothalamus
  and, 101
Carbon dioxide; *see also* Capnography
  arterial pressure, respiratory compromise
    and, 736
  central chemoreceptors in breathing
    regulation and, 179-180
  cerebral blood flow and, 525-526
  coronary blood flow and, 131
  end tidal
    for CPR assessment, 743
    for trauma patient assessment, 719
  gas embolus, pneumoperitoneum and,
    638t
  for laser surgery, 630t
  oxygen transport and, 171-172
  pH, muscle relaxants and, 330
  for pneumoperitoneum in laparoscopy,
    635, 636t
  rising end-tidal level of, malignant
    hyperthermia and, 678
Carbon dioxide dissociation curve, 172,
  173
Carbon dioxide response curve, 181, 181
Carbon dioxide transport, 172-174, 174
  carbaminohemoglobin and, 172-173
  pulse oximetry interpretation and, 364
  in solution, 172
Carbon monoxide poisoning,
  carboxyhemoglobin and, 365
Carbon tetrachloride
  malignant hyperthermia and, 710b
  toxic jaundice and, 226
Carbonic anhydrase inhibitors, 195, 197
Carboxyhemoglobin, 365, 400, 652
Cardene, 261t
Cardiac antiarrhythmics, during ambulatory
  surgery, 619b
Cardiac arrest
  anaphylactic shock and, 726
  definition of, 125
  Stage II anesthesia and, 276
Cardiac catheterization, definition of, 475

Cardiac compression, for cardiopulmonary
  resuscitation, 739-741, 740
  rates for newborn, infant, child, or adult,
    741t
Cardiac cycle, 126-127, 127
Cardiac disease
  anesthetics and, 131
  epidural block for, 351
  functional classification of, 132b
  neostigmine and, 326
  thoracic surgery and, 471
Cardiac dysrhythmias; *see also* Ventricular
    dysrhythmias
  alcohol abuse and, 701
  anaphylactic shock and, 726
  cardiogenic shock and, 724-725, 725
  during laparoscopy, 635
  malignant hyperthermia and, 712
  procainamide and, 710
  shock and, 723
  as transfusion reaction, 398
  vascular surgery and, 501-502
Cardiac index
  aging and, 682
  cardiac surgery and, 486
  cardiogenic shock and, 725
  postoperative monitoring, 384
Cardiac inotropic agents, for hypotension,
  144
Cardiac output, 127-128
  aging and, 682
  burn injuries and, 610
  cardiac surgery and, 486
  cardiac surgery complications and, 487,
    488
  cardiogenic shock and, 724-725
  definition of, 125
  during laparoscopy, 635
  neurogenic shock and, 726
  obesity and, 649
  postoperative monitoring, 384
  during pregnancy, 688
  pulmonary circulation and, 167
  septic shock and, 727
Cardiac reflexes, medulla oblongata and, 102
Cardiac surgery, 473-492
  anesthesia for, 485
  complications, 487-491
  definitions, 473-483
  gastrointestinal system and, 491
  intraoperative considerations, 484-485
  nervous system and, 491
  PACU care after, 485-487
  patient transition from operating room to
    PACU after, 356-357, 485
  physiologic changes with CPB, 484-485
  renal system and, 491
  respiratory system and, 490-491
Cardiac surgical intensive care unit
  (CSICU), 473
Cardiac tamponade, 716, 718t
  cardiac surgery complications and, 487,
    488-489
  cardiogenic shock and, 725
  cardiopulmonary arrest and, 744
  obstructive shock and, 723, 728
  pulseless electrical activity and, 720

Cardiogenic shock, 716, 717t, 723, 724-725
Cardiomegaly, obesity and, 651
Cardiomyopathies, cardiogenic shock and,
  725
Cardiomyotomy, 559
Cardioplegia, definition of, 475
Cardiopulmonary bypass (CPB), 476
  for cardiac surgery, 484
  definition of, 475-476
  physiologic changes associated with, 484-
    485
  for thoracic aneurysms, after vascular
    surgery, 503
Cardiopulmonary resuscitation (CPR), 83-
  85, 735-746
  asystole, 744
  emergency equipment, 736-737
  ethical issues, 735
  indications for, 736
  pharmacological therapy, 744-746
  primary ABCD survey, 737-743
    airway, 737-738
    breathing, 738-739
    circulation, 739-741
    defibrillation, 741-743
  secondary ABCD survey, 743-744
    airway, 743
    breathing, 743
    circulation, 743
    differential diagnosis, 743-744
  steps in, 737
  urgency of, 735-736
Cardiovascular disease
  drug effects and, 265
  PET scans and diagnosis of, 520
Cardiovascular function, postoperative,
  371-374
  blood pressure monitoring, 371-373
    clinical issues, 373
    invasive, 373
    noninvasive automatic, 372-373
    noninvasive manual, 371-372
  clinical assessment, 371
  hypothermia in children, 673-674
  prostate surgery and, 576
  pulse pressure monitoring, 373-374
Cardiovascular system
  adrenergic and cholinergic receptors,
    135-148
  aging and, 682
  circulatory system, 133-135
  heart, 126-133
  in infants and young children, 662,
    664
  laparoscopy and, 634
  methylxanthines and, 141
  morphine and, 306
  obesity and, 649-650
  pregnancy and, 689b, 690b
  rheumatoid arthritis and, 647-648
  smoking and, 652-653
  succinylcholine effects on, 327
Cardioversion
  diazepam and, 295
  for supraventricular arrhythmias, 376-
    377
  for ventricular arrhythmias, 377, 377

Cardizem, 141, 143, 254t
Carina, 155
Carotid arteries, 112, *113*
    arterial blood pressure and, 128
    rupture after radical neck surgery, 449
Carotid blowout, 449
Carotid bodies, breathing regulation and,
    179-180
Carotid bypass, 496
Carotid endarterectomy, 496, 499-500
    cranial nerve assessment for, 500, 500t
Carotid pulse, in trauma patient, 720
Carpopedal spasm, hypomagnesemia and,
    207
Cast care
    after amputation, 515
    after orthopedic surgery, 509
Catapres; *see* Clonidine
Cataracts
    definition of, 453
    surgery for, 452, 456-457
Catecholamines, 213
    action of, *142*
    adrenalectomy and, 578
    adrenergic receptors and, 140
    beta₁ receptors and, 140
    enflurane contraindication with, 286
    muscle relaxants and, 330
    potassium loss and, 206
    regulation of, 217
    see also Epidural catheter pumps;
    Foley catheter(s); Retention catheters
    for airway management, 413-414
    bladder injuries and, 639
    bulb, after abdominal resection, 561
    central venous, for infants or children,
        671-672
    coudé-tip, for tracheostomy suctioning,
        443
    fiberoptic, 531
    grenade, after abdominoperineal
        resection, 561
    indwelling, for infants and children, 673
    infections related to, 40b
    placement for premature infants, 665
    pulmonary artery
        flow-directed, 379
        myocardial infarction and, 133
    suprapubic, 569-570, 575
        mushroom, *576*
    Swan-Ganz, 133
        for malignant hyperthermia treatment,
            712b
        severe chest injuries and, 719
    ureteral, 570
    urethral, 569
        postoperative use of, 198, 568-569,
            570
        after C-section, 584
    ventricular, 530, *530*, 531
Cations
    definition of, 201
    fluid distribution and, 204
Caudal block, for regional anesthesia in
    children, 675
Caudate nucleus, 95-96, *96*, 96, *100*
Caveoli, 167

Cavernous sinus, *108*
Cecostomy, definition of, 551
Celiotomy, definition of, 554
Cell membrane stabilizers, for pain
    management, 424
Cell Saver blood recovery systems, for
    severe chest injuries, 719
Cellular/cell-mediated immunity, 239, 241-
    242
    definition of, 238
Centers for Disease Control and Prevention
    (CDC), 40, 55
    bioterrorism response planning, 731
    bioterrorism response systems, 731-732
    on postoperative infection control, 405
    Universal Precautions, 233
Central compartment in compartmental
    model of pharmacokinetics, 250
Central cord syndrome (CCS) 539
Central nervous system, 93-124
    blood-brain and blood-CSF barriers of,
        111-112
    brain, 93-115
        oxygen toxicity and, 187
        postoperative monitoring of, 385
    spinal cord, 115-123
Central nervous system depressants, abuse
    of, 697, 700-701
    effects and signs of, 698-699t
Central nervous system sympathomimetics,
    abuse of, 697, 702
    effects and signs of, 699t
Central sulcus, 94, 95, 97
Central venous pressure (CVP), *199*
    during laparoscopy, 635
    monitor, 133
Cephalosporins, muscle relaxants and,
    330b
Cerclage procedure, 584-585
    definition of, 581
Cerebellar ataxia, 102
Cerebellar nuclei, 102
Cerebellum, 94, *94*, 95, *100*
    brainstem and, *102*
    CSF circulation through, *107*, *110*
    functional description of, 102, 104
    pyramidal cell axons and, 97
Cerebral anoxia, vomiting center excitation
    and, 656
Cerebral aqueduct, 94, 101, *102*, *111*
    CSF circulation through, *107*, *109*, *110*
Cerebral atrophy, diagnosis of, 519
Cerebral blood flow (CBF)
    inhalant anesthetic agents and, 527
    intracranial pressure and, 525-526
Cerebral cortex, 94-95, *109*
    breathing regulation and, 182-183
    functional areas of, 97
Cerebral hypoperfusion, progressive phase
    hemorrhage and, 723-724
Cerebral nuclei, 94, 95-96
Cerebral peduncles, 94, *101*
    functional description of, 101
Cerebral perfusion pressure (CPP), 113-
    114
    autoregulation and, 526
    intracranial pressure and, 525

Cerebrospinal fluid (CSF), 94, 109, 203-
    204
    cerebral aqueduct and, 101
    drainage from nose or ears, 720
    in fourth ventricle, 104
    intracranial pressure monitoring and,
        529-531
    nasal suctioning caution, 106
Cerebrospinal fluid (CSF) system, 109-111
    intercranial pressure and, 113-115, *115*
Cerebrovascular accidents, internal capsule
    and, 98
Cerebrovascular resistance (CVR),
    intracranial pressure and, 525
Cerebrum, 93-94, *94*
    coronal section in front of thalamus, 96
    coronal view from anterior backward,
        100
    CSF circulation through, *107*, *110*
    functional aspects of, 96
Certified Ambulatory Perianesthesia nurse
    (CAPA), 12, 14b
    expertise development and, 20
Certified Postanesthesia Nurse (CPAN),
    12, 14b
    expertise development and, 20
Certified Registered Nurse Anesthetist,
    medical malpractice claims study by,
    66-67
Cervical conization, definition of, 581
Cervical plexus, 121
Cervical spine
    injuries to, 537
        in children, 679, 679-680
    segments of, 118, *119*
    surgery on, 514
Cervical vertebrae, 115, *116*
    skull and, *105*
Cervicodorsal sympathectomy, 498-499
Cesarean hysterectomy, definition of, 581
Cesarean section (C-section)
    care after, 583-584
    definition of, 581
    epidural block for, 351, 693
    postoperative pain management, 694-695
    spinal anesthesia for, 693
Chalazion, definition of, 453
Checklists, electronic, risk management
    and, 73
Chemical burns, 236, 609-610, 715
Chemical regulation
    arterial blood pressure and, 128
    cardiac muscle excitability and
        contractility and, 130b
Chemoreceptor trigger zone (CTZ),
    vomiting and, 656
Chemoreceptors, for breathing regulation
    central, 180-181
    peripheral, 179-180
Chemotactic factor
    cellular immunity and, 242
    immediate hypersensitivity reaction and,
        242
Chest compression for cardiopulmonary
    resuscitation, 739-741
    rates for newborn, infant, child, or adult,
        741t

Chest drainage systems, 469-470, 470
Chest tubes
    after cardiac surgery, 486
    for cardiac surgery, 484
    cardiac surgery complications and quality
        of drainage from, 488
    definition of, 465
    management after thoracic surgery, 469,
        469-470
Chest wall
    integrity of, in trauma patient, 719, 720-
        721
    reconstruction, definition of, 465
Cheyne-Stokes respirations, 534t
    definition of, 150
Chilblains, 236
    definition of, 231
Children; see also Infants
    age-specific pain measurement tools for,
        676t
    airway equipment for, 663t
    ambulatory surgery for, 619
        fasting, 620
    anatomic and physiologic considerations
        body fluids composition and
            regulation, 664-665
        cardiovascular system, 662, 664
        respiratory system, 661-662
    anesthesia for, 661
        administration techniques, 666-667
    cardiac compression for CPR, 739-741
    cardiovascular age-related changes in,
        662t
    development stage theories, 669t
    discharge from PACU, 680
    eye hit with BB, 463
    eye surgery and, 457
    gynecomastia, 597, 598
    inhalant abuse by, 703
    intravenous fluids for, 387
    intravenous premedications before
        surgery, 620
    ketamine anesthesia and, 301, 302
    otolaryngologic surgery for, 679
    pain management for, 429
        age-specific measurement tools for, 676t
    postoperative care for, 667-675
        monitoring procedures, 669-673
        pain management and regional
            analgesia, 674-675
        problems after ambulatory surgery,
            622
        psychosocial considerations, 668-669
        thermal regulation in PACU, 673-674
        safety considerations, 674
    postoperative concerns, 675
        airway obstruction, 677
        laryngospasm, 675
        malignant hyperthermia, 678
        nausea and vomiting, 677-678
    succinylcholine contraindications for,
        327-328
    tonsillectomy and adenoidectomy for,
        438
    tracheostomy complications in, 445
    trauma care for, 679-680
Chin lift, for airway opening, 737, 738

Chirocaine, 341, 344; see also
    Levobupivacaine
Chloramphenicol
    muscle relaxants and, 330b
    for plague, 733
Chlordiazepoxide, geriatric patients and,
    685t
Chloride shift, carbon dioxide transport
    and, 173
Chloroform, 283-284
    abuse of, 703
    toxic jaundice and, 226
Chloroprocaine (Nesacaine), 253t, 341,
    342t; see also Nesacaine
    C-section and, 693, 695
    malignant hyperthermia and, 711b
Chlorothiazide, 195
Chlorpromazine (Thorazine)
    after ear surgery, 435
    droperidol and, 299
    extrapyramidal reactions and, 98
    for LSD bad trips, 703
    muscle relaxants and, 269t
Chlorpropamide (Diabinese), 253t
Cholecystectomy
    biliary lithotripsy versus, 227-228
    definition of, 551
    laparoscopic, 564, 634
        care after, 564-565
    meperidine for pain management in, 423
Cholecystostomy, definition of, 551
Cholelithiasis, 227-228
    definition of, 221
Cholinergic, definition of, 125
Cholinergic nerves, 136b
    acetylcholine and, 135-136
    drugs that interfere with transmission by,
        142t
Cholinergic neurotransmitters,
    biochemistry, 136, 137b
Cholinergic receptors, 137-139
    neuromuscular transmission and, 317, 318
    organs stimulated by, 139t
Cholinesterase
    LSD and, 703
    plasma, 226
    pregnancy and, 691
Chordae tendineae, 129
Chordee, definition of, 566
Choroid plexuses, 100, 102, 109, 110
    blood-CSF barrier and, 112
Chronic obstructive pulmonary disease
    (COPD), 162, 642-644
    cardiac surgery complications and, 487
    description of, 642
    geriatric patients and, 686
    midazolam and, 296
    perianesthetic care, 643-644
    smoking and, 652
    surgical considerations, 642
    water loss and, 202
Chronic subdural hematoma, 522
Chronotropic, definition of, 125
Chronotropism, 129
Chvostek's sign, 207
    after thyroid surgery, 550
    definition of, 201

Chyme, definition of, 221
Cigar smoking, 652
Cigarette smoking; see also Smoking
    chronic bronchitis and, 642
    postoperative pulmonary complications
        and, 184
Cilia, nasal, 151-152, 152
    immunologic defense and, 238-239
Cimetidine (Tagamet), 253t
    for aspiration pneumonitis in pregnant
        patients, 692
    pharmacologic effects on latter drugs
        from, 271
    tetracaine and, 344
    for vomiting/regurgitation, 223-224
Cineplastic amputation, definition of, 506
Cingulate gyrus, 99
Cingulum, 99
Ciprofloxacin, for anthrax, 732
Circle of Willis, 111
Circle system, for inhalation anesthesia
    administration, 281
Circulatory system, 133-135
    blood platelets, 134-135
    blood vessels, 135
    for cardiopulmonary resuscitation
        primary survey, 739-741
        secondary survey, 743
    carotid endarterectomy and, 499-500
    microcirculation, 135
    overload, as transfusion reaction, 398
    red blood cells, 133-134
    in trauma patient, 719-720
    vascular surgery and, 496-498, 502
    white blood cells, 134
Circumcision, 578
    definition of, 566
    regional anesthesia and, 675
Circumflex arteries, 131
Circus movement
    definition of, 126
    reduction of, 141
Cisatracurium (Nimbex), 253t, 324
Cistern, definition of, 93
Cistern magna, 109-110
Citanest, 262t, 343; see also Prilocaine
Citrate intoxication, as transfusion
    reaction, 398
Claustrophobia, MRI and, 519
Claustrum, 96, 96
Clinical nurse specialists (CNS), PACU
    role for, 15-16
Clinical practice guidelines
    definitions of, 71-72
    risk management and, 73
Clinitest, for insulin and glucose
    monitoring, 646, 646t
Clones
    definition of, 238
    humoral immunity and, 239-240
Clonidine (Catapres, Dixarit), 253t
    alpha$_2$ receptors and, 140
    Inapsine interaction with, 267t
    withdrawal
        for opiate detoxification in PACU,
            315
        syndrome, 140

Closed (tension) pneumothorax, 164
Closing capacity (CC), 161
  pregnancy and, 691
Closing volume (CV), 161
Clostridium botulinum, 733
Clotting; *see* Coagulation system
Club drugs, abuse of, 697, 703-704
Cluster breathing, 534t
CO_2; *see* Carbon dioxide
Coagulation system
  assessment of, 207-208
  burn injuries and, 611
  cardiac surgery and, 489-490
  during cardiopulmonary bypass, 485
  hypothermia in newborns and infants
    and, 673-674
  liver and, 227
  liver surgery and, 563
  partial thromboplastin time and, 134
  pregnancy and, 691
Coagulopathy, consumption, multiple
  trauma and, 718
Coarctation of the aorta, 477
  definition of, 476
Cocaine, 253t, 339, 341, 342t
  abuse of, 697, 702
    effects and signs of, 699t
  neurohumoral transmission and, 142t
Coccygeal spinal segment, 118, *119*
Coccyx, 115, 116-117
Cochlear branch of acoustic nerves (VII),
  103t
Cochlear implant, 436
  definition of, 433
Codeine, 304
  abuse of, effects and signs of, 698t
  for oral analgesia, 431
Cogentin; *see* Benztropine
Cold burns, 609
Colfosceril (Exosurf), respiratory care and,
  266t
Colistin, muscle relaxants and, 268t, 271,
  330b
Collecting ducts, renal, 190, *191*
Colliculi, 101
Colloid oncotic pressure, 208
Colloid osmotic pressure, 204-205
Colloid solutions, for fluid resuscitation in
  multiple trauma, 718
Colloids, 208-209
  definition of, 201
  thyroid gland and, 216
Colon, 225
  laparoscopic perforation of, 639
Color analog scales, for pain measurement
  in children, 676t
Colorimetric sensor, direct-reading liquid
  crystal, 706-707
Colostomy, *561*
  abdominoperineal resection and, 561-
    562
  care after, 560
  definition of, 551
  site of, 225
Colpocleisis, 587
Colporrhaphy, definition of, 581
Column of fornix, 99

Coma
  from anthrax, 732
  brain injuries and, 520
  diabetic, 646
    characteristics, 647t
  gamma hydroxybutyrate and, 704
Comminuted fractures, of skull, 520
Commission on Medical Malpractice, 65
Commissural fibers, 95
Commissure, definition of, 93
Commissurotomy, definition of, 476
Committee on Quality of Health Care in
  America, 71
Communication
  ERR WATCH principles on, 50-51
  informed consent/refusal and, 81, 82
  medical malpractice suits and, 69
  perioperative and perianesthesia nurses,
    354-358
  resuscitation orders and, 84-85
Compartment syndrome
  after orthopedic surgery, 510
    on arm or forearm, 511
  blunt trauma and, 715-716
  from trauma injury, 720
Compartmental model of
  pharmacokinetics, 249-250, *250*
Compazine, 262t, 460, 658t
Competitive antagonists, definition of, 248
Complement split-products, septic shock
  and, 727
Complement system
  during cardiopulmonary bypass, 484
  humoral immunity and, 240, 241
Compliance, definition of, 517
Compliance (lung), definition of, 150
Compliance (lung) (C_L), 161-165
Compound fractures, of skull, 520
Compresses, after ophthalmic surgery, 461
Compression forces, trauma and, 715
Compression fracture, of spine, 537, *538*
Computed tomography (CT), for vascular
  disease diagnosis, 493
Concentration effect, for inhalation
  anesthetic, 278
Concussions, 520
  neurogenic shock and, 726
Conduction, definition of, 125, 317
Conduction anesthesia, 339
  recovery from, 340b
Conductor pads, adhesive, for defibrillation,
  742
Condyles
  of knee joint, 512
  of lower jaw, temporal bones and, 104
Confidentiality, medical ethics and, 78
Congestive heart failure, cardiac surgery
  complications and, 487, 488
Conjugate gaze, cranial surgery and, 535
Conjunctivitis, anaphylactic shock and,
  726
Consciousness; *see also* Level of
  consciousness
  as anesthetic stage, 276
  arteriovenous malformations and, 524
  asystole and, 744
  Class IV hemorrhage and, 724

Consciousness (*Continued*)
  concussions and, 520
  epidural hematoma and, 521
  intracranial pressure assessment and,
    532-533
  progressive phase hemorrhage and, 724
  reticular formation and, 104
  shock and, 723
Constipation, opioids for pain management
  and, 424
Contact dermatitis, local anesthetics and,
  344
Contact lenses, trauma nurse's check for,
  720
Contact-transmission precautions, 40b
Continuous passive motion (CPM)
  machines
  knee surgery and, 507
  LiteLift, *514*
Continuous positive airway pressure, 401,
  402, 402t
  after cardiac surgery, 485-486
Continuous quality improvement, 41-43,
  43
Contraceptives, oral, insulin interaction
  with, 270t
Contrast media, anaphylactic shock and,
  726
Contusions
  blunt trauma and, 715
  cardiac, shock from, 717t
  of skull, 520
  from trauma injury, 720, 721
Convection warming, postanesthetic
  warming and, 707
Convolutions, in cerebral cortex, 95
Convulsions; *see* Seizures
COPD; *see* Chronic obstructive pulmonary
  disease
Cor pulmonale
  definition of, 125
  emphysema and, 642
Corlopam, 256t
Corneal transplant surgery, *455*
Coronal suture, *105*
Coronary arteries, 131
  dilators, during ambulatory surgery, 619b
  obesity and, 651
Coronary artery steal, 131
Coronary cardiogenic shock, 724
Corpora quadrigemina, 94, 101
Corpus callosum, 94, 95, 96, *100*
  blood supplies for, 112
Corpus striatum, 96
  blood supplies for, 112
Corpuscles, renal, 190
Cortex, 96
  basal ganglia and, 96
  renal, 189
    steroids regulation by, 217
Corticobulbar tracts, in the pons, 102
Corticospinal tracts, in the pons, 102
Corticosteroids, 266t
  for anaphylactic shock, 726-727
  for cardiogenic shock, 725
  for immunosuppression, 246
  insulin interaction with, 270t

Corticosteroids (*Continued*)
  intracranial pressure and, 529
  for postintubation croup, 677
  respiratory care and, 266t
Corticotropin-releasing hormone (CRH),
    ACTH and, 215, 217
Cortisol, 217
  in blood, during laparoscopy, 637
Cortisone, after adrenalectomy, 578
Cost containment; *see also* Managed care
  perianesthesia nursing and, 11, 59
Cost-benefit analysis, managed care and, 61
Cost-effectiveness analysis, managed care
  and, 61-62
Coudé-tip catheter, for tracheostomy
  suctioning, 443
Cough, nonproductive, anthrax and, 732
Cough/coughing reflex, 102
  after abdominal surgery, 559
  after eye surgery, 459
  after geriatric surgery, 686
  after hip or femoral surgery, 512
  after laryngoscopy, 441
  after pediatric surgery, 670
  after thoracic surgery, 468
  for geriatric patients, 683
  nausea and, 658
  perianesthesia nursing care, 186
  postoperative, 362, 394
    smoking and, 653
Countershock
  external direct current (DC), 378, *378*
  myocardial infarction and, 133
Covert (ibutilide fumarate), 257t
COX-2 NSAIDs, for pain management, 423
CPR; *see* Cardiopulmonary resuscitation
Cranial bones, 104, 106
  lateral view of, *105*
Cranial dura, 106
Cranial nerve(s), *100, 101, 101*
  assessment for carotid endarterectomy
    patient, 500t
  basal view of, *95*
  brainstem and, 104
  names and functions of, 103t
  parasympathetic nervous system and,
    123
  in the pons, 102
Cranial surgery, 518-535
  brain injuries and pathologic conditions,
    520-524
  definition of, 517
  diagnostic tools, 518-520
  intracranial pressure assessment, 531-532
  intracranial pressure dynamics, 524-531
  PACU nursing care after, 535, 536b
  postoperative nursing management, 532-
    535
Craniectomy, definition of, 517
Craniotomy, definition of, 517
Cranium, 104
  interior of, *105*
Creatine phosphokinase (CPK), 132
  malignant hyperthermia and, 708, 709b
Creatinine, 193, 194t
  after kidney transplantation, 573
Creatinine clearance, 198, *199*

Crepitus, 469; *see also* Emphysema,
  subcutaneous
  definition of, 517
Crew Resource Management, 45
Cribriform palate, *105*
Cribriform plate, 106
Cricoid cartilage, 152, 153, *153*
  in newborns, edema near, 661
Cricoid pressure, anesthesia induction in
  pregnant patients and, 692
Crisis Resource Management (CRM), 45-
  53
  ERR WATCH principles, 47-51, 48b
  human factors in, 45-47
  simulated patient for training in, 52-53
  training, 45
  training format, 51-52
Crista galli, *105*
Cromolyn (Intal), respiratory care and,
  266t
"Crossing the Quality Chasm: A New
  Health System for the 21st Century"
  (Committee on Quality of Health
  Care in America), 71
Cross-tolerance, definition of, 248
Croup, postintubation, 677
Crowing, postoperative, 362
Cruciate ligaments, 512
Cruzan, Nancy, 79, 85-86
Crying, heart rate after pediatric surgery
  and, 670
CryoCuff system, *513*
Cryoprecipitate, 211
  definition of, 201
Cryotherapy, of eye, *458*
Cryptorchidism, malignant hyperthermia
  and, 708
Crystalloids, 208-209
  after cardiac surgery, 490
  for blood loss hemorrhage, 724
  definition of, 201
  for fluid resuscitation in multiple trauma,
    718
CT scanning; *see also* Computed
  tomography
  for cranial surgery diagnosis, 518-519,
    519
  for spinal surgery diagnosis, 535
Culdoscopy, definition of, 581
Curare; *see also* d-Tubocurarine chloride
  kidney disease and, 198
Cushing's reflex, 533
Cushing's triad, 533
Cutaneous anthrax, 732
Cyanosis
  from anthrax, 732
  definition of, 125, 150
  evaluation for postoperative, 362
  malignant hyperthermia and, 709, 709b
  orthopedic surgery and, 508
  shock and, 723
  surgery with COPD and, 644
Cyclic adenosine monophosphate (cAMP),
  213
Cyclohexyl nitrite, abuse of, 703
Cyclophosphamide (Cytoxan), for
  immunosuppression, 246, 573

Cyclopropane, 284
Cyclosporine (Sandimmune), 253t
  for immunosuppression, 573
Cystectomy, definition of, 566
Cystitis, definition of, 189
Cystocele, definition of, 581
Cystolithotomy, definition of, 566
Cystoscopy, 568, 574, 578
  definition of, 566
  history of, 634
Cystotomy, definition of, 566
Cytal, for bladder irrigation, 205
Cytochrome P-450 microsomal enzyme
  system, 227
  liver and, 226
Cytotoxic hypersensitivity reaction, 242

D

Dacron bypass, aortoiliac, *502*
Dacron graft, crimped, for aneurysm of
  distal aorta, *501*
Dacryocystitis, definition of, 453
Dacryocystorhinostomy, definition of, 453
Dalgan, 310-311, 310t
Dalton's law of partial pressure, 169
Dantrolene (Dantrium), 253t
  for malignant hyperthermia, 8b, 678,
    709, 710, 711b, 712b
Date-rape drugs, abuse of, 697, 704
Day of Surgery/Procedure, perianesthesia
  nursing role in, 13b
DDAVP, 254t
De Weese caval grid filter, *494*
Dead-space air, 158, 367
Deafness, loop diuretics and, 196
Decadron; *see* Dexamethasone
Decamethonium bromide (Syncurine), 329
  kidney disease and, 197
Deceleration forces, trauma and, 715
Decerebrate rigidity, 535
Decompensation, definition of, 517
Decompression laminectomy, for spinal
  cord injuries, 539
Decorticate posturing, 535
Decortication of the lung, definition of, 465
Decussate, definition of, 93
Deep vein thrombosis
  during laparoscopy, 637
  orthopedic surgery and, 510
Deep-dermal burns, 236
Deep-dermal partial-thickness burns, 608
Defense, U.S. Department of, bioterrorism
  response system, 731-732
Defensive medicine, 65
Defibrillation, for primary CPR, 741-743,
  742
  asystole and, 744
Defibrillator/monitor, for cardiopulmonary
  resuscitation, 737, 741, *742*
Deglutition, definition of, 221
Delirium
  emergence, 385, 395, 622
    in children, 667
  Stage II anesthesia and, 276
Delirium tremens, alcohol withdrawal and,
  701
Delta opioid receptors, 304-305

Demadex, 264t
Demerol; *see* Meperidine
Dentate gyrus, 99
Deodorant sprays, abuse of, 703
Depressed skull fractures, 520
Dermatitis
    contact, as delayed hypersensitivity
        reaction, 243
    thiazide diuretics and, 196
Dermatochalasis, definition of, 453
Dermatomes
    craniad to caudad sequence, 349
    pregnancy and, 688
    spinal or regional anesthesia and, 121,
        348-349
Dermis, 231, 607
Desaturation on exercise, 166-167
Desensitization, succinylcholine and, 336
Desflurane (Suprane), 253t, 287-288
    intracranial pressure and, 528
    for pediatric anesthesia, 666, 667
Desmopressin (DDAVP), 254t
Desquamation, definition of, 231
Dexamethasone (Decadron, Respihaler,
        Turbinaire), 254t
    intracranial pressure and, 529
    for nausea, 658-659, 658t
    phenobarbital interaction with, 270t
    for postintubation croup, 677
    respiratory care and, 266t
Dextran
    as synthetic colloid, 209
    transfusion of, 399
Dextrostix, for insulin monitoring, 646
Dezocine (Dalgan), 310-311, 310t
Diabetes insipidus, 215
    definition of, 215
Diabetes mellitus, 218, 645-646
    anesthesia and, 645-646
    cardiac surgery complications and, 487
    complications, 647t
    enflurane contraindication in, 286
    eye surgery and, 452
    nursing care, 646
    obesity and, 650
Diabinese, 253t
Diagnostic testing, before ambulatory
        surgery, 620
Diamox, 197
Diaphoresis
    alcohol abuse and, 701
    from anthrax, 732
Diaphragm muscle, spinal surgery and, 514
Diaphragmatic herniorrhaphy, definition of,
        552
Diarrhea
    bloody, from gastrointestinal anthrax, 732
    definition of, 221
    sodium depletion and, 225
    water loss and, 202, 203
Diastasis, 126
Diastole, 126-127
    definition of, 125
    valve cusps and, 129
Diastolic blood pressure, 128-129, 371, 372,
        372
    cardiac compression for CPR and, 740
    cardiogenic shock and, 725

Diastolic blood pressure
    hemorrhage and, 723
    in infants and young children, 662, 662t
    during pregnancy, 688
Diazepam (Valium), 254t, 295-296
    abuse of, 700-701
        effects and signs of, 699t
    after ear surgery, 435
    alcohol withdrawal and, 701
    bupivacaine and, 343
    geriatric patients and, 685t
    ketamine with, 301
    kidney disease and, 197
    for local anesthetic overdose, 344-345
    for LSD bad trips, 703
    malignant hyperthermia and, 711b
    physostigmine salicylate and, 138
    for postoperative anxiety, 390
    respiratory and cardiovascular depression
        monitoring and, 227
Diazoxide, for hypertension, 145, 146t
Dibucaine (Nupercaine), 342t
Dicumarol, tolbutamide interaction with,
        269t
Diencephalon, 94, 100-101
    reticular formation and, 104
Diethyl ether, 276, 284
Diethylstilbestrol (Stilphostrol),
        succinylcholine interaction with,
        270t
Digestive fluids, 203
Digestive system, 222; *see also*
        Gastrointestinal tract
    associated structures and, 552
Digitalis
    calcium chloride interaction with, 269t
    for cardiogenic shock, 725
    myocardial infarction and, 133
    quinidine interaction with, 267t
    succinylcholine interaction with, 267t
    thiazide diuretics interaction with, 267t
    d-tubocurarine interaction with, 267t
Digoxin (Lanoxin), 254t
    geriatric patients and, 685t
    kidney disease and, 197
Dihydrostreptomycin, muscle relaxants and,
        268t, 271, 330b
Dilantin, 262t; *see also* Phenytoin
Dilatation of cervix and curettage of uterus
        (D&C), 585
    definition of, 581-582
Dilaudid; *see* Hydromorphone
Diltiazem (Cardizem), 141, 143, 254t
Dimenhydrinate (Dramamine), after ear
        surgery, 435
Diode (laser), 631t
Diphenhydramine (Benadryl), 254t
    after pediatric surgery, 678
    for anaphylactic shock, 726
    for nausea, 657t, 658
    for pruritus, 695
    for urticarial wheals with meperidine,
        305
2,3-Diphosphoglycerate (2,3-DPG)
    in donated blood, 209
    oxygen transport and, 172
    pulse oximetry interpretation and, 364
Diplopia, myasthenia gravis and, 644

Diprivan; *see* Propofol
Direct-vision nasotracheal intubation, 416
Disarticulation, definition of, 506
Discectomy, definition of, 506
Discharge planning, 624
Diskectomy, definition of, 506
Disopyramide, d-tubocurarine interaction
        with, 267t
Disorientation
    physostigmine salicylate and, 138-139
    postoperative, 395
        geriatric patients and, 683
Dissection tonsillectomy, 439
Disseminated intravascular coagulation
        (DIC), 208
    malignant hyperthermia and, 712
Dissociative anesthetics, 301-302
Distribution, of inhalation anesthetics, 278,
        280
Distributive shock, 717t, 723, 725-728; *see
        also* Neurogenic shock
Diuretics
    after cardiac surgery, 487
    aldosterone antagonists, 196
    carbonic anhydrase inhibitors, 197
    geriatric patients and, 685t
    halothane interaction with, 267t
    intracranial pressure and, 529
    loop, 196
    osmotic, 195
    potassium-sparing, 196
    thiazide, 195-196
    transfusion reactions and, 398
Diuril, 195
Diverticulum, definition of, 551
Diverting capnographs, 366
Dixarit; *see* Clonidine
DNR (do not resuscitate) orders, 83, 84
    ethics committees and, 87
Do Not Attempt Resuscitation (DNAR)
        orders, cardiopulmonary resuscitation
        and, 735
Do not resuscitate (DNR) orders, 83, 84
Dobutamine (Dobutrex), 143, 254t
    action of, 144t
    for cardiogenic shock, 725
    for septic shock, 728
"Documentation of Perioperative Nursing
        Care" (AORN), 355
Dolasetron (Anzement), for nausea, 657t,
        658
L-Dopa, 136; *see also* Levodopa
Dopamine (Intropin), 136, 143, 254t
    action of, 144t
    for cardiogenic shock, 725
    in chemoreceptor trigger zone, 656, 658
    for septic shock, 728
Dopaminergic receptors, 140
Doppler device, ultrasonic, 498, 498
Dopram, 254t
Dornase alfa (Pulmozyme), respiratory care
        and, 266t
Dorsal, definition of, 93
Dorsal fornix, 99
Dorsal gray horn, 121, *122*
Dorsal respiratory group (DRG) neurons,
        183
Dorsal root, spinal nerve, *120*, 121, *122*

Dorsal spinal segments, *119*
Dorsalis pedis pulse, 512
Dose-response relationships, 249
Down syndrome children, anesthesia for, 667
Doxacurium chloride (Nuromax), 254t, 320t, 322-323
Doxapram (Dopram), 254t
Doxycycline
  for anthrax, 732
  for plague, 733
DPG; *see* 2,3-Diphosphoglycerate
Drainage; *see also* Chest drainage systems; Hemovac drainage device; Penrose drain
  after abdominal gynecologic surgery, 588
  after abdominal surgery, 556, 559
  after abdominoperineal resection, 561
  after breast biopsy, 592
  after genital surgery, 587
  after genitourinary surgery, 571
  after herniorrhaphy, 562
  after laparoscopic cholecystectomy, 564
  after laparoscopy, 586
  after liver surgery, 562
  after mammoplasty, 598
  after mastopexy, 597
  after pediatric surgery, 667-668
  after radical mastectomy, 594-595
  after trauma injuries, 719, 720
  after vaginal surgery, 587
Dressings
  after abdominal gynecologic surgery, 588
  after abdominal surgery, 556
  after abdominoperineal resection, 561
  after adrenalectomy, 579
  after appendectomy or herniorrhaphy, 562
  after breast biopsy, 592
  after C-section, 583-584
  after genital surgery, 587
  after genitourinary surgery, 570, 571
  after kidney transplantation, 573
  after laparoscopic cholecystectomy, 564-565
  after laparoscopy, 586
  after large bowel surgery, 560
  after lumpectomy, 593-594
  after mammoplasty, 598
  after mastopexy, 597
  after pediatric surgery, 667-668, 673
  after radical mastectomy, 594
  after thyroid surgery, 549
  after trauma injuries, 720
  after vaginal surgery, 587
  after vascular surgery, 498, 504
Dromotropic, definition of, 125
Dromotropism, 129
Droperidol (Inapsine), 255t, 299-301; *see also* Innovar
  after ear surgery, 435
  clonidine interaction with, 267t
  extrapyramidal reactions and, 98
  ketamine with, 301
  kidney disease and, 198
  malignant hyperthermia and, 711b
  for nausea, 657t, 658, 695
  for ophthalmic surgery patients, 460

Droperidol (Inapsine) *(Continued)*
  physostigmine salicylate and, 138
  postoperative excitement from, 395
  renal function and, 197
Droplet-transmission precautions, 40b
Drug abuse
  analgesic comparison for, 310t
  definition of, 697
  with nalbuphine, 310
  with rophy, 297-298
Drug advancements, medical errors and, 68
Drug biotransformation, 270-271
  liver and, 226, 227
Drug response(s), 248
  dose-response relationships and, 249
  pharmacokinetic, 249-250
  physiologic dysfunction effects on, 251, 265
  removal from systemic circulation and, 251
  systemic absorption by administration routes, 250-251
Drug-drug interactions, 265, 270-271
  aging and, 684
  antibiotics, 268t
  antihypersensitive drugs, 267t
  PACU and, 271-272
  pharmacodynamic, 271
  pharmacokinetic, 265, 270-271
Drug-induced parkinsonism, 98
Dry powder inhalers (DPIs), 251
Dual block, succinylcholine and, 336
Ductal carcinoma in situ (DCIS), definition of, 590
Ducts of Bellini, 190-191
Dumbbell tumors, 545
Duodenum, 225
  laparoscopic perforation of, 639
Dura mater
  cranial, *106, 106-108, 109, 110*
  spinal, *107, 110, 117, 122,* 346
  termination, *118*
Duramorph, 260t; *see also* Morphine
Duranest; *see* Etidocaine
Dwarfism, 215
Dyazide, 196
Dye (laser), 631t
Dyrenium, 196
Dyspnea
  after laryngoscopy, 440
  from anthrax, 732
  definition of, 150
  myasthenia gravis and, 644
  obesity and, 649
Dystonic reactions, acute, 98
Dysuria, definition of, 189

E

Ear(s)
  divisions of, *435*
  fluids of, 203
  frontal section through outer, middle, and inner, *434*
  inner, cerebellum and vestibular apparatus of, 102
  meperidine and labyrinthine apparatus of, 305

Ear(s) *(Continued)*
  surgery on, 434-436
  surgery on middle, nitrous oxide contraindication in, 288-289
  trauma nurse's evaluation of, 720
Early (septic) shock, 727
"Easy lay," abuse of, 704
Eaton-Lambert syndrome, smoking and, 652
Ebola, as biological warfare agent, 731b
Ecchymosis
  around mastoid area, basilar skull fractures and, 520
  from trauma wounds, 720, 721
Echothiophate iodide, succinylcholine interaction with, 269t
"Ecstasy," abuse of, 703-704
Ectopic, definition of, 125
Ectopic pacemaker, definition of, 125
Ectopic pregnancy
  care after, 584
  definition of, 581
Ectropion, definition of, 453
Edecrin; *see* Ethacrynic acid
Edema, 204-205; *see also* Interstitial edema; Laryngeal edema; Pulmonary edema
  angioneurotic, local anesthetics and, 344
  blunt trauma and, 715
  definition of, 201
  pedal, obesity and, 650
  peripheral, after cardiac surgery, 490
  postoperative laryngeal, 363
  radical neck surgery and, 449
  spinal cord, 537
  from trauma injury, 720, 721
Edrophonium chloride (Tensilon, Enlon), 255t, 317
  acetylcholinesterase and, 138
  for muscle relaxant reversal, 325
  myasthenia gravis and, 644
Education
  by clinical nurse specialists, 15-16
  grand rounds on ethical issues, 87
Effective dose
  for inhalation anesthetics, 280-281
  median, 249
Effective filtration pressure, 205
Effector phase, of anaphylactic shock, 726
Effector T lymphocytes, in cellular immunity, 242
Efferent, definition of, 93
Efferent arterioles, renal, 190, *191*
Efferent impulses
  of reticular formation, 104
  spinal cord and, 117-118
Efficacy, drug, definition of, 248
Elasticity, of lung
  functional residual capacity and, 159
  pulmonary hysteresis and, 160
Electrical burns, 236, 609, 610, 715
Electrical shock, from defibrillators, *742*
Electrocardiogram, *127*
  in acute renal failure, 198
  hyperkalemia diagnosis and, 199
  malignant hyperthermia and, 708
  myocardial infarction and, 132
  pulse oximetry and, 365, 366

Electrocardiographic monitoring
amphetamines abuse and, 702
CPR and, 736
defibrillation, 741
secondary circulation survey, 743
for malignant hyperthermia, 711, 711b
postoperative, 374-378
cardiac surgery and, 486
geriatric surgery and, 684
lead placement, 374, 375
obesity and, 651
pediatric surgery and, 669, 672
hypothermia and, 674
sinus arrhythmias, 375-376
supraventricular arrhythmias, 376,
376-377, 377
ventricular arrhythmias, 377, 377-378,
378
straight-line waves, 744
Electroencephalography (EEG), for cranial
surgery diagnosis, 520
Electrolytes, 205-207
abdominal surgery and balance of, 556-
557
acute imbalance signs and symptoms,
390t
for alcohol withdrawal, 701
burn injuries and redistribution of, 610
crystalloid fluids and, 208
definition of, 125
drug-drug interactions in PACU and,
268-269t
fluid distribution and, 204
imbalance in
loop diuretics and, 196
malignant hyperthermia and, 678
muscle relaxants and, 329
inhalation agents and balance of, 290
kidney transplantation and, 573
large bowel surgery and, 560
malignant hyperthermia and, 711
muscle relaxants and, 268t
pediatric surgery and, 673
postoperative monitoring of, 386-388
small bowel surgery and, 560
vomiting and, 655, 656
Electromyography
for botulism diagnosis, 733
for spinal surgery diagnosis, 535
Electronic checklists, risk management and,
73
Electronic contact cleaners, abuse of, 703
Electroshock therapy, succinylcholine for,
326
Electrosurgery, thermal injuries from, 639
Elimination, of inhalation anesthetics,
278
Elimination clearance, of drug, 250
Embolectomy, 496, 500
definition of, 493
Embolism
cardiac surgery and, 491
definition of, 125
pulmonary, after orthopedic surgery, 510
surgical techniques for prevention of,
494
Embolus, definition of, 493

Emergence excitement, 395; see also
Delirium, emergence
Emergency Medical Treatment and Active
Labor Act, 79
Emergency Nurses Association
certification by, 15t
on psychological aspects of trauma care,
722
Emergency surgery; see also ERR WATCH
principles
vomiting/regurgitation after, 224
Emergent equipment, 7
EMLA, 339
Emotional disturbances, malignant
hyperthermia and, 709, 710b
Emotional processes
association fibers and, 96
in cerebral cortex, 97
diencephalon and, 100
hypothalamus and, 101
limbic system and, 99
Emphysema, 642
preexisting, postoperative complications
and, 183
senile, 683
smoking and, 652
subcutaneous
chest tube placement and, 469
laryngofissure and, 446
tracheostomy and, 445
trauma injury and, 720
Enalapril (Vasotec), 255t
Enalaprilat (Vasotec IV), 255t
Encephalitides, as biological warfare agent,
731b
Encephalon, 93
Encephalopathy, hypertension and, 147
End of life, ethical dilemmas during, 85-88
End plate potential (EPP), neuromuscular
transmission and, 318
Endarterectomy, 496
definition of, 493
End-diastolic volume, 127
Endocardium
of heart ventricles, 129
rheumatoid arthritis and, 647
Endocrine glands
definition of, 213
physiology of, 214-218
Endocrine system, 213
arterial blood pressure and, 128
hormones, 213-214
hypoadrenocorticism, 218-219
hypothalamus and, 101
pituitary gland, 214
Endorphins, 304
septic shock and, 727
Endoscopic retrograde
cholangiopancreatography (ERCP),
definition of, 551
Endoscopic thyroidectomy, definition of, 548
Endoscopy
ambulatory surgery and, 615
definition of, 433, 551
diagnostic, 558
early carcinoma of vocal cord, 446b
history of, 633

Endosteal dura, 109
Endotracheal intubation; see also Tracheal
intubation
for anesthesia induction in pregnant
patients, 692
balloon-cuffed, as artificial airway, 362
bronchial bifurcation angles and, 155-
156
for cardiopulmonary resuscitation
ventilation
primary, 739
secondary, 743
laryngoscopy and, 440
laryngospasm and, 155
nasotracheal, 416-417
after maxillofacial surgery, 450
balloon-cuffed, as artificial airway, 362
obesity and, 651
oral, 414-416
for pediatric anesthesia, 662
laryngeal mask airway and, 666
Endotracheal tube(s), 413-414, 736
for children, 661
fire safety during laser surgery and, 633
recommended sizes for, 412t
Endovascular stent-grafting, 495
End-systolic volume, 127
Enflurane (Ethrane), 255t, 285-286
for anesthesia maintenance in pregnant
patients, 692
cardiac dysrhythmias and, 131
drug-drug interactions with, 272
fluid preloading during pregnancy and,
690
intracranial pressure and, 527
kidney disease and, 197
lacrimation and, 278
malignant hyperthermia and, 710b
oil-gas partition coefficient of, 280
pulmonary vascular resistance and, 167
Enlon; see Edrophonium chloride
Enoxaparin (LMW Heparin), 255t
Enteric system, definition of, 221
Enterocele, definition of, 582
Entropion, definition of, 453
Enucleation, 456
definition of, 453
firm pressure dressing after, 462
oculocardiac reflex after, 459
Enuresis, definition of, 189
Enzyme inducers
drug biotransformation and, 227
enflurane contraindication with, 286
Ependyma, 102
Ephedra, anesthesia interaction with, 274t
Ephedrine, 255t
action of, 144t
for neurogenic shock, 726
respiratory care and, 266t
Epidermis, 231, 607
layers of, 232
Epididymectomy, definition of, 566
Epidural (EPI) administration of drugs
after thoracic surgery, 467
of opioids for pain management, 425
for pain management, 423, 424, 426,
721

Epidural anesthetics, 339, 351
  after laparoscopic cholecystectomy, 565
  sickle cell anemia and, 654
Epidural catheter pumps, 422, 425
Epidural hematoma, 521-522, *522*
Epidural space, *109*, 117, 346
Epigastric and hypogastric herniorrhaphy,
    definition of, 552
Epiglottis, 152, *153*
  in newborns, 661
  raising, for oral endotracheal intubation,
    414-415
Epilepsy
  flumazenil and, 298
  PET scans and diagnosis of, 520
Epinephrine (Adrenalin), 255t
  action of, 144t
  for anaphylactic shock, 726
  for asystole, 744
  biochemistry, 136-137
  for cardiogenic shock, 725
  during cardiopulmonary bypass, 484
  for cardiopulmonary resuscitation, 743, 745
  for cesarean section, 693
  drug absorption and, 270
  drug-drug interactions in PACU and,
    268t, 271-272
  halothane and, 286
  during laparoscopy, 637
  local anesthetics and, 341
    overdose of, 345
  metabolism of, *138*
  nebulized racemic, for postintubation
    croup, 677
  renal function and, 197
  respiratory care and, 266t
  for shock after adrenalectomy, 578
Epipharynx, sniff or aspiration reflex and,
    181-182
Epiphora, definition of, 453
Epispadias, 578
  definition of, 566
Epistaxis
  definition of, 150
  nasal trauma and, 152
Epithalamus, functional description of, 100-
    101
Epithelial cells, 135
Epithelium, immunologic defense and, 238-
    239
Equal pressure point (EPP), 162, *163*
  COPD and, 643
Equilibrium, cerebellum and, 102
Erbium:YAG (laser), 630t
ERR WATCH principles, 47-51, 48b
  attention allocation, 49-50
  call for help, 51
  communication, 50-51
  environment, 47-48
  reevaluation, 49
  resources, 48-49
  simulation in CRM training, 51
  teamwork, 50
  workload, 49
Error
  human, 45-47
  medical, technology and, 68

Erythrocytes, 209
  during cardiopulmonary bypass, 485
  shock and, 723
Esidrix, 196
Esmolol (Brevibloc), 255t
  for hypertension, 145, 146t, 148
Esophagectomy, 559
Esophagogastroduodenoscopy (EGD),
    definition of, 551
Esophagomyotomy, 559
Esophagoscopy
  definition of, 551
  diagnostic, 558
Esophagus, 221
  care after surgery of, 558-559
  disorders of, 221-222
Esters, local anesthetic, 341, 342t
Estrogen, 218
Estrus
  definition of, 93
  melatonin and, 100-101
Ethacrynic acid (Edecrin), 196, 198, 255t
  muscle relaxants and, 269t
Ethanol, malignant hyperthermia and,
    710b
Ether(s); *see also* Diethyl ether
  abuse of, 703
  anesthesia signs and stages with, 276,
    277-278
Ethics; *see also* Medical ethics
  end of life dilemmas, 85-88
Ethics committees, 87-88
Ethics consultation services, 87-88
Ethics in Patient Referrals Act, 79
Ethmoid bone, 104
Ethmoid sinuses, 104
Ethmoidectomy, definition of, 433
Ethrane; *see* Enflurane
Ethylene, 284
Ethylenediaminetetraacetic acid,
    chloroprocaine and, 695
Etidocaine (Duranest), 255t, 341, 342t,
    344
  malignant hyperthermia and, 710b
Etomidate (Amidate), 255t, 292, 293-294
  intracranial pressure and, 528
  for pregnant patients, 692
Eutonyl, sympathetic hyperactivity and,
    137
Evacuation procedures, for bioterrorism
    response, 731
Evidence-based medicine, 60
  medical practice guidelines and, 72
Evisceration, of eye, definition of, 454
Excimer (laser), 631t
Excitability, definition of, 125
Excitation-contraction (E-C) coupling
  malignant hyperthermia and, 709
  neuromuscular transmission and, 708
Excitatory and conductive muscle, 129,
    318-319
Exenteration, of eye, definition of, 454
Exercise, malignant hyperthermia and,
    710b
Exna, 196
Exogenous surfactants, 266t
  respiratory care and, 266t

Exosurf, respiratory care and, 266t
Expiratory reserve volume (ERV), 157-158,
    158t
  functional residual capacity and, 159
  obesity and, 649
  pregnancy and, 691
External direct current (DC) countershock,
    378, *378*
External fixators, definition of, 506
Extracellular fluid (ECF)
  distribution of, 203-204
  sodium and chloride ions in, 204
Extracellular fluid volume and osmolality
  kidney regulation of, 192-193, *199*
  in geriatric patients, 683
Extracorporeal shock wave lithotripsy,
    definition of, 566
Extradural hematoma, 521
Extradural-extramedullary tumors, 545
Extraocular surgery, 456
Extrapyramidal cell axons, 97-98, 101
Eye(s); *see also* Lid reflex
  anatomy of, *453*
  of child hit with BB, 463
  depth of anesthesia and movement of,
    278
  fluids of, 203
  oxygen toxicity and, 187
  protection during laser surgery, 633
  trauma nurse's evaluation of, 720
Eye muscle surgery, 456
Eye surgery, 452-464
  anesthesia, 456-458
  cardiorespiratory assessment and care for,
    459-460
  dressings, *462*, 462-463
  PACU issues and, 459b
  pain management, 460-461
  postoperative intraocular pressure, 461
  psychologic aspects of, 463

F

F_1O_2, definition of, 150
Fabric protector sprays, abuse of, 703
Face masks, for ventilation of children,
    661
Faces scales, for pain measurement in
    children, 676t
Facets, of vertebrae, 115
Facial block, for eye surgery, 456
Facial grimacing, psychotropic drugs and,
    98
Facial nerves (VII), 102
  ear surgery and, 434
  type and functions of, 103t
Fade, in recovery from neuromuscular
    blockade, 333
Falls, trauma from, 715
Falx cerebelli, 107
Falx cerebri, 107, *109*
Family needs, bioethics and, 87
Famotidine (Pepcid), 255t; *see also* Pepcid
  for vomiting/regurgitation, 224
Fascia; *see* Compartment syndrome
Fasciculation, muscle, succinylcholine and,
    327, 328
Fasciotomy, definition of, 506

Fasting
  before ambulatory procedures, 619-620
  gastric emptying and, 223
Fasttracking
  collaborative plan for, 39b
  perianesthesia nursing and, 11
  policies, 39
Fat embolism syndrome, after orthopedic
    surgery, 510
Fat metabolism
  glucocorticoids and, 217
  hypothalamus and, 101
Fatigue, malignant hyperthermia and, 709
Fatty acids, free, septic shock and, 727
Fear
  limbic system and, 99
  stomach physiology and, 223
Federal Bureau of Investigation,
    bioterrorism response system, 731-732
Federal Energy Management Agency,
    bioterrorism response system, 731-732
Federal government, managed care and, 55-
    56, 79
Federated Ambulatory Surgery Association
    (FASA), Outcomes Monitoring
    Project, 619
Feeding behavioral responses, limbic system
    and, 99
Fee-for-service (FFS) systems, 54-55
Feet, perianesthesia care after surgery on,
    514
Felt-tip marker fluid, abuse of, 703
Femoral herniorrhaphy, definition of, 552
Femoral nerve, 122
Femoral pulse, in trauma patient, 720
Femoral-popliteal bypass graft, 496, 497
Fenestration, 436
  definition of, 433
Fenoldopam (Corlopam), 256t
Fentanyl (Sublimaze), 256t, 304; see also
    Innovar; Sublimaze
  abuse of, effects and signs of, 698t
  administration of, 306-307
  after anesthesia with enflurane, 285
  after ophthalmic surgery, 460-461
  droperidol and, 299, 300
  epidural administration of, 313, 351
  for eye surgery, 456
  intracranial pressure and, 528
  as lollipop for children, 667
  malignant hyperthermia and, 711b
  mu opioid receptors and, 304
  for pain management, 424, 425-426
    after C-section, 695
    after pediatric surgery, 674
  patient-controlled analgesia with, 315t
  transdermal administration of, 425
Fetal monitoring, 693-694, 693t
  indirect, 694
Fever
  from anthrax, 732
  hemolytic reactions to transfusions and,
    211, 397-398
  from plague, 732
  surgery with COPD and, 644
Feverfew, anesthesia interaction with, 274t
Fiberoptic catheters, 531

Fibrillation
  atrial, postoperative monitoring of, 377,
    377
  definition of, 125
  ventricular
    CPR after, 737, 741, 742, 743
    lidocaine for, 745
    postoperative monitoring of, 378, 378
Fibrinogen, coagulation and, 208
Fibrinolytic therapy, 494, 495
  definition of, 493
Fick technique, for cardiac output, 127-128
Field block anesthesia, 339
Filtration, renal, 191, 192t
Filum terminale, 118, 346
Fimbria of fornix, 99
Final common pathway, 122-123
Fingers, motor control of, 96
Fink phenomenon, nitrous oxide
    contraindication and, 289
Fire safety, laser procedures and, 633
First ventricle, 109; see also Lateral
    ventricles
Fissure of Rolando, 95; see also Central
    sulcus
Fissure of Sylvius, 95; see also Lateral sulcus
Fissures; see also Sylvian fissure
  in cerebral cortex, 95
Fixed chest syndrome, 307, 309
Fixed costs, PACU, 58
Flaxedil; see Gallamine
Flexeril, for spinal cord injuries, 540
Flexion, postoperative, 394
Flexion fracture, of spine, 537, 538
Flonase, respiratory care and, 266t
Flovent, respiratory care and, 266t
Fluids
  acute imbalance signs and symptoms,
    390t
  alcohol abuse and balance of, 701
  blood component therapy, 209-210
    types, 210-211
  blood fluid balance, 201-203
  burn injury management and, 610
  crystalloids/colloids administration, 208-
    209
  distribution in body, 203-204
  edema, 204-205
  gastric emptying and, 223
  hourly maintenance in infants and
    children, 664t
  for hypovolemic shock treatment, 724
  imbalances from abnormal output of,
    389t
  muscle relaxants and balance of, 329
  obesity and, 651
  perioperative replacement of, 207-208
  postoperative balance, 386-388
    abdominal surgery, 556-557
    adrenalectomy and, 578-579
    cystoscopy and, 568
    genitourinary surgery and, 568
    intake of, 386-387
      cerclage procedure and, 584-585
      C-section and, 583
      genital or vaginal surgery and, 587
      genitourinary surgery and, 570, 571

Fluids (Continued)
    geriatric surgery and, 684
    oral, 387-388
    intravenous, 387
    large bowel surgery and, 560
    management after thoracic surgery,
      469
    management after thyroid surgery, 549
    myasthenia gravis and, 645
    output, 388
      prostate surgery and, 576
      trauma injuries and, 720
    pediatric surgery and, 669, 673
    pregnancy and preloading of, 690-691
    rheumatoid arthritis and, 649
    small bowel surgery and, 560
    vascular surgery and, 498, 503-504
  in premature infants, 665
  transfusion reactions, 211
  volume status assessment, 211-212
Flumazenil (Romazicon), 256t, 298-299
  abuse of, 701
  for ambulatory surgery, 621
  benzodiazepine receptors and, 292
  in children, 666, 670
  for pain management side effects, 424
Flunisolide (AeroBid), respiratory care and,
    266t
Flunitrazepam (Rohypnol), 297-298
  abuse of, 704
Fluorescent-antibody test, for plague, 732
Fluoromar, 284-285
Fluoroscopy, for spinal surgery diagnosis,
    535
Fluothane; see Halothane
Flurazepam, geriatric patients and, 685t
Fluroxene, 284-285
Fluticasone (Flonase/Flovent), respiratory
    care and, 266t
Flutter, atrial
  definition of, 125
  postoperative monitoring of, 376, 376-
    377
Flutter valve closure, 221
Focal deficit, definition of, 517
Foley catheter(s), 569, 571
  after gynecologic surgery, 588
  bladder injuries and, 639
  fluid management in trauma patients
    and, 719
  prostate surgery and, 575-576, 576
Follicles, thyroid gland, 216
Follicle-stimulating hormone, 218
Fontanelles, assessment after pediatric
    surgery, 673
Food and Drug Administration (FDA), 55
  on droperidol, 300
  on laser procedures, 632
Foot surgery, perianesthesia care after, 514
Foot-drop, peroneal nerve compression and,
    512
Foramen magnum, 105, 106, 112
  medulla oblongata and, 102
Foramen of Magendie, 107, 109, 110, 111
Foramen of Monro, 109, 110, 111
Foramen ovale, 105
Foramina of Luschka, 109, 110

Forane; *see* Isoflurane
Force, in trauma injuries, 715
Forearm, perianesthesia care after surgery on, 511
Forebrain, 93-101
  association areas, 99
  basal ganglia, 95-96, *96*
  cerebral cortex, 94-95
  cerebrum, 94
    functional aspects of, 96
  diencephalon, 100-101
  limbic system, 99, *99*-100
  motor areas, 96-98
  sensory areas, 98-99
Forehead, 104
Fortral, 309
Fothergill-Hunter procedure, 587
Fourth ventricle, 94, 104
  in brain stem, *101*, *102*
  cerebral aqueduct and, 101
  CSF circulation through, 109, *110*
  lateral and superior views, *111*
  median aperture of, *107*
Fractional inspired concentration of oxygen (FIO₂)
  for laryngospasm, 440
  oxygen transport and, 171
Frank-Starling law of the heart, 128
Fredet-Ramstedt operation, definition of, 554
Free radicals, blunt trauma and, 715
Free-electron (laser), 632t
Frequency-doubled (KTP) YAG (laser), 630t
Fresh frozen plasma (FFP), 211
Friction injuries of skin, postsurgical, 357
Friction rub, myocardial infarction and, 132
Frontal bone, 104, *105*
Frontal lobe, 94, *94*, 95
  blood supplies for, 112
  premotor area in, 97
Frontal sinuses, 104
Frostbite, 236, 609
  definition of, 231
Full-thickness burns, 236, 608
  excision of, 611, *612*
Full-thickness skin grafts, 612
Functional residual capacity (FRC), 158t, 159
  aging and, 683
  obesity and, 649
  postoperative, 185, 402
    composite curve of mean values of, *186*
  pregnancy and, 691
Fundus
  examination after C-section, 584
  of stomach, 222, *222*
Fungal mycotoxins, as biological warfare agent, 731b
Funiculi, spinal, 121
Furosemide (Lasix), 196, 198, 256t
  intracranial pressure and, 529
  for malignant hyperthermia cart, 8b
  for malignant hyperthermia treatment, 712b
  muscle relaxants and, 269t

G
Gallamine (Flaxedil), 322
  geriatric surgery and, 684
  kidney disease and, 197
  myasthenia gravis and, 644
  recurarization and, 336
Gallbladder, 227, *227*-228
  care after surgery of, 564-565
  removal of drugs from systemic circulation and, 251
Gallstones, obesity and, 650
Gamma globulin, during cardiopulmonary bypass, 485
Gamma hydroxybutyrate (GHB), abuse of, 704
Gamma knife, 527
Gamma-aminobutyric acid (GABA), nonopioid drug interaction with, 292
Ganglion, spinal nerve, 121
Ganglionic blocking agents, nicotinic receptor responses and, 137
Garlic, anesthesia interaction with, 274t
Gas exchange, 165-167
  respiration and, 169-170
Gaseous anesthetic agents, 283
Gastrectomy, 559
  definition of, 551
Gastric decompression, after abdominal surgery, 557
Gastric emptying, 223
  pregnancy and, 691
Gastric resection, 559
Gastrin, stomach physiology and, 222, 223
Gastritis, definition of, 221
Gastroduodenostomy, *553*
Gastroenterostomy, *553*
  definition of, 551
Gastrointestinal anthrax, 732
Gastrointestinal tract, 221-230; *see also* specific parts, e.g. *Esophagus*
  burn injuries and, 610-611
  cardiac surgery and, 491
  care after surgery of, 558-562
  pregnancy and, 689b, 691-692
  spinal cord injuries and, 544
  water balance in, 202
Gastrojejunostomy, *553*
Gastroscopy, definition of, 551
Generation X, 21, 22-24t
Genital surgery
  care for female, 586-587
  terms for female, 581-583
Genitofemoral nerve, 122
Genitourinary surgery, 566-580
  abdominal distention after, 570-571
  care after diagnostic procedures, 567-568
  dressings care, 570
  fluid intake, 570
  general postoperative care, 568-569
  pain management, 571
  suprapubic catheters, 569-570
  of ureter for stone removal, *571*
  ureteral catheters, 570
Gentamicin
  muscle relaxants and, 268t, 271, 330b
  for plague, 733
"Georgia home boy," abuse of, 704

Geriatric patients, 682-687
  age-related problems
    Alzheimer's disease, 684-685
    cardiovascular system, 682
    drug interactions, 684, 685t
    hepatobiliary system, 684
    neuromuscular system, 683
    psychologic aspects, 684
    renal system, 683-684
    respiratory system, 683
  definition of, 682
  perianesthesia care, 686
Giantism, 215
Gilliam procedure, 587
Ginger, anesthesia interaction with, 274t
Ginkgo, anesthesia interaction with, 274t
Ginseng, anesthesia interaction with, 274t
Glasgow coma scale, 486, 533t
  hypertonic solutions, for fluid resuscitation in multiple trauma, 718
  intracranial pressure assessment and, 532
Glaucoma
  acute, after ophthalmic surgery, 461
  definition of, 454
  postoperative care after surgery for, 459
  surgery for, 456
Glipizide (Glucotrol), 256t
Globus pallidus, 96, *96*
Glomerular filtration rate (GFR), 199
  in geriatric patients, 684
  in infants and children, 664
  pregnancy and, 692
Glomerulus, 190
Glossectomy, definition of, 433
Glossopharyngeal nerve (IX), *101*
  medulla oblongata and, 102
  type and functions of, 103t
Glottis, 153
Glucagon, 217-218, 256t
  malignant hyperthermia and, 709
  pancreas and, 228
Glucocorticoids, 217
Glucogenesis, septic shock and, 727
Gluconeogenesis, 217
  definition of, 213
  pancreas and, 228
Glucose
  diabetes mellitus, anesthesia and, 645-646, 646t
  monitoring
    after pancreatic surgery, 564
    after pediatric surgery, 673
  pancreatic production of insulin and, 228
Glucotrol, 256t
Glutamic-oxaloacetic transaminase, myocardial infarction and, 132
Glycogenesis, 217
Glycogenolysis, 217
Glycolysis
  malignant hyperthermia and, 709
  shock and, 723
Glycopyrrolate (Robinul), 256t
  for bradycardia
    in aging patients, 682
    in high spinal block, 350

Glycopyrrolate (Robinul) (*Continued*)
　heart rate after pediatric surgery and, 670
　for hypotension, 144
　for muscle relaxant reversal, 325, 326
　nasal intubation and, 181
　for nausea, 657t, 658
　pediatric anesthesia and, 666
　physostigmine salicylate and, 139
　succinylcholine for children/adolescents and, 328
Glycosuria
　definition of, 189
　diabetes mellitus and, 645
　opioid abuse and, 697
Golden hour, trauma treatment and, 714, 724
Golden seal, anesthesia interaction with, 274t
Gonadotropic hormones, 215
Gonads, 218
　melatonin and development of, 100-101
Goniotomy, definition of, 454
Gonorrhea, multidrug resistant, 41
Graded drug response, 249
Graft-*versus*-host disease, as transfusion reaction, 398
Granisetron (Kytril), 256t
　for nausea, 657t
Gray matter, 94
　on cerebellum cortex, 102
　pontine nuclei of pons, 102
　in spinal cord, *107*, 120-121
Grenade catheters, after abdominoperineal resection, 561
Grimacing, facial, psychotropic drugs and, 98
Growth, hypothalamus and, 101
Growth hormone, 214-215
Growth hormone-releasing hormone, 214
Guanethidine
　for hypertension, 147
　neurohumoral transmission and, 142t
　norepinephrine inhibition by, 141
Gun shot wounds, 715
Gustatory area, in cerebral cortex, 99
Gynecologic surgery
　care after, 585-587
　　abdominal, 587-588
　terms used in, 583
Gynecomastia, 597, 598
Gyrus
　in cerebral cortex, 95
　precentral, motor functions and, 96
Gyrus fasciolaris, 99

H

Hair sprays, abuse of, 703
Haldane effect, 172-173
Hallucinations; *see also* Delirium
　alcohol abuse and, 701
　ketamine anesthesia and, 301-302
　LSD and, 702-703
Halo traction, 514
Haloperidol (Haldol), 256t, 299
　agitation treatment guidelines for, 299b
　extrapyramidal reactions and, 98

Halothane (Fluothane), 256t, 286
　abuse of, 703
　for anesthesia maintenance in pregnant patients, 692
　calcium channel blockers and, 143
　cardiac dysrhythmias and, 131
　diuretics interaction with, 267t
　drug-drug interactions with, 271-272
　gallamine with, 322
　geriatric patients and, 685t
　intracranial pressure and, 527
　lacrimation and, 278
　malignant hyperthermia and, 678, 709, 710b
　morphine addiction and, 697
　oil-gas partition coefficient of, 280
　for pediatric anesthesia, 666, 667
　physostigmine salicylate and, 138
　potency of, 280, 281
　pulmonary vascular resistance and, 167
　succinylcholine and, 328
　thiopental interactions in obesity with, 270
　verapamil interaction with, 267t
Hands
　motor control of, 96
　perianesthesia care after surgery on, 511
　positioning after surgery on, 507
Hapten, definition of, 238
Harrington rods, 515
　definition of, 506
　for spinal cord injuries, 539
Harvard Medical Practice Study, 65-66, 69
Hashish; *see* Marijuana
Head and neck cancer, reconstructive surgery in, 449-450
Head trauma
　in children, 679-680
　concomitant spinal cord injuries, 543
　PET scans and diagnosis of, 520
Headache
　from plague, 732
　postspinal, 350-351
Head-tilt maneuver, for airway opening, 737-738, *738*
Health and Human Services, U.S. Department of (DHHS), 55
　medical malpractice databank of, 66, 67
　operating divisions of, 55
　on pain management, 426
Health Care Quality Improvement Act (1986), 66
Health departments
　bioterrorism response planning, 731
　bioterrorism response systems, 731-732
Health, Education, and Welfare, U.S. Secretary of, Commission on Medical Malpractice, 65
Health personnel, latex allergies and, 244
Healthcare financing, 54
Healthcare provider organizations, 56
Healthcare-associated infections, 40b
Hearing
　area in cerebral cortex, 97, 99
　cerebellum and, 102
　inferior colliculi, 101

Hearing (*Continued*)
　loss, inhalant abuse and, 703
　postoperative, 389
Heart, 126-133; *see also* Arrhythmias; *entries under* Cardiac; Ventricular dysrhythmias
　anesthetics and, 131-132
　arterial blood pressure, 128-129
　cardiac cycle, 126-127, *127*
　cardiac output, 127-128
　circulation in, 131
　conduction of impulses in, 129-131
　obesity and, 650
　perianesthesia nursing care for, 133
　rheumatoid arthritis and, 647-648
　stunned, defibrillation for CPR and, 744
　surgery with COPD and, 643
　surgery with myasthenia gravis and, 645
　syncytial nature of, *130*
　trauma injuries and, 720-721
　valves, 129
　　abnormalities of, cardiogenic shock and, 725
Heart block (complete), definition of, 125
Heart failure, malignant hyperthermia and, 712
Heart rate
　Class IV hemorrhage and, 724
　fetal, 693, 693t
　　indirect, 694
　in infants and young children, 662, 662t, 664
　limbic system and, 99
　moderate phase hemorrhage and, 723
　pediatric surgery and, 670
　during pregnancy, 688
　progressive phase hemorrhage and, 724
Heat stroke, 707; *see also* Malignant hyperthermia
Helium, for pneumoperitoneum in laparoscopy, 635, 636t
Helper T lymphocytes, in cellular immunity, 241-242
Hematocrit
　burn injuries and, 611
　in infants and children after surgery, 673
　measure of, 134
　rheumatoid arthritis and postoperative, 648
　splenic contraction and, 228
Hematomas
　blunt trauma and, 715
　from brain injury, 520, 521
　　diagnosis of, 519
　　epidural, 521-522, *522*
　　intracerebral, *522*, 523
　　subdural, 522-523
　　types of, *522*
　carotid endarterectomy and, 500
Hematuria
　definition of, 189
　trauma injury and, 721
Hemiarthroplasty, definition of, 506
Hemicholinium, neurohumoral transmission and, 142t
Hemilaryngectomy, 446b
Heminephrectomy, definition of, 566

Hemodialysis
kidney transplantation and, 572
social worth and, 79
Hemodynamic parameters, 378-385
invasive monitoring methods, 379t
potential problems with, 380-384t
in left-atrial pressure, 380, 384
line placement in, 380
in pulmonary artery pressure, 380
in pulmonary capillary wedge pressure, 384
in right-atrial pressure, 380
Hemoglobin; see also Oxyhemoglobin
bilirubin and, 226
dysfunctional, 365, 400
in newborns, 664
oxygen depletion, inhalant abuse and, 703
in red blood cells, 134
rheumatoid arthritis and postoperative, 648
sickle cell anemia and, 653
Hemolysis
definition of, 201
sickle cell anemia and, 655
transfusions and, 211, 397
Hemolytic jaundice, 226
Hemorrhage
abdominal gynecologic surgery and, 588
adrenalectomy and, 578
cardiac surgery and, 487, 489-490
cerebral, 521
classifications, 723-724
early phase, 723
ectopic pregnancy and, 584
epidural block contraindication for, 351
eye surgery and, 462
fluid resuscitation after multiple trauma and, 718
gynecologic surgery and, 585
head injuries and, 523-525
hypovolemic shock and, 723
intraventricular, 523
laparoscopy and, 639
laryngectomy and, 447
laryngoscopy and, 441
liver surgery and, 562
moderate phase, 723
nasal surgery and, 437
ophthalmic surgery and, 460
pediatric surgery and, 673
postpartum, after inhalation anesthetic agents, 692
progressive phase, 723-724
radical neck surgery and, 449
subarachnoid, 523
diagnosis of, 519
surgically related, bleeding time and, 134
trauma injury and, 721
shock from, 717t
uterine aspiration and, 585
Hemorrhoidectomy, definition of, 552
Hemostasis, definition of, 201
Hemostatic plug, 134
Hemothorax
cardiac surgery and, 490
definition of, 465

Hemovac drainage device, 447, 448
after hip or femoral surgery, 512
after knee surgery, 514
after lumpectomy, 593-594
after radical mastectomy, 595
Heparin, 255t, 256t
partial thromboplastin time and, 134
propranolol interaction with, 267t
for sickle cell anemia and hemolysis, 655
Hepatitis B virus, transmission prevention, 41, 233
Hepatitis, halothane and, 286
Hepatobiliary system, 221-230; see also specific parts, e.g. Esophagus
aging and, 684
Hepatocytes, 226
Herbal medicines, 273
anesthesia interactions with, 274t
Hering-Breuer reflex, 182
Hernia
abdominal wall, laparoscopy and, 634
definition of, 552
hiatal, 222, 224, 558
obesity and, 650
repair with gastric wrap, 555
regional anesthesia for pediatric repair of, 675
Herniated nucleus pulposus, 544-545, 545
Herniation, supratentorial, 523
Herniorrhaphy
care after, 562
definition of, 552-553
Heroin, abuse of, effects and signs of, 697, 698t
Herpes, genital, trauma nurse's assessment of, 721
Hetastarch (Hespan), 209, 256t
transfusion of, 399
Hexafluorenium bromide (Mylaxen), 329
Hilum, renal, 189
Hindbrain, 94, 102, 104
basal ganglia and, 96
pons, 102
Hip
perianesthesia care after surgery on, 512
positioning after surgery on, 507
Hippocampus, 99, 100
Histamine
blunt trauma and, 715
in chemoreceptor trigger zone, 656, 658
immediate hypersensitivity reaction and, 242
pain and, 422
septic shock and, 727
Histamine$_2$ receptors, stomach physiology and, 222, 223
HIV/AIDs
perianesthesia nursing and, 11
transmission prevention, 41, 233
tuberculosis and, 40
Hives, as latex allergic reaction, 245b
Hoarseness, after tracheal intubation, 417-418
Hofmann elimination, atracurium and, 324
Holium:YAG (laser), 630t

Home care, after ambulatory surgery, 616, 617
instructions for, 624-625
Homeostasis, kidney role in, 192
Hormonal-metabolic measures, for pain measurement in children, 676t
Hormones
definition of, 213
fixed-receptor model, 213-214
mobile-receptor model, 213, 214
Hospital Infection Control Practices Advisory Committee, 40
Hospitalization plans, for bioterrorism response, 731
"Hug," abuse of, 703-704
Human error, 45-47
Human Services Operating Division, DHHS, 55
Humid weather, malignant hyperthermia and, 710b
Humidification; see also Mist therapy
nasal mucus and, 151-152
postoperative ventilation and, 400
Humoral immunity, 239-241
definition of, 238
Hyaline membrane disease, 665-666
Hyaluronidase (Wydase), 256t
Hydralazine (Apresoline), 257t
for hypertension, 145, 146t, 147
Hydrocelectomy, definition of, 566
Hydrocephalus, 524
diagnosis of, 519
Hydrochloric acid
immunologic defense and, 239
stomach physiology and, 222
Hydrochlorothiazide, 196
Hydrocodone, for oral analgesia, 431
Hydrocortisone, 217, 272
phenobarbital interaction with, 270t
Hydrocortisone sodium succinate (Solu-Cortef), 257t
Hydrodiuril, 196
Hydromorphone (Dilaudid), 257t
dosing for, 429b
for pain management, 423, 424, 426
Hydrostatic pressure, 168, 204
edema and, 204-205
Hydroxyapatite orbital implants, 452
definition of, 454
Hydroxyzine (Atarax or Vistaril), for nausea, 658t
Hyoid bone, 105
larynx and, 152, 153
Hyoscyamine, kidney disease and, 197
Hyperactivity, after pediatric surgery, 668
Hypercalcemia, definition of, 201
Hypercapnia
chronic
acid-base imbalances and, 175
hyperventilation and, 180-181
definition of, 150
Hypercarbia
COPD and, 643
hypertension and, 145
infant respiratory distress syndrome and, 665-666
during laparoscopy, 637

Hypercarbia (*Continued*)
  pneumoperitoneum and, 638t
  rheumatoid arthritis and, 647
Hyperdynamic stage
  of burn injuries, 610
  of septic shock, 727
Hyperemia, postischemic, 128-129
Hyperextension fracture, of spine, 537, 538
Hyperglycemia
  during cardiopulmonary bypass, 484
  diabetes mellitus and, 645, 646
Hyperglycemic factor, 217
Hyperkalemia
  aldosterone antagonists and, 196
  cardiopulmonary arrest and, 744
  definition of, 201
  electrocardiographic evidence of, *199*
  malignant hyperthermia and, 709b, 712
  potassium chloride IV push caution,
    206
  potassium-sparing diuretics and, 196
  sodium bicarbonate and, 746
Hypermagnesemia, 207
  definition of, 201
  potassium loss and, 206
Hypernatremia
  definition of, 201
  dilutional, 205
Hyperosmotic solutions, definition of, 201
Hyperoxemia
  definition of, 150
  infant respiratory distress syndrome and,
    665-666
Hyperoxia, retinopathy of prematurity and,
    665
Hyperpnea, definition of, 150
Hyperpyrexia, alcohol abuse and, 701
Hyperreactivity, definition of, 248
Hypersensitivity reactions, 242, 243t; *see*
    also Allergies
  definition of drug-induced, 248
  Type I (anaphylactic, immediate), 241,
    242 (*see also* Anaphylaxis)
    latex and, 244
  Type II (cytotoxic), 242
  Type III (arthus), 243
  Type IV (delayed), 242
  Type IV (delayed or cell-mediated), 243
Hyperstat, for hypertension, 145, 146t
Hypertension
  aging and, 682
  alcohol and, 701
  burn injuries and pulmonary, 610
  cardiac surgery complications and, 487,
    489
  club drugs abuse and, 703
  cocaine and, 702
  definition of, 125
  drug-drug reactions in PACU and, 267t,
    272
  drugs for, 146t
  LSD and, 702
  malignant hyperthermia and, 678
  obesity and, 651
  postoperative, 135
  pregnancy-induced, hypermagnesemia
    and, 207
  systolic, intraocular pressure and, 461

Hypertension (*Continued*)
  therapy, 144-148
  vascular surgery and, 502
Hyperthermia; *see also* Body temperature
  malignant (*see* Malignant hyperthermia)
  physiologic alterations with, 386b
  postoperative monitoring, 385-386
  sickle cell anemia and, 654
Hypertonic solutions
  crystalloid, 208
  definition of, 201
  for fluid resuscitation in multiple trauma,
    718
Hypertriglyceridemia, propofol and, 295
Hypertrophic subaortic stenosis, 474
Hyperventilation
  acute, acid-base imbalances and, 176
  carbon dioxide elimination and, 175b
  definition of, 150
Hypervolemia
  after cardiac surgery, 490-491
  definition of, 125
  hypertension and, 145
  sodium excess and, 205
Hypnosis
  anesthesia and, 276
  for pain management, 426
Hypoadrenocorticism, 218-219
Hypoalbuminemia, septic shock and, 727
Hypocalcemia, 206
  definition of, 201
  thyroid surgery and, 549-550
Hypocapnia, definition of, 150
Hypocarbia, hypothermia-related, during
    cardiopulmonary bypass, 485
Hypochlorhydria, definition of, 221
Hypodermis, 231, 607
  burns of, 608
Hypodynamic stage
  of burn injuries, 610
  of septic shock, 727
Hypoglossal nerve (XII), *101*
  medulla oblongata and, 102
  type and functions of, 103t
Hypoglycemia, diabetes mellitus and,
    646
Hypokalemia
  cardiopulmonary arrest and, 744
  definition of, 201
  diuretics and, 196, 205
  treatment for, 206
Hypomagnesemia, 207
  definition of, 201
Hyponatremia, definition of, 201
Hypoosmotic solutions, definition of, 201
Hypoparathyroidism, thyroid surgery and,
    549-550
Hypophyseal fossa, *107*
Hyporeactivity, definition of, 248
Hypospadias, 578
  definition of, 566
Hypotension
  aging and, 682
  ambulatory surgery and, 622
  anaphylactic shock and, 726
  calcium channel blockers and, 143
  Class IV hemorrhage and, 724
  enflurane and, 285

Hypotension (*Continued*)
  hemolytic reactions to transfusions and,
    211
  laparoscopy and, 639
  malignant hyperthermia and, 712
  maternal, after inhalation anesthetic
    agents, 692
  nausea, vomiting and, 656
  PACU ventilation and, 181
  rheumatoid arthritis and, 648
  septic shock and, 727
  spinal anesthesia and, 350
  spinal cord injuries and, 540, 544
  steroids, anesthesia and, 272
  supine, during pregnancy, 688
  therapy for, 143-144
Hypotensive effect, ocular, after eye surgery,
    459
Hypothalamus, 95, 96, 100
  functional description of, 101
  inhalation agents, body temperature and,
    290
  limbic system and, 99
  physiological responses to feelings and,
    98
  pituitary gland and, 214
  thirst center in, 202
Hypothermia; *see also* Body temperature
  from anthrax, 732
  burn injuries and, 613
  cardiopulmonary arrest and, 744
  definition of, 476
  geriatric patients and, 685, 686
  hypertension and, 145
  muscle relaxants and, 331
  in newborns, 662
  pediatric surgery and, 673-674
  physiologic alterations with, 386b
  postoperative monitoring, 385-386, 406,
    706-707
  pulseless electrical activity and, 720
  radical mastectomy and, 595
Hypotonic solutions, definition of, 201
Hypoventilation
  carbon dioxide retention and, 175b
  definition of, 150
  flumazenil and benzodiazepine-induced,
    298
  hypertension and, 145
  hypoxemia and, 177
  in newborns, 662
  obesity and, 649
  postoperative, 361, 400
Hypovolemia
  ambulatory surgery and, 622
  cardiac surgery and, 490
  cardiopulmonary arrest and, 744
  loop diuretics and, 196
  myocardial infarction and, 133
  postoperative, 143
  pulseless electrical activity and, 720
  third space fluid loss and blood loss after
    surgery, 203-204
Hypovolemic shock, 716, 717t, 723-724
Hypoxemia, 131
  cardiogenic shock and, 725
  causes, 177-179
  definition of, 150

Hypoxemia (*Continued*)
  in geriatric patients, 686
  hypertension and, 145
  in newborns, 662, 664
  obesity and, 649, *650*, 651
  postoperative, 362
  prostaglandins and chronic, 167
  pulmonary edema and, 169
  rheumatoid arthritis and, 647
  sickle cell anemia and, 654
Hypoxia
  alcohol withdrawal and, 701
  alveolar, pulmonary vascular resistance
    and, 167
  cardiopulmonary arrest and, 744
  COPD and, 643
  definition of, 150
  diffusion, nitrous oxide contraindication
    with, 289
  malignant hyperthermia and, 710b
  myocardial, smoking and, 652
  in newborns, 662
  pediatric surgery and, 670
  pneumoperitoneum and, 638t
  progressive phase hemorrhage and,
    724
  shock and, 722-723
  sickling and, 653
Hysterectomy
  ambulatory laparoscopically-assisted
    vaginal, 616
  care after, 588
  definition of, 582
    Cesarean, 581
    radical, 583
    total abdominal, 583
    total laparoscopic, 586
Hysterical reactions, acute dystonic
  reactions *versus*, 98
Hysteroscopy
  care after, 588
  definition of, 582

I

Ibuprofen, after pediatric surgery, 674
Ibutilide fumarate (Covert), 257t
Ice therapy, for pain management, 426
Idiosyncrasy, definition of, 249
Ileal conduit procedure; *see also*
    Ureterostomy
  anastomosed ureters and, *567*
Ileostomy
  care after, 560
  definition of, 553
Ileus, spinal surgery and, 514
Iliac arteries, bypass procedures on, 500
Ilioinguinal nerve, 122
Imagery, guided, for trauma patients, 721
Immersion foot, 236
  definition of, 231
Immobilization, for spinal cord injuries,
    539, 540
Immobilization devices care, after
  orthopedic surgery, 509
  on shoulder, 511
Immune system, 238-247
  acquired immunity, 239-242
    cellular, *240*, 241-242

Immune system (*Continued*)
    humoral, 239-241, *240*
  after burn injuries, 611
  hypersensitivity reactions, 242-243, 243t
  immunosuppression, 245-246
  innate, 239
  latex allergy, 243-245
  physical and chemical barriers, 238-239
Immunity, definition of, 238
Immunodeficiency disease, definition of,
    238
Immunoglobulin A (IgA), 240, 240-241
Immunoglobulin D (IgD), 240, *240*, 241
Immunoglobulin E (IgE), 240, *240*, 241
Immunoglobulin G (IgG), 240, *240*, 241
Immunoglobulin M (IgM), 240, *240*, 241
Immunoglobulins, humoral immunity and,
    239, 240-241
Immunosuppression, 245
  definition of, 238
  forms of, 245-246
Implantable cardioverter-defibrillator
    (ICD), definition of, 476-477
In situ, definition of, 591
Inapsine; *see* Droperidol
Incisional herniorrhaphy, definition of, 552
Incisions, abdominopelvic, 555, *556*
  for laparoscopy, 586
  obesity and, 651
  in prostate surgery, 575-576
  in renal and ureteral surgery, 571, *571*
Increased abdominal pressure, during
    laparoscopy, 637
Inderal; *see* Propranolol
Induced immunosuppression, 245, 246
Indusium griseum, 99
Infant respiratory distress syndrome, 665-666
Infants
  cardiac compression for CPR, 739-741,
    740
  eye surgery and, 457
  newborn
    body temperature, 664-665
    inhalation agents and, 290
    Hering-Breuer reflex and, 182
    intravenous fluids for, 387
    nitrous oxide and pulmonary vascular
      resistance in, 167
    pediatric circle system and, 666
    premature, 665-666
      infant respiratory distress syndrome,
        665-666
      oxygen toxicity and retrolental
        fibroplasia in, 187
      pressure cycled ventilators for, 670
      retinopathy, 665
      thermal regulation in, 665
  pain management for, 429
  postoperative psychosocial support for,
    668
  primary CPR pulse survey, 739
  primary CPR ventilation for, 739
  pyloric stenosis surgery for, 560
  tracheostomy complications in, 445
Infarction; *see also* Myocardial infarction
  definition of, 125
  pulmonary, smoking and, 653
  sickle cell anemia and, 654

Infection; *see also* Septic shock
  malignant hyperthermia and, 710b
Infection control, 40-41
  adrenalectomy and, 579
  antiinfective agents for, 266t
  aseptic technique for, 233-234, 236
  burn injuries and, 611, 613
  cystoscopy and, 568
  immunosuppression and, 246
  for kidney transplantation, 573
  laparoscopy and, 639
  mouth-to-mouth ventilation and, 739
  PACU interior design and, 3
  postoperative, 405
  for premature infants, 665
  smoking and, 653
  thoracic surgery and, 471
  thyroid surgery and, 550
  trauma care and, 722
Infectious disease agents, bioterrorism and,
    730
Inferior cerebellar peduncle, *101*
Inferior colliculi, 101, *101*
Inferior, definition of, 93
Inferior gluteal nerve, 122
Inferior petrosal sinus, *108*
Inferior sagittal sinus, *108*
Inferior vena cava; *see* Vena cava, inferior
Infiltrating ductal carcinoma (IDC),
    definition of, 590
Infiltration anesthesia, 339
Infiltrative lobular carcinoma (ILC),
    definition of, 590-591
Inflammatory breast cancer, definition of,
    591
Informed consent/refusal, 80-88
  for ambulatory surgery, 619
  communication skills for, 82
  ethics committees and policies on, 87
  life expectancy probabilities and, 80-81
  patient capacity for, 82
  standard of medical care determination
    and, 73
  therapeutic privilege and, 81
  treatment options discussion and, 82-83
Infratentorial, definition of, 517
Inguinal herniorrhaphy, 554
  definition of, 552-553
Inhalants
  abuse of, 697, 703
  respiratory, during ambulatory surgery,
    619b
Inhalation anesthesia, 276-278; *see also*
    Anesthesia, inhalation
Inhalational anthrax, 732
Inhaled partial pressure, 278
Innate immunity, 239
  definition of, 238
Innovar; *see also* Droperidol; Fentanyl
  intracranial pressure and, 528
  kidney disease and, 198
  renal function and, 197
  sustained maximum inspiration after, 300
Inocor, for hypotension, 144
Inotropic, definition of, 126
Inotropism, 129
Inspiratory capacity (IC), 158t, 159
  pregnancy and, 691

Inspiratory reserve volume (IRV), 158-159, 158t
  pregnancy and, 691
Institute of Medicine
  on medical practice guidelines, 72
  report on human error, 45
Insufflation, for inhalation anesthesia administration, 281
Insulin, 217, 218
  during cardiopulmonary bypass, 484
  diabetes mellitus and, 645-646, 646t
  drug-drug interactions in PACU with, 270t
  for hyperkalemia with malignant hyperthermia, 8b, 712, 712b
  pancreatic production of, 228
  time of action of various preparations of, 647t
Insulin-lente, 257t
Insulin-NPH, 257t
Insulin-NPH 70/Reg30, 257t
Insulin-regular, 257t
Insulin-semilente, 257t
Insulin-ultralente, 257t
Insurance companies
  managed care and, 56-57
  medical malpractice and, 68
  medical malpractice studies and, 66
Intal, respiratory care and, 266t
Integumentary system, 231-237
  anatomy of, 607
  aseptic technique, 233
    for burn injuries, 233-234, 236
    for intravenous therapy, 233
  functions, 231-233
Intellectual processes
  association fibers and, 96
  in cerebral cortex, 97, 98
Intensive care unit (ICU)
  ASPAN clinical guidelines on, 60
  bioethics and needs of, 87-88
  DNR orders and, 84
  PACU care for, 30
Intercalated disks, of cardiac muscle, 129
Intercellular junctions, blood-brain barrier and, 112
Intercondylar notch, 512
Intercostal paralysis, Stage III anesthesia and, 277
Interferon, cellular immunity and, 242
Interlobar arteries, renal, 189-190, 191
Intermaxillary fixation (IMF), 450
Intermittent mandatory ventilation (IMV), 401, 402, 402t
Internal capsule, 95, 96, 96
  blood supplies for, 112
  primary motor and premotor fibers through, 98
Internal fixation, definition of, 506
International Guidelines 2000 Conference on Cardiopulmonary Resuscitation and Emergency Cardiovascular Care, 735
Internet, patient information sources on, 618, 618b
Intersegmental tracts, spinal, 121

Interstitial edema, 169
  during cardiopulmonary bypass, 484-485
  septic shock and, 727
Interstitial fluid (ISF), 203-204
  edema and, 204-205
Interstitial fluid hydrostatic pressure (P$_{is}$), 168, 204-205
Interventricular foramen, 109, 110, 111
Intervertebral disk, 115
Intervertebral foramen (foramina), 115, 120, 121
Intervertebral notches, 115
Intestinal obstruction, nitrous oxide contraindication with, 288
Intestinal surgery, vomiting/regurgitation after, 224
Intestinal tubes
  irrigation, 557-558
  patency, 557
Intestines, 225
Intraaortic balloon pump, for cardiogenic shock, 725
Intraarterial catheter, blood pressure monitoring with, 373
Intracellular fluid (ICF)
  distribution of, 203
  potassium and phosphate ions in, 204
Intracerebral hematoma, 522, 523
Intracranial pressure (ICP), 113-115
  anesthetic agents and
    inhalation, 527-528
    intravenous, 528-529
  assessment, 531-532
  barbiturates and, 529
  diuretics and, 529
  dynamics, 524-531
    with failed compensatory mechanisms, 526
  enflurane and, 285, 286
  etomidate and, 294
  head injuries and, 521
  ketamine contraindication with, 301
  midazolam and, 296
  monitoring, 529-531
    devices for, 530, 530-531
  neurosurgical procedures and, 527
  postoperative nursing management, 532-535
  pressure waves in, 531
  pressure-volume curve, 524-525, 525
  spinal subarachnoid space and, 117
  supratentorial herniation and, 523
  vomiting center excitation and, 656
Intradural-extramedullary tumors, 545
Intraluminal pressure, 162
Intramedullary tumors, 545
Intramuscular administration of drugs
  for pain management, 423, 424
  systemic absorption of, 251
Intranasal antrostomy (antral window), definition of, 433
Intraocular lens (IOL) implant, definition of, 454, 454
Intraocular pressure, 461
  succinylcholine and, 329
Intraocular surgery, 456

Intraoperative blood scavenging, autologous blood transfusions and, 210
Intrapulmonary shunt, 177, 177-178
Intrathecal (IT) administration of drugs, for pain management, 423, 425
Intratracheal tube, 413-414
Intravascular fluid, 203
Intravenous lines; see also Patient-controlled analgesia
  administration of drugs
    for pain management, 423, 424-425, 721
    systemic absorption of, 251
  for anesthetics
    nonopioid, 292-303
    opioid, 304-316
  for cardiopulmonary resuscitation, 743
  for postoperative fluids in infants and children, 671
  sterile technique for, 233
  for trauma patients, 720
Intraventricular catheters (IVCs), 530, 531
Intraventricular hemorrhage, 523
Intropin; see Dopamine
Intussusception, definition of, 553
Invasive ductal carcinoma (IDC), definition of, 590
Invasive lobular carcinoma (ILC), definition of, 590-591
Involuntary movements, subthalamus and, 101
Involuntary repetitive movements, tardive dyskinesia and, 98
Iodine, protein-bound, 216
Iodine plaque irradiation, 462
  for cranial surgery diagnosis, 518-519
  lead shield after, 462
Ipran; see also Propranolol
  for hypertension, 146t, 148
Ipratropium (Atrovent, Itrop), 257t
  respiratory care and, 266t
Irrational behavior
  after ketamine anesthesia, 301-302
  postoperative, 395
Irritant receptors, breathing regulation and, 182, 183
Ischemia
  brain, 521, 526
  definition of, 126, 493
  postanesthesia shivering and, 707
  shock and, 723
  visceral organ, pneumoperitoneum and, 638t
Islet of Langerhans cells, 217-218, 228
Isocarboxazid, sympathetic hyperactivity and, 137
Isoetharine (Bronkosol), respiratory care and, 266t
Isoflurane (Forane), 257t, 286-287
  for anesthesia maintenance in pregnant patients, 692
  cardiac dysrhythmias and, 131
  coronary artery steal and, 131
  drug-drug interactions with, 272
  intracranial pressure and, 527-528
  lacrimation and, 278

Isoflurane (Forane) (*Continued*)
  malignant hyperthermia and, 710b
  oil-gas partition coefficient of, 280
  for pediatric anesthesia, 666, 667
  pulmonary vascular resistance and,
    167
Isometric relaxation, 126
Isoproterenol (Isuprel), 143, 257t
  action of, 144t
  beta receptors and, 140
  procainamide and, 710
  respiratory care and, 266t
Isoptin; *see* Verapamil
Isotonic solutions
  crystalloid, 208
  definition of, 201
Isthmus, 99
Isuprel; *see* Isoproterenol
Itching; *see* Pruritus
Itrop, 257t; *see also* Ipratropium
IV PCA pumps, 422, 425; *see also* Patient-
  controlled analgesia

J

J (juxtapulmonary capillary) receptors, 182,
  183
Jackson-Pratt closed drainage system
  abdominoperineal resection and, 561
  lumpectomy and, 594
  radical mastectomy and, 595
Jaundice, bilirubin and, 226
Jaw thrust, for airway opening, 737-738,
  738
Jejunum, 225
Joint Commission on Accreditation of
  Healthcare Organizations (JCAHO)
  on discharge planning, 624
  on ethical issues processes, 87
  quality improvement standards of, 42
  on Sentinel Event Alert, 619
Joint replacement
  definition of, 506
  hip, 512
  knee, 512, 514
  shoulder, 511
Journal of the American Medical
  Association (JAMA), on "standard of
  care," 72
Jugular foramen, 105
Jugular veins, 107-108, 108
Justice, medical ethics and, 78
Juxtaglomerular apparatus, 191, 192

K

Kanamycin, muscle relaxants and, 268t,
  271, 330b
Kappa opioid receptors, 304-305
Kava, anesthesia interaction with, 274t
Kenalog, respiratory care and, 266t
Keratoplasty, definition of, 454
Ketamine (Ketalar), 257t, 301-302
  abuse of, 704
  for burn injuries, 612
  diazepam and, 295
  intracranial pressure and, 528, 529
  intraocular pressure and, 461
  malignant hyperthermia and, 711b

Ketamine (Ketalar) (*Continued*)
  for pediatric anesthesia, 667, 674
  phencyclidine and, 191
  physostigmine and, 298
  postoperative excitement from, 395
  for pregnant patients, 692
Ketorolac (Toradol), 257t, 310t, 311
  for analgesia in pregnant patient, 695
  ophthalmic surgery and, 461
  for pain management, 313, 423
  pediatric surgery and, 674
Kidney(s)
  anatomy of, 189-191
  anesthetic effects on, 197
  arterial supply to, 191
  autoregulation, 192
  countercurrent mechanism, 191-192
  extracellular fluid regulation by, 204
  homeostasis regulation and, 192-193
  hormone control, 192
  inhalant abuse and, 703
  obesity and, 650
  physiology of, 191, 192t
  pregnancy and, 692
  removal of drugs from systemic
    circulation and, 251
  sickle cell anemia and, 654
  surgery with COPD and, 643
  water balance and, 203
Kidney disease, drug effects and, 197-198,
  251, 265
Kidney failure, 198
  during laparoscopy, 637
  malignant hyperthermia and, 712
  opioids for pain management and, 424
Kidney stones, hypocalcemia and, 206
Kidney transplantation, 572, 572-574
  definition of, 566
  donors for, 572-573
  graft rejection in, 573-574, 574b
Kiesselbach's plexus, 152
Killer T cells, cellular immunity and, 242
Kineplastic amputation, definition of,
  506
Kinetic beds, spinal cord injuries and, 543,
  543
Knee surgery
  continuous passive motion (CPM)
    machines and, 507
  CryoCuff system after, 513, 513
  perianesthesia care after, 512-514
Korotkoff sounds, in blood pressure
  monitoring, 371, 373
Krypton (laser), 631t
Kussmaul respirations, definition of, 150
Kyphosis
  malignant hyperthermia and, 708
  thoracic, obesity and, 649
Kytril, 256t, 657t

L

Labetalol (Normodyne, Trandate), 258t
  for hypertension, 145, 146t, 148
Labor, premature, 693-694
Labyrinthectomy, definition of, 433
Lacerations, of brain, 520
Lacrimal bone, 105

Lacrimation, depth of anesthesia and, 278
Lactate
  coronary blood flow and, 131
  in donated blood, 209
Lactic acid
  malignant hyperthermia and, 709
  oxygen debt and, 722-723
Lactic dehydrogenase (LDH), myocardial
  infarction and, 132
Lactogenic hormone, 215
Laennec's cirrhosis, 701
Lambda, 105
Lambdoid suture, 105
Laminae, of vertebrae, 115, 116
Laminectomy, 116
  decompression, for spinal cord injuries,
    539
  definition of, 506, 517
  for intraspinal neoplasms, 545
Lanatoside C, kidney disease and, 197
Lanoxin; *see* Digoxin
Lansoprazole (Prevacid), 258t
Laparoscopy, 627, 633-641
  ambulatory surgery and, 615
  anatomy of, 586
  for appendectomy or herniorrhaphy,
    562
  bladder injuries, 639
  bowel injuries, 639
  complications, 638-639
  contraindications to, 635t
  definition of, 553-554
  diagnostic, 558
  for ectopic pregnancy, 584
  gasless, 637
  gynecologic
    care after, 585-586
    terms, 581-583
  history of, 633-634
  patient position and, 637, 637t
  pneumoperitoneum, 634-635
    cardiopulmonary effects of, 636t
    cardiovascular changes, 635
    complications, 638, 638t
    insufflation gases for, 636t
    other system effects, 636-637
    respiratory changes, 635-636
  postoperative issues, 637-639
  preoperative issues, 634
  therapeutic and diagnostic indications
    for, 634t
  trocar placement during, 585
  vascular injuries, 639
Laparotomy
  definition of, 554
  for ectopic pregnancy, 584
  terms used in, 581-583
Lapses, human error as, 46
Large bowel surgery
  care after, 560-562
  resection for malignancy, 561
Larodopa, for drug-induced parkinsonism,
  98
Laryngeal edema
  anaphylactic shock and, 726
  postoperative, 363
    in children, 677

Laryngeal mask airway (LMA), 418-420, 666, 736
Laryngeal nerve injury, 549
Laryngeal pharynx, 152
Laryngeal sinus, 153
Laryngeal stridor, after laryngoscopy, 440
Laryngectomy, 445-447
  definition of, 433
  total, 446b, 447
  types of, 446b
Laryngofissure, 445-446, 446b
  definition of, 433
Laryngoscope, 411-412, 412
  direct-vision nasotracheal intubation with, 416
  for newborns, 661
Laryngoscopy, 440-441
  definition of, 433
Laryngospasm, 154-155
  hypocalcemia and, 206
  laryngoscopy and, 440
  LMA removal and, 419
  pediatric surgery and, 675
  postoperative, 362-363
  rectal examination and, 225
  respiratory compromise and, 736
  Stage II anesthesia and, 276, 277
  succinylcholine for, 326
  T&A and, 440
  tracheal intubation and, 418
Larynx, 152-155, 153
  in newborns, 661
  recurrent laryngeal nerves, 154
Laser deepithelialization, for reduction mammoplasty, 597
Laser neurosurgery, 527
Laser plume, 633
Laser surgery, 627-633
  about, 627
  benefits of, 628b
  intraoperative issues, 632-633
  laser light, 627
  postoperative care, 633
  preoperative care for, 629, 632
  tissue interaction, 627-629, 629
    temperature increases and, 629t
  types of, 629, 630-632t
Laser-assisted percutaneous transluminal angioplasty, 494-495
LASIK (laser-assisted in situ keratomileusis)
  definition of, 455
  speculum for, 460
Lasix; see Furosemide
Late (septic) shock, 727
Lateral apertures, 110
Lateral gray horn, 121, 122
Lateral (ventral) horn, 100
Lateral sulcus, 95; see also Sylvian fissure
Lateral ventricles, 96, 100
  CSF circulation through, 107, 109, 110
  lateral and superior views, 111
Latex allergy, 243-245
  Home Page (website), 244
  patients at risk for, 244b
  perianesthesia care for, 245b

LeFort operation, 587
Left occipital cortex, 99
Left parietal bone, 104
Left temporal bone, 104
Left-atrial catheter, 379
Left-atrial pressure, 380, 384
  after cardiac surgery, 486
Left-ventricular end-diastolic pressure (LVEDP), myocardial infarction and, 133
Legal issues; see also Medical malpractice
  medical ethics and, 77
Legs
  motor control of, 96
  perianesthesia care after surgery on, 512
  positioning after surgery on, 507
Lentiform nucleus, 95-96, 96
Leukemia, immunosuppression and, 245
Leukocytes, 134, 209
  during cardiopulmonary bypass, 485
  shock and, 723
Leukocytosis, definition of, 126
Leukopenia, 134
  definition of, 126
Levallorphan (Lorfan), 312
Level of consciousness; see also Consciousness
  assessment of, 533, 533t
Levobupivacaine (Chirocaine), 342t, 344; see also Chirocaine
Levodopa (Larodopa), for drug-induced parkinsonism, 98
Levophed; see Norepinephrine
Librium, abuse of, effects and signs of, 699t
Licensed practical nurses (LPNs), 16
Licensed vocational nurses (LVNs), 16
Lid block, for eye surgery, 456
Lid reflex, Stage II anesthesia and, 276, 277
Lidocaine (Xylocaine), 258t, 341, 342t, 343
  for alcohol withdrawal, 701
  for cardiopulmonary resuscitation, 743, 745
  for cesarean section, 693
  for eye surgery, 456
  for laryngospasm in children, 675
  malignant hyperthermia and, 709, 710b, 712
  for malignant hyperthermia cart, 8b
  muscle relaxants and, 269t, 330-331
  myocardial infarction and, 133
  propranolol interaction with, 267t
  for thoracic surgery, 467
  d-tubocurarine interaction with, 267t
Ligation; see also Tubal ligation
  definition of, 493
  inferior vena cava, 494
  of veins, 496
  vena cava, 500
Light
  coherent versus incoherent, 627, 628
  collimated versus uncollimated, 627, 628
  laser light versus, 627
Limbic lobe, 99
Limbic system, 99-100
  anatomy of, 99
Lincomycin, muscle relaxants and, 268t, 271, 330b

Linear accelerator (LINAC) units, 527
Linear skull fractures, 520
Lipolysis
  definition of, 213
  glucocorticoids and, 217
Liquaemin sodium, 256t; see also Heparin
"Liquid Ecstasy," abuse of, 704
LiteLift continuous passive motion (CPM) machine, 514
Lithium
  geriatric patients and, 685t
  pancuronium and succinylcholine interactions with, 269t
Lithotripsy
  ambulatory surgery and, 615
  definition of, 221
  extracorporeal shock wave, 572
Little's area, 152
Liver
  anatomy and physiology of, 225-226
  cardiogenic shock and, 725
  care after surgery of, 562-563
  geriatric surgery and, 684
  inhalant abuse and, 703
  obesity and, 650
  pregnancy and, 691
  removal of drugs from systemic circulation and, 251
  thiazide diuretics and, 196
  T-tube placement in common bile duct, 563, 563
Liver cirrhosis, alcoholic, 701
Liver diseases
  alcohol abuse and, 701
  drug effects and, 265
  opioid abuse and, 697
Liver failure
  acute, 227
  opioids for pain management and, 424
Living wills
  cardiopulmonary resuscitation and, 735
  end-of-life preferences and, 86
  enforcement of, 79
  ethics committees and policies on, 87
  information about, 87
LMA-Classic, for airway management, 418, 418
LMA-Fastrach, 419, 419
LMA-Flexible, 419
LMA-ProSeal, 419
LMA-Unique, 419
Loading dose, 250
  patient-controlled analgesia and, 313-314
Lobar bronchi, 156, 156
Lobectomy
  definition of, 465
  positioning after, 467
Lobular carcinoma in situ (LCIS), definition of, 591
Local anesthesia; see Anesthesia, local
Local governments, managed care and, 56
Logrolling, 515
Longitudinal fissure, 100
  in cerebral cortex, 95
Longitudinal striae, 99
Long-term outcomes, managed care and, 62

Loop diuretics, 195, 196, 198
  insulin interaction with, 270t
Loop of Henle, 190, *191*
Lopressor, for hypertension, 148
Lorazepam (Ativan), 258t, 297
  abuse of, effects and signs of, 699t
  agitation treatment guidelines for, 298b
  for postoperative anxiety, 390
Lordosis
  definition of, 506
  lumbar, obesity and, 649
  malignant hyperthermia and, 708
Lorfan, 312
"Love drug," abuse of, 703-704
Low segment C-section, definition of, 581
Lower extremity nerve injuries,
    postsurgical, 358
Lower motor neurons, definition of, 93
LSD (lysergic acid diethylamide), abuse of,
    697, 702-703
  effects and signs of, 700t
Lumbar myelogram, *537*
Lumbar plexus, 121, *122*
Lumbar puncture, 117
  administration techniques, 346-348, *347*
  intracranial pressure monitoring and, 529
Lumbar spinal nerves, 122
Lumbar spinal segments, 118, *119*
Lumbar spine
  injuries to, 537
  surgery on, 515
Lumbar sympathectomy, 499
Lumbar vertebrae, 115, 116-117
Lumbosacral nerve injuries, postsurgical, 358
Lumpectomy, 592-594, *593*
  definition of, 591
Lund and Browder age-adjusted burn injury
    chart, 608, *609*
Lung(s); *see also under* Pulmonary; Thoracic
    surgery
  capacities, 157, 158t, 159
    graphic representation of, *157*
  infant respiratory distress syndrome, 665-
      666
  inhalation injuries to, 610
  laparoscopy and, 634
  mechanics, 159-161
  oxygen toxicity and, 187
  pregnancy and mechanics of, 691
  pressure-volume (P-V) curve, *159*, 159-
      160
    inflation and deflation paths of, *160*
    lung compliance and, 161-162
  protection by, 167
  pulmonary circulation, 165-167
  rheumatoid arthritis and dysfunction of,
      647
  septic shock and, 727
  water balance in, *168*, 168-169, 202
Lung compliance (C$_L$), 161-165
  combined P-V of lung and chest wall, 165
  equal pressure point (EPP), 162, *163*
  mechanical features of chest wall, 164
  perianesthesia patient and, 165, *166*
  pulmonary time constant, 162-164
Lung disease, preexisting, postoperative
    complications and, 183

Lung elastic recoil (Pst$_L$), 162
Lung injury, acute, septic shock and, 727
Lung receptors, in breathing regulation,
    182
Lung volume, 157-159, 158t
  graphic representation of, *157*
  postoperative complications in, 183-185
  preoperative *versus* postoperative, 184-
      185, *185*
Lupus erythematosus, as hypersensitivity
    reaction, 243
Luque rods, 515
  definition of, 506
Luteinizing hormone, 218
Lymph, 203
Lymph node dissection, after lumpectomy,
    593, *593*
Lymphocytes, 134
  humoral immunity and, 239-240
Lymphoma, immunosuppression and, 245
Lymphopenia, definition of, 238
Lymphotoxin, cellular immunity and, 242
Lysergic acid diethylamide; *see* LSD
Lysosomal enzymes, immediate
    hypersensitivity reaction and, 242

M

MAC awake, 281
MAC hours, 281
MAC-BAR, 281
Maceration of skin, postsurgical, 357-358
Macintosh blade, for laryngoscope, 411,
    413
  positioning for insertion of, *416*
Macroglossia, in children, 679
Macrophages, cellular immunity and, 241-
    242
Magill attachment, for anesthesia machine,
    282, *283*
Magill forceps, for nasotracheal intubation,
    416-417, *417*
Magnesium, 207, 258t
  calcium and, 216
  for cardiopulmonary resuscitation, 743,
      745
  muscle relaxants and, 269t, 329-330
  for sickle cell anemia and hemolysis,
      655
Magnetic resonance imaging (MRI), 519
  cerebral blood flow studies with, 112-113
  normal cranial, *519*
  for spinal surgery diagnosis, 535
  for vascular disease diagnosis, 493
Main arterial pressure (MAP), cerebral
    perfusion pressure and, 525, 526
Mainstream capnographs, 366
Malaise, hemolytic reactions to transfusions
    and, 211
Malecot catheter, 569
Malignant hyperthermia (MH), 7, 678,
    707-712
  club drugs and, 703
  complications after, 712
  emergency supplies for, 7, 8b
  eye surgery and, 459-460
  genetic susceptibility to, 708
  pathophysiology of, 709

Malignant hyperthermia (MH) (*Continued*)
  perioperative management of patient
      susceptible to, 710-711
  pharmacologic agents associated with, 710
  signs and symptoms of, 709b
  succinylcholine and, 328
  susceptibility evaluation, 708
  treatment, 711-712
  triggering, 709, 710b
Malpractice crisis, 64-66
Mamillary body, 99
Mamillothalamic tract, 99
Mammoplasty, 597-598
  definition of, 590
Managed care, 54-63
  about, 54-55
  ambulatory surgery and, 615
  case managers role in, 58
  clinical guidelines and, 60
  cost-benefit analysis and, 61
  cost-effectiveness analysis and, 61-62
  evidence-based strategies for, 60
  gag orders under, 79
  healthcare delivery structure, 55-56
  long-term outcomes and, 62
  outcomes research and, 60-61
  PACU cost of care, 58-59
  patient education and, 59
  payment for, 56-57
  perianesthesia nurses and, 58, 59
  short-term outcomes and, 62
  strategy, 57-58
Mandible, *105*
  hypoplastic, malignant hyperthermia
      and, 708
Mandibular branch of trigeminal nerve
    (V), 103t
Mannitol (Osmitrol), 198, 258t
  in bladder irrigation fluid, 205
  intracranial pressure and, 529
  for malignant hyperthermia treatment,
      712b
  for ocular hypotensive effect, 459
  as osmotic diuretic, 195
Mapleson D breathing circuit, for pediatric
    anesthesia, 666
Marburg virus, as biological warfare agent,
    731b
Marcaine; *see* Bupivacaine
Marijuana
  abuse of, 697, 702
    effects and signs of, 699t
  benzodiazepines and, 700
Marplan, sympathetic hyperactivity and,
    137
Marshall-Marchetti operation, definition of,
    567
Mastectomy, 594; *see also* Breast
    reconstruction
  ambulatory, 616
  modified radical, *593*, 594
    definition of, 591
  radical, *593*, 594-595
    definition of, 592
Master gland; *see* Pituitary gland
Mastoid portions of temporal bones, inner
    ear and air cells of, 104, *106*

Mastoid process, 105
Mastoidectomy, 435-436
   definition of, 433
Mastoiditis, 106
Mastopexy, 591, 596-597
   definition of, 591
Mathematical model of pharmacokinetics, 249-250
Mature generation of workers, 21, 22-24t
Maxair, respiratory care and, 266t
Maxillary branch of trigeminal nerve (V), 103t
Maxillofacial injuries, trauma nurse's check for, 720
Maxillofacial surgery, 450-451
Mazicon; see Flumazenil
McDonald procedure, 584-585
MDMA, abuse of, 703-704
MDR-TB, 40
MEAC (minimum effective analgesic concentration), 313
Mean arterial pressure, 128, 372
   cardiac surgery and, 486
   during laparoscopy, 635
Mean systemic arterial pressure (MSAP), 114
Mechanical assist devices, definition of, 477-478
Mechanical heart valves, 482
Medial temporal lobe, olfactory area in, 99
Mediastinal widening, from anthrax, 732
Mediastinoscopy, definition of, 466
Medicaid, 55, 57
   gag orders under, 79
   medical malpractice and, 65
Medical error
   reporting, 73
   systematic approach to analyzing, 69-71
   technology and, 68
Medical ethics, 77-92
   court cases on, 77
   ethics committees/consult services role in, 88-90
   informed consent/refusal, 80-88
      Arato v. Avedon case, 80-82
      end-of-life and, 85-88
      resuscitation, 83-85
   physician paternalism and, 78-79
   resources on, 77
   roots of law and, 78
Medical malpractice, 64-76
   new approach to, 68-69
   perspective on, 64-66
   risk management suggestions, 72-74
   sources for identifying PACU, 66-67
   standard of care, individual liability and, 71-72
   systems approach to, 69-71
   traditional approach to, 67-68
Medical malpractice insurance, coverage provisions, 73
Medicare, 55, 57
   ambulatory surgery and, 615
   gag orders under, 79
   medical malpractice and, 65
Medicine, U.S. regulation of, 78
Meditation, for pain management, 426

Medulla, renal, 189
Medulla oblongata, 94, 110
   in basal view of brain, 95
   in brainstem, 101, 102
   functional description of, 102
   in lateral view of brain, 94
Medullary carcinoma, definition of, 591
Melanocyte-stimulating hormone, 215
Melatonin, 100-101
Mendelson's syndrome, 224
Meningeal dura, 106, 109
Meninges, 106-108
   coronal section, 109
Meniscal cartilage, 512
Meniscectomy, definition of, 506
Mental foramen, 105
Mental retardation, midazolam with ketamine for pediatric anesthesia and, 667
Meperidine (Demerol), 258t, 305-306, 310t
   abuse of, effects and signs of, 698t
   drug-drug interactions in PACU and, 268t
   geriatric patients and, 685t
   mu opioid receptors and, 304
   myocardial infarction and, 133
   for pain management, 423
      pediatric surgery and, 674
   respiratory and cardiovascular depression monitoring and, 227
   vomiting center excitation and, 656
Mephentermine (Wyamine), 259t
   action of, 144t
Mepivacaine (Carbocaine), 259t, 341, 342t, 343
   for eye surgery, 456
   malignant hyperthermia and, 710b
Meptazinol, mu-1 opioid receptor and, 304
Mescalin, respiratory care and, 266t
Mesencephalon, 94, 95, 100
   in brainstem, 101, 102
   description of, 101
Meshed autograft skin, 612
Mestinon; see Pyridostigmine
Metabolic acidosis, 176, 176b, 176t, 194
   cardiogenic shock and, 725
   diabetes mellitus and, 646
   malignant hyperthermia and, 709, 709b
   pneumoperitoneum and, 638t
   progressive phase hemorrhage and, 724
   shock and, 723
Metabolic alkalosis, 176, 176t
   kidney regulation of, 194, 195
Metabolic regulation
   cerebral blood flow and, 525-526
   definition of, 93
Metabolism
   body heat and, 706
   of inhalation anesthetics, 278
   in newborns and infants, 673
      hypothermia and, 673-674
   oxygen consumption and, 722-723
   septic shock and, 727
Metaproterenol (Metaprel), 259t
   respiratory care and, 266t

Metaraminol (Aramine), 259t
   action of, 144t
   for hypotension, 144
Metareactivity, definition of, 249
Metarterioles, 135
Metered dose inhalers (MDIs), 251
Methadone (Dolophine), 259t
   abuse of, effects and signs of, 698t
   opiate abuse and, 700
   withdrawal, for opiate detoxification in PACU, 315
Methemoglobin, 400
   definition of, 150
Methemoglobinemia, 365
Methicillin-Resistant Staphylococcus aureus (MRSA), 41
Methohexital (Brevital), 259t, 293
Methoxamine (Vasoxyl), 259t
   action of, 144t
   for hypotension, 144, 148
Methoxyflurane (Penthrane), 285
   kidney disease and, 197
Methyldopa
   geriatric patients and, 685t
   for hypertension, 147
   neurohumoral transmission and, 142t
   sympathetic nerve stimulation and, 141
Methylene blue (Urolene Blue), 259t
Methylergonovine (Methergine), 259t
Methylprednisolone
   intracranial pressure and, 529
   for spinal cord injuries, 540
Methylxanthines, bronchodilatation and, 141
Metoclopramide (Reglan), 259t
   for aspiration pneumonitis in pregnant patients, 224
   esophageal resting pressure and, 221
   for nausea, 657t, 658
   for ophthalmic surgery patients, 460
   for opiate detoxification in PACU, 315
   postoperative excitement from, 395
   for postoperative nausea and vomiting in children, 678
   for vomiting/regurgitation, 224
Metocurine iodide (Metubine), 320t, 322
Metoprolol (Toprol), 260t
   for hypertension, 145, 148
Metubine, 320t, 322
Microangiopathy, diabetes mellitus and, 645
Microcirculation, 135
Micrognathia, in children, 679
Microsomal enzymes, 227
Midamor, 196
Midazolam (Versed), 260t, 296-297
   abuse of, 700-701
      effects and signs of, 699t
   agitation treatment guidelines for, 297b
   breast biopsy and, 592
   for eye surgery, 456
   with ketamine for pediatric anesthesia, 667
   for opiate detoxification in PACU, 315
   for postoperative anxiety, 390, 395
   for premedication with pediatric anesthesia, 666
   propofol and, 294

Midbrain, 94, 101; *see also* Mesencephalon

Middle cerebellar peduncle, *101*

Migration inhibitory factor, cellular immunity and, 242

Miles (Teflon) serrated caval clip, *494*

Miller blade, for laryngoscope, 411-412, *413*
  positioning for insertion of, *416*

Milrinone (Primacor), 260t
  for hypotension, 144

Mineralocorticoids, 217

Minimally invasive coronary artery bypass grafting, definition of, 478

Minimally invasive radio-guided parathyroidectomy (MIRP), definition of, 548

Minimum alveolar concentration (MAC), 279, 279t
  anesthetic agent potency and, 280-281
  Stage III anesthesia and, 276-277

Minimum effective analgesic concentration (MEAC), 313

Minute ventilation V_E, definition of, 150

Mist therapy, 152; *see also* Humidification
  COPD and postoperative oxygen, 643-644
  myasthenia gravis and postoperative, 645
  for postintubation croup, 677
  sickle cell anemia and, 654

Mistakes
  human error as, 46
  reportable, 70

Mitral regurgitation, definition of, 478

Mitral stenosis, definition of, 478

Mitral valve, 129, *129*

Mivacurium (Mivacron), 260t, 320t, 324-325
  for children and adolescents, 327-328

Mobilization, postoperative, 394; *see also* Ambulation
  cardiac surgery and, 491
  cranial surgery and, 533-534
  orthopedic surgery and, 508
  spinal surgery and, 545
  thoracic surgery and, 468

Modulation, of pain, 422

Monitored anesthesia care (MAC), for eye surgery, 456

Monoamine oxidase (MAO) inhibitors, hypertension and, 147

Montelukast (Singulair), respiratory care and, 266t

Morbid obesity
  definition of, 649
  surgery for, 650

Moretz (Teflon) vena caval clip, *494*

Morphine, 260t, 304, 306, 310t
  abuse of, effects and signs of, 698t
  dosing for, 429b
  drug-drug interactions in PACU and, 268t
  epidural administration of, 351
  malignant hyperthermia and, 711b
  mu opioid receptors and, 304
  myocardial infarction and, 133
  opiate abuse and, 700

Morphine (*Continued*)
  for pain management, 313, 423, 425-426
    burn injuries and, 613
    C-section and, 695
    ophthalmic surgery and, 460-461
    pediatric surgery and, 674, 675
    surgery with myasthenia gravis and, 645
  for spinal cord injuries, 540
  vomiting center excitation and, 656

Motion sickness, nausea, vomiting and history of, 656

Motivation, limbic system and, 100

Motor areas, in cerebral cortex, 96-98
  premotor, 97-98
  primary, 96-97
  speech, 98

Motor cortex, 97

Motor function, after cranial surgery, 533-534

Motor neurons
  of reticular formation, 104
  spinal, 121

Motor root, 121

Motor vehicle crashes, trauma from, 715

Mouth-to-patient barrier device, for primary CPR ventilation, 739

MRI; *see* Magnetic resonance imaging

Mu opioid receptors, 304-305

Mucinous carcinoma, definition of, 591-592

Mucoactive agents, 266t
  respiratory care and, 266t

Mucomyst, respiratory care and, 266t

Mucosa, hydration of, after pediatric surgery, 673

Mucus, pulmonary, immunologic defense and, 238-239

Multidrug resistant organisms, 41

Murmur, definition of, 126

Muscarine, 137
  neurohumoral transmission and, 142t

Muscarinic receptors
  in chemoreceptor trigger zone, 658
  neuromuscular transmission and, 317, 318
  overdose signs and, 326, 326b

Muscle activity, 317-319, *318, 319*
  basal ganglia and, 96
  cerebellum and, 102, 104
  postoperative, 394
  skeletal, motor cortex and, 96

Muscle myopathies, malignant hyperthermia and, 708

Muscle pain, from anthrax, 732

Muscle relaxants, 317-338
  antibiotics and, 268t, 330, 330b
  body temperature and, 331
  calcium deficiency and, 330
  carbon dioxide and, 330
  cardiac antidysrhythmic drugs and, 330-331
  catecholamines and, 330
  chlorpromazine interaction with, 269t
  depolarizing, 326-329
  depth of anesthesia and, 278
  electrolytes and, 268t
  enflurane and, 285

Muscle relaxants (*Continued*)
  factors influencing, 329-331
  fluid balance and, 329
  inhalation anesthetics and, 270t, 331
  lidocaine interaction with, 269t
  magnesium deficiency and, 329-330
  neuromuscular blockade and, 331-334
  neuromuscular disorders and response to, 334, 335t, 336
  neuromuscular transmission physiology, 317-319, 708
  nondepolarizing
    intermediate-acting, 323-324
    long-acting, 321-323
    neuromuscular blockade and, 271
    for pregnant patients, 692
    reversal of, 325-326
    short-acting, 324-325
  for pain management, 424
  pH and, 330
  pharmacologic overview of, 319, 320t, 321
  potassium deficiency and, 329
  Procaine interaction with, 269t
  quinidine interaction with, 267t
  recovery from, 332b
  sodium deficiency and, 329
  special problems in PACU with, 334, 336

Muscle relaxation, anesthesia and, 276

Muscle tension
  club drugs abuse and, 703
  malignant hyperthermia and, 708

Muscle tone
  after surgery with COPD, 644
  cerebellum and, 102
  depth of anesthesia and, 278
  thermal regulation and, 706

Muscles, skeletal; *see also* Rigidity, muscular
  injury to, malignant hyperthermia and, 710b
  neuromuscular transmission physiology, 317-319, 708

Muscle-skin flaps, in breast reconstruction, 595-596, *596*

Musculoskeletal system
  patient transition from operating room to PACU and, 358
  physiology of, 708
  trauma nurse's assessment of, 721

Music therapy, for trauma patients, 721

Mustache dressings, for nasal surgery, 437

Myalgia, succinylcholine and, 328

Myasthenia gravis, 644-645
  pancuronium and, 322

Myasthenic syndrome, smoking and, 652

Mycobacterium tuberculosis, antibiotic-resistant, 41

Myelogram, lumbar, *537*

Myelography, for spinal surgery diagnosis, 535, 537

Mylaxen, 329

Myocardial depression, in newborns, 664

Myocardial infarction, 132-133
  atropine contraindications with, 746
  cardiac surgery complications and, 487, 488

Myocardial infarction (*Continued*)
  cardiogenic shock and, 724-725
  obesity and, 651
  pneumoperitoneum and, 638t
  postanesthesia shivering and, 707
Myocardial ischemia
  midazolam and, 296
  pancuronium and, 322
Myocardial protection techniques, definition of, 478
Myocardial revascularization, definition of, 478-479
Myocardium
  definition of, 126
  rheumatoid arthritis and, 647
Myoglobin, halothane, succinylcholine and, 328
Myoglobinemia, malignant hyperthermia and, 709b
Myomectomy, abdominal, definition of, 583
Myoplasm
  malignant hyperthermia and, 709
  neuromuscular transmission and, 708
Myosin, neuromuscular transmission and, 319
Myringoplasty, definition of, 434
Myringotomy, 435
  definition of, 433

N

Nalbuphine (Nubain), 309-310, 310t
  for analgesia and reversing respiratory depression, 272, 313
  kappa opioid receptors and, 305
Nalmefene HCL (Revex), 260t
Naloxone (Narcan), 260t, 312
  for ambulatory surgery, 621
  for fentanyl reversal, 307
    pediatric surgery and, 670
  nausea, vomiting and, 658
  opiate abuse and, 700
  for opiate detoxification in PACU, 315-316
  for opioid overdose, 305
  for pain management, after C-section, 695
  for pain management side effects, 424
  for respiratory depression by opioids, 272, 313
  sigma opioid receptors and, 305
  for sufentanil reversal, 308
Naltrexone (ReVia, Trexan), 260t, 312
  withdrawal, for opiate detoxification in PACU, 315
Narcan; see Naloxone
Narcotic antagonists, 311-312
Narcotics; see Opioids
Nardil, sympathetic hyperactivity and, 137
Naropin; see Ropivacaine
Nasal bone, 105; see also Nose
Nasal cavities, frontal sinuses and, 104
Nasal suctioning, 403, 404
  cranial surgery caution, 106
Nasogastric tubes, 557-558
  after abdominal surgery, 559
  after cardiac surgery, 487

Nasogastric tubes (*Continued*)
  after herniorrhaphy, 562
  after laparoscopic cholecystectomy, 564
  after vascular surgery, 504
  irrigation, 557-558
  patency, 557
  patient comfort, 558
Nasopharyngeal airway, 362, 411, 719
Nasopharynx, 152
Nasotracheal intubation, 416-417
  after maxillofacial surgery, 450
  balloon-cuffed, as artificial airway, 362
National Institute for Occupational and Health, latex allergies web site, 244
National Institutes of Health (NIH), 55
National Patient Safety Foundation, 46
National Practitioner Databank (NPDB), 67
Nausea; see also Postoperative nausea and vomiting syndrome
  adrenalectomy and, 579
  club drugs abuse and, 703
  definition of, 221
  ear surgery and, 435
  enflurane and, 286
  eye surgery and, 460
  from gastrointestinal anthrax, 732
  laparoscopy and, 638
  management
    cost-benefit analysis on, 61
    evidence-based strategies for, 60
  morphine and, 306
  nasal surgery and, 437
  nursing care, 658
  spinal anesthesia and, 350
  trauma injuries and, 721-722
Navoban, 657t
Nd:YAG (laser), 630t
Near total thyroidectomy, definition of, 548
Necessary equipment, 7
Neck, trauma nurse's evaluation of, 720
Neck injury, head-tilt maneuver and, 737
Neck surgery
  radical, 447, 448, 449
    complications of, 449
  reconstruction, 449-450
Neck vein distension
  cardiogenic shock and, 725
  trauma nurse's assessment of, 720
Nedrocromil (Tilade), respiratory care and, 266t
Needle biopsy
  definition of, 466
  topical anesthesia for, 467
Neisseria gonorrhoeae, 41
Nembutal, 262t
  abuse of, effects and signs of, 698t
Neomycin, muscle relaxants and, 268t, 271, 330b
Neoplasms; see Tumors
Neostigmine (Prostigmin), 260t, 317
  acetylcholinesterase and, 138
  doxacurium chloride reversal with, 323
  for muscle relaxant reversal, 325, 326
  for myasthenia gravis, 644
Neo-Synephrine; see Phenylephrine
Nephrectomy, definition of, 566

Nephritis, definition of, 189
Nephrons, renal, 190, *191*
Nephrosis, definition of, 189
Nephrostomy, definition of, 566
Nephrotomy, definition of, 566
Nephrotoxicity, 198
Nephroureterectomy, definition of, 566
Nerves, physiology of, 339-341
Nervous system
  arterial blood pressure and, 128
  autonomic (*see* Autonomic nervous system)
  cardiac surgery and, 491
  central (*see* Central nervous system)
  patient transition from operating room to PACU and, 358
  pituitary gland and, 214
Nesacaine, 253t, 341; *see also* Chloroprocaine
  succinylcholine interaction with, 269t
Neural pathways, 94
Neuraxial opioids, 312-313
Neuroblastoma, 137
  adrenalectomy for, 578
Neurogenic shock, 716, 717t, 723, 725-726
Neuroglia, definition of, 93
Neuroglia cells, in spinal cord, 120
Neurohumoral transmission, 317
Neurohypophysis, 214
  hormones of, 215
Neuroleptanalgesia, 198
  definition of, 300
  etomidate and, 294
Neuroleptanesthesia, extrapyramidal reactions and, 98
Neuroleptic agents, extrapyramidal reactions and, 98
Neurologic status
  cardiac surgery and, 486
  carotid endarterectomy and, 500
  trauma injury and, 720
  vascular surgery and, 504
Neuromuscular blockade
  assessment of, 331-334
  atracurium and, 324
  criteria for recovery from, 332b
  inhalation anesthetics and, 331
  thiazide and, 271
  trauma injuries and, 721
  vecuronium and, 323
Neuromuscular blocking drugs (NMBDs), 317; *see also* Muscle relaxants
  nicotinic receptor responses and, 137
  sickle cell anemia and, 654
  smoking and, 652
Neuromuscular system, aging and, 683
Neuromuscular transmission, physiology of, 317-319, *318*, *319*
Neurons, 94
Neurosurgical patient care, 517-547
  cranial surgery, 518-535
  spinal surgery, 535-546
Neurovascular assessment in orthopedic patients, 507-508
  after foot surgery, 514
  after knee surgery, 513
  after spinal surgery, 515

Neutralization, antibody, 241
Newborns; see Infants, newborn
Nexters, 21, 22-24t, 24
Nicardipine (Cardene), 261t
Nicotine, neurohumoral transmission and,
    142t
Nicotinic receptors, 137
    neuromuscular transmission and, 317-318
    overdose signs and, 326, 326b
Nifedipine (Procardia), 141, 143, 261t
    for hypertension, 145, 146t
Nimbex, 253t, 324
Nines, Rule of, for burns, 608, 608
Nipple, Paget's disease of, definition of, 592
Nipple-areola reconstruction, 595-596, 596
Nipride, 261t; see also Nitroprusside;
        Sodium nitroprusside
    for hypertension, 145-147, 146t
    for septic shock, 728
Nissen fundoplication, 555
Nitroglycerin, 261t
    for hypertension, 146t, 148
    myocardial infarction and, 133
    for septic shock, 728
    for cardiac surgery complications, 488
Nitrol IV, for hypertension, 146t
Nitropress, 261t; see also Nitroprusside;
        Sodium nitroprusside
    for hypertension, 146t
Nitroprusside (Nipride, Nitropress), 261t;
        see also Nipride; Sodium nitroprusside
    coronary artery steal and, 131
Nitrostat IV, for hypertension, 146t
Nitrous oxide, 261t, 288-289
    abuse of, 703
    for anesthesia maintenance in pregnant
        patients, 692
    intracranial pressure and, 528
    malignant hyperthermia and, 711b
    for pneumoperitoneum in laparoscopy,
        635, 636t
    potency of, 280
    pulmonary vascular resistance and, 167
    as Stage I anesthetic agent, 276
    thiopental, oxygen combination
        anesthetic with, 292
Nitrous-narcotic technique
    fentanyl in, 307
    nausea, vomiting and, 658
    pentazocine in, 309
Nizatidine (Axid), 261t
    for opiate detoxification in PACU, 315
    for vomiting/regurgitation, 224
Nociception, 340; see also Pain
No-CPR program, 735
Nodule, in cerebellum, 102
Noncoronary cardiogenic shock, 724, 725
Nondiverting capnographs, 366
Nonmaleficence, medical ethics and, 77, 78
Nonopioid intravenous anesthetics, 292-
    303
Nonsteroidal anti-inflammatory drugs
    (NSAIDs)
    narcotics and, 431
    for pain management, 423
        in children, 674
    surgical bleeding and, 207

Norcuron; see Vecuronium bromide
Norepinephrine (Levophed), 136, 261t
    action of, 144t
    alpha$_1$ receptors and, 140
    biochemistry, 136
    during cardiopulmonary bypass, 484
    for high spinal block, 350
    inhibitors of, 141
    during laparoscopy, 637
    metabolism of, 138
    pulmonary epithelium and, 167
    renal function and, 197
    for septic shock, 728
    for shock after adrenalectomy, 578
Normodyne; see Labetalol
Normotensive, definition of, 126
Normothermia, evidence-based strategies
        for return to, 60
Noscapine, 304
Nose; see also under Nasal; Nasogastric
        tubes; Nasopharyngeal airway
    anatomy of, 151-152
    intubation for
        perianesthesia nursing care, 186
        upper airways receptors and, 181
    mucus blanket of, 152
    sagittal section through, 151, 437
    surgery on, 436-438
    trauma nurse's evaluation of, 720
Nosocomial infections, 40b
Novocain, 341; see also Procaine
NSAIDs; see Nonsteroidal anti-
        inflammatory drugs
Nubain; see Nalbuphine
Nuclear magnetic resonance imaging, 519;
        see also Magnetic resonance imaging
Nucleus pulposus, 115-116
    herniated, 544-545, 545
Nupercaine, 342t
Nuromax; see Doxacurium chloride
Nurse anesthetists, medical malpractice
        and, 67
Nurse manager, 12
Nurses, questioning doctor's orders by, 73
Nurses' aides, PACU and, 16
Nutrition
    albumin production and, 226
    bronchial, pulmonary circulation and,
        167
Nystagmus
    cerebellum and, 102
    cranial surgery and, 535
    ear surgery and, 435
    ketamine for pediatric anesthesia and,
        667
    myasthenia gravis and, 644

O

Obesity, 649-651
    cardiac surgery complications and, 487
    cardiovascular system and, 649-650, 651
    in children, obstructive sleep apnea and,
        679
    definition of, 649
    lung volume and, 158
    MRI and, 519
    nausea, vomiting and, 656

Obesity (Continued)
    nursing care for, 650-651
        fluid dynamics, 651
        psychologic aspects, 651
    postoperative pulmonary complications
        and, 184
    pregnancy and, 650
    respiratory system and, 649, 650-651
    thiopental-halothane interactions and,
        270
Obesity-hypoventilation syndrome, 649
Obstetric surgery
    care after, 583-585
    terms used in, 581
Obstructive jaundice, 226
Obstructive shock, 716, 718t, 723, 728
Obturator nerve, 122
Occipital bone, 104, 105
Occipital lobe, 94, 94, 95
    blood supplies for, 112
Occipital plexus, 108
Occlusion, definition of, 126
Occupational Health and Safety
        Administration (OSHA)
    on bloodborne pathogens exposure, 41
    on postoperative infection control,
        405
    on protective gloves, 244
    universal standards overview, 233, 235-
        236b
Ocularist, definition of, 455
Oculocardiac reflex
    compresses after ophthalmic surgery and,
        461
    definition of, 455
    during eye surgery, 459
Oculogyric crises, psychotropic drugs and,
        98
Oculomotor nerve (III), 101
    pupillary activity, cranial surgery and,
        535
    type and functions of, 103t
    uncal herniation and, 523
Oculoplastic surgery, 456
Oddi's sphincter, 227
Oil-gas partition coefficient, 279-280, 279t,
        289-290
    of specific anesthetics, 280
Olfactory area, in cerebral cortex, 99
Olfactory bulb, 99
    and tract, 95
Olfactory nerve (I), type and functions of,
        103t
Oliguria, 195
    acute hepatic failure and, 227
    definition of, 189
    kidney failure and, 198, 199
Olive, in brain stem, 101
Omeprazole (Prilosec), 261t
Oncotic pressure, 204, 205
Ondansetron (Zofran), 261t
    for nausea, 657t, 658
    for ophthalmic surgery patients, 460
    for opiate detoxification in PACU, 315
    for postoperative nausea and vomiting in
        children, 678, 679
Oophorectomy, definition of, 583

Oophorocystectomy, definition of, 583
Open channel block, succinylcholine and, 336
Open drop method, for inhalation anesthesia administration, 282
Open (simple) pneumothorax, 164
Open reduction, definition of, 506
Open skull fractures, 520
Open systems, for inhalation anesthesia administration, 282
Operating room
   cardiopulmonary resuscitation in, 735
   DNR orders in, 83, 84
   transition to PACU from, 354-359
      communication in, 354-358
      perianesthesia nursing, 354
      perioperative nursing, 354
Ophthalmic branch of trigeminal nerve (V), 103t
Opiate receptors, limbic system and, 99
Opioid intravenous anesthetics, 304-316
   as surgical premedications, 620
Opioid receptors, concept of, 304-305
Opioids, 305-312
   abuse of, 697, 700
      effects and signs of, 698t
   for analgesia, 422, 423-424, 429, 568
      in children, 674
   antagonists, 311-312, 621
   burn injuries and, 613
   in chemoreceptor trigger zone, 656
   concept of, 304-305
   definition of, 304
   descriptions, 305-311
   detoxification in PACU from, 315-316
   droperidol contraindication with, 300-301
   drug-drug interactions in PACU and, 268t, 272
   genitourinary surgery and, 571
   intracranial pressure and, 528-529
   intrathecal and epidural administration of, 312-313, 425
   LSD and, 703
   nausea, vomiting and, 658
   NSAIDs and, 431
   for pain management with tolerance to, 425
   pediatric surgery and, 674
   for post C-section pain relief, 695
   postoperative excitement from, 395
   rheumatoid arthritis and, 647
   stomach physiology and, 223
   surgery with COPD and, 644
   surgery with myasthenia gravis and, 645
   as surgical premedications, 620
Opium, abuse of, effects and signs of, 698t
Opium suppositories, after cystoscopy, 568
Opsonin, phagocytosis and, 239
Optic chiasma, 95
Optic nerve, 95, 99
Optic nerve (II), type and functions of, 103t
Optic reflexes, 101
Optic tract, 96, 101
Oral airway assessment and management, 409-411
Oral analgesia, 424
Oral drugs, systemic absorption of, 250-251
Oral suctioning, 403

Oralet lollipop, for pediatric sedation, 667
Orbitofrontal cortex, 99
Orchiectomy, definition of, 566
Orchiopexy
   definition of, 566
   postoperative nausea and vomiting after, 677
Orderlies, PACU and, 16
Oretic, 196
Organ donors, kidney, 572-573
Oropharyngeal airway, 362, 409-411, 410, 719
Oropharynx, 152
Orthopedic patients, 506-516
   compartment syndrome, 510
   complications, 509-511
   deep vein thrombosis, 510
   fat embolism syndrome, 510
   general perianesthesia care, 507-511
   immobilization devices care, 509
   neurovascular assessment, 507-508
   perianesthesia care
      after amputation, 515
      after arm and forearm surgery, 511
      after femoral surgery, 512
      after foot surgery, 514
      after hand surgery, 511
      after hip surgery, 512
      after knee surgery, 512-514
      after shoulder surgery, 511-512
      spinal surgery, 514-515
   positioning, 507
   range-of-motion exercises, 509
   shock, 510-511
   urinary retention, 511
   wound care, 509
Orthopnea
   definition of, 151
   obesity and, 649
Orthotripsy, 615
Osmitrol; see Mannitol
Osmolality
   after kidney transplantation, 573
   after pediatric surgery, 673
   crystalloid fluids and, 208
   definition of, 201
Osmosis, of CSF, 111
Osmotic diuretics, 195, 198
Osmotic pressure, 204
Ossiculoplasty, definition of, 433
Osteoporosis
   definition of, 506
   spinal cord injuries and, 544
Osteotomy, definition of, 506
Oswald solubility coefficient, 279
Otolaryngologic surgery, for children, 679
Otologic surgery, 434-436
Outcomes research, 60-61
Outpatient surgery; see Ambulatory surgery
Overdose
   anesthetic, 276, 277
      opioids and, 305
   cardiopulmonary arrest and, 744
   gamma hydroxybutyrate and, 704
   patient-controlled analgesia in children, 675
Oxazepam (Serax), 261t
   abuse of, effects and signs of, 699t

Oxychodone, for oral analgesia, 431
Oxygen; see also Mist therapy; Pulse oximetry
   balanced technique and, 305
   carbon dioxide transport and, 172-173
   in patient-controlled analgesia, 315
   post anesthesia administration of, 185-187, 400, 401t
      for children, 667
   postoperative, 399-400
      ambulatory surgery, 622
      cerclage procedure, 584
      for children, 673
      COPD and, 643
      for geriatric patients, 686
      myasthenia gravis and, 645
      nasal surgery, 438
      prostate surgery, 576
   saturation time, 166, 622
      sickle cell anemia and, 654
   toxicity, 186-187, 400
Oxygen dissociation curve, pulse oximetry and, 172
Oxygen saturation monitor
   after pediatric surgery, 670
   for CPR assessment, 743
Oxygen transport, 170-172
Oxyhemoglobin, 151, 170
Oxyhemoglobin dissociation curve, 170-172, 171, 364, 365
   in newborns, 664
Oxyntic glands, definition of, 221
Oxytocin (Pitocin), 215, 261t
   after C-section, 584

P

Pacemaker, definition of, 126
PACU; see Postanesthesia Care Unit
Paddles, defibrillator, 742
Paget's disease of the nipple, definition of, 592
Pain; see also Myalgia
   ketamine control of, 301
   meperidine and, 305
   pediatric measurement tools for, 676t
   physiology of, 339-341
   postoperative
      cranial surgery and motor response to, 534-535
      hypertension and, 145
      nausea and, 656
      orthopedic surgery, 508
      pediatric surgery, heart rate and, 670
      spinal surgery, 515
      trauma injuries, 721
   quality of, 428
   rating scales for, 427-428, 428
      children and, 675
   sensations of, 98
   stomach physiology and, 223
   transfusion reactions and, 211
   understanding, 422-426
Pain management, 4, 9, 422-432
   after abdominal surgery, 559
   after abdominoperineal resection, 562
   after adrenalectomy, 579
   after ambulatory surgery, 429, 431, 622
   after anal or rectal surgery, 562

Pain management (*Continued*)
  after bladder surgery, 574
  after burn injuries, 613
  after extracorporeal shock wave
      lithotripsy, 572
  after genital or vaginal surgery, 587
  after genitourinary surgery, 571
  after laparoscopic cholecystectomy, 565
  after laparoscopy, 586, 637-638
  after liver surgery, 563
  after mammoplasty, 598
  after nasal surgery, 438
  after ophthalmic surgery, 460-461
  after pediatric surgery, 674-675
  after penile surgery, 578
  after radical mastectomy, 595
  after surgery with myasthenia gravis, 645
  after thoracic surgery, 468-469
  after thyroid surgery, 549
  after transurethral resection of prostate,
      575
  after trauma injuries, 721
  after vascular surgery, 498, 502, 504
  alfentanil for, 308
  ASPAN clinical guidelines on, 60
  care procedures for, 426-429, 431
      analgesia during surgery, 427
      analgesia in PACU, 429
      assessment with pain scales, 427-428,
          428
      nursing assessment, 428-429
      PACU environment, 427
      preoperative interview and exam, 426-
          427
      withdrawal syndrome, 429
  dezocine for, 311
  end-of-life preferences for, 86, 87
  evidence-based strategies for, 60
  fentanyl for, 307
  morphine for, 306
  myocardial infarction and, 133
  neuraxial opioids for, 312-313
  postoperative, 394
  sickle cell anemia and, 654
  for spinal cord injuries, 540
Paint thinners, abuse of, 703
Paletouvuloplasty, definition of, 433
Palpation
  of chest
      postoperative, 362
      for trauma assessment, 362
  for pulse in peripheral arteries, 497, 719-
      720
Palpitation, definition of, 126
Palsies, spinal anesthesia and, 350
Pancreas, 217-218, 228, 229
  care after surgery of, 563-564
Pancreatic juice, 228
Pancreaticoduodenectomy
  care after, 563-564
  definition of, 554
Pancreatitis, 228
  definition of, 221
  meperidine for pain management in, 423
Pancuronium (Pavulon), 261t, 319, 320t,
    321-322
  aminophylline interaction with, 269t
  geriatric patients and, 685t

Pancuronium (Pavulon) (*Continued*)
  kidney disease and, 198
  lithium interaction with, 269t
  malignant hyperthermia and, 711b
  muscle paralysis and, 142t
Panheparin, 256t; *see also* Heparin
Panhypopituitarism, 218
Papaverine, 304
Papillary muscles, 129
Paradoxical second heart sound (S_2),
    myocardial infarction and, 132
Parahippocampal gyrus, 99
Paralysis
  botulism and, 733
  spinal anesthesia and, 350
Parasympathetic nerve endings, 130-131
Parasympathetic nervous system, 123
  bronchi and, 156-157
  coronary blood flow and, 131
  skeletal muscle of pelvic floor and, 225
  spinal nerves and, 121
  stomach physiology and, 223
Paraterminal gyrus, 99
Parathormone, 213
  calcium and, 216-217
Parathyroid glands, 216-217
  surgery of, 548-550
      anesthesia, 548
      complications, 549-550
Parathyroidectomy, definition of, 548
Paresthesia, definition of, 506
Pargyline, sympathetic hyperactivity and,
    137
Parietal bones, 104, *105*
Parietal lobe, 94, *94, 95*
  blood supplies for, 112
  sensory areas in, 98
Parietal pleura, 157
Parietooccipital sulcus, 95
Parkinsonism, drug-induced, 98
Parnate, sympathetic hyperactivity and, 137
Parolfactory area, 99
Paromomycin, muscle relaxants and, 268t
Paroxysmal nocturnal dyspnea (PND),
    definition of, 151
Paroxysmal tachycardia, definition of, 126
Partial pressure, 169
  arterial oxygen, sickle cell anemia and,
      654
  definition of, 151
  of inhalation anesthetics, 278
Partial thromboplastin time (PTT), 134, 207
Partial-thickness burns, 234, 236, 608
Passive acquired immunity, definition of, 238
Patent ductus arteriosus (PDA), definition
    of, 479
Paternalism, medical
  ethical issues in, 78-79
  patient autonomy *versus*, 78
  respect for patient autonomy and, 80
Patient(s); *see also* Patient assessment;
    Patient position; Patient-controlled
    analgesia
  after cerclage procedure, 584
  after vascular surgery on large vessels,
      501
  autonomy of, respect for, 77-78
  informed consent and, 80

Patient(s) (*Continued*)
  resuscitation orders and, 83-85
  treatment option discussions and, 87
  as consumers
      bioethics and, 87
      medical products and services
          marketing to, 68
      standard of medical care
          determination and, 73
  discharge from PACU, 33, 38-39, 406-407
      summary, 37
  education for, managed care and, 59
  perianesthesia care
      for acute pancreatitis, 228
      for biliary lithotripsy, 228
      for burns, 234, 236
      endocrine system monitoring, 218-219
      for eye surgery, 459-463
      fluid volume monitoring, 211-212
      for high spinal block, 349-350
      for immunosuppressed, 246
      of intubated patient, 417
      for latex allergic reactions, 245b
      oxygen therapy for, 179, 185-187
      renal function monitoring, 198
      syndrome of inappropriate secretion of
          antidiuretic hormone and, 219
      vomiting/regurgitation monitoring,
          224-225
  post anesthesia care, 393-408
      after droperidol administration, 300-301
      after intravenous regional anesthesia,
          353
      after ketamine anesthesia, 301-302
      after lorazepam and narcotic
          administration, 297
      after midazolam anesthesia, 296-297
      after propofol anesthesia, 295
      after thiopental anesthesia, 293
      delayed emergence, 395, 685
      ear surgery, 434-436
      emergence excitement, 395
      general safety and comfort, 405-406
      infection control, 405
      intravenous therapy, 395
      oxygen therapy, 399-403
          administration of, 400, 401t
          humidity and, 400
          mechanical ventilation, 401-403,
              402, 402t
      radical neck surgery, 449
      respiratory function maintenance, 399-
          405
      stir-up regimen, 393-395
      suctioning, 403-404
      tracheostomy, 441, 443-445
      transfer from PACU, 406-407, 429
      transfusion therapy, 395-399
  postoperative care for, comfort, anxiety
      and, 389-390
  privacy for, 3
  records, 33, *34-37*
  safety of, systems approach to, 69-71
  simulated, 52-53
Patient assessment, 360-392
  of cardiovascular function and perfusion,
      371-374
  of central nervous system, 385

Patient assessment (*Continued*)
clinical, 361-363
electrocardiographic monitoring, 374-378
of fluid and electrolyte balance, 386-388
hemodynamic monitoring, 378-385
at PACU admission, 361
preoperative, 360-361
psychosocial, 388-390
of respiratory function, 361-371
of thermal balance, 385-386
Patient bays, minimum square footage for, 3
Patient classification system (PCS), 32-33
Patient position
after abdominal surgery, 555-556, 559
after adrenalectomy, 578
after ambulatory surgery, 622
after bladder surgery, 574
after carotid endarterectomy, 499
after C-section, 583
after cystoscopy, 568
after ear surgery, 435
after gastrointestinal surgery, 559
after genital surgery, 587
after gynecologic surgery, 588
after herniorrhaphy, 562
after hip or femoral surgery, 512
after knee surgery, 512
after laparoscopic cholecystectomy, 564
after mammoplasty, 598
after mastopexy, 596-597
after ophthalmic surgery, 461-462
after orthopedic surgery, 507
after pediatric surgery, 667, 668, 670
laryngospasm and, 675
after prostate surgery, 576
after radical mastectomy, 595
after shock trauma, 719
after sympathectomy, 499
after thoracic surgery, 467, 468
after thyroid surgery, 548-549
after tonsillectomy, 679
after vaginal surgery, 587
after vascular surgery, 496
for geriatric patients, 683
for kidney transplantation, 573
during laparoscopy, 635, 637, 637t
for laryngeal mask airway, 418-419
morphine effects on changes in, 306, 512
nausea, vomiting and changes in, 656
of newborns, ventilation and, 662
obesity and, 650
for oral endotracheal intubation, 414, *415*
postoperative, 394, 406
with COPD, 643
pregnancy and, 688, 691, 693
of pregnant patient, 692
respiratory compromise and, 736
sample reporting on, 355-356
Patient Self-Determination Act, 79, 86
Patient-controlled analgesia (PCA), 313-314, 425; *see also* IV PCA pumps
after abdominal surgery, 559
after C-section, 694-695
after gastrointestinal surgery, 559
after laparoscopic cholecystectomy, 565
after trauma injuries, 721
education on, 426-427

Patient-controlled analgesia (PCA)
(*Continued*)
epidural, 314, 426
loading bolus for, 429
protocol for, 314t
Pavulon; *see* Pancuronium
PCP; *see* Phencyclidine
Pectus carinatum, malignant hyperthermia and, 708
Pediatric advanced cardiac life support (PALS), 15
Pediatric Advanced Life Support (PALS), eye surgery and, 452
Pediatric circle system, for anesthesia, 666
Pedicle deepithelialization, for reduction mammoplasty, 597
Pedicles, of vertebrae, 115
PEEP (positive end-expiratory pressure), 162, 401, 402t
definition of, 151
spinal cord injuries and, 543
Pelvis, 189
anatomy of female, 588
trauma injury to, 721
Penetrating trauma, 715
Penicillin
muscle relaxants and, 330b
probenecid interaction with, 271
Penicillin G, for anthrax, 732
Penicillin-resistant *Streptococcus pneumoniae*, 41
Penile implant, definition of, 566
Penile prostheses, 578
Penis, care after surgery on, 577-578
Penrose drain, 576
in prostate surgery, 575
Pentamidine, respiratory care and, 266t
Pentazocine (Talwin), 309, 310t, 312
opiate abuse and, 700
Penthrane, 285; *see also* Methoxyflurane
Pent-nitrous technique, 292
Pentobarbital (Nembutal), 262t
Pentothal; *see* Thiopental
Pepcid, 255t; *see also* Famotidine
for anaphylactic shock, 727
Peptic ulcer, definition of, 221
Perception, of pain, 422
Percussion, of chest, postoperative, 362
Percutaneous endoscopic gastrostomy (PEG), definition of, 554
Percutaneous nephrolithotomy, definition of, 566
Percutaneous transluminal angioplasty (PTA), 494-495
definition of, 493
laser-assisted, 494-495
Percutaneous transluminal coronary angioplasty (PTCA), definition of, 479-480
Perforated ulcers, 560
Perfusion; *see also* Ventilation-perfusion matching
distribution of, 176
pulse oximetry and, 365
to ventilation
decreased, *177*, 177-178
increased, *177*, 178-179

Perianesthesia nursing
definition of, 354
as specialty, 11-29
scope of, 13-14b
Peribulbar block, for eye surgery, 456
Pericardiectomy, definition of, 480
Pericarditis, definition of, 126
Perineal incision, in prostate surgery, 575, 576
Period of ejection, 126
Period of isometric contraction, 126
Period of rapid filling of the ventricles, 126
Perioperative nurses, patient reports by, 356b
Perioperative nursing, definition of, 354
Periorbital ecchymosis, basilar skull fractures and, 520
Periosteal dura, 106
Peripheral arterial catheter (A-line), 379
Peripheral artery embolectomy, 496
Peripheral circulation, 135; *see also* Peripheral vascular dilation
Peripheral compartment in compartmental model of pharmacokinetics, 250
Peripheral nerve stimulator (PNS), 332, *332*
Peripheral neuropathies, inhalant abuse and, 703
Peripheral resistance, definition of, 126
Peripheral vascular dilation
marijuana abuse and, 702
septic shock and, 727
Peritoneal fluid, 203
Peritoneoscopy, definition of, 553-554
Peritubular capillaries, renal, 190
Peroneal nerve, compression after hip or femoral surgery of, 512
Perspiration, insensible and sensible, 203
Pezzer catheter, 569
pH
acid-base relationships and, 174-176
carbon dioxide, muscle relaxants and, 330
kidney regulation of, 194-195
oxygen transport and, 171
pulse oximetry interpretation and, 364
Phacoemulsification, definition of, 455
Phagocytosis
definition of, 238
innate immunity and, 239
Pharmacodynamics
definition of, 249
drug-drug interactions, 271
in geriatric patients, 684
Pharmacokinetics, 249-250
definition of, 249
drug-drug interactions, 265, 267-270t, 270-271
in geriatric patients, 684
of inhalation anesthetics, 278-280
Pharmacology, 248-275; *see also* Anesthetic agents
drug responses, 248, 249-251, 265
drug-drug interactions, 265, 267-270t, 270-271
drugs used in PACU, 252-265t, 273
major drug groups and intended physiologic response, 266t

Pharmacology (*Continued*)
  postoperative nausea and vomiting
      interventions, 658-659
  special considerations, 272-273, 273t
Pharynx, 152
Phenanthrenes, 304
Phencyclidine (PCP), abuse of, 697, 702
  effects and signs of, 700t
Phenelzine sulfate, sympathetic
    hyperactivity and, 137
Phenergan; *see* Promethazine
Phenobarbital (Barbital)
  abuse of, effects and signs of, 698t
  drug-drug interactions in PACU with,
      270t
  kidney disease and, 197
Phenothiazines
  acute dystonic reactions and, 98
  extrapyramidal reactions and, 98
  malignant hyperthermia and, 710-711
  physostigmine salicylate and, 138
  for postoperative nausea and vomiting in
      children, 677-678
  sickle cell anemia and, 655
Phenoxybenzamine, neurohumoral
    transmission and, 142t
Phentolamine (Regitine), 262t
  clonidine withdrawal syndrome and, 140
  for hypertension, 146t, 147
  myocardial infarction and, 133
Phenylalanine, 136
Phenylephrine (Neo-Synephrine), 262t
  action of, 144t
  for high spinal block, 350
  for hypotension, 144
  hypotension detection and, 143
  respiratory care and, 266t
Phenylethanolamine-N-methyltransferase,
    136
Phenytoin (Dilantin), 262t
  d-tubocurarine interaction with, 267t
Pheochromocytoma, 137
  adrenalectomy for, 578
  clonidine withdrawal syndrome and, 140
  hypertension and, 147
Phimosis, 578
  definition of, 566
Phonocardiogram, *127*
Phosphate, 206
Phosphodiesterase, cyclic AMP and, 140,
    141
Phosphorus, calcium and, 216
Phrenic nerve, 121
Phrenic nucleus, definition of, 517
Phyllodes tumor, definition of, 592
Physical dependence
  definition of, 697
  by opioids, 697
Physicians
  medical ethics *versus* legal system and, 88
  medical malpractice insurance and, 68
  therapeutic privilege, informed consent
      doctrine and, 81
Physiologic model of pharmacokinetics,
    249
Physiologic positive end-expiratory pressure
    (PEEP), 162

Physostigmine (Antilirium), 138, 262t, 298
  blood-brain barrier effects of, 138
  for geriatric patients, 686
  for postoperative anxiety, 395
Physostigmine (Antilirium), neurohumoral
    transmission and, 142t
Pia mater
  cranial, *102, 106, 108, 109, 110*
  spinal, *107, 110, 117, 122,* 346
Pickwickian syndrome, 649
Pineal body (or gland), 100, *101*
Pineal gland, 216
Pinocytosis, adrenergic neurotransmitters
    and, 136-137
Pipe smoking, 652
Pipecuronium (Arduran), 262t, 320t, 323
Pirbuterol (Maxair), respiratory care and,
    266t
Pitocin; *see* Oxytocin
Pitressin; *see* Vasopressin
Pituitary gland, 112
  dysfunction, 215-216
  hypothalamus and, 101
  limbic system and, 100
  physiology of, 214
  sella turcica and, 104
  surgical access to, 106
Plague, as biological warfare agent, 730,
    731b, 732-733
Plaque, definition of, 455
Plasma, 209
  fresh frozen (FFP), 211, 718
  redistribution, after pediatric surgery,
      673
  single donor, 211
  volume loss, hypovolemic shock and,
      717t, 723
Plasma concentration curve, 250, *250*
Plasma protein fraction (PPF), 399
Plastic surgery, 600-606
Plateau wave, 531
Platelet count (PC), 134, 207
Platelet-activating factor, septic shock and,
    727
Platelets, 209
  during cardiopulmonary bypass, 485
  shock and, 723
  for thrombocytopenia, 211
  transfusion of, 399, 718
Plavix, surgical bleeding and, 207
Plethysmography, 159, 363-364
Pleural effusion, smoking and, 653
Plexus, definition of, 93
Plication, definition of, 493
Plication ring, *474*
Pneumatic stockings, spinal surgery and,
    515
Pneumonectomy
  definition of, 466
  positioning after, 467
Pneumonia
  after thoracic surgery, 471
  from plague, 732
Pneumonic plague, 732-733
Pneumoperitoneum
  cardiopulmonary effects of, 636t
  laparoscopy and, 634-635

Pneumotaxic center, 183
Pneumothorax, 164
  cardiac surgery and, 490
  cardiopulmonary arrest and, 744
  chest tube clamping and, 471
  chest tube placement and, 469, *469*
  definition of, 466
  nitrous oxide contraindication with, 288
  postoperative, 363
  tension
    as obstructive shock, 716, 718t, 723,
        728
    pneumoperitoneum and, 638t
Poisoning, with gamma hydroxybutyrate,
    704
Polycythemia, definition of, 126, 151
Polymorphonuclear leukocytes (PMNs),
    134
Polymyxin
  interactions with anesthetic agents by,
      271
  muscle relaxants and, 330b
Polymyxin A, muscle relaxants and, 268t
Polymyxin B, muscle relaxants and, 268t
Polyuria, 198
Pons, 94, *94, 95, 100, 110*
  in brain stem, *101, 102*
  functional description of, 102
  medulla oblongata and, 102
Pontocaine, 342t, 344; *see also* Tetracaine
  succinylcholine interaction with, 269t
Position; *see* Patient position
Positive end-expiratory pressure (PEEP),
    162, 401, 402t
  definition of, 151
  spinal cord injuries and, 543
Positive pleural pressure (Ppl), 162
Positron emission tomography (PET)
  cerebral blood flow studies with, 112-113
  for cranial surgery diagnosis, 519-520
Postanesthesia Care Unit (PACU)
  aging nursing population and, 24-25
  basic staff orientation program, 17, *19*
    content, 18-19
    suggested topics, 18-19b
  body substance isolation in, 3
  competency assessment for, 20-21
  drugs used in, 252-265t, 273
  electrical outlets in, 4
  emergency bag contents, 6b
  ergonomics and efficiency in, 5, 7
  expertise development, 19-20
  generation gap, 21, 24
    diversity, 22-24t
  layout of, 5
  lighting for, 4
    pulse oximetry readings and, 366
  management and policies, 30-44
    fasttracking, 39, 39b
    infection control, 40-41
    OSHA requirements and, 42b
    patient classification, 32-33
    patient discharge, 33, 38-39
      summary, *37*
    patient records, 33, *34-36*
    quality improvement, 41-43, *42, 43*
    self-scheduling, 32

Postanesthesia Care Unit (PACU)
(*Continued*)
shared governance, 32
staffing, 30-32
standards of care, 39-40
suggested procedures and, 31b
visitors, 33
medical gases location in, 4
negative pressure isolation in, 3
organizational structure, 12
pain service, 4, 9
Phase I, 1
malignant hyperthermia emergency
supplies, 7
perianesthesia nursing role in, 13b
recovery from ambulatory surgery and,
621-622
space
components, 2
location, 2
storage areas and equipment for, 6b
Phase II, 1
after ambulatory surgery, goals of, 621-
625
perianesthesia nursing role in, 13b
space
components, 2-5
location, 2
storage areas and equipment for, 6b
Phase III, perianesthesia nursing role in,
13b
purpose of, 30
reception and waiting area, 7
space
components of, 2-5, 7
definition of, 1-2
location, 2
staffing, 3-4, 12, 14-17
nurse manager, 12
nurse selection, 12, 14-15
nursing personnel, 15-16
patterns, 16-17
retention practices, 30-32, 32b
standard equipment for, 7, 9
storage in, 4, 5
stress and burnout in, 25-27
telephone and data jacks in, 4
Postanesthesia recovery score (PARS), 33,
38, 38b
for cardiac surgery, 496
for pediatric surgery, 680, 680t
Postcentral gyrus, gustatory area and, 99
Postcommissural fornix, 99
Postdischarge follow-up, 625
Posterior clinoid process, 105
Posterior cord syndrome, 539
Posterior gray horns, 121
Posterior median fissure, 120
Posterior perforated substance, 95
Posterior tibial pulse, 512
Postischemic hyperemia, 128-129
Postoperative nausea and vomiting
syndrome (PONV), 655-659
after tonsillectomy, 679
in children, 677-678
incidence of, 656, 658
mechanism of action, 655, 655-656, 656

Postoperative nausea and vomiting
syndrome (PONV) (*Continued*)
nursing care, 658
airway management, 659
pharmacologic interventions, 658-659
Post-TURP syndrome, 575
Postural reflexes, 101
cerebellum and, 102
definition of, 93
Posturing, decorticate, 535
Potassium, 205-206
coronary blood flow and, 131
geriatric patients and, 683-684
malignant hyperthermia and, 678
muscle relaxants and, 268t, 329
Potassium chloride, for malignant
hyperthermia, 712b
Potassium-sparing diuretics, 195, 196
Potency, drug, definition of, 249
Preanesthesia phase, perianesthesia nursing
role in, 13b
Precapillary sphincter, 135
Precentral gyrus
motor functions and, 96
premotor area and, 97
Precipitation, antibody, 241
Precommissural septum, 99
Precordial pulsations, abnormal
malignant hyperthermia and, 711
myocardial infarction and, 132
Prednisolone, phenobarbital interaction
with, 270t
Preeclampsia, hypertension and, 145
Preexcitation syndrome, definition of, 126
Prefrontal area, 97, 98
Pregnancy; *see also* Aortocaval compression
bupivacaine contraindication in, 343
ectopic
care after, 584
definition of, 581
enflurane contraindication in, 286
laparoscopy and, 634
obesity and, 650
physiologic changes of, 688, 689b
cardiovascular
hematologic alterations, 691
hemodynamic alterations, 688, 690-
691
gastrointestinal, 691-692
respiratory, 691
stomach physiology and, 223
Pregnant patient
intraoperative anesthesia care of, 692-693
medication issues for, 695
perianesthesia care of fetus and, 693-694
post-cesarean section pain management,
694-695
Prehippocampal rudiment, 99
Preload, definition of, 126
Premature atrial contractions (PACs),
postoperative monitoring of, 374, 376,
376
Premature infants; *see* Infants, newborn,
premature
Premature ventricular contractions (PVCs),
postoperative monitoring of, 374, 377,
377-378

Premotor area, 97-98
Premotor cortex, 97
Preoperative patients
pain management interview, 426-427
staffing for, 4
Presaril, 264t
Pressure at mouth (Pao), 162
Pressure injuries of skin, postsurgical, 357
Pressure transfusions, 397
Pressure waves, intracranial pressure and,
531
Pressure-volume (P-V) curve, *159*, 159-160
of chest wall during deflation, *164*
inflation and deflation paths of, *160*
lung compliance and, 161-162
of lungs and chest wall, *165*
perianesthesia patient and, *166*
Priapism, after trauma injury, 721
Prilocaine (Citanest), 262t, 341, 343
Prilosec, 261t
Primacor, 260t; *see also* Milrinone
Primary ABCD survey, for cardiopulmonary
resuscitation, 737
Primary hearing, area in cerebral cortex, 97
Primary plague pneumonia, 732
Primary somesthetic sensations, in cerebral
cortex, 97
Primary vision area in cerebral cortex, 97
Priming technique, for vecuronium
administration, 323-324
Private healthcare organizations, managed
care and, 56
Probenecid, penicillin interaction with,
271
Procainamide (Procamide, Procapan,
Pronestyl), 262t
for cardiopulmonary resuscitation, 743,
745
for malignant hyperthermia, 710
for malignant hyperthermia treatment,
712b
Procaine (Novocain), 262t, 339, 341, 342t
for eye surgery, 456
malignant hyperthermia and, 711b
muscle relaxants and, 269t
succinylcholine interaction with, 269t
Procardia; *see* Nifedipine
Procaterol (Mescalcin), respiratory care
and, 266t
Prochlorperazine (Compazine), 262t
for nausea, 658t
for ophthalmic surgery patients, 460
Procidentia, definition of, 582
Proctocolectomy, total, with ileoanal
anastomosis, 560
Proctosigmoidectomy, *561*
Progesterone, 218
Projection fibers, 95
Prolactin, 215
Promethazine (Phenergan), 262t
for nausea, 657t, 658
physostigmine salicylate and, 138
Promotility agents, for pain management
side effects, 424
Pronestyl, 262t
Propane gas, abuse of, 703
Propanidid, 302

Propofol (Diprivan), 263t, 294-295
   for eye surgery, 456
   intracranial pressure and, 528-529
   for opiate detoxification in PACU, 315-316
   for pediatric anesthesia, 667, 678, 679
Propoxyphene (Darvon), 312
   for analgesia in pregnant patient, 695
Propranolol (Inderal, Ipran), 263t
   for alcohol withdrawal, 701
   geriatric patients and, 685t
   heparin interaction with, 267t
   for hypertension, 145, 146t, 148
   inhalation anesthetics interaction with, 267t
   lidocaine interaction with, 267t
   neurohumoral transmission and, 142t
   pseudocholinesterase deficiencies and, 327
   d-tubocurarine interaction with, 267t
Proprioception, 98-99
   definition of, 93
Propriospinal tracts, 121
Proptosis
   definition of, 455
   intraocular pressure and, 461
Prosencephalon, 93-94
Prostaglandins
   pain management and, 423
   septic shock and, 727
Prostate
   postoperative care, 574-576, 576
   transurethral resection of, 575
      irrigation fluids for, 205
Prostatectomy
   complications, 576
   definition of, 567
Prostigmin; see Neostigmine
Protamine sulfate, 263t
Protein
   in body fluids, 204
   shock and synthesis of, 723
   synthesis of, 226-227
Protein hormones, 213
Proteinuria, opioid abuse and, 697
Proteolysis, septic shock and, 727
Prothrombin time (PT), 134-135
   coagulation assessment and, 207-208
Protodiastole, 126
Pruritus
   from anthrax, 732
   from morphine for pain management, 423-424
Pseudocholinesterase, 226
   deficiencies, succinylcholine and, 327
   propanidid and, 302
Psychedelic drugs, abuse of, 697, 702-703
   effects and signs of, 700t
Psychologic dependence, definition of, 697
Psychosocial assessment; see also Anxiety
   after trauma injuries, 722
   postoperative, 388-390
Psychosocial comfort, postoperative, 406
   assessment of, 388-390
   for children, 668-669
   for geriatric patients, 684, 686
   for pregnant patient, 693

Psychotropic drugs, acute dystonic reactions from, 98
Pterygium, definition of, 455
Pterygoid plexus, 108
Ptosis
   bilateral, 454
   definition of, 455
   malignant hyperthermia and, 708
   myasthenia gravis and, 644
Public Health Service, United States, 55
   Tuskegee Syphilis Study, 79
Pudendal nerve, 122
Pudendal plexus, 121, 122
Pulmonary arteries, 157
   colloids and, 209
Pulmonary arteriography, 496
Pulmonary artery banding, definition of, 480
Pulmonary artery catheter
   flow-directed, 379
   myocardial infarction and, 133
Pulmonary artery pressure, 380
   after cardiac surgery, 486
   cardiogenic shock and, 725
Pulmonary capillary wedge pressure, 380
   after cardiac surgery, 486
   cardiogenic shock and, 725
Pulmonary circulation, 135, 165-167
   nutrition and, 167
Pulmonary diseases, epidural block for, 351
Pulmonary edema, 168-169
   after laryngospasm in children, 675
   cardiogenic shock and, 725
   hypertension and, 145
   loop diuretics for, 196
   malignant hyperthermia and, 712
   mannitol and, 195
   noncardiac, respiratory compromise and, 736
   opioid abuse and, 697
   shock and, 723
   ventilation rate and, 182
Pulmonary embolism
   after orthopedic surgery, 510
   after prostate surgery, 576
   obstructive shock and, 728
Pulmonary fibrosis
   functional residual capacity and, 159
   gas exchange and, 166-167
   preexisting, postoperative complications and, 184
Pulmonary hysteresis, 160, 160-161
Pulmonary stenosis, definition of, 480
Pulmonary stretch receptors (PSRs), 182
Pulmonary time constant, 162-164
Pulmonary valves, 129
Pulmonary vascular resistance, 166, 167
   infant respiratory distress syndrome and, 666
   postoperative monitoring of, 384-385
Pulmonary veins, 157
   left ventricle and, 167
Pulmozyme, respiratory care and, 266t
Pulse; see also Precordial pulsations
   amphetamines abuse and, 702
   cardiac compression for CPR and, 741
   cardiopulmonary resuscitation and, 739

Pulse (Continued)
   malignant hyperthermia and, 711b, 712
   moderate phase hemorrhage and, 723
   peripheral
      after cardiac surgery, 487, 491
      after hip or femoral surgery, 512
      after orthopedic surgery, 508
      after vascular surgery, 496-498
      palpation for, 497, 719-720
   phencyclidine abuse and, 702
   rate, hypothalamus and, 101
   rate and character of, 374
      after pediatric surgery, 672, 673
Pulse deficit, definition of, 126
Pulse oximeter, 363
   placement for premature infants, 665
Pulse oximetry, 363-366
   applications, 364
   clinical issues, 364-366
   CPR and, 736
   for desaturation monitoring, 166-167
   interpretations of measurements, 364
   for oxyhemoglobin dissociation curve determination, 172
   for patient assessment, 362
      in trauma, 719
   during patient transport and in PACU, 179, 358
   in patient-controlled analgesia, 315
   postoperative oxygen saturation monitoring with, 400
      orthopedic surgery, 508
      pediatric surgery, 669, 670
      radical mastectomy, 594
      thoracic surgery, 468
   technology overview, 363-364
Pulse pressure monitoring, 373-374
   after vascular surgery, 496-497
Pulseless electrical activity, in trauma patient, 720
Pupillary light reflex, 101
   cranial surgery and, 535
Purkinje fibers, 129, 130, 130
Putamen, 96, 96
Pyelitis, definition of, 189
Pyelonephritis, obesity and, 650
Pyeloplasty, definition of, 567
Pyelostomy, definition of, 567
Pyelotomy, definition of, 567
Pyloric antrum of stomach, 222, 222-223
   obstruction of, 559
Pyloric stenosis, 560
Pyloromyotomy, definition of, 554
Pyloroplasty, 553
   definition of, 554
Pyramidal cell axons, 97-98
Pyramidal signs, definition of, 517
Pyridostigmine (Regonol, Mestinon), 263t, 317
   acetylcholinesterase and, 138
   muscle relaxant reversal and, 325, 326
   for myasthenia gravis, 644
Pyrogallol, neurohumoral transmission and, 142t
Pyrosis, definition of, 221
Pyruvate, coronary blood flow and, 131

Q

Q fever, as biological warfare agent, 731b
Q waves, cardiac surgery complications and, 488
QRS voltage, obesity and, 650
Q-T interval, obesity and, 650
Quadriceps muscle, knee and, 512, 513
Quality assurance (QA), 41-43
Quality improvement demarcated intermittent interaction model, 42, 42
Quality improvement seamless continuous interaction model, 43
Quality of care *versus* cost of care, 59
Quantal drug response, 249
Quarantine plans, for bioterrorism response, 731
Queckenstedt test, 537
Quelicin; *see* Succinylcholine
Quinidine
    digitalis interaction with, 267t
    malignant hyperthermia and, 710b
    muscle relaxants and, 267t, 331
    myocardial infarction and, 133
    pseudocholinesterase deficiencies and, 327
    d-tubocurarine interaction with, 267t
Quinine, sickle cell anemia and, 655

R

Raccoon's eyes, basilar skull fractures and, 520, 720
Radial pulse
    after arm and forearm surgery, 511
    after shoulder surgery, 511
    in trauma patient, 720
Radial traction, 160-161
Radiant burns, 715
Radiography, conventional, 518
    of lateral skull, 518
    for spinal surgery diagnosis, 535
Rales, definition of, 151
Ramsay Sedation Scoring System, 273, 273t
Ramus/rami
    definition of, 93
    spinal, 121, 122
Range-of-motion exercises
    after hip or femoral surgery, 512
    after knee surgery, 513
    for orthopedic patients, 509
    after arm surgery, 511
Ranitidine (Zantac), 263t
    for aspiration pneumonitis in pregnant patients, 692
    for ophthalmic surgery patients, 460
    for vomiting/regurgitation, 224
Rapacuronium (Raplon), 263t, 325
Rapid repetitive movements, tardive dyskinesia and, 98
Rapid respiratory decompensation, from morphine for pain management, 423
Ratchet effect, in neuromuscular transmission, 319
Reabsorption, renal, 191, 192t
Reach to Recovery, 595
Readily available equipment, 7
Reagins, 242
Rebetron, respiratory care and, 266t

Receptors, definition of, 249
Recovery; *see also* Postanesthesia recovery score
    from ambulatory surgery, 621-622
    from conduction anesthesia, 340b
    from neuromuscular blockade, 333
        criteria for, 332b
Rectal temperature, 707
Rectal thermometers, immunosuppression and, 246
Rectocele, definition of, 583
Rectum, 225
    care after surgery of lower, 562
    trauma nurse's assessment of, 721
Recurarization, muscle relaxants and, 336
Recurrent laryngeal nerves, 153-154, 154
Red blood cells (RBCs), 133-134, 209; *see also* Sickle cell anemia
    after burn injuries, 611
    oxygen saturation time, 166
    packed, 210-211
        transfusion of, 399, 718
    pregnancy and, 689b, 691
Red nucleus, 100, 101
    basal ganglia and, 96
Reduced hemoglobin, definition of, 151
Reduction mammoplasty, 597-598
Re-entry, definition of, 126
Reflection, laser beam, 628
Reflexes
    midbrain as control center for, 101
    reticular formation and, 104
Refusal, medical treatment, 82; *see also* Informed consent/refusal
Regional anesthesia, 339, 346-353; *see also* Anesthesia, regional
Regitine; *see* Phentolamine
Reglan; *see* Metoclopramide
Regonol; *see* Pyridostigmine
Regurgitation, stomach physiology and, 223-225
Relaxation exercises
    after gynecologic surgery, 587
    after laparoscopic cholecystectomy, 565
Releasing factor (RF), definition of, 213
Releasing hormones (RH), 214
    definition of, 213
Remifentanil (Ultiva), 263t, 308-309
Renal artery, 189
    bypass procedures on, 500
Renal capsule, 190
Renal system, 189; *see also* Diuretics; Kidney(s)
    acid-base balance, 194-195
    aging and, 683-684
    anatomy of, 190
    angiography, 567
    arterial blood pressure and, 128
    biopsy, 567-568
    cardiac surgery and, 491
    kidney anatomy, 189-191
    shutdown or failure of, 198
    urine components, 193-194, 194t
Renal vein, 189
Renin-angiotensin-aldosterone mechanism
    aldosterone regulation by, 217
    arterial blood pressure and, 128, 192, 193
    renal function and, 197

Receptors, definition of, 249
Repetitive movements, tardive dyskinesia and, 98
Reports; *see also* Written patient reports
    anesthesia for trauma patient, 719
    bioterrorism disease incidents, 731
    medical error, 73
    from OR to PACU, 355-356, 356b
    of trauma nurse's assessment, 721
Research
    by clinical nurse specialists, 16
    on medical malpractice, 68-69
    outcomes, 60-61
Resectoscope, for transurethral surgery, 574
Reserpine
    neurohumoral transmission and, 142t
    norepinephrine inhibition by, 141, 267t
Residual volume (RV), 158, 158t
    functional residual capacity and, 159
    pregnancy and, 691
Respihaler; *see* Dexamethasone
Respiration; *see also* Breathing; Respiratory function
    blood gas transport and, 169-170
    buprenorphine and, 311
    carbon dioxide transport, 172-174
    Cheyne-Stokes, 534t
        definition of, 150
    definition of, 151
    morphine and rapid decompensation of, 423
    myasthenia gravis and, 644, 645
    opioids for pain management and, 424
    oxygen transport and, 170-172
    pons and, 102
    postoperative, 362-363
    Stage III and IV anesthesia and, 277
    trauma nurse assessment of, 719
Respiratory acidosis, 175-176, 175b, 176t, 194
    cardiogenic shock and, 725
    diabetes mellitus and, 646
    emphysema and, 642
    malignant hyperthermia and, 709, 709b
    pneumoperitoneum and, 638t
Respiratory alkalosis, 175-176, 175b, 176t
    pregnancy and, 691
Respiratory compromise, 736
Respiratory distress syndrome, acute, septic shock and, 727
Respiratory exchange ratio, 169-170
Respiratory function, 361-371
    after abdominal surgery, 556, 559
    after cranial surgery, 533
    after liver surgery, 562
    after pediatric surgery, 667, 670
    assessment and care after thoracic surgery, 467-468
    cardiac surgery and, 490-491
    complications after spinal cord injury, 543
    inspection for, 361-362
    patient transition from operating room to PACU and, 358
    spinal surgery and, 514
Respiratory rate
    after pediatric surgery, 669
    after thoracic surgery, 468
    Class IV hemorrhage and, 724

Respiratory rate (*Continued*)
 in infants and young children, 662, 662t
 limbic system and, 99
 in patient-controlled analgesia, 314
 trauma nurse assessment of, 719
 water loss and, 202
Respiratory reflexes, medulla oblongata
  and, 102
Respiratory system
 aging and, 683
 anatomy of, 151-157
 anesthetic agents and, 150
 balance of forces and, 159
 botulism and, 733
 breathing regulation, 179-183
 obesity and, 649, 650-651
 physiology, 157-179
 postoperative lung volumes, 183-185
 pregnancy and, 689b, 691
Respondeat superior, medical malpractice
  and, 68
Restlessness; *see also* Delirium, emergence
 adrenalectomy and, 579
 alcohol abuse and, 701
 moderate phase hemorrhage and, 723
 physostigmine salicylate and, 138-139
 postoperative, 362, 395
 pulse oximetry and, 365-366
 shock and, 723
Resuscitation
 ethical considerations in, 83-85
 information about, 87
Resuscitation not indicated (RNI) policies,
  84
Retention catheters
 after cardiac surgery, 487
 after genitourinary surgery, 568-569, 569,
  570
Reticular activating system (RAS), 104
 uncal herniation and, 523
Reticular formation, 101
 functional description of, 104
 pons and, 102
 premotor area neurons and, 97
Retinal detachment
 positioning after surgery for, 462
 postoperative nausea and vomiting after
  surgery for, 460
 surgery for, 457
Retinoblastoma, definition of, 455
Retinopathy of prematurity, 665
Retinopexy
 definition of, 455
 pneumatic, 457
Retrobulbar block
 for eye surgery, 456
 traditional, 458
Retrognathia, in children, 679
Retrograde incision, in prostate surgery, 575
Retrolental fibroplasia, in premature
 infants, 187, 665
Retropubic incision, in prostate surgery,
  575, 576
Reverse Trendelenburg position, for
 laparoscopy, 637, 637t
Revex, 260t
ReVia, 260t
Rh blood groups, 209, 211

Rhabdomyolysis
 after trauma injury, 721
 succinylcholine and, 328
Rheumatoid arthritis, 646-649
 airway management, 647
 corrective surgery for, 648t
 perianesthesia hazards with, 648t
Rhinencephalon, 99; *see also* Limbic system
Rhinitis, allergic, as immediate
 hypersensitivity reaction, 243
Rhinocort, respiratory care and, 266t
Rhizotomy, definition of, 518
Rhombencephalon, 94, 102; *see also*
 Hindbrain
Rhonchi, definition of, 151
Rhythmic repetitive movements, tardive
 dyskinesia and, 98
Ribavirin (Rebetron), respiratory care and,
  266t
Ribonucleic acid (RNA), 213-214
Right occipital cortex, 99
Right parietal bone, 104
Right temporal bone, 104
Right-atrial catheter, 379
Right-atrial pressure, 380
 after cardiac surgery, 486
 intracranial pressure and, 525
Righting reflexes, 101
 definition of, 93
Rigidity
 cerebral control of, 97
 decerebrate, 535
 drug-induced parkinsonism and, 98
 muscular, malignant hyperthermia and,
  678, 709, 709b
 reticular formation and, 104
Rima glottis, 153
Ringer's solution, lactated, for fluid
 resuscitation in multiple trauma, 718
Risk management, 72-74; *see also* Medical
 malpractice
Ritodrine HCL (Yutopar), 263t
RNI (resuscitation not indicated) policies,
  84
"Roach," abuse of, 704
Robert Wood Johnson Foundation,
 SUPPORT study on end-of-life
 preferences, 86-87
Robinul; *see* Glycopyrrolate
Rocuronium (Zemuron), 263t, 324
Rohypnol, 297-298
 abuse of, 704
Romazicon; *see* Flumazenil
"Roofies," abuse of, 704
"Rope," abuse of, 704
Rophy, abuse of, 297-298, 704
Ropivacaine (Naropin), 263t, 341, 342t,
  344
Rostral spread, opioids and, 313, 314
Rotational beds, spinal cord injuries and,
  543, 543
Ruby laser, 630t
Rule of Nines, for burns, 608, 608
Russell's skin traction, 508

S

Sacral plexus, 121, 122
Sacral spinal segments, 118, *119*

Sacrum, 115
Safety
 laser use, 632-633
 margin of, for drug response, 249
Saline solution, for fluid resuscitation in
 multiple trauma, 718
Salingooophorectomy, definition of, 583
Salmeterol (Serevent), 263t
 respiratory care and, 266t
Salpingectomy, definition of, 583
Salpingostomy, definition of, 583
Sandimmune, 253t
Sarcolemma, neuromuscular transmission
  and, 708
Sarcoplasmic reticulum
 malignant hyperthermia and, 709
 neuromuscular transmission and, 708
Scattering, laser beam, 628-629
Schizophrenia, PET scans and diagnosis of,
  520
Scleral buckle/buckling, *457*
 definition of, 455
 surgery for, 456
Scoliosis, 515
 definition of, 506
Scopolamine (Transderm-Scop), 263t
 Alzheimer's disease and, 685
 for nausea, 657t, 658
 physostigmine and, 298
Scott's syndrome, 688
Scrotal surgery, 576-577, *577*
Seattle God Committee, 79
Second ventricle, 109; *see also* Lateral
 ventricles
Secondary ABCD survey, for
 cardiopulmonary resuscitation, 737
Secondary hearing, area in cerebral cortex,
  97
Secondary injury, to spinal cord, 537-
  538
Secondary somesthetic sensations, in
 cerebral cortex, 97
Secondary vision, area in cerebral cortex,
  97
Secretary-clerk, for PACU, 16
Secretion, renal, 191, 192t
Sedative drugs; *see also* Ramsay Sedation
 Scoring System; Tranquilizers
 anesthesia and, 272-273
Sedimentation rate, myocardial infarction
 and, 132
Segmentectomy/segmental resection
 definition of, 466
 positioning after, 467
Seizure disorders
 enflurane contraindication in, 286
 gamma hydroxybutyrate and, 704
Seizures
 acute dystonic reactions *versus*, 98
 diazepam and, 295
 thiopental and, 292
Self-antigens, immunosuppression and, 245,
  246
Self-Care Deficit Nursing Theory (Orem),
  616
Self-fulfilling prophecy concept, 616
Self-retaining catheter, 569
Self-scheduling, 30-32

Sella turcica, 104, *105*
Sellick maneuver, anesthesia induction in pregnant patients and, 692
Semilunar valves, 129
Semiopen systems, for inhalation anesthesia administration, 282-283
Senile dementia of the Alzheimer type, 684-685
Sensitization phase, of anaphylactic shock, 726
Sensitized lymphocytes, definition of, 238
Sensorcaine, 342t, 343; *see also* Bupivacaine
Sensors, breathing regulation and, 179-182
Sensory areas, 98-99
in cerebral cortex, 96, 97
Sensory function, after cranial surgery, 533-534
Sensory root, 121
Sentinel Event Alert, 619
Sepsis, from gastrointestinal anthrax, 732
Septic shock, 718t, 723, 727-728
cardiogenic shock and, 724
Septum pellucidum, 99
Sequestration crisis, in sickle cell anemia, 655
Sequestrectomy, definition of, 506
Serax, 261t
abuse of, effects and signs of, 699t
Serevent, 263t
respiratory care and, 266t
Serotonin
in chemoreceptor trigger zone, 656, 658
pain and, 422
pulmonary epithelium and, 167
Serum sickness
as hypersensitivity reaction, 243
local anesthetics and, 344
Sevoflurane, 287
intracranial pressure and, 528
for pediatric anesthesia, 666, 667
Sexual behavior, limbic system and, 100
Sexual maturity, hypothalamus and, 101
Shape, recognition of, 99
Shearing forces, trauma and, 715
Shearing injuries of skin, postsurgical, 357
Sheet skin grafts, 612, 613
Shirodkar procedure, 584-585
Shivering
postanesthesia, 706, 707
postpartum, 584
Shock; *see also* Trauma
adrenalectomy and, 578-579
after abdominal gynecologic surgery, 588
after ectopic pregnancy, 584
after orthopedic surgery, 510-511
cardiogenic, 724-725
in children, 664
distributive, 725-728
anaphylactic, 726-727
neurogenic, 725-726
septic, 727-728
epidural block contraindication for, 351
gynecologic surgery and, 585
hypovolemic, 723-724
immediate hypersensitivity reaction and, 242

Shock (*Continued*)
obstructive, 728
trauma and, 716, 722-728
types of, 717-718t
Short-term memory, 97
Short-term outcomes, managed care and, 62
Shoulder
ambulatory surgery on, 616
immobilization of, 507
perianesthesia care after surgery on, 511-512
Shunt(s), in ventilation-perfusion mismatching, *177*, 177-178
Sickle cell anemia
about, 653
anesthesia and, 654
crisis types, 654-655
nursing care, 654
pathogenesis of, 653-654
Sickle cell disease, homozygous, 653
Sickle cell trait, 653
Sickle cell-beta thalassemia, 653
Sickle cell-hemoglobin C disease, 653
Sickle cell-thalassemia, 653
Siderosis, transfusion, 398
Sidestream capnographs, 366, 367
Sigh mechanism, 185
Sigma opioid receptors, 304, 305
Sigmoid sinus, 108
Sigmoid sinus depression, *105*
Simmonds' disease, 215
Simple fractures, of skull, 520
Simple obesity, 649
Simulation training
for emergency and urgent situations, 45, 51
format, 51-52
simulated patient, 52-53
Single donor plasma, 211
Singulair, respiratory care and, 266t
Sinoatrial (SA) node, 129-130, *130*
Sinus arrest, postoperative monitoring for, 376
Sinus bradycardia, postoperative monitoring for, 375
Sinus tachycardia, postoperative monitoring for, 375
Sinuses
ethmoid, 104
frontal, 104
sphenoid, 104
surgery on, 436-437, 438
Sinusoids, hepatic, 226
Size, recognition of, 99
Skilled movements
area in cerebral cortex, 97
cerebral control of, 96-97
control and coordination of, 97
pyramidal and extrapyramidal structure/function and, 97-98
Skin, 231; *see also* Integumentary system
anatomy of, 607
assessment in trauma patient, 720
breakdown of, spinal cord injuries and, 543-544
Class IV hemorrhage and, 724
color of, after cardiac surgery, 487, 491

Skin (*Continued*)
cutaneous anthrax and, 732
neurogenic shock and, 726
protective nature of, 233
septic shock and, 727
shock and, 723
thermoregulation and, 232, *232*
water balance and, 203
Skin grafting
after burn injuries, 612, 613
after radical mastectomy, 595
Skin injuries, patient transition from operating room to PACU and, 357
Skull
coronal section, *109*
lateral view of, *105*
lateral x-ray of, *518*
Skull fractures, categories of, 520, *522*
Sleep
club drugs abuse and, 703
diencephalon and, 100
hypothalamus and, 101
Sleeve resection, definition of, 466
Slips, human error as, 46
Slow codes, 83-84
Slow lung units, 163-164
Small bowel, care after surgery of, 560
Small volume nebulizers (SVNs), 251
Smallpox, as biological warfare agent, 730, 731b, 733
Smell, area in cerebral cortex, 99
SMI; *see* Sustained maximum inspiration
Smoke evacuation system, laser procedures and, 633
Smoking
carboxyhemoglobin and, 365
cardiovascular effects of, 652-653
nursing care, 653
respiratory effects of, 651-652
Sneezing reflex, 102; *see also* Cough/coughing reflex
Sniffing position, after pediatric surgery, 670
"Soap," abuse of, 704
Social Security, managed care and, 57
Social worth, hemodialysis and, 79
Society of Critical Care Medicine, Ethics Committee guidelines on resuscitation in ICU, 84
Sodium, 205
geriatric patients and, 683
muscle relaxants and, 329
Sodium bicarbonate, 264t
for cardiopulmonary resuscitation, 746
for malignant hyperthermia, 8b, 711-712, 712b
Sodium citrate (Bicitra), 263t, 264t
for aspiration pneumonitis in pregnant patients, 692
for vomiting/regurgitation, 223
Sodium nitroprusside (SNP), 264t; *see also* Nipride; Nitroprusside
for hypertension, 145-147, 146t
myocardial infarction and, 133
Sodium pentothal, 292-293; *see also* Thiopental
Solcotrans Plus Orthopaedic Autotransfusion System, 509

Solu-Cortef, 257t
Somatomedin, 214
Somatostatin (Zecnil), 217, 263t
  growth hormone and, 214
Somatotropin, 214-215
Somesthetic sensations; see also Sensory
      areas
  area in cerebral cortex, 97
Sorbitol, in bladder irrigation fluid, 205
Sore throat, after tracheal intubation, 417-
      418
Sotalol hydrochloride (Betapace), 264t
Sound level in PACU, analgesics and,
      60
Soviet Union, biological warfare program,
      730
"Special K" (ketamine), abuse of, 704
Speculums, 633
Speech, cerebral cortex center for, 97, 98
Spencer vena caval plication, 494
Spermatocelectomy, definition of, 567
Sphenoid bone, 104, 105
  surgical access to pituitary gland and,
      106
Sphenoid sinuses, 104
Spinal accessory nerve (XI), 101
  type and functions of, 103t
Spinal administration of drugs, for pain
      management, 424
Spinal anesthesia; see Anesthesia, spinal
Spinal arteries, 123
Spinal block, high, in spinal anesthesia,
      349-350
Spinal bones, 115-117
Spinal cord, 94, 95, 115-123, 346; see also
      Spinal cord injuries; Spine
  ascending and descending tracts of, 120
  axons in, 97
  basal ganglia and, 96
  CSF circulation through, 107, 110
  foramen magnum and, 106
  medulla oblongata and, 102
  protection of, 115-117
  structure and function of, 117-118, 120-
      123
  structure and nerve connections of, 122
  vascular network, 123
  vertebrae and, 119
Spinal cord injuries, 537-538, 538
  anesthetic considerations with, 544
  assessment tool, 541-542
  bone demineralization, 544
  care and considerations with, 539-540
  complications, 540-544
  gastrointestinal complications, 544
  head injury and, 543
  neurogenic shock and, 723, 726
  pain management, 540
  respiratory complications, 543
  shock from, 716, 717t
  skin breakdown, 543-544
  trauma nurse's assessment of, 721
  urological complications, 544
Spinal fusion
  definition of, 506
  for herniated nucleus pulposus, 545
  for spinal cord injuries, 539

Spinal meninges, 117, 122
Spinal nerves, 115, 346
  arrangement of, 121
  spinal cord segments and, 118, 119,
      120
Spinal respiratory neurons, 183
Spinal shock, 540
  definition of, 518
Spinal surgery, 535-546
  diagnostic tools, 535, 537
  herniated nucleus pulposus, 544-545,
      545
  intraspinal neoplasms, 545, 546
  postoperative care, 545-546
  for spine injuries, 537-540
      complete spinal cord lesion, 538-539
      complications, 540, 543-544
      decompression and fusion in, 539
      incomplete spinal cord lesion, 538,
          539
      nursing care with, 539-540, 541-542
Spine, 115
  anatomy of, 346, 347
  care after surgery on, 514-515
  injuries of, 537-538
      in children, 679, 679-680
Spinous process, of vertebrae, 115, 116
Spirometry, incentive, 185
  after hip or femoral surgery, 512
  after spinal surgery, 515
  patient education on, 426-427
  stir-up regimen, 393-394
Spironolactone, 196
Spleen, 228
Splenectomy, 228
  care after, 563
  definition of, 554
Splinting, for pain management, 426
Split-thickness skin grafts, 612
Spray paints, abuse of, 703
Squamous cell cancer, 231
St. John's wort, anesthesia interaction with,
      274t
Stab wounds, 715
Stacked shocks, for defibrillation, 743
Stadol; see Butorphanol
Staff facilities, PACU, 5
Staffing, PACU
  ASPAN clinical guidelines on, 60
  ASPEN Standards on, 3-4
Standard of care
  individual liability and, 71-72
  PACU, 39-40
Standard Precautions, 40
Stapedectomy, 436, 436
  definition of, 433
Stark Act, on Ethics in Patient Referrals,
      79
Starling equation, 168, 169
State governments, managed care and, 56
Stem cells, definition of, 238
Stereotactic radiosurgery, 527
Stereotaxis, 527
Sternotomy
  for cardiac surgery, 484
  definition of, 466
Steroid anesthesia, 302

Steroid hormones, 213; see also
      Corticosteroids
  anesthesia and, 272
  etomidate and, 294
  hypoadrenocorticism and, 218-219
Stethoscope, hypotension detection and,
      143
Stewart technique, for cardiac output, 127,
      128
Stiff lungs, 647
Stilphostrol, succinylcholine interaction
      with, 270t
Stir-up regimen, 393-395
  after thoracic surgery, 468
  atelectasis and, 167
  central nervous system and, 385
  coughing, 394
  deep-breathing exercises, 393-394
  for geriatric patients, 683
  hypoxemia and, 177
  lung volumes and capacities and, 157,
      159
  mobilization, 394
  modifications of, 394-395
      COPD and, 643
      for geriatric patients, 686
  pain management, 394
  positioning, 394
  preexisting lung disease and, 184
Stomach
  anatomy and physiology of, 222, 222-
      223
  care after surgery on, 559-560
  laparoscopic perforations of, 639
  perforated ulcers of, 560
  pregnancy and, 691
Stool softeners, for pain management side
      effects, 424
Strabismus
  definition of, 455-456
  oculocardiac reflex during repair of, 459
  postoperative nausea and vomiting after
      surgery for, 460, 677
Straight catheter, 569
Straight sinus, 108
Streptococcus pneumoniae, penicillin-
      resistant, 41
Streptokinase, fibrinolytic therapy and, 495
Streptomycin
  interactions with anesthetic agents by,
      271
  muscle relaxants and, 268t, 330b
  for plague, 733
Stress
  behavioral symptoms of, 25-27, 25b
  definition of, 213
  during laparoscopy, 637
  PACU causes of, 26b, 427
  response to anesthesia and biochemical
      products of, 197
Stress ulcers, spinal cord injuries and, 544
Stria medullaris thalami, 99
Stria terminalis, 99
Stricture, definition of, 189
Styloid process, 105
Subarachnoid blocks (anesthetic), 339
  definition of, 518

Subarachnoid bolts or screws, 530, 531
Subarachnoid cisternae (reservoirs), 108
Subarachnoid hemorrhage, 523
    diagnosis of, 519
Subarachnoid space, 106, 109, 117, 122
    anesthetic agents in, 346
    CSF circulation through, 107, 110, 110
    intercranial pressure and, 113, 114
Subcallosal gyrus, 99
Subconjunctival block, for eye surgery, 456
Subcutaneous administration of drugs,
    systemic absorption of, 251
Subdigital arteriography, definition of, 493-
    494
Subdural catheters, 530
Subdural hematoma, 522, 522-523
Subdural space, 108, 109, 117
Sublimaze; see also Fentanyl
    droperidol and, 299
    drug-drug interactions in PACU and, 268t
Sublingual administration of drugs, systemic
    absorption of, 251
Subluxation, definition of, 518
Submucosal resection, definition of, 433-
    434
Substance abuse; see also Drug abuse
    among trauma patients, 721
    with cannabinoids, 702
    with club drugs, 703-704
    with CNS depressants, 700-701
    with CNS sympathomimetics, 702
    with date-rape drugs, 704
    effects and signs of, 698-700t
    with inhalants, 703
    with opioids, 697, 700
    with psychedelics, 702-703
Substance P, pain and, 422
Substantia nigra, 100
    basal ganglia and, 96
Substituted judgment test, informed
    consent/refusal and, 82
Subthalamic nucleus, 100
Subthalamus, 100
    functional description of, 101
Subvalvular aortic stenosis, 474
Succinylcholine (Anectine, Quelicin,
    Sucostrin), 264t, 320t
    about, 326-327
    advantages and uses, 327
    in aging patients, 682
    antibiotics interactions with, 271
    contraindications with spinal cord
        injuries, 544
    diethylstilbestrol interaction with, 270t
    digitalis interaction with, 267t
    disadvantages and side effects, 327-329
    echothiophate iodide interaction with,
        269t
    for fixed chest syndrome, 307
    hyperkalemia and, 206
    kidney disease and, 198
    for laryngospasm, 155
    lithium interaction with, 269t
    liver dysfunction and, 226-227
    LSD and, 703
    malignant hyperthermia and, 678, 710b
    nasal intubation and, 181

Succinylcholine (Anectine, Quelicin,
    Sucostrin) (Continued)
    neurohumoral transmission and, 142t
    pediatric anesthesia and, 666
    phase II block, 336
    pregnancy and recovery from, 691
    for pregnant patients, 692
    prolonged response to, 334
    d-tubocurarine interaction with, 269t
    untoward reactions, 327
Sucostrin; see Succinylcholine
Suction catheter, patient control of, 450
Suction curettage, definition of, 581
Suction lipectomy, for gynecomastia, 598
Suctioning, 403-404
    after abdominal surgery, 557-558
    after tonsillectomy, 679
    after vascular surgery, 501
    for geriatric patients, 683
    for postoperative nausea and vomiting,
        659
    smoking and, 653
    tracheal, for geriatric patients, 686
    tracheostomy care, 443-444
Sufentanil (Sufenta), 264t, 307-308
    drug-drug interactions in PACU and,
        268t
    epidural administration of, 313
    intracranial pressure and, 528
    for pain management, after pediatric
        surgery, 674
    patient-controlled analgesia with, 315t
Sulcus, 106
    in cerebral cortex, 95
Sulfite, dezocine contraindication for
    allergy to, 311
Sulfonamides, sickle cell anemia and, 655
Sump catheters, after abdominoperineal
    resection, 561
Superficial burns, 608
Superficial partial-thickness burns, 608
Superficial temporal artery, 113
Superior cerebellar peduncle, 101
Superior colliculi, 101, 101
Superior gluteal nerve, 122
Superior laryngeal nerves, 153
Superior petrosal sinus, 108
Superior sagittal sinus, 107, 108, 110
    coronal section, 109
Superior sagittal suture, 109
SUPPORT study on end-of-life preferences,
    86-87
Suppressor T lymphocytes, in cellular
    immunity, 241-242
Supracommissural septum, 99
Supraglottic laryngectomy, 446, 446b
Suprane; see Desflurane
Suprapubic catheters, 569-570, 575
    mushroom, 576
Suprapubic incision, in prostate surgery,
    575
Suprapubic prostatectomy, drainage tube
    placement after, 576
Supratentorial, definition of, 517
Supratentorial herniation, 523
Supravalvular aortic stenosis, 474
Surface tension phenomenon, 161

Surfactant, on lung tissue, 161
Surgeons, patient reports by, 356b
Surgical plume, 633
Surgical site infections, 40b
Surital, 264t
Survanta, respiratory care and, 266t
Sustained maximum inspiration (SMI),
    159
    airway closure and, 161
    for geriatric patients, 683
    nausea and, 658
    perianesthesia nursing care, 186
    postoperative
        with COPD, 643
        droperidol anesthesia and, 300
        geriatric surgery, 686
        hip or femoral surgery, 512
        incentive spirometer and, 185
        pediatric surgery, 670
        thoracic surgery, 468
    smoking and, 653
    in stir-up regimen, 393
Sustained tetanus, as graded drug response,
    332-333
Swallowing reflex, 102
    Stage II anesthesia and, 277
Sweat glands, 232
Sweating, 203, 232
    club drugs abuse and, 703
    malignant hyperthermia and, 678, 709b
    nausea and, 658
Sylvian fissure, 94, 95, 97
Syme amputation, definition of, 506
Sympathectomy, definition of, 494
Sympathetic nerves, 131
    stimulators, 141
Sympathetic nervous system, 123
    bronchi and, 157
    spinal nerves and, 121
    stimulation of, 139
    sweat glands and, 232
Sympatholysis, anesthesia and, 276
Sympathomimetic amines, drug-drug
    interactions in PACU and, 268t
Syncope, definition of, 126
Syncurine, 329; see also Decamethonium
    bromide
Syncytium, functional, 129
Syndrome of inappropriate secretion of
    antidiuretic hormone (SIADH), 219
Synergistic effect, definition of, 249
Synovial fluid, 203
Syphilis tests, opioid abusers and, 697
Systemic circulation, 135
Systemic vascular resistance
    during laparoscopy, 635
    postoperative monitoring of, 384
Systems approach to patient safety, 69-71
Systole
    AV valves and, 129
    definition of, 126
Systolic blood pressure, 128-129, 371, 372,
    372
    aging and, 682
    cardiac compression for CPR and, 740
    in infants and young children, 662, 662t
    during pregnancy, 688

T

T lymphocytes
  cellular immunity and, 241-242
  definition of, 238
  humoral immunity and, 239-240
Tachycardia
  after laparoscopy, 639
  after nasal surgery, 437
  after surgery with COPD, 644
  alcohol abuse and, 701
  amphetamines abuse and, 702
  atrial, postoperative monitoring of, 376,
    376
  club drugs abuse and, 703
  CPR and, 736
  during laparoscopy, 635
  malignant hyperthermia and, 678, 709,
    709b
  marijuana abuse and, 702
  nausea and, 658
  paroxysmal, definition of, 126
  shock and, 723
  sinus, postoperative monitoring for, 375,
    375
  ventricular
    CPR after, 737, 741, 742, 743
    lidocaine for, 745
    postoperative monitoring of, 378, 378
Tachyphylaxis, definition of, 249
Tachypnea
  malignant hyperthermia and, 678, 709,
    709b
  nausea and, 658
Tagamet; see Cimetidine
Talwin; see Pentazocine
Tangential excision, in burn injuries, 611-
  612
Tardive dyskinesia, 98
Target organ, definition of, 213
T-binder, for scrotal support, 577, 577
Technology
  medical errors and, 68
  perianesthesia nursing and, 11
Teeth, pediatric surgery and loose, 668
Tegmentum, 101
Telemetry patients, PACU care for, 30
Telencephalon, 93-94; see also Cerebrum
Temperature; see also Body temperature
  sensations of, 98
Temporal bones, 104, 105
Temporal lobe, 94, 94, 95
  blood supplies for, 112
Tenormin, 252t
Tensilon; see Edrophonium chloride
Tension pneumothorax, 164, 638t, 716, 718t
  obstructive shock and, 723, 728
Tentorium, 102, 107
Tentorium cerebelli, 107
Terbutaline (Brethine), 264t
  cyclic AMP and, 140
  respiratory care and, 266t
Testosterone, 218
Tetanic stimulus, 332-334, 333
Tetanus
  succinylcholine contraindications in, 328
  succinylcholine for convulsions from,
    326

Tetany, 206
  after thyroid surgery, 549-550
  definition of, 201
Tetracaine (Pontocaine), 264t, 341, 342t,
    344; see also Pontocaine
  for cesarean section, 693
  for eye surgery, 456
  malignant hyperthermia and, 711b
Tetracycline
  aluminum-containing antacid and, 270
  muscle relaxants and, 268t, 271, 330b
  for plague, 733
Tetrahydrocannabinol (THC), 702
Tetralogy of fallot, 480
  definition of, 480-481
Texture of objects, recognition of, 99
Thalamus, 100, 101
  functional description of, 100
  intellectual processes and, 98
Thallium-201 scans, 632
Thebaine, 304
Theophylline, for apnea in premature
  infants, 665
Therapeutic index, for drug response, 249,
  308
Therapeutic privilege, informed consent
  doctrine and, 81, 82
Thermal burns, 236, 715
Thermal imbalance
  definition of, 706
  malignant hyperthermia, 707-712
  postoperative, 706-707
Thermistor, 706
Thermocouple, 706
Thermodilution measurement of cardiac
  output, 127
Thermometry, infrared tympanic
  membrane, 386
Thermoregulation; see Body temperature
Thiamylal (Surital), 264t
Thiazide diuretics, 195-196
  digitalis interaction with, 267t
  insulin interaction with, 270t
  muscle relaxants and, 269t
Thiocyanate toxicity, 147
Thiopental (Pentothal), 264t, 292-293
  alcoholism and, 701
  balanced technique and, 305
  halothane interactions in obesity with,
    270
  intracranial pressure and, 528
  kidney disease and, 197-198
  malignant hyperthermia and, 711b
  for pregnant patients, 692
  respiratory and cardiovascular depression
    monitoring and, 226, 227
Third space
  colloid solutions and, 209
  crystalloid solutions and, 208
  definition of, 201
  fluid distribution and, 203-204
  hypovolemic shock and, 717t, 723
Third ventricle, 96, 100, 100
  in brain stem, 101
  cerebral aqueduct and, 101
  CSF circulation through, 107, 109,
    110

Thoracentesis
  definition of, 466
  topical anesthesia for, 467
Thoracic spinal nerves, 122
Thoracic spinal segments, 118
Thoracic spine
  injuries to, 537
  surgery on, 515
Thoracic surgery, 465-472
  anesthesia for, 466-467
  chest tube management, 469, 469-470
  complications, 471
  COPD and, 643
  fluid management, 469
  pain management, 468-469
  Pleur-Evac chest drainage systems, 470
  positioning after, 467
  respiratory assessment and care, 467-468
  respiratory management after, 468
Thoracic vertebrae, 115, 116
Thoracoplasty/thoracostomy, definition of,
  466
Thoracotomy
  for cardiac surgery, 484
  definition of, 466
Thora-Drain, severe chest injuries and, 719
Thorazine; see Chlorpromazine
Throat surgery, 438-447
  laryngectomy, 445-447
  laryngoscopy, 440-441
  tonsillectomy and adenoidectomy, 438-
    440
  tracheostomy, 441, 442-443, 443-445
Thrombectomy, 496, 500
  definition of, 494
Thrombocytopenia, coagulation and, 208
Thrombolytic agents, for cardiogenic shock,
  725
Thrombosis
  cardiopulmonary arrest and, 744
  deep vein
    after orthopedic surgery, 510
    during laparoscopy, 637
    definition of, 126
    smoking and, 652
    spinal cord injuries and, 540
  venous
    cardiac surgery and, 491
    obesity and, 651
Thrombus
  definition of, 494
  sickle cell anemia and, 654
Thymectomy, for myasthenia gravis, 644-
  645
Thymoma, myasthenia gravis and, 644
Thymosin, cellular immunity and, 241
Thyrocalcitonin, 216
Thyroglobulin, 216
Thyroid cartilage, 152, 153, 153
Thyroid gland, 108, 216
  surgery of, 548-550
    anesthesia, 548
    cardiopulmonary assessment and care,
      549
    complications, 549-550
Thyroid lobectomy with isthmusectomy,
  definition of, 548

Thyroid storm, 550
Thyroidectomy, definition of, 548
Thyroid-stimulating hormone (TSH), 215, 216
Thyrotropin, 215
Thyroxine (T$_4$), 216
Tidal volume (V$_T$), 157, 158t
   pregnancy and, 691
   for primary CPR ventilation, 739
Tigan, for ophthalmic surgery patients, 460
Tilade, respiratory care and, 266t
To Err is Human: Building a Safer Health System (Institute of Medicine), 69
Tobramycin (TOBI), respiratory care and, 266t
Tolbutamide, Dicumarol interaction with, 269t
Tolerance
   definition of, 249, 697
   for opioids, 697
Tomography, computed, for vascular disease diagnosis, 493
Tongue
   motor control of, 96
   postoperative airway obstruction and, 409, 410, 737
   respiratory compromise and, 736
   surgery on, 438
"Tongue tied," definition of, 433
Tonoclonic movements, definition of, 518
Tonometer
   definition of, 456
   intraocular pressure measurement with, 461, 461
Tonsil tray, 440, 440b
Tonsillectomy and adenoidectomy (T&A), 438-440, 679
   definition of, 434
   discharge from PACU after, 680
   dissection, 439
   nausea and vomiting after, 677
Topical anesthesia, 339
   definition of, 456
   for eye surgery, 456-457
   for thoracic surgery, 467
Toprol; *see* Metoprolol
Toradol; *see* Ketorolac
Tornalate, respiratory care and, 266t
Torr, definition of, 151
Torsades de pointes (TdP), droperidol and, 300
Torsemide (Demadex, Presaril), 264t
Torsion spasms, psychotropic drugs and, 98
Tort reform, for medical malpractice, 65
Torticollis, psychotropic drugs and, 98
Total lung capacity (TLC), 158t, 159
   aging and, 683
Touch, sensations of, 98
Toxemia, obesity and, 650
Toxic jaundice, 226
Trabeculectomy, definition of, 456
Trachea, 155-156
   in newborns, 661
   trauma injuries of, 720
Tracheal dilator and hook, 444
Tracheal edema, postoperative, in children, 677

Tracheal intubation, 411-420; *see also* Endotracheal intubation
   adverse sequelae after, 417-418
   aspiration of gastrointestinal contents after, 418
   cardiac compression for CPR and, 741
   equipment for, 411-414, 412, 412b, 413
   hoarseness after, 417-418
   laryngeal mask airway, 418-420
   nasotracheal, 416-417
      after maxillofacial surgery, 450
      balloon-cuffed, as artificial airway, 362
   oral
      blade insertion for, 414, 416
      head positioning for, 414
      patient assessment in, 415-416
      patient positioning for, 414
      patient ventilation in, 416
      raising epiglottis and visualizing vocal cords in, 414-415
      tube placement, 415
   sore throat after, 417-418
   tube removal in, 417
   upper airways receptors and, 181-182
Tracheal suctioning, 403-405, 404
Tracheal tube, 413, 413-414
   placement of, 415
Tracheal tug, depth of anesthesia and, 277
Trachelorrhaphy, definition of, 583
Tracheostomy, 152, 441, 443-445
   bedside equipment for, 443b
   complications of, 444-445
   definition of, 434
   dressings, 444, 444
   incision for, 441
   laryngectomy and, 445-446
   laryngoscopy and, 440
   nursing care after, 559
   suctioning, 443-444
   tray contents for, 441b
   tube positions and, 445
   tubes and obturators for, 441, 442, 443
Traction
   after hip or femoral surgery, 512
   after orthopedic surgery, 507
   halo, for cervical spine surgery, 514
   Russell's, 508
Tracrium, 252t, 320t, 324; *see also* Atracurium
Traditional generation of workers, 21
Train-of-four
   as graded drug response, 249
   neuromuscular blockade assessment with, 332, 334, 334
Trandate; *see* Labetalol
Tranquilizers; *see also* Sedative drugs
   sufentanil with, 308
Transcellular fluids, 203
Transcutaneous electric nerve stimulation (TENS)
   after gastrointestinal surgery, 559
   after laparoscopic cholecystectomy, 565
   for pain management, 426
Transdermal administration of drugs, for pain management, 424, 425
Transderm-Scop; *see* Scopolamine
Transduction, of pain, 422

Transduodenal sphincterotomy, definition of, 554-555
Transfer factor, cellular immunity and, 242
Transfusions, 209-210
   anaphylactic shock and, 726
   for anemia with rheumatoid arthritis, 648
   for fluid resuscitation in multiple trauma, 718
   postoperative, 395-399
      on nonblood substitutes, 399
      of packed red blood cells, 399, 718
      of plasma proteins, 399
      of platelets, 399
      of whole blood, 395-397
   reactions to, 211
      allergic, 398
      delayed, 398-399
      febrile, 397-398
      hemolytic, 397
      treatment of immediate, 398
Transit time, RBC, 166
Transmission
   definition of, 317
   laser beam, 629
   of pain, 422
Transmission-Based Precautions, 40, 40b
Transmyocardial laser revascularization (TMLR), 632
Transplantation
   definition of, 466
   definition of cardiac, 481
Transposition of the great arteries (TGA), definition of, 481
Transsphenoidal hypophysectomy, 106
Transurethral resection of the prostate (TURP), 575
   irrigation fluids for, 205
Transurethral surgery, definition of, 567
Transverse fissure, in brain, 95
Transverse foramen (foramina), 112, 116
Transverse process, of vertebrae, 115, 116
Transverse sinus, 108
Tranylcypromine
   neurohumoral transmission and, 142t
   sympathetic hyperactivity and, 137
Trauma
   about, 714
   blunt, 715
   in children, 679-680
   collaborative approach to, 718-719
   contusion of tissues in, 715-716
   diagnostic studies and protocols, 718
   mechanisms of injury, 714-715
   penetrating, 715
   perianesthesia phase, 719-722
      anesthesia report, 719
      infectious risk, 722
      nausea, 721-722
      nursing assessment, 719-721
      nursing diagnosis, 722
      psychologic assessment, 722
   prehospital phase, 714
   scoring systems, 716
   shock as complication to, 722-728
   stabilization phase, 716, 718
   succinylcholine contraindications in, 328

Travel box, ICU, 7
  contents, 9t
Trembling
  after C-section, 584
  droperidol and, 299
Tremors
  cerebral control of, 97
  oscillatory, drug-induced parkinsonism
    and, 98
Trench foot, 236
Trendelenburg position, for laparoscopy,
  637, 637t
Trexan, 260t
Triamcinolone (Kenalog), respiratory care
  and, 266t
Triamterene, 196
Trichlormethane; see Chloroform
Trichloroethylene, 285
Tricuspid regurgitation, definition of, 481
Tricuspid stenosis, definition of, 481
Tricuspid valves, 129
Tricyclic antidepressants, physostigmine
  salicylate and, 138
Tricylic/phenobarbitone overdose, sodium
  bicarbonate and, 746
Tridil, for hypertension, 146t
Trifluoroethyl vinyl ether, 284-285
Trigeminal nerve (V), 101, 101, 102
  type and functions of, 103t
Trihexyphenidyl (Artane)
  for acute dystonic reactions, 98
  droperidol extrapyramidal excitation and,
    300
  for drug-induced parkinsonism, 98
Triiodothyronine (T₃), 216
Trilene, 285
Trimethaphan camsylate (Arfonad), 264t
  for hypertension, 146t, 147-148
Trimethobenzamide (Tigan), for
  ophthalmic surgery patients, 460
Trochlear nerve (IV), 101, 101
  type and functions of, 103t
Tropic hormones, definition of, 213
Tropisetron (Navoban), for nausea, 657t
Troponin C, neuromuscular transmission
  and, 708
Troponin-tropomyosin, neuromuscular
  transmission and, 319
Trousseau test, after thyroid surgery, 550
Trousseau's sign, 207
  definition of, 201
Trunk, motor control of, 96
Truth-telling, medical ethics and, 78
T-tube, placement in common bile duct,
  563, 563, 564
Tubal ligation, 586
  definition of, 583
  laparoscopic, 634
Tubal plasty, definition of, 583
Tuberculin skin tests, delayed
  hypersensitivity reactions and, 243
Tuberculosis (TB), 40
d-Tubocurarine chloride (Curare), 264t,
  319, 320t, 321
  aminophylline interaction with, 269t
  kidney disease and, 198
  lidocaine interaction with, 267t

d-Tubocurarine chloride (Curare)
    (Continued)
  myasthenia gravis and, 644
  recurarization and, 336
  succinylcholine interaction with, 269t
Tubular capillaries, renal, 190
Tubular carcinoma, definition of, 592
Tubular necrosis, 198
Tubules, renal, 190, 191, 191
Tuffier's line, for lumbar puncture, 348
Tuinal, abuse of, effects and signs of, 698t
Tularemia, as biological warfare agent, 731b
Tumors
  diagnosis of cranial, 519
  intracranial, 524
  intraspinal, 545, 546
Tunica adventitia, 135
Tunica intima, 135
Tunica media, 135
Turbinaire; see Dexamethasone
TURP (transurethral resection of the
  prostate), 575
  irrigation fluids for, 205
Tuskegee Syphilis Study, 79
12-10 concept, 177; see also Respiratory
  exchange ratio
Tympanic probe, for temperature
  assessment, 707
Tympanoplasty, 436
  definition of, 434
Tympanoplasty grafts, nitrous oxide
  contraindication with, 288
Type IV reaction, lymphocytes and, 134
Typhus, as biological warfare agent, 731b
Tyrosine, 136

U

Ulcers
  from gastrointestinal anthrax, 732
  peptic, definition of, 221
  perforated gastric, 560
  from stress, spinal cord injuries and, 544
Ulnar nerve injuries, postsurgical, 358
Ultiva; see Remifentanil
Ultrasonic Doppler device, 498, 498
Ultrasonography, for vascular disease
  diagnosis, 493
Umbilical herniorrhaphy, definition of,
  553
Uncal herniation, 523
Uncrossed pyramidal tracts, 97
Uncus, 99
Uninsured persons, 57
United States, biological warfare program,
  730
United States Center for Medicare and
  Medicaid Services (CMS), 54-63
Universal donor blood, 718
Universal precautions, 40, 233, 234b
  trauma care and, 722
Universal Standards Overview, OSHA,
  235-236b
Unlicensed Assistive Personnel (UAPs), 16
Upper motor neurons, definition of, 93
Uptake
  adrenergic neurotransmitters and, 137
  of inhalation anesthetics, 278

Urea, 193, 194t
  as osmotic diuretic, 195
Uremia, definition of, 189
Ureter(s), 189
  ileal conduit with anastomosed, 567
Ureteral catheters, 570
Ureteral surgery, care after, 571-574
Ureterectomy, definition of, 567
Ureteroileostomy, definition of, 567
Ureterolithotomy, definition of, 567
Ureteroneocystostomy, definition of, 567
Ureteroplasty, definition of, 567
Ureterostomy; see also Ileal conduit
  procedure
  cutaneous, definition of, 567
Ureterovesical anastomosis, definition of,
  567
Urethra, care after surgery on, 577-578
Urethral catheters, 569
  postoperative use of, 198, 568-569, 570
  after C-section, 584
Urethral dilation and internal urethrotomy,
  definition of, 567
Urethral meatotomy, definition of, 567
Urethrocele, definition of, 583
Urethroplasty, definition of, 567
Uric acid, 193, 194t
Urinary incontinence, definition of, 189
Urinary output
  malignant hyperthermia and, 711b,
    712
  moderate phase hemorrhage and, 723
  postoperative, 388
    adrenalectomy, 579
    genital or vaginal surgery, 587
    geriatric surgery, 684, 686
    gynecologic surgery, 588
    kidney transplantation, 573
    pediatric surgery, 673
    penile surgery, 578
    trauma injury, 721
    vascular surgery, 498, 503-504
  progressive phase hemorrhage and, 724
  shock and, 723
Urinary retention, 189
  after abdominal surgery, 559-560
  after anal or rectal surgery, 562
  after appendectomy or herniorrhaphy,
    562
  after cystoscopy, 568
  after orthopedic surgery, 511
  spinal anesthesia and, 350
Urinary system
  anatomy of, 190
  complications of, spinal cord injuries
    and, 544
  gynecologic surgery and, 585
Urine
  carbon dioxide transport and, 174
  components of, 193-194, 194t
  formation of, 191
  renal function monitoring and, 198
  retention catheters after cardiac surgery
    for, 487
Urine/plasma (U/P), 199
Urokinase, fibrinolytic therapy and, 495
Urolene Blue, 259t

Urticaria
  anaphylactic shock and, 726
  as immediate hypersensitivity reaction, 243, 244
  local anesthetics and, 344
Uterine aspiration, 585
  definition of, 581
Uterine perforation, 585
Uterus
  massage after C-section, 584
  prolapse of, definition of, 582

V
V wave, 126
Vacuum for suction, PACU construction and, 4
Vagina, trauma nurse's assessment of, 721
Vaginal plastic operation, definition of, 583
Vaginal surgery, 586-587
  terms used in, 581-583
Vagotomy, 553, 559
  definition of, 555
Vagus nerve (X), 101
  breathing regulation and, 183
  bronchi and, 156-157
  laryngeal nerves and, 153
  medulla oblongata and, 102
  parasympathetic nervous system and, 123
  stomach function and, 223
  type and functions of, 103t
Valerian, anesthesia interaction with, 274t
Valium; see Diazepam
Valleculae, 152
Valsalva's maneuver
  definition of, 518
  intraocular pressure and, 461
Valve cusps, 129
Valve replacement
  definition of, 481-483
  types of, 482
Valvular aortic stenosis, 474
Vanceril, respiratory care and, 266t
Vancomycin (Vancocin), 264t
Vancomycin-Resistant Enterococci (VRE), 41
Vanillylmandelic acid, 137
Varicocelectomy, 577
  definition of, 567
Varicose veins, obesity and, 650
Vasa recta, 190
Vasa vasorum, 135
Vascular resistance
  arterial blood pressure and, 128
  pulmonary, 166, 167
    postoperative monitoring of, 384-385
  systemic, postoperative monitoring of, 384
Vascular surgery patients, 493-505
  diagnostic procedures, 496
  general considerations, 495-496
  on large vessels, 500-504
    body temperature, 502-503
    cardiopulmonary status, 501-502
    circulatory status, 502
    dressings, 504
    input and output, 503-504
    neurologic status, 504

Vascular surgery patients (Continued)
    pain management, 504
    positioning and initial care, 501
  noninvasive alternatives to, 494-495
  perianesthesia care, 496-498
  on peripheral vessels, 496-500
    carotid endarterectomy, 499-500
    sympathectomy, 498
      cervicodorsal, 498-499
      lumbar, 499
Vasectomy, definition of, 567
Vasoconstriction
  cerebral blood flow and, 526
  peripheral, cardiac surgery complications and, 489
  septic shock and, 727
Vasoconstrictors, pulse oximetry and, 365
Vasodilatation
  cardiogenic shock and, 725
  cerebral blood flow and, 526
  neurogenic shock and, 726
  septic shock and, 727
Vasoepididymostomy, definition of, 567
Vasogenic shock; see Distributive shock
Vasomotion, 135
Vasomotor center, arterial blood pressure and, 128
Vasomotor reflexes, medulla oblongata and, 102
Vasoocclusive crisis, in sickle cell anemia, 654-655
Vasopressin (Pitressin), 215, 264t; see also Antidiuretic hormone
  for cardiopulmonary resuscitation, 743, 745
Vasopressors
  for cardiogenic shock, 725
  for high spinal block, 350
  for neurogenic shock, 726
Vasospasms, subarachnoid hemorrhage and, 523
Vasotec, 255t
Vasotec IV, 255t
Vasovagal syncope, after eye surgery, 459
Vasovasostomy, definition of, 567
Vasoxyl; see Methoxamine
Vecuronium bromide (Norcuron), 265t, 320t, 323-324
  for anesthesia maintenance in pregnant patients, 692
Veins, 135
  cosmetic surgery on, 615
  laparoscopic perforation of, 639
  ligation and stripping of, 496
  varicose, obesity and, 650
Velocity, in trauma injuries, 715
Velpeau bandage, after mammoplasty, 598
Vena cava
  inferior
    ligation, 494
    ligation and plication of, 500
    Miles (Teflon) serrated caval clip, 494
    Moretz (Teflon) vena caval clip, 494
    obstructive shock and, 728
    partially occluding Teflon clip on, 503
    pregnancy and obstruction of, 688
Venous blood pressure, cerebral blood flow and, 525

Venous pooling, neurogenic shock and, 726
Venous pulsations, pulse oximetry and, 366
Venous sinuses, 106, 106-108
  CSF circulation through, 110, 110
Venous stasis/thromboembolism, pneumoperitoneum and, 638t
Venous thrombosis
  cardiac surgery and, 491
  obesity and, 651
Ventilation; see also Capnography
  after cardiac surgery, 485
  after vascular surgery, 501
  cardiac compression for CPR and, 740-741
  cardiopulmonary resuscitation and, 739
  definition of, 151
  distribution of, 176
  in geriatric patients, 683
  laryngospasm and, 154-155
  malignant hyperthermia and, 711
  mechanical, 401-403, 402
  in newborns, 661
    pressure cycled, 670
  with oral tracheal intubation, 416
  to perfusion
    decreased, 177, 177-178
    increased, 177, 178-179
  pregnancy and mechanics of, 691
  pressure support, spinal cord injuries and, 543
  propofol and, 294-295
  respiration and, 169-170
Ventilation-perfusion matching, 176-177, 177
  hypoxemia and, 177
  obesity and, 649
Ventolin, 252t
  respiratory care and, 266t
Ventral, definition of, 93
Ventral corticospinal tracts, 97
Ventral gray horn, 121, 122
Ventral respiratory group (VRG) neurons, 183
Ventral root, spinal nerve, 120, 121, 122
Ventricles
  in brain, 94, 109
  in heart, 126, 129
    left, pulmonary veins and, 167
Ventricular aneurysm repair, 484
  definition of, 483
Ventricular catheters, 530, 531
Ventricular contraction, premature, 374, 377, 377-378
Ventricular dysrhythmias; see also Arrhythmias; Cardiac dysrhythmias
  hypomagnesemia and, 207
  malignant hyperthermia and, 709
Ventricular ectomy, lidocaine for, 745
Ventricular fluid pressure, intracranial pressure monitoring and, 529
Ventricular gallop, myocardial infarction and, 132
Ventricular muscle, 129
Ventricular septal defect, 484
  definition of, 483
Ventricular syncytia, 129
Venules, 135

Verapamil (Isoptin), 141, 143, 265t
  halothane interaction with, 267t
  for hypertension, 146t
Verbal patient reports, 355
Versed; see Midazolam
Vertebrae, 115-117, 116
  spinal cord and, 119
  structure, 118
Vertebral arteries, 112, 123
Vertebral foramen, 115
Vertigo, after ear surgery, 435
Vesicopsoas hitch procedure, definition of, 567
Vesicourethral suspension, definition of, 567
Vestibular branch of acoustic nerves (VII), 103t
Vestibulocochlear nerve (VIII), 101
Veterans Health Administration, 56
Vigilance, medical malpractice and, 66-67
Viomycin, muscle relaxants and, 268t
VISA (S. aureus intermediately resistant to vancomycin), 41
Visceral pleura, 157
Vision
  area in cerebral cortex, 97, 99
  blurred
    club drugs abuse and, 703
    myasthenia gravis and, 644
  botulism and, 733
  cerebellum and, 102
  subthalamus and, 101
  superior colliculi and, 101
  trauma nurse's evaluation of, 720
Visitors, PACU policy on, 33
Vistaril, 658t
Visual Analog Scale, for pain measurement in children, 675, 676t
Visual reflexes, 101
Visualization, for pain management, 426
Vital capacity (VC), 158t, 159
  aging and, 683
Vital signs
  after ambulatory surgery, 622
  after liver surgery, 562, 563
  after pediatric surgery, 667, 669
  after prostate surgery, 576
  intracranial pressure and, 532-533
  kidney transplantation and, 573
  spinal cord injuries and, 540
Vitamin D, calcium and, 216, 217
"Vitamin K" (ketamine), abuse of, 704
Vitamins, alcohol withdrawal and, 701
Vitrectomy, 456, 457
  definition of, 456
Vocal cords
  laryngectomy and, 445-447
  motor control of, 96
  nasotracheal suctioning and, 404
  in newborns, 661
  visualizing, for oral endotracheal intubation, 414-415

Vocal process, 153
Voice box, 152-155
Volatile inhalation agents, 283
Volkmann contracture, definition of, 506
Volume reduction surgery, definition of, 466
Voluntary movements
  cerebellum and, 102
  reticular formation and, 104
Volvulus, definition of, 555
Vomiting; see also Postoperative nausea and vomiting syndrome
  afferent connections of, 655
  after adrenalectomy, 579
  after laparoscopy, 638
  after nasal surgery, 437
  definition of, 221
  enflurane and, 286
  eye surgery and, 460
  from gastrointestinal anthrax, 732
  hiatal hernia and, 222
  intermaxillary facial fixation and, 450
  morphine and, 306
  pregnancy and, 691
  spinal anesthesia and, 350
  Stage II anesthesia and, 276, 277
  stomach physiology and, 223-225
  trauma injuries and, 721-722
  water loss and, 202, 203
Vomiting center, 655-656, 656
  afferent connections of, 655
Vomiting reflex, 102
Vulvectomy, 587

W

Warfarin, geriatric patients and, 685t
Warm air therapy, postanesthetic warming and, 707
Warmed blankets, for postpartum trembling, 584
Warming mattresses, water-circulating, postanesthetic warming and, 707
Water; see also Fluids
  Alzheimer's disease and anesthesia emergence, 685
  in body, 201-202
  distribution in infants and children, 664
  in gastrointestinal tract, 202
  intoxication, TURP and, 575
  loss, average 24-hour, 193t
  in lungs, 202
  normal daily intake and output of, 202b
  in skin, 203
Water balance
  during cardiopulmonary bypass, 484-485
  hypothalamus and, 101
  inhalation agents and, 290
  in lung, 168, 168-169
  muscle relaxants and, 329
  redistribution with burn injuries, 610
Water-circulating warming mattresses, postanesthetic warming and, 707

Wedge resection
  definition of, 466
  positioning after, 467
Wernicke's area, 97
Wheeze/wheezing
  definition of, 151
  postoperative, 363
  pulmonary edema and, 195
Whipping cream aerosols, abuse of, 703
Whipple procedure
  care after, 563-564
  definition of, 554
White blood cells, 134, 209
  myocardial infarction and, 132
White fiber tracts
  in cerebellum, 102
  in the pons, 102
White matter, 94, 95, 96, 109
  in spinal cord, 107, 120, 121, 122
Withdrawal syndrome; see also Drug abuse
  alcohol, 701
  benzodiazepines, 701
  definition of, 697
  Naloxone and, 312
  opioids, 697, 700
  pain management and, 429
Wound care
  after large bowel surgery, 560-561
  after orthopedic surgery, 509
  aseptic technique and, 233
  in burn injury management, 610-613
  vomiting and, 655
Wound dehiscence and infection, after cardiac surgery, 487, 490
Written patient reports, 355
  after cardiac surgery, 487
  on discharge after ambulatory surgery, 624
  on PACU discharge, 407
Wyamine, 259t
  action of, 144t
Wydase, 256t

X

"XTC," abuse of, 703-704
Xylocaine; see Lidocaine

Y

Yawn maneuver, airway closure and, 161
Yawn mechanism, 185
Yersinia pestis, 732
Yutopar, 263t

Z

Zafirlukast (Accolate), respiratory care and, 266t
Zantac; see Ranitidine
Zecnil; see Somatostatin
Zemuron, 263t, 324
Zidovudine, 41
Zileuton (Zyflo), respiratory care and, 266t
Zofran; see Ondansetron
Zygomatic bone, 105